The NutriBase Complete Book of

FOOD COUNTS

The NutriBase Complete Book of

FOOD COUNTS

AVERY
a member of Penguin Group (USA) Inc.
NEW YORK

Every effort has been made to ensure that the information contained in this book is complete and accurate. However, neither the publisher nor the author is engaged in rendering professional advice or services to the individual reader. The ideas, procedures, and suggestions contained in this book are not intended as a substitute for consulting with your physician. All matters regarding health require medical supervision. Neither the author nor the publisher shall be liable or responsible for any loss, injury, or damage allegedly arising from any information or suggestion in this book.

Most Avery books are available at special quantity discounts for bulk purchase for sales promotions, premiums, fund-raising, and educational needs. Special books or book excerpts also can be created to fit specific needs. For details, write Putnam Special Markets, 375 Hudson Street, New York, NY 10014.

a member of
Penguin Group (USA) Inc.
375 Hudson Street
New York, NY 10014
www.penguin.com

Library of Congress Cataloging-in-Publication Data

The NutriBase complete book of food counts.
p. cm.
ISBN 1-58333-107-7
1. Food—Composition—Tables.   2. Nutrition—Tables.

TX551 .N743   2001   2001046264
613.2'8—dc21

Printed in the United States of America
13 15 17 19 20 18 16 14 12

CONTENTS

INTRODUCTION

For thousands of years, people have recognized the life-sustaining nature of food. But only during the last four or five decades have we begun to understand the many ways in which our choices of foods can affect the quality of our health and the length of our lives. And only during the last five or ten years have we really begun to appreciate how profound the effects of those choices can be.

Now we know that some of the so-called "inevitable" diseases, such as atherosclerosis, osteoporosis, and even cancer are often the consequences of poor nutritional choices. Research has clearly shown the relationship between poor nutritional intake and many of these diseases. The studies prove that a high-fat diet can—and often does—contribute to the development of coronary artery disease; that low fiber intake promotes the development of colon cancer; that folic acid deficiency increases the risk of birth defects; and that inadequate calcium intake fosters the onset of osteoporosis and bone fractures. The list of nutrition-related disorders goes on and on.

There is a hopeful side to this story. Studies have clearly demonstrated the positive effects that good nutritional choices can have on our health. Many cases of cardiovascular disease can be prevented, and even reversed, through dietary changes. The incidence of cancer can be reduced with diets that are low in fat and high in cruciferous vegetables (broccoli and cauliflower, for instance) and through the use of the antioxidant nutrients, such as vitamins C and E. Bone strength can be increased and fracture rates decreased with a diet rich in calcium and vitamin D. Blood cholesterol levels can be reduced with dietary fiber, niacin, and garlic. Blood pressure can be lowered with sodium restriction and calcium and magnesium supplementation. The list of health-promoting nutritional interventions is lengthy and is growing constantly.

THE NEW NUTRITION

Modern research studies are giving rise to a "new" nutrition, one that is both scientifically sound and practical. The new nutrition differs from the old in at least two important ways. First, the old nutrition dealt in generalities, such as the four food groups, and created minimum dietary recommendations designed to prevent deficiency-related disorders. The new nutrition seeks to achieve *optimal* levels of health and creates specific recommendations based on individual differences, such as age, sex, lifestyle, and medical factors. Second, the old nutrition left many nutritional decisions up to the health professionals and food marketers, while the new nutrition puts *you* in control. It empowers you with the information necessary to evaluate confusing and conflicting claims, and it enables you to reject foods that do not meet your nutritional needs and goals.

This book is designed to provide you with that empowering information. It will help you make wiser choices when you buy food and when you dine out. It will help you interpret nutritional stories in the media so you can distinguish useful information from nonsense. It will give you the control you need over your personal nutrition.

As you take more control over the foods you are eating and put more thought into your choices, keep in mind that good nutrition is just one element of a healthy lifestyle. To achieve maximum benefits from the new nutrition, your life should be filled with physical activity and free of cigarette smoke and other toxic substances. In addition, the stress in your life should be under control. Even the best diet can't overcome the problems caused by smoking, an immoderate use of alcohol, poorly managed stress, or other health-compromising habits.

Finally, be aware that research is constantly adding to our knowledge of nutrition and in the process changing some of our beliefs. As best you can, try to keep up with the new information and, when appropriate, make whatever dietary changes are necessary. But also be skeptical about nutritional news that seems too good to be true. (More often than not, it isn't true.) Be wary of nutritional claims made by people who are trying to sell you something. And be cautious—don't make any drastic changes in your nutritional program without first talking to a health professional who is knowledgeable about nutrition and about your particular medical circumstances. Don't forget: If the right nutritional choices are powerful enough to keep you well, it is only logical that the wrong ones could make you sick.

The following section will explain some of the basics of nutrition. After that, you will learn how to use this book to locate the information you need to improve your diet.

A QUICK LOOK AT THE BASIC NUTRIENTS

Water, carbohydrates, protein, and fat are the basic building blocks of a healthy diet. Each works in different ways to fuel the body, to build and repair the cells that make up the body, and to provide the environment in which the cells live.

Water

The human body is two-thirds water by weight. Indeed, water is an essential nutrient that is involved in every function of the body. It helps transport nutrients and waste products into and out of cells. It is necessary for all digestive, absorptive, circulatory, and excretory functions, and for the utilization of the water-soluble vitamins. And it is needed to maintain proper body temperature.

Carbohydrates

Carbohydrates provide the body with the energy it needs to function. There are two primary types of carbohydrates, generally referred to as *simple* and *complex.* Sugars such as glucose, fructose (fruit sugar), and sucrose (table sugar) are examples of simple carbohydrates. Starch, on the other hand, is a complex carbohydrate.

One type of carbohydrate you may have heard a good deal about is fiber. Referred to in the past as roughage, fiber is actually the part of plant material that our body cannot digest. Yet fiber is known to perform a number of important functions. It promotes feelings of fullness; prevents constipation, hemorrhoids, and other intestinal problems; and is associated with a reduced incidence of colon cancer. In addition, fiber may help lower blood cholesterol levels, reducing the risk of heart disease.

Protein

Protein is essential for growth and development. It provides the body with energy, and is needed for the manufacture of hormones, antibodies, enzymes, and muscle tissues. It also helps maintain the proper acid-alkali balance.

Fat

Much attention has been focused on the need to limit dietary fat intake. Nevertheless, the body does need fats—but the right fats, and in appropriate quantities. Specifically, it needs essential fatty acids, which perform a variety of vital bodily functions. Essential fatty acids carry the fat-soluble vitamins.

They are essential for growth and development, and for the maintenance of healthy skin, hair, and nails. And they provide the body with energy.

Most of us are aware that there are several kinds of dietary fat—saturated, polyunsaturated, and monounsaturated—and that some are better than others. To understand the difference between these three types of fats, it is helpful to first learn a little about cholesterol.

Cholesterol is a white, waxy, fatty substance produced by the liver. It is essential to our well-being, as it helps to build cell membranes, to produce hormones, and to manufacture bile acids. The liver is capable of manufacturing all of the cholesterol needed for good health.

The cholesterol manufactured by the liver is carried through the bloodstream by molecules known as low-density lipoproteins, or LDLs. High levels of LDLs in the bloodstream are associated with clogged arteries, high blood pressure, stroke, and heart disease. This is why LDL is sometimes referred to as "bad cholesterol." Fortunately, many people can reduce their LDL levels through proper diet.

High-density lipoproteins, or HDLs, are molecules that carry excess cholesterol from different body tissues back to the liver, where it is converted into bile acids and then eliminated through the intestines. High levels of HDLs are linked with a decreased risk of cardiovascular disease. This is why HDL is often called "good cholesterol." To a limited extent, HDL levels can be raised through regular exercise.

How are the three types of fat related to cholesterol? Saturated fats—which come from foods of animal origin such as meat, fish, poultry, milk, butter, and cheese, as well as from palm, coconut, and palm kernel oil—have been shown to increase total blood cholesterol levels, especially the undesirable LDL portion. Polyunsaturated fats—found mainly in vegetable oils like corn, sunflower, safflower, and soybean—tend to lower levels of both HDL and LDL. Monounsaturated fats—found mainly in certain vegetable and nut oils, including olive, peanut, and Canola—have been shown to reduce total blood cholesterol without lowering levels of the good cholesterol, HDL. Indeed, some monounsaturated fats have been shown to raise HDL levels.

One other element, *trans-fatty acids,* might also play a role in blood cholesterol levels. Trans-fatty acids occur when polyunsaturated oils are altered through hydrogenation, a process used to harden liquid vegetable oils into solid foods like margarine and shortening. One recent study found that trans-monounsaturated fatty acids raise LDL cholesterol levels, behaving much like saturated fats. Simultaneously, these trans-fatty acids reduced HDL cholesterol readings. Much more research is necessary, since some studies have not produced clear-cut conclusions about these substances. But your dietary choices could become less matter-of-fact than they now appear. For now, however, it is clear that when your goal is to lower cholesterol, polyunsaturated and monounsaturated are much more desirable than saturated fats, and are probably more desirable than any kind of hydrogenated fats.

A Word About Calories

When we talk about foods, we often mention the number of calories a certain food has. Calories are not among the four basic nutrients, nor are they considered micronutrients. What, then, are calories?

A calorie is an energy unit. As already discussed, carbohydrates, protein, and fat provide the body with the energy it needs to function. This energy is measured in calories. There are, for instance, approximately four calories in every gram of protein, four calories in every gram of carbohydrate, and nine calories in every gram of fat. It is no wonder, then, that people who are trying to lose weight are often advised to cut down on fatty foods. On a gram-for-gram basis, fat is more than twice as fattening as carbohydrates or protein.

In addition to having more calories than protein or carbohydrates, dietary fat is metabolized differently. Because dietary fat is similar in chemical composition to body fat, it takes less energy to convert it to body fat. In fact, it takes only 3 percent of the calories in the fat we eat to turn that food into body fat, while it takes at least 25 percent of the calories in the carbohydrates and proteins we eat to convert them into body fat. Remember, though, that if you eat more calories than your body needs, regardless of the nutrient source of these calories, the excess will be stored as body fat.

Being Sodium Wise

Not even a brief look at nutrition would be complete without a word or two about sodium. The mineral sodium is necessary for health. It helps to maintain normal fluid levels in the body, is involved in healthy muscle functioning, and supports the blood and lymphatic systems.

It is important to note, however, that most people get too much sodium in their diets. We need less than 500 milligrams of sodium a day to stay healthy. This is enough to accomplish the functions that sodium performs in the body. A quick glance through some randomly selected pages of this book will show you how easy it is to reach the 500-milligram mark. You may be surprised by the amount of salt present in the foods you eat regularly, and by your typical daily intake.

If you are trying to reduce your intake of sodium, it is important to be aware of two hidden sources of this mineral. One source includes a number of food ingredients and additives other than salt itself. For instance, both baking powder and baking soda contain sodium, as does the flavor enhancer monosodium glutamate (MSG). In general, by looking for the word *sodium* among ingredient listings, you should be able to identify most sodium sources.

Medications—including over-the-counter cough, antacid, and pain relief preparations—constitute the second hidden source of sodium. Again, any ingredient that contains the word *sodium*—for example, sodium salicylate—should alert you to a possible problem.

THE FOOD GUIDE PYRAMID

The U.S. Department of Agriculture (USDA) encourages Americans to eat a well-balanced diet, which it illustrates with a diagram known as the Food Guide Pyramid. At the base of the pyramid are breads, cereals, rice, and pasta. Six to eleven servings from this group are recommended daily—more servings than from any other group of foods in the pyramid. The next level is occupied by vegetables, with three to five daily servings recommended, and by fruit, with two to four servings recommended. Moving upward, the next level is shared by milk, yogurt, and cheese—two to three servings—and meat, poultry, fish, dry beans, eggs, and nuts—two to three servings. Finally, at the peak of the pyramid are fats, oils, and sweets, for which there are no recommended amounts, only a note that they should be consumed sparingly.

To ensure that you have adequate servings of healthful foods, it is best to follow the Food Guide Pyramid and, within each group, to choose foods that are high in the nutrients needed for good health. The remainder of this book shows how each food rates in terms of its nutrient values. The following guidelines should help you design and stick to a well-balanced diet:

■ When choosing breads, cereals, rice, and pasta, always choose whole-grain, high-fiber, low-fat varieties, preferably without added sugar, coloring, or unnecessary preservatives. Choose brown rice over white rice, and whole-grain pastas over pastas made from white flour.

FOOD GUIDE PYRAMID
A Guide to Daily Food Choices

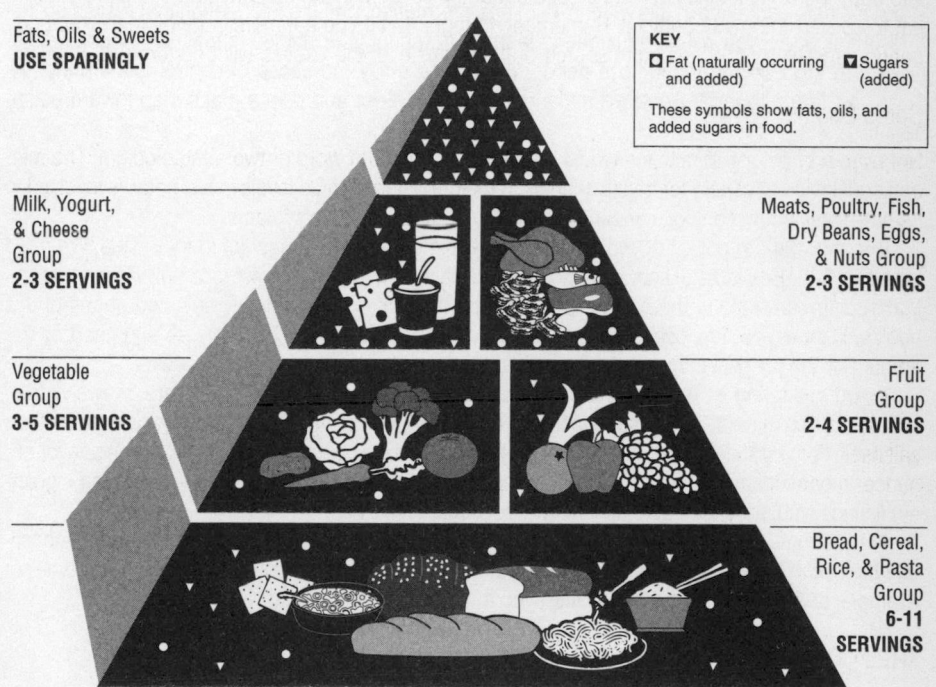

Fats, Oils & Sweets
USE SPARINGLY

KEY
☐ Fat (naturally occurring   ▼ Sugars
and added)   (added)

These symbols show fats, oils, and
added sugars in food.

Milk, Yogurt,
& Cheese
Group
2-3 SERVINGS

Meats, Poultry, Fish,
Dry Beans, Eggs,
& Nuts Group
2-3 SERVINGS

Vegetable
Group
3-5 SERVINGS

Fruit
Group
2-4 SERVINGS

Bread, Cereal,
Rice, & Pasta
Group
**6-11
SERVINGS**

Source: U.S. Department of Agriculture &
U.S. Department of Health and Human Services

■ Eat your vegetables and fruits fresh and, preferably, raw as often as possible. Water-soluble vitamins such as vitamin C may leach out of foods during cooking, be damaged by overprocessing, or be destroyed when foods are overcooked. Even fat-soluble vitamins, which are fairly stable during low-temperature cooking, can be affected by frying. For this reason, it is best to steam or microwave vegetables rather than boiling or frying them. And, unless produce is organically grown, be sure to peel or thoroughly wash it before eating to reduce such unwanted elements as waxes and pesticide residue.

■ Select low-fat and nonfat varieties of milk, yogurt, and cheese. These provide the most nutrients and the least amount of fat. When eating meat, poultry, or fish, choose the leanest cuts available, trim off any excess fat, and bake or broil the foods instead of frying them.

■ Select as few foods as possible from the fats, oils, and sweets category. When you do use fats and oils, choose monounsaturated and polyunsaturated fats instead of saturated ones. Limit your intake of sweets. Choose fresh fruits instead of cakes, cookies, and other high-fat desserts.

The following section should provide you with the details you need to better access and understand the data contained in this volume. With this information, and the information that makes up the bulk of this book, you will be equipped to learn more about your unique nutritional needs and the foods you are using to meet those needs. You should enjoy the sense of control this knowledge gives you. More important, you will make better food choices and take a major step toward better health.

How to Use
This Book

This book was designed to provide comprehensive nutritional information on a wide range of foods, both generic and brand name, raw and prepared. The information provided here was gleaned from a number of government agencies, from hundreds of manufacturers, and from food trade associations. This information was compiled and later supplemented through countless hours of follow-up that involved hundreds of additional sources. Because scientific techniques are continually being improved, this book will be continually updated to reflect the most current nutritional data available.

This easy-to-use guide is divided into two parts. The first part is an A-to-Z reference to the nutrients provided by foods. In this section, you will find the amount of calories, fat, saturated fat, and cholesterol, as well as the percentage of calories that come from fat. The second is an A-to-Z reference to the nutrient values of restaurant-chain foods. In this section, foods are listed alphabetically under the name of the appropriate restaurant, and each food item is accompanied by the amounts of the general nutrients found in that item.

All of the foods in this reference have been listed alphabetically. For instance, if you are looking for the nutrient values of ground beef, you would turn to the *B's* and look under *Beef.* For convenience, similar foods have sometimes been grouped together in categories such as *Baby Foods, Breads, Candies, Cereals, Cheese, Cookies, Pasta,* and *Sauces.* Therefore, if the food you are looking for is not listed individually by its own name, you should try looking it up under a logical category.

Some foods are known by two or more names. In most cases, the food is listed under just one name, and cross-references have been provided to guide you to the proper listing. For instance, chickpeas are also called garbanzo and ceci beans. In this book, you will find the nutrient information under *Chickpeas,* with cross-references under *Ceci* and *Garbanzo.*

If you are unable to find a particular food, look for the entry for a similar food. The nutritional data should be close, if not exact, for any product not listed.

After you locate the listing for the food you are interested in, you may find that abbreviations have been used to provide you with the information you need. Refer to page xv for a key to the abbreviations used throughout this book.

When examining the nutrient values of cooked generic foods, keep in mind that unless otherwise noted, no additional ingredients have been added during cooking. For processed foods such as cake or pancake mixes, the term "prepared" signifies that the item has been prepared according to the directions on the package, with whatever additional ingredients that requires. Unless otherwise noted, the food values for fish, meats, and poultry are for meat only, and do not include skin or bones.

Codes and Abbreviations

To provide the most comprehensive nutritional information possible, a number of codes and abbreviations have been used throughout this book. A complete translation is given below.

>	greater than
<	less than
approx	approximately
cal	calories
calc	calcium
carbs	carbohydrates
fl	fluid
fol	folic acid
gm	gram
IU	international unit[1]
lb	pound
mag	magnesium
mcg	microgram(s)
med	medium-sized
mg	milligram(s)
(mq)	may contain a measurable quantity[2]
na	not available

nia	niacin
pkg	package
pot	potassium
prep	prepared according to directions
prot	protein
rib	riboflavin
sat fat	saturated fat
sod	sodium
tbsp	tablespoon
thi	thiamine
tr	trace
(tr)	may contain a trace amount
tsp	teaspoon
w/	with
w/o	without
wt	weight
zn	zinc

[1] International units, which are used throughout this book to express vitamin A content, are a measure of fat-soluble vitamin activity. The amounts of all other nutrients are expressed in grams or milligrams, which are units of mass and weight.

[2] The food item may contain a quantity ranging from a trace amount to a substantial amount. This quantity depends upon any one of a number of variables—such as soil condition and mineral content of fertilizer used—that may have affected the food item during growing, processing, and/or preparation.

A-to-Z Listing of Foods

A

Food Name	Serv. Size	Total Cal.	Prot. gms	Carbs gms	Sod. mgs	Fiber gms	Fat gms	Chol. mgs
ABALONE, mixed species, raw	3 oz	89	15	5	256	0	0.6	72
ABALONE MUSHROOM. See MUSHROOM, OYSTER.								
ACEROLA, RAW/Barbados cherry/Puerto Rican cherry/West Indian cherry								
raw, trimmed	1 medium	2	0	0	0	0	0.0	0
raw, untrimmed	1 cup	31	0	8	7	1	0.3	0
ACEROLA JUICE								
	1 cup	56	1	12	7	1	0.7	0
	1 fl oz	7	0	1	1	0	0.1	0
ACORN								
dried	1 oz	144	2	15	0	na	8.9	0
raw	1 oz	110	2	12	0	na	6.8	0
ACORN FLOUR. See under FLOUR.								
ACORN SQUASH. See SQUASH, ACORN.								
ADZUKI BEAN. See BEAN, ADZUKI.								
AGAR. See under SEA VEGETABLE.								
AHI. See under TUNA, YELLOWFIN.								
AKU. See under TUNA, SKIPJACK.								
ALARIA. See under SEA VEGETABLE.								
ALASKA KING CRAB. See under CRAB.								
ALBACORE. See under TUNA.								
ALCOHOLIC BEVERAGES. See BEER AND ALE; COCKTAIL; COCKTAIL MIXER; SHERRY; VERMOUTH; WINE; WINE, COOKING; WINE COOLER; and individual listings.								
ALE. See BEER, ALE, AND MALT LIQUOR.								
ALFALFA SEEDS								
(Arrowhead Mills)	1 cup	40	5	4	0	0	1.0	0
sprouted, raw	1 cup	10	1	1	2	1	0.2	0
sprouted, raw	1 tbsp	1	0	0	0	0	0.0	0
ALFALFA TABLETS *(Shaklee)*	10 tablets	5	0	0	2	0	0.0	0
ALGAE								
blue-green, Klamath lake algae	1 gram	3	1	0	3	na	0.0	0
spirulina, dried	1 cup	44	9	4	157	1	1.2	0
ALLIGATOR	1 oz	41	8.3	na	na	na	0.8	18
ALLSPICE								
ground	1 tbsp	16	0	4	5	1	0.5	0
ground	1 tsp	5	0	1	1	0	0.2	0
ground *(Durkee)*	1 tsp	7	0	0	0	0	0.0	0
ground *(Laurel Leaf)*	1 tsp	7	0	0	0	0	0.0	0
ground *(McCormick/Schilling)*	1 tsp	6	0	1	1	1	0.0	0
ground *(Spice Islands)*	1 tsp	6	0	1	1	0	0.1	0
ground *(Tone's)*	1 tsp	5	0	1	2	0	0.2	0
ALMOND								
ground	1 cup	549	20	19	1	11	48.1	0
whole kernels, approx 24	1 oz	164	6	6	0	3	14.4	0
(Beer Nuts)	1 oz	180	5	7	51	0	14.4	0
(Dole)	1 oz	170	6	12	4	0	14.0	0
(Fisher)	1 oz	170	3	3	0	0	15.0	0
natural, chopped *(Blue Diamond)*	1 oz	172	6	6	0	4	14.3	0
natural, sliced *(Blue Diamond)*	1 oz	172	6	6	0	4	14.3	0
natural, unsalted *(Flanigan Farms)*	1 oz	170	6	5	4	na	14.0	0
natural, whole *(Blue Diamond)* natural	1 oz	172	6	6	0	4	14.3	0
natural, whole or sliced *(Azar)*	2 oz	340	12	12	6	5	30.0	0
Barbecue *(Blue Diamond)*	1 oz	167	6	5	243	4	15.0	0
Blanched								
pieces	1 oz	165	6	6	8	3	14.4	0

Food Name	Serv. Size	Total Cal.	Prot. gms	Carbs gms	Sod. mgs	Fiber gms	Fat gms	Chol. mgs
pieces	1 tbsp	53	2	2	3	1	4.6	0
whole kernels	1 cup	842	32	29	41	15	73.4	0
(Blue Diamond)	1 oz	175	6	5	2	4	14.5	0
(Planters)	1 oz	170	6	6	0	0	15.0	0
slivered (Azar)	2 oz	330	11	10	4	5	29.0	0
slivered (Blue Diamond)	1 oz	175	6	5	2	4	14.5	0
whole (Blue Diamond)	1 oz	175	6	5	2	4	14.5	0
Chili w/lemon (Blue Diamond)	1 oz	172	6	4	245	3	16.0	0
Dry-roasted								
whole kernels, salted	1 cup	824	30	27	468	16	72.9	0
whole kernels, salted, approx 22	1 oz	169	6	5	96	3	15.0	0
whole kernels, unsalted	1 cup	824	30	27	1	16	72.9	0
whole kernels, unsalted, approx 22	1 oz	169	6	5	0	3	15.0	0
California, whole (Flanigan Farms)	1/4 cup	170	6	6	0	3	15.0	0
chopped, unsalted (Flanigan Farms)	1/4 cup	170	6	6	0	3	15.0	0
(Planters)	1 oz	170	6	6	200	0	15.0	0
sliced, unsalted (Flanigan Farms)	1/4 cup	170	6	6	0	3	15.0	0
slivered, unsalted (Flanigan Farms)	1/4 cup	170	6	5	0	3	15.0	0
unsalted (Blue Diamond)	1 oz	170	6	5	1	3	15.1	0
w/tamari (Eden Foods)	1 oz	170	8	8	35	4	12.0	0
Honey-roasted								
unblanched	1 oz	168	5	8	37	4	14.1	0
whole kernels, unblanched	1 cup	855	26	40	187	20	71.9	0
(Blue Diamond)	1 oz	170	5	8	37	3	14.2	0
(Planters)	1 oz	170	5	9	180	0	13.0	0
Oil-roasted								
whole kernels, salted	1 cup	953	33	28	532	16	86.6	0
whole kernels, salted, approx 22	1 oz	172	6	5	96	3	15.6	0
whole kernels, unsalted	1 cup	953	33	28	2	16	86.6	0
whole kernels, unsalted, approx 22	1 oz	172	6	5	0	3	15.6	0
Raw								
sliced (Planters)	1 oz	170	6	6	0	0	15.0	0
slivered (Planters)	1 oz	170	6	6	0	0	15.0	0
whole (Planters)	1 oz	170	6	6	0	0	15.0	0
Roasted (Dole)	1 oz	170	6	5	4	0	14.0	0
Smokehouse (Blue Diamond)	1 oz	173	6	5	169	3	15.8	0
Unblanched								
sliced	1 cup	549	20	19	1	11	48.1	0
slivered	1 cup	624	23	21	1	13	54.7	0
whole	1 cup	821	30	28	1	17	71.9	0
Yogurt-coated, made w/real fruit juice (Fruit Source)	9 pieces	210	4	19	40	2	14.0	5
ALMOND BUTTER								
salted	1 cup	1583	38	53	1125	9	147.8	0
salted	1 tbsp	101	2	3	72	1	9.5	0
unsalted	1 cup	1583	38	53	28	9	147.8	0
unsalted	1 tbsp	101	2	3	2	1	9.5	0
(Hain)								
blanched, toasted	2 tbsp	220	8	3	10	0	19.0	0
raw, 'Natural'	2 tbsp	190	8	3	5	0	18.0	0
(Maranatha Natural)								
organic, raw	2 tbsp	190	7	8	5	0	15.0	0
roasted	2 tbsp	190	7	8	5	0	15.0	0
(Roaster Fresh)								
gourmet	1 oz	184	5	6	4	0	16.0	0
roasted fresh, creamy, salted	1 oz	184	5	6	4	0	16.0	0
(Westbrae)								
crunchy, unsalted, 'Natural'	2 tbsp	190	7	7	0	0	17.0	0

Food Name	Serv. Size	Total Cal.	Prot. gms	Carbs gms	Sod. mgs	Fiber gms	Fat gms	Chol. mgs
smooth, unsalted, 'Natural'	2 tbsp	190	7	7	0	0	17.0	0
ALMOND DRINK original flavor *(Almond Mylk)*	8 fl oz	80	2	8	190	2	4.0	0
ALMOND MEAL								
partially defatted	4 oz	463	44.8	32.8	8	>2,6c	20.8	0
partially defatted, salted	4 oz	463	44.8	32.8	846	>2,6c	20.8	0
ALMOND OIL								
	1 cup	1927	0	0	0	0	218.0	0
	1 tbsp	120	0	0	0	0	13.6	0
(Hain)	1 tbsp	120	0	0	0	0	14.0	0
pure-pressed organic *(Spectrum)*	1 tbsp	120	0	0	0	0	14.0	0
sweet *(International Collection)*	1 tbsp	120	0	0	0	0	14.0	0
ALMOND PASTE								
	1 oz	130	3	14	3	1	7.9	0
firmly packed	1 cup	1040	20	109	20	11	63.0	0
ALOE VERA JUICE								
sodium-free, certified 100% juice *(Sunburst)*	2 fl oz	5	0	1	3	0	0.0	0
AMARANTH								
	1 cup	729	28	129	41	30	12.7	0
(Arrowhead Mills) whole-grain, organic	1/4 cup	170	7	29	0	3	2.0	0
AMARANTH DISH/ENTRÉE								
(Health Valley) w/vegetables, fat-free, 'Fast Menu'	1 cup	160	8	31	290	9	0.0	0
AMARANTH FLOUR. See under FLOUR.								
AMARANTH LEAVES								
boiled, drained	1 cup	28	3	5	28	na	0.2	0
raw	1 cup	6	1	1	6	na	0.1	0
raw	1 leaf	3	0	1	3	na	0.0	0
AMARANTH SEED *(Arrowhead Mills)*	2 oz	200	8	35	1	4	3.0	0
ANASAZI BEAN. See BEAN, ANASAZI.								
ANCHO PEPPER. See PEPPER, ANCHO.								
ANCHOVY								
Canned								
European, in oil, boneless, drained	1 oz	60	8	0	1040	0	2.8	24
European, in oil, drained	2 oz	95	13	0	1651	0	4.4	38
European, in oil, drained	5 medium	42	6	0	734	0	1.9	17
European, in oil, drained	1 medium	8	1	0	147	0	0.4	3
flat fillets, in olive oil *(Crown Prince)*	9 fillets	35	4	0	1050	0	2.5	15
flat fillets, in olive oil, salt added *(Reese)*	6 fillets	25	4	0	750	0	1.5	15
Fresh, European, raw	3 oz	111	17	0	88	0	4.1	51
ANCHOVY PASTE								
(Reese)	1 tbsp	30	2	0	940	0	2.5	55
(Roland)	1 tbsp	30	2	0	1140	0	2.5	24
ANGEL HAIR. See under PASTA; PASTA DISH/ENTRÉE.								
ANGLER FISH. See MONKFISH.								
ANISE, dried *(McCormick/Schilling)*	1 serving	18	1	2	0	1	0.8	0
ANISE SEED								
	1 tbsp	23	1	3	1	1	1.1	0
	1 tsp	7	0	1	0	0	0.3	0
(Tone's)	1 tsp	7	0	1	2	0	0.3	0
ANTELOPE								
raw	1 oz	32	6	0	14	0	0.6	27
roasted	3 oz	128	25	0	46	0	2.3	107
roasted, boneless, yield from 1 lb raw	11.9 oz	510	100	0	184	0	9.1	428
APPLE								
Canned, sweetened slices, drained	1 cup	137	0	34	6	4	0.9	0
Dehydrated, sulfured								
low moisture, stewed	1 cup	143	1	38	50	5	0.2	0
low moisture, uncooked	1 cup	208	1	56	74	7	0.3	0

Food Name	Serv. Size	Total Cal.	Prot. gms	Carbs gms	Sod. mgs	Fiber gms	Fat gms	Chol. mgs
rings, uncooked	1 ring	16	0	4	6	1	0.0	0
stewed	1 cup	145	1	39	51	5	0.2	0
uncooked	1 cup	209	1	57	75	7	0.3	0
Fresh								
boiled, peeled, sliced	1 cup	91	0	23	2	4	0.6	0
microwaved, peeled, sliced	1 cup	95	0	24	2	5	0.7	0
raw, peeled, quartered or chopped	1 cup	74	0	19	0	3	0.5	0
raw, peeled, sliced	1 cup	63	0	16	0	2	0.3	0
raw, peeled, whole, medium, approx 3 per lb	1 apple	73	0	19	0	2	0.4	0
raw, unpeeled, whole, large, approx 2 per lb	1 apple	125	0	32	0	6	0.8	0
raw, unpeeled, whole, medium, approx 3 per lb	1 apple	81	0	21	0	4	0.5	0
raw, unpeeled, whole, small, approx 4 per lb	1 apple	63	0	16	0	3	0.4	0
Frozen								
unsweetened slices, heated	1 cup	97	1	25	6	4	0.7	0
unsweetened slices, unheated	1 cup	83	0	21	5	3	0.6	0
APPLE BUTTER								
(Bama)	2 tsp	25	0	6	5	0	0.0	0
(Eden Foods)	1 tbsp	25	0	3	0	0	0.0	na
(Knudsen & Sons) organic	2 tbsp	25	0	6	0	0	0.0	0
(Lucky Leaf)	4 oz	200	0	49	15	0	1.0	0
(Musselman's)	4 oz	200	0	49	15	0	1.0	0
(Smucker's)								
'Autumn Harvest'	1 tsp	12	0	3	0	0	0.0	0
cider	1 tsp	12	0	3	0	0	0.0	0
natural	1 tsp	12	0	3	0	0	0.0	0
'Simply Fruit'	1 tsp	16	0	4	0	0	0.0	0
spiced	1 tsp	12	0	3	0	0	0.0	0
(Tap'n Apple)	1 oz	45	1	13	1	1	0.1	0
(White House)	1 oz	50	0	12	5	0	0.0	0
APPLE DISH								
escalloped, frozen *(Stouffer's)*	2/3 cup	182	0	37	71	3	3.0	0
escalloped, frozen *(Stouffer's)*	1 oz	31	0	7	1	1	0.5	0
fried *(Luck's)*	1/2 cup	130	0	33	0	2	0.0	0
APPLE JUICE. See also CIDER; CIDER MIX; FRUIT DRINK; FRUIT DRINK MIX; FRUIT JUICE BLEND; FRUIT JUICE DRINK.								
Canned, bottled, or boxed								
w/added vitamin C	1 cup	117	0	29	7	0	0.3	0
w/added vitamin C	1 fl oz	15	0	4	1	0	0.0	0
w/o added vitamin C	1 cup	117	0	29	7	0	0.3	0
w/o added vitamin C	1 fl oz	15	0	4	1	0	0.0	0
w/o added vitamin C	8.45 fl oz	123	0	31	8	0	0.3	0
(Flav-R-Pac)	1 cup	120	0	29	15	0	0.0	0
(Indian Summer)	6 fl oz	90	1	21	10	0	1.0	0
(J. Hungerford)								
	9.03 fl oz	128	0	32	6	0	0.0	0
50% juice	9.03 fl oz	119	0	30	8	0	0.0	0
100% juice	9.03 fl oz	112	0	28	17	0	0.0	0
(Juicy Juice)	6 fl oz	90	0	21	5	0	0.0	0
(Knudsen)								
clear	8 fl oz	110	0	28	5	na	0.0	0
Gravenstein	8 fl oz	110	1	28	0	0	0.0	0
natural	8 fl oz	120	0	30	25	na	0.0	0
(Kraft) 'Pure 100%'	6 fl oz	80	0	20	5	0	0.0	0
(Lucky Leaf)								
'Individual Portion Control'	3.8 fl oz	60	0	14	0	0	0.0	0
100% vitamin-C enriched	6 fl oz	90	0	21	0	0	0.0	0
(McCain) 100% juice 'Junior'	4.2 fl oz	50	0	13	5	0	0.0	0

Food Name	Serv. Size	Total Cal.	Prot. gms	Carbs gms	Sod. mgs	Fiber gms	Fat gms	Chol. mgs
(Mott's)	6 fl oz	88	0	22	13	0	0.0	0
(Musselman's)								
'Individual Portion Control'	3.8 fl oz	60	0	14	0	0	0.0	0
100% vitamin-C enriched	6 fl oz	90	0	21	0	0	0.0	0
(Ocean Spray)	6 fl oz	90	0	23	15	0	0.0	0
(Red Cheek)								
'Natural'	6 fl oz	97	0	24	16	0	0.0	0
'100% Pure'	6 fl oz	97	0	24	7	0	0.0	0
(S&W)								
	8 fl oz	120	0	30	0	0	0.0	0
'100% Pure Unsweetened'	6 fl oz	85	0	20	5	0	0.0	0
(S. Martinelli) 'Sparkling'	6 fl oz	100	0	25	5	0	0.0	0
(Sippin' Pak) 100% pure	8.45 fl oz	110	0	28	25	0	0.0	0
(Tree Top) 100%	8 fl oz	120	0	29	25	0	0.0	0
(TreeSweet)	6 fl oz	90	0	22	15	0	0.0	0
(Tropicana)								
100% pure	8 fl oz	116	0	29	17	0	0.0	0
100% pure	6 fl oz	80	1	20	15	0	1.0	0
'Pure Premium' 'Orchardstand'	8 fl oz	110	1	27	0	na	0.0	na
'Season's Best'	8 fl oz	120	0	29	25	1	0.0	na
(Ultra Slim Fast) golden	8 fl oz	153	5	29	167	3	1.0	7
(Veryfine) '100%'	8 fl oz	107	0	27	10	0	0.0	0
(Welch's)								
'Orchard Cocktail'	10 fl oz	170	0	42	95	0	0.0	0
sparkling	6 fl oz	100	0	24	5	0	0.0	0
(White House)	6 fl oz	87	0	22	5	0	0.0	0
Chilled or frozen								
concentrate, w/o added vitamin C, prepared	1 cup	112	0	28	17	0	0.2	0
concentrate, w/o added vitamin C, prepared	1 fl oz	14	0	3	2	0	0.0	0
concentrate, w/added vitamin C, prepared	1 cup	112	0	28	17	0	0.2	0
concentrate, w/added vitamin C, prepared	1 fl oz	14	0	3	2	0	0.0	0
concentrate, w/added vitamin C, undiluted	6-oz can	350	1	87	53	na	0.8	0
concentrate, w/o added vitamin C, undiluted	6-oz can	350	1	87	53	1	0.8	0
(A&P) diluted as directed	6 fl oz	90	1	22	0	0	1.0	0
(Sunkist) diluted as directed	8 fl oz	79	0	19	12	0	0.2	0
APPLE KIT								
(Concord)								
candy, microwaveable, prepared	1 apple	50	0	14	0	0	0.0	0
caramel, microwaveable, prepared	1 apple	150	2	27	105	0	3.0	5
APPLE PIE SPICE. See under SEASONING MIX.								
APPLE SPREAD, no sugar added *(Fifty 50)*	1 tsp	2	0	1	5	0	0.0	0
APPLE SYRUP *(Knudsen)*	1 oz	75	1	15	0	0	1.0	0
APPLE TOPPING *(Flav-R-Pac)*	2 tbsp	40	0	10	45	0	0.0	0
APPLESAUCE								
canned, sweetened, w/salt	1 cup	194	0	51	71	3	0.5	0
canned, sweetened, w/o salt	1 cup	194	0	51	8	3	0.5	0
canned, sweetened, w/o salt	1 cup	194	0	51	8	3	0.5	0
canned, unsweetened, w/added vitamin C	1 cup	105	0	28	5	3	0.1	0
canned, unsweetened w/o added vitamin C	1 cup	105	0	28	5	3	0.1	0
cinnamon *(Tree Top)*	1/2 cup	83	0	21	0	1	0.0	0
cranberry, 'CranFruit' *(Ocean Spray)*	2 oz	100	0	23	10	0	0.0	0
original *(Tree Top)*	1/2 cup	83	0	21	0	1	0.0	0
unsweetened *(Tree Top)*	1/2 cup	58	0	15	0	1	0.0	0
APRICOT								
Canned								
halves, peeled, in extra light syrup, w/liquid	1 cup	121	1	31	5	4	0.2	0
halves, peeled, in heavy syrup, w/liquid	1 cup	214	1	55	10	4	0.2	0

Food Name	Serv. Size	Total Cal.	Prot. gms	Carbs gms	Sod. mgs	Fiber gms	Fat gms	Chol. mgs
halves, unpeeled, in juice, w/liquid	1 cup	117	2	30	10	4	0.1	0
halves, unpeeled, in light syrup, w/liquid	1 cup	159	1	42	10	4	0.1	0
halves, unpeeled, in water, w/liquid	1 cup	66	2	16	7	4	0.4	0
whole, peeled, in heavy syrup, w/o pits, w/liquid	1 cup	236	1	61	32	4	0.1	0
whole, peeled, in water, w/o pits, w/liquid	1 cup	50	2	12	25	2	0.1	0
whole, unpeeled, in heavy syrup, w/liquid	1 cup	199	1	52	10	4	0.2	0
whole, unpeeled, in heavy syrup, w/liquid	1/2 apricot	33	0	9	2	1	0.0	0
whole, unpeeled, in juice, w/liquid	1/2 apricot	17	0	4	1	1	0.0	0
whole, unpeeled, in light syrup, w/liquid	1/2 apricot	25	0	7	2	1	0.0	0
whole, unpeeled, in water, w/liquid	1/2 apricot	10	0	2	1	1	0.1	0
Dehydrated/sulfured								
halves, stewed	1 cup	213	3	55	8	8	0.4	0
halves, uncooked	1 cup	309	5	80	13	12	0.6	0
low-moisture, stewed	1 cup	314	5	81	12	na	0.6	0
low-moisture, uncooked	1 cup	381	6	99	15	na	0.7	0
uncooked	1/2 apricot	8	0	2	0	0	0.0	0
Fresh								
raw, halved	1 cup	74	2	17	2	4	0.6	0
raw, sliced	1 cup	79	2	18	2	4	0.6	0
raw, whole	1 med	17	0	4	0	1	0.1	0
Frozen								
sweetened	1 cup	237	2	61	10	5	0.2	0
sliced (Flav-R-Pac)	2/3 cup	70	1	18	0	1	0.0	0
APRICOT KERNEL OIL								
	1 cup	1927	0	0	0	0	218.0	0
	1 tbsp	120	0	0	0	0	13.6	0
(Hain)	1 tbsp	120	0	0	0	0	14.0	0
ARBORIO RICE. See under RICE.								
ARROWHEAD								
boiled, drained	1 medium	9	1	2	2	na	0.0	0
powdered (Tone's)	1 tsp	10	0	2	1	0	0.0	0
raw	1 large	25	1	5	6	na	0.1	0
raw	1 medium	12	1	2	3	na	0.0	0
ARROWROOT								
raw, whole	1 med root	21	1	4	9	0	0.1	0
raw, sliced	1 cup	78	5	16	31	2	0.2	0
ARROWROOT FLOUR. See under FLOUR.								
ARTICHOKE. See also ARTICHOKE, JERUSALEM.								
Canned								
globe, bottoms (Reese)	2 pieces	35	2	7	260	1	0.0	0
globe, hearts (C&W)	1/2 cup	25	2	4	60	5	0.0	0
globe, hearts, 5-7 per can (Reese)	2 pieces	30	2	6	240	1	0.0	0
globe, hearts, quartered (Maria)	1/2 cup	35	2	6	330	3	0.0	0
globe, hearts, 10-12 per can (Reese)	4 pieces	30	2	6	240	1	0.0	0
hearts, marinated (Progresso)	1/3 cup	160	1	6	290	1	14.0	0
Fresh								
globe, fresh (Dole)	1 large	23	2	5	65	3	0.1	0
globe or French, boiled, drained	1 medium	60	4	13	114	6	0.2	0
globe or French, hearts, boiled, drained	1/2 cup	42	3	9	80	5	0.1	0
globe or French, raw	1 large	76	5	17	152	9	0.2	0
globe or French, raw	1 medium	60	4	13	120	7	0.2	0
Frozen								
globe or French, unprepared	9-oz pkg	97	7	20	120	10	1.1	0
globe or French, w/salt, drained	9-oz pkg	108	7	22	694	11	1.2	0
globe or French, w/salt, drained	1 cup	76	5	15	486	8	0.8	0
globe or French, w/salt, drained, 1/3 of 10-oz pkg	1 serving	36	2	7	231	4	0.4	0
globe or French, w/o salt, drained	1 cup	76	5	15	89	8	0.8	0

Food Name	Serv. Size	Total Cal.	Prot. gms	Carbs gms	Sod. mgs	Fiber gms	Fat gms	Chol. mgs
globe or French, w/o salt, drained	9-oz pkg	108	7	22	127	11	1.2	0
globe or French, w/o salt, drained, 1/3 of 10-oz pkg	1 serving	36	2	7	42	4	0.4	0
hearts (Seabrook)	3 oz	25	3	4	6	1	0.0	0
hearts, 'Deluxe' (Birds Eye)	3 oz	30	2	7	140	0	0.0	0
ARTICHOKE, JERUSALEM/sunchoke								
raw, sliced	1 cup	114	3	26	6	2	0.0	0
ARUGULA/rucola/rugula								
raw	1 leaf	1	0	0	1	0	0.0	0
raw	1/2 cup	3	0	0	3	0	0.1	0
(Frieda of California)	1 oz	7	1	1	4	0	0.1	0
ASIAN PEAR/Chinese pear/sand pear								
Fresh								
raw, whole, approx 2.25 x 2.5-inch diam	1 fruit	51	1	13	0	4	0.3	0
raw, whole, approx 3-3/8 x 3-inch diam	1 fruit	116	1	29	0	10	0.6	0
ASPARAGUS								
Canned								
cuts, green, drained	1 cup	46	5	6	695	4	1.6	0
cuts, green, w/liquid	1/2 cup	18	2	3	346	1	0.2	0
cuts, green, 50% less salt, w/liquid (Green Giant)	1/2 cup	20	2	3	210	1	0.0	0
cuts, green (Stokely)	1/2 cup	20	2	3	380	0	0.0	0
cuts, green, w/liquid (Green Giant)	1/2 cup	20	2	3	420	1	0.0	0
cuts, green 'No Salt or Sugar Added' (Stokely)	1/2 cup	20	2	3	5	0	0.0	0
cuts, white, w/liquid (Green Giant)	1/2 cup	16	2	3	410	1	0.0	0
cuts and tips (Finast)	1 cup	35	4	6	720	0	0.0	0
points, green (S&W)	1/2 cup	17	4	3	10	0	0.0	0
spears, drained	1 med spear	3	0	0	52	0	0.1	0
green, cut (Green Giant)	1/2 cup	18	2	3	420	1	0.0	0
green, cut, 50% less salt (Green Giant)	1/2 cup	18	2	3	210	1	0.0	0
green, cut 'No Salt Added' (Pathmark)	1/2 cup	20	3	2	5	0	0.0	0
green, cut (Pathmark)	1/2 cup	20	3	2	450	0	0.0	0
green, extra large 'LeSueur' (Green Giant)	4.5 oz	20	2	3	440	1	0.0	0
green, extra long (Green Giant)	4.5 oz	20	2	3	400	1	0.0	0
green 'Fancy' (S&W)	1/2 cup	18	2	3	320	0	0.0	0
spears, colossal (S&W)	3 pieces	10	1	3	170	1	0.0	0
white (Green Giant)	1/2 cup	16	2	3	410	1	0.0	0
Fresh								
cuts, boiled, drained	1/2 cup	22	2	4	10	1	0.3	0
cuts, raw	1 cup	31	3	6	3	3	0.3	0
spears, boiled, drained, whole	4 med spears	14	2	3	7	1	0.2	0
spears, fresh (Dole)	5 spears	18	2	2	0	2	0.0	0
spears, raw, extra large, 8.75 to 10-inch long	1 spear	6	1	1	0	1	0.0	0
spears, raw, large, 7.25 to 8.5-inch long	1 spear	5	0	1	0	0	0.0	0
spears, raw, medium, 5.25 to 7-inch long	1 spear	4	0	1	0	0	0.0	0
spears, raw, small, up to 5-inch long	1 spear	3	0	1	0	0	0.0	0
tips, raw, 2 inches long or less	1 spear tip	1	0	0	0	0	0.0	0
Frozen								
cuts (Birds Eye)	3.3 oz	25	3	4	5	0	0.0	0
cuts (Flav-R-Pac)	3/4 cup	20	3	3	5	2	0.0	0
cuts (Seabrook)	3.3 oz	25	3	4	6	0	0.0	0
cuts, unprepared	10-oz pkg	68	9	12	23	5	0.7	0
cuts, w/salt, boiled, drained	10-oz pkg	82	9	14	703	5	1.2	0
cuts, w/salt, boiled, drained	1 cup	50	5	9	432	3	0.8	0
cuts, w/o salt, boiled, drained	10-oz pkg	82	9	14	12	5	1.2	0
cuts, w/o salt, boiled, drained	1 cup	50	5	9	7	3	0.8	0
cuts and spears (Frosty Acres)	3.3 oz	25	3	4	6	0	0.0	0
spears (Birds Eye)	3.3 oz	25	3	4	0	0	0.0	0
spears (Finast)	3.3 oz	25	3	4	5	0	0.0	0

Food Name	Serv. Size	Total Cal.	Prot. gms	Carbs gms	Sod. mgs	Fiber gms	Fat gms	Chol. mgs
spears *(Frosty Acres)*	3.3 oz	25	3	4	4	1	0.0	0
spears *(Seabrook)*	3.3 oz	25	3	4	4	1	0.0	0
spears *(Southern)*	3.5 oz	27	3	4	20	0	0.2	0
spears, boiled, drained	4 spears	17	2	3	2	1	0.3	0
spears, unprepared	4 spears	14	2	2	5	1	0.1	0

ATLANTIC COD. See under COD.
ATLANTIC MACKEREL. See under MACKEREL.
ATLANTIC OCEAN PERCH. See OCEAN PERCH.
ATLANTIC POLLACK. See POLLACK.
ATLANTIC SALMON. See under SALMON.
AUBERGINE. See EGGPLANT.
AVOCADO
ALL COMMERCIAL VARIETIES
Fresh

Food Name	Serv. Size	Total Cal.	Prot. gms	Carbs gms	Sod. mgs	Fiber gms	Fat gms	Chol. mgs
raw, cubed	1 cup	242	3	11	15	8	23.0	0
raw, puréed	1 cup	370	5	17	23	12	35.2	0
raw, sliced	1 cup	235	3	11	15	7	22.4	0
raw, whole	1 medium	324	4	15	20	10	30.8	0

CALIFORNIA
Fresh

raw, puréed	1 cup	407	5	16	28	11	39.9	0
raw, whole, peeled and pitted	1 medium	306	4	12	21	8	30.0	0

FLORIDA
Fresh

raw, puréed	1 cup	258	4	20	12	12	20.4	0
raw, whole, peeled and pitted	1 medium	340	5	27	15	16	27.0	0

AVOCADO OIL

	1 cup	1927	0	0	0	0	218.0	na
	1 tbsp	124	0	0	0	0	14.0	na
(Hain)	1 tbsp	120	0	0	0	0	14.0	0
pure-pressed, organic *(Spectrum)*	1 tbsp	120	0	0	0	0	14.0	0

AWA/milkfish

baked, broiled, grilled, or microwaved	3 oz	162	22	0	78	0	7.3	57
raw	3 oz	126	17	0	61	0	5.7	44

B

Food Name	Serv. Size	Total Cal.	Prot. gms	Carbs gms	Sod. mgs	Fiber gms	Fat gms	Chol. mgs

BABASSU OIL. See PALM KERNEL OIL.
BABY FOOD
CEREAL
Barley

dry	1/2 oz	55	2	11	7	1	0.5	0
dry	1 tbsp	9	0	2	1	0	0.1	0
instant *(Heinz)*	3.5 oz	370	9	79	15	0	3.7	0
instant, prepared w/0.5 oz cereal and 2.4 oz whole milk *(Gerber)*	2.9 oz	100	3	14	0	0	4.0	0
instant, prepared w/2.4 oz formula '1st Foods' *(Gerber)*	1/2 oz	110	2	16	0	0	4.0	0
prepared w/whole milk	1 oz	31	1	5	14	na	0.9	na
Cereal w/applesauce and bananas, '3rd Foods' *(Gerber)*	7 tbsp	82	1	18	3	0	0.6	0
Cereal w/egg yolks								
junior	1 jar	88	3	12	56	2	3.1	107
strained	1 oz	14	1	2	9	0	0.5	18
w/eggs	1 oz	16	1	2	11	na	0.4	15
Cereal w/egg yolks and bacon, junior	1 oz	22	1	2	14	0	1.4	27

Food Name	Serv. Size	Total Cal.	Prot. gms	Carbs gms	Sod. mgs	Fiber gms	Fat gms	Chol. mgs
Corn								
instant, dry 'Tropical Foods' *(Gerber)*	3.5 oz	390	6	81	55	0	4.6	0
instant, prepared w/milk 'Tropical Foods' *(Gerber)*	2.4 oz	110	3	15	0	0	4.0	0
High-protein								
instant, dry	1/2 oz	54	5	7	7	1	0.9	0
instant, dry	1 tbsp	9	1	1	1	0	0.1	0
instant, prepared w/whole milk	1 oz	31	2	3	14	na	1.1	na
w/apple and orange, instant, dry	1/2 oz	53	4	8	15	1	0.9	0
w/apple and orange, instant, dry	1 tbsp	9	1	1	2	0	0.2	0
w/apple and orange, instant, prepared w/whole milk	1 oz	32	2	4	16	na	1.1	na
Mixed								
dry	1/2 oz	57	2	11	6	1	0.7	0
dry	1 tbsp	9	0	2	1	0	0.1	0
prepared w/whole milk	1 oz	32	1	5	13	0	1.0	3
instant, dry *(Earth's Best)*	0.5 oz	60	2	11	0	0	0.0	0
instant, dry, '2nd Foods' *(Gerber)*	0.5 oz	60	1	11	0	0	1.0	0
instant *(Heinz)*	3.5 oz	373	13	72	12	0	4.9	0
instant, prepared w/apple juice, '2nd Foods' *(Gerber)*	2.4 oz	90	1	20	0	0	1.0	0
instant, prepared w/0.5 oz cereal, 2.4 oz formula, 'Stages 2' *(Beech-Nut)*	0.5 oz	120	2	17	25	0	4.0	0
instant, prepared w/0.5 oz cereal, 2.5 oz formula *(Earth's Best)*	3 oz	110	3	16	15	0	3.0	0
instant, prepared w/0.5 oz cereal, 2.4 oz whole milk, 'Stages 2' *(Beech-Nut)*	2.9 oz	100	4	14	50	0	3.0	0
w/apple and bananas, 'Stages 2' *(Beech-Nut)*	4.5 oz	90	2	19	0	0	1.0	0
w/apple and bananas, strained *(Heinz)*	3.5 oz	70	1	16	3	0	0.3	0
w/apple 'Stages 2' *(Beech-Nut)*	4 oz	70	0	16	0	1	0.0	na
w/applesauce and bananas, junior	1 oz	24	0	5	10	0	0.1	0
w/applesauce and bananas, strained	1 oz	23	0	5	1	0	0.1	0
w/applesauce and bananas, '3rd Foods' *(Gerber)*	7 tbsp	82	1	19	3	0	0.6	0
w/banana, dry	1/2 oz	59	2	12	18	1	0.7	0
w/banana, dry	1 tbsp	10	0	2	3	0	0.1	0
w/bananas, dry, '2nd Foods' *(Gerber)*	0.5 oz	60	1	11	0	0	1.0	0
w/fruit and nuts, no sugar added, 1-4 yr, dry *(Familia)*	1.5 oz	170	4	31	4	0	3.0	0
w/fruit and nuts, 100% natural, 1-4 yr, dry *(Familia)*	1.5 oz	170	4	32	1	0	3.0	0
w/fruit and nuts, 1-4 yr, prepared w/whole milk *(Familia)*	1.5 oz	270	9	38	77	0	8.0	0
w/fruit and nuts, 1-4 yr, prepared w/2/3 cup milk *(Familia)*	1.5 oz	270	9	39	74	0	8.0	0
Oatmeal								
dry	1/2 oz	60	2	10	5	1	1.2	0
dry	1 tbsp	10	0	2	1	0	0.2	0
prepared w/whole milk	1 oz	33	1	4	13	0	1.2	3
w/apple, 'Stages 2' *(Beech-Nut)*	4 oz	70	1	16	0	1	0.0	na
w/apple and bananas 'Stages 2' *(Beech-Nut)*	4.5 oz	90	2	17	5	0	1.0	0
w/apple and bananas, strained *(Heinz)*	3.5 oz	76	2	16	3	1	0.6	0
w/apple and cinnamon, instant, '3rd Foods' *(Gerber)*	1 pkt	90	2	16	50	0	2.0	0
w/applesauce and bananas, junior	1 oz	21	0	4	9	0	0.2	0
w/applesauce and bananas, strained	1 oz	21	0	4	1	0	0.2	0
w/applesauce and bananas, '3rd Foods' *(Gerber)*	7 tbsp	80	1	17	3	0	0.8	0
w/bananas, dry	1/2 oz	59	2	11	18	1	0.9	0
w/bananas, dry	1 tbsp	10	0	2	3	0	0.1	0
w/bananas, prepared w/whole milk	1 oz	33	1	5	17	na	1.1	na
w/bananas, instant '3rd Foods' *(Gerber)*	1 pkt	90	2	16	50	0	2.0	0
w/bananas, 100% natural, organic, dry *(Healthy Times)*	0.5 oz	60	2	12	0	0	0.0	0
w/bananas, organic, prepared w/2.4 oz formula *(Healthy Times)*	0.5 oz	100	3	17	15	0	3.0	0

Food Name	Serv. Size	Total Cal.	Prot. gms	Carbs gms	Sod. mgs	Fiber gms	Fat gms	Chol. mgs
w/fruit, toddler, instant, dry	0.75 oz	84	2	16	42	2	1.5	0
w/fruit, toddler, instant, dry	1 tbsp	21	1	4	11	0	0.4	0
w/honey, dry	1/2 oz	56	2	10	7	na	1.0	na
w/honey, dry	1 tbsp	9	0	2	1	na	0.2	na
w/honey, prepared w/whole milk	1 oz	33	1	4	14	na	1.1	na
Rice								
dry	1/2 oz	59	1	12	5	0	0.7	0
dry	1 tbsp	10	0	2	1	0	0.1	0
prepared w/whole milk	1 oz	33	1	5	13	0	1.0	3
prepared w/formula '1st Foods' (Gerber)	2.4 oz	110	2	16	0	0	4.0	0
(Heinz)	3.5 oz	376	8	78	12	0	4.1	0
brown, dry (Earth's Best)	0.5 oz	60	1	12	0	0	0.0	0
brown, prepared w/0.5 oz cereal, 2.5 oz formula (Earth's Best)	3 oz	110	2	17	15	0	3.0	0
instant, prepared w/0.5 oz cereal, 2.4 oz whole milk, 'Stage 1' (Beech-Nut) 'Stage 1'	2.9 oz	110	2	17	30	0	3.0	0
instant, prepared w/0.5 oz cereal, 2.4 oz formula, 'Stage 1' (Beech-Nut)	0.5 oz	120	2	18	20	0	4.0	0
sprouted (Health Valley)	1 tbsp	60	1	10	5	2	1.0	0
w/apple, instant, prepared w/0.5 oz cereal, 2.4 oz formula (Beech-Nut)	2.9 oz	120	1	19	20	0	4.0	0
w/apple, instant, prepared w/0.5 oz cereal, 2.4 oz whole milk (Beech-Nut)	2.9 oz	110	3	17	50	0	3.0	0
w/apple, 'Stage 2' (Beech-Nut)	4 oz	70	0	16	0	1	0.0	na
w/apple and bananas, 'Stage 2' (Beech-Nut)	4.5 oz	100	2	24	25	0	0.0	0
w/apple and bananas, strained (Heinz)	3.5 oz	70	1	16	5	0	0.2	0
w/applesauce and bananas, '2nd Foods' (Gerber)	7 tbsp	79	1	18	9	0	0.2	0
w/applesauce and bananas, strained	1 oz	22	0	5	8	0	0.1	0
w/applesauce and bananas, strained	1 tbsp	13	0	3	4	0	0.1	0
w/applesauce and bananas, strained, '2nd Foods' (Gerber)	4 oz jar	89	1	19	32	1	0.5	0
w/applesauce and bananas, strained, 'Strained 2' (Heinz)	4.25 oz jar	95	1	21	34	1	0.5	0
w/bananas, dry	1 tbsp	10	0	2	2	0	0.1	0
w/bananas, dry	1/2 oz	61	1	12	14	0	0.6	0
w/bananas, prepared w/whole milk	1 oz	33	1	5	16	0	1.0	3
w/bananas, dry, '2nd Foods' (Gerber)	0.5 oz	60	1	11	0	0	1.0	0
w/bananas, prepared w/0.5 oz cereal, 2.4 oz formula (Beech-Nut)	0.5 oz	120	1	19	20	0	4.0	0
w/bananas, prepared w/0.5 oz cereal, 2.4 oz whole milk (Beech-Nut)	2.9 oz	100	3	17	50	0	3.0	0
w/honey, prepared w/whole milk	1 oz	33	1	5	14	na	0.9	na
w/mango, dry, 'Tropical Foods' (Gerber)	3.5 oz	386	6	84	20	0	2.6	0
w/mango, prepared w/milk, 'Tropical Foods' (Gerber)	2.4 oz	100	3	15	0	0	3.0	0
w/mixed fruit, junior	1 oz	22	0	5	3	0	0.1	0
w/mixed fruit, junior	1 tbsp	12	0	3	2	0	0.0	0
w/mixed fruit, junior (Gerber)	6 oz	140	1	31	17	0	1.0	0
w/mixed fruit, '3rd Foods' (Gerber)	6-oz jar	134	2	31	17	1	0.3	0
DESSERTS AND SNACKS								
Apple-strawberry dessert, 'Stage 2' (Beech-Nut)	4 oz	100	0	23	0	1	0.0	na
Apple-peach-strawberry dessert, 'Stage 2' (Beech-Nut)	4 oz	100	0	22	0	1	0.0	na
Banana-pineapple dessert, 'Stage 2' (Beech-Nut)	4 oz	100	0	23	15	0	0.0	0
Banana-vanilla dessert, (Gerber) 'Tropical Foods'	7 tbsp	85	1	19	11	0	0.9	0
Cereal snack								
apple-banana, finger snacks, 'Graduates' (Gerber)	3.2 oz	405	8	83	86	0	4.8	0
apple-cinnamon, finger snacks 'Graduates' (Gerber)	3.2 oz	407	8	83	84	0	5.0	0

Food Name	Serv. Size	Total Cal.	Prot. gms	Carbs gms	Sod. mgs	Fiber gms	Fat gms	Chol. mgs
Cookies and crackers								
animal-shaped, baked, chunky *(Gerber)*	3.5 oz	443	7	75	187	0	13.1	0
apple, organic, 'Hugga Bears' *(Healthy Times)*	1 oz	120	2	17	38	0	3.0	0
arrowroot	1 oz	125	2	20	105	0	4.1	0
arrowroot	1 cookie	22	0	4	19	0	0.7	0
arrowroot, baked finger snacks, 'Graduates' *(Gerber)*	3.5 oz	452	8	70	324	0	15.3	0
arrowroot, maple, wheat-free *(Healthy Times)*	1 cookie	120	2	17	38	0	3.0	0
cinnamon animal cracker, baked 'Graduates' *(Gerber)*	3.5 oz	449	6	79	369	0	12.3	0
pretzel	1 oz	113	3	23	76	1	0.6	0
pretzel, baked, finger snacks, 'Graduates' *(Gerber)*	3.5 oz	403	11	83	597	0	3.3	0
strawberry, organic, 'Hugga Bears' *(Healthy Times)*	1 oz	120	2	17	38	0	3.0	0
teething biscuit	1 oz	111	3	22	103	0	1.2	0
teething biscuit	1 biscuit	43	1	8	40	0	0.5	0
teething, biscuit, baked, chunky, 'Biter Biscuit' *(Gerber)*	1 biscuit	50	1	9	0	0	1.0	0
teething toast *(Zings!)*	1 serving	35	1	5	10	1	1.0	0
zwieback	1 oz	121	3	21	66	1	2.8	6
zwieback	1 piece	30	1	5	16	0	0.7	1
zwieback toast *(Gerber)*	1 cracker	30	1	5	16	0	0.7	1
zwieback toast, baked, chunky *(Gerber)*	3.5 oz	432	13	69	210	0	11.5	0
Cottage cheese								
w/pineapple, 'Stage 2' *(Beech-Nut)*	4.5 oz	130	2	26	15	0	1.0	0
w/pineapple 'Stage 3' *(Beech-Nut)*	6 oz	170	3	36	20	0	2.0	0
w/pears, 'Stage 2' *(Beech-Nut)*	4 oz	120	2	24	15	1	1.0	na
w/pears, 'Stage 3' *(Beech-Nut)*	6 oz	180	3	37	20	1	2.0	na
Custard/pudding								
banana pudding, 'Stage 2' *(Beech-Nut)*	4 oz	110	0	26	0	0	0.0	na
banana pudding, strained *(Heinz)*	3.5 oz	74	1	17	9	0	0.5	0
cherry-vanilla pudding, strained	1 oz	19	0	5	5	0	0.1	3
cherry-vanilla pudding, strained *(Gerber)*	4.5 oz	90	0	21	12	0	1.0	3
cherry-vanilla pudding, junior	1 oz	20	0	5	4	0	0.1	3
custard pudding, junior *(Heinz)*	3.5 oz	75	2	14	27	0	1.2	0
custard pudding, strained *(Heinz)*	3.5 oz	75	2	14	27	0	1.2	0
orange pudding, strained	1 oz	23	0	5	6	0	0.3	1
pineapple pudding, junior	1 oz	25	0	6	6	0	0.1	0
pineapple pudding, junior	1 tbsp	13	0	3	3	0	0.1	0
pineapple pudding, junior, '3rd Foods' *(Gerber)*	6-oz jar	148	2	37	37	1	0.7	0
pineapple pudding, strained	1 oz	23	0	6	5	0	0.1	0
pineapple pudding, strained	1 tbsp	12	0	3	3	0	0.0	0
pineapple pudding, strained, '2nd Foods'	4 oz jar	92	1	23	21	1	0.3	0
tutti frutti pudding, junior *(Heinz)*	3.5 oz	67	0	16	12	0	0.4	0
vanilla custard, 'Stage 2' *(Beech-Nut)*	4 oz	120	2	23	60	0	3.0	0
vanilla custard, 'Stage 3' *(Beech-Nut)*	6 oz	180	3	30	80	0	5.0	0
vanilla custard, '3rd Foods' *(Gerber)*	6 oz	190	2	32	85	0	6.0	0
vanilla custard, junior *(Gerber)*	6 oz	150	3	31	41	0	2.0	23
vanilla custard, strained *(Gerber)*	4.5 oz	100	2	22	32	0	1.0	14
vanilla pudding, junior	1 cup	197	4	40	60	0	2.2	87
vanilla pudding, junior	1 oz	24	0	5	7	0	0.3	11
vanilla pudding, junior	1 tbsp	12	0	2	4	0	0.1	5
vanilla pudding, junior, 'Junior 3' *(Heinz)*	6 oz jar	146	3	30	44	0	1.7	65
vanilla pudding, junior, 'Stage 3' *(Beech-Nut)*	6 oz jar	146	3	30	44	0	1.7	65
vanilla pudding, junior, '3rd Foods' *(Gerber)*	6 oz jar	146	3	30	44	0	1.7	65
vanilla pudding, strained	1 cup	195	4	37	64	0	4.6	18
vanilla pudding, strained	1 oz	24	0	5	8	0	0.6	2
vanilla pudding, strained	1 tbsp	12	0	2	4	0	0.3	1
vanilla pudding, strained, '2nd Foods' *(Gerber)*	4 oz jar	96	2	18	32	0	2.3	9

Food Name	Serv. Size	Total Cal.	Prot. gms	Carbs gms	Sod. mgs	Fiber gms	Fat gms	Chol. mgs
vanilla pudding, strained, 'Stages 2' *(Beech-Nut)*	4 oz jar	96	2	18	32	0	2.3	9
vanilla pudding, strained, 'Strained 2' *(Heinz)*	4 oz jar	96	2	18	32	0	2.3	9
Dutch apple dessert								
junior	1 oz	22	0	5	1	0	0.0	0
junior *(Heinz)*	3.5 oz	69	0	16	5	0	0.4	0
'Stage 2' *(Beech-Nut)*	4 oz	100	0	22	10	0	0.0	0
strained	1 oz	19	0	5	5	0	0.3	0
strained *(Heinz)*	3.5 oz	69	0	16	5	0	0.4	0
'3rd Foods' *(Gerber)*	7 tbsp	77	0	17	14	0	0.9	0
Fruit dessert								
junior *(Gerber)*	6 oz	130	0	30	12	0	1.0	0
junior *(Heinz)*	3.5 oz	65	0	16	14	0	0.2	0
junior, w/o added vitamin C	1 oz	18	0	5	4	0	0.0	0
junior, w/o added vitamin C	1 tbsp	9	0	3	2	0	0.0	0
junior, w/o added vitamin C, '3rd Foods' *(Gerber)*	6-oz jar	107	1	29	22	1	0.0	0
junior, w/o added vitamin C 'Junior 3' *(Heinz)*	6-oz jar	107	1	29	22	1	0.0	0
nonfat, 'Stage 3' *(Beech-Nut)*	6 oz	120	0	28	0	2	0.0	0
strained *(Gerber)*	4.5 oz	100	0	24	13	0	1.0	0
strained *(Heinz)*	3.5 oz	66	0	16	11	0	0.2	0
strained, w/o added vitamin C	1 oz	17	0	5	4	0	0.0	0
strained, w/o added vitamin C	1 tbsp	9	0	2	2	0	0.0	0
strained, w/o added vitamin C, '2nd Foods' *(Gerber)*	4-oz jar	67	0	18	16	1	0.0	0
strained, w/o added vitamin C, 'Strained 2' *(Heinz)*	4.25-oz jar	71	0	19	17	1	0.0	0
'3rd Foods' *(Gerber)*	7 tbsp	73	0	18	7	0	0.2	0
Guava dessert								
tropical fruit, 'Stage 2' *(Beech-Nut)*	4 oz	90	0	22	10	2	0.0	na
w/tapioca 'Tropical Foods' *(Gerber)*	7 tbsp	69	0	17	3	0	0.1	0
Hawaiian dessert								
Hawaiian delight, '3rd Foods' *(Gerber)*	7 tbsp	87	1	20	15	0	0.1	0
Hawaiian delight, junior *(Gerber)*	6 oz	150	2	33	32	0	1.0	3
strained *(Gerber)*	4.5 oz	120	2	25	23	0	1.0	2
Mango dessert								
tropical fruit dessert, 'Stage 2' *(Beech-Nut)*	4.5 oz	100	0	25	15	0	0.0	0
w/tapioca, 'Tropical Foods' *(Gerber)*	7 tbsp	75	0	18	2	0	0.2	0
Mango-banana dessert, w/passionfruit, 'Tropical Foods'								
(Gerber)	7 tbsp	73	0	18	9	0	0.1	0
Papaya dessert, w/tapioca, 'Tropical Foods' *(Gerber)*	7 tbsp	62	0	15	7	0	0.2	0
Papaya-pineapple dessert, 'Tropical Foods' *(Gerber)*	7 tbsp	76	0	19	8	0	0.0	0
Peach cobbler								
junior	1 oz	19	0	5	3	0	0.0	0
junior	1 tbsp	10	0	3	1	0	0.0	0
junior *(Gerber)*	6 oz	130	1	30	15	0	1.0	0
'2nd Foods' *(Gerber)*	4-oz jar	73	0	20	8	1	0.0	0
strained	1 oz	18	0	5	2	0	0.0	0
strained	1 tbsp	10	0	3	1	0	0.0	0
strained *(Gerber)*	4.5 oz	100	1	23	9	0	1.0	0
strained *(Heinz)*	3.5 oz	72	1	17	6	0	0.3	0
'Strained 2' *(Heinz)*	4-oz jar	73	0	20	8	1	0.0	0
'3rd Foods' *(Gerber)*	6-oz jar	114	1	31	15	1	0.0	0
'3rd Foods' *(Gerber)*	7 tbsp	77	1	18	9	0	0.1	0
Peach-mango dessert, 'Tropical Foods' *(Gerber)*	7 tbsp	60	0	17	7	0	0.2	0
Pineapple-banana dessert, 'Tropical Foods' *(Gerber)*	7 tbsp	79	0	19	9	0	0.1	0
Tropical dessert								
island fruit dessert, 'Stage 2' *(Beech-Nut)*	4 oz	100	0	23	10	0	0.0	na
mango dessert, 'Stage 2' *(Beech-Nut)*	4 oz	110	0	26	10	1	0.0	na
medley, 'Tropical Foods' *(Gerber)*	7 tbsp	64	0	15	6	0	0.1	0
papaya dessert, 'Stage 2' *(Beech-Nut)*	4 oz	100	0	22	10	0	0.0	na

Food Name	Serv. Size	Total Cal.	Prot. gms	Carbs gms	Sod. mgs	Fiber gms	Fat gms	Chol. mgs
w/tapioca, strained *(Gerber)*	4.5 oz	80	0	20	6	0	0.0	0
Yogurt								
apple, 'Stage 2' *(Beech-Nut)*	4 oz	100	1	22	25	0	1.0	0
apple, 'Breakfast' *(Earth's Best)*	4.5 oz	100	3	17	20	0	2.0	0
banana, 'Stage 2' *(Beech-Nut)*	4 oz	120	1	24	25	0	2.0	0
banana, strained *(Heinz)*	3.5 oz	83	1	19	20	0	0.5	0
blueberry, 'Breakfast' *(Earth's Best)*	4.5 oz	100	3	16	20	0	2.0	0
mixed fruit, 'Stage 2' *(Beech-Nut)*	4 oz	100	1	21	15	1	0.0	na
mixed fruit, 'Stage 3' *(Beech-Nut)*	6 oz	170	1	30	30	1	0.0	na
peach, '2nd Foods' *(Gerber)*	7 tbsp	76	1	17	14	0	0.4	0
peach, 'Stage 2' *(Beech-Nut)*	4.5 oz	120	1	25	30	0	2.0	0
pear, 'Stage 2' *(Beech-Nut)*	4.5 oz	130	1	29	35	0	2.0	0
pear, strained *(Heinz)*	3.5 oz	80	1	18	19	0	0.4	0
tropical, 'Breakfast' *(Earth's Best)*	4.5 oz	110	3	19	20	0	2.0	0
DINNERS AND MAIN DISHES								
Apple and chicken dinner								
'Simple Recipe' '2nd Foods' *(Gerber)*	4 oz	70	3	12	15	2	1.5	0
'Simple Dinner' 'Stage 2' *(Beech-Nut)*	4 oz	73	2	12	14	2	1.6	6
strained	1 oz	18	1	3	3	1	0.4	1
Apple and ham dinner								
'Simple Recipe' '2nd Foods' *(Gerber)*	4 oz	80	3	12	15	2	2.0	0
strained	1 tbsp	9	0	2	1	0	0.1	1
Apple and turkey dinner								
'Simple Recipe' '2nd Foods' *(Gerber)*	4 oz	80	3	13	20	0	2.0	0
strained	1 tbsp	10	0	2	2	0	0.2	1
Beans and rice dinner, 'Tropical Foods' *(Gerber)*	7 tbsp	52	2	7	8	0	1.5	0
Beef and rice dinner, toddler	1 oz	23	1	2	101	na	0.8	na
Beef and vegetable dinner								
lean meat, junior *(Gerber)*	4.5 oz	100	8	10	29	0	3.0	12
lean meat, strained *(Gerber)*	4.5 oz	90	7	9	32	0	3.0	11
'Stage 2' *(Beech-Nut)*	4.5 oz	90	2	10	35	0	4.0	0
'Stage 3' *(Beech-Nut)*	6 oz	160	6	16	70	0	7.0	0
Beef dinner								
junior *(Gerber)*	2.5 oz	80	11	1	38	0	4.0	20
'Stage 1' *(Beech-Nut)*	2.8 oz	90	10	0	40	0	5.0	0
'Stage 3' *(Beech-Nut)*	6 oz	150	6	14	45	0	8.0	0
'3rd Foods' *(Gerber)*	7 tbsp	103	15	0	52	0	4.6	0
Beef lasagna dinner, toddler	1 oz	22	1	3	129	na	0.6	na
Beef noodle dinner								
chunky, 'Homestyle' *(Gerber)*	7 tbsp	88	4	10	216	0	3.5	0
junior	1 oz	16	1	2	5	0	0.5	2
junior	1 tbsp	9	0	1	3	0	0.3	1
'Step 3' *(Heinz)*	6 oz	97	4	13	29	2	3.2	14
strained	1 oz	18	1	2	4	0	0.6	2
strained	1 tbsp	10	0	1	2	0	0.4	1
w/egg noodles, '2nd Foods' *(Gerber)*	7 tbsp	62	3	8	10	0	2.0	0
w/egg noodles, 'Stage 2' *(Beech-Nut)*	4 oz	100	1	8	50	2	6.0	na
w/egg noodles, 'Stage 3' *(Beech-Nut)*	6 oz	130	3	13	50	2	6.0	na
w/egg noodles, 'Step 2' *(Heinz)*	3.5 oz	49	2	6	15	0	1.8	0
w/egg noodles, '3rd Foods' *(Gerber)*	6 oz	130	4	18	45	3	1.9	0
Beef stew								
'Table Time' *(Beech-Nut)*	6 oz	150	10	16	380	0	6.0	0
toddler	1 oz	14	1	2	98	0	0.3	4
Broccoli and chicken dinner								
'Simple Recipe' '2nd Foods' *(Gerber)*	4 oz	45	4	3	30	2	2.0	7
'Step 2' *(Heinz)*	4 oz	47	4	4	21	3	1.7	7
strained	1 oz	12	1	1	5	1	0.4	2

Food Name	Serv. Size	Total Cal.	Prot. gms	Carbs gms	Sod. mgs	Fiber gms	Fat gms	Chol. mgs
Carrot and beef dinner								
'Simple Recipe' '2nd Foods' *(Gerber)*	4 oz	70	4	6	80	2	3.5	0
strained	1 tbsp	9	1	1	9	0	0.4	1
Chicken and rice dinner					-			
'Stage 2' *(Beech-Nut)*	4 oz	80	1	9	70	1	3.0	0
'Tropical Foods' *(Gerber)*	7 tbsp	48	2	7	14	0	1.3	0
Chicken and vegetable dinner								
'Stage 2' *(Beech-Nut)*	4.5 oz	90	3	14	65	0	3.0	0
'Stage 3' *(Beech-Nut)*	6 oz	90	7	13	70	0	2.0	0
w/broccoli, simple recipe, '2nd Foods' *(Gerber)*	7 tbsp	42	4	3	20	0	1.5	0
Chicken dinner								
junior *(Gerber)*	2.5 oz	110	11	1	28	0	7.0	42
'3rd Foods' *(Gerber)*	7 tbsp	132	15	0	39	0	7.9	0
w/vegetables, lean meat, junior *(Gerber)*	4.5 oz	90	7	10	32	0	3.0	19
w/vegetables, lean meat, strained *(Gerber)*	4.5 oz	90	7	8	31	0	3.0	18
Chicken noodle dinner								
junior	1 oz	16	1	2	22	0	0.3	3
junior	1 tbsp	9	0	1	12	0	0.2	1
'2nd Foods' *(Gerber)*	4 oz	80	3	11	35	2	2.5	18
'Step 2' *(Heinz)*	4 oz	75	3	10	26	2	2.3	18
'Step 3' *(Heinz)*	6 oz	94	4	15	133	2	2.0	15
'Stage 2' *(Beech-Nut)*	4 oz	70	1	7	45	2	4.0	na
'Stage 3' *(Beech-Nut)*	6 oz	110	3	14	55	1	4.0	na
strained	1 oz	19	1	3	7	1	0.6	5
strained	1 tbsp	11	0	1	4	0	0.3	3
'3rd Foods' *(Gerber)*	6 oz	110	4	16	65	4	3.5	0
w/carrots and peas, chunky *(Gerber)*	7 tbsp	65	4	9	207	0	1.5	0
Chicken stew								
toddler	1 oz	22	1	2	57	0	1.0	8
toddler	1 tbsp	12	1	1	32	0	0.6	5
w/noodles 'Graduates' *(Gerber)*	3.2 oz	69	4	9	308	0	2.0	0
Green bean and rice dinner *(Earth's Best)*	4.5 oz	70	2	14	0	0	0.0	0
Green bean and turkey dinner								
'Simple Recipe' '2nd Foods' *(Gerber)*	7 tbsp	55	4	7	11	0	1.5	0
'Step 2' *(Heinz)*	4 oz	60	4	6	12	3	2.1	9
strained	1 oz	15	1	2	3	1	0.5	2
Ham and vegetable dinner								
lean meat, junior *(Gerber)*	4.5 oz	110	8	11	27	0	4.0	11
lean meat, strained *(Gerber)*	4.5 oz	100	7	10	26	0	4.0	12
'Stage 2' *(Beech-Nut)*	4.5 oz	80	3	12	30	0	3.0	0
Lamb and vegetable dinner, 'Stage 2' *(Beech-Nut)*	4.5 oz	90	2	13	40	0	4.0	0
Macaroni and beef dinner								
in sauce, 'Graduates' *(Gerber)*	3.2 oz	78	5	11	302	0	1.7	0
'Stage 2' *(Beech-Nut)*	4.5 oz	90	2	13	40	0	4.0	0
'Stage 3' *(Beech-Nut)*	6 oz	130	3	14	60	2	6.0	0
Macaroni and cheese								
(Earth's Best)	4.5 oz	100	4	12	10	0	4.0	0
junior	1 oz	17	1	2	22	0	0.6	2
strained	1 oz	19	1	3	25	0	0.6	2
'Table Time' *(Beech-Nut)*	6 oz	200	3	21	320	0	12.0	na
Macaroni, tomato, and beef dinner								
junior	1 oz	17	1	3	5	0	0.3	1
junior	1 tbsp	9	0	2	3	0	0.2	1
'2nd Foods' *(Gerber)*	4 oz	70	3	11	40	1	1.0	8
strained	1 oz	17	1	3	11	0	0.4	2
strained	1 tbsp	10	0	2	6	0	0.2	1
'Step 2' *(Heinz)*	4 oz	69	3	11	43	1	1.7	8

Food Name	Serv. Size	Total Cal.	Prot. gms	Carbs gms	Sod. mgs	Fiber gms	Fat gms	Chol. mgs
'3rd Foods' *(Gerber)*	7 tbsp	60	3	10	12	0	0.9	0
Pasta dinner								
alphabet pasta w/beef and tomato sauce, chunky								
(Gerber)	7 tbsp	80	4	11	199	0	2.0	0
(Earth's Best)	4.5 oz	90	3	13	20	0	3.0	0
pasta w/vegetables *(Gerber)*	4 oz	68	2	9	12	2	2.4	6
seashells in tomato sauce, 'Table Time' *(Beech-Nut)*	6 oz	150	3	25	170	1	4.0	na
Potato and green bean dinner *(Earth's Best)*	4.5 oz	100	4	13	25	0	3.0	0
Ravioli								
w/beef and sauce, 'Graduates' *(Gerber)*	3.2 oz	97	3	16	322	0	2.0	0
w/beef and sauce, micro cup, 'Graduates' *(Gerber)*	6 oz	170	6	28	590	0	4.0	0
w/cheese and sauce, 'Graduates' *(Gerber)*	3.2 oz	99	4	16	297	0	2.2	0
w/cheese and sauce, micro cup, 'Graduates' *(Gerber)*	6 oz	170	6	28	510	0	4.0	0
Rice and beef dinner, w/tomato sauce, chunky *(Gerber)*	7 tbsp	79	4	12	202	0	1.9	0
Rice and chicken dinner, saucy, chunky *(Gerber)*	7 tbsp	67	3	10	222	0	1.5	0
Rice and lentil dinner *(Earth's Best)*	4.5 oz	80	3	13	25	0	2.0	0
Spaghetti								
in tomato sauce w/beef, '3rd Foods' *(Gerber)*	6 oz	140	5	20	80	2	4.5	9
rings w/meat sauce, 'Table Time' *(Beech-Nut)*	6 oz	160	7	20	180	0	6.0	na
w/beef, chunky *(Gerber)*	7 tbsp	85	4	13	223	0	1.9	0
w/beef, junior *(Gerber)*	6 oz	120	5	19	41	0	3.0	7
w/beef, 'Stage 3' *(Beech-Nut)*	6 oz	130	3	16	70	1	6.0	0
w/beef, '3rd Foods' *(Gerber)*	7 tbsp	64	3	11	20	0	1.2	0
w/meat, junior *(Heinz)*	3.5 oz	58	2	10	19	1	1.3	0
w/mini meatballs, 'Graduates' *(Gerber)*	6 oz	160	7	21	590	0	5.0	0
w/tomato and meat, junior	1 oz	19	1	3	21	0	0.4	1
w/tomato and meat, junior	1 tbsp	11	0	2	12	0	0.2	1
w/tomato and meat, 'Step 3' *(Heinz)*	6 oz	116	4	19	128	2	2.3	9
w/tomato and meat, toddler	1 oz	21	2	3	101	na	0.3	na
Sweet potato and chicken dinner								
(Earth's Best)	4.5 oz	90	3	13	30	0	2.0	0
'Stage 2' *(Beech-Nut)*	4 oz	84	3	12	25	1	2.5	12
strained	1 tbsp	12	0	2	4	0	0.3	2
Turkey and barley dinner *(Gerber)*	4-oz jar	60	3	9	23	2	1.2	5
Turkey and rice dinner								
junior	1 oz	16	1	3	23	0	0.3	1
junior	1 tbsp	9	0	2	13	0	0.1	1
'2nd Foods' *(Gerber)*	4 oz	60	2	9	30	1	1.5	6
'Stage 2' *(Beech-Nut)*	4 oz	70	1	8	50	1	3.0	0
'Stage 3' *(Beech-Nut)*	6 oz	100	3	13	60	1	3.0	0
strained	1 oz	15	1	2	6	0	0.4	1
strained	1 tbsp	8	0	1	3	0	0.2	1
w/vegetables, 'Step 2' *(Heinz)*	4 oz	59	3	9	23	1	1.4	6
w/vegetables, 'Step 3' *(Heinz)*	6 oz	95	4	16	136	2	1.6	7
'3rd Foods' *(Gerber)*	6 oz	100	4	14	45	2	3.5	7
Turkey and vegetable dinner								
lean meat, junior *(Gerber)*	4.5 oz	100	7	10	31	0	4.0	16
lean meat, strained *(Gerber)*	4.5 oz	100	7	9	31	0	4.0	17
Turkey dinner								
junior *(Gerber)*	2.5 oz	100	10	1	37	0	6.0	38
supreme, 'Stage 2' *(Beech-Nut)*	4 oz	90	3	9	45	1	4.0	0
Turkey stew								
w/rice, 'Graduates' *(Gerber)*	3.2 oz	59	5	8	298	0	1.0	0
w/rice, 'Table Time' *(Beech-Nut)*	6 oz	150	6	14	200	1	7.0	na
Vegetable and bacon dinner								
junior	1 oz	20	1	2	13	0	1.1	1
junior	1 tbsp	11	0	1	7	0	0.6	0

Food Name	Serv. Size	Total Cal.	Prot. gms	Carbs gms	Sod. mgs	Fiber gms	Fat gms	Chol. mgs
'Step 2' *(Heinz)*	4 oz	80	2	10	55	2	3.3	5
'Step 3' *(Heinz)*	6 oz	121	3	13	77	2	6.6	5
'2nd Foods' *(Gerber)*	4 oz	80	2	10	60	1	3.5	5
strained	1 oz	20	1	2	14	0	0.8	1
strained	1 tbsp	11	0	1	8	0	0.5	1
Vegetable and beef dinner								
chunky *(Gerber)*	7 tbsp	70	4	9	201	0	2.0	0
(Earth's Best)	4.5 oz	90	3	11	15	0	3.0	0
junior	1 oz	18	1	3	21	0	0.5	2
junior	1 tbsp	10	0	1	12	0	0.3	1
'2nd Foods' *(Gerber)*	4 oz	70	3	10	35	3	2.5	7
'Stage 2' *(Beech-Nut)*	4 oz	80	1	8	45	1	4.0	na
'Stage 3' *(Beech-Nut)*	6 oz	130	3	14	60	2	6.0	na
'Step 2' *(Heinz)*	4 oz	71	3	9	21	2	2.7	7
'Step 3' *(Heinz)*	6 oz	105	4	15	128	2	3.1	14
strained	1 oz	18	1	2	5	1	0.7	2
strained	1 tbsp	10	0	1	3	0	0.4	1
'3rd Foods' *(Gerber)*	6 oz	110	4	15	65	3	3.5	14
Vegetable and chicken dinner								
junior	1 oz	15	1	2	22	0	0.3	2
junior	1 tbsp	8	0	1	12	0	0.2	1
'2nd Foods' *(Gerber)*	4 oz	70	3	10	35	2	2.0	12
'Stage 2' *(Beech-Nut)*	4 oz	80	2	8	40	1	4.0	na
'Stage 3' *(Beech-Nut)*	6 oz	110	4	14	55	1	4.0	na
'Step 2' *(Heinz)*	4-oz jar	67	3	10	27	2	2.0	12
strained	1 oz	17	1	2	7	1	0.5	3
strained	1 tbsp	9	0	1	4	0	0.3	2
'3rd Foods' *(Gerber)*	6 oz	100	4	15	75	3	3.0	12
Vegetable and dumpling dinner								
w/beef, 'Step 2' *(Heinz)*	3.5 oz	49	2	9	15	0	1.3	0
w/beef, 'Step 3' *(Heinz)*	3.5 oz	47	2	7	16	0	1.2	0
Vegetable and ham dinner								
chunky *(Gerber)*	7 tbsp	70	4	9	200	0	2.3	0
junior	1 oz	17	1	2	25	0	0.5	1
junior	1 tbsp	10	0	1	14	0	0.3	0
'2nd Foods' *(Gerber)*	4 oz	70	2	10	20	1	2.5	6
'Stage 2' *(Beech-Nut)*	4 oz	80	2	9	30	1	3.0	na
'Step 2' *(Heinz)*	4 oz	67	2	9	18	2	2.4	6
'Step 3' *(Heinz)*	6 oz	102	3	15	148	2	3.2	5
strained	1 oz	17	1	2	5	0	0.6	1
strained	1 tbsp	9	0	1	3	0	0.3	1
'3rd Foods' *(Gerber)*	6 oz	120	4	16	55	3	4.0	5
Vegetable and lamb dinner								
junior	1 oz	14	1	2	4	0	0.5	1
strained	1 oz	15	1	2	6	0	0.6	2
strained	1 tbsp	8	0	1	3	0	0.3	1
'Step 2' *(Heinz)*	4 oz	59	2	8	23	1	2.3	7
Vegetable and noodle dinner								
w/chicken, 'Step 2' *(Heinz)*	3.5 oz	54	2	8	24	0	1.7	0
w/chicken, 'Step 3' *(Heinz)*	3.5 oz	57	2	9	21	0	1.8	0
w/turkey, 'Step 2' *(Heinz)*	3.5 oz	47	1	7	22	0	1.6	0
w/turkey, 'Step 3' *(Heinz)*	3.5 oz	48	1	6	21	0	2.0	0
Vegetable and turkey dinner								
(Earth's Best)	4.5 oz	60	3	11	15	0	1.0	0
junior	1 oz	15	0	2	25	0	0.5	1
junior	1 tbsp	8	0	1	14	0	0.3	1
strained	1 oz	14	1	2	6	0	0.3	1

Food Name	Serv. Size	Total Cal.	Prot. gms	Carbs gms	Sod. mgs	Fiber gms	Fat gms	Chol. mgs
strained	1 tbsp	8	0	1	3	0	0.1	1
'2nd Foods' *(Gerber)*	4 oz	60	3	10	30	2	1.0	5
'3rd Foods' *(Gerber)*	6 oz	110	4	16	75	3	3.5	7
toddler	1 oz	23	1	2	95	na	1.0	na
Vegetable dinner, 'Summer' *(Earth's Best)*	4.5 oz	90	3	12	15	0	3.0	0
Vegetable stew								
w/beef, 'Graduates' *(Gerber)*	6 oz	120	8	15	420	3	2.5	0
w/beef, 'Table Time' *(Beech-Nut)*	6 oz	110	4	16	170	1	3.0	na
w/chicken, 'Table Time' *(Beech-Nut)*	6 oz	190	5	23	340	0	8.0	0
Vegetable and beef dinner								
w/macaroni 'Stage 2' *(Beech-Nut)*	4 oz	110	2	9	50	1	6.0	na
w/dumpling, junior	1 oz	14	1	2	15	na	0.2	na
w/dumpling, strained	1 oz	14	1	2	14	na	0.3	na
Vegetable, noodle, and chicken dinner								
junior	1 oz	18	0	3	7	0	0.6	na
strained	1 oz	18	1	2	6	0	0.7	na
Vegetable, noodle, and turkey dinner								
junior	1 oz	15	1	2	5	0	0.4	na
strained	1 oz	12	0	2	6	0	0.3	na
EGG YOLKS								
(Gerber) '2nd Foods'	7 tbsp	193	10	1	42	0	16.8	0
FORMULA								
Infant formula, mix								
liquid, w/iron 'Enfamil' *(Mead Johnson)*	1 fl oz	41	1	4	11	0	2.2	0
liquid concentrate, low-iron, 'Enfamil' *(Mead Johnson)*	1 fl oz	41	1	4	11	0	2.2	0
liquid concentrate, low-iron *(Gerber)*	1 fl oz	40	1	4	12	0	2.1	1
liquid concentrate, low-iron, 'Similac' *(Ross)*	1 fl oz	40	1	4	10	0	2.2	1
liquid concentrate, low-iron, 'SMA' *(Wyeth-Ayerst)*	1 fl oz	41	1	4	9	0	2.2	2
liquid concentrate, w/iron, 'Alsoy' *(Carnation)*	1 fl oz	41	1	4	17	0	2.3	0
liquid concentrate, w/iron, 'Enfamil Nutramigen' *(Mead Johnson)*	1 fl oz	41	1	5	20	0	2.1	0
liquid concentrate, w/iron, 'Enfamil ProSobee' *(Mead Johnson)*	1 fl oz	40	1	4	14	0	2.1	0
liquid concentrate, w/iron, 'Follow-Up' *(Carnation)*	1 fl oz	41	1	5	16	0	1.7	1
liquid concentrate, w/iron, 'Follow-Up Soy' *(Carnation)*	1 fl oz	42	1	4	18	0	2.3	0
liquid concentrate, w/iron *(Gerber)*	1 fl oz	40	1	4	12	0	2.1	1
liquid concentrate, w/iron, 'Good Start' *(Carnation)*	1 fl oz	40	1	4	10	0	2.0	4
liquid concentrate, w/iron, 'Isomil' *(Ross)*	1 fl oz	40	1	4	18	0	2.2	0
liquid concentrate, w/iron, 'Isomil DF' *(Ross)*	1 fl oz	40	1	4	18	0	2.2	0
liquid concentrate, w/iron, 'Nursoy' *(Wyeth-Ayerst)*	1 fl oz	41	1	4	11	0	2.2	0
liquid concentrate, w/iron, 'Similac with Iron' *(Ross)*	1 fl oz	40	1	4	10	0	2.2	1
liquid concentrate, w/iron, 'SMA' *(Wyeth-Ayerst)*	1 fl oz	41	1	4	9	0	2.2	3
powder, low-iron, 'Enfamil' *(Mead Johnson)*	1 scoop	44	1	5	12	0	2.3	0
powder, low-iron *(Gerber)*	1 scoop	44	1	5	13	0	2.4	0
powder, low-iron 'Similac' *(Ross)*	1 scoop	46	1	5	11	0	2.5	1
powder, low-iron 'SMA' *(Wyeth-Ayerst)*	1 scoop	45	1	5	10	0	2.4	3
powder, soy, w/iron, milk-free, prepared *(Gerber)*	5 fl oz	100	3	10	47	0	5.3	0
powder, soy, w/iron, milk-free, prepared 'ProSobee' *(Mead Johnson)*	5 fl oz	100	3	10	36	0	5.3	0
powder, soy, w/iron, milk-free (Isomil), prepared	5 fl oz	100	3	10	44	0	5.5	0
powder, w/iron, 'Alsoy' *(Carnation)*	1 scoop	22	1	2	9	0	1.2	0
powder, w/iron, 'Enfamil' *(Mead Johnson)*	1 scoop	44	1	5	12	0	2.3	0
powder, w/iron, 'Enfamil Nutramigen' *(Mead Johnson)*	1 scoop	48	1	5	22	0	2.4	0
powder, w/iron, 'Follow-Up' *(Carnation)*	1 scoop	44	1	6	17	0	1.8	1
powder, w/iron, *(Gerber)*	1 scoop	44	1	5	13	0	2.4	0
powder, w/iron, 'Good Start' *(Carnation)*.	1 scoop	45	1	5	10	0	2.3	4
powder, w/iron, 'Isomil' *(Ross)*	1 scoop	45	1	5	20	0	2.5	0

Food Name	Serv. Size	Total Cal.	Prot. gms	Carbs gms	Sod. mgs	Fiber gms	Fat gms	Chol. mgs
powder, w/iron, 'Lofenalac' *(Mead Johnson)*	1 scoop	44	1	6	21	0	1.7	0
powder, w/iron, 'Nursoy' *(Wyeth-Ayerst)*	1 scoop	44	1	5	13	0	2.4	0
powder, w/iron, 'Portagen' *(Mead Johnson)*	1 scoop	44	2	5	24	0	2.2	1
powder, w/iron, 'Pregestimil' *(Mead Johnson)*	1 scoop	44	1	4	17	0	2.5	0
powder, w/iron, prepared, 'Lofenalac' *(Mead Johnson)*	1 fl oz	20	1	3	10	0	0.8	0
powder, w/iron, prepared 'Portagen' *(Mead Johnson)*	1 fl oz	20	1	2	11	0	1.0	0
powder, w/iron, prepared 'Enfamil Pregestimil' *(Mead Johnson)*	1 fl oz	20	1	2	8	0	1.1	0
powder, w/iron, 'ProSobee' *(Mead Johnson)*	1 scoop	44	1	4	16	0	2.3	0
powder, w/iron, 'SAM' *(Wyeth-Ayerst)*	1 scoop	45	1	5	10	0	2.4	3
powder, w/iron, 'Similac' *(Ross)*	1 scoop	46	1	5	11	0	2.5	1
powder, w/iron, 'Soylac' *(Carnation)*	1 scoop	22	1	2	10	0	1.2	0
Infant formula, ready to use								
low-iron 'Alimentum' *(Ross)*	1 fl oz	20	1	2	9	0	1.1	0
low-iron, 'Enfamil' *(Mead Johnson)*	1 fl oz	20	0	2	5	0	1.1	0
low-iron *(Gerber)*	1 fl oz	20	0	2	6	0	1.1	0
low-iron 'Similac' *(Ross)*	1 fl oz	20	0	2	5	0	1.1	1
low-iron, 'SMA' *(Wyeth-Ayerst)*	1 fl oz	20	0	2	4	0	1.1	1
low-iron 'Similac Natural Care' *(Ross)*	1 fl oz	24	1	3	10	0	1.3	1
w/iron, 'Similac with Iron' *(Ross)*	1 fl oz	24	1	3	10	0	1.3	1
soy, w/iron, 'Alsoy' *(Carnation)*	1 fl oz	20	1	2	9	0	1.1	0
soy, w/iron, 'Follow-Up Soy' *(Carnation)*	1 fl oz	20	1	2	9	0	1.1	0
soy, w/iron, milk-free, 'Enfamil ProSobee' *(Mead Johnson)*	5 fl oz	100	3	10	36	0	5.3	0
soy, w/iron, milk-free *(Gerber)*	5 fl oz	100	3	10	47	0	5.3	0
soy, w/iron, milk-free, 'Isomil' *(Ross)*	5 fl oz	100	3	10	44	0	5.4	0
soy, w/iron, milk-free, 'Nursoy' *(Wyeth-Ayerst)*	5 fl oz	100	3	10	30	0	5.3	0
soy, w/iron, 'Nursoy' *(Wyeth-Ayerst)*	1 fl oz	20	1	2	5	0	1.1	0
w/iron, 'Enfamil Nutramigen' *(Mead Johnson)*	1 fl oz	20	1	2	10	0	1.0	0
w/iron, 'Enfamil with Iron' *(Mead Johnson)*	1 fl oz	20	0	2	5	0	1.1	0
w/iron, 'Follow-Up' *(Carnation)*	1 fl oz	20	1	3	8	0	0.8	0
w/iron *(Gerber)*	1 fl oz	20	0	2	6	0	1.1	0
w/iron, 'Good Start' *(Carnation)*	1 fl oz	20	0	2	5	0	1.0	2
w/iron, 'Isomil' *(Ross)*	1 fl oz	20	0	2	9	0	1.1	0
w/iron, 'Isomil DM' *(Ross)*	1 fl oz	20	1	2	9	0	1.1	0
w/iron, 'Similac' *(Ross)*	1 fl oz	20	0	2	5	0	1.1	1
w/iron, 'SMA' *(Wyeth-Ayerst)*	1 fl oz	20	0	2	4	0	1.1	1
Toddler formula, mix								
liquid, prepared, 'Next Step' *(Mead Johnson)*	1 fl oz	20	1	2	7	0	1.1	0
powder, soy, prepared, 'Next Step Soy' *(Mead Johnson)*	1 fl oz	20	1	2	9	0	0.9	0
Toddler formula, ready to use								
w/iron *(Pediasure)*	1 fl oz	29	1	3	11	0	1.5	1
FRUIT								
Apple *(Earth's Best)*	4.5 oz	60	0	14	5	0	1.0	0
Apple and apricot								
'Stage 2' *(Beech-Nut)*	4 oz	70	0	17	0	1	0.0	na
(Earth's Best)	4.5 oz	70	0	15	5	0	1.0	0
strained *(Heinz)*	3.5 oz	55	0	13	3	0	0.3	0
Apple and banana								
(Earth's Best)	4.5 oz	80	0	18	15	0	1.0	0
'2nd Foods' *(Gerber)*	4 oz	60	0	15	0	0	0.0	0
'Stage 2' *(Beech-Nut)*	4 oz	60	0	14	0	1	0.0	na
'Stage 3' *(Beech-Nut)*	6 oz	90	0	21	0	1	0.0	na
Apple and blueberry								
(Earth's Best)	4.5 oz	60	0	14	0	0	1.0	0
junior	1 oz	18	0	5	4	1	0.1	0

Food Name	Serv. Size	Total Cal.	Prot. gms	Carbs gms	Sod. mgs	Fiber gms	Fat gms	Chol. mgs
'2nd Foods' *(Gerber)*	4 oz	60	0	14	1	5	2.0	0
'Stage 2' *(Beech-Nut)*	4 oz	70	0	17	0	1	0.0	na
strained	1 oz	17	0	5	1	1	0.1	0
'3rd Foods' *(Gerber)*	6 oz	80	0	19	2	0	1.0	0
Apple and cherry, 'Stage 3' *(Beech-Nut)*	6 oz	110	0	26	0	1	0.0	na
Apple and cranberry, w/tapioca, strained *(Heinz)*	3.5 oz	66	0	16	6	0	0.3	0
Apple and pear								
'Stage 2' *(Beech-Nut)*	4 oz	80	0	19	0	1	0.0	na
'Step 3' *(Heinz)*	3.5 oz	57	0	13	1	1	0.2	0
Apple and plum, *(Earth's Best)*	4.5 oz	70	0	16	10	0	1.0	0
Apple and raspberry								
w/sugar, junior	1 oz	16	0	4	1	1	0.1	0
w/sugar, strained	1 oz	16	0	4	1	1	0.1	0
Apple and sweet potato, 'Tender Harvest' *(Gerber)*	4 oz	71	0	17	3	2	0.2	0
Applesauce								
(Earth's Best)	4.5 oz	52	0	14	3	2	0.3	0
'1st Foods' *(Gerber)*	2.5 oz	35	0	9	0	0	0.0	0
golden delicious, 'Stage 1' *(Beech-Nut)*	2.5 oz	50	0	11	0	0	0.0	0
junior *(Heinz)*	3.5 oz	53	0	12	2	0	0.2	0
junior	1 oz	10	0	3	1	0	0.0	0
junior	1 tbsp	6	0	2	0	0	0.0	0
'2nd Foods' *(Gerber)*	4 oz	60	0	14	3	0	1.0	0
'Stage 3' *(Beech-Nut)*	6 oz	100	0	23	0	2	0.0	0
'Step 1' *(Heinz)*	3.5 oz	73	0	18	1	0	0.1	0
'Step 2' *(Heinz)*	4 oz	46	0	12	2	2	0.2	0
'Step 3' *(Heinz)*	6 oz	63	0	18	3	3	0.0	0
strained	1 oz	12	0	3	1	0	0.1	0
strained	1 tbsp	7	0	2	0	0	0.0	0
'3rd Foods' *(Gerber)*	6 oz	90	0	20	3	0	1.0	0
w/apricot	1 oz	13	0	4	1	1	0.1	0
w/apricot	1 tbsp	8	0	2	0	0	0.0	0
w/apricot, '2nd Foods' *(Gerber)*	7 tbsp	53	0	13	1	0	0.2	0
w/apricot, 'Stage 2' *(Beech-Nut)*	4.5 oz	80	0	19	0	0	0.0	0
w/apricot, 'Step 2' *(Heinz)*	4 oz	51	0	13	3	2	0.2	0
w/apricot, 'Step 3' *(Heinz)*	6 oz	80	0	21	5	3	0.3	0
w/apricot, strained *(Earth's Best)*	4.5 oz	58	0	15	4	2	0.3	0
w/apricot, strained	1 oz	13	0	3	1	1	0.1	0
w/apricot, strained	1 tbsp	7	0	2	0	0	0.0	0
w/banana, 'Stage 2' *(Beech-Nut)*	4.5 oz	80	0	18	0	0	0.0	0
w/banana, 'Stage 3' *(Beech-Nut)*	6 oz	100	0	25	0	0	0.0	0
w/banana, strained	1 tbsp	11	0	3	0	0	0.0	0
w/cherry, 'Stage 2' *(Beech-Nut)*	4.5 oz	70	0	18	5	0	0.0	0
w/cherry, 'Stage 3' *(Beech-Nut)*	6 oz	100	0	24	0	0	0.0	0
w/cherry, junior	1 oz	16	0	4	0	0	0.0	0
w/cherry, strained	1 oz	14	0	4	0	0	0.0	0
w/pineapple, junior	1 oz	11	0	3	1	0	0.0	0
w/pineapple, strained	1 oz	10	0	3	1	0	0.0	0
Apricot								
w/pear, 'Stage 3' *(Beech-Nut)*	6 oz	120	1	27	0	0	0.0	0
w/pear and apple, 'Stage 3' *(Beech-Nut)*	6 oz	130	0	32	0	3	0.0	na
w/pear and applesauce, 'Stage 2' *(Beech-Nut)*	4.5 oz	90	0	21	0	0	0.0	0
w/tapioca, junior	3.5 oz	66	0	16	10	0	0.2	0
w/tapioca, junior	1 tbsp	9	0	3	1	0	0.0	0
w/tapioca, '2nd Foods' *(Gerber)*	4 oz	90	0	20	8	0	1.0	0
w/tapioca, 'Step 2' *(Heinz)*	4.25 oz	72	0	20	10	2	0.0	0
w/tapioca, 'Step 3' *(Heinz)*	6 oz	107	1	29	10	3	0.0	0
w/tapioca, strained	3.5 oz	64	0	15	7	0	0.2	0

Food Name	Serv. Size	Total Cal.	Prot. gms	Carbs gms	Sod. mgs	Fiber gms	Fat gms	Chol. mgs
w/tapioca, strained	1 tbsp	9	0	2	1	0	0.0	0
w/tapioca, '3rd Foods' *(Gerber)*	6 oz	130	1	29	9	0	1.0	0
Banana								
(Earth's Best)	4.5 oz	100	2	22	60	0	0.0	0
'1st Foods' *(Gerber)*	2.5 oz	70	1	17	0	0	0.0	0
Chiquita, 'Baby's First' *(Beech-Nut)*	2.5 oz	70	0	16	0	0	0.0	0
Chiquita, 'Stage 3' *(Beech-Nut)*	6 oz	160	1	33	0	3	0.0	na
'Step 1' *(Heinz)*	3.5 oz	107	1	25	3	0	0.2	0
w/pineapple and tapioca, '2nd Foods' *(Gerber)*	7 tbsp	52	0	12	0	0	0.1	0
w/pineapple and tapioca, '3rd Foods' *(Gerber)*	7 tbsp	52	0	12	4	0	0.1	0
w/tapioca, junior	1 oz	19	0	5	3	0	0.1	0
w/tapioca, junior	1 tbsp	10	0	3	1	0	0.0	0
w/tapioca, '2nd Foods' *(Gerber)*	4 oz	110	1	24	12	0	1.0	0
w/tapioca, 'Step 2' *(Heinz)*	3.5 oz	73	0	18	8	0	0.2	0
w/tapioca, 'Step 3' *(Heinz)*	3.5 oz	73	0	18	8	0	0.2	0
w/tapioca, strained	1 oz	16	0	4	3	0	0.0	0
w/tapioca, strained	1 tbsp	9	0	2	1	0	0.0	0
w/tapioca, '3rd Foods' *(Gerber)*	6 oz	140	1	31	15	0	1.0	0
Banana and apple, strained *(Gerber)*	4.5 oz	90	0	20	9	0	1.0	0
Banana and pear, w/applesauce, 'Stage 2' *(Beech-Nut)*	4.5 oz	100	0	24	0	0	0.0	0
Banana and pineapple								
'Stage 2' *(Beech-Nut)*	4.5 oz	110	0	27	15	0	0.0	0
w/tapioca, junior	1 oz	19	0	5	2	0	0.0	0
w/tapioca, junior	1 tbsp	10	0	3	1	0	0.0	0
w/tapioca, '2nd Foods' *(Gerber)*	4.5 oz	60	1	15	5	0	0.0	0
w/tapioca, 'Step 2' *(Heinz)*	3.5 oz	64	0	15	8	0	0.2	0
w/tapioca, 'Step 3' *(Heinz)*	6 oz	116	0	31	14	3	0.2	0
w/tapioca, strained	1 oz	18	0	5	2	0	0.0	0
w/tapioca, '3rd Foods' *(Gerber)*	6 oz	90	1	20	7	0	1.0	0
Guava								
w/tapioca, '2nd Foods' *(Gerber)*	4 oz	90	0	20	3	0	1.0	0
w/tapioca, 'Stage 2' *(Beech-Nut)*	4.5 oz	100	0	24	10	0	0.0	0
w/tapioca, strained	1 oz	19	0	5	1	1	0.0	na
Guava and papaya, w/tapioca, strained	1 oz	18	0	5	na	0	0.0	na
Mango								
w/tapioca, '2nd Foods' *(Gerber)*	4 oz	90	0	21	4	0	1.0	0
w/tapioca, strained	1 oz	23	0	6	1	0	0.1	0
w/tapioca, strained	1 tbsp	12	0	3	1	0	0.0	0
Mango and banana								
w/passionfruit and tapioca, '2nd Foods' *(Gerber)*	4.5 oz	100	0	25	12	0	0.0	0
Mixed fruit								
apple, peach, and strawberries 'Stage 2' *(Beech-Nut)*	4.5 oz	100	0	24	0	0	0.0	0
apple, pear, and banana 'Stage 2' *(Beech-Nut)*	4.5 oz	100	0	24	0	0	0.0	0
Papaya								
'Stage 2' *(Beech-Nut)*	4.5 oz	100	0	24	15	0	0.0	0
w/tapioca, '2nd Foods' *(Gerber)*	4 oz	80	0	19	9	0	1.0	0
Papaya and applesauce, w/tapioca, strained	1 oz	20	0	5	1	0	0.0	na
Peach								
'1st Foods' *(Gerber)*	2.5 oz	30	0	7	0	0	0.0	0
'2nd Foods' *(Gerber)*	4 oz	90	1	19	4	0	1.0	0
'Stage 3' *(Beech-Nut)*	6 oz	100	0	21	0	4	0.0	0
'Step 1' *(Heinz)*	3.5 oz	80	1	18	2	0	0.2	0
'Step 2' *(Heinz)*	3.5 oz	68	1	15	7	1	0.3	0
'Step 3' *(Heinz)*	3.5 oz	68	1	15	7	1	0.3	0
'3rd Foods' *(Gerber)*	6 oz	110	1	25	5	0	1.0	0
w/banana, 'Stage 2' *(Beech-Nut)*	4 oz	70	0	15	0	3	0.0	na
w/mango and tapioca, '2nd Foods' *(Gerber)*	4 oz	100	0	24	9	0	1.0	0

Food Name	Serv. Size	Total Cal.	Prot. gms	Carbs gms	Sod. mgs	Fiber gms	Fat gms	Chol. mgs
w/oatmeal and banana *(Earth's Best)*	4.5 oz	70	2	15	5	0	1.0	0
w/sugar, '1st Foods' *(Gerber)*	2.5 oz	30	<1	7	0	1	0.0	0
w/sugar, junior	1 oz	20	0	5	1	0	0.1	0
w/sugar, junior	1 tbsp	11	0	3	1	0	0.0	0
w/sugar, '2nd Foods' *(Gerber)*	4 oz	70	<1	17	10	1	0.0	0
w/sugar, 'Stage 1' *(Beech-Nut)*	2.5 oz	50	0	13	4	1	0.1	0
w/sugar, 'Stage 3' *(Beech-Nut)*	6 oz	121	1	32	9	3	0.3	0
w/sugar, 'Step 1' *(Heinz)*	2.5 oz	50	0	13	4	1	0.1	0
w/sugar, 'Step 2' *(Heinz)*	4 oz	80	1	21	7	2	0.2	0
w/sugar, 'Step 3' *(Heinz)*	6 oz	121	1	32	9	3	0.3	0
w/sugar, strained	1 oz	20	0	5	2	0	0.1	0
w/sugar, strained	1 tbsp	11	0	3	1	0	0.0	0
w/sugar, '3rd Foods' *(Gerber)*	6 oz	110	1	26	10	2	0.0	0
w/yogurt 'Stage 2' *(Beech-Nut)*	4.5 oz	120	1	25	30	0	2.0	0
yellow cling, 'Stage 1' *(Beech-Nut)*	2.5 oz	45	0	10	0	0	0.0	0
Pear								
Bartlett, 'Stage 1' *(Beech-Nut)*	2.5 oz	50	0	12	0	0	0.0	0
Bartlett, 'Stage 3' *(Beech-Nut)*	6 oz	110	0	27	0	5	0.0	0
Bartlett, w/applesauce, 'Stage 2' *(Beech-Nut)*	4 oz	80	0	20	0	0	0.0	0
(Earth's Best)	4.5 oz	60	0	14	11	0	0.0	0
'1st Foods' *(Gerber)*	2.5 oz	40	0	11	2	0	0.0	0
junior	1 oz	12	0	3	1	1	0.0	0
junior	1 tbsp	7	0	2	0	1	0.0	0
'2nd Foods' *(Gerber)*	4 oz	80	1	16	3	0	1.0	0
'Step 1' *(Heinz)*	3.5 oz	76	1	18	3	0	0.2	0
'Step 2' *(Heinz)*	3.5 oz	60	0	14	3	0	0.2	0
'Step 3' *(Heinz)*	3.5 oz	60	0	14	3	0	0.2	0
strained	1 oz	12	0	3	1	1	0.1	0
strained	1 tbsp	7	0	2	0	1	0.0	0
'3rd Foods' *(Gerber)*	6 oz	100	1	21	2	0	1.0	0
Pear and pineapple								
junior	1 oz	12	0	3	0	1	0.1	0
junior	1 tbsp	7	0	2	0	0	0.0	0
'2nd Foods' *(Gerber)*	7 tbsp	55	0	13	1	0	0.2	0
'Stage 2' *(Beech-Nut)*	4 oz	46	0	12	5	3	0.1	0
'Step 2' *(Heinz)*	4 oz	46	0	12	5	3	0.1	0
strained	1 oz	12	0	3	1	1	0.0	0
strained	1 tbsp	7	0	2	1	0	0.0	0
'3rd Foods' *(Gerber)*	6 oz	100	1	21	3	0	1.0	0
Pear and raspberry, *(Earth's Best)*	4.5 oz	60	0	15	0	0	0.0	0
Plum								
w/tapioca, junior	1 oz	21	0	6	2	0	0.0	0
w/tapioca, junior	1 tbsp	11	0	3	1	0	0.0	0
(Gerber) '3rd Foods'	6 oz	120	0	28	10	3	0.0	0
w/tapioca, '2nd Foods' *(Gerber)*	4 oz	80	0	19	10	2	0.0	0
w/tapioca, strained	1 oz	20	0	6	2	0	0.0	0
w/tapioca, strained	1 tbsp	11	0	3	1	0	0.0	0
w/tapioca, 'Step 2' *(Heinz)*	4 oz	80	0	22	7	1	0.0	0
Prune								
'1st Foods' *(Gerber)*	2.5 oz	70	1	17	0	0	0.0	0
w/oatmeal *(Earth's Best)*	4.5 oz	100	1	24	20	0	0.0	0
w/pear, 'Stage 2' *(Beech-Nut)*	4 oz	110	0	24	10	3	0.0	0
w/tapioca, junior	1 oz	20	0	5	1	1	0.0	0
w/tapioca, '2nd Foods' *(Gerber)*	4 oz	100	1	22	5	0	1.0	0
w/tapioca, 'Step 2' *(Heinz)*	3.5 oz	90	1	22	8	0	0.2	0
w/tapioca, strained	1 oz	20	0	5	1	1	0.0	0

Food Name	Serv. Size	Total Cal.	Prot. gms	Carbs gms	Sod. mgs	Fiber gms	Fat gms	Chol. mgs
w/tapioca, strained .... 1 tbsp	1 tbsp	11	0	3	1	0	0.0	0
Tropical fruit, junior .... 1 oz	1 oz	17	0	5	2	na	0.0	na
JUICE								
Apple								
.... 1 fl oz	1 fl oz	15	0	4	1	0	0.0	0
beginner, 'Step 1' *(Heinz)* .... 4 fl oz	4 fl oz	59	0	15	4	0	0.1	0
(Earth's Best) .... 4.2 fl oz	4.2 fl oz	62	0	15	4	0	0.1	0
(Gerber) .... 4 fl oz	4 fl oz	60	<1	14	0	0	0.1	0
100% juice, 'Junior' *(McCain)* .... 4.2 fl oz	4.2 fl oz	50	0	13	5	0	0.0	0
'Stage 1' *(Beech-Nut)*............................. 4 fl oz	4 fl oz	60	0	15	4	0	0.1	0
strained, 'Saver Size' *(Heinz)* .... 4.2 fl oz	4.2 fl oz	70	0	17	15	0	0.0	0
Apple-apricot, strained, 'Step 2' *(Heinz)* .... 3.5 fl oz	3.5 fl oz	47	0	11	8	0	0.2	0
Apple-banana								
.... 1 fl oz	1 fl oz	16	0	4	1	0	0.0	0
(Earth's Best) .... 4.2 fl oz	4.2 fl oz	60	0	14	2	0	0.0	0
(Gerber) .... 4 fl oz	4 fl oz	60	<1	15	10	0	0.1	0
strained, 'Step 2' *(Heinz)* .... 3.5 fl oz	3.5 fl oz	52	0	13	6	0	0.2	0
w/calcium, 'Graduates' *(Gerber)*..................... 6 fl oz	6 fl oz	100	<1	24	20	1	0.0	0
w/vitamin C, 'Stage 2' *(Beech-Nut)* .... 4 fl oz	4 fl oz	70	0	16	0	0	0.0	na
Apple-cherry								
.... 1 fl oz	1 fl oz	13	0	3	1	0	0.1	0
'Graduates' *(Gerber)* .... 6 fl oz	6 fl oz	80	0	21	25	0	0.0	0
100% juice, 'Junior' *(McCain)* .... 4.2 fl oz	4.2 fl oz	50	0	13	5	0	0.0	0
strained, 'Step 2' *(Heinz)* .... 3.5 fl oz	3.5 fl oz	45	0	11	7	0	0.2	0
w/vitamin C., 'Stage 2' *(Beech-Nut)* .... 4 fl oz	4 fl oz	70	0	17	10	0	0.0	0
Apple-cranberry, strained, 'Step 2' *(Heinz)* .... 3.5 fl oz	3.5 fl oz	48	0	12	7	0	0.2	0
Apple-grape								
.... 1 fl oz	1 fl oz	14	0	4	1	0	0.1	0
(Earth's Best) .... 4.2 fl oz	4.2 fl oz	60	0	15	4	0	0.3	0
(Gerber) .... 4 fl oz	4 fl oz	60	<1	15	20	0	0.0	0
strained, 'Step 2' *(Heinz)* .... 4 fl oz	4 fl oz	58	0	14	4	0	0.3	0
w/calcium, 'Graduates' *(Gerber)* .... 6 fl oz	6 fl oz	98	0	24	8	1	0.2	0
Apple-peach								
.... 1 fl oz	1 fl oz	13	0	3	0	0	0.0	0
(Gerber) .... 3.2 fl oz	3.2 fl oz	47	0	11	5	0	0.1	0
strained, 'Step 2' *(Heinz)* .... 3.5 fl oz	3.5 fl oz	44	0	10	7	0	0.2	0
Apple-pineapple, strained, 'Step 2' *(Heinz)* .... 3.5 fl oz	3.5 fl oz	47	0	11	6	0	0.2	0
Apple-plum								
.... 1 fl oz	1 fl oz	15	0	4	0	0	0.0	0
(Gerber) .... 3.2 fl oz	3.2 fl oz	48	0	12	8	0	0.1	0
Apple-prune								
.... 4 fl oz	4 fl oz	91	0	23	6	0	0.1	0
.... 1 fl oz	1 fl oz	23	0	6	2	0	0.0	0
strained, 'Step 2' *(Heinz)* .... 3.5 fl oz	3.5 fl oz	50	0	12	7	0	0.2	0
Apple-white grape, 'Stage 2' *(Beech-Nut)* .... 4 fl oz	4 fl oz	58	0	14	4	0	0.3	0
Fruit punch, w/calcium, 'Graduates' *(Gerber)* .... 6 fl oz	6 fl oz	98	0	24	8	1	0.2	0
Grape								
'Juice Plus' 'Stage 2' *(Beech-Nut)* .... 4 fl oz	4 fl oz	100	0	23	10	0	0.0	0
white *(Gerber)* .... 4 fl oz	4 fl oz	80	0	20	10	0	0.0	0
white, 'Stage 1' *(Beech-Nut)*...................... 4 fl oz	4 fl oz	100	0	23	10	0	0.0	0
white, strained, 'Step 2' *(Heinz)* .... 3.5 fl oz	3.5 fl oz	58	0	14	6	0	0.2	0
Guava, w/mixed fruit, 'Tropical Foods' *(Gerber)* .... 3.2 fl oz	3.2 fl oz	58	0	14	6	0	0.1	0
Mango								
w/mixed fruit, 'Tropical Foods' *(Gerber)* .... 3.2 fl oz	3.2 fl oz	59	0	14	5	0	0.1	0
nectar, w/grape and pear juice, 'Stage 2' *(Beech-Nut)* .... 4 fl oz	4 fl oz	80	0	19	5	0	0.0	0
Mixed fruit								
.... 1 fl oz	1 fl oz	15	0	4	1	0	0.0	0
.... 4 fl oz	4 fl oz	59	0	15	5	0	0.1	0

Food Name	Serv. Size	Total Cal.	Prot. gms	Carbs gms	Sod. mgs	Fiber gms	Fat gms	Chol. mgs
100% juice, 'Junior' *(McCain)*	4.2 fl oz	60	0	15	5	0	0.0	0
strained, 'Step 2' *(Heinz)*	3.5 fl oz	50	0	12	6	0	0.2	0
Orange								
	1 fl oz	14	0	3	0	0	0.1	0
'2nd Foods' *(Gerber)*	4 fl oz	60	<1	13	10	0	0.4	0
strained, 'Step 2' *(Heinz)*	4 fl oz	55	1	13	1	0	0.4	0
Orange-apple								
	1 fl oz	13	0	3	1	na	0.1	na
strained, 'Step 2' *(Heinz)*	3.5 fl oz	50	0	11	8	0	0.3	0
Orange-apple-banana								
	1 fl oz	15	0	4	1	0	0.0	0
strained, 'Step 2' *(Heinz)*	4 fl oz	59	1	14	5	0	0.1	0
Orange-apricot	1 fl oz	14	0	3	2	0	0.0	0
Orange-banana	1 fl oz	16	0	4	1	na	0.0	na
Orange-carrot, '3rd Foods' *(Gerber)*	3.2 fl oz	43	1	10	10	0	0.1	0
Orange-pineapple	1 fl oz	15	0	4	1	0	0.0	0
Papaya								
nectar, w/pear and grape juice 'Stage 2' *(Beech-Nut)*	4 fl oz	70	0	17	10	0	0.0	0
Pear								
(Earth's Best)	4.2 fl oz	60	0	15	0	0	0.0	0
'1st Foods' *(Gerber)*	3.2 fl oz	46	0	11	1	0	0.1	0
'Stage 1' *(Beech-Nut)*	4 fl oz	60	0	15	0	0	0.0	0
strained, 'Saver Size' *(Heinz)*	4.2 fl oz	70	0	15	25	0	1.0	0
strained, 'Step 2' *(Heinz)*	3.5 fl oz	49	0	12	9	0	0.2	0
Pineapple-carrot, '3rd Foods' *(Gerber)*	3.2 fl oz	47	0	11	10	0	0.1	0
Prune-orange	1 fl oz	22	0	5	1	na	0.1	na
Tropical blend								
nectar, 'Stage 2' *(Beech-Nut)*	4 fl oz	90	0	21	10	0	0.0	0
'Stage 2' *(Beech-Nut)*	4 fl oz	90	0	19	5	0	0.0	0
MEAT								
Beef								
and beef gravy, '2nd Foods' *(Gerber)*	2.5 oz	70	8	3	30	0	3.5	21
junior	1 oz	30	4	0	19	0	1.4	8
junior	1 tbsp	16	2	0	10	0	0.7	4
junior, 'Step 3' *(Heinz)*	2.5 oz	75	10	0	47	0	3.5	20
strained	1 oz	30	4	0	23	0	1.5	8
strained	1 tbsp	16	2	0	12	0	0.8	4
strained, 'Step 2' *(Heinz)*	2.5 oz	76	10	0	58	0	3.8	21
'3rd Foods' *(Gerber)*	7 tbsp	103	15	0	52	0	4.6	0
w/broth, 'Stage 1' *(Beech-Nut)*	2.5 oz	76	10	0	58	0	3.8	21
w/broth, strained, 'Step 2' *(Heinz)*	3.5 oz	123	15	0	53	0	7.2	0
w/egg yolks *(Gerber)*	2.5 oz	80	10	0	38	0	4.0	21
Chicken								
and chicken gravy, '2nd Foods' *(Gerber)*	2.5 oz	80	8	2	35	0	4.5	44
junior	1 oz	42	4	0	14	0	2.7	17
junior	1 tbsp	22	2	0	8	0	1.4	9
'Stage 1' *(Beech-Nut)*	2.8 oz	80	10	0	55	0	4.0	0
strained	1 oz	37	4	0	13	0	2.2	17
strained	1 tbsp	20	2	0	7	0	1.2	9
strained, 'Step 2' *(Heinz)*	2.5 oz	92	10	0	33	0	5.6	44
'3rd Foods' *(Gerber)*	7 tbsp	132	15	0	39	0	7.9	0
w/broth, junior, 'Step 3' *(Heinz)*	3.5 oz	143	14	1	59	0	9.7	0
Chicken stick, 'Graduates' *(Gerber)*	2.5 oz	100	11	1	300	0	5.0	65
Ham								
and ham gravy, '2nd Foods' *(Gerber)*	2.5 oz	79	10	0	29	0	4.1	17
junior	1 oz	35	4	0	19	0	1.9	8
strained	1 oz	31	4	0	12	0	1.6	7

Food Name	Serv. Size	Total Cal.	Prot. gms	Carbs gms	Sod. mgs	Fiber gms	Fat gms	Chol. mgs
strained	1 tbsp	17	2	0	6	0	0.9	4
'3rd Foods' *(Gerber)*	7 tbsp	123	15	0	42	0	7.2	0
w/egg yolks, strained *(Gerber)*	2.5 oz	90	10	1	30	0	5.0	17
Lamb								
and lamb gravy, '2nd Foods' *(Gerber)*	2.5 oz	70	8	2	30	0	3.0	27
junior	1 oz	32	4	0	21	0	1.5	11
'Stage 1' *(Beech-Nut)*	2.8 oz	70	9	0	50	0	3.0	0
strained	1 oz	29	4	0	18	0	1.3	11
strained	1 tbsp	15	2	0	9	0	0.7	6
strained, 'Step 2' *(Heinz)*	2.5 oz jar	73	10	0	44	0	3.3	27
w/broth, strained, 'Step 2' *(Heinz)*	3.5 oz	129	15	0	59	0	7.6	0
w/egg yolks, strained *(Gerber)*	2.5 oz	70	10	1	36	0	3.0	27
Liver, w/broth, strained, 'Step 2' *(Heinz)*	3.5 oz	100	14	4	49	0	3.2	0
Meat stick								
'Graduates' *(Gerber)*	2.5 oz	100	10	1	340	0	7.0	35
junior	1 stick	18	1	0	55	0	1.5	7
Pork, strained	1 oz	35	4	0	12	0	2.0	14
Turkey								
and turkey gravy, '2nd Foods' *(Gerber)*	2.5 oz	70	7	2	35	0	4.0	42
'Stage 1' *(Beech-Nut)*	2.8 oz	100	9	0	50	0	6.0	0
strained, 'Step 2' *(Heinz)*	2.5 oz	81	10	0	39	0	4.1	42
junior	1 oz	37	4	0	20	0	2.0	15
junior	1 tbsp	19	2	0	11	0	1.1	8
strained	1 oz	32	4	0	16	0	1.6	17
strained	1 tbsp	17	2	0	8	0	0.9	9
'3rd Foods' *(Gerber)*	7 tbsp	115	15	0	52	0	6.1	0
w/egg yolks, strained *(Gerber)*	2.5 oz	100	10	1	38	0	6.0	42
Turkey stick								
'Graduates' *(Gerber)*	2.5 oz	100	10	1	300	0	7.0	60
junior	1 stick	18	1	0	48	0	1.4	7
Veal								
and veal gravy, '2nd Foods' *(Gerber)*	2.5 oz	90	8	2	35	0	6.0	18
junior	1 oz	31	4	0	20	0	1.4	8
'Stage 1' *(Beech-Nut)*	2.8 oz	60	10	0	50	0	2.0	0
strained, 'Step 2' *(Heinz)*	2.5 oz	72	10	0	45	0	3.4	18
strained	1 oz	29	4	0	18	0	1.4	7
strained	1 tbsp	15	2	0	10	0	0.7	4
'3rd Foods' *(Gerber)*	7 tbsp	108	16	0	56	0	5.0	0
w/broth, strained, 'Step 2' *(Heinz)*	3.5 oz	130	15	0	57	1	7.9	0
w/egg yolks, strained *(Gerber)*	2.5 oz	80	10	1	38	0	4.0	18
Veal and beef								
junior *(Gerber)*	6 oz	110	4	16	31	0	3.0	7
strained *(Gerber)*	4.5 oz	90	3	11	17	0	4.0	5
Veal and ham								
junior *(Gerber)*	6 oz	120	3	17	24	0	4.0	7
strained *(Gerber)* strained	4.5 oz	80	2	11	14	0	3.0	4
Veal and turkey								
junior *(Gerber)*	6 oz	100	3	15	24	0	3.0	19
strained *(Gerber)*	4.5 oz	70	2	10	17	0	2.0	12
SOUP								
Chicken								
'Stage 2' *(Beech-Nut)*	4 oz jar	57	2	8	18	1	1.9	5
strained	1 oz	14	0	2	5	0	0.5	1
strained, 'Step 2' *(Heinz)*	3.5 oz	49	2	7	20	0	1.7	0
w/stars, 'Table Time' *(Beech-Nut)*	6 oz	150	7	17	170	1	6.0	0
Cream of broccoli, '3rd Foods' *(Gerber)*	3.2 oz	26	1	3	83	0	1.1	0
Cream of potato, '3rd Foods' *(Gerber)*	3.2 oz	33	1	5	69	0	0.8	0

Food Name	Serv. Size	Total Cal.	Prot. gms	Carbs gms	Sod. mgs	Fiber gms	Fat gms	Chol. mgs
Cream of tomato, '3rd Foods' *(Gerber)*	3.2 oz	41	1	7	73	0	0.7	0
Cream of vegetable, '3rd Foods' *(Gerber)*	3.2 oz	29	1	4	48	0	0.8	0
VEGETABLES								
Beets								
'2nd Foods' *(Gerber)*	7 tbsp	39	1	8	91	0	0.2	0
strained	1 oz	10	0	2	24	1	0.0	0
strained	1 tbsp	5	0	1	12	0	0.0	0
strained *(Gerber)*	4.5 oz	60	1	11	115	0	1.0	0
strained, 'Step 2' *(Heinz)*	3.5 oz	40	1	8	34	0	0.2	0
Carrots								
beginner, 'Step 1' *(Heinz)*	2.5 oz	19	1	4	26	1	0.1	0
(Earth's Best)	1 tbsp	4	0	1	5	0	0.0	0
(Earth's Best)	4.5 oz	40	1	7	70	0	0.0	0
'1st Foods' *(Gerber)*	2.5 oz	25	1	5	0	0	0.0	0
junior	1 oz	9	0	2	14	0	0.1	0
junior	1 tbsp	4	0	1	7	0	0.0	0
junior, 'Step 3' *(Heinz)*	6 oz	54	1	12	83	3	0.3	0
'2nd Foods' *(Gerber)*	4 oz	35	1	7	85	2	0.0	0
'Stage 1' *(Beech-Nut)*	2.5 oz	25	0	6	80	0	0.0	0
'Stage 3' *(Beech-Nut)*	6 oz	70	1	15	170	5	0.0	0
strained	1 oz	8	0	2	10	0	0.0	0
strained, 'Step 2' *(Heinz)*	4 oz	31	1	7	42	2	0.1	0
'3rd Foods' *(Gerber)*	6 oz	50	1	11	150	3	0.0	0
'Vegetable Dices' 'Graduates' *(Gerber)*	2.5 oz	22	1	4	35	1	0.0	0
Carrots and parsnips *(Earth's Best)*	4.5 oz	60	0	14	30	0	0.0	0
Carrots and peas *(Beech-Nut)*	4 oz	50	2	10	25	3	0.0	na
Corn and butternut squash *(Earth's Best)*	4.5 oz	90	2	15	0	0	2.0	0
Corn, creamed								
junior	1 oz	18	0	5	15	1	0.1	0
junior	1 tbsp	10	0	2	8	0	0.1	0
junior, 'Step 3' *(Heinz)*	6 oz	111	2	28	88	4	0.7	2
'Stage 2' *(Beech-Nut)*	4 oz	90	1	18	20	2	0.0	0
'2nd Foods' *(Gerber)*	4 oz	70	2	14	15	0	0.5	1
strained	1 oz	16	0	4	12	1	0.1	0
strained	1 tbsp	9	0	2	6	0	0.1	0
strained, 'Step 2' *(Heinz)*	4 oz	64	2	16	49	2	0.5	1
Beans, green								
beginner, 'Step 1' *(Heinz)*	2.5 oz	18	1	4	1	1	0.1	0
creamed, junior	1 oz	9	0	2	3	0	0.1	0
creamed, junior	1 tbsp	5	0	1	2	0	0.1	0
creamed, junior *(Gerber)*	6 oz	80	3	16	14	0	1.0	0
creamed, junior, 'Step 3' *(Heinz)*	6 oz	54	2	12	20	3	0.7	2
creamed, '3rd Foods' *(Gerber)*	7 tbsp	45	2	9	8	0	0.2	0
'1st Foods' *(Gerber)*	2.5 oz	25	1	4	1	1	0.0	0
junior	1 oz	7	0	2	1	1	0.0	0
junior	1 tbsp	4	0	1	0	0	0.0	0
'2nd Foods' *(Gerber)*	4 oz	40	1	6	10	1	0.0	0
'Stage 1' *(Beech-Nut)*	4 oz	35	1	6	0	3	0.0	0
'Stage 3' *(Beech-Nut)*	6 oz	50	1	10	0	4	0.0	0
strained	1 oz	7	0	2	1	1	0.0	0
strained	1 tbsp	4	0	1	0	0	0.0	0
strained, 'Step 2' *(Heinz)*	3.5 oz	25	1	5	2	1	0.2	0
'Vegetable Dices' 'Graduates' *(Gerber)*	2.5 oz	21	1	4	23	0	0.1	0
w/potatoes *(Gerber)*	4 oz	71	2	11	20	2	2.1	6
w/rice, '3rd Foods' *(Gerber)*	6 oz	70	2	15	20	1	0.0	0
Garden vegetables								
(Earth's Best)	4.5 oz	70	1	15	15	0	0.0	0

Food Name	Serv. Size	Total Cal.	Prot. gms	Carbs gms	Sod. mgs	Fiber gms	Fat gms	Chol. mgs
strained	1 oz	10	1	2	10	0	0.1	0
'2nd Foods' (Gerber)	4 oz	45	2	7	26	2	0.5	0
'Stage 2' (Beech-Nut)	4.5 oz	60	2	11	35	0	0.0	0
Mixed vegetables								
junior	1 oz	12	0	2	10	0	0.1	0
junior	1 tbsp	6	0	1	5	0	0.1	0
'2nd Foods' (Gerber)	4 oz	45	1	9	20	2	0.0	0
'Stage 2' (Beech-Nut)	4.5 oz	50	1	12	30	0	0.0	0
strained	1 oz	12	0	2	4	0	0.1	0
strained, 'Step 2' (Heinz)	3.5 oz	44	1	9	21	0	0.4	0
'3rd Foods' (Gerber)	6 oz	70	2	14	32	0	1.0	0
'Vegetable Dices' 'Graduates' (Gerber)	2.5 oz	35	1	6	55	2	0.0	0
Peas								
beginner, 'Step 1' (Heinz)	2.5 oz	28	2	6	3	1	0.2	0
creamed, strained	1 oz	15	1	3	4	1	0.5	1
creamed, strained	1 tbsp	8	0	1	2	0	0.3	1
creamed, strained, 'Step 2' (Heinz)	4 oz	60	2	10	16	2	2.1	5
'1st Foods' (Gerber)	2.5 oz	30	2	6	0	0	0.0	0
'2nd Foods' (Gerber)	4 oz	60	4	10	6	0	1.0	0
strained	1 oz	11	1	2	1	1	0.1	0
strained	1 tbsp	6	1	1	1	0	0.0	0
strained, 'Step 2' (Heinz)	4 oz	45	4	9	5	2	0.3	0
tender, sweet, 'Stage 1' (Beech-Nut)	2.5 oz	28	2	6	3	1	0.2	0
tender, sweet, 'Stage 1' (Beech-Nut)	4 oz	45	4	9	5	2	0.3	0
w/brown rice (Earth's Best)	4.5 oz	80	5	16	10	0	0.0	0
w/rice, '3rd Foods' (Gerber)	6 oz	90	5	16	5	0	1.0	0
Potato								
'Graduates' (Gerber)	3.2 oz	38	1	9	6	0	0.1	0
toddler	1 tbsp	5	0	1	6	0	0.0	0
Spinach								
creamed, '2nd Foods' (Gerber)	4 oz	50	3	8	55	2	1.0	0
creamed, strained	1 oz	10	1	2	14	1	0.4	1
creamed, strained	1 tbsp	6	0	1	7	0	0.2	1
w/potato (Earth's Best)	4.5 oz	60	2	8	25	0	2.0	0
Squash								
beginner, 'Step 1' (Heinz)	2.5 oz	17	1	4	1	1	0.1	0
butternut, 'Stage 1' (Beech-Nut)	2.5 oz	30	0	7	0	0	0.0	0
'1st Foods' (Gerber)	2.5 oz	25	1	5	0	0	0.0	0
junior	1 oz	7	0	2	0	1	0.1	0
junior	1 tbsp	3	0	1	0	0	0.0	0
'2nd Foods' (Gerber)	4 oz	35	1	7	5	1	0.0	0
'Stage 1' (Beech-Nut)	4 oz jar	27	1	6	2	2	0.2	0
strained	1 oz	7	0	2	1	1	0.1	0
strained (Earth's Best)	4.5 oz	31	1	7	3	3	0.3	0
strained, 'Step 2' (Heinz)	4 oz	27	1	6	2	2	0.2	0
'3rd Foods' (Gerber) junior	6 oz	60	1	11	3	0	1.0	0
w/corn (Gerber)	4 oz	57	2	11	6	2	0.7	0
winter (Earth's Best)	4.5 oz	50	1	12	10	0	0.0	0
Sweet potato								
beginner, 'Step 1' (Heinz)	2.5 oz	40	1	9	14	1	0.1	0
(Earth's Best)	4.5 oz	60	1	12	15	0	1.0	0
'1st Foods' (Gerber)	2.5 oz	45	1	10	0	0	0.0	0
junior	1 oz	17	0	4	6	0	0.0	0
junior	1 tbsp	8	0	2	3	0	0.0	0
junior, 'Step 3' (Heinz)	6 oz	102	2	24	37	3	0.2	0
'2nd Foods' (Gerber)	4.5 oz	70	1	16	20	1	0.0	0
'Stage 1' (Beech-Nut)	2.5 oz	50	0	11	10	0	0.0	0

Food Name	Serv. Size	Total Cal.	Prot. gms	Carbs gms	Sod. mgs	Fiber gms	Fat gms	Chol. mgs
'Stage 3' *(Beech-Nut)*	6 oz	110	1	25	15	1	0.0	0
strained	1 oz	16	0	4	6	0	0.0	0
strained *(Earth's Best)*	1 tbsp	8	0	2	3	0	0.0	0
strained, 'Step 2' *(Heinz)*	4 oz	64	1	15	23	2	0.1	0
'3rd Foods' *(Gerber)* junior	6 oz	110	1	24	39	0	1.0	0
WATER, w/fluoride, sodium-free *(Beech-Nut)*	4 oz	0	0	0	0	0	0.0	0
BACON								
cured, approx 12 slices per lb, raw	1 slice	211	3	0	277	0	21.9	25
cured, approx 20 slices per lb, raw	3 slices	378	6	0	496	0	39.1	46
cured, broiled, pan-fried, or roasted	3 med slices	109	6	0	303	0	9.4	16
(Hormel)								
'Black Label'	1 oz	142	3	2	192	0	14.0	18
'Black Label' low-salt	1.76 oz	250	5	2	260	0	25.0	32
'Black Label' sliced, cooked	2 slices	60	4	0	298	0	5.0	0
'Range' thick-sliced	1 oz	152	2	2	199	0	16.0	17
(Hickory Ridge) cured, hickory flavor	2 slices	80	5	0	340	0	6.0	15
(JM)								
cooked	2 slices	100	4	1	370	0	9.0	12
'Lower Sodium' cooked	2 slices	100	4	1	260	0	9.0	0
'Lower Sodium' raw	2 slices	290	5	1	250	0	30.0	0
raw	2 slices	280	4	1	530	0	29.0	38
(Jones Dairy Farm) raw	1 slice	165	2	0	187	0	17.0	25
(Louis Rich) turkey, cooked	1 slice	34	2	0	184	0	2.7	12
(Oscar Mayer)								
	1 slice	70	4	0	290	0	6.0	15
approx 0.2-oz slices, cooked	1 slice	33	2	0	138	0	2.8	5
'Center Cut' approx 0.2-oz slices, cooked	1 slice	25	2	0	113	0	1.8	6
'Center Cut' cooked, yield from 1 lb raw	6 oz	852	69	4	3813	0	62.5	189
cooked, yield from 16-oz pkg, raw	5 oz	784	47	3	3236	0	64.9	127
lower salt	1 slice	70	5	1	200	0	5.0	15
thick-cut, cooked	1 slice	60	4	0	250	0	5.0	10
(Range Brand) 'Sliced' cooked	2 slices	110	6	0	392	0	9.0	0
(Red Label) cooked	3 slices	110	6	0	0	0	10.0	0
(West Virginia)								
cured, smoked flavor, cooked	2 slices	80	4	0	340	0	7.0	10
thick-sliced, cooked	1 slice	80	3	0	260	0	7.0	10
BACON, CANADIAN STYLE								
cured, grilled, yield from 6-oz pkg	5.9 oz	257	34	2	2149	0	11.7	81
cured, raw	6 oz	267	35	3	2395	0	11.8	85
cured, 6 slices per 6 oz, grilled	2 slices	86	11	1	719	0	3.9	27
cured, 6 slices per 6 oz, raw	2 slices	89	12	1	799	0	4.0	28
(Hormel) sliced	1 oz	45	6	0	315	0	2.0	0
(Jones Dairy Farm) unheated	1 slice	25	3	0	144	0	1.0	7
(Light & Lean)	2 slices	35	6	0	0	0	1.0	0
(Oscar Mayer)	1 slice	50	8	0	620	0	1.5	25
BACON BITS								
*(Bac*Os)*								
imitation	2 tsp	25	2	2	90	0	1.0	0
imitation, bits, cholesterol-free	1 tbsp	30	3	2	120	0	1.0	0
(Bac' N Pieces) imitation, chips cholesterol-free	1 1/2 tbsp	30	3	2	240	0	1.0	0
(Hormel)								
	1 oz	117	12	1	1008	0	7.0	16
	1 tbsp	30	3	0	313	0	2.0	0
50% less fat	1 tsp	30	3	0	250	0	1.5	5
(Oscar Mayer) real	1 tbsp	25	3	0	220	0	1.5	5
(Schilling) imitation, 'Bac'N Pieces'	1 tsp	26	2	2	51	0	0.4	0
(Tone's) imitation	1 tsp	7	1	0	59	0	0.3	0

Food Name	Serv. Size	Total Cal.	Prot. gms	Carbs gms	Sod. mgs	Fiber gms	Fat gms	Chol. mgs
BACON DISH/ENTRÉE (Stouffer's) strata, frozen .... 1 oz		52	3	3	125	0	3.5	31
BACON PIECES (Hormel) .... 1 oz		94	12	2	654	0	5.0	26
BACON SUBSTITUTE								
(Healthy Favorites) turkey, w/pork 'Breakfast Strips' .... 11 grams		18	2	0	145	0	1.0	9
(Heartline)								
Canadian style, vegetarian, nonfat, lite .... 0.5 oz		22	5	1	135	3	0.0	0
Canadian style, vegetarian, yield from 4 oz cooked .... 2 oz		176	19	9	260	0	7.0	0
(JM)								
beef, heated .... 2 slices		100	7	1	320	0	7.0	20
beef, raw .... 2 slices		200	9	1	430	0	18.0	53
(Louis Rich) turkey .... 1 slice		30	2	0	190	0	2.5	10
(Morningstar Farms) vegetarian, 'Breakfast Strips' ...... 2 strips		56	2	2	220	1	4.4	0
(Mr. Turkey) turkey, 70% less fat .... 1 slice		25	3	0	170	0	2.0	10
(Sizzlean)								
beef, heated .... 2 strips		70	6	0	480	0	5.0	0
pork, brown sugar cured, heated .... 2 strips		110	6	2	490	0	9.0	0
pork, heated .... 2 strips		90	6	0	530	0	8.0	0
(White Wave SoyFood) vegetarian, 'Healthy' .... 1 oz		27	4	4	310	3	1.0	0
(Worthington) vegetarian, 'Stripples' .... 2 strips		56	2	2	220	1	4.4	0
BAGEL								
BLUEBERRY								
(Earth Grains) 3 oz .... 1 bagel		245	9	48	210	0	0.0	0
(Lender's)								
4-inch diam, frozen, 'Bagel Shop' .... 1 bagel		264	11	53	427	2	1.5	0
3.13 oz, frozen, 'Big'n Crusty' .... 1 serving		214	8	46	409	2	0.8	0
3-inch diam, 'Premium' .... 1 bagel		209	8	43	409	2	1.3	0
2.5 oz, frozen .... 1 bagel		190	7	38	250	0	1.0	0
(Western Bagel) .... 1 bagel		240	8	43	410	2	4.0	0
CINNAMON-RAISIN								
(Earth Grains) 3 oz .... 1 bagel		245	9	48	210	0	0.0	0
(Finast) w/cinnamon & honey, 2.5 oz .... 1 bagel		200	8	40	305	0	1.0	0
(Lender's) 'Big'n Crusty' 3 1/8 oz .... 1 bagel		250	8	49	370	0	2.0	0
(Sara Lee)								
2.5 oz .... 1 bagel		200	7	39	230	0	2.0	0
3.1 oz .... 1 bagel		240	8	48	280	0	2.0	0
(Thomas')								
.... 1 bagel		160	6	36	290	1	1.0	0
'Deli Style' .... 1 bagel		170	6	33	230	2	2.0	0
(Western Bagel) .... 1 bagel		230	8	40	410	4	4.0	0
EGG								
4.5-inch diam .... 1 bagel		306	12	58	556	3	2.3	26
3-inch diam .... 1 bagel		158	6	30	288	1	1.2	14
(Lender's)								
'Bakery Style' .... 1 bagel		210	9	41	450	2	2.0	5
3.13 oz, frozen, 'Big'n Crusty' .... 1 bagel		250	9	47	380	0	2.0	15
2 oz, frozen .... 1 bagel		160	6	32	340	0	1.0	0
(Sara Lee)								
3.1 oz, frozen .... 1 bagel		250	9	48	450	0	2.0	20
2.5 oz, frozen .... 1 bagel		200	8	38	360	0	2.0	15
(Thomas') .... 1 bagel		170	7	35	280	2	1.5	15
HONEY RAISIN (Lender's) 2.5 oz .... 1 bagel		200	8	40	310	0	1.0	0
HONEY WHEAT (Earth Grains) 3 oz .... 1 bagel		240	9	45	210	0	0.0	0
MULTIGRAIN (Thomas') .... 1 bagel		170	6	35	310	1	1.5	0
OAT BRAN								
(Lender's) 2.5 oz, frozen .... 1 bagel		170	7	36	290	3	2.0	0
(Sara Lee)								
3 oz, frozen .... 1 bagel		220	9	47	450	0	1.0	0

Food Name	Serv. Size	Total Cal.	Prot. gms	Carbs gms	Sod. mgs	Fiber gms	Fat gms	Chol. mgs
2.5 oz, frozen	1 bagel	180	8	38	360	0	1.0	0
ONION								
4.5-inch diam	1 bagel	303	12	59	587	3	1.8	0
3-inch diam	1 bagel	157	6	30	304	1	0.9	0
(Earth Grains) 3-oz bagel	1 bagel	240	9	45	210	0	0.0	0
(Lender's)								
3.13 oz, frozen, 'Big'n Crusty'	1 bagel	230	9	46	480	0	1.0	0
2 oz, frozen	1 bagel	160	7	31	290	0	1.0	0
0.9 oz, frozen, 'Bagelettes'	1 bagel	70	3	14	135	0	1.0	0
(Sara Lee) 3.1 oz, frozen	1 bagel	230	9	45	560	0	1.0	0
2.5 oz, frozen	1 bagel	190	7	37	450	0	1.0	0
(Sprouted Wheat Bagels) w/poppy seeds, organic	1 bagel	250	6	50	320	0	1.0	0
(Thomas')	1 bagel	170	6	35	300	2	1.5	0
(Western Bagel)	1 bagel	220	8	39	430	4	4.0	0
ORGANIC *(Bible Bagels)*	1 bagel	180	11	29	130	4	2.0	0
PLAIN								
4.5-inch diam	1 bagel	303	12	59	587	3	1.8	0
4-inch diam	1 bagel	245	9	48	475	2	1.4	0
3-inch diam	1 bagel	157	6	30	304	1	0.9	0
2.5-inch diam	1 bagel	72	3	14	139	1	0.4	0
(Earth Grains) 3-oz bagel	1 bagel	240	9	45	210	0	0.0	0
(Lender's)								
'Bakery Style'	1 bagel	210	8	42	450	2	2.0	0
soft, 2.5 oz, frozen	1 bagel	210	7	36	350	0	3.0	12
3.13 oz, frozen, 'Big'n Crusty'	1 bagel	240	9	47	450	0	1.0	0
2 oz, frozen	1 bagel	150	6	30	320	0	1.0	0
0.9 oz, frozen, 'Bagelettes'	1 bagel	70	3	13	170	0	1.0	0
(Sara Lee)								
3.1 oz, frozen	1 bagel	230	9	46	580	0	1.0	0
2.5 oz, frozen	1 bagel	190	8	38	460	0	1.0	0
(Thomas')	1 serving	160	6	35	320	2	1.0	0
POPPY SEED								
4.5-inch diam	1 bagel	303	12	59	587	3	1.8	0
4-inch diam	1 bagel	245	9	48	475	2	1.4	0
3-inch diam	1 bagel	157	6	30	304	1	0.9	0
(Lender's) 2 oz, frozen	1 bagel	160	7	29	370	0	1.0	0
(Sara Lee)								
3.1 oz, frozen	1 bagel	230	9	46	560	0	1.0	0
2.5 oz, frozen	1 bagel	190	8	37	450	0	1.0	0
PUMPERNICKEL *(Lender's)* 2 oz, frozen	1 bagel	160	6	31	330	0	1.0	0
RAISIN								
(Lender's)								
'Bakery Style'	1 bagel	220	8	44	380	2	2.0	0
0.9 oz, frozen, 'Bagelettes'	1 bagel	70	2	14	110	0	1.0	0
RYE *(Lender's)* 2 oz, frozen	1 bagel	150	6	30	310	0	1.0	0
SESAME SEED								
4.5-inch diam	1 bagel	303	12	59	587	3	1.8	0
4-inch diam	1 bagel	245	9	48	475	2	1.4	0
3-inch diam	1 bagel	157	6	30	304	1	0.9	0
(Sprouted Wheat Bagels)	1 bagel	250	6	50	320	0	1.0	0
SPELT *(Rudi's)* organic	1 bagel	280	11	54	440	0	2.0	0
WATER *(Western Bagel)*	1 bagel	230	8	41	420	2	4.0	0
WHEAT *(Lender's)* w/raisin, 2.5 oz	1 bagel	190	6	39	310	0	1.0	0
WHOLE GRAIN (Natural Ovens)	1 bagel	190	8	36	210	8	2.0	0
BAGEL CHIPS								
cinnamon raisin *(Original Bagel Crisps)*	1 oz	130	4	20	170	1	4.0	0
garlic *(Original Bagel Crisps)*	1 oz	130	4	20	190	1	4.0	0

Food Name	Serv. Size	Total Cal.	Prot. gms	Carbs gms	Sod. mgs	Fiber gms	Fat gms	Chol. mgs
BAGEL MIX gluten-free *(Gluten Free Pantry)* .... 1 serving		150	2	36	170	1	0.0	0
BAKED BEANS, CANNED.								
(B&M)								
red kidney .... 8 oz		250	15	42	640	11	7.0	5
yellow eye .... 8 oz		326	15	50	770	15	7.0	4
(Beanee Weenee) w/sliced hot dogs .... 1 cup		30	16	35	1240	8	14.0	40
(Bearitos)								
black beans, nonfat .... 1/2 cup		110	6	22	360	3	0.0	0
vegetarian, organic, fat-free, original .... 1/2 cup		130	6	26	360	3	0.0	0
(Green Giant)								
barbecue, dry beans in brine .... 1/2 cup		140	6	28	460	5	0.5	0
dry beans in brine .... 1/2 cup		160	6	31	580	7	1.5	5
honey bacon, dry beans in brine .... 1/2 cup		160	6	34	490	6	0.5	0
w/onion, dry beans in brine .... 1/2 cup		150	5	28	620	5	1.5	0
(Friends)								
red kidney .... 8 oz		340	17	57	1060	11	4.0	4
red kidney, w/pork .... 8 oz		270	14	55	990	11	4.0	4
(Health Valley) honey baked, nonfat .... 1/2 cup		110	7	24	135	7	0.0	0
(Heinz) vegetarian, in tomato sauce .... 8 oz		230	13	41	880	11	1.0	0
(Homestyle) pork and beans, food service product ...... 1/2 cup		157	6	27	621	11	4.8	2
(Joan of Arc)								
barbecue, dry beans in brine .... 1/2 cup		140	6	28	460	5	0.5	0
dry beans in brine .... 1/2 cup		160	6	31	580	7	1.5	5
honey bacon, dry beans in brine .... 1/2 cup		160	6	34	490	6	0.5	0
w/onion, dry beans in brine .... 1/2 cup		150	5	28	620	5	1.5	0
(Luck's)								
October, seasoned w/pork .... 1/2 cup		140	8	20	340	7	3.0	3
pork and beans in tomato sauce .... 1/2 cup		150	6	28	630	6	1.0	0
(Ranch Style) pork & beans .... 1/2 cup		140	6	28	740	6	0.5	5
(S&W) 'Brick Oven' .... 1/2 cup		160	7	32	620	7	0.5	0
(Van Camp's)								
nonfat, seasoned w/brown sugar .... 1/2 cup		130	7	28	430	5	0.0	0
w/brown sugar and bacon .... 1/2 cup		140	7	29	520	5	1.0	0
w/pork, in tomato sauce .... 1/2 cup		110	6	24	490	6	1.5	0
w/beef .... 1 cup		322	17	45	1264	na	9.2	59
w/franks .... 1 cup		368	17	40	1114	18	17.0	16
w/pork .... 1 cup		268	13	51	1047	14	3.9	18
w/pork and sweet sauce .... 1 cup		281	13	53	850	13	3.7	18
w/pork and tomato sauce .... 1 cup		248	13	49	1113	12	2.6	18
w/pork and tomato sauce .... 1 tbsp		15	1	3	70	1	0.2	1
BAKER'S YEAST. See under YEAST.								
BAKING CHOCOLATE. See CHOCOLATE, BAKING.								
BAKING MIX								
general purpose, whole wheat, dry *(Insta-Bake)* .... 1/3 cup		150	4	25	540	3	5.0	0
BAKING POWDER								
Double-acting								
(Clabber Girl) .... 1/4 tsp		3	0	1	138	0	0.0	0
(Rumford) .... 1/4 tsp		3	0	1	109	0	0.0	0
sodium aluminum sulfate .... 1 tsp		2	0	1	488	0	0.0	0
sodium aluminum sulfate .... 1/2 tsp		1	0	1	244	0	0.0	0
straight phosphate .... 1 tsp		2	0	1	363	0	0.0	0
straight phosphate .... 1/2 tsp		1	0	1	182	0	0.0	0
Low-sodium								
.... 1 tsp		5	0	2	5	0	0.0	0
.... 1/2 tsp		2	0	1	2	0	0.0	0
(Featherweight) .... 1 tsp		8	0	2	2	0	0.0	0

Food Name	Serv. Size	Total Cal.	Prot. gms	Carbs gms	Sod. mgs	Fiber gms	Fat gms	Chol. mgs
Regular								
(Calumet)	1/4 tsp	0	0	0	100	0	0.0	0
(Davis)	1 tsp	6	0	2	450	0	0.0	0
(Tone's)	1 tsp	5	0	1	290	0	0.0	0
BAKING SODA								
	1 tsp	0	0	0	1259	0	0.0	0
	1/2 tsp	0	0	0	629	0	0.0	0
(Arm & Hammer)	1/2 tsp	0	0	0	476	0	0.0	0
(Tone's)	1 tsp	0	0	0	821	0	0.0	0
BALSAM PEAR/bitter gourd								
Leafy tips								
boiled, drained	1 cup	20	2	4	8	1	0.1	0
raw	1/2 cup	7	1	1	3	na	0.2	0
raw	1 med leaf	1	0	0	0	na	0.0	0
Pods								
boiled, drained, 1/2-inch pieces	1 cup	24	1	5	7	2	0.2	0
boiled, drained 1/2-inch pieces	1/2 cup	12	1	3	4	1	0.1	0
raw	1 medium	21	1	5	6	0.2	0	8%
raw, 1/2-inch pieces	1 cup	16	1	3	5	3	0.2	0
BAMBOO SHOOTS								
Canned								
(La Choy)	2 tbsp	3	0	1	0	0	0.1	0
drained, 1/8-inch slices	1 cup	25	2	4	9	2	0.5	0
sliced (China Boy)	1/2 cup	15	1	3	10	1	0.0	0
Fresh								
boiled, drained	1 med shoot	17	2	3	6	1	0.3	0
boiled, drained, 1/2-inch slices	1 cup	14	2	2	5	1	0.3	0
raw, 1/2-inch pieces	1/2 cup	21	2	4	3	2	0.2	0
raw, 1/2-inch slices	1 cup	41	4	8	6	3	0.5	0
BANANA								
Dehydrated or powdered								
	1 cup	346	4	88	3	8	1.8	0
	1 tbsp	21	0	5	0	0	0.1	0
Fresh, raw								
mashed	1 cup	207	2	53	2	5	1.1	0
sliced	1 cup	138	2	35	2	4	0.7	0
whole, extra large, 9 inches long and up	1 banana	140	2	36	2	4	0.7	0
whole, extra small, up to 6 inches long	1 banana	75	1	19	1	2	0.4	0
whole, large, 8 to 8 7/8 inches long	1 banana	125	1	32	1	3	0.7	0
whole, medium, 7 to 7 7/8 inches long	1 banana	109	1	28	1	3	0.6	0
whole, small, 6 to 6 7/8 inches long	1 banana	93	1	24	1	2	0.5	0
BANANA CHIPS								
	3 oz	441	2	50	5	7	28.6	0
	1.5 oz	218	1	25	3	3	14.1	0
	1 oz	147	1	17	2	2	9.5	0
BANANA PEPPER. See PEPPER, BANANA.								
BANANA SQUASH. See SQUASH, BANANA.								
BARBADOS CHERRY. See ACEROLA.								
BARBECUE SPICE. See under SEASONING MIX.								
BARLEY								
	1 cup	651	23	135	22	32	4.2	0
pearled, cooked	1 cup	193	4	44	5	6	0.7	0
pearled, cooked (Tone's)	1 tsp	8	0	2	1	0	0.1	0
pearled, quick, raw, 'Scotch Brand' (Quaker)	1/3 cup	172	6	36	0	5	0.5	0
pearled, raw	1 cup	704	20	155	18	31	2.3	0
pearled, raw (Arrowhead Mills)	2 oz	200	5	45	1	7	1.0	0

Food Name	Serv. Size	Total Cal.	Prot. gms	Carbs gms	Sod. mgs	Fiber gms	Fat gms	Chol. mgs
BARLEY FLAKES rolled *(Arrowhead Mills)* .... 1/3 cup		110	4	28	0	5	1.0	0
BARLEY FLOUR. See under FLOUR.								
BARLEY MALT, natural, organic *(Eden Foods)* .... 1/2 tsp		10	0	2	1	0	0.0	0
BARLEY MALT FLOUR. See under FLOUR.								
BARLEY MIX, organic *(Ener-G Foods)* .... 1 cup		396	15	85	503	8	1.6	0
BASELLA. See SPINACH, VINE.								
BASIL								
Dried								
(Golden Dipt) .... 2 grams		8	0	1	36	0	0.0	0
(McCormick/Schilling) .... 1 tsp		3	0	0	0	0	0.0	0
crumbled *(Spice Islands)* .... 1 tsp		3	0	1	1	0	0.1	0
crumbled *(Tone's)* .... 1 tsp		4	0	1	1	0	0.1	0
ground .... 1 tbsp		11	1	3	2	2	0.2	0
ground .... 1 tsp		4	0	1	0	1	0.1	0
Fresh								
chopped .... 2 tbsp		1	0	0	0	0	0.0	0
ground *(Durkee)* .... 1 tsp		5	0	0	0	0	0.0	0
ground *(Laurel Leaf)* .... 1 tsp		5	0	0	0	0	0.0	0
whole leaves .... 5 med leaves		1	0	0	0	0	0.0	0
BASMATI RICE. See under RICE.								
BASS, CALICO. See SUNFISH.								
BASS, FRESHWATER								
mixed species, baked, broiled, grilled, or microwaved ..... 3 oz		124	21	0	77	0	4.0	74
mixed species, raw .... 3 oz		97	16	0	60	0	3.1	58
BASS, SEA								
mixed species, baked, broiled, grilled, or microwaved ..... 3 oz		105	20	0	74	0	2.2	45
mixed species, raw .... 3 oz		82	16	0	58	0	1.7	35
BASS, STRIPED								
mixed species, baked, broiled, grilled, or microwaved ..... 3 oz		105	19	0	75	0	2.5	88
mixed species, raw .... 3 oz		82	15	0	59	0	2.0	68
BATTER MIX, ALL PURPOSE								
all-purpose, no MSG, dry mix *(Don's Chuck Wagon)* ... 1/4 cup		100	4	20	580	1	0.0	0
beer, dry mix *(Golden Dipt)* .... 1 oz		100	2	22	650	0	0.0	0
corn dog, dry mix *(Golden Dipt)* .... 1 oz		100	3	22	490	0	0.0	0
fish and chips, no MSG, dry mix								
(Don's Chuck Wagon) .... 1/4 cup		100	3	21	740	1	0.0	0
fish and chips, dry mix *(Golden Dipt)* .... 1.25 oz		120	2	27	910	0	0.0	0
golden mushroom, no MSG, dry mix								
(Don's Chuck Wagon) .... 1/4 cup		95	3	21	990	1	0.0	0
onion ring, no MSG, dry mix *(Don's Chuck Wagon)* .... 1/4 cup		100	3	21	690	1	0.0	0
onion ring, dry mix *(Golden Dipt)* .... 1 oz		100	2	22	570	0	0.0	0
tempura, dry mix *(Golden Dipt)* .... 1 oz		100	3	22	130	0	0.0	0
BAY LEAF								
dried *(McCormick/Schilling)* .... 1 tsp		2	0	0	0	0	0.0	0
dried, crumbled .... 1 tbsp		6	0	1	0	0	0.2	0
dried, crumbled .... 1 tsp		2	0	0	0	0	0.1	0
dried, crumbled *(Durkee)* .... 1 tsp		2	0	0	0	0	0.0	0
dried, crumbled *(Laurel Leaf)* .... 1 tsp		2	0	0	0	0	0.0	0
dried, crumbled *(Spice Islands)* .... 1 tsp		5	0	0	1	0	0.1	0
dried, crumbled *(Tone's)* .... 1 tsp		2	0	1	0	0	0.1	0
BEAN, ADZUKI								
Canned								
mature seeds, sweetened .... 1 cup		702	11	163	645	na	0.1	0
organic, no salt added, very low sodium								
(Eden Foods) .... 1/2 cup		80	7	18	10	5	1.0	0
organic, w/liquid *(Eden Foods)* .... 1/2 cup		100	6	17	20	4	1.0	0

Food Name	Serv. Size	Total Cal.	Prot. gms	Carbs gms	Sod. mgs	Fiber gms	Fat gms	Chol. mgs
Fresh								
mature seeds, boiled	1 cup	294	17	57	18	17	0.2	0
mature seeds, raw	1 cup	648	39	124	10	25	1.0	0
raw *(Arrowhead Mills)*	2 oz	190	13	35	3	14	1.0	0
Jarred, organic *(Eden Foods)*	1/2 cup	90	6	16	35	4	0.0	0
BEAN, ANASAZI, dry *(Arrowhead Mills)*	1/4 cup	150	10	27	0	9	0.5	0
BEAN, BLACK/black turtle bean								
Canned								
(Green Giant)	1/2 cup	90	7	21	580	6	0.0	0
(Joan of Arc)	1/2 cup	90	7	21	580	6	0.0	0
(Old El Paso)	1/2 cup	100	7	17	400	7	1.0	0
(Progresso)	1/2 cup	100	7	17	400	7	1.0	0
(Ranch Style)	1/2 cup	100	6	19	380	5	0.0	0
(S&W)	1/2 cup	70	5	17	520	6	0.0	0
'Fiesta' style *(Stokely)*	1/2 cup	100	6	17	600	4	0.5	0
50% less salt *(S&W)*	1/2 cup	70	5	17	260	6	0.0	0
'Sun Vista' *(S&W)*	1/2 cup	70	5	20	630	7	1.0	0
organic, no salt added, very low sodium								
(Eden Foods)	1/2 cup	70	7	17	15	6	1.0	0
Dry								
mature seeds, boiled	1 cup	227	15	41	2	15	0.9	0
mature seeds, raw	1 cup	662	42	121	10	29	2.8	0
mature seeds, raw	1 tbsp	41	3	8	1	2	0.2	0
raw *(Arrowhead Mills)*	2 oz	190	13	35	9	11	1.0	0
BEAN, BLACK TURTLE. See BEAN, BLACK.								
BEAN, BROAD. See BEAN, FAVA.								
BEAN, CANNELLINI, CANNED								
(Progresso)	1/2 cup	100	5	18	270	5	0.5	0
white *(Pathmark)*	1/2 cup	100	6	18	390	0	0.0	0
BEAN, CRANBERRY/borlotti/Roman bean/rose coco bean								
Canned *(Progresso)*	1/2 cup	110	7	18	420	12	1.0	0
Dried								
mature seeds, boiled	1 cup	241	17	43	2	18	0.8	0
mature seeds, canned	1 cup	216	14	39	863	16	0.7	0
mature seeds, raw	1 cup	653	45	117	12	48	2.4	0
BEAN, FAVA/broad bean/horse bean/jack bean								
Canned								
(Progresso)	1/2 cup	110	6	20	250	5	0.5	0
mature seeds	1 cup	182	14	32	1160	9	0.6	0
Fresh								
immature seeds, raw	1 med bean	6	0	1	4	0	0.0	0
immature seeds, raw	1 cup	78	6	13	55	5	0.7	0
mature seeds, boiled	1 cup	187	13	33	9	9	0.7	0
mature seeds, raw	1 cup	512	39	87	20	38	2.3	0
mature seeds, raw	1 tbsp	32	2	5	1	2	0.1	0
raw, in pod	1 cup	111	10	22	32	na	0.9	0
raw, in pod	1 med pod	5	0	1	2	na	0.0	0
BEAN, FRENCH/haricots. See also BEAN, GREEN.								
Fresh								
boiled	1 cup	228	12	43	11	17	1.3	0
raw	1 cup	631	35	118	33	46	3.7	0
BEAN, GARBANZO. See CHICKPEA.								
BEAN, GOA. See BEAN, WINGED.								
BEAN, GREAT NORTHERN								
Canned								
(A&P)	1 cup	210	14	38	0	0	1.0	0
(Allens)	1/2 cup	105	5	17	440	0	1.0	0
(Bush's Best)	1/2 cup	70	5	16	380	5	0.0	0

Food Name	Serv. Size	Total Cal.	Prot. gms	Carbs gms	Sod. mgs	Fiber gms	Fat gms	Chol. mgs
(Green Giant)	1/2 cup	80	6	18	290	5	1.0	0
(Joan of Arc)	1/2 cup	80	6	18	290	5	1.0	0
mature seeds	1 cup	299	19	55	10	13	1.0	0
mature seeds, no salt added	1 cup	209	15	37	4	12	0.8	0
organic, w/liquid *(Eden Foods)*	1/2 cup	110	6	20	15	6	1.0	0
seasoned, w/pork *(Luck's)*	1/2 cup	140	7	20	290	6	3.0	3
'Sun-Vista' *(S&W)*	1/2 cup	70	6	17	490	6	0.0	0
w/pork *(Allens)*	1/2 cup	100	5	19	320	0	1.0	0
w/pork *(Luck's)*	7.25 oz	220	12	32	645	13	5.0	0
Dried								
mature seeds, boiled	1 cup	209	15	37	4	12	0.8	0
mature seeds, raw	1 cup	620	40	114	26	37	2.1	0

BEAN, GREEN/string bean/snap bean
Canned

Food Name	Serv. Size	Total Cal.	Prot. gms	Carbs gms	Sod. mgs	Fiber gms	Fat gms	Chol. mgs
(Pathmark)	1/2 cup	20	1	5	350	0	0.0	0
(Stokely)	1/2 cup	20	1	4	360	0	0.0	0
almandine *(Green Giant)*	1/2 cup	45	2	5	300	2	3.0	0
Blue Lake, cut *(Bush's Best)*	1/2 cup	20	1	5	360	2	0.0	0
Blue Lake, cut *(Pathmark)*	1/2 cup	20	1	4	430	0	0.0	0
Blue Lake, cut, 'Premium' *(S&W)*	1/2 cup	20	1	4	385	0	0.0	0
Blue Lake, French style, *(Pathmark)*	1/2 cup	20	1	4	430	0	0.0	0
Blue Lake, French style, 'Premium' *(S&W)*	1/2 cup	20	1	4	385	0	0.0	0
cut *(A&P)*	1/2 cup	20	1	4	350	0	1.0	0
cut *(Allens)*	1/2 cup	20	1	4	350	0	1.0	0
cut *(Bush's Best)*	1/2 cup	20	1	5	360	2	0.0	0
cut *(Featherweight)*	1/2 cup	25	1	5	10	0	0.0	0
cut *(Finast)*	1/2 cup	20	1	4	400	0	0.0	0
cut *(Freshlike)*	1/2 cup	20	1	4	340	0	0.0	0
cut *(Green Giant)*	1/2 cup	16	1	4	300	1	0.0	0
cut *(IGA)*	1/2 cup	20	1	5	10	0	0.0	0
cut *(Pathmark)*	1/2 cup	20	1	4	430	0	0.0	0
cut *(S&W)*	1/2 cup	20	1	4	340	2	0.0	0
cut *(Stokely)*	1/2 cup	20	1	4	400	1	0.0	0
cut *(Veg-All)*	1/2 cup	20	1	4	340	0	0.0	0
cut, 'No Frills' *(Pathmark)*	1 cup	35	2	8	640	0	0.0	0
cut, 'Pantry Express' *(Green Giant)*	1/2 cup	12	1	3	20	1	0.0	0
cut, 'Veri-Green' *(Finast)*	1/2 cup	20	1	4	320	0	0.0	0
cut, 50% less salt *(Green Giant)*	1/2 cup	16	1	4	195	1	0.0	0
cut, no salt added *(Finast)*	1/2 cup	20	1	4	10	0	0.0	0
cut, no salt added *(Freshlike)*	1/2 cup	20	1	4	5	0	0.0	0
cut, stringless, w/liquid *(S&W)*	1/2 cup	20	1	4	3850	0	0.0	0
cut, water packed, w/o salt *(Freshlike)*	1/2 cup	20	1	4	5	0	0.0	0
cut, water packed, w/o sugar or salt *(Freshlike)*	1/2 cup	20	1	4	5	0	0.0	0
cut, w/liquid *(Del Monte)*	1/2 cup	20	1	4	355	0	0.0	0
cut, w/liquid, no salt added *(Del Monte)*	1/2 cup	20	1	4	10	0	0.0	0
dilled *(S&W)*	1 oz	20	0	5	125	1	0.0	0
European, slender, whole *(Stokely)*	1/2 cup	20	1	4	370	1	0.0	0
50% less salt *(Green Giant)*	1/2 cup	18	1	4	150	1	0.0	0
French style *(A&P)*	1/2 cup	20	1	4	350	0	1.0	0
French style *(Allens)*	1/2 cup	20	1	4	350	0	1.0	0
French style *(Bush's Best)*	1/2 cup	20	1	5	360	2	0.0	0
French style *(Finast)*	1/2 cup	20	1	4	400	0	0.0	0
French style *(Freshlike)*	1/2 cup	20	1	4	340	0	0.0	0
French style *(Green Giant)*	1/2 cup	16	1	4	390	1	3.0	0
French style *(Stokely)*	1/2 cup	20	1	4	400	1	0.0	0
French style *(Veg-All)*	1/2 cup	20	1	4	340	0	0.0	0
French style, 'No Frills' *(Pathmark)*	1 cup	35	2	8	640	0	0.0	0

Food Name	Serv. Size	Total Cal.	Prot. gms	Carbs gms	Sod. mgs	Fiber gms	Fat gms	Chol. mgs
French style, cut *(TenderSweet)*	1/2 cup	20	1	4	400	1	0.0	0
French style, cut, no salt added *(TenderSweet)*	1/2 cup	20	1	4	5	0	0.0	0
French style, no salt added *(A&P)*	1/2 cup	20	1	4	10	0	1.0	0
French style, no salt added *(Freshlike)*	1/2 cup	20	1	4	5	0	0.0	0
French style, no salt added *(Pathmark)*	1/2 cup	20	1	5	10	0	0.0	0
French style, seasoned, w/liquid *(Del Monte)*	1/2 cup	20	1	4	355	0	0.0	0
French style, stringless, w/liquid *(S&W)*	1/2 cup	20	1	4	3850	0	0.0	0
French style, water packed, no salt added *(Freshlike)*	1/2 cup	20	1	4	5	0	0.0	0
Italian, flat, cut *(Stokely)*	1/2 cup	20	1	4	370	1	0.0	0
Italian style *(Allens)*	1/2 cup	18	1	3	260	0	1.0	0
Italian style, cut *(Del Monte)*	1/2 cup	25	1	6	355	0	0.0	0
kitchen-sliced *(Green Giant)*	1/2 cup	16	1	4	390	1	0.0	0
kitchen-sliced, 50% less salt *(Green Giant)*	1/2 cup	20	1	4	200	1	0.0	0
no salt added *(A&P)*	1/2 cup	20	1	4	10	0	1.0	0
no salt added *(Pathmark)*	1/2 cup	20	1	5	10	0	0.0	0
no salt added, cut, drained	1 cup	27	2	6	3	3	0.1	0
no salt added, whole, drained	10 med beans	12	1	3	1	1	0.1	0
no salt or sugar *(Stokely)*	1/2 cup	20	1	4	5	0	0.0	0
regular pack, cut, drained	1 cup	27	2	6	354	3	0.1	0
regular pack, cut, w/liquid	1/2 cup	18	1	4	311	2	0.1	0
w/shelly beans, cut *(Bush's Best)*	1/2 cup	35	3	8	290	4	0.0	0
whole *(A&P)*	1/2 cup	20	1	4	350	0	1.0	0
whole *(Bush's Best)*	1/2 cup	20	1	5	360	2	0.0	0
whole *(Finast)*	1/2 cup	25	1	4	400	0	0.0	0
whole *(Freshlike)*	1/2 cup	20	1	4	340	0	0.0	0
whole *(IGA)*	1 cup	45	2	8	640	0	0.0	0
whole *(Pathmark)*	1/2 cup	20	1	4	430	0	0.0	0
whole, stringless, w/liquid *(S&W)*	1/2 cup	20	1	4	3850	0	0.0	0
whole, w/liquid *(Del Monte)*	1/2 cup	20	1	4	355	0	0.0	0
Freeze-Dried *(Mountain House)* prepared as directed	1/2 cup	35	1	6	0	0	0.0	0
Fresh								
boiled, drained	1 cup	44	2	10	4	4	0.3	0
raw, cut	1 cup	34	2	8	7	4	0.1	0
raw, whole, approx 4-inch long	10 beans	17	1	4	3	2	0.1	0
Frozen								
(Flav-R-Pac)	2/3 cup	25	1	4	10	2	0.0	0
cut *(A&P)*	3 oz	25	1	6	140	0	1.0	0
cut *(Birds Eye)*	3 oz	25	1	6	0	2	0.0	0
cut *(Finast)*	3 oz	25	1	6	5	0	0.0	0
cut *(Freshlike)*	3 oz	25	1	6	5	0	0.0	0
cut *(Frosty Acres)*	3 oz	25	1	6	3	1	0.0	0
cut *(Green Giant)*	3/4 cup	25	1	5	0	2	0.0	0
cut *(Pictsweet)*	2/3 cup	25	1	4	10	2	0.0	0
cut *(Seabrook)*	3 oz	25	1	6	3	1	0.0	0
cut *(Veg-All)*	3 oz	25	1	6	5	0	0.0	0
cut, 'Portion Pack' *(Birds Eye)*	3 oz	25	1	6	0	2	0.0	0
cut, 'Singles' *(Stokely)*	3 oz	30	2	6	5	0	1.0	0
French cut *(C&W)*	2/3 cup	30	1	5	0	2	0.0	0
French cut *(Flav-R-Pac)*	1 cup	25	1	4	10	2	0.0	0
French style *(A&P)*	3 oz	25	1	6	0	0	1.0	0
French style *(Birds Eye)*	3 oz	25	1	6	0	2	0.0	0
French style *(Finast)*	3 oz	25	1	6	5	0	0.0	0
French style *(Freshlike)*	3 oz	25	1	6	5	0	0.0	0
French style *(Frosty Acres)*	3 oz	25	1	6	3	1	0.0	0
French style *(Pictsweet)*	1 cup	25	1	4	10	2	0.0	0
French style *(Seabrook)*	3 oz	25	1	6	3	1	0.0	0
French style *(Southern)*	3.5 oz	34	2	7	20	0	0.1	0

Food Name	Serv. Size	Total Cal.	Prot. gms	Carbs gms	Sod. mgs	Fiber gms	Fat gms	Chol. mgs
French style *(Veg-All)*	3 oz	25	1	6	5	0	0.0	0
French style, w/almonds, 'Combination Vegetable' *(Birds Eye)*	3 oz	50	3	8	340	2	2.0	0
Italian cut *(C&W)*	3/4 cup	25	1	4	10	2	0.0	0
Italian cut *(Finast)*	3 oz	30	2	7	5	0	0.0	0
Italian style *(Birds Eye)*	3 oz	30	2	7	0	3	0.0	0
Italian style *(Freshlike)*	3 oz	30	2	7	5	0	0.0	0
Italian style *(Frosty Acres)*	3 oz	30	2	7	3	1	0.0	0
Italian style *(Seabrook)*	3 oz	30	2	7	3	1	0.0	0
Italian style *(Veg-All)*	3 oz	30	2	7	5	0	0.0	0
no salt added, drained	1 cup	38	2	9	12	4	0.2	0
petite, 'Deluxe' *(Birds Eye)*	2.6 oz	20	1	5	0	2	0.0	0
petite, whole *(C&W)*	3/4 cup	25	1	4	10	2	0.0	0
petite, whole *(Flav-R-Pac)*	3/4 cup	25	1	4	10	2	0.0	0
'Plain Polybag' *(Green Giant)*	1/2 cup	14	1	4	10	1	0.0	0
whole *(Flav-R-Pac)*	3/4 cup	25	1	4	10	2	0.0	0
whole *(Freshlike)*	3 oz	25	1	5	5	0	0.0	0
whole *(Seabrook)*	3 oz	25	1	5	1	1	0.0	0
whole *(Southern)*	3.5 oz	33	2	7	20	0	0.1	0
whole *(Veg-All)*	3 oz	25	1	5	5	0	0.0	0
whole 'Farm Fresh' *(Birds Eye)*	4 oz	30	2	7	0	2	0.0	0
whole, 'Deluxe' *(Birds Eye)*	3 oz	25	1	5	0	2	0.0	0
w/almonds 'Harvest Fresh' *(Green Giant)*	2/3 cup	60	2	5	95	2	3.0	0
w/creamy mushroom 'Garden Gourmet' *(Green Giant)*	1 pkg	220	6	29	860	4	11.0	25
w/salt, drained	1 cup	38	2	9	331	4	0.2	0
BEAN, HORSE. See BEAN, FAVA.								
BEAN, HYACINTH								
immature seeds, boiled, drained	1 cup	44	3	8	2	na	0.2	0
immature seeds, raw	1 cup	37	2	7	2	na	0.2	0
mature seeds, boiled, drained	1 cup	227	16	40	14	na	1.1	0
mature seeds, raw	1 cup	722	50	128	44	na	3.5	0
BEAN, ITALIAN								
dry beans in brine *(Green Giant)*	1/2 cup	130	5	24	480	5	1.0	0
dry beans in brine *(Joan of Arc)*	1/2 cup	130	5	24	480	5	1.0	0
BEAN, JACK. See BEAN, FAVA.								
BEAN, KIDNEY								
CALIFORNIA RED								
Dried								
mature seeds, boiled	1 cup	219	16	40	7	16	0.2	0
mature seeds	1 cup	607	45	110	20	46	0.5	0
DARK RED								
Canned								
(Allens)	1/2 cup	105	5	20	290	0	1.0	0
(Bush's Best)	1/2 cup	70	6	17	300	6	0.0	0
(Finast)	1/2 cup	110	6	20	350	0	2.0	0
(Green Giant)	1/2 cup	90	7	20	330	5	1.0	0
(Joan of Arc)	1/2 cup	90	7	20	330	5	1.0	0
(Pathmark)	1/2 cup	110	8	18	370	0	0.0	0
(Progresso)	1/2 cup	110	7	20	280	8	0.5	0
(Stokely)	1/2 cup	120	7	21	380	5	0.5	0
(Stokely)	1/2 cup	110	7	20	360	0	1.0	0
(Van Camp's)	1 cup	182	12	35	830	0	0.5	0
50% less salt *(Green Giant)*	1/2 cup	90	7	20	165	5	1.0	0
50% less salt *(Joan of Arc)*	1/2 cup	90	7	20	165	5	1.0	0
50% less salt, 'Lite' *(S&W)*	1/2 cup	120	7	22	355	0	1.0	0
'Premium' *(S&W)*	1/2 cup	120	6	22	596	0	1.0	0

Food Name	Serv. Size	Total Cal.	Prot. gms	Carbs gms	Sod. mgs	Fiber gms	Fat gms	Chol. mgs
LIGHT RED								
Canned								
(Allens)	1/2 cup	105	5	2	290	0	1.0	0
(Bush's Best)	1/2 cup	70	6	17	300	6	0.0	0
(Finast) light	1/2 cup	110	6	20	350	0	2.0	0
(Green Giant)	1/2 cup	90	7	20	330	5	1.0	0
(Joan of Arc)	1/2 cup	90	7	20	330	5	1.0	0
(Stokely)	1/2 cup	110	7	20	360	0	1.0	0
(Stokely)	1/2 cup	120	7	21	380	5	0.5	0
(Van Camp's)	1 cup	184	12	36	650	0	0.5	0
50% less salt (Green Giant)	1/2 cup	90	7	20	165	5	1.0	0
50% less salt (Joan of Arc)	1/2 cup	90	7	20	165	5	1.0	0
RED								
Canned								
(A&P)	1/2 cup	110	7	20	440	0	1.0	0
(Green Giant)	1/2 cup	90	7	20	250	6	0.0	0
(Hunt's)	1/2 cup	95	6	20	484	5	0.5	0
(Joan of Arc)	1/2 cup	90	7	20	250	6	0.0	0
(Pathmark)	1/2 cup	110	7	20	350	0	0.0	0
(Pathmark)	1/2 cup	110	8	18	370	0	0.0	0
(Progresso)	1/2 cup	100	9	21	210	7	1.0	0
(Stokely)	1/2 cup	110	7	20	360	0	1.0	0
(Van Camp's)	1 cup	184	12	36	650	0	0.5	0
50% less salt, 'Lite' (S&W)	1/2 cup	120	7	22	355	0	1.0	0
mature seeds	1 cup	218	13	40	873	16	0.9	0
mature seeds	1 tbsp	14	1	2	55	1	0.1	0
New Orleans style (Van Camp's)	1 cup	178	12	34	940	0	0.6	0
'Nutradiet' (S&W)	1/2 cup	90	7	16	1	0	1.0	0
organic, very low-sodium, no salt added								
(Eden Foods)	1/2 cup	60	8	18	20	10	1.0	0
'Premium' (S&W)	1/2 cup	120	6	22	596	0	1.0	0
Dried								
boiled (A&P)	1 cup	230	17	41	5	0	1.0	0
mature seeds, boiled	1 cup	225	15	40	4	13	0.9	0
mature seeds, boiled	1 tbsp	14	1	3	0	1	0.1	0
mature seeds, raw	1 cup	613	43	110	44	46	1.5	0
mature seeds, raw	1 cup	620	41	113	22	28	1.9	0
mature seeds, raw	1 tbsp	41	3	7	1	2	0.1	0
raw (Arrowhead Mills)	2 oz	190	13	35	3	12	1.0	0
Sprouted, mature seeds	1 cup	53	8	8	11	na	0.9	0
ROYAL RED								
Dried								
mature seeds, boiled	1 cup	218	17	39	9	16	0.3	0
mature seeds, raw	1 cup	605	47	107	24	46	0.8	0
BEAN, LIMA/butterbean								
Canned								
(A&P)	1/2 cup	110	7	20	380	0	1.0	0
(Featherweight)	1/2 cup	80	5	16	25	0	0.0	0
(Freshlike)	1/2 cup	80	5	16	320	0	0.0	0
(Green Giant)	1/2 cup	80	6	16	420	4	0.0	0
(Joan of Arc)	1/2 cup	80	6	16	420	4	0.0	0
(S&W)	1/2 cup	100	6	19	440	0	1.0	0
(Stokely)	1/2 cup	80	5	16	390	0	0.0	0
(Van Camp's)	1 cup	162	11	30	710	0	0.5	0
(Veg-All)	1/2 cup	80	5	16	320	0	0.0	0
baby (Bush's Best)	1/2 cup	70	5	16	370	5	0.0	0
all green (Bush's Best)	1/2 cup	90	4	17	400	4	0.0	0

Food Name	Serv. Size	Total Cal.	Prot. gms	Carbs gms	Sod. mgs	Fiber gms	Fat gms	Chol. mgs
baby (C&W)	1/2 cup	90	6	15	80	5	0.5	0
Fordhook (Stokely)	1/2 cup	80	5	14	300	0	0.0	0
gem, green and white (Bush's Best)	1/2 cup	80	5	17	300	4	0.0	0
green (A&P)	1/2 cup	80	5	15	320	0	1.0	0
giant, seasoned w/pork (Luck's)	1/2 cup	150	8	23	340	5	3.0	3
green, small, 'Fancy' (S&W)	1/2 cup	80	6	16	390	0	0.0	0
green, small, w/pork (Luck's)	7.5 oz	220	10	33	640	8	7.0	0
green, tiny (Allens)	1/2 cup	90	5	15	350	0	1.0	0
green, w/liquid (Del Monte)	1/2 cup	70	4	14	355	0	0.0	0
green and white (Allens)	1/2 cup	90	5	15	370	0	1.0	0
'Harvest Fresh' (Green Giant)	1/2 cup	80	4	15	130	4	0.0	0
immature seeds, no salt added, w/liquid	1/2 cup	88	5	17	5	4	0.4	0
immature seeds, regular pack, w/liquid	1/2 cup	88	5	17	312	4	0.4	0
large (Allens)	1/2 cup	110	5	18	370	0	1.0	0
large (Bush's Best)	1/2 cup	70	5	16	370	5	0.0	0
large, mature seeds	1 cup	190	12	36	810	12	0.4	0
'No Salt or Sugar Added' (Stokely)	1/2 cup	80	5	16	5	0	0.0	0
seasoned w/pork (Luck's)	1/2 cup	140	6	23	350	5	2.0	0
speckled (Bush's Best)	1/2 cup	70	5	17	310	5	0.0	0
speckled, seasoned w/pork (Luck's)	1/2 cup	140	6	22	320	5	3.0	3
water packed, w/o salt (Freshlike)	1/2 cup	80	5	16	5	0	0.0	0
w/ham (Dennison's)	7.5 oz	250	14	33	935	9	7.0	0
w/pork (Luck's)	7.5 oz	230	12	34	720	9	7.0	0
Dried
baby, boiled	1 cup	229	15	42	435	14	0.7	0
baby, boiled (A&P)	1 cup	230	16	40	15	0	1.0	0
baby, raw	1 cup	677	42	127	26	42	1.9	0
immature seeds, boiled, drained	1 cup	209	12	40	29	9	0.5	0
immature seeds, raw	1 cup	176	11	31	12	8	1.3	0
large, mature seeds, boiled	1 cup	216	15	39	4	13	0.7	0
large, mature seeds, boiled	1 tbsp	13	1	2	0	1	0.0	0
mature seeds, raw	1 cup	602	38	113	32	34	1.2	0
mature seeds, raw	1 tbsp	38	2	7	2	2	0.1	0
Frozen
(Flav-R-Pac)	1/2 cup	100	6	20	130	4	0.0	0
(Green Giant)	1/2 cup	100	6	19	30	5	0.0	0
(Health Valley)	1/2 cup	94	6	18	26	3	0.0	0
baby (Birds Eye)	3.3 oz	130	7	24	115	0	0.0	0
baby (Freshlike)	3.3 oz	130	7	24	100	0	1.0	0
baby (Frosty Acres)	3.3 oz	130	7	24	125	2	0.0	0
baby (Seabrook)	3.3 oz	130	7	24	125	2	0.0	0
baby (Southern)	3.5 oz	135	7	25	125	0	0.5	0
baby (Veg-All)	3.3 oz	130	7	24	100	0	1.0	0
baby, butter (Seabrook)	3.3 oz	140	7	26	213	2	1.0	0
baby, green (A&P)	3.3 oz	130	7	24	130	0	1.0	0
Fordhook (A&P)	3.3 oz	100	6	19	70	0	1.0	0
Fordhook (Birds Eye)	3.3 oz	100	6	19	100	0	0.0	0
Fordhook (Flav-R-Pac)	1/2 cup	90	6	17	110	5	0.0	0
Fordhook (Frosty Acres)	3.3 oz	100	6	19	71	2	0.0	0
Fordhook (Seabrook)	3.3 oz	100	6	19	71	2	0.0	0
Fordhook, immature seeds, no salt added, boiled, drained	1/2 cup	85	5	16	45	5	0.3	0
Fordhook, immature seeds, no salt added, boiled, drained	10-oz pkg	311	19	58	165	18	1.1	0
Fordhook, immature seeds, unprepared	1/2 cup	85	5	16	46	4	0.3	0
Fordhook, immature seeds, unprepared	10-oz pkg	301	18	56	165	16	1.0	0
'Harvest Fresh' (Green Giant)	1/2 cup	80	6	18	170	4	0.0	0

Food Name	Serv. Size	Total Cal.	Prot. gms	Carbs gms	Sod. mgs	Fiber gms	Fat gms	Chol. mgs
immature seeds, drained	1/2 cup	95	6	18	239	5	0.3	0
immature seeds, drained, 10-oz pkg	1 pkg	327	21	60	824	19	0.9	0
immature seeds, no salt added, drained	1/2 cup	95	6	18	26	5	0.3	0
immature seeds, no salt added, drained	10-oz pkg	327	21	60	90	19	0.9	0
speckled *(Seabrook)*	3.3 oz	120	7	23	19	2	0.0	0
speckled *(Southern)*	3.5 oz	135	8	25	30	0	0.4	0
tiny *(Seabrook)*	3.3 oz	110	6	21	144	2	1.0	0
BEAN, MARROW								
regular, boiled	4 oz	158	11.0	28.5	7	7.2	0.4	0
regular, boiled	1/2 cup	125	8.6	22.5	6	5.7	0.3	0
regular, raw	1/2 cup	337	23.6	60.9	16	15.4	0.9	0
regular, raw	1 oz	94	6.6	17.1	5	4.3	0.2	0
small, boiled	4 oz	161	10.2	29.3	2	5.0	0.7	0
small, boiled	1/2 cup	127	8.1	23.2	2	3.7	0.6	0
small, raw	1/2 cup	363	22.8	67.2	13	11.1	1.3	0
small, raw	1 oz	95	6.0	17.6	3	2.9	0.3	0
BEAN, MOTH								
mature seeds, boiled	1 cup	207	14	37	18	na	1.0	0
mature seeds, raw	1 cup	672	45	121	59	na	3.2	0
BEAN, MUNG								
Canned								
mature seeds, sprouted, drained	1 cup	15	2	3	175	1	0.1	0
sprouted *(La Choy)*	2 oz	8	1	1	20	1	0.1	0
Dried								
mature seeds, boiled	1 cup	212	14	39	4	15	0.8	0
mature seeds, raw	1 cup	718	49	130	31	34	2.4	0
mature seeds, raw	1 tbsp	45	3	8	2	2	0.1	0
Sprouted								
mature seeds, raw	1 cup	31	3	6	6	2	0.2	0
mature seeds, raw	12-oz pkg	102	10	20	20	6	0.6	0
mature seeds, stir-fried	1 cup	62	5	13	11	2	0.3	0
BEAN, MUNGO								
mature seeds, boiled	1 cup	189	14	33	13	12	1.0	0
mature seeds, raw	1 cup	706	52	122	79	38	3.4	0
BEAN, NAVY								
Dry								
mature seeds, boiled	1 cup	258	16	48	2	12	1.0	0
mature seeds raw	1 cup	697	46	126	29	51	2.7	0
'Michigan #1' cooked *(A&P)*	1 cup	220	15	40	15	0	1.0	0
Canned								
(Allens)	1/2 cup	160	8	24	440	0	1.0	0
(Bush's Best)	1/2 cup	60	5	17	370	7	0.0	0
flavored w/bacon *(Trappey's)*	1/2 cup	130	7	28	430	5	0.0	0
mature seeds	1 cup	296	20	54	1174	13	1.1	0
organic, no salt added, very low sodium *(Eden Foods)*	1/2 cup	70	6	18	15	7	1.0	0
seasoned w/pork *(Luck's)*	1/2 cup	140	7	19	310	5	4.0	3
w/ham, 'Homestyle' *(Hunt's)*	9.03 oz	239	16	38	737	10	2.7	10
Sprouted, mature seeds, raw	1 cup	70	6	14	14	na	0.7	0
BEAN, PINK								
mature seeds, boiled	1 cup	252	15	47	3	9	0.8	0
mature seeds, raw	1 cup	720	44	135	17	27	2.4	0
BEAN, PINTO								
Dried								
boiled *(A&P)*	1 cup	230	17	42	5	0	1.0	0
mature seeds, boiled	1 cup	234	14	44	3	15	0.9	0
mature seeds, boiled	1 tbsp	15	1	3	0	1	0.1	0
mature seeds, raw	1 cup	656	40	122	19	47	2.2	0

Food Name	Serv. Size	Total Cal.	Prot. gms	Carbs gms	Sod. mgs	Fiber gms	Fat gms	Chol. mgs
mature seeds, raw	1 tbsp	41	3	8	1	3	0.1	0
raw (Arrowhead Mills)	2 oz	200	13	36	3	11	1.0	0
raw (Evans)	1 cup	660	43	121	19	0	2.0	0
Canned								
(Allens)	1/2 cup	105	5	18	480	0	1.0	0
(Bush's Best)	1/2 cup	60	5	15	350	5	0.0	0
(Gebhardt)	1/2 cup	92	7	18	505	7	1.2	0
(Green Giant)	1/2 cup	90	6	20	280	5	1.0	0
(Joan of Arc)	1/2 cup	90	6	20	280	5	1.0	0
(Old El Paso)	1/2 cup	100	6	19	320	8	0.0	0
(Progresso)	1/2 cup	110	7	7	250	7	1.0	0
(Ranch Style)	1/2 cup	100	6	19	580	5	0.0	5
baked style, w/pork, 15-oz can (Luck's)	7.5 oz	220	12	30	787	7	6.0	0
baked style, w/pork, 29-oz can (Luck's)	7.25 oz	220	11	30	520	11	6.0	0
mature seeds	1 cup	206	12	37	706	11	1.9	0
organic, no salt added, very low sodium (Eden Foods)	1/2 cup	70	6	17	15	6	1.0	0
organic, w/liquid (Eden Foods)	1/2 cup	110	6	20	20	6	1.0	0
picante style (Green Giant)	1/2 cup	100	7	21	580	7	1.0	0
picante style (Joan of Arc)	1/2 cup	100	7	21	580	7	1.0	0
seasoned w/pork (Luck's)	1/2 cup	140	7	19	310	6	4.0	3
'Sun-Vista' (S&W)	1/2 cup	80	3	12	530	3	0.5	0
w/jalapeño peppers (Ranch Style)	1/2 cup	110	5	21	700	6	0.0	5
w/onions, seasoned w/pork (Luck's)	1/2 cup	150	7	24	300	6	3.0	3
Frozen								
(Seabrook)	3.2 oz	160	9	29	0	0	0.0	0
immature seeds, frozen, no salt added, drained 10-oz pkg	1 pkg	460	26	88	236	24	1.4	0
immature seeds, unprepared, 10-oz pkg	1 pkg	483	28	92	261	16	1.4	0
immature seeds, w/salt, drained, 10-oz pkg	1 pkg	460	26	88	906	24	1.4	0
Jarred, organic, low-sodium (Eden Foods)	1/2 cup	120	7	22	30	6	0.0	0
BEAN, RED								
Canned								
(A&P)	1/2 cup	120	7	23	400	0	1.0	0
(Allens)	1/2 cup	115	7	20	350	0	1.0	0
(Bush's Best)	1/2 cup	70	5	17	350	6	0.0	0
(Green Giant)	1/2 cup	90	6	19	340	5	1.0	0
(Joan of Arc)	1/2 cup	90	6	19	340	5	1.0	0
(Van Camp's)	1 cup	194	11	38	928	0	0.6	0
small (Hunt's)	4 oz	91	6	18	578	0	0.0	0
small, baked-style (B&M)	8 oz	223	9	36	725	11	5.0	5
BEAN, ROMAN. See BEAN, CRANBERRY.								
BEAN, ROSE COCO. See BEAN, CRANBERRY.								
BEAN, SHELLY								
Canned								
(Allens)	1/2 cup	35	2	6	395	0	1.0	0
(Stokely)	1/2 cup	35	2	7	470	0	0.0	0
w/liquid	1 cup	74	4	15	818	8	0.5	0
BEAN, SNAP. See BEAN, GREEN; BEAN, WAX.								
BEAN, SOYA. See SOYBEAN.								
BEAN, STRING. See BEAN, GREEN; BEAN, WAX.								
BEAN, WAX/yellow snap bean								
Canned								
(Allens)	1/2 cup	15	1	3	260	0	1.0	0
(Stokely)	1/2 cup	20	1	4	360	0	0.0	0
cut (S&W)	1/2 cup	20	1	4	400	1	0.0	0
cut, 'Premium Golden' (S&W)	1/2 cup	20	1	5	385	0	0.0	0
cut, water packed, w/o salt (Freshlike)	1/2 cup	18	1	4	5	0	0.0	0

Food Name	Serv. Size	Total Cal.	Prot. gms	Carbs gms	Sod. mgs	Fiber gms	Fat gms	Chol. mgs
cut, water packed, w/o sugar or salt *(Freshlike)*	1/2 cup	18	1	4	5	0	0.0	0
golden, cut *(Del Monte)*	1/2 cup	20	0	4	355	0	0.0	0
golden, French style *(Del Monte)*	1/2 cup	20	0	4	355	0	0.0	0
no salt added, cut, drained	1/2 cup	14	1	3	1	1	0.1	0
no salt added, w/liquid	1/2 cup	18	1	4	17	2	0.1	0
no salt or sugar *(Stokely)*	1/2 cup	20	1	4	5	0	0.0	0
regular pack, cut, drained	1 cup	27	2	6	339	2	0.1	0
regular pack, whole, drained	10 med beans	12	1	3	156	1	0.1	0
regular pack, cut, w/liquid	1/2 cup	18	1	4	311	2	0.1	0
Fresh								
boiled, drained	1 cup	44	2	10	4	4	0.3	0
raw	1 cup	34	2	8	7	4	0.1	0
Frozen								
(Flav-R-Pac)	2/3 cup	25	1	4	10	2	0.0	0
(Frosty Acres)	3 oz	25	2	5	1	1	0.0	0
cut *(Seabrook)*	3 oz	25	2	5	1	1	0.0	0
no salt added, drained	1 cup	38	2	9	12	4	0.2	0
w/salt, drained	1 cup	38	2	9	331	4	0.2	0
BEAN, WHITE. See also BEAN, CANNELLINI.								
Dried								
mature seeds, boiled	1 cup	249	17	45	11	11	0.6	0
mature seeds, boiled	1 tbsp	16	1	3	1	1	0.0	0
mature seeds, raw	1 cup	673	47	122	32	31	1.7	0
mature seeds, raw	1 tbsp	42	3	8	2	2	0.1	0
small white, mature seeds, boiled	1 cup	254	16	46	4	19	1.1	0
small white, mature seeds, raw	1 cup	722	45	134	26	54	2.5	0
Canned, mature seeds	1 cup	307	19	57	13	13	0.8	0
BEAN, WINGED/goa bean								
immature seeds, boiled, drained	1 cup	24	3	2	2	na	0.4	0
immature seeds, raw	1 med pod	8	1	1	1	na	0.1	0
immature seeds, raw, sliced	1 cup	22	3	2	2	na	0.4	0
mature seeds, boiled	1 cup	255	16	45	9	18	1.9	0
mature seeds, boiled	1 cup	253	18	26	22	na	10.0	0
mature seeds, raw	1 cup	744	54	76	69	na	29.7	0
BEAN, YARDLONG								
boiled, drained	1 med pod	7	0	1	1	na	0.0	0
boiled, drained, sliced	1 cup	49	3	10	4	na	0.1	0
boiled, mature seeds	1 cup	202	14	36	9	6	0.8	0
mature seeds, raw	1 cup	579	41	103	28	18	2.2	0
raw	1 med pod	6	0	1	0	na	0.0	0
raw, sliced	1 cup	43	3	8	4	na	0.4	0
BEAN, YELLOW, dried, mature seeds, raw	1 cup	676	43	119	24	49	5.1	0
BEAN DISH/ENTRÉE. See also BAKED BEANS, CANNED; BEAN SALAD; BEANS, CHILI; BURRITO; CHILI; ENCHILADA.								
(Amy's Kitchen)								
meatless 'Salisbury steak,' 'Country Dinner'	1 entrée	420	12	63	700	9	16.0	20
(Banquet) beans and frankfurters, frozen	10 oz	520	17	57	1230	0	25.0	35
(Bearitos)								
refried beans, low-fat, no salt	1 serving	80	5	14	10	2	2.0	0
refried beans, nonfat	1 serving	70	4	14	350	2	0.0	0
refried beans, organic, canned	1 oz	30	2	5	61	0	0.5	0
refried beans, organic, no salt, canned	1 oz	29	2	5	2	0	0.5	0
refried beans, spicy, organic, canned	1 oz	31	2	5	56	1	0.6	0
refried beans, vegetarian, spicy, low-fat, canned	3.2 oz	80	5	14	280	2	2.0	0
refried beans, w/black beans, low-fat	1 serving	80	6	14	320	1	1.0	0
refried beans, w/green chilies, nonfat	1/2 cup	40	3	8	245	3	0.0	0
(Bush's Best) mixed, canned	1/2 cup	70	6	17	410	6	0.0	0

Food Name	Serv. Size	Total Cal.	Prot. gms	Carbs gms	Sod. mgs	Fiber gms	Fat gms	Chol. mgs
(Chi-Chi's) refried beans	7.5 oz	250	9	29	930	0	11.0	5
(Del Monte)								
refried beans, canned	1/2 cup	130	6	20	530	0	2.0	0
refried beans, spicy, canned	1/2 cup	130	6	20	480	0	2.0	0
(Flav-R-Pac)								
beans Parisian, frozen	1 cup	25	1	4	10	2	0.0	0
beans Parisian w/buttery sauce, frozen	1/2 cup	50	2	8	450	2	2.5	0
beans supreme, frozen	2/3 cup	50	3	9	95	4	0.0	0
four bean salad, frozen	1/3 cup	70	2	17	370	2	0.5	0
green beans w/onions and ham, 'Grande Classics'	1/2 cup	40	2	6	460	2	2.0	5
Oregon bean medley, frozen	2/3 cup	45	3	8	65	3	0.0	0
(Gebhardt)								
refried beans	1/2 cup	109	6	20	497	6	2.8	1
refried beans, food service product	1/2 cup	109	6	20	497	6	2.8	1
refried beans, jalapeño	1/2 cup	105	7	19	380	6	3.0	1
(refried beans, nonfat	1/2 cup	92	7	20	480	6	0.5	0
refried beans, vegetarian	1/2 cup	118	8	21	550	7	2.3	0
(Green Giant)								
Mexican beans, canned, dry beans in brine	1/2 cup	120	6	21	530	5	1.5	0
three bean salad, canned	1/2 cup	70	2	16	470	3	0.0	0
(Health Valley)								
black beans w/garden vegetables, western, 'Fast Menu'	7.5 oz	120	13	14	170	15	1.0	0
(Homestyle)								
beans 'n fixins, food service product	1/2 cup	125	2	30	575	8	2.8	1
country kettle beans, food service product	1/2 cup	131	6	26	365	6	2.0	1
(Hunt's) beans and fixin's, 'Big John's'	1/2 cup	127	7	23	590	6	3.5	3
(Joan of Arc) Mexican beans, canned, dry beans in brine	1/2 cup	120	6	21	530	5	1.5	0
(Kid's Kitchen) beans and wieners, microwave cup	7.5 oz	310	13	36	750	0	13.0	45
(Lean Cuisine) three bean chili w/rice	1 entrée	210	8	32	460	7	6.0	10
(Libby's)								
beans and frankfurters in sauce, micro cup, 'Diner'	7.75 oz	330	15	38	930	4	15.0	55
(Lipton)								
beans and chicken w/sauce, mix, dry	1/4 pkg	120	6	26	470	0	1.0	0
beans and chicken w/sauce, mix, prepared	1/2 cup	150	6	26	500	0	4.0	0
(Little Pancho)								
refried beans, w/green chilies, nonfat, canned	1/2 cup	80	6	15	330	0	0.0	0
(Luck's) pinto and great northern, seasoned w/pork	1/2 cup	130	7	22	370	8	2.0	3
(Morningstar Farms) 'Spicy Black Bean Burger'	1 patty	110	11	16	470	5	1.0	0.0
(Morton) beans and frankfurters, frozen	10 oz	350	11	46	1490	0	13.0	30
(Natural Touch)								
'Spicy Black Bean Burger'	1 patty	110	11	15	330	5	1.0	0
'Nine Bean Loaf'	1 slice	160	8	14	350	0	8.0	0
(Old El Paso)								
refried beans, canned	1/4 cup	55	3	8	200	3	1.0	1
refried beans, nonfat	1/2 cup	110	6	20	480	6	0.0	0
refried beans, spicy, canned	1/4 cup	35	1	5	280	2	1.0	1
refried beans, vegetarian, spicy, canned	1/4 cup	70	6	15	730	5	1.0	0
refried beans, w/cheese, canned	1/4 cup	36	2	4	280	2	1.0	2
refried beans, w/green chilies, canned	1/4 cup	49	3	8	252	3	1.0	0
refried beans, w/sausage, canned	1/2 cup	200	7	14	360	8	13.0	10
(Rice A Roni) red beans and rice	2.5 oz	158	5	29	675	3	4.0	0
(Rosarita)								
refried beans	1/2 cup	125	7	22	585	8	2.7	0
refried beans, nacho cheese	1/2 cup	137	8	24	703	7	3.2	0
refried beans, no fat	1/2 cup	123	7	28	574	6	0.5	0

Food Name	Serv. Size	Total Cal.	Prot. gms	Carbs gms	Sod. mgs	Fiber gms	Fat gms	Chol. mgs
refried beans, original, food service product	1/2 cup	109	6	20	497	6	2.8	1
refried beans, quick cooking, food service product	1/2 cup	185	11	31	704	10	6.7	0
refried beans, spicy	1/2 cup	118	7	22	574	6	2.7	0
refried beans, spicy, food service product	1/2 cup	109	6	20	530	6	2.6	1
refried beans, vegetarian	1/2 cup	121	7	23	562	6	2.1	0
refried beans, vegetarian, food service product	1/2 cup	118	8	21	550	6	2.3	0
refried beans, vegetarian, spicy, canned	4 oz	120	7	19	470	0	2.0	0
refried beans, vegetarian, w/canola oil	4 oz	100	7	18	480	6	2.0	0
refried beans, vegetarian, w/soybean oil	4 oz	100	7	18	480	6	2.0	0
refried beans, w/bacon	1/2 cup	116	8	19	489	8	3.1	1
refried beans, w/black beans, low-fat	1/2 cup	107	8	23	569	7	0.6	0
refried beans, w/green chilies	1/2 cup	110	6	20	495	7	2.9	1
refried beans, w/green chilies, no fat	1/2 cup	101	8	22	565	8	0.1	0
refried beans, w/onions	1/2 cup	114	6	21	508	6	2.8	1
salsa refried beans, no fat	1/2 cup	99	6	22	554	8	0.5	0
(S&W)								
bean salad, deli style, canned	1/2 cup	80	4	20	670	4	0.0	0
kidney, garbanzo and green beans in vinaigrette,								
canned	1/2 cup	90	4	17	726	0	1.0	0
(Santiago)								
refried beans, smooth	1/2 cup	174	7	24	469	10	5.8	3
refried beans, whole bean style	1/2 cup	174	7	24	469	10	5.8	0
(Stouffer's) green bean-mushroom casserole	1/2 cup	140	3	13	530	2	8.0	10
(Swanson) beans and frankfurters frozen	10.5 oz	440	14	53	900	0	19.0	0
(Weight Watchers) white beans and								
vegetables Parisian	1 entrée	220	13	23	690	13	9.0	20

BEAN DISH/ENTRÉE MIX
(Fantastic Foods)

black beans, instant, prepared	1/3 cup	160	10	29	310	7	1.5	0
refried beans, instant, prepared	1/3 cup	160	9	29	320	11	1.0	0
refried beans, instant, prepared w/o added ingredients . . .	1/2 cup	157	10	28	400	0	2.0	0

BEAN SALAD. See under BEAN DISH/ENTRÉE.

BEAN SPROUTS
Canned

(Chun King)	85 grams	5	1	0	15	0	0.0	0
(La Choy)	1 cup	14	1	1	17	1	0.1	0
(La Choy) food service product	1 cup	12	1	2	20	1	0.1	0

BEANS, CHILI
Canned

(Gebhardt)	1/2 cup	134	7	31	630	7	1.0	0
(Hunt's)	1/2 cup	87	6	17	597	6	1.0	0
(S&W)	1/2 cup	110	7	23	580	6	1.0	1
(Sun Vista)	1/2 cup	110	7	24	360	7	1.0	0
extra spicy *(Green Giant)*	1/2 cup	100	7	21	580	6	1.0	0
extra spicy *(Joan of Arc)*	1/2 cup	100	7	21	580	6	1.0	0
50% less salt *(Green Giant)*	1/2 cup	100	7	21	310	7	1.0	0
50% less salt *(Joan of Arc)*	1/2 cup	100	7	21	310	7	1.0	0
hot *(Bush's Best)*	1/2 cup	70	5	20	420	6	0.0	0
spiced *(Gebhardt)*	1/2 cup	100	7	19	654	8	1.6	0

BEANS, REFRIED. See under BEAN DISH/ENTRÉE.
BEAR

raw	1 oz	46	6	0	na	0	2.4	na
simmered	3 oz	220	28	0	60	0	11.4	83
simmered, yield from 1 lb raw, boneless	8 oz	717	90	0	197	0	37.1	271

BEAVER, RAW

raw	1 oz	41	7	0	14	0	1.4	na
roasted	3 oz	180	30	0	50	0	5.9	99
roasted, yield from 1 lb raw, boneless	11 oz	664	109	0	185	0	21.8	366

Food Name	Serv. Size	Total Cal.	Prot. gms	Carbs gms	Sod. mgs	Fiber gms	Fat gms	Chol. mgs
BEECHNUT, dried	1 oz	163	2	9	11	na	14.2	0
BEEF. See also under LUNCHEON MEAT.								
(NOTE: TRIMMED = Lean; separable fat removed after cooking. UNTRIMMED = Separable fat not removed.)								
BRAIN								
pan-fried	3 oz	167	11	0	134	0	13.5	1696
raw	4 oz	142	11	0	116	0	10.5	1889
simmered	3 oz	136	9	0	102	0	10.7	1746
BRISKET								
choice, shredded *(Cripple Creek)*	3 oz	180	18	6	570	0	12.0	60
choice, sliced *(Cripple Creek)*	3 oz	120	12	6	540	0	6.0	60
chopped *(Cripple Creek)*	3 oz	180	15	6	375	0	12.0	60
BRISKET, FLAT HALF								
Trimmed								
all grades, 0-inch fat, braised	3 oz	162	27	0	54	0	5.3	81
all grades, 1/4-inch fat, braised	3 oz	189	27	0	54	0	8.2	81
all grades, 1/4-inch fat, raw	1 oz	42	6	0	21	0	1.8	17
Untrimmed								
all grades, 0-inch fat, braised	3 oz	183	26	0	53	0	8.0	81
all grades, 1/8-inch fat, braised	3 oz	263	23	0	50	0	18.0	81
all grades, 1/8-inch fat, raw	4 oz	266	22	0	76	0	19.1	75
all grades, 1/4-inch fat, braised	3 oz	309	21	0	48	0	24.2	81
all grades, 1/4-inch fat, raw	4 oz	328	20	0	70	0	26.7	79
BRISKET, POINT HALF								
Trimmed								
all grades, 0-inch fat, braised	3 oz	207	24	0	65	0	11.7	77
all grades, 1/4-inch fat, braised	3 oz	222	24	0	65	0	13.3	77
all grades, 1/4-inch fat, raw	1 oz	46	6	0	24	0	2.4	18
Untrimmed								
all grades, 0-inch fat, braised	3 oz	304	20	0	58	0	24.2	78
all grades, 1/8-inch fat, braised	3 oz	297	21	0	59	0	23.1	78
all grades, 1/8-inch fat, raw	1 oz	75	5	0	20	0	5.9	20
all grades, 1/4-inch fat, braised	3 oz	343	19	0	55	0	29.1	78
all grades, 1/4-inch fat, raw	1 oz	94	5	0	18	0	8.2	22
BRISKET, WHOLE								
Trimmed								
all grades, 0-inch fat, braised, ...	3 oz	185	25	0	60	0	8.6	79
all grades, 1/4-inch fat, braised	3 oz	206	25	0	60	0	10.8	79
all grades, raw	1 oz	44	6	0	22	0	2.1	18
Untrimmed								
all grades, 0-inch fat, braised	3 oz	247	23	0	55	0	16.6	79
all grades, 1/8-inch fat, braised	3 oz	281	22	0	54	0	20.8	79
all grades, 1/8-inch fat, raw	1 oz	71	5	0	20	0	5.4	19
all grades, 1/4-inch fat, braised	3 oz	327	20	0	52	0	26.8	80
all grades, 1/4-inch fat, raw	1 oz	88	5	0	18	0	7.5	21
CHOPPED, canned *(Armour)*	3 oz	280	11	3	1290	0	24.0	0
CHUCK, ARM POT ROAST								
Trimmed								
all grades, 0-inch fat, braised	3 oz	179	28	0	56	0	6.5	86
all grades, 1/4-inch fat, braised	3 oz	184	28	0	56	0	7.1	86
all grades, 1/4-inch fat, raw	1 oz	37	6	0	19	0	1.2	17
choice, 0-inch fat, braised	3 oz	186	28	0	56	0	7.4	86
choice, 1/4-inch fat, braised	3 oz	191	28	0	56	0	7.9	86
choice, 1/4-inch fat, raw	1 oz	39	6	0	19	0	1.4	17
prime, 1/2-inch fat, braised	3 oz	222	28	0	56	0	11.4	86
prime, 1/2-inch fat, raw	1 oz	44	6	0	19	0	2.0	17
select, 0-inch fat, braised	3 oz	168	28	0	56	0	5.4	86
select, 1/4-inch fat, braised	3 oz	175	28	0	56	0	6.1	86

Food Name	Serv. Size	Total Cal.	Prot. gms	Carbs gms	Sod. mgs	Fiber gms	Fat gms	Chol. mgs
select, 1/4-inch fat, raw	1 oz	35	6	0	19	0	1.0	17
Untrimmed								
all grades, 0-inch fat, braised	3 oz	238	25	0	53	0	14.5	85
all grades, 1/8-inch fat, braised	3 oz	263	24	0	52	0	17.6	85
all grades, 1/8-inch fat, raw	1 oz	69	5	0	17	0	5.2	19
all grades, 1/4-inch fat, braised	3 oz	282	23	0	51	0	20.2	84
all grades, 1/4-inch fat, raw	1 oz	69	5	0	17	0	5.2	19
choice, 1/4-inch fat, braised	3 oz	296	23	0	50	0	21.9	84
choice, 1/4-inch fat, raw	1 oz	72	5	0	17	0	5.5	20
prime, 1/2-inch fat, braised	3 oz	332	22	0	49	0	26.3	84
prime, 1/2-inch fat, raw	1 oz	83	5	0	16	0	6.8	20
select, 1/8-inch fat, raw	1 oz	62	5	0	17	0	4.4	19
select, 1/4-inch fat, braised	3 oz	268	24	0	51	0	18.5	85
select, 1/4-inch fat, raw	1 oz	66	5	0	17	0	4.8	19
CHUCK, BLADE ROAST								
Trimmed								
all grades, 0-inch fat, braised	3 oz	215	26	0	60	0	11.3	90
all grades, 1/4-inch fat, braised	3 oz	213	26	0	60	0	11.1	90
all grades, 1/4-inch fat, raw	1 oz	42	5	0	22	0	2.1	18
choice, 0-inch fat, braised	3 oz	225	26	0	60	0	12.5	90
choice, 1/4-inch fat, braised	3 oz	224	26	0	60	0	12.2	90
choice, 1/4-inch fat, raw	1 oz	45	5	0	22	0	2.4	18
prime, 1/2-inch fat, braised	3 oz	270	26	0	60	0	17.5	90
prime, 1/2-inch fat, raw	1 oz	58	5	0	22	0	3.8	18
select, 0-inch fat, braised	3 oz	202	26	0	60	0	9.9	90
select, 1/4-inch fat, braised	3 oz	201	26	0	60	0	9.9	90
select, 1/4-inch fat, raw	1 oz	39	5	0	22	0	1.8	18
Untrimmed								
all grades, 0-inch fat, braised	3 oz	284	23	0	55	0	20.5	88
all grades, 1/8-inch fat, braised	3 oz	290	23	0	55	0	21.4	88
all grades, 1/8-inch fat, raw	1 oz	70	5	0	19	0	5.5	20
all grades, 1/4-inch fat, braised	3 oz	293	23	0	54	0	21.8	88
all grades, 1/4-inch fat, raw	1 oz	72	5	0	19	0	5.7	20
choice, 1/8-inch fat, braised	3 oz	305	22	0	54	0	23.2	88
choice, 1/8-inch fat, raw	1 oz	75	5	0	19	0	6.0	20
choice, 1/4-inch fat, braised	3 oz	309	22	0	54	0	23.6	88
choice, 1/4-inch fat, raw	1 oz	77	5	0	19	0	6.3	20
prime, 1/2-inch fat, braised	3 oz	354	22	0	54	0	29.0	88
prime, 1/2-inch fat, raw	1 oz	93	5	0	18	0	8.1	21
select, 1/8-inch fat, braised	3 oz	270	23	0	56	0	19.0	88
select, 1/8-inch fat, raw	1 oz	65	5	0	20	0	4.9	20
select, 1/4-inch fat, braised	3 oz	277	23	0	55	0	19.8	88
select, 1/4-inch fat, raw	1 oz	67	5	0	19	0	5.1	20
CUBE STEAK, lean cuts, raw *(Lean and Free)*	4 oz	109	24	0	0	0	1.0	61
FLANK								
Trimmed								
choice, 0-inch fat, broiled	3 oz	176	23	0	71	0	8.6	57
choice, 0-inch fat, raw	1 oz	44	6	0	21	0	2.1	14
Untrimmed								
choice, 0-inch fat, braised	3 oz	201	24	0	61	0	11.1	60
choice, 0-inch fat, broiled	3 oz	192	22	0	69	0	10.7	58
choice, 0-inch fat, raw	4 oz	203	22	0	80	0	12.0	59
GROUND								
Extra lean, 17% fat								
baked, medium	3 oz	213	21	0	42	0	13.7	70
baked, well done	3 oz	233	26	0	54	0	13.6	91
broiled, medium	3 oz	218	22	0	60	0	13.9	71

Food Name	Serv. Size	Total Cal.	Prot. gms	Carbs gms	Sod. mgs	Fiber gms	Fat gms	Chol. mgs
broiled, well done	3 oz	225	24	0	70	0	13.4	84
pan-fried, medium	3 oz	217	21	0	60	0	14.0	69
pan-fried, well done	3 oz	224	24	0	69	0	13.6	79
raw	4 oz	264	21	0	75	0	19.3	78
raw	1 oz	66	5	0	19	0	4.8	20
Lean, 21% fat								
baked, medium	3 oz	228	20	0	48	0	15.6	66
baked, well done	3 oz	248	25	0	60	0	15.6	84
broiled, medium	3 oz	231	21	0	65	0	15.7	74
broiled, well done	3 oz	238	24	0	76	0	15.0	86
lean cuts, raw (Lean and Free)	4 oz	161	22	0	0	0	7.5	67
pan-fried, medium	3 oz	234	21	0	65	0	16.2	71
pan-fried, well done	3 oz	235	23	0	74	0	15.0	81
raw	4 oz	298	20	0	78	0	23.4	85
raw	1 oz	75	5	0	20	0	5.9	21
Regular, 27% fat								
baked, medium	3 oz	244	20	0	51	0	17.8	74
baked, well done	3 oz	269	24	0	64	0	18.2	92
broiled, medium	3 oz	246	20	0	71	0	17.6	77
broiled, well done	3 oz	248	23	0	79	0	16.5	86
1/4-pound patties (Bar-S)	1 patty	330	18	0	80	0	28.0	85
1/4-pound patties (Chuck Wagon)	1 patty	400	9	5	750	2	35.0	95
1/4-pound patties (Manor House)	1 patty	330	18	0	65	0	28.0	60
pan-fried, medium	3 oz	260	20	0	71	0	19.2	76
pan-fried, well done	3 oz	243	23	0	79	0	16.1	83
raw	4 oz	350	19	0	77	0	30.0	96
raw	1 oz	88	5	0	19	0	7.5	24
HEART								
raw	4 oz	132	19	3	71	0	4.3	158
simmered	3 oz	149	24	0	54	0	4.8	164
KIDNEY								
raw	1 oz	30	5	1	51	0	0.9	81
simmered	3 oz	122	22	1	114	0	2.9	329
LIVER								
braised	3 oz	137	21	3	60	0	4.2	331
pan-fried	3 oz	184	23	7	90	0	6.8	410
raw	4 oz	162	23	7	82	0	4.4	400
LOIN, TOP								
Trimmed								
all grades, 0-inch fat, broiled	3 oz	168	24	0	58	0	7.1	65
all grades, 1/4-inch fat, broiled	3 oz	176	24	0	58	0	8.0	65
all grades, 1/4-inch fat, raw	1 oz	40	6	0	17	0	1.6	17
choice, 0-inch fat, broiled	3 oz	178	24	0	58	0	8.2	65
choice, 1/4-inch fat, broiled	3 oz	182	24	0	58	0	8.6	65
choice, 1/4-inch fat, raw	1 oz	43	6	0	17	0	1.8	17
prime, 1/4-inch fat, broiled	3 oz	208	24	0	58	0	11.6	65
prime, 1/4-inch fat, raw	1 oz	54	6	0	17	0	3.0	17
prime, 1/2-inch fat, raw	3 oz	208	24	0	58	0	11.6	65
select, 0-inch fat, broiled	3 oz	156	24	0	58	0	5.9	65
select, 1/4-inch fat, broiled	3 oz	164	24	0	58	0	6.6	65
select, 1/4-inch fat, raw	1 oz	38	6	0	17	0	1.3	17
Untrimmed								
all grades, 0-inch fat, broiled	3 oz	180	24	0	57	0	8.7	65
all grades, 1/8-inch fat, broiled	3 oz	228	22	0	54	0	14.7	66
all grades, 1/4-inch fat, broiled	3 oz	244	22	0	54	0	16.8	67
choice, 0-inch fat, broiled	3 oz	194	24	0	57	0	10.2	65
choice, 1/8-inch fat, broiled	3 oz	241	22	0	54	0	16.3	67

Food Name	Serv. Size	Total Cal.	Prot. gms	Carbs gms	Sod. mgs	Fiber gms	Fat gms	Chol. mgs
choice, 1/4-inch fat, broiled	3 oz	253	22	0	54	0	17.8	67
prime, 1/8-inch fat, broiled	3 oz	264	22	0	54	0	18.8	67
prime, 1/4-inch fat, broiled	3 oz	275	22	0	54	0	20.2	67
prime, 1/2-inch fat, broiled	3 oz	288	21	0	53	0	22.0	68
select, 0-inch fat, broiled	3 oz	169	24	0	57	0	7.5	65
select, 1/8-inch fat, broiled	3 oz	215	22	0	55	0	13.2	66
select, 1/4-inch fat, broiled	3 oz	226	22	0	54	0	14.6	67
LUNGS								
braised	3 oz	102	17	0	86	0	3.1	235
raw	4 oz	104	18	0	224	0	2.8	273
PANCREAS								
braised	3 oz	230	23	0	51	0	14.6	223
raw	4 oz	266	18	0	76	0	21.0	232
PORTERHOUSE								
Trimmed								
all grades, 0-inch fat, broiled	3 oz	183	22	0	59	0	9.9	54
all grades, 1/4-inch fat, broiled	3 oz	180	22	0	59	0	9.3	56
all grades, 1/4-inch fat, raw	1 oz	45	6	0	16	0	2.1	16
choice, 0-inch fat, broiled	3 oz	190	22	0	59	0	10.9	55
choice, 1/4-inch fat, broiled	3 oz	183	22	0	59	0	9.8	59
choice, 1/4-inch fat, raw	1 oz	45	6	0	16	0	2.3	17
select, 0-inch fat, broiled	3 oz	165	23	0	59	0	7.5	49
select, 1/4-inch fat, broiled	3 oz	173	23	0	59	0	8.2	49
select, 1/4-inch fat, raw	1 oz	42	6	0	16	0	1.6	14
Untrimmed								
all grades, 0-inch fat, broiled	3 oz	237	20	0	55	0	16.7	57
all grades, 1/8-inch fat, broiled	3 oz	252	20	0	54	0	18.6	60
all grades, 1/8-inch fat, raw	1 oz	70	5	0	15	0	5.2	18
all grades, 1/4-inch fat, broiled	3 oz	273	19	0	54	0	21.1	62
all grades, 1/4-inch fat, raw	1 oz	73	5	0	14	0	5.6	18
choice, 1/8-inch fat, broiled	3 oz	254	20	0	54	0	18.8	63
choice, 1/8-inch fat, raw	1 oz	73	5	0	15	0	5.7	19
choice, 1/4-inch fat, broiled	3 oz	278	19	0	53	0	21.8	64
choice, 1/4-inch fat, raw	1 oz	73	5	0	15	0	5.7	19
select, 0-inch fat, broiled	3 oz	227	21	0	55	0	15.3	54
select, 1/8-inch fat, broiled	3 oz	250	20	0	54	0	18.0	55
select, 1/8-inch fat, raw	1 oz	63	6	0	15	0	4.2	16
select, 1/4-inch fat, broiled	3 oz	262	20	0	54	0	19.6	56
select, 1/4-inch fat, raw	1 oz	63	6	0	15	0	4.2	16
RIB, LARGE END								
Trimmed								
all grades, ribs 6-9, 0-inch fat, roasted	3 oz	202	23	0	62	0	11.4	69
all grades, ribs 6-9, 1/4-inch fat, broiled	3 oz	190	21	0	61	0	11.0	65
all grades, ribs 6-9, 1/4-inch fat, raw	1 oz	47	6	0	19	0	2.6	17
all grades, ribs 6-9, 1/4-inch fat, roasted	3 oz	201	23	0	62	0	11.2	69
choice, ribs 6-9, 0-inch fat, roasted	3 oz	215	23	0	62	0	12.8	69
choice, ribs 6-9, 1/4-inch fat, broiled	3 oz	204	21	0	61	0	12.5	65
choice, ribs 6-9, 1/4-inch fat, raw	1 oz	50	6	0	19	0	2.9	17
choice, ribs 6-9, 1/4-inch fat, roasted	3 oz	213	23	0	62	0	12.5	69
prime, ribs 6-9, 1/4-inch fat, broiled	3 oz	250	21	0	60	0	17.7	70
prime, ribs 6-9, 1/4-inch fat, raw	1 oz	60	6	0	19	0	4.0	17
prime, ribs 6-9, 1/4-inch fat, roasted	3 oz	241	23	0	62	0	15.6	69
prime, ribs 6-9, 1/2-inch fat, broiled	3 oz	250	21	0	60	0	17.7	70
prime, ribs 6-9, 1/2-inch fat, roasted	3 oz	241	23	0	62	0	15.6	69
select, ribs 6-9, 0-inch fat, roasted	3 oz	187	23	0	62	0	9.7	69
select, ribs 6-9, 1/4-inch fat, broiled	3 oz	175	21	0	61	0	9.3	65
select, ribs 6-9, 1/4-inch fat, raw	1 oz	43	6	0	19	0	2.2	17

Food Name	Serv. Size	Total Cal.	Prot. gms	Carbs gms	Sod. mgs	Fiber gms	Fat gms	Chol. mgs
select, ribs 6-9, 1/4-inch fat, roasted	3 oz	187	23	0	62	0	9.7	69
Untrimmed								
all grades, ribs 6-9, 0-inch fat, roasted	3 oz	300	20	0	55	0	24.0	72
all grades, ribs 6-9, 1/8-inch fat, broiled	3 oz	287	18	0	54	0	23.1	68
all grades, ribs 6-9, 1/8-inch fat, raw	1 oz	90	5	0	16	0	7.7	20
all grades, ribs 6-9, 1/8-inch fat, roasted	3 oz	302	20	0	54	0	24.2	72
all grades, ribs 6-9, 1/4-inch fat, broiled	3 oz	295	18	0	54	0	24.2	69
all grades, ribs 6-9, 1/4-inch fat, raw	1 oz	92	5	0	16	0	8.0	20
all grades, ribs 6-9, 1/4-inch fat, roasted	3 oz	310	19	0	54	0	25.3	72
choice, ribs 6-9, 0-inch fat, roasted	3 oz	316	19	0	54	0	25.9	72
choice, ribs 6-9, 1/8-inch fat, broiled	3 oz	315	18	0	54	0	26.5	69
choice, ribs 6-9, 1/8-inch fat, raw	1 oz	94	5	0	15	0	8.3	20
choice, ribs 6-9, 1/8-inch fat, roasted	3 oz	334	19	0	54	0	27.8	72
choice, ribs 6-9, 1/4-inch fat, broiled	3 oz	312	18	0	54	0	26.2	69
choice, ribs 6-9, 1/4-inch fat, raw	1 oz	98	4	0	15	0	8.7	21
choice, ribs 6-9, 1/4-inch fat, roasted	3 oz	326	19	0	54	0	27.2	72
prime, ribs 6-9, 1/8-inch fat, broiled	3 oz	343	18	0	53	0	29.7	73
prime, ribs 6-9, 1/8-inch fat, raw	1 oz	104	4	0	15	0	9.4	21
prime, ribs 6-9, 1/4-inch fat, broiled	3 oz	351	17	0	52	0	30.8	73
prime, ribs 6-9, 1/4-inch fat, raw	1 oz	107	4	0	15	0	9.8	21
prime, ribs 6-9, 1/4-inch fat, roasted	3 oz	342	19	0	54	0	28.8	72
prime, ribs 6-9, 1/2-inch fat, broiled	3 oz	361	17	0	51	0	32.1	74
prime, ribs 6-9, 1/2-inch fat, raw	1 oz	109	4	0	15	0	10.0	21
prime, ribs 6-9, 1/2-inch fat, roasted	3 oz	346	19	0	54	0	29.4	72
select, ribs 6-9, 1/8-inch fat, broiled	3 oz	275	18	0	54	0	21.9	68
select, ribs 6-9, 1/8-inch fat, raw	1 oz	84	5	0	16	0	7.0	20
select, ribs 6-9, 1/8-inch fat, roasted	3 oz	283	20	0	55	0	22.0	71
select, ribs 6-9, 1/4-inch fat, broiled	3 oz	275	18	0	54	0	21.9	68
select, ribs 6-9, 1/4-inch fat, raw	1 oz	86	5	0	16	0	7.4	20
select, ribs 6-9, 1/4-inch fat, roasted	3 oz	289	20	0	55	0	22.7	72
RIB, SHORTRIB								
Trimmed								
choice, braised	3 oz	251	26	0	49	0	15.4	79
choice, raw	1 oz	49	5	0	18	0	2.9	17
Untrimmed								
choice, braised	3 oz	400	18	0	43	0	35.7	80
choice, raw	1 oz	110	4	0	14	0	10.3	22
RIB, SMALL END								
Trimmed								
all grades, ribs 10-12, 0-inch fat, broiled	3 oz	181	24	0	59	0	8.8	68
all grades, ribs 10-12, 1/4-inch fat, broiled	3 oz	188	24	0	59	0	9.5	68
all grades, ribs 10-12, 1/4-inch fat, raw	1 oz	43	6	0	18	0	2.1	17
all grades, ribs 10-12, 1/4-inch fat, roasted	3 oz	185	23	0	60	0	9.8	67
choice, ribs 10-12, 0-inch fat, broiled	3 oz	191	24	0	59	0	9.9	68
choice, ribs 10-12, 1/4-inch fat, broiled	3 oz	198	24	0	59	0	10.7	68
choice, ribs 10-12, 1/4-inch fat, raw	1 oz	46	6	0	18	0	2.4	17
choice, ribs 10-12, 1/4-inch fat, roasted	3 oz	197	23	0	60	0	11.1	67
prime, ribs 10-12, 1/4-inch fat, broiled	3 oz	221	24	0	59	0	13.2	68
prime, ribs 10-12, 1/4-inch fat, raw	1 oz	57	6	0	18	0	3.6	17
prime, ribs 10-12, 1/4-inch fat, roasted	3 oz	258	23	0	64	0	17.9	68
prime, ribs 10-12, 1/2-inch fat, broiled	3 oz	221	24	0	59	0	13.2	68
prime, ribs 10-12, 1/2-inch fat, roasted	3 oz	258	23	0	64	0	17.9	68
select, ribs 10-12, 0-inch fat, broiled	3 oz	168	24	0	59	0	7.4	68
select, ribs 10-12, 1/4-inch fat, broiled	3 oz	176	24	0	59	0	8.2	68
select, ribs 10-12, 1/4-inch fat, raw	1 oz	40	6	0	18	0	1.8	17
select, ribs 10-12, 1/4-inch fat, roasted	3 oz	173	23	0	60	0	8.3	67

Food Name	Serv. Size	Total Cal.	Prot. gms	Carbs gms	Sod. mgs	Fiber gms	Fat gms	Chol. mgs
Untrimmed								
all grades, ribs 10-12, 0-inch fat, broiled	3 oz	252	21	0	54	0	17.9	71
all grades, ribs 10-12, 1/8-inch fat, broiled	3 oz	281	20	0	53	0	21.4	71
all grades, ribs 10-12, 1/8-inch fat, raw	1 oz	82	5	0	15	0	6.9	20
all grades, ribs 10-12, 1/8-inch fat, roasted	3 oz	290	19	0	54	0	23.1	71
all grades, ribs 10-12, 1/4-inch fat, broiled	3 oz	286	20	0	53	0	22.1	71
all grades, ribs 10-12, 1/4-inch fat, raw	1 oz	84	5	0	15	0	7.1	20
all grades, ribs 10-12, 1/4-inch fat, roasted	3 oz	295	19	0	54	0	23.8	71
choice, ribs 10-12, 1/8-inch fat, broiled	3 oz	292	20	0	53	0	22.8	71
choice, ribs 10-12, 1/8-inch fat, raw	1 oz	86	5	0	15	0	7.3	20
choice, ribs 10-12, 1/8-inch fat, roasted	3 oz	305	19	0	54	0	24.8	71
choice, ribs 10-12, 1/4-inch fat, broiled	3 oz	297	20	0	53	0	23.5	71
choice, ribs 10-12, 1/4-inch fat, raw	1 oz	89	5	0	15	0	7.7	20
choice, ribs 10-12, 1/4-inch fat, roasted	3 oz	312	19	0	53	0	25.7	71
prime, ribs 10-12, 1/8-inch fat, broiled	3 oz	301	21	0	54	0	23.7	71
prime, ribs 10-12, 1/8-inch fat, raw	1 oz	95	5	0	15	0	8.3	20
prime, ribs 10-12, 1/8-inch fat, roasted	3 oz	349	19	0	55	0	29.9	71
prime, ribs 10-12, 1/4-inch fat, broiled	3 oz	307	20	0	53	0	24.4	71
prime, ribs 10-12, 1/4-inch fat, raw	1 oz	97	5	0	15	0	8.5	20
prime, ribs 10-12, 1/4-inch fat, roasted	3 oz	354	19	0	55	0	30.5	71
prime, ribs 10-12, 1/2-inch fat, broiled	3 oz	309	20	0	53	0	24.8	71
prime, ribs 10-12, 1/2-inch fat, raw	1 oz	99	5	0	15	0	8.8	20
prime, ribs 10-12, 1/2-inch fat, roasted	3 oz	357	19	0	54	0	30.8	72
select, ribs 10-12, 1/8-inch fat, broiled	3 oz	268	20	0	54	0	20.0	71
select, ribs 10-12, 1/8-inch fat, raw	1 oz	78	5	0	15	0	6.4	20
select, ribs 10-12, 1/8-inch fat, roasted	3 oz	275	19	0	54	0	21.3	71
select, ribs 10-12, 1/4-inch fat, broiled	3 oz	273	20	0	53	0	20.6	71
select, ribs 10-12, 1/4-inch fat, raw	1 oz	81	5	0	15	0	6.7	20
select, ribs 10-12, 1/4-inch fat, roasted	3 oz	281	19	0	54	0	22.2	71
RIB, WHOLE								
Trimmed								
all grades, ribs 6-12, 1/4-inch fat, broiled	3 oz	190	22	0	60	0	10.4	65
all grades, ribs 6-12, 1/4-inch fat, raw	1 oz	45	6	0	18	0	2.4	17
all grades, ribs 6-12, 1/4-inch fat, roasted	3 oz	195	23	0	61	0	10.6	68
choice, ribs 6-12, 1/4-inch fat, broiled	3 oz	201	22	0	60	0	11.7	65
choice, ribs 6-12, 1/4-inch fat, raw	1 oz	48	6	0	18	0	2.7	17
choice, ribs 6-12, 1/4-inch fat, roasted	3 oz	207	23	0	61	0	11.9	68
prime, ribs 6-12, 1/4-inch fat, broiled	3 oz	238	22	0	60	0	15.9	69
prime, ribs 6-12, 1/4-inch fat, raw	1 oz	58	6	0	18	0	3.8	17
prime, ribs 6-12, 1/4-inch fat, roasted	3 oz	248	23	0	63	0	16.5	69
prime, ribs 6-12, 1/2-inch fat, broiled	3 oz	238	22	0	59	0	15.9	70
prime, ribs 6-12, 1/2-inch fat, roasted	3 oz	248	23	0	63	0	16.5	69
select, ribs 6-12, 1/4-inch fat, broiled	3 oz	175	22	0	60	0	8.9	65
select, ribs 6-12, 1/4-inch fat, raw	1 oz	42	6	0	18	0	2.0	17
select, ribs 6-12, 1/4-inch fat, roasted	3 oz	181	23	0	61	0	9.1	68
Untrimmed								
all grades, ribs 6-12, 1/8-inch fat, broiled	3 oz	286	19	0	54	0	22.7	70
all grades, ribs 6-12, 1/8-inch fat, raw	1 oz	87	5	0	16	0	7.4	20
all grades, ribs 6-12, 1/8-inch fat, roasted	3 oz	298	19	0	54	0	23.9	71
all grades, ribs 6-12, 1/4-inch fat, broiled	3 oz	291	19	0	54	0	23.3	70
all grades, ribs 6-12, 1/4-inch fat, raw	1 oz	89	5	0	15	0	7.6	20
all grades, ribs 6-12, 1/4-inch fat, roasted	3 oz	304	19	0	54	0	24.7	71
choice, ribs 6-12, 1/8-inch fat, broiled	3 oz	299	19	0	54	0	24.2	70
choice, ribs 6-12, 1/8-inch fat, raw	1 oz	91	5	0	15	0	7.9	20
choice, ribs 6-12, 1/8-inch fat, roasted	3 oz	310	19	0	54	0	25.3	71
choice, ribs 6-12, 1/4-inch fat, broiled	3 oz	306	19	0	53	0	25.1	70
choice, ribs 6-12, 1/4-inch fat, raw	1 oz	94	5	0	15	0	8.3	20
choice, ribs 6-12, 1/4-inch fat, roasted	3 oz	320	19	0	54	0	26.5	72

Food Name	Serv. Size	Total Cal.	Prot. gms	Carbs gms	Sod. mgs	Fiber gms	Fat gms	Chol. mgs
prime, ribs 6-12, 1/8-inch fat, broiled	3 oz	328	19	0	53	0	27.5	72
prime, ribs 6-12, 1/8-inch fat, raw	1 oz	101	5	0	15	0	9.0	20
prime, ribs 6-12, 1/8-inch fat, roasted	3 oz	340	19	0	55	0	28.6	72
prime, ribs 6-12, 1/4-inch fat, broiled	3 oz	333	18	0	53	0	28.2	72
prime, ribs 6-12, 1/4-inch fat, raw	1 oz	103	5	0	15	0	9.3	21
prime, ribs 6-12, 1/4-inch fat, roasted	3 oz	348	19	0	54	0	29.6	72
prime, ribs 6-12, 1/2-inch fat, broiled	3 oz	347	18	0	51	0	29.9	73
prime, ribs 6-12, 1/2-inch fat, raw	1 oz	105	4	0	15	0	9.5	21
prime, ribs 6-12, 1/2-inch fat, roasted	3 oz	361	18	0	54	0	31.4	73
select, ribs 6-12, 1/8-inch fat, broiled	3 oz	268	19	0	54	0	20.6	69
select, ribs 6-12, 1/8-inch fat, raw	1 oz	82	5	0	16	0	6.8	20
select, ribs 6-12, 1/8-inch fat, roasted	3 oz	281	20	0	55	0	21.8	71
select, ribs 6-12, 1/4-inch fat, broiled	3 oz	275	19	0	54	0	21.4	70
select, ribs 6-12, 1/4-inch fat, raw	1 oz	84	5	0	16	0	7.1	20
select, ribs 6-12, 1/4-inch fat, roasted	3 oz	286	19	0	54	0	22.5	71
RIB EYE, SMALL END								
Trimmed								
choice, ribs 10-12, 0-inch fat, broiled	3 oz	191	24	0	59	0	9.9	68
choice, ribs 10-12, 0-inch fat, raw	1 oz	46	6	0	18	0	2.4	17
lean cuts, raw *(Lean and Free)*	4 oz	121	25	0	59	0	2.6	71
Untrimmed								
choice, ribs 10-12, 0-inch fat, broiled	3 oz	261	21	0	54	0	18.9	71
choice, ribs 10-12, 0-inch fat, raw	1 oz	78	5	0	16	0	6.3	19
choice, ribs 10-12, 1/8-inch fat, broiled	3 oz	255	21	0	54	0	18.1	70
choice, ribs 10-12, 1/8-inch fat, raw	1 oz	74	5	0	16	0	5.8	19
ROLLED, lean cuts, raw *(Lean and Free)*	4 oz	125	25	0	60	0	2.8	0
ROUND, BOTTOM								
Trimmed								
all grades, 0-inch fat, braised	3 oz	173	27	0	43	0	6.5	82
all grades, 0-inch fat, roasted	3 oz	156	24	0	56	0	5.7	66
all grades, 1/4-inch fat, braised	3 oz	178	27	0	43	0	7.0	82
all grades, 1/4-inch fat, raw	1 oz	41	6	0	17	0	1.6	17
all grades, 1/4-inch fat, roasted	3 oz	161	24	0	56	0	6.3	66
choice, 0-inch fat, braised	3 oz	181	27	0	43	0	7.4	82
choice, 0-inch fat, roasted	3 oz	164	24	0	56	0	6.6	66
choice, 1/4-inch fat, braised	3 oz	187	27	0	43	0	8.0	82
choice, 1/4-inch fat, raw	1 oz	43	6	0	17	0	1.8	17
choice, 1/4-inch fat, roasted	3 oz	168	24	0	56	0	7.0	66
prime, 1/2-inch fat, broiled	3 oz	212	27	0	43	0	10.8	82
prime, 1/2-inch fat, raw	1 oz	45	6	0	17	0	2.1	17
select, 0-inch fat, braised	3 oz	163	27	0	43	0	5.4	82
select, 0-inch fat, roasted	3 oz	145	24	0	56	0	4.6	66
select, 1/4-inch fat, braised	3 oz	167	27	0	43	0	5.8	82
select, 1/4-inch fat, raw	1 oz	39	6	0	17	0	1.3	17
select, 1/4-inch fat, roasted	3 oz	152	24	0	56	0	5.3	66
Untrimmed								
all grades, 0-inch fat, braised	3 oz	181	26	0	43	0	7.5	82
all grades, 0-inch fat, roasted	3 oz	160	24	0	56	0	6.2	66
all grades, 1/8-inch fat, braised	3 oz	218	25	0	43	0	12.2	82
all grades, 1/8-inch fat, raw	1 oz	54	6	0	16	0	3.2	18
all grades, 1/8-inch fat, roasted	3 oz	195	23	0	54	0	10.6	67
all grades, 1/4-inch fat, braised	3 oz	234	24	0	43	0	14.4	82
all grades, 1/4-inch fat, raw	1 oz	59	6	0	16	0	3.8	18
all grades, 1/4-inch fat, roasted	3 oz	211	23	0	54	0	12.7	68
choice, 0-inch fat, braised	3 oz	193	26	0	43	0	9.0	82
choice, 0-inch fat, roasted	3 oz	173	24	0	55	0	7.7	66
choice, 1/8-inch fat, braised	3 oz	228	25	0	43	0	13.5	82

Food Name	Serv. Size	Total Cal.	Prot. gms	Carbs gms	Sod. mgs	Fiber gms	Fat gms	Chol. mgs
choice, 1/8-inch fat, raw	1 oz	57	6	0	16	0	3.5	18
choice, 1/8-inch fat, roasted	3 oz	205	23	0	54	0	11.8	67
choice, 1/4-inch fat, braised	3 oz	241	24	0	43	0	15.2	82
choice, 1/4-inch fat, raw	1 oz	62	6	0	16	0	4.2	18
choice, 1/4-inch fat, roasted	3 oz	221	22	0	54	0	13.9	68
prime, 1/2-inch fat, braised	3 oz	252	25	0	43	0	16.2	82
prime, 1/2-inch fat, raw	1 oz	64	6	0	16	0	4.4	18
select, 0-inch fat, braised	3 oz	171	26	0	43	0	6.4	82
select, 0-inch fat, roasted	3 oz	150	24	0	56	0	5.1	66
select, 1/8-inch fat, braised	3 oz	208	25	0	43	0	11.2	82
select, 1/8-inch fat, raw	1 oz	51	6	0	16	0	2.9	18
select, 1/8-inch fat, roasted	3 oz	186	23	0	54	0	9.6	67
select, 1/4-inch fat, braised	3 oz	220	25	0	43	0	12.8	82
select, 1/4-inch fat, raw	1 oz	55	6	0	16	0	3.4	18
select, 1/4-inch fat, roasted	3 oz	199	23	0	54	0	11.3	68
ROUND, EYE OF								
Trimmed								
all grades, 0-inch fat, roasted	3 oz	141	25	0	53	0	4.0	59
all grades, 1/4-inch fat, raw	1 oz	37	6	0	15	0	1.2	15
all grades, 1/4-inch fat, roasted	3 oz	143	25	0	53	0	4.2	59
choice, 0-inch fat, roasted	3 oz	149	25	0	53	0	4.8	59
choice, 1/4-inch fat, raw	1 oz	39	6	0	15	0	1.4	15
choice, 1/4-inch fat, roasted	3 oz	149	25	0	53	0	4.8	59
prime, 1/2-inch fat, raw	1 oz	42	6	0	15	0	1.8	15
prime, 1/2-inch fat, roasted	3 oz	168	25	0	53	0	7.0	59
select, 0-inch fat, roasted	3 oz	132	25	0	53	0	3.0	59
select, 1/4-inch fat, raw	1 oz	35	6	0	15	0	1.0	15
select, 1/4-inch fat, roasted	3 oz	136	25	0	53	0	3.4	59
Untrimmed								
all grades, 0-inch fat, roasted	3 oz	145	24	0	53	0	4.6	59
all grades, 1/8-inch fat, raw	1 oz	47	6	0	14	0	2.4	16
all grades, 1/8-inch fat, roasted	3 oz	165	24	0	52	0	6.9	60
all grades, 1/4-inch fat, raw	1 oz	60	6	0	14	0	4.1	17
all grades, 1/4-inch fat, roasted	3 oz	195	23	0	50	0	10.8	61
choice, 0-inch fat, roasted	3 oz	153	24	0	53	0	5.4	59
choice, 1/8-inch fat, raw	1 oz	49	6	0	14	0	2.6	16
choice, 1/8-inch fat, roasted	3 oz	170	24	0	52	0	7.6	60
choice, 1/4-inch fat, raw	1 oz	62	6	0	14	0	4.2	17
choice, 1/4-inch fat, roasted	3 oz	205	23	0	50	0	12.0	61
select, 1/8-inch fat, raw	1 oz	45	6	0	15	0	2.2	16
select, 1/8-inch fat, roasted	3 oz	158	24	0	52	0	6.2	60
select, 1/4-inch fat, raw	1 oz	57	6	0	14	0	3.7	17
select, 1/4-inch fat, roasted	3 oz	184	23	0	51	0	9.6	61
prime, 1/2-inch fat, raw	1 oz	63	6	0	14	0	4.3	17
prime, 1/2-inch fat, roasted	3 oz	213	23	0	50	0	12.7	61
ROUND, FULL CUT								
Trimmed								
choice, 1/4-inch fat, broiled	3 oz	162	25	0	54	0	6.2	66
choice, 1/4-inch fat, raw	1 oz	39	6	0	16	0	1.4	16
select, 1/4-inch fat, broiled	3 oz	146	25	0	54	0	4.4	66
select, 1/4-inch fat, raw	1 oz	36	6	0	16	0	1.0	16
Untrimmed								
choice, 1/8-inch fat, broiled	3 oz	200	23	0	53	0	11.0	67
choice, 1/8-inch fat, raw	1 oz	55	6	0	15	0	3.4	18
choice, 1/4-inch fat, broiled	3 oz	204	23	0	52	0	11.6	68
choice, 1/4-inch fat, raw	1 oz	58	6	0	15	0	3.6	18
select, 1/8-inch fat, broiled	3 oz	185	23	0	53	0	9.4	67

Food Name	Serv. Size	Total Cal.	Prot. gms	Carbs gms	Sod. mgs	Fiber gms	Fat gms	Chol. mgs
select, 1/8-inch fat, raw	1 oz	52	6	0	15	0	3.0	18
select, 1/4-inch fat, broiled	3 oz	190	23	0	53	0	10.0	47
select, 1/4-inch fat, raw	1 oz	54	6	0	15	0	3.3	18
ROUND, TOP								
Trimmed								
all grades, 0-inch fat, braised	3 oz	169	31	0	38	0	4.3	77
all grades, 1/4-inch fat, braised	3 oz	174	31	0	38	0	4.8	77
all grades, 1/4-inch fat, broiled	3 oz	153	27	0	52	0	4.2	71
all grades, 1/4-inch fat, raw	1 oz	36	6	0	15	0	0.9	16
choice, 0-inch fat, braised	3 oz	176	31	0	38	0	4.9	77
choice, 1/4-inch fat, braised	3 oz	181	31	0	38	0	5.5	77
choice, 1/4-inch fat, broiled	3 oz	161	27	0	52	0	5.0	71
choice, 1/4-inch fat, pan-fried	3 oz	193	30	0	60	0	7.3	82
choice, 1/4-inch fat, raw	1 oz	37	6	0	15	0	1.1	16
prime, 1/2-inch fat, broiled	3 oz	183	27	0	52	0	7.5	71
prime, 1/4-inch fat, broiled	3 oz	183	27	0	52	0	7.5	71
prime, 1/4-inch fat, raw	1 oz	43	6	0	15	0	1.8	16
lean cuts, raw *(Lean Limousin)*	4 oz	134	25	0	49	0	4.5	0
select, 0-inch fat, braised	3 oz	162	31	0	38	0	3.4	77
select, 1/4-inch fat, braised	3 oz	167	31	0	38	0	3.9	77
select, 1/4-inch fat, broiled	3 oz	144	27	0	52	0	3.1	71
select, 1/4-inch fat, raw	1 oz	34	6	0	15	0	0.7	16
Untrimmed								
all grades, 0-inch fat, braised	3 oz	178	30	0	38	0	5.4	77
all grades, 1/8-inch fat, braised	3 oz	202	29	0	38	0	8.6	77
all grades, 1/8-inch fat, broiled	3 oz	176	26	0	51	0	7.2	72
all grades, 1/8-inch fat, raw	1 oz	46	6	0	14	0	2.2	17
all grades, 1/4-inch fat, braised	3 oz	211	29	0	38	0	9.7	77
all grades, 1/4-inch fat, broiled	3 oz	184	26	0	51	0	8.2	72
all grades, 1/4-inch fat, raw	1 oz	50	6	0	14	0	2.7	17
choice, 0-inch fat, braised	3 oz	184	30	0	38	0	6.0	77
choice, 1/8-inch fat, braised	3 oz	213	29	0	38	0	9.9	77
choice, 1/8-inch fat, broiled	3 oz	184	26	0	51	0	8.0	72
choice, 1/8-inch fat, pan-fried	3 oz	226	28	0	58	0	11.8	82
choice, 1/8-inch fat, raw	1 oz	48	6	0	14	0	2.4	17
choice, 1/4-inch fat, braised	3 oz	221	29	0	38	0	10.9	77
choice, 1/4-inch fat, broiled	3 oz	190	26	0	51	0	9.0	72
choice, 1/4-inch fat, pan-fried	3 oz	235	28	0	58	0	13.1	82
choice, 1/4-inch fat, raw	1 oz	51	6	0	14	0	2.8	17
prime, 1/2-inch fat, broiled	3 oz	201	26	0	51	0	9.9	72
prime, 1/2-inch fat, raw	1 oz	53	6	0	14	0	3.0	17
prime, 1/8-inch fat, broiled	3 oz	191	27	0	52	0	8.6	71
prime, 1/8-inch fat, raw	1 oz	49	6	0	14	0	2.5	17
prime, 1/4-inch fat, broiled	3 oz	195	26	0	51	0	9.1	71
prime, 1/4-inch fat, raw	1 oz	51	6	0	14	0	2.7	17
select, 0-inch fat, braised	3 oz	170	30	0	38	0	4.5	77
select, 1/8-inch fat, braised	3 oz	191	29	0	38	0	7.3	77
select, 1/8-inch fat, broiled	3 oz	167	26	0	51	0	6.2	72
select, 1/8-inch fat, raw	1 oz	44	6	0	14	0	2.0	17
select, 1/4-inch fat, braised	3 oz	199	29	0	38	0	8.4	77
select, 1/4-inch fat, broiled	3 oz	175	26	0	51	0	7.2	72
select, 1/4-inch fat, raw	1 oz	46	6	0	14	0	2.3	17
ROUND TIP								
Trimmed								
all grades, 0-inch fat, roasted	3 oz	150	24	0	55	0	5.0	69
all grades, 1/4-inch fat, raw	1 oz	35	6	0	18	0	1.1	17
all grades, 1/4-inch fat, roasted	3 oz	157	24	0	55	0	5.9	69

Food Name	Serv. Size	Total Cal.	Prot. gms	Carbs gms	Sod. mgs	Fiber gms	Fat gms	Chol. mgs
choice, 0-inch fat, roasted	3 oz	153	24	0	55	0	5.4	69
choice, 1/4-inch fat, raw	1 oz	37	6	0	18	0	1.2	17
choice, 1/4-inch fat, roasted	3 oz	160	24	0	55	0	6.2	69
prime, 1/4-inch fat, raw	1 oz	41	6	0	18	0	1.7	17
prime, 1/2-inch fat, roasted	3 oz	181	24	0	55	0	8.6	69
prime, 1/4-inch fat, roasted	3 oz	181	24	0	55	0	8.6	69
select, 0-inch fat, roasted	3 oz	145	24	0	55	0	4.5	69
select, 1/4-inch fat, raw	1 oz	34	6	0	18	0	0.9	17
select, 1/4-inch fat, roasted	3 oz	153	24	0	55	0	5.4	69
Untrimmed								
all grades, 0-inch fat, roasted	3 oz	162	24	0	54	0	6.7	69
all grades, 1/8-inch fat, raw	1 oz	54	6	0	16	0	3.3	18
all grades, 1/8-inch fat, roasted	3 oz	186	23	0	54	0	9.6	70
all grades, 1/4-inch fat, raw	1 oz	57	5	0	16	0	3.7	18
all grades, 1/4-inch fat, roasted	3 oz	199	23	0	54	0	11.3	70
choice, 0-inch fat, roasted	3 oz	170	24	0	54	0	7.6	70
choice, 1/8-inch fat, raw	1 oz	56	6	0	16	0	3.6	18
choice, 1/8-inch fat, roasted	3 oz	194	23	0	54	0	10.5	70
choice, 1/4-inch fat, raw	1 oz	60	5	0	16	0	4.1	19
choice, 1/4-inch fat, roasted	3 oz	210	23	0	53	0	12.6	71
prime, 1/4-inch fat, raw	1 oz	61	6	0	16	0	4.1	18
prime, 1/4-inch fat, roasted	3 oz	233	22	0	53	0	15.2	71
prime, 1/2-inch fat, raw	1 oz	63	5	0	16	0	4.6	19
prime, 1/2-inch fat, roasted	3 oz	241	22	0	52	0	16.3	71
select, 1/8-inch fat, raw	1 oz	50	6	0	16	0	2.9	18
select, 1/8-inch fat, roasted	3 oz	179	23	0	54	0	8.7	70
select, 1/4-inch fat, raw	1 oz	53	6	0	16	0	3.2	18
select, 1/4-inch fat, roasted	3 oz	191	23	0	54	0	10.3	70
ROUND STEAK, lean cuts, raw *(Lean and Free)*	4 oz	111	26	0	60	0	1.1	0
SHANK CROSSCUTS								
Trimmed								
choice, 1/4-inch fat, raw	1 oz	36	6	0	18	0	1.1	11
choice, 1/4-inch fat, simmered	3 oz	171	29	0	54	0	5.4	66
Untrimmed								
choice, 1/4-inch fat, raw	3 oz	150	17	0	51	0	8.4	37
choice, 1/4-inch fat, simmered	3 oz	224	26	0	52	0	12.5	68
SIRLOIN, TOP								
Trimmed								
all grades, 0-inch fat, broiled	3 oz	162	26	0	56	0	5.8	76
all grades, 1/4-inch fat, broiled	3 oz	166	26	0	56	0	6.1	76
all grades, 1/4-inch fat, raw	1 oz	37	6	0	16	0	1.2	17
choice, 0-inch fat, broiled	3 oz	170	26	0	56	0	6.6	76
choice, 1/4-inch fat, broiled	3 oz	172	26	0	56	0	6.8	76
choice, 1/4-inch fat, pan-fried	3 oz	202	28	0	65	0	9.3	84
choice, 1/4-inch fat, raw	1 oz	39	6	0	16	0	1.4	17
select, 0-inch fat, broiled	3 oz	153	26	0	56	0	4.8	76
select, 1/4-inch fat, broiled	3 oz	158	26	0	56	0	5.3	76
select, 1/4-inch fat, raw	1 oz	35	6	0	16	0	1.0	17
Untrimmed								
all grades, 0-inch fat, broiled	3 oz	183	25	0	55	0	8.5	76
all grades, 1/8-inch fat, broiled	3 oz	211	24	0	54	0	12.0	77
all grades, 1/8-inch fat, raw	1 oz	58	6	0	15	0	3.8	19
all grades, 1/4-inch fat, broiled	3 oz	219	24	0	54	0	13.1	77
all grades, 1/4-inch fat, raw	1 oz	62	5	0	15	0	4.3	19
choice, 0-inch fat, broiled	3 oz	195	25	0	54	0	9.8	76
choice, 1/8-inch fat, broiled	3 oz	220	24	0	54	0	13.2	77
choice, 1/8-inch fat, pan-fried	3 oz	266	24	0	60	0	17.9	83

Food Name	Serv. Size	Total Cal.	Prot. gms	Carbs gms	Sod. mgs	Fiber gms	Fat gms	Chol. mgs
choice, 1/8-inch fat, raw	1 oz	60	5	0	15	0	4.1	19
choice, 1/4-inch fat, broiled	3 oz	229	23	0	53	0	14.2	77
choice, 1/4-inch fat, pan-fried	3 oz	277	24	0	60	0	19.4	83
choice, 1/4-inch fat, raw	1 oz	64	5	0	15	0	4.6	19
select, 0-inch fat, broiled	3 oz	166	25	0	55	0	6.4	76
select, 1/8-inch fat, broiled	3 oz	204	24	0	54	0	11.3	77
select, 1/8-inch fat, raw	1 oz	55	6	0	15	0	3.5	19
select, 1/4-inch fat, broiled	3 oz	208	24	0	54	0	11.8	77
select, 1/4-inch fat, raw	1 oz	59	5	0	15	0	3.9	19
SIRLOIN STEAK, lean cuts, raw *(Lean and Free)*	4 oz	111	24	0	67	0	1.8	66
SIRLOIN TIP, lean cuts, raw *(Lean and Free)*	4 oz	110	23	0	62	0	1.2	66
SPLEEN								
braised	3 oz	123	21	0	48	0	3.6	295
raw	4 oz	119	21	0	96	0	3.4	297
STRIP LOIN STEAK, lean cuts, raw *(Lean and Free)*	4 oz	113	25	0	61	0	1.8	67
T-BONE								
Trimmed								
all grades, 0-inch fat, broiled	3 oz	163	22	0	60	0	7.6	44
all grades, 1/4-inch fat, broiled	3 oz	173	23	0	60	0	8.3	48
all grades, 1/4-inch fat, raw	1 oz	42	6	0	16	0	1.8	14
choice, 0-inch fat, broiled	3 oz	168	22	0	60	0	8.2	44
choice, 1/4-inch fat, broiled	3 oz	174	23	0	60	0	8.5	50
choice, 1/4-inch fat, raw	1 oz	44	6	0	16	0	2.1	16
lean cuts, raw *(Lean and Free)*	4 oz	125	26	0	54	0	2.7	0
select, 0-inch fat, broiled	3 oz	150	22	0	60	0	6.3	46
select, 1/4-inch fat, broiled	3 oz	168	23	0	60	0	7.6	43
select, 1/4-inch fat, raw	1 oz	37	6	0	16	0	1.3	11
Untrimmed								
all grades, 0-inch fat, broiled	3 oz	210	21	0	57	0	13.5	48
all grades, 1/8-inch fat, broiled	3 oz	238	21	0	56	0	16.5	53
all grades, 1/8-inch fat, raw	1 oz	62	5	0	15	0	4.3	16
all grades, 1/4-inch fat, broiled	3 oz	256	20	0	55	0	18.8	54
all grades, 1/4-inch fat, raw	1 oz	64	5	0	15	0	4.5	16
choice, 0-inch fat, broiled	3 oz	217	21	0	57	0	14.4	48
choice, 1/8-inch fat, broiled	3 oz	243	20	0	56	0	17.3	55
choice, 1/8-inch fat, raw	1 oz	66	5	0	15	0	4.8	18
choice, 1/4-inch fat, broiled	3 oz	263	20	0	54	0	19.8	57
choice, 1/4-inch fat, raw	1 oz	67	5	0	15	0	4.9	18
select, 0-inch fat, broiled	3 oz	194	21	0	58	0	11.6	49
select, 1/8-inch fat, broiled	3 oz	225	21	0	56	0	14.9	48
select, 1/8-inch fat, raw	1 oz	54	6	0	16	0	3.4	13
select, 1/4-inch fat, broiled	3 oz	238	21	0	56	0	16.5	49
select, 1/4-inch fat, raw	1 oz	56	6	0	15	0	3.5	13
TENDERLOIN								
Trimmed								
all grades, 0-inch fat, broiled	3 oz	175	24	0	54	0	8.1	71
all grades, 1/4-inch fat, broiled	3 oz	179	24	0	54	0	8.5	71
all grades, 1/4-inch fat, raw	1 oz	45	6	0	15	0	2.2	18
all grades, 1/4-inch fat, roasted	3 oz	189	24	0	52	0	9.8	71
choice, 0-inch fat, broiled	3 oz	180	24	0	54	0	8.6	71
choice, 1/4-inch fat, broiled	3 oz	189	24	0	54	0	9.5	71
choice, 1/4-inch fat, raw	1 oz	47	6	0	15	0	2.4	18
choice, 1/4-inch fat, roasted	3 oz	196	24	0	61	0	10.6	71
fillet steak, lean cuts, raw *(Lean and Free)*	4 oz	116	24	0	68	0	2.4	61
prime, 1/4-inch fat, broiled	3 oz	197	24	0	54	0	10.5	71
prime, 1/4-inch fat, raw	1 oz	48	6	0	15	0	2.5	18
prime, 1/4-inch fat, roasted	3 oz	217	23	0	50	0	13.0	73

Food Name	Serv. Size	Total Cal.	Prot. gms	Carbs gms	Sod. mgs	Fiber gms	Fat gms	Chol. mgs
prime, short loin, 1/2-inch fat, broiled	3 oz	197	24	0	54	0	10.5	71
prime, short loin, 1/2-inch fat, roasted	3 oz	217	23	0	50	0	13.0	73
select, 0-inch fat, broiled	3 oz	170	24	0	54	0	7.5	71
select, 1/4-inch fat, broiled	3 oz	169	24	0	54	0	7.4	71
select, 1/4-inch fat, raw	1 oz	43	6	0	15	0	2.0	18
select, 1/4-inch fat, roasted	3 oz	179	24	0	52	0	8.8	71
Untrimmed								
all grades, 0-inch fat, broiled	3 oz	200	23	0	53	0	11.2	72
all grades, 1/8-inch fat, broiled	3 oz	239	22	0	51	0	16.2	73
all grades, 1/8-inch fat, raw	1 oz	77	5	0	14	0	6.2	20
all grades, 1/8-inch fat, roasted	3 oz	275	20	0	48	0	20.9	72
all grades, 1/4-inch fat, broiled	3 oz	247	21	0	50	0	17.2	73
all grades, 1/4-inch fat, raw	1 oz	80	5	0	14	0	6.5	20
all grades, 1/4-inch fat, roasted	3 oz	282	20	0	48	0	21.8	73
choice, 0-inch fat, broiled	3 oz	207	23	0	52	0	12.2	72
choice, 1/8-inch fat	3 oz	251	22	0	50	0	17.6	73
choice, 1/8-inch fat, raw	1 oz	79	5	0	14	0	6.3	20
choice, 1/8-inch fat, roasted	3 oz	281	20	0	55	0	21.6	72
choice, 1/4-inch fat, broiled	3 oz	258	21	0	50	0	18.6	73
choice, 1/4-inch fat, raw	1 oz	82	5	0	14	0	6.7	20
choice, 1/4-inch fat, roasted	3 oz	288	20	0	55	0	22.4	73
prime, 1/8-inch fat, broiled	3 oz	262	21	0	50	0	18.9	73
prime, 1/8-inch fat, raw	1 oz	78	5	0	14	0	6.2	20
prime, 1/8-inch fat, roasted	3 oz	292	20	0	47	0	22.7	75
prime, 1/4-inch fat, broiled	3 oz	269	21	0	50	0	19.9	73
prime, 1/4-inch fat, raw	1 oz	81	5	0	14	0	6.5	20
prime, 1/4-inch fat, roasted	3 oz	300	20	0	47	0	23.7	75
prime, short loin, 1/2-inch fat, broiled	3 oz	270	21	0	50	0	19.9	73
prime, short loin, 1/2-inch fat, roasted	3 oz	304	20	0	47	0	24.4	75
select, 0-inch fat, broiled	3 oz	195	23	0	53	0	10.6	72
select, 1/8-inch fat, broiled	3 oz	226	22	0	51	0	14.7	73
select, 1/8-inch fat, raw	1 oz	76	5	0	14	0	6.0	20
select, 1/8-inch fat, roasted	3 oz	269	20	0	48	0	20.1	72
select, 1/4-inch fat, broiled	3 oz	230	22	0	51	0	15.2	73
select, 1/4-inch fat, raw	1 oz	79	5	0	14	0	6.4	20
select, 1/4-inch fat, roasted	3 oz	275	20	0	48	0	21.0	73
THYMUS								
braised	3 oz	271	19	0	99	0	21.2	250
raw	4 oz	267	14	0	108	0	23.0	252
TONGUE								
raw	4 oz	253	17	4	78	0	18.2	98
raw	1 oz	64	4	1	20	0	4.6	25
simmered	3 oz	241	19	0	51	0	17.6	91
TRIPE								
canned *(Armour)*	6 oz	180	33	1	230	0	4.0	0
raw	4 oz	111	16	0	52	0	4.5	107
raw	1 oz	28	4	0	13	0	1.1	27
BEEF, CORNED. See also under HASH.								
Canned								
cured	1 oz	71	8	0	285	0	4.2	24
cured, sliced, 0.75-oz slices	1 slice	53	6	0	211	0	3.1	18
(Dinty Moore)	2 oz	130	15	0	0	0	8.0	0
Fresh								
brisket, cured, cooked	3 oz	213	15	0	964	0	16.1	83
brisket, cured, raw	1 oz	56	4	0	35	0	4.2	15
(Eckrich) 'Slender Sliced'	1 oz	40	6	1	270	0	1.0	0
(Healthy Deli)	1 oz	35	6	1	210	0	1.0	11

Food Name	Serv. Size	Total Cal.	Prot. gms	Carbs gms	Sod. mgs	Fiber gms	Fat gms	Chol. mgs
(Healthy Deli) 'St. Paddy's'	1 oz	24	4	1	290	0	0.4	7
(Hillshire Farm)	1 oz	31	6	1	230	0	0.4	0
(Oscar Mayer)	0.6 oz	17	3	0	204	0	0.3	8
BEEF, CORNED, SPREAD, canned *(Hormel)*	0.5 oz	35	2	0	0	0	3.0	0
BEEF, DRIED, SLICED								
(Armour)	1.1 oz	60	8	2	0	0	2.0	0
ground and formed, extra lean *(Hormel)*	10 slices	50	8	1	1240	0	1.5	25

BEEF DINNER/ENTRÉE. See also BEEF, CORNED; BURRITO; CHILI; CHIMICHANGA; HAMBURGER ENTRÉE MIX; MEAT LOAF DINNER/ENTRÉE; RAVIOLI DISH/ENTRÉE; SANDWICH.

Food Name	Serv. Size	Total Cal.	Prot. gms	Carbs gms	Sod. mgs	Fiber gms	Fat gms	Chol. mgs
(Armour)								
pepper steak, frozen, 'Classics Lite'	11.25 oz	220	17	29	970	0	4.0	35
pot roast, Yankee, frozen, 'Classics'	10 oz	310	25	26	670	0	12.0	85
Salisbury steak, frozen, 'Classics'	11.25 oz	350	22	26	1430	0	17.0	55
Salisbury steak, frozen, 'Classics Lite'	11.5 oz	300	21	29	1020	0	2.0	35
Salisbury steak, Parmigiana frozen, 'Classics'	11.5 oz	410	22	32	1120	0	21.0	60
sirloin, roast, frozen, 'Classics'	10.45 oz	190	19	21	970	0	4.0	55
sirloin tips, frozen, 'Classics'	10.25 oz	230	22	20	820	0	7.0	70
stew, canned	8 oz	210	11	16	1200	0	11.0	0
stew, microwave	7.5 oz	150	10	15	870	0	5.0	0
Stroganoff, 'Classics Lite'	11.25 oz	250	18	33	510	0	6.0	55
(Banquet)								
barbecue beef, homestyle 'Healthy Balance'	10.25 oz	270	14	43	680	0	5.0	25
barbecue beef, sliced, w/sauce, 'Cookin' Bags'	4 oz	100	9	11	0	0	2.0	0
beef enchilada and tamale entrée	1 entrée	400	10	56	1530	9	15.0	30
beef entrée, frozen, 'Extra Helping'	16 oz	870	34	50	810	0	61.0	120
beef entrée, frozen, 'Platters'	10 oz	460	22	20	630	0	34.0	75
beef pie, frozen	7 oz	510	12	39	870	0	33.0	25
beef pie, frozen, 'Supreme Microwave'	7 oz	440	14	30	730	0	29.0	35
beef w/gravy, potatoes, peas in sauce	1 pkg	270	26	19	742	4	10.0	71
chicken-fried steak	1 entrée	420	15	39	1200	4	23.0	35
chopped beef entrée, frozen	11 oz	420	21	14	600	0	32.0	80
creamed, chipped beef, frozen, 'Cook in' Bags'	4 oz	100	7	9	0	0	4.0	0
meat loaf entrée (Banquet)	1 entrée	280	12	23	1020	3	16.0	60
patty, charbroiled, w/mushroom and onion gravy, frozen	8 oz	300	12	14	0	0	21.0	0
patty, charbroiled, w/mushroom gravy, frozen	8 oz	290	13	13	0	0	21.0	0
patty, w/country-style vegetables	1 entrée	310	11	22	1090	3	20.0	40
patty, Western style	1 entrée	380	14	28	1400	5	23.0	40
pot roast 'Yankee'	1 entrée	231	14	20	1134	4	10.0	60
Salisbury steak, frozen	1 entrée	380	12	28	1140	4	24.0	60
Salisbury steak, frozen	11 oz	500	23	26	600	0	34.0	80
Salisbury steak, frozen, 'Extra Helping'	18 oz	910	50	49	740	0	60.0	175
Salisbury steak, w/gravy, frozen, 'Cookin' Bags'	5 oz	190	9	8	0	0	14.0	0
Salisbury steak, w/gravy, frozen, 'Family Entrées'	8 oz	300	13	12	0	0	22.0	0
Salisbury steak, w/gravy, potatoes, corn in sauce	1 pkg	398	15	28	na	3	25.0	51
Salisbury steak, w/gravy, potatoes, corn in sauce, 'Extra Helping'	1 pkg	782	27	47	2195	7	54.1	131
Salisbury steak, w/mushroom gravy, frozen, 'Extra Helping'	18 oz	890	51	48	685	0	58.0	169
Salisbury steak, charbroiled, frozen, 'Healthy Balance'	10.5 oz	270	14	34	800	0	8.0	35
sliced beef entrée	1 entrée	270	26	19	740	4	10.0	70
sliced beef, w/gravy, frozen, 'Cookin' Bags'	4 oz	100	8	5	0	0	5.0	0
stew, frozen, 'Family Entrées'	7 oz	140	6	18	0	0	5.0	0
Stroganoff, homestyle, 'Healthy Balance'	11.3 oz	360	13	49	710	0	12.0	30
Stroganoff sauce, w/noodles, 'Family Entrées'	7 oz	190	17	18	0	0	6.0	0
(Budget Gourmet)								
beef Stroganoff	1 entrée	250	16	30	580	4	7.0	35
beef Stroganoff, 'Light'	1 entrée	290	20	32	580	3	7.0	35

Food Name	Serv. Size	Total Cal.	Prot. gms	Carbs gms	Sod. mgs	Fiber gms	Fat gms	Chol. mgs
beef Stroganoff, frozen, 'Special Selections'	1 entrée	260	18	28	500	3	8.0	35
meatballs w/gravy, 'Light & Healthy'	1 dinner	310	22	37	540	5	8.0	35
Mexicana, frozen	12.8 oz	560	33	56	1290	0	23.0	50
Oriental, 'Light'	1 entrée	270	16	35	1070	3	8.0	35
pepper steak, w/rice	1 entrée	290	18	38	1060	4	8.0	40
pot roast, Yankee	1 entrée	230	15	30	650	4	5.0	30
pot roast, Yankee, frozen	11 oz	380	27	22	690	0	21.0	70
roast beef w/mashed potato and gravy, frozen	1 entrée	340	15	33	890	3	17.0	40
sirloin, roast, frozen	9.5 oz	330	13	36	700	0	14.0	85
sirloin, roast, frozen, 'Supreme'	1 entrée	300	16	32	850	3	13.0	65
Salisbury steak	1 entrée	240	16	27	550	2	8.0	40
Salisbury steak, beef sirloin, 'Light'	1 entrée	240	21	28	550	2	5.0	40
Salisbury steak, w/seasoned potatoes	1 entrée	240	16	30	570	4	6.0	45
sirloin, in herb sauce, 'Light'	1 entrée	260	19	30	850	5	7.0	30
sirloin entrée, frozen, 'Light & Healthy'	1 dinner	330	23	40	430	5	8.0	35
sirloin of beef, special recipe	1 entrée	270	19	36	510	5	5.0	25
sirloin tips, in burgundy sauce, frozen	11 oz	310	24	28	720	0	11.0	65
sirloin tips, w/country style vegetables, frozen	10 oz	310	16	21	570	0	18.0	40
sirloin-cheddar melt w/potato wedges, frozen	1 entrée	370	17	29	800	3	21.0	85
stir-fry w/red potato and vegetables, 'Light & Healthy'	1 dinner	261	18	34	494	7	5.9	44
(Bryan Foods) puréed beef	1/3 cup	120	12	0	40	0	7.0	40
(Castleberry Premium)								
stew	1 pkg	918	42	56	2781	6	58.5	156
stew	1 serving	331	15	20	1002	2	21.1	56
(Chun King)								
teriyaki beef, frozen	13 oz	380	22	68	2200	0	2.0	0
pepper beef Oriental, frozen	13 oz	310	17	53	1300	0	3.0	0
Szechwan beef, frozen	13 oz	340	20	57	1810	0	3.0	0
(Cripple Creek)								
beef brisket, choice, chopped, w/sauce	3 oz	150	15	6	510	0	9.0	45
(Dining Lite)								
pepper steak, frozen	9 oz	260	18	33	1050	0	6.0	40
Salisbury steak, frozen	9 oz	200	18	14	1000	0	8.0	55
teriyaki beef, frozen	9 oz	270	20	36	850	0	5.0	45
(Dinty Moore)								
beef entrée, packaged, 'Micro Meal'	1 bowl	260	15	21	1160	3	13.0	45
meat loaf, w/gravy and mashed potatoes, canned	1 bowl	300	18	27	1160	3	13.0	40
meat loaf w/mashed potatoes and gravy, 'American Classics'	10 oz	262	18	26	0	0	9.0	0
roasted beef, w/gravy and mashed potatoes, canned	1 bowl	240	24	25	860	2	5.0	35
roasted beef, w/gravy and potatoes, microwave, 'Classics'	10 oz	260	26	26	910	0	6.0	45
stew, canned	1 cup	222	11	16	984	3	13.1	38
stew, microwave bowl	10 oz	260	15	19	1180	0	14.0	45
stew, microwave cup	7.5 oz	180	11	15	830	0	9.0	30
(Estee) stew, canned	7.5 oz	210	14	17	65	0	11.0	30
(Featherweight) stew, canned	7.5 oz	160	17	17	400	0	3.0	35
(Freezer Queen)								
beef patty, charbroiled, frozen	10 oz	300	17	20	1260	0	17.0	0
beef patty, charbroiled, w/mushroom and onion gravy, frozen	7 oz	200	13	10	960	0	12.0	0
beef patty, charbroiled, w/mushroom gravy, frozen	7 oz	180	12	9	1050	0	11.0	0
beef w/peppers in sauce, w/rice, 'Single Serve'	9 oz	260	21	38	810	0	3.0	0
creamed, chipped beef, frozen, 'Cook-In-Pouch'	5 oz	80	5	11	500	0	2.0	0
meat loaf, w/tomato sauce, frozen, 'Family Suppers'	7 oz	230	12	15	850	0	13.0	0
Salisbury steak, frozen	10 oz	380	18	28	1260	0	22.0	0
Salisbury steak, w/gravy, frozen, 'Cook-In-Pouch'	5 oz	160	9	7	850	0	11.0	0

Food Name	Serv. Size	Total Cal.	Prot. gms	Carbs gms	Sod. mgs	Fiber gms	Fat gms	Chol. mgs
Salisbury steak, w/gravy, frozen 'Family Suppers' .... 7 oz		200	13	9	1110	0	13.0	0
Salisbury steak, charbroiled, w/vegetable medley, frozen ... 9 oz		330	22	14	990	0	22.0	0
sliced beef w/gravy, frozen .... 10 oz		210	18	18	1010	0	7.0	0
sliced beef w/gravy, frozen, 'Cook-In-Pouch' .... 4 oz		60	9	4	500	0	1.0	0
sliced beef w/gravy, 'Deluxe Family Suppers' .... 7 oz		130	15	10	870	0	3.0	0
sliced beef w/mashed potatoes and carrots .... 1 pkg		207	15	26	648	4	4.8	31
stew, frozen, 'Family Suppers' .... 7 oz		150	9	15	820	0	6.0	0
(Gebhardt)								
beef tamale .... 1 serving		134	2	9	385	1	10.3	14
beef tamale, food service product .... 1 serving		321	3	26	819	3	24.2	13
(Green Giant)								
burgers, Italian style, frozen .... 1 burger		140	17	8	370	5	4.5	0
burgers, original, frozen .... 1 burger		140	18	8	380	5	4.0	0
burgers, Southwest style, frozen .... 1 burger		140	16	9	370	5	4.0	0
(Healthy Choice)								
barbecue beef, sirloin w/sauce .... 11 oz		280	17	44	240	0	4.0	25
beef Bejing, w/broccoli .... 1 entrée		300	21	45	420	6	4.5	25
beef Cantonese, w/peppers .... 1 entrée		280	22	32	480	5	7.0	55
beef casserole w/macaroni .... 1 entrée		220	12	34	450	5	4.0	20
beef dinner w/mesquite, w/barbecue sauce, mashed potato, corn .... 1 pkg		320	21	38	491	5	9.0	3
beef macaroni, frozen .... 1 serving		211	14	33	444	5	2.2	14
beef patty, charbroiled .... 1 entrée		280	16	41	550	7	6.0	25
beef ribs, boneless, w/barbecue sauce, frozen, 11 oz .... 1 serving		330	28	40	530	0	6.0	70
beef Stroganoff .... 1 entrée		310	19	44	440	3	7.0	60
beef tips, 'Traditional' .... 1 entrée		260	20	32	390	6	6.0	40
beef tips Francais .... 1 entrée		300	20	40	520	4	7.0	40
meat loaf, 'Traditional' .... 1 entrée		330	15	52	460	6	7.0	35
mesquite barbecue beef .... 1 entrée		320	21	38	490	5	9.0	55
pepper steak, frozen .... 9.5 oz		250	18	36	560	0	4.0	40
pepper steak, Oriental (Healthy Choice) .... 1 entrée		260	9	34	520	2	5.0	35
peppercorn steak patty, grilled .... 1 entrée		220	16	26	470	5	6.0	30
pot roast 'Yankee' .... 1 entrée		290	19	38	460	4	7.0	55
roasted beef, chopped and formed, 'Fresh Trak' .... 1 slice		30	5	1	240	0	1.0	10
Salisbury steak, w/mushroom gravy, mashed potato, corn, frozen .... 1 entrée		326	18	48	466	6	6.9	49
sirloin tips, traditional, frozen .... 1 meal		260	20	32	390	6	5.0	40
(Hereford)								
roasted beef w/gravy, canned, ready-to-serve .... 2/3 cup		165	23	12	810	0	3.0	74
(Hormel)								
beef steak, breaded, frozen .... 4 oz		370	14	13	0	0	30.0	0
beef w/mushrooms, micro cup, 'Health Selections' .... 7 oz		210	21	25	390	0	3.0	45
dried beef, sliced, ground and formed, extra lean ..... 10 slices		50	8	1	1240	0	1.5	25
stew, microwave cup .... 7.5 oz		230	13	11	1140	0	15.0	45
(La Choy)								
beef chow mein, bi-pack .... 1 cup		105	9	15	756	3	1.7	12
beef chow mein, canned *(LaChoy)* .... 3/4 cup		40	5	5	960	2	2.0	16
beef pepper Oriental, bi-pack .... 1 cup		104	11	11	1065	3	2.7	22
beef pepper Oriental, frozen, food service product ...... 1 cup		150	8	30	714	2	0.7	10
beef w/broccoli and rice, frozen, 'Fresh & Lite' .... 11 oz		260	17	42	1299	5	5.0	51
pepper beef, canned .... 3/4 cup		100	7	12	1340	2	4.0	9
pepper steak .... 1 serving		175	10	37	4710	7	0.8	0
pepper steak, frozen .... 3.81 oz		36	2	7	942	1	0.2	0
pepper steak, frozen, w/rice and vegetables, 'Fresh & Lite' .... 10 oz		280	21	33	1082	2	8.0	36

Food Name	Serv. Size	Total Cal.	Prot. gms	Carbs gms	Sod. mgs	Fiber gms	Fat gms	Chol. mgs
teriyaki beef, w/rice and vegetables, frozen, 'Fresh & Lite'	10 oz	240	17	40	1198	2	5.0	57
(Le Menu)								
pepper steak, frozen	11.5 oz	370	26	36	1020	0	13.0	0
Salisbury steak, frozen	10.5 oz	370	20	28	880	0	20.0	0
Salisbury steak, frozen, 'Lightstyle'	10 oz	280	18	31	400	0	9.0	0
sirloin, chopped, frozen	12.25 oz	430	25	28	1010	0	24.0	0
sirloin tips, frozen	11.5 oz	400	30	29	760	0	18.0	0
Stroganoff	10 oz	430	26	28	980	0	24.0	0
(Lean Cuisine)								
beef chop suey, frozen	1 oz	16	2	2	85	0	0.5	4
beef Oriental	1 entrée	250	14	30	480	4	8.0	30
beef patty and whipped potatoes, 'Hearty Portions'	1 entrée	370	28	43	790	7	9.0	50
beef tips barbecue	1 entrée	290	13	47	560	7	6.0	30
beef w/peppercorns	1 entrée	220	15	23	580	2	7.0	35
homestyle beef and noodles, 'Hearty Portions'	1 entrée	330	20	46	780	6	7.0	45
meat loaf	1 entrée	250	18	30	590	4	6.0	50
meat loaf, w/macaroni and cheese, frozen	9 3/8 oz	280	26	26	540	0	8.0	55
meat loaf, w/whipped potatoes	1 entrée	250	22	25	570	5	7.0	45
Oriental beef, w/vegetables and rice, frozen	1 entrée	242	14	36	497	na	4.8	23
oven roasted beef	1 entrée	260	18	28	590	4	8.0	50
pot roast	1 entrée	210	13	25	570	6	6.0	30
pot roast w/whipped potatoes	1 entrée	210	16	21	570	3	7.0	40
Salisbury steak, w/gravy, frozen, food service product	1 oz	34	3	2	105	0	1.4	10
Salisbury steak, w/gravy and scalloped potatoes, frozen	9.5 oz	240	23	22	580	0	7.0	45
Salisbury steak, w/macaroni and cheese, frozen	1 entrée	270	23	27	590	4	8.0	60
sirloin, peppercorn, frozen, 'Cafe Classics'	1 pkg	210	13	24	480	4	7.0	25
(Lean Magic)								
mesquite beef patty, flame-broiled	1 piece	138	18	3	218	1	6.4	42
Salisbury steak, flame broiled	1 piece	148	17	4	400	1	7.2	41
Salisbury steak, flame broiled, '30'	1 piece	110	15	4	449	1	3.7	35
(Libby's)								
beef and macaroni, microwave cup, 'Diner'	7.75 oz	230	10	34	670	3	6.0	20
roasted beef w/gravy	2/3 cup	140	26	2	801	0	3.0	70
stew, canned, 15 oz package	7.5 oz	160	12	18	870	0	5.0	0
stew, microwave cup, 'Diner'	7.75 oz	240	12	22	790	0	12.0	40
stew, hearty, 'Microeasy' prepared	1/4 pkg	370	31	14	800	0	20.0	0
(Lunch Bucket) stew, hearty, microwave cup	7.5 oz	180	8	13	870	0	11.0	40
(Lunch Express) beef Oriental	1 entrée	290	12	43	880	4	8.0	15
(Lloyd's) barbecue beef, w/hickory smoked sauce	1/2 cup	200	15	21	980	1	7.0	35
(Marie Callender's)								
meat loaf, w/mashed potatoes and gravy	14 oz	540	23	42	1570	6	30.0	95
pot roast, old fashioned, w/gravy	1 cup	260	17	31	790	3	7.0	45
Salisbury steak, sirloin, w/gravy	14 oz	550	30	51	1680	6	25.0	85
Yankee pot pie	10-oz pie	690	16	57	1390	3	44.0	25
(Michelina's) Cantonese chow mein, 'Lean 'n Tasty'	1 entrée	250	8	42	1340	3	4.5	5
(Morton)								
Salisbury steak, frozen	10 oz	300	12	23	1420	0	17.0	40
sliced beef, frozen	10 oz	220	24	20	950	0	5.0	65
(Mountain House)								
beef w/rice and onions, freeze-dried, prepared	1 cup	330	11	42	265	0	12.0	0
stew, freeze-dried, prepared	1 cup	260	16	26	75	0	9.0	0
Stroganoff, freeze-dried, prepared	1 cup	270	10	26	118	0	13.0	0
(Myers)								
beef pie, frozen	3.5 oz	123	7	10	343	0	6.0	0
creamed, chipped beef, frozen	3.5 oz	136	9	7	863	0	8.0	0

Food Name	Serv. Size	Total Cal.	Prot. gms	Carbs gms	Sod. mgs	Fiber gms	Fat gms	Chol. mgs
Stroganoff	3.5 oz	112	8	7	346	0	6.0	0
(Nalley's)								
stew, canned, 'Big Chunk'	7.5 oz	200	10	24	790	0	7.0	0
stew, canned, 'Homestyle'	8 oz	180	11	22	810	0	5.0	0
(Nestlé)								
stew, 'Chef-Mate'	1 pkg	2305	181	228	14285	39	74.0	394
stew, 'Chef-Mate'	1 cup	192	15	19	1187	3	6.1	33
(Pathmark) stew, canned, 'No Frills'	8 oz	190	10	25	625	0	4.0	0
(Pierre)								
beef and onion patty, breaded, flame-broiled, frozen, 'Two-Fers'	1 piece	96	6	1	129	0	7.8	18
beef and onion patty, flame-broiled, frozen, product 3879	1 piece	161	16	2	317	1	9.8	42
beef and onion patty, flame-broiled, frozen, product 9675	1 piece	177	15	2	265	1	11.7	43
beef and onion patty, flame-broiled, frozen, product 9680	1 piece	473	28	4	636	2	38.4	90
beef finger, country-fried, frozen, product 3714	1 piece	79	4	3	114	0	5.5	11
beef finger, country-fried, frozen, product 3813	1 piece	82	4	4	126	0	5.5	10
beef finger, country-fried, frozen, product 3814	1 piece	100	5	4	121	0	7.0	15
beef nugget, country-fried, frozen, product 1910	1 piece	54	2	2	54	0	4.0	8
beef nugget, country-fried, frozen, product 1935	1 piece	49	2	2	71	0	3.4	5
beef nugget, country-fried, frozen, product 3711	1 piece	47	3	2	76	0	3.1	8
beef nugget, country-fried, frozen, product 3811	1 piece	51	3	2	74	0	3.1	9
beef patty, country-fried, frozen, product 1840	1 piece	356	18	16	519	2	24.8	42
beef patty, country-fried, frozen, product 1845	1 piece	292	15	14	427	1	20.3	31
beef patty, country-fried, frozen, product 3712	1 piece	306	17	16	364	1	20.1	41
beef patty, country-fried, frozen, product 3713	1 piece	360	18	17	401	1	24.6	46
beef patty, country-fried, frozen, product 3812	1 piece	304	17	15	479	1	19.9	38
beef patty, deluxe, flame-broiled, frozen, product 9100	1 piece	216	16	2	323	1	15.9	47
beef patty, deluxe, flame-broiled, frozen, product 9110	1 piece	160	12	1	239	1	11.8	35
beef patty, flame-broiled, frozen, product 3771	1 piece	153	16	2	248	1	8.9	41
beef patty, flame-broiled, frozen, product 3774	1 piece	211	23	2	367	1	12.3	57
beef patty, flame-broiled, frozen, product 3781	1 piece	154	17	2	250	1	9.0	41
beef patty, flame-broiled, frozen, product 3871	1 piece	158	16	2	291	1	9.5	41
beef patty, flame-broiled, frozen, product 3874	1 piece	218	22	2	401	1	13.1	57
beef patty, flame-broiled, frozen, product 3881	1 piece	158	16	2	293	1	9.6	42
beef patty, flame-broiled, frozen, product 9220	1 piece	186	11	2	313	1	15.1	31
beef patty, flame-broiled, frozen, product 9230	1 piece	229	13	2	386	2	18.6	38
beef patty, jalapeño, flame-broiled, product 3778	1 piece	154	16	2	340	1	9.0	41
beef patty, jalapeño, flame-broiled, frozen, product 3878	1 piece	159	16	2	335	1	9.6	41
beef patty, less fat, flame-broiled, product 3772	1 piece	143	16	2	298	1	7.9	36
beef patty, mesquite, deluxe, flame-broiled, frozen, product 9103	1 piece	216	15	2	277	1	16.3	42
beef patty, mesquite, flame-broiled, frozen, product 3870	1 piece	158	16	2	246	1	9.5	41
beef patty, mesquite, flame-broiled, frozen, product 3880	1 piece	159	16	2	247	1	9.6	42
beef patty, mesquite, flame-broiled, product 3770	1 piece	153	16	2	248	1	8.9	41
beef patty, mesquite, flame-broiled, product 3780	1 piece	154	17	2	250	1	9.0	41
beef patty w/onions, flame-broiled, product 3779	1 piece	153	16	2	315	1	8.8	41
beef steak, country-fried, frozen, product 3710	1 piece	315	17	14	494	0	21.0	59
beef steak, country-fried, frozen, product 1610	1 piece	356	17	14	377	0	25.6	52
beef steak, country-fried, frozen, product 3810	1 piece	343	21	16	498	0	21.1	64
beef steak, flame-broiled, frozen, product 9010	1 piece	249	18	0	285	0	18.9	64
beef steak, flame-broiled, frozen, product 9017	1 piece	237	18	1	360	0	17.4	64

Food Name	Serv. Size	Total Cal.	Prot. gms	Carbs gms	Sod. mgs	Fiber gms	Fat gms	Chol. mgs
beef steak, flame-broiled, frozen, product 9503	1 piece	177	16	1	309	0	12.0	52
beef steak, flame-broiled, product 3760	1 piece	164	16	1	259	0	10.2	47
beef steak, flame-broiled, product 3765	1 piece	164	16	1	259	0	10.2	47
beef steak, flame-broiled, product 3860	1 piece	189	17	1	261	0	12.8	56
beef steak, mesquite, flame-broiled, frozen, product 3863	1 piece	194	17	1	297	0	13.1	57
beef steak, mesquite, flame-broiled, product 3763	1 piece	169	17	1	295	0	10.5	48
flame-broiled, frozen, 'Two-Fers' product 9684	1 piece	98	6	1	130	0	7.8	19
meat loaf, flame-broiled, product 3724	1 piece	162	16	4	363	1	9.1	41
meat loaf, flame-broiled, product 3725	1 piece	152	16	4	360	1	8.2	36
meat loaf, flame-broiled, frozen, product 3824	1 piece	170	16	4	364	1	10.1	44
mesquite beef patty, flame-broiled, less fat, product 3773	1 piece	145	16	3	231	1	7.9	36
New York strip, flame-broiled, frozen, product 3877	1 piece	164	16	2	340	1	10.2	44
New York strip, flame-broiled, product 3777	1 piece	159	17	2	345	0	9.5	44
Salisbury steak, flame-broiled, frozen, product 3820	1 piece	161	16	3	500	1	9.8	42
Salisbury steak, flame-broiled, frozen, product 9600	1 piece	186	16	2	553	1	12.4	45
Salisbury steak, flame-broiled, less fat	1 piece	147	16	3	512	1	8.2	36
Salisbury steak, flame-broiled, product 3720	1 piece	157	16	2	503	0	9.3	42
(Pillsbury) casserole, frozen, 'Microwave Classic'	1 pkg	430	16	34	1100	0	25.0	0
(Rib-B-Q)								
beef and onion patty, flame-broiled, frozen, 'Lean Magic'	1 piece	138	17	2	313	1	6.7	42
beef and turkey barbecue, flame-broiled, frozen, product 9126, 'Lean Magic 30'	1 piece	116	14	8	560	1	3.1	29
beef and turkey patty, flame-broiled, w/tangy glaze, 'Lean Magic 30'	1 piece	120	17	7	541	1	3.1	35
beef and turkey patty, flame-broiled, w/teriyaki sauce, 'Lean Magic 30'	1 piece	28	4	2	127	0	0.7	8
beef barbecue, flame-broiled, frozen, product 3732, 'Lean Magic 30'	1 piece	139	15	4	398	1	7.3	33
beef patty, flame-broiled, 'Lean Magic'	1 piece	136	18	2	280	1	6.5	42
beef rib barbecue, flame-broiled, frozen, product 3733 ...	1 piece	154	16	3	403	1	8.6	39
beef rib barbecue, flame-broiled, frozen, product 3833 ...	1 piece	175	16	3	405	1	10.7	47
beef rib barbecue, flame-broiled, frozen, product 4150 ...	1 piece	204	12	3	387	1	15.9	35
beef rib barbecue, flame-broiled, frozen, product 3832, 'Lean Magic'	1 piece	156	15	3	400	1	9.0	39
(Rice A Roni)								
beef and mushroom rice dish, prepared	2.5 oz	164	4	29	714	1	3.4	0
(Right Course)								
Dijon beef, w/pasta and vegetables, frozen	9.5 oz	290	20	31	580	0	9.0	40
fiesta, w/corn pasta	8 7/8 oz	270	18	33	590	0	7.0	30
pot roast, homestyle, frozen	9.25 oz	220	17	22	550	0	7.0	35
ragout, w/rice pilaf, frozen	10 oz	300	19	38	550	0	8.0	50
(Steak-Umm) sandwich steak	2 oz	180	9	0	50	0	16.0	0
(Stouffer's)								
beef pie	1 entrée	450	19	36	1140	3	26.0	65
beef pot pie	1 pie	415	11	41	740	2	23.0	25
beef stew, frozen, food service product	1 oz	23	2	2	103	0	1.0	5
beef Stroganoff, frozen, food service product	1 oz	41	3	1	116	0	2.7	10
beef Stroganoff w/noodles	1 entrée	390	23	30	1100	2	20.0	85
creamed chipped beef entrée	1 entrée	160	10	6	690	1	11.0	40
creamed chipped beef, frozen	1 pkg	435	25	18	1546	na	29.5	109
creamed chipped beef, frozen	1 serving	175	10	7	621	na	11.9	44
creamed chipped beef, frozen, food service product	1 oz	40	2	1	156	0	2.8	9
homestyle beef w/noodles, gravy, vegetable	8 3/8 oz	230	16	26	720	0	7.0	0
meat loaf, w/whipped potatoes, 'Homestyle'	1 entrée	390	20	24	910	3	24.0	80

Food Name	Serv. Size	Total Cal.	Prot. gms	Carbs gms	Sod. mgs	Fiber gms	Fat gms	Chol. mgs
pepper steak, beef w/rice, frozen	10.5 oz	310	20	35	700	0	10.0	0
Salisbury steak, w/gravy, macaroni and cheese, frozen	9 5/8 oz	350	25	23	1130	0	17.0	0
Salisbury steak w/gravy, macaroni and cheese, 'Homestyle'	1 pkg	386	23	26	1015	na	21.2	63
steak w/green pepper	1 entrée	330	17	45	650	3	9.0	35
(Swanson)								
barbecue beef w/sauce	11 oz	460	30	51	860	0	17.0	0
beef enchilada entrée	1 entrée	500	21	68	1220	11	16.0	25
beef entrée, frozen	11.25 oz	310	26	38	770	0	6.0	0
beef pot pie, 'Hungry Man'	1 pie	660	24	70	1590	6	31.0	50
beef w/gravy	1 entrée	370	19	40	700	6	15.0	40
chopped beef steak, frozen, 'Hungry Man'	16.75 oz	640	35	41	1600	0	37.0	0
chopped sirloin w/gravy	1 entrée	380	19	37	730	5	14.0	40
meat loaf	1 entrée	380	19	37	730	5	14.0	35
Salisbury steak	1 entrée	340	16	35	920	6	15.0	30
Salisbury steak, frozen, 'Homestyle Recipe'	10 oz	320	21	22	980	0	16.0	0
Salisbury steak, in gravy, w/mashed potatoes, frozen	1 entrée	330	17	24	1040	3	18.0	30
Salisbury steak, frozen, 'Hungry Man'	1 entrée	610	34	46	1620	10	33.0	80
sirloin, chopped, frozen	10.75 oz	340	20	28	790	0	16.0	0
sirloin tips, in burgundy sauce, frozen, 'Homestyle Recipe'	7 oz	160	12	16	550	0	5.0	0
sirloin tips, w/noodles and beef gravy, frozen	1 entrée	290	16	34	530	5	11.0	50
sliced beef, frozen, 'Hungry Man'	15.25 oz	450	37	49	1060	0	12.0	0
(Top Shelf)								
beef and potatoes, microwave bowl	1 serving	254	29	22	1211	0	6.0	88
beef entrée, packaged	10 oz	320	25	22	910	0	15.0	70
beef ribs, boneless, packaged, microwave bowl	1 serving	440	28	29	550	0	24.0	90
beef sukiyaki, packaged, microwave bowl	1 serving	330	24	36	1700	0	10.0	45
Oriental beef entrée, packaged, microwave bowl	1 serving	290	25	25	1700	0	10.0	45
roasted beef, tender, frozen	10 oz	240	28	19	880	0	6.0	60
roasted beef, tender, packaged, microwave bowl	1 serving	240	27	18	980	0	7.0	65
Stroganoff, microwave bowl	1 serving	320	29	24	1250	0	12.0	48
(Tyson)								
champignon, frozen, 'Gourmet Selection'	10.5 oz	370	27	31	830	0	15.0	0
pepper steak, beef, frozen, 'Gourmet Selection'	11.25 oz	330	20	38	1130	0	11.0	0
pot roast w/potatoes, 'Homestyle'	1 entrée	270	19	25	640	4	10.0	40
Salisbury steak, supreme, frozen, 'Gourmet Selection'	10 oz	430	16	34	810	0	26.0	0
short ribs in gravy, frozen	9 oz	350	30	12	900	0	20.0	0
short ribs, frozen, 'Gourmet Selection'	11 oz	470	25	38	950	0	24.0	0
stir-fry, w/rice, Oriental vegetables, frozen	1 pkg	867	52	142	3167	na	10.0	na
stir-fry, w/rice, Oriental vegetables, frozen	1 serving	433	26	71	1584	na	5.0	na
(Ultra Slim-Fast)								
beef w/mushroom gravy, frozen	10.5 oz	290	19	44	830	0	5.0	35
meat loaf, beef, w/tomato sauce, frozen	10.5 oz	340	19	52	780	0	9.0	35
pepper steak, beef, w/parsley rice, frozen	12 oz	270	22	36	690	0	4.0	45
(Weight Watchers)								
beef Cantonese, w/rice, frozen, 'Stir Fry'	9 oz	200	14	27	530	0	4.0	15
beef Romanoff, supreme, w/pasta and vegetables, frozen	9 oz	230	12	29	540	0	7.0	20
beef stir-fry, frozen, 'Jade Garden'	9 oz	150	13	17	490	0	3.0	20
London broil, frozen, 'Ultimate 200'	7.5 oz	110	17	4	320	0	3.0	25
London broil, in mushroom sauce, frozen	7.37 oz	140	18	9	510	0	3.0	40
pepper steak	1 entrée	240	18	33	690	4	4.5	35
Salisbury steak, grilled, w/gravy	1 entrée	260	19	24	620	3	10.0	40
sirloin tips, frozen, 'Ultimate 200'	7.5 oz	200	20	20	560	0	6.0	30
stew, chunky, microwave cup	7.5 oz	120	14	14	450	0	2.0	20

Food Name	Serv. Size	Total Cal.	Prot. gms	Carbs gms	Sod. mgs	Fiber gms	Fat gms	Chol. mgs
(Wolf Brand) stew, canned .... 1 cup		179	10	18	1043	1	7.5	0
(Yu Sing)								
beef and pepper Oriental, w/rice .... 1 container		230	8	38	820	2	5.0	10
BEEF DINNER/ENTRÉE MIX. See also HAMBURGER ENTRÉE MIX.								
(Hamburger Helper) meat loaf mix, prepared .... 1 slice		270	24	11	580	0	14.0	110
(Lipton)								
meat loaf mix, homestyle, mix only, 'Microeasy' .... 1/4 pkg		90	4	15	630	0	1.0	0
meat loaf mix, homestyle, prepared w/ground beef, 'Microeasy' .... 1/4 pkg		390	31	15	700	0	22.0	0
BEEF JERKY								
chopped and formed .... 1 oz		116	9	3	627	1	7.3	14
cured, dried .... 1 oz		47	8	0	984	0	1.1	12
(Eagle)								
kippered beefsteak .... 0.8 oz		50	10	1	550	0	0.5	20
kippered beefsteak, hot .... 0.8 oz		50	9	2	560	0	0.5	20
kippered turkey steak .... 0.8 oz		60	9	2	580	0	1.5	20
(Frito-Lay's)								
.... 0.21-oz piece		25	3	1	200	0	1.0	10
'Tender' .... 0.7 oz		120	5	2	370	0	10.0	25
(Hickory Farms) .... 1 oz		100	16	4	1360	0	3.0	73
(Hormel) 'Lumberjack' .... 1 oz		101	5	0	304	0	9.0	0
(Pemmican)								
'Arrowhead' .... 0.7-oz piece		70	8	2	580	0	3.0	0
'Steakers' .... 0.14-oz piece		40	5	2	160	0	1.0	0
jalapeño .... 0.25 oz		25	3	1	220	0	1.0	0
natural .... 0.25 oz		25	3	1	220	0	1.0	0
peppered .... 0.25 oz		25	3	1	220	0	1.0	0
Tabasco .... 0.25 oz		25	3	1	220	0	1.0	0
'Tender Brave' .... 1 oz		80	14	2	830	0	2.0	0
'Tender Chief' .... 1 oz		80	14	2	830	0	2.0	0
'Tender Tomahawk' .... 0.25 oz		20	3	1	210	0	1.0	0
'Tender Trail' .... 1 oz		80	14	2	830	0	2.0	0
'Tender Tribe' .... 1 oz		80	14	2	830	0	2.0	0
teriyaki .... 0.25 oz		20	3	1	200	0	1.0	0
(Rustlers Roundup) .... 5 servings		20	2	1	115	1	1.5	5
(Slim Jim)								
'Big Jerk' .... 0.25-oz piece		25	3	1	220	0	1.0	0
'Giant Jerk' .... 0.63-oz piece		60	7	2	510	0	2.0	0
.... 0.14-oz piece		20	2	1	120	0	1.0	0
regular, 'Super Jerk' .... 0.31-oz piece		30	4	1	250	0	1.0	0
Tabasco 'Super Jerk' .... 0.31-oz piece		30	4	1	250	0	1.0	0
(Tumen)								
hot pepperoni style .... 1/2 oz		50	5	2	125	1	2.0	0
smoked ham style .... 1/2 oz		50	5	2	125	1	2.0	0
spicy Italian style .... 1/2 oz		50	5	2	125	1	2.0	0
BEEF SEASONING. See under HAMBURGER ENTRÉE MIX; MARINADE; MARINADE MIX; SEASONING MIX.								
BEEF SPREAD								
(Hormel) roast beef, canned .... 0.5 oz		31	2	0	0	0	2.0	0
(Underwood)								
roast beef, canned .... 2 1/8 oz		140	9	1	360	0	11.0	45
roast beef, canned, 'Light' .... 2 1/8 oz		90	9	2	210	0	6.0	30
roast beef, canned, mesquite smoked .... 2 1/8 oz		126	9	1	300	0	11.0	45
BEEF STEW. See under BEEF DINNER/ENTRÉE.								
BEEF STICK								
(Eagle) .... 1 oz		110	7	1	480	0	9.0	20
(Eagle) pepperoni sausage .... 1.25 oz		150	10	3	740	0	11.0	25

Food Name	Serv. Size	Total Cal.	Prot. gms	Carbs gms	Sod. mgs	Fiber gms	Fat gms	Chol. mgs
BEEF SUBSTITUTE								
(Heartline)								
lite, vegetarian, 'Beef Fillet Style'	0.5 oz	22	5	1	135	3	0.0	0
lite, vegetarian, 'Ground Beef Style'	0.5 oz	22	2	1	135	3	0.0	0
vegetarian, 'Beef Fillet Style'	2 oz	176	19	9	480	0	7.0	0
vegetarian, 'Ground Beef Style'	2 oz	176	19	9	480	0	7.0	0
vegetarian, 'Teriyaki Beef Style'	2 oz	176	19	9	450	0	7.0	0
(Morningstar Farms)								
ground beef substitute, vegetarian, 'Burger Style Recipe Crumbles'	2/3 cup	80	10	4	210	2	2.5	0
ground beef substitute, vegetarian, 'Ground Meatless'	1/2 cup	60	10	4	260	2	0.0	0
(Worthington)								
beef style, vegetarian, meatless	1 slice	113	9	4	624	3	6.8	0
corned beef style, vegetarian, roll, frozen	2.5 oz	150	12	9	660	0	7.0	0
corned beef style, vegetarian, frozen, approx 2-oz slices	4 slices	120	9	8	740	0	6.0	0
ground beef style, vegetarian, 'Burger Crumbles'	1 pkg	3809	365	109	7855	83	213.1	0
ground beef style, vegetarian, 'Burger Crumbles'	1 cup	231	22	7	476	5	12.9	0
ground beef style, vegetarian, 'Burger Crumbles'	1 serving	116	11	3	238	3	6.5	0
roll, vegetarian, frozen, approx 2.5-oz slices	4 slices	130	12	7	750	0	6.0	0
smoked, roll, frozen, approx. 2-oz slices	3 slices	120	10	7	790	0	6.0	0
steak style, 'Stakelets'	1 serving	144	12	6	484	2	8.0	2
(White Wave)								
roast beef style, vegetarian, sandwich sliced	1 slice	90	14	8	270	1	0.0	0
BEEF SUBSTITUTE DINNER/ENTRÉE								
(Amy's Kitchen)								
burger, vegetarian, 'California'	1 serving	100	4	17	290	3	3.0	0
burger, vegetarian, organic, frozen	2.5-oz burger	173	6	22	181	1	4.0	0
Salisbury steak, meatless, 'Country Dinner'	1 entrée	420	12	63	700	9	16.0	20
(Boca Burger)								
burger, vegetarian, frozen, 'Chef Max's Favorite'	1 burger	110	14	9	296	4	0.0	0
burger, vegetarian, original, frozen	1 burger	84	12	9	227	5	0.0	0
(Fantastic Foods)								
burger, tofu, vegetarian, prepared w/o cooking fat	3.4-oz burger	133	11	14	320	0	5.0	0
(Gardenburger)								
burger, vegetarian, original	2.5 oz	130	8	18	290	5	2.9	11
burger, vegetarian, soy-free	2.5 oz	140	8	21	180	5	2.5	0
burger, Greek, classic, vegetarian, 'Gourmet'	2.5 oz	121	6	17	306	2	2.9	8
hamburger style, vegetarian, low-fat	2.5 oz	115	16	7	381	3	2.6	4
veggie medley patty, vegetarian	2.5 oz	100	6	17	280	3	0.7	0
zesty bean patty, vegetarian	2.5 oz	120	7	19	290	5	2.5	10
(Green Giant)								
burger, vegetable protein, vegetarian, original, 'Harvest Burger'	1 pkg	552	72	28	1654	23	16.7	0
burger, vegetable protein, vegetarian, original, 'Harvest Burger'	1 patty	137	18	7	411	6	4.1	0
burger, vegetarian, all-vegetable, Southwestern style, 'Harvest Burger'	1 patty	140	16	9	370	5	4.0	0
(Heartline) burger, vegetarian, meatless	4 oz	176	19	9	480	5	7.0	0
(Ken & Robert's)								
burger, vegetarian	1 serving	130	5	26	260	3	1.0	0
burger, vegetarian, frozen, 2.5 oz, 'Truly Amazing'	1 patty	110	5	19	390	0	2.0	0
(Legume)								
stew, beef style	1 cup	150	10	29	450	5	0.0	0
tamale, beef style, vegetarian, low-fat	3 tamales	220	10	40	350	3	2.5	0
(Loma Linda)								
burger, vegetarian, dry mix, 'Patty Mix'	1/3 cup	90	14	7	480	5	1.0	0

Food Name	Serv. Size	Total Cal.	Prot. gms	Carbs gms	Sod. mgs	Fiber gms	Fat gms	Chol. mgs
dinner loaf, dry mix, 'Savory Dinner Loaf'	1/3 cup	90	14	7	560	5	1.5	0
(Love Natural Foods)								
burger, vegetarian, prepared, 'Loveburger'	4-oz burger	245	17	20	224	8	11.0	0
(Morningstar Farms)'								
burger, vegetarian, 'Better'N Burgers'	1 patty	80	13	8	360	3	0.0	0
burger, vegetarian, 'Grillers'	1 patty	140	15	5	260	2	6.0	0
burger, vegetarian, 'Hard Rock Café All-Natural Veggie Burgers'	1 patty	170	6	18	340	3	8.0	0
burger, vegetarian, 'Harvest Burgers' Italian style	1 patty	140	17	8	370	5	4.5	0
burger, vegetarian, 'Harvest Burgers' original flavor	1 patty	140	18	8	370	5	4.0	0
burger, vegetarian, 'Harvest Burgers' Southwestern style	1 patty	140	16	9	370	5	4.0	0
burger, vegetarian, 'Harvest Burgers' recipe crumbles	1/2 cup	70	12	5	200	3	0.0	0
burger, vegetarian, frozen, 'Oven Roasted Veggie Burgers'	1 patty	120	14	40	400	2	8.0	10
burger, vegetarian, 'Quarter Prime'	1 patty	140	24	6	370	3	2.0	0
burger, vegetarian, and cheese, 'Stuffed Sandwiches'	1 sandwich	290	14	10	400	2	8.0	10
(Natural Touch)								
burger, vegetarian, 'Hard Rock Cafe All Natural Veggie Burgers'	1 patty	170	%6	18	340	3	8.0	0
burger, vegetarian, 'Vegan Burger'	1 patty	70	11	6	370	3	0.0	0
'Loaf Mix' dry mix	4 tbsp	100	14	10	700	7	0.5	0
'Stroganoff Mix' dry mix	4 tbsp	90	5	10	610	3	3.5	10
(Naturally Tofu) burger, vegetarian, meatless	4 oz	165	20	25	52	9	2.0	0
(Nature's Burger)								
burger, vegetarian, prepared w/o cooking fat, 'Original'	3-oz burger	152	7	21	228	0	4.0	0
burger, barbecue, vegetarian, prepared w/o cooking fat	3-oz burger	117	4	24	423	0	0.8	0
burger, pizza, vegetarian, prepared w/o cooking fat	3-oz burger	121	5	24	406	0	1.0	0
(Tempeh) burger, soy and rice, vegetarian, frozen	2 2/3 oz	140	12	13	0	5	5.0	0
(White Wave)								
burger, vegetarian, 'Veggielife'	1 serving	130	6	20	250	3	3.5	0
tempeh burger, vegetarian	1 serving	110	12	10	270	6	2.5	0
(Worthington)								
burger, vegetarian, 'FriPats'	1 patty	132	15	4	323	4	6.3	2
burger, vegetarian, 'Vegetarian Burger'	1/4 cup	60	9	2	270	1	2.0	0
'Meatless Corned Beef' 72-oz roll	3/8-inch slice	130	9	4	510	2	9.0	0
'Meatless Corned Beef' 8-oz carton	4 slices	140	10	5	520	2	9.0	0
'Meatless Smoked Beef'	6 slices	120	11	6	730	3	6.0	0
pie, vegetarian, frozen	8 oz	360	9	44	1940	0	16.0	0
stew, vegetarian, 'Country Stew'	1 cup	210	13	20	830	5	9.0	0
roast, vegetarian, 'Dinner Roast'	3/4-inch slice	180	12	5	580	3	12.0	<5
sliced, vegetarian, 'Savory Slices'	3 slices	150	10	6	540	3	9.0	0
steak, vegetarian, 'Prime Stakes'	1 piece	136	9	4	445	4	9.3	2
steak, vegetarian, 'Stakelets'	1 piece	140	12	6	480	2	8.0	0
steak, vegetarian, 'Vegetable Steaks'	2 slices	80	15	3	300	3	1.5	0

BEEF SUBSTITUTE DINNER/ENTRÉE MIX

Food Name	Serv. Size	Total Cal.	Prot. gms	Carbs gms	Sod. mgs	Fiber gms	Fat gms	Chol. mgs
(Fantastic Foods)								
Stroganoff, creamy, 'Tofu Classics' mix only	1/2 cup	190	10	35	660	3	5.0	5
(Loma Linda) vegetarian 'Vita-Burger Chunks'	1/4 cup	75	10	6	353	4	1.1	0
(Tofu Classics)								
Stroganoff, creamy, vegetarian, prepared w/tofu	1/2 cup	94	7	11	264	0	3.0	0

Food Name	Serv. Size	Total Cal.	Prot. gms	Carbs gms	Sod. mgs	Fiber gms	Fat gms	Chol. mgs
Stroganoff, creamy, vegetarian, prepared w/tofu,								
2 tbsp salted butter .... 1/2 cup		127	7	11	310	0	7.0	0
BEEF SUBSTITUTE JERKY								
original flavor, meatless *(Pemmican)* .... 1 pkg		420	17	59	90	9	13.0	0
vegetarian, 'Spicy Italian Style' *(Cajun Jerky)* .... 0.5 oz		50	5	2	125	1	2.0	0
vegetable protein, 'Jerquee' *(Stonewall's)* .... 0.5 oz		50	5	2	125	1	2.0	0
BEEF TALLOW								
.... 1 cup		1849	0	0	0	0	205.0	223
.... 1 tbsp		115	0	0	0	0	12.8	14
BEEFALO								
composite of cuts, raw .... 1 oz		41	7	0	22	0	1.4	12
composite of cuts, roasted .... 3 oz		160	26	0	70	0	5.4	49
BEER, ALE, AND MALT LIQUOR								
ALE								
(McSorley's) .... 12 fl oz		166	2	15	6	0	0.0	0
(Tiger Head) .... 12 fl oz		166	2	15	6	0	0.0	0
BEER								
.... 12 fl oz		146	1	13	18	1	0.0	0
light .... 12 fl oz		99	1	5	11	0	0.0	0
(Anheuser Marzen) .... 12 fl oz		168	2	15	12	0	0.0	0
(Beck's) .... 12 fl oz		148	2	10	14	0	0.0	0
(Budweiser)								
.... 12 fl oz		144	1	11	12	0	0.0	0
light, 'Bud Light' .... 12 fl oz		110	1	7	12	0	0.0	0
(Busch) .... 12 fl oz		144	1	12	12	0	0.0	0
(Carlsberg)								
.... 12 fl oz		149	1	12	12	0	0.0	0
light .... 12 fl oz		110	1	7	12	0	0.0	0
(Coors)								
.... 12 fl oz		137	1	12	1	0	0.0	0
'Coors Dry' .... 12 fl oz		119	0	6	1	0	0.0	0
'Extra Gold' .... 12 fl oz		151	1	13	1	0	0.0	0
light, 'Coors Light' .... 12 fl oz		103	1	5	1	0	0.0	0
3.2% .... 12 fl oz		119	1	10	1	0	0.0	0
3.2%, 'Coors Dry' .... 12 fl oz		101	1	5	1	0	0.0	0
3.2%, 'Extra Gold' .... 12 fl oz		121	1	10	1	0	0.0	0
3.2%, light, 'Coors Light' .... 12 fl oz		98	1	5	1	0	0.0	0
(Cutter) nonalcoholic .... 12 fl oz		76	1	20	1	0	0.0	0
(Dribeck's) .... 12 fl oz		94	1	7	14	0	0.0	0
(Kaliber) nonalcoholic .... 12 fl oz		71	1	11	3	0	0.0	0
(Keystone)								
.... 12 fl oz		121	1	7	1	0	0.0	0
'Keystone Dry' .... 12 fl oz		121	1	6	1	0	0.0	0
light, 'Keystone Light' .... 12 fl oz		100	1	4	1	0	0.0	0
3.2% .... 12 fl oz		104	1	6	1	0	0.0	0
3.2%, light, 'Keystone Light' .... 12 fl oz		99	0	5	1	0	0.0	0
(Killian's)								
.... 12 fl oz		161	1	15	1	0	0.0	0
3.2% .... 12 fl oz		128	1	11	1	0	0.0	0
(Knickerbocker) .... 12 fl oz		140	1	12	9	0	0.0	0
(LA) light alcohol .... 12 fl oz		114	1	16	12	0	0.0	0
(Lite)								
.... 12 fl oz		96	1	3	6	0	0.0	0
'Genuine Draft' .... 12 fl oz		98	1	4	6	0	0.0	0
(Lowenbrau)								
'Dark Special' .... 12 fl oz		158	1	14	7	0	0.0	0
'Special' .... 12 fl oz		158	1	14	7	0	0.0	0

Food Name	Serv. Size	Total Cal.	Prot. gms	Carbs gms	Sod. mgs	Fiber gms	Fat gms	Chol. mgs
(Meister Brau)								
....	12 fl oz	141	1	13	6	0	0.0	0
light	12 fl oz	98	1	4	6	0	0.0	0
(Michelob)								
....	12 fl oz	156	2	14	12	0	0.0	0
'Classic Dark'	12 fl oz	158	2	14	12	0	0.0	0
'Dry'	12 fl oz	133	1	8	12	0	0.0	0
light	12 fl oz	134	1	12	12	0	0.0	0
(Miller)								
'Genuine Draft'	12 fl oz	147	1	13	7	0	0.0	0
'High-Life'	12 fl oz	147	1	13	7	0	0.0	0
'Magnum'	12 fl oz	162	1	10	8	0	0.0	0
(Milwaukee)								
'Milwaukee's Best'	12 fl oz	133	1	11	6	0	0.0	0
'Milwaukee's Best Light' ...	12 fl oz	98	1	4	6	0	0.0	0
(Natural Light) light	12 fl oz	110	1	7	12	0	0.0	0
(O'Doul's) nonalcoholic ...	12 fl oz	70	1	15	0	0	0.0	0
(Prior) 'Double Dark'	12 fl oz	171	1	15	10	0	0.0	0
(Rheingold)								
....	12 fl oz	148	1	13	9	0	0.0	0
light	12 fl oz	96	1	3	7	0	0.0	0
(Rolling Rock)								
light	12 fl oz	104	0	8	1	0	0.0	0
'Premium'	12 fl oz	145	0	10	1	0	0.0	0
(Schmidt's)								
....	12 fl oz	148	1	13	9	0	0.0	0
'Classic'	12 fl oz	144	1	13	10	0	0.0	0
light	12 fl oz	96	1	3	7	0	0.0	0
(Sharp's) nonalcoholic ...	12 fl oz	86	1	10	5	0	0.0	0
BEET								
Fresh								
boiled, drained, whole, approx 2-inch diam	2 med beets	44	2	10	77	2	0.2	0
boiled, drained, sliced	1/2 cup	37	1	8	65	2	0.2	0
raw, sliced	1 cup	58	2	13	106	4	0.2	0
raw, whole, approx 2-inch diam	1 med beet	35	1	8	64	2	0.1	0
Canned								
cut *(Stokely)*	1/2 cup	40	1	8	300	0	0.0	0
diced *(S&W)*	1/2 cup	40	1	9	270	0	0.0	0
diced *(Stokely)*	1/2 cup	35	1	7	300	0	0.0	0
diced, drained	1 cup	49	1	11	305	3	0.2	0
Harvard *(Green Giant)*	1/3 cup	60	1	15	270	2	0.0	0
Harvard *(Stokely)*	1/2 cup	70	1	18	135	0	0.0	0
Harvard, sliced, w/liquid	1 cup	180	2	45	399	6	0.1	0
no salt, 'No Salt or Sugar Added' *(Stokely)* ...	1/2 cup	40	1	8	40	0	0.0	0
no salt, w/liquid	1 cup	69	2	16	52	3	0.2	0
pickled *(Freshlike)*	1/2 cup	40	1	9	650	0	0.0	0
pickled *(Stokely)*	1/2 cup	100	1	25	400	0	0.0	0
pickled *(Veg-All)*	1/2 cup	100	1	25	650	0	0.0	0
pickled, crinkle sliced, w/liquid *(Del Monte)*	1/2 cup	80	1	19	375	0	0.0	0
pickled, sliced, w/liquid	1 cup	148	2	37	599	6	0.2	0
pickled, sliced, w/red wine vinegar, 'Party' *(S&W)*	1 oz	15	0	4	50	1	0.0	0
pickled, sliced, w/red wine vinegar, regular *(S&W)*	1/2 cup	70	1	16	215	0	0.0	0
pickled, whole *(S&W)*	1 oz	15	0	4	50	1	0.0	0
pickled, whole, extra small *(S&W)*	1/2 cup	70	1	16	215	0	0.0	0
regular pack, w/liquid	1 cup	69	2	16	620	3	0.2	0
shredded, drained	1 cup	60	2	14	378	3	0.3	0
sliced *(A&P)*	1/2 cup	40	1	9	300	0	1.0	0

Food Name	Serv. Size	Total Cal.	Prot. gms	Carbs gms	Sod. mgs	Fiber gms	Fat gms	Chol. mgs
sliced *(Featherweight)*	1/2 cup	45	1	10	55	0	0.0	0
sliced *(Finast)*	1/2 cup	40	1	9	390	0	0.0	0
sliced *(Green Giant)*	1/2 cup	35	1	8	260	2	0.0	0
sliced *(Pathmark)*	1/2 cup	45	1	10	330	0	0.0	0
sliced *(Stokely)*	1/2 cup	40	1	8	300	0	0.0	0
sliced, no salt added *(Finast)*	1/2 cup	40	1	9	40	0	0.0	0
sliced, no salt added *(A&P)*	1/2 cup	35	1	8	50	0	1.0	0
sliced, no salt added *(Green Giant)*	1/2 cup	35	1	8	60	2	0.0	0
sliced, no salt added *(Pathmark)*	1/2 cup	35	1	7	35	0	0.0	0
sliced, 'Nutradiet' *(S&W)*	1/2 cup	35	1	9	40	0	0.0	0
sliced, drained	1 cup	53	2	12	330	3	0.2	0
sliced, drained	1 slice	2	0	1	16	0	0.0	0
sliced, small *(Freshlike)*	1/2 cup	40	1	9	260	0	0.0	0
sliced, small, tender, 'Premium' *(S&W)*	1/2 cup	40	1	9	270	0	0.0	0
sliced, water packed, w/o salt *(Freshlike)*	1/2 cup	40	1	9	50	0	0.0	0
sliced, water packed, w/o sugar or salt *(Freshlike)*	1/2 cup	40	1	9	50	0	0.0	0
sliced, w/liquid, no salt added *(Del Monte)*	1/2 cup	35	1	8	100	0	0.0	0
whole *(A&P)*	1/2 cup	40	1	9	300	0	1.0	0
whole *(Green Giant)*	1/2 cup	35	1	8	260	2	0.0	0
whole *(IGA)*	1/2 cup	40	1	9	275	0	0.0	0
whole *(Stokely)*	1/2 cup	40	1	8	300	0	0.0	0
whole, baby, 'LeSueur' *(Green Giant)*	1/2 cup	35	1	8	260	2	0.0	0
whole, drained	1 beet	7	0	2	47	0	0.0	0
whole, drained	1 cup	51	1	12	316	3	0.2	0
whole, small *(Freshlike)*	1/2 cup	40	1	9	260	0	0.0	0
Jarred								
pickled *(Stokely)*	1/2 cup	90	1	22	280	0	0.0	0
pickled, sliced *(Stokely)*	1 oz	25	0	6	100	0	0.0	0
pickled, whole *(Stokely)*	1 oz	25	0	6	100	0	0.0	0
BEET GREENS								
boiled, drained, 1-inch pieces	1 cup	39	4	8	347	4	0.3	0
boiled, drained, 1-inch pieces	1/2 cup	19	2	4	174	2	0.1	0
raw	1 cup	7	1	2	76	1	0.0	0
raw	1 med leaf	6	1	1	64	1	0.0	0
raw, 1-inch pieces	1/2 cup	4	0	1	38	1	0.0	0
BEET ROOT JUICE *(Biotta)* bottled	6 fl oz	75	2	16	128	0	0.1	0
BELL PEPPER. See PEPPER, BELL.								
BELLYFISH. See MONKFISH.								
BERRIES. See also individual listings.								
mixed, Oregon, frozen *(Flav-R-Pac)*	4.9 oz	70	1	16	20	6	0.0	0
BISCOTTI								
chocolate chip, gluten-free *(Ener-G Foods)*	1 serving	122	1	17	136	0	5.1	0
orange walnut, gluten-free *(Gluten Free Pantry)*	1 serving	110	1	22	25	1	2.5	0
plain, gluten-free *(Ener-G Foods)*	1 serving	81	1	11	96	0	3.3	0
BISCUIT								
dough, mixed-grain	1 oz	75	2	13	190	na	1.6	0
dough, mixed-grain, baked, 2.25-inch diam	1 biscuit	116	3	21	295	na	2.5	0
dough, plain or buttermilk	1 oz	90	2	12	314	0	3.8	0
dough, plain or buttermilk, baked	1 oz	98	2	13	341	0	4.2	0
dough, plain or buttermilk, baked, 2.25-inch diam	1 biscuit	93	2	13	325	0	4.0	0
dough, plain or buttermilk, less fat	1 oz	73	2	13	354	0	1.3	0
dough, plain or buttermilk, less fat, baked	1 oz	85	2	16	411	1	1.5	0
dough, plain or buttermilk, less fat, baked, 2.25-inch diam	1 biscuit	63	2	12	305	0	1.1	0
(Awrey's)								
2-inch square	1 oz	80	2	12	260	0	3.0	0
3-inch square	2 oz	160	4	23	520	1	5.0	0

Food Name	Serv. Size	Total Cal.	Prot. gms	Carbs gms	Sod. mgs	Fiber gms	Fat gms	Chol. mgs
(Bridgford) frozen	2 oz	180	4	28	632	0	6.0	1
(Ballard)								
light, oven-ready, 'Extra Lights'	1 piece	50	1	10	180	0	0.0	0
(Big Country)								
butter	1 biscuit	100	2	13	300	0	4.0	0
'Butter Tastin"	1 piece	100	2	14	320	0	4.0	0
buttermilk	1 biscuit	100	2	14	300	0	4.0	0
Southern style	1 biscuit	100	2	14	300	0	4.0	0
(1869 Brand)								
baking powder	1 biscuit	100	2	12	300	0	5.0	0
'Butter Tastin"	1 piece	100	2	12	300	0	5.0	0
buttermilk	1 biscuit	100	2	12	300	0	5.0	0
(Good 'N Buttery)								
fluffy	1 biscuit	90	1	11	270	0	5.0	0
(Hungry Jack)								
buttermilk, 'Extra Rich'	1 piece	50	1	9	180	0	1.0	0
flaky	2 biscuits	170	3	23	600	1	7.0	0
flaky, 'Honey Tastin"	2 biscuits	180	3	25	580	1	7.0	0
flaky, Southern style	1 biscuit	80	2	12	300	0	4.0	0
fluffy	2 biscuits	180	3	23	570	1	8.0	0
(Lite Fluff) buttermilk, ready to bake, Texas style	1 biscuit	90	2	16	250	0	2.5	0
(Mrs. Wright's)								
butter-flavored, ready to bake, 'Jumbos'	1 biscuit	180	4	24	360	2	9.0	0
butter-flavored, ready to bake, Texas style	1 biscuit	100	2	15	260	1	3.0	0
buttermilk, ready to bake, 'Jumbos'	1 biscuit	180	4	23	360	2	9.0	0
buttermilk, ready to bake, Texas style	1 biscuit	90	2	16	250	0	2.5	0
(Pillsbury)								
'Big Premium Heat 'n Eat'	2 biscuits	280	5	32	610	0	15.0	0
butter, 'Grands'	1 biscuit	200	4	23	580	1	10.0	0
buttermilk, 'Grands'	1 biscuit	200	4	23	570	1	10.0	0
buttermilk, 'Heat 'n Eat'	2 biscuits	170	4	27	530	0	5.0	0
buttermilk, light, 'Extra Lights'	3 biscuits	150	4	29	490	1	2.0	0
cinnamon-raisin	1 biscuit	200	4	28	580	1	8.0	0
flaky, 'Grands'	1 biscuit	190	4	23	530	0	8.0	0
home style, 'Grands'	1 biscuit	190	4	24	600	1	9.0	0
Southern style 'Grands'	1 biscuit	200	4	23	580	1	10.0	0
w/cinnamon and raisin, 'Grands'	1 biscuit	190	3	27	540	0	7.0	0
(Roman Meal)								
	2 biscuits	180	4	32	456	1	3.8	0
oat bran, w/honey and nuts	1 biscuit	131	2	20	278	1	4.7	0
white, 'Premium'	1 biscuit	127	2	19	308	0	4.7	0
(Stilwell) buttermilk, 3-inch diam	1 biscuit	210	4	30	370	0	9.0	0
(Wonder)	1 piece	80	2	14	140	1	1.0	0
BISCUIT, TOASTER								
(Northridge) English muffin	1 muffin	80	2	16	135	0	1.0	0
(Oroweat) 'Australian'	1 biscuit	180	6	30	440	1	5.0	0
(Oroweat) w/cinnamon and raisin	1 biscuit	200	5	34	410	1	5.0	0
BISCUIT DOUGH								
buttermilk, artificial flavor, refrigerated *(Pillsbury)*	1 serving	154	5	30	547	na	1.4	na
BISCUIT MIX								
plain or buttermilk, dry mix	1 cup	548	10	81	1633	3	19.7	3
plain or buttermilk, dry mix	1 oz	121	2	18	362	1	4.4	1
plain or buttermilk, prepared	1 oz	95	2	14	271	1	3.4	1
plain or buttermilk, prepared, 3-inch diam	1 biscuit	191	4	28	544	1	6.9	2
(Arrowhead Mills)	2 oz	100	4	19	96	0	1.0	0
(Bisquick)	1/2 cup	240	4	37	700	0	8.0	0
(Bisquick)	1/3 cup	170	3	25	481	1	6.0	0

Food Name	Serv. Size	Total Cal.	Prot. gms	Carbs gms	Sod. mgs	Fiber gms	Fat gms	Chol. mgs
(Gold Medal)	1/3 cup	170	3	26	470	1	6.0	0
(Health Valley) buttermilk, 'Biscuit & Pancake Mix'	1 oz	100	4	20	170	3	1.0	0
(Kentucky Kernel) all natural, dry mix	1/4 cup	171	3	28	659	1	5.0	0
(Krusteaz)								
prepared, 2-inch diam	1 biscuit	90	2	14	260	0	3.0	1
w/cinnamon and raisin, glazed, prepared, 3-inch diam	1 biscuit	200	2	39	150	1	4.0	0
(Martha White)								
'BixMix' prepared w/2% milk	1 biscuit	90	2	15	240	0	2.0	2
buttermilk, dry mix	1 serving	171	3	26	504	na	5.9	na
(Robin Hood) 'Pouch Mix' 0.7 oz mix prepared w/skim milk	1/8 mix	90	2	14	270	0	3.0	0
(Tone's) buttermilk	1 tsp	1	0	0	1	0	0.0	0
BISON/American buffalo								
raw	1 oz	31	6	0	15	0	0.5	18
ribeye, trimmed to 0-inch fat, raw	1 oz	33	6	0	14	na	0.7	18
ribeye, trimmed to 0-inch fat, raw	4 oz	131	25	0	54	na	2.7	70
roasted	3 oz	122	24	0	48	0	2.1	70
roasted, boneless, yield from 1 lb raw	11.9 oz	486	97	0	194	0	8.2	279
shoulder, trimmed to 0-inch fat	4 oz	123	24	0	67	na	2.4	75
shoulder, trimmed to 0-inch fat, raw	1 oz	31	6	0	17	na	0.6	19
top round, trimmed to 0-inch fat, raw	1 oz	31	6	0	14	na	0.5	19
top round, trimmed to 0-inch fat, raw	4 oz	124	25	0	58	na	1.8	75
BITTER GOURD. See BALSAM PEAR.								
BITTER LEMON. See under SOFT DRINKS AND MIXERS.								
BLACK BEAN. See BEAN, BLACK.								
BLACK CHERRY JUICE								
(Knudsen)	8 fl oz	180	2	43	40	na	0.0	0
(Smucker's) 'Naturally 100%'	8 fl oz	130	0	31	10	0	0.0	0
BLACK CURRANT. See under CURRANT.								
BLACK PEPPER. See PEPPER, GROUND, BLACK.								
BLACK TURTLE BEAN. See BEAN, BLACK.								
BLACKBERRIES								
Canned, in heavy syrup, w/liquid	1 cup	236	3	59	8	9	0.4	0
Fresh, raw	1 cup	75	1	18	0	8	0.6	0
Frozen								
Marion *(Flav-R-Pac)*	1 cup	80	2	19	5	7	0.0	0
unsweetened	18-oz pkg	326	6	80	5	26	2.2	0
unsweetened	1 cup	97	2	24	2	8	0.6	0
BLACKBERRY SYRUP. See under SYRUP.								
BLACK-EYED PEAS/cowpeas								
Canned								
(Allens)	1/2 cup	100	7	18	370	0	1.0	0
Crowder, 'Fresh' *(Allens)*	1/2 cup	80	5	15	370	0	1.0	0
Crowder, frozen *(Seabrook)*	3 oz	130	8	23	0	1	1.0	0
Crowder, seasoned w/pork, canned *(Luck's)*	1/2 cup	120	6	18	280	4	3.0	3
Crowder, Southern, mature seeds, boiled, drained	1 cup	200	13	36	7	11	0.9	0
Crowder, Southern, mature seeds, w/pork	1 cup	199	7	40	840	8	3.8	17
immature seeds, drained	1 cup	160	5	34	7	8	0.6	0
mature *(A&P)*	7.5 oz	120	7	20	410	0	1.0	0
mature *(Allens)*	1/2 cup	105	5	18	300	0	1.0	0
mature *(Green Giant)*	1/2 cup	90	7	18	300	4	1.0	0
mature *(Joan of Arc)*	1/2 cup	90	7	18	300	4	1.0	0
packed from fresh shelled *(Bush's Best)*	1/2 cup	70	5	16	350	3	0.0	0
packed from soaked dry *(Bush's Best)*	1/2 cup	70	5	16	350	3	0.0	0
seasoned w/bacon *(Bush's Best)*	1/2 cup	90	7	16	420	3	1.0	0
seasoned w/pork *(Luck's)*	1/2 cup	130	6	18	280	3	3.0	3

Food Name	Serv. Size	Total Cal.	Prot. gms	Carbs gms	Sod. mgs	Fiber gms	Fat gms	Chol. mgs
'Sun-Vista' *(S&W)*	1/2 cup	70	6	15	550	4	0.0	0
w/jalapeño peppers *(Ranch Style)*	1/2 cup	110	6	19	660	4	0.5	5
w/snaps *(Allens)*	1/2 cup	100	5	20	370	0	1.0	0
Dried								
Catjang, mature seeds, boiled, drained	1 cup	200	14	35	32	6	1.2	0
Catjang, mature seeds, uncooked	1 cup	573	40	100	97	18	3.5	0
Crowder, Southern, mature seeds, uncooked	1 cup	561	39	100	27	18	2.1	0
Crowder, Southern, mature seeds, uncooked	1 tbsp	35	2	6	2	1	0.1	0
immature seeds, uncooked	1 cup	131	4	27	6	7	0.5	0
mature, boiled *(A&P)*	1 cup	230	15	41	15	0	1.0	0
Fresh								
leafy tips, boiled, drained, chopped	1 cup	12	2	1	3	na	0.1	0
leafy tips, raw, chopped	1 cup	10	1	2	3	na	0.1	0
leafy tips, raw, whole	1 med leaf	1	0	0	0	na	0.0	0
young pods w/seeds, boiled, drained	1 cup	32	2	7	3	na	0.3	0
young pods w/seeds, raw, chopped	1 cup	41	3	9	4	na	0.3	0
young pods w/seeds, raw, whole	1 med pod	5	0	1	0	na	0.0	0
Frozen								
(Flav-R-Pac)	1/2 cup	110	7	21	10	4	1.0	0
(Freshlike)	3.3 oz	130	9	23	5	0	1.0	0
(Frosty Acres)	3.3 oz	130	9	23	6	1	1.0	0
(Pictsweet)	1/2 cup	110	7	21	10	4	1.0	0
(Seabrook)	3.3 oz	130	9	23	6	1	1.0	0
(Southern)	3.5 oz	136	9	24	20	0	0.7	0
(Veg-All)	3.3 oz	130	9	23	5	0	1.0	0
immature seeds, drained	1 cup	224	14	40	9	11	1.1	0
immature seeds, unprepared	10-oz pkg	395	26	71	17	14	2.0	0
immature seeds, unprepared	1 cup	222	14	40	10	8	1.1	0
BLINTZ								
apple, kosher *(Empire Kosher)*	2 blintzes	220	6	36	260	5	5.5	5
blueberry *(Golden)*	1 crepe	90	2	18	150	0	1.0	10
blueberry, kosher *(Empire Kosher)*	2 blintzes	190	4	36	260	2	4.0	10
cheese, kosher *(Empire Kosher)*	2 blintzes	200	11	29	310	3	6.0	20
cheese, low-fat *(Golden)*	1 crepe	80	6	13	135	0	2.0	13
cherry *(Golden)*	1 crepe	95	3	18	145	0	1.0	5
cherry, kosher *(Empire Kosher)*	2 blintzes	200	5	38	280	3	4.0	10
potato, kosher *(Empire Kosher)*	2 blintzes	190	6	32	530	3	6.0	10
BLUE CRAB. See under CRAB.								
BLUEBERRIES								
Canned, in heavy syrup, w/liquid	1 cup	225	2	56	8	4	0.8	0
Fresh								
raw	1 pint	225	3	57	24	11	1.5	0
raw	50 berries	38	0	10	4	2	0.3	0
Frozen								
sweetened	10-oz pkg	230	1	62	3	6	0.4	0
sweetened, thawed	1 cup	186	1	50	2	5	0.3	0
unsweetened	20-oz pkg	289	2	69	6	15	3.6	0
unsweetened, unthawed	1 cup	79	1	19	2	4	1.0	0
(Flav-R-Pac)	1 cup	70	1	16	10	4	0.0	0
BLUEBERRY JUICE. See also FRUIT DRINK, FRUIT DRINK MIX; FRUIT JUICE BLEND.								
mountain blueberry, organic *(Mountain Sun)*	8 fl oz	108	0	27	0	0	0.0	0
BLUEBERRY TOPPING *(Flav-R-Pac)*	2 tbsp	40	0	10	5	1	0.0	0
BLUEFIN TUNA. See under TUNA.								
BLUEFISH								
baked, broiled, grilled, or microwaved	3 oz	135	22	0	65	0	4.6	65
raw	3 oz	105	17	0	51	0	3.6	50

Food Name	Serv. Size	Total Cal.	Prot. gms	Carbs gms	Sod. mgs	Fiber gms	Fat gms	Chol. mgs
BOAR, WILD								
raw	1 oz	35	6	0	na	0	0.9	na
roasted	3 oz	136	24	0	51	0	3.7	65
roasted, boneless, yield from 1 lb raw	11.9 oz	544	96	0	204	0	14.9	262
BOBWHITE. See QUAIL.								
BOK CHOY/Chinese cabbage/napa cabbage/pak-choi/pe-tsai								
boiled, drained	1 leaf	2	0	0	1	0	0.0	0
boiled, drained, shredded	1 cup	20	3	3	58	3	0.3	0
fresh, shredded *(Dole)*	1/2 cup	5	1	1	23	0	0.1	0
raw	1 head	109	13	18	546	8	1.7	0
raw	1 leaf	2	0	0	9	0	0.0	0
raw, shredded	1 cup	12	1	2	7	2	0.2	0
BONITO. See under TUNA.								
BORAGE, raw, 1-inch pieces	1 cup	19	2	3	71	na	0.6	0
BORECOLE. See KALE.								
BORLOTTI. See BEAN, CRANBERRY.								
BOYSENBERRIES								
Canned, in heavy syrup	1 cup	225	3	57	8	7	0.3	0
Frozen								
(Flav-R-Pac)	1 cup	59	2	20	18	7	0.0	0
unsweetened	10-oz pkg	142	3	35	3	11	0.7	0
unsweetened	1 cup	66	1	16	1	5	0.3	0
BOYSENBERRY JUICE (Smucker's) 'Naturally 100%'	8 fl oz	120	0	30	10	0	0.0	0
BRAMBLE. See RASPBERRY.								
BRATWURST. See under SAUSAGE.								
BRAZIL NUT/paranut								
dried, unblanched, approx 6-8 kernels	1 oz	186	4	4	1	2	18.8	0
dried, unblanched, shelled, approx 32 kernels	1 cup	918	20	18	3	8	92.7	0
BREAD								
ALFALFA SPROUT								
(Vermont Bread Company)								
	1 slice	80	2	15	115	2	1.0	0
'Sandwich'	1 slice	90	3	17	130	2	1.5	0
APPLE WALNUT *(Arnold)*	1 slice	64	2	13	103	1	1.3	1
APPLE HONEY *(Brownberry)* wheat	1 slice	69	2	11	148	2	1.9	0
AUSTRIAN *(Du Jour)* brown and serve	1 oz	70	3	13	140	1	1.0	0
BARBECUE *(Colombo Brand)* 'BBQ Loaf'	2 oz	139	8	24	318	0	1.6	0
BRAN								
(Brownberry)								
'Bran'nola'	1 slice	85	4	18	137	3	1.4	0
whole, 'Natural'	1 slice	58	2	12	167	2	1.4	0
w/raisins	1 slice	61	2	12	108	2	1.3	0
(Earth Grains) 'Gold'N Bran'	1 oz	70	3	12	150	0	1.0	0
(Oroweat) original, natural, 'Bran'nola'	1 slice	100	4	19	160	2	1.0	0
(Pepperidge Farm) honey, 1.5-lb loaf	1 slice	90	3	18	160	1	1.0	0
BROWN								
canned	1 slice	88	2	19	284	2	0.7	0
canned	1 oz	55	1	12	179	1	0.4	0
(B&M)								
plain, 1/2-inch slice	1 slice	92	2	21	345	2	0.0	0
w/raisins, 1/2-inch slice *(B&M)*	1 slice	94	2	22	320	2	0.0	0
(Friends)								
plain, 1/2-inch slice	1 slice	92	2	21	345	2	0.0	0
w/raisins, 1/2-inch slice *(Friends)*	1 slice	94	2	22	320	2	0.0	0
(S&W) canned, 'New England'	2 slices	76	2	17	172	0	0.0	0
BROWN RICE								
(Ener-G Foods)								
gluten free	1 slice	122	1	20	25	1	4.3	1

Food Name	Serv. Size	Total Cal.	Prot. gms	Carbs gms	Sod. mgs	Fiber gms	Fat gms	Chol. mgs
gluten free, yeast-free	1 slice	154	1	25	282	3	3.5	0
(Mystic Lake Dairy) wheat gluten-free	1 slice	155	2	22	0	0	6.0	0
BUTTERMILK								
(Grant's Farm)	1 slice	70	3	12	190	0	1.0	0
(Oroweat)	1 slice	100	4	20	210	1	1.0	0
CINNAMON RAISIN								
(Arizona Original Homestyle) 100% stone ground	1 slice	116	4	23	130	2	0.0	0
(Arnold)	1 slice	67	2	13	86	1	1.4	2
(Pepperidge Farm)	1 slice	90	2	16	100	2	2.0	0
CINNAMON OATMEAL *(Oatmeal Goodness)*	1 slice	90	4	15	140	1	2.0	0
CINNAMON SWIRL *(Pepperidge Farm)*	1 slice	90	2	15	110	2	3.0	0
DARK *(Hollywood)*	1 slice	70	3	13	160	1	1.0	0
DATE								
(Dromedary) date nut roll	1/2-inch slice	80	1	13	160	0	2.0	0
(Thomas') date nut loaf	1 oz	80	1	15	160	1	2.5	5
EGG								
5 x 3 x 1/2-inch slices	1 slice	115	4	19	197	1	2.4	20
(Ener-G Foods) gluten-free	1 slice	176	3	23	83	1	6.8	7
FLAXSEED *(Natural Ovens)* 'Flax 'N Honey'	1 slice	70	3	15	70	3	0.5	0
FRENCH								
large slices, approx 5 x 2-1/2 x 1 inch	1 slice	96	3	18	213	1	1.1	0
medium slices, approx 4-3/4 x 4 x 1/2 inch	1 slice	69	2	13	152	1	0.8	0
small slices, approx 2-1/2 x 2 x 1/2 inch	1 slice	41	1	8	91	0	0.5	0
(Colombo Brand)								
extra sour	2 oz	150	8	27	311	0	1.3	0
sweet, 'French Stick'	2 oz	154	7	27	331	0	1.9	0
(DiCarlo) 'Parisian'	1 slice	70	3	13	180	1	1.0	0
(Du Jour) brown and serve	1 oz	70	3	13	140	1	1.0	0
(Farm Hearth) twin loaves	1 oz	80	3	15	160	0	1.0	0
(Monterey Baking) high-fiber, low-calorie	1 slice	48	2	10	98	3	0.1	0
(Pepperidge Farm)								
enriched	1 slice	130	4	25	280	1	1.5	0
enriched, twin loaves	1 slice	130	4	26	270	1	1.5	0
'Hearth'	1 oz	75	3	14	160	1	1.0	0
(Pillsbury)	1 slice	150	6	28	370	1	1.0	0
GARLIC								
(Campione) frozen	1 serving	101	2	12	154	1	4.7	na
(Cole's) mini-loaf, ready-to-serve	1.8 oz	180	4	21	290	1	8.0	2
(Colombo Brand)	2 oz	185	6	17	331	0	10.1	0
(Mamma Bella)								
frozen	2 slices	150	3	16	240	1	8.0	0
sliced	2 slices	160	3	16	260	1	9.0	5
(Marie Callender's) original	1 piece	190	4	25	290	2	8.0	0
(Pepperidge Farm)								
crusty, Italian	1 serving	186	4	21	200	na	9.6	5
heat and serve	1.7 oz	170	4	19	240	3	9.0	20
HAWAIIAN *(King's Hawaiian Bread)*	2 oz	180	6	30	160	2	4.0	20
HEALTH *(Brownberry)* 'Health Nut'	1 slice	71	2	12	158	3	2.6	0
HONEY BRAN *(Pepperidge Farm)*	1 slice	90	3	18	160	1	1.0	0
HONEY NUT *(Roman Meal)* w/rice bran	1 slice	71	3	13	127	1	1.6	0
HONEY WHEAT BERRY *(Arnold)*	1 slice	77	3	17	143	2	1.2	0
INDIAN FRY								
Navajo, 10.5-inch diam	1 serving	526	11	85	1112	3	15.2	0
Navajo, 5-inch diam	1 serving	296	6	48	626	2	8.6	0
ITALIAN								
large slices, approx 4-1/2 x 3-1/4 x 3/4 inch	1 slice	81	3	15	175	1	1.1	0
medium slices	1 slice	54	2	10	117	1	0.7	0

Food Name	Serv. Size	Total Cal.	Prot. gms	Carbs gms	Sod. mgs	Fiber gms	Fat gms	Chol. mgs
small slices, approx 3-1/4 x 2-1/2 x 1/2 inch	1 slice	27	1	5	58	0	0.3	0
(Arnold)								
'Francisco International'	1 slice	72	3	14	190	1	1.1	0
'Francisco International' sliced thick	1 slice	66	2	14	111	1	0.8	0
light, 'Bakery'	1 slice	45	2	10	90	2	0.5	0
(Brownberry) 'Light'	1 slice	44	2	10	89	2	0.5	0
(Monk's) 'Hi-Fibre'	1 slice	70	3	13	80	1	1.0	0
(Monterey Baking) twist	1 slice	71	2	15	148	0	0.2	0
(Pepperidge Farm)								
enriched, brown and serve	1 slice	130	4	24	260	1	2.0	0
'Hearth'	1 oz	80	2	14	150	0	1.0	0
(Wonder) 'Family'	1 slice	70	2	13	160	1	1.0	0
LIGHT *(Hollywood)*	1 slice	70	3	13	150	1	1.0	0
MILLET, 'Sunny Millet' *(Natural Ovens)*	1 slice	50	3	15	80	7	0.0	0
MIXED GRAIN								
7-grain, w/whole grain, large slices	1 slice	80	3	15	156	2	1.2	0
7-grain, w/whole-grain, medium slices	1 slice	65	3	12	127	2	1.0	0
(Arizona Original Homestyle) 9-grain,								
100% stone-ground	1 slice	94	4	23	102	2	0.0	0
(Arnold) bran, nutty, 'Bran'nola'	1 slice	85	4	17	144	3	1.6	0
(Aunt Hattie's) 7-grain	1 slice	100	4	17	200	0	2.0	0
(Beefsteak) multigrain	1 slice	70	3	11	130	2	1.0	0
(BreadMill Bakery) 5-grain, organic	1 slice	122	6	23	298	0	1.0	0
(Brownberry) bran, 'Bran'nola Nutty Grains'	1 slice	85	4	17	144	3	1.6	0
(Colonial) w/honey, 'Family Recipe'	1 slice	70	3	14	180	0	1.0	0
(Earth Grains) 12-grain	1 oz	70	3	13	140	0	1.0	0
(Food for Life) multigrain, w/wheat, rice, and almond,								
gluten-free	1 slice	120	5	22	5	0	2.5	0
(Grant's Farm)								
7-grain	1 slice	60	3	13	140	0	1.0	0
7-grain, 'Light'	1 slice	40	2	9	115	0	1.0	0
w/honey	1 slice	70	3	13	170	0	1.0	0
(Healthy Choice)								
multigrain	1 slice	60	3	12	120	2	0.5	0
7-grain	1 slice	80	4	18	170	3	1.0	0
(Home Pride) 7-grain	1 slice	70	3	12	140	1	1.0	0
(Kilpatrick's) w/honey, 'Family Recipe'	1 slice	70	3	14	180	0	1.0	0
(Monterey Baking)								
9-grain	1 slice	111	4	23	220	1	0.4	0
9-grain, low salt	1 slice	111	4	23	50	1	0.4	0
(Natural Ovens)								
7-grain	1 slice	70	3	15	70	3	0.5	0
whole wheat, flax, millet, and soy, 'Stay Trim'	1 slice	50	2	15	90	7	0.0	0
(Oroweat)								
9-grain, 'Light'	1 slice	40	2	10	135	2	0.0	0
12-grain	1 slice	110	5	20	210	1	2.0	0
(Pepperidge Farm)								
multigrain, granola, w/oat and honey	1 slice	60	2	12	105	2	2.0	0
7-grain, 'Hearty Slice'	2 slices	180	5	36	340	2	2.0	0
(Rainbo) w/honey, 'Family Recipe'	1 slice	70	3	14	180	0	1.0	0
(Roman Meal)								
multigrain, 'Round Top'	1 slice	67	3	13	140	1	0.8	0
multigrain, sliced, sandwich thin	1 slice	55	2	11	114	1	0.7	0
multigrain, 'Sun Grain'	1 slice	68	3	12	140	2	1.4	0
(Rudi's) 'Ancient Grain Bread'	1 slice	85	3	14	215	0	2.0	0
(Vermont Bread Company) 'Soft 10'	1 piece	90	3	16	130	2	2.0	0
(Weight Watchers) multigrain	1 slice	40	2	9	100	0	1.0	0

Food Name	Serv. Size	Total Cal.	Prot. gms	Carbs gms	Sod. mgs	Fiber gms	Fat gms	Chol. mgs
NUT *(Orowoat)* 'Health Nut'	1 slice	110	4	20	200	2	2.0	0
OAT								
(Colonial) split top, 'Family Recipe'	1 slice	70	3	13	140	0	1.0	0
(Earth Grains) w/honey and nuts	1 oz	80	3	14	85	0	2.0	0
(Kilpatrick's) split top, 'Family Recipe'	1 slice	70	3	13	140	0	1.0	0
(Oroweat) light, 'Country Oat'	1 slice	40	2	10	135	2	0.0	0
(Pepperidge Farm)								
hearty, crunchy	1 slice	100	4	17	180	2	2.0	0
honey granola	1 slice	60	2	12	105	2	2.0	0
(Rainbo) split top 'Family Recipe'	1 slice	70	3	13	140	0	1.0	0
OAT BRAN								
	1 slice	71	3	12	122	1	1.3	0
lower calorie	1 slice	46	2	9	81	3	0.7	0
(Awrey's)	1 slice	50	2	10	130	1	0.0	0
(BreadMill Bakery)								
organic, 'Light'	1 slice	113	4	22	229	0	1.0	0
w/honey, whole wheat, organic	1 slice	121	5	23	315	0	1.0	0
(Earth Grains) w/honey	1 oz	80	3	13	105	0	1.0	0
(Grant's Farm)	1 slice	70	3	14	140	0	1.0	0
(Monterey Baking)								
	1 slice	100	3	18	160	3	1.5	0
low-salt	1 slice	99	4	16	50	3	4.1	0
(Oatmeal Goodness) 'Light'	1 slice	40	2	6	90	0	1.0	0
(Oroweat) natural, 'Bran'nola Country'	2 slices	230	8	39	390	3	4.0	0
(Roman Meal)								
'Split-Top'	1 slice	68	3	13	140	1	0.9	0
w/honey	1 slice	71	3	13	130	1	1.2	0
w/honey and nut	1 slice	72	3	12	130	1	1.6	0
(Vermont Bread Company)								
w/oatmeal, low-sodium	1 slice	70	2	14	120	2	1.0	0
w/oatmeal, 'Sandwich Bread'	1 slice	100	3	18	120	2	1.5	0
(Weight Watchers)	1 slice	40	1	10	100	0	1.0	0
OATMEAL								
	1 slice	73	2	13	162	1	1.2	0
lower calorie	1 slice	48	2	10	89	na	0.8	0
(Arnold) light, 'Bakery'	1 slice	44	2	10	98	2	0.6	0
(Grant's Farm) w/toasted almonds	1 slice	80	3	14	135	0	1.0	0
(Hearty Grains) twists	1 serving	80	2	15	120	1	2.0	0
(Oatmeal Goodness)								
cinnamon	1 slice	90	4	15	140	1	2.0	0
w/bran	1 slice	90	4	15	140	1	2.0	0
w/sunflower seeds	1 slice	90	4	15	140	1	2.0	0
	1 slice	90	3	17	200	1	1.0	0
'Light Style'	1 slice	45	2	9	95	1	0.0	0
1.5 lb. loaf	1 slice	90	3	17	200	1	1.0	0
'Very Thin'	1 slice	40	1	8	80	0	1.0	0
OATNUT *(Oroweat)*	1 slice	100	3	18	200	1	2.0	0
ORANGE RAISIN *(Brownberry)*	1 slice	67	2	13	83	1	1.2	0
PITA								
white, large, 6.5-inch diam	1 pita	165	5	33	322	1	0.7	0
white, small, 4-inch diam	1 pita	77	3	16	150	1	0.3	0
whole wheat, large, 6.5-inch diam	1 pita	170	6	35	340	5	1.7	0
whole wheat, small, 4-inch diam	1 pita	74	3	15	149	2	0.7	0
(Kangaroo) w/onion, nonfat, sliced, no oils	1 pita	75	4	15	160	0	0.0	0
(Sahara)								
oat bran	1/2 piece	66	2	15	163	2	0.3	0
100% whole wheat	1 pita	130	7	28	310	5	1.0	0

Food Name	Serv. Size	Total Cal.	Prot. gms	Carbs gms	Sod. mgs	Fiber gms	Fat gms	Chol. mgs
original	1 pita	150	6	31	290	1	1.0	0
sourdough	1 pita	150	5	33	320	2	0.5	0
white	1/2 piece	79	3	16	147	0	0.5	0
white, mini	1 slice	79	3	16	147	0	0.5	0
whole wheat	1 piece	150	6	28	320	1	2.0	0
(Vermont Bread Company)	1/2 pita	80	3	16	90	3	0.5	0
POTATO *(Ener-G Foods)* gluten-free	1 slice	170	3	24	77	1	5.4	0
PROTEIN, w/gluten	1 slice	47	2	8	104	1	0.4	0
PUMPERNICKEL								
regular slices	1 slice	65	2	12	174	2	0.8	0
snack size	1 slice	18	1	3	47	0	0.2	0
thick slices, approx 5 x 4 x 3/8 inch	1 slice	80	3	15	215	2	1.0	0
thin slices	1 slice	50	2	10	134	1	0.6	0
(Arnold)	1 slice	70	3	15	198	1	0.9	0
(Pepperidge Farm)								
'Family'	1 slice	80	3	15	230	2	1.0	0
small, 'Party'	4 slices	60	2	12	160	1	1.0	0
RAISIN								
large slices	1 slice	88	3	17	125	1	1.4	0
medium slices	1 slice	71	2	14	101	1	1.1	0
thin slices	1 slice	63	2	12	90	1	1.0	0
(BreadMill Bakery) whole wheat, organic	1 slice	120	5	24	327	0	1.0	0
(Brownberry)								
bran	1 slice	61	2	12	108	2	1.3	0
cinnamon	1 slice	66	1	13	107	1	1.3	0
walnut	1 slice	68	2	11	96	2	2.7	0
(Ener-G Foods)								
gluten-free, egg-free	1 slice	116	1	20	139	1	2.7	0
gluten-free, w/egg	1 slice	154	3	32	56	2	1.5	0
(Monk's) cinnamon	1 slice	70	3	10	85	0	2.0	0
(Northridge) walnut, royal	1 slice	90	2	16	90	0	2.0	0
(Pepperidge Farm)								
cinnamon swirl	1 slice	90	2	16	100	1	2.0	0
(Pillsbury) oatmeal, 'Hearty Grain'	1 serving	90	2	16	210	1	2.0	0
(Vermont Bread Company)								
cinnamon, low-fat, low-sodium	1 slice	80	3	17	115	2	0.5	0
RICE								
(Ener-G Foods)								
gluten-free, 'Papa's Loaf'	1 slice	144	1	19	98	3	5.9	0
white rice, yeast free, gluten-free	1 slice	147	1	24	272	3	3.1	0
(French Meadow)								
sourdough, whole grain, yeast-free, organic	1.35 oz	84	4	17	180	3	1.0	0
RICE BRAN								
	1 slice	66	2	12	119	1	1.2	0
(Monk's) golden	1 slice	70	3	14	80	2	1.0	0
(Roman Meal)								
	1 slice	70	3	12	132	1	1.5	0
w/honey and nuts	1 slice	71	3	13	127	1	1.6	0
RICE STARCH *(Med Diet)* low-protein	1 slice	155	0	29	25	6	4.0	0
RYE								
lower calorie, medium slices	1 slice	47	2	9	93	3	0.7	0
lower calorie, thick slices	1 slice	65	3	13	130	4	0.9	0
lower calorie, thin slices	1 slice	41	2	8	81	2	0.6	0
regular, medium slices	1 slice	83	3	15	211	2	1.1	0
regular, snack size	1 slice	18	1	3	46	0	0.2	0
regular, thin slices	1 slice	52	2	10	132	1	0.7	0
(Arnold) w/dill	1 slice	71	3	14	187	1	1.0	0

Food Name	Serv. Size	Total Cal.	Prot. gms	Carbs gms	Sod. mgs	Fiber gms	Fat gms	Chol. mgs
(Beefsteak)								
'Hearty'	1 slice	70	3	13	180	1	1.0	0
'Mild'	1 slice	70	3	13	180	1	1.0	0
'Soft'	1 slice	70	3	13	170	1	1.0	0
w/onion	1 slice	70	3	12	170	1	1.0	0
w/wheat berries	1 slice	70	3	13	160	1	1.0	0
(Braun's) 'Old Allegheny'	1 slice	70	3	13	160	1	1.0	0
(Brownberry)								
seedless, natural, sliced thin	1 slice	45	2	10	118	1	0.6	0
w/caraway, 'Natural'	1 slice	73	3	15	185	1	0.8	0
(Earth Grains) sliced very thin, 'Light'	1 oz	70	3	14	230	0	1.0	0
(Food for Life) white, 100% wheat-free,								
no preservatives	2 slices	217	4	42	257	0	4.0	0
(Grant's Farm) cracked rye, w/honey	1 slice	70	3	13	190	0	1.0	0
(Levy's)								
Jewish, seeded	1 slice	76	3	16	181	1	0.9	0
Jewish, seedless	1 slice	75	3	16	178	1	0.8	0
(Mrs. Wright's) Jewish, w/seeds	2 slices	110	3	20	320	1	1.5	0
(Natural Ovens) mild	1 slice	70	3	13	70	4	0.5	0
(Oroweat) hearty, 'Light'	1 slice	40	2	10	135	2	0.0	0
(Pepperidge Farm)								
Dijon	1 slice	50	2	9	170	1	1.0	0
Dijon, 'Hearty'	1 slice	70	3	15	260	2	1.0	0
seedless, 'Family'	1 slice	80	3	16	210	2	1.0	0
small, 'Party'	4 slices	60	2	12	250	1	1.0	0
w/seeds, 'Family'	1 slice	80	3	16	220	2	1.0	0
(Vermont Bread Company)								
	1 slice	70	2	14	115	2	1.0	0
'Black Russian'	1 slice (1/2")	110	3	23	120	3	0.0	0
'Sandwich'	1 slice	100	3	18	120	3	1.5	0
(Weight Watchers)	1 slice	40	2	10	100	0	1.0	0
(Wonder)	1 slice	70	2	13	150	1	1.0	0
SOURDOUGH								
(Boudin)	2 slices	130	5	27	297	0	1.0	0
(DiCarlo)	1 slice	70	3	12	140	1	1.0	0
(Earth Grains) 'Light'	1 slice	40	2	9	115	0	1.0	0
(French Meadow) yeast-free, organic	2 oz	132	7	29	0	0	0.9	0
(Monterey Baking)	1 slice	75	3	16	152	1	0.2	0
(Rainbo) 'Light'	1 slice	40	2	9	110	2	1.0	0
SPELT *(French Meadow)* sprouted, yeast-free, organic	1.5 oz	93	5	18	160	4	0.0	0
SPLIT TOP *(Healthy Choice)*	1 slice	60	3	12	120	2	0.5	0
SUNFLOWER								
(BreadMill Bakery) w/whole wheat, organic	1 slice	129	6	21	287	0	2.0	0
(Monk's) w/bran	1 slice	70	3	12	80	2	1.0	0
SUNFLOWER SESAME *(Vermont Bread Company)*	1 slice	70	3	14	120	2	1.0	0
SWEET *(Vermont Bread Company)*	1 slice	70	3	15	120	2	0.0	0
TAPIOCA								
(Ener-G Foods)								
gluten free	1 slice	141	1	19	175	4	6.0	0
gluten free, thin sliced	1 slice	88	0	12	109	2	3.7	0
THREE SEED *(Monterey Baking)*	1 slice	100	4	16	220	na	2.5	0
VIENNA								
(Pepperidge Farm)								
'Light Style'	1 slice	45	2	10	100	1	0.0	0
sliced thick, 'Hearth'	1 slice	70	2	13	125	0	1.0	0
WHEAT								
(Arizona Original Homestyle)								
w/honey, 100% stone ground	1 slice	110	5	23	380	2	0.0	0

Food Name	Serv. Size	Total Cal.	Prot. gms	Carbs gms	Sod. mgs	Fiber gms	Fat gms	Chol. mgs
(Arnold)								
'Brick Oven'	1 slice	57	2	11	104	2	1.5	0
light, golden, 'Bakery'	1 slice	44	2	10	86	2	0.5	0
(Aunt Hattie's)								
buttertop	1 slice	70	3	13	140	0	1.0	5
w/buttermilk	1 slice	70	3	12	130	0	1.0	0
(Beefsteak)								
light, 'Hearty'	1 slice	70	3	11	160	1	1.0	0
'Soft'	1 slice	70	3	12	160	2	1.0	0
(BreadMill Bakery)								
w/oat bran and honey, all-natural, organic	1 slice	120	5	23	400	1	1.0	0
w/sunflower, all natural, organic	1 slice	130	6	1	380	2	2.0	0
(Brownberry)								
	1 slice	74	3	13	127	1	1.8	0
'Hearth'	1 oz	70	3	14	150	2	1.4	0
'Natural'	1 slice	80	3	17	183	2	1.3	0
w/apple and honey	1 slice	69	2	11	148	2	1.9	0
(Colonial)								
'Family Recipe'	1 slice	70	3	14	150	0	1.0	0
honey buttered, split top	1 slice	70	3	14	140	0	1.0	0
stone ground, 'Family Recipe'	1 slice	70	3	14	150	0	1.0	0
(Country Grain)	1 slice	70	3	12	160	1	1.0	0
(Earth Grains)								
cracked wheat	1 oz	70	2	12	180	0	1.0	0
'Light 35'	1 oz	35	2	8	100	0	1.0	0
sliced very thin	1 oz	70	2	13	150	0	1.0	0
(Fresh and Natural)	1 slice	70	3	13	140	2	1.0	0
(Grant's Farm)								
'Light'	1 slice	40	2	9	115	0	1.0	0
stone ground	1 slice	60	3	12	150	0	1.0	0
(Healthy Choice) honey wheat	1 slice	60	3	12	120	2	0.5	0
(Hearty Grains) cracked wheat, w/honey, twists	1 serving	80	2	14	120	1	2.0	0
(Home Pride)								
butter top wheat	1 slice	80	2	14	190	1	1.0	0
stone ground	1 slice	70	3	12	140	2	1.0	0
(Kamut) stone-ground, yeast-free, organic, frozen	1 slice	120	7	23	140	4	0.0	0
(Kilpatrick's)								
'Family Recipe'	1 slice	70	3	14	150	0	1.0	0
stone ground, 'Family Recipe'	1 slice	70	3	14	150	0	1.0	0
(Mrs. Wright's)								
	2 slices	100	4	18	240	2	1.5	0
crushed wheat, sliced, round top	1 slice	70	2	15	160	1	0.5	0
crushed wheat, sliced, sandwich thin	1 slice	60	2	12	130	1	0.5	0
dark wheat, 'Bran'nola'	1 slice	83	4	18	166	3	1.0	0
(Natural Ovens) cracked wheat	1 slice	80	4	16	70	3	0.5	0
(Oatmeal Goodness)								
w/oatmeal	1 slice	90	4	15	140	1	2.0	0
w/oatmeal, 'Light'	1 slice	40	2	6	90	0	1.0	0
(Pepperidge Farm)								
cracked wheat	1 slice	70	2	13	140	1	1.0	0
'Light Style'	1 slice	45	2	9	90	1	0.0	0
1.5-lb loaf	1 slice	90	3	18	190	2	2.0	0
sprouted	1 slice	70	3	11	100	2	2.0	0
2-lb loaf, 'Family'	1 slice	70	2	13	130	2	1.0	0
w/sesame, 'Hearty'	2 slices	190	7	36	340	3	3.0	0
(Pipin' Hot) thick sliced	1 slice	70	2	12	170	0	2.0	0
(Rainbo)								
'Family Recipe'	1 slice	70	3	14	150	0	1.0	0

Food Name	Serv. Size	Total Cal.	Prot. gms	Carbs gms	Sod. mgs	Fiber gms	Fat gms	Chol. mgs
honey buttered, split top	1 slice	70	3	14	140	0	1.0	0
'Light'	1 slice	40	2	9	100	2	1.0	0
stone ground, 'Family Recipe'	1 slice	70	3	14	150	0	1.0	0
(Vermont Bread Company)								
low-sodium	1 slice	80	2	15	115	2	1.0	0
sodium-free	1 slice	90	3	15	0	2	2.0	0
sprouted	1 slice	70	3	15	115	2	0.5	0
(Weight Watchers)	1 slice	40	2	9	100	0	1.0	0
(Wonder)								
nonfat, 'Light'	1 slice	40	3	7	120	0	1.0	0
sliced	1 slice	80	2	14	160	0	1.0	0
sliced, 'Family'	1 slice	80	2	13	160	1	1.0	0
WHEAT BERRY								
(Arizona Original Homestyle) cracked, stone-ground	1 slice	93	4	23	135	2	0.0	0
(Arnold) w/honey	1 slice	77	3	17	143	2	1.2	0
(Earth Grains) w/honey	1 oz	70	3	12	160	1	1.0	0
(Grant's Farm)	1 slice	70	3	13	150	0	1.0	0
(Healthy Choice)	1 slice	80	4	18	170	3	1.0	0
(Oroweat) w/honey	1 slice	90	3	17	180	2	1.0	0
WHEAT BRAN *(Grant's Farm)* w/honey	1 slice	70	3	14	120	0	1.0	0
WHEAT GERM	1 slice	73	3	14	155	1	0.8	0
WHITE								
medium slices	1 slice	67	2	12	135	1	0.9	0
medium slices, crust removed	1 slice	32	1	6	65	0	0.4	0
thick slices	1 slice	80	2	15	161	1	1.1	0
thin slices	1 slice	53	2	10	108	0	0.7	0
very thin slices	1 slice	40	1	7	81	0	0.5	0
(Arnold)								
'Brick Oven'	1 slice	61	2	11	134	1	1.2	0
'Country White'	1 slice	98	3	19	204	1	1.8	0
extra fiber, 'Brick Oven'	1 slice	55	2	12	93	2	0.8	0
'Light Premium'	1 slice	42	2	10	89	2	0.5	0
(Aunt Hattie's)								
buttertop, 'Homestyle'	1 slice	70	3	13	140	0	1.0	0
w/buttermilk, 'Homestyle'	1 slice	80	3	13	140	0	1.0	0
(Beefsteak) 'Robust'	1 slice	70	3	13	140	1	1.0	0
(Brownberry)								
'Light Premium'	1 slice	42	2	10	89	2	0.5	0
'Natural'	1 slice	59	2	11	136	1	1.1	0
(Colonial) honey buttered, split top	1 slice	80	3	14	140	0	1.0	0
(Earth Grains)								
'Light 35'	1 oz	35	2	8	105	0	1.0	0
very thin sliced	1 oz	80	2	14	160	0	1.0	0
(Grant's Farm) 'Light'	1 slice	40	2	9	115	0	1.0	0
(Holsum)								
enriched, 'Country Style'	1 slice	70	2	14	135	0	1.0	0
thin sliced	1 slice	70	2	14	160	0	1.0	0
(Kilpatrick's) honey buttered, split top	1 slice	80	3	14	140	0	1.0	0
(Monk's)	1 slice	60	3	10	95	0	1.0	0
(Mrs. Wright's)								
enriched	2 slices	100	3	20	190	1	1.0	0
sliced, Sandwich style, 'Winners'	1 slice	70	3	13	160	2	1.0	0
(Northridge) 'Old Fashioned'	1 slice	70	2	13	125	0	1.0	0
(Pepperidge Farm)								
'Hearty Country'	2 slices	190	7	38	340	2	2.0	0
sliced, sandwich style	2 slices	130	4	24	260	0	2.0	0
thin sliced, 1-lb loaf	1 slice	80	2	14	130	0	2.0	0

Food Name	Serv. Size	Total Cal.	Prot. gms	Carbs gms	Sod. mgs	Fiber gms	Fat gms	Chol. mgs
'Toasting'	1 slice	90	3	17	200	1	1.0	0
2-lb loaf, 'Large Family'	1 slice	70	2	13	150	0	1.0	0
very thin sliced	1 slice	40	1	8	80	0	0.0	0
(Pipin' Hot) loaf, thick sliced	1 slice	70	2	12	170	0	2.0	0
(Rainbo)								
honey buttered, split top	1 slice	80	3	14	140	0	1.0	0
'Light'	1 slice	40	2	9	100	2	1.0	0
thin sliced, special recipe, 'Iron Kids'	1 slice	60	3	13	140	2	1.0	0
(Vermont Bread Company)								
'Old Fashioned Sandwich'	1 slice	70	2	14	100	1	1.0	0
'Soft'	1 piece	80	2	15	115	1	1.0	0
(Weight Watchers)	1 slice	40	2	10	100	0	1.0	0
(Wonder)								
'High-Fiber'	1 slice	40	2	6	80	3	0.0	0
'Light'	1 slice	40	3	7	110	2	0.0	0
sliced	1 slice	70	2	14	150	0	1.0	0
sliced thin	1 slice	50	2	10	120	1	1.0	0
w/buttermilk	1 slice	70	2	13	160	1	1.0	0
WHOLE GRAIN								
(Healthy Choice)	1 slice	80	4	18	170	3	1.0	0
(Natural Ovens)	1 slice	70	4	13	70	5	0.5	0
WHOLE WHEAT								
	1 slice	69	3	13	148	2	1.2	0
(Arnold) 100%, stone ground	1 slice	48	2	10	97	2	0.7	0
(Aunt Hattie's)	1 slice	90	4	14	170	0	2.0	0
(BreadMill Bakery)								
w/orange, organic	1 slice	130	5	24	420	1	1.0	0
w/poppyseed, organic	1 slice	120	6	22	340	1	1.0	0
w/raisin, organic	1 slice	120	5	24	410	1	1.0	0
(Daily)	1 piece	140	6	26	0	0	0.0	0
(Earth Grains)	1 oz	70	3	11	150	0	1.0	0
(Monk's) 100% stone ground	1 slice	70	3	13	110	0	1.0	0
(Northridge) 100%	1 slice	60	3	11	120	2	1.0	0
(Oroweat) 100% stone ground	1 slice	60	3	11	125	2	1.0	0
(Pepperidge Farm)								
thin sliced, 1-lb loaf	1 slice	60	2	12	110	2	1.0	0
very thin sliced	1 slice	35	2	7	75	0	0.0	0
(Vermont Bread Company)								
'Sandwich'	1 slice	90	3	18	120	3	1.0	0
'Soft Whole Wheat'	1 piece	80	3	15	110	2	1.0	0
sourdough	1 slice	80	3	16	120	3	0.5	0
(Wonder)								
'High-Fiber'	1 slice	40	2	6	80	3	0.0	0
'Light'	1 slice	40	3	7	120	2	0.0	0
100%	1 slice	70	3	12	160	2	1.0	0
'Soft 100%'	1 slice	70	4	10	140	2	1.0	0
BREAD, QUICK								
cornbread *(Ballard)*	1 piece	130	4	23	520	2	2.5	25
cornbread *(Marie Callender's)*	1 piece	150	2	27	310	2	3.0	5
raisin loaf, fat-free, cholesterol-free *(Entenmann's)*	1 slice	140	2	33	150	1	0.0	0
BREAD, QUICK, MIX								
APPLE CINNAMON								
(Pillsbury)								
mix only	1/12 pkg	140	2	30	160	0	1.0	0
prepared w/1/4 cup oil, 1/4 cup egg substitute	1/12 loaf	190	2	31	170	0	6.0	0
prepared w/water, 1/4 cup oil, 1 egg	1/12 loaf	180	2	31	170	0	6.0	20

Food Name	Serv. Size	Total Cal.	Prot. gms	Carbs gms	Sod. mgs	Fiber gms	Fat gms	Chol. mgs
BANANA								
(Keebler) individual, 'Elfin Loaf' prepared w/margarine . . . . . 1 loaf	1 loaf	186	2	31	172	1	6.0	25
(Krusteaz) w/nuts, prepared . . . . 3/4-inch slice	3/4-inch slice	190	3	33	300	2	6.0	3
(Pillsbury)								
mix only . . . . 1/12 pkg	1/12 pkg	120	2	27	190	0	1.0	0
prepared, regular recipe . . . . 1/12 loaf	1/12 loaf	170	3	27	220	0	6.0	0
prepared w/water, 3 tbsp oil, 1/2 cup egg substitute . . . 1/12 loaf	1/12 loaf	170	3	27	210	0	6.0	0
prepared w/water, 3 tbsp oil, 2 eggs . . . . 1/12 loaf	1/12 loaf	170	3	27	200	0	5.0	35
BLUEBERRY								
(Pillsbury)								
mix only . . . . 1/12 pkg	1/12 pkg	130	2	29	160	0	1.0	0
nut, prepared . . . . 1/12 loaf	1/12 loaf	150	2	26	150	0	4.0	0
prepared, regular recipe . . . . 1/12 loaf	1/12 loaf	150	2	26	150	0	4.0	0
prepared w/water, 1/4 cup oil, 1 egg . . . . 1/12 loaf	1/12 loaf	180	2	30	160	0	6.0	20
prepared w/water, 1/4 cup oil, 1/4 cup egg substitute . . . 1/12 loaf	1/12 loaf	180	2	30	170	0	6.0	0
CHERRY *(Pillsbury)* prepared, regular recipe . . . . 1/12 loaf	1/12 loaf	180	3	29	150	0	5.0	0
CORNBREAD								
(Aunt Jemima) 'Easy' . . . . 1/3 cup	1/3 cup	150	2	26	450	1	4.0	0
(Ballard)								
mix only . . . . 1/16 pkg	1/16 pkg	120	2	24	560	0	2.0	0
prepared . . . . 1 serving	1 serving	110	2	21	500	1	1.5	0
(Dromedary)								
mix only . . . . 3 tbsp	3 tbsp	100	2	19	280	0	2.0	0
prepared, 2 x 2-inch pieces . . . . 1 piece	1 piece	130	3	20	480	0	3.0	0
(Gluten Free Pantry) gluten-free, prepared . . . . 1 serving	1 serving	130	3	29	290	2	0.0	0
(Gold Medal)								
white, 'Pouch Mix' prepared w/egg, whole milk . . . . 1/6 pan	1/6 pan	150	4	22	490	0	5.0	0
yellow, 'Pouch Mix' prepared w/egg, whole milk . . . . 1/6 pan	1/6 pan	150	4	23	500	0	5.0	0
(Hodgson Mill)								
Mexican, w/jalapeño, mix only . . . . 1/4 cup	1/4 cup	100	4	21	310	1	1.0	0
and muffin mix, whole-grain cornmeal . . . . 1/4 cup	1/4 cup	130	4	28	240	3	1.0	0
(Kentucky Kernel) sweet, all-natural, mix only . . . . 1/4 cup	1/4 cup	120	2	24	310	0	2.0	0
(Krusteaz)								
Southern, prepared, 2 x 2-inch pieces . . . . 1 piece	1 piece	140	3	27	450	0	3.0	8
w/honey, prepared . . . . 1/16 loaf	1/16 loaf	120	2	21	230	0	3.0	17
(Martha White)								
'Cotton Pickin' prepared w/water . . . . 1/6 pan	1/6 pan	110	2	21	360	0	2.0	0
'Cotton Pickin' prepared . . . . 1/4 pan	1/4 pan	170	3	31	540	0	3.0	2
Mexican, prepared w/2% milk . . . . 1/6 pan	1/6 pan	140	2	24	410	0	4.0	25
w/buttermilk, prepared w/water . . . . 1/6 pan	1/6 pan	110	2	21	360	0	2.0	0
yellow, 'Light Crust' prepared . . . . 2 oz	2 oz	140	4	21	400	0	4.0	26
yellow, prepared w/water . . . . 1/6 pan	1/6 pan	130	2	27	310	0	2.0	0
(Pillsbury)								
prepared . . . . 1/18 pkg	1/18 pkg	130	4	23	520	1	2.5	25
twists, prepared . . . . 1 serving	1 serving	130	3	17	320	0	6.0	0
(Robin Hood)								
white, 'Pouch Mix' prepared w/egg, whole milk . . . . 1/6 pan	1/6 pan	150	4	22	490	0	5.0	0
yellow, 'Pouch Mix' prepared w/egg, whole milk . . . . 1/6 pan	1/6 pan	150	4	23	500	0	5.0	0
CRANBERRY								
(Pillsbury)								
mix only . . . . 1/12 pkg	1/12 pkg	140	2	30	150	0	1.0	0
prepared w/water, 2 tbsp oil, 1 egg . . . . 1/12 loaf	1/12 loaf	160	2	30	150	0	4.0	20
prepared w/water, 2 tbsp oil 1/4 cup egg substitute . . . . 1/12 loaf	1/12 loaf	170	3	30	160	0	4.0	0
CRANBERRY-ORANGE								
(Gluten Free Pantry) gluten-free, prepared . . . . 1 serving	1 serving	150	1	35	150	1	0.0	0
DATE NUT								
(Dromedary)								
mix only . . . . 1/12 pkg	1/12 pkg	166	2	26	242	0	7.0	0

Food Name	Serv. Size	Total Cal.	Prot. gms	Carbs gms	Sod. mgs	Fiber gms	Fat gms	Chol. mgs
prepared	1/12 loaf	183	2	26	248	0	8.0	0
(Pillsbury)								
mix only	1/12 pkg	140	2	31	140	0	1.0	0
prepared	1/12 loaf	180	3	32	160	1	4.0	20
prepared w/water, 1 tbsp oil, 1/4 cup egg substitute	1/12 loaf	160	2	32	150	0	3.0	0
IRISH SODA *(Gluten Free Pantry)* gluten-free	1 serving	130	3	28	270	1	1.0	5
NUT								
(Pillsbury)								
mix only	1/12 pkg	150	3	27	180	0	3.0	0
prepared w/water, 2 tbsp oil, 1 egg	1/12 loaf	170	3	27	190	0	6.0	20
prepared w/water, 2 tbsp oil, 1/4 cup egg substitute	1/12 loaf	170	3	28	190	0	6.0	0
OATMEAL-RAISIN								
(Pillsbury)								
mix only	1/12 pkg	140	3	30	170	0	2.0	0
prepared w/water, 1/4 cup oil, 1 egg	1/12 loaf	190	3	30	180	0	7.0	20
prepared w/1/4 cup oil, 1/4 cup egg substitute	1/12 loaf	190	3	30	180	0	7.0	0
PUMPKIN								
(Pillsbury)								
mix only	1/12 pkg	130	2	26	190	1	1.5	0
prepared	1/12 loaf	170	3	27	200	1	6.0	35
BREAD CRUMBS								
Italian, dry, grated *(Tone's)*	1 tsp	8	0	2	15	0	0.1	1
Italian or plain, whole wheat, organic *(Jaclyn's)*	14 grams	28	4	13	5	0	1.0	0
Italian style *(Devonsheer)*	1 oz	104	4	21	408	1	1.3	0
Italian style *(Progresso)*	1/4 cup	110	4	20	430	1	1.5	0
Italian style *(Progresso)*	2 tbsp	60	2	11	240	0	1.0	0
Italian style, whole wheat *(Jaclyn's)*	0.5 oz	28	4	13	5	0	1.0	0
plain *(Contadina)*	1/3 cup	100	3	19	701	1	1.5	0
plain *(Devonsheer)*	1 oz	108	4	22	272	1	1.4	0
plain *(Progresso)*	1/4 cup	100	4	19	210	1	1.5	0
plain *(Progresso)*	2 tbsp	60	2	11	110	0	1.0	0
plain, dry, grated	1 cup	427	14	78	931	3	5.8	0
plain, dry, grated	1 oz	112	4	21	244	1	1.5	0
plain, dry, grated *(Tone's)*	1 tsp	8	0	2	15	0	0.1	1
seasoned, dry, grated	1 cup	440	17	84	3180	5	3.1	1
seasoned, dry, grated	1 oz	104	4	20	751	1	0.7	0
BREAD DOUGH								
cracked wheat, unbleached, high-protein, frozen *(Rhodes)*	1 oz	75	3	15	0	0	1.0	0
French, crusty, refrigerated, prepared, 1-inch slice *(Pillsbury)*	1 slice	60	2	11	120	0	1.0	0
raisin, unbleached flour, no preservatives, frozen, prepared *(Rhodes)*	1 slice	70	2	13	0	0	1.0	0
refrigerated *(Roman Meal)*	1 oz	85	2	13	199	1	2.8	0
wheat, refrigerated, prepared, thick sliced *(Pipin' Hot)*	1 slice	70	0	12	170	0	2.0	0
white, enriched, frozen *(Bridgford)*	2 oz	150	5	28	325	0	2.0	0
white, frozen *(Bridgford)*	1 oz	76	3	14	156	0	1.2	0
white, frozen *(Rhodes)*	1 slice	139	5	26	280	2	2.3	0
white, frozen *(Rich's)*	2 slices	120	4	23	300	0	1.0	0
white, refrigerated, prepared, 1-inch slice *(Pipin' Hot)*	1 slice	70	3	12	170	0	2.0	0
w/honey, frozen *(Bridgford)*	2 oz	150	6	27	304	0	2.0	0
w/honey, unbleached high-protein flour, frozen *(Rhodes)*	1 slice	125	6	23	219	3	2.0	0
w/walnuts and honey, frozen *(Bridgford)*	1 oz	76	3	14	152	0	0.9	0
BREAD MIX								
caraway rye, mix only *(Hodgson Mill)*	1/4 cup	120	5	22	190	3	2.0	0
caraway rye, gluten-free *(Gluten Free Pantry)*	1 serving	110	4	23	170	1	0.0	0

Food Name	Serv. Size	Total Cal.	Prot. gms	Carbs gms	Sod. mgs	Fiber gms	Fat gms	Chol. mgs
cracked wheat, for bread machines *(Pillsbury)*	1/12 pkg	130	4	25	260	2	2.0	0
European cheese and herb, low-fat, cholesterol-free, mix only *(Hodgson Mill)*	1/4 cup	130	5	21	250	1	2.0	0
French, country, gluten-free, prepared *(Gluten Free Pantry)*	1 slice	110	1	25	115	1	0.0	0
Italian, frozen *(Rhodes)*	1 slice	130	5	23	280	1	2.0	0
9-grain, low-fat, mix only *(Hodgson Mill)*	1/4 cup	130	5	22	150	2	2.0	0
oatmeal, w/raisin, mix only *(Pillsbury)*	1/12 pkg	140	3	30	170	0	2.0	0
oatmeal, w/raisin, prepared w/water, 1/4 cup oil, 1 egg *(Pillsbury)*	1/12 pkg	190	3	30	180	0	7.0	20
oatmeal, w/raisin, prepared w/water, 1/4 cup oil, 1/4 cup egg substitute *(Pillsbury)*	1/12 pkg	190	3	30	180	0	7.0	0
potato, fat free, cholesterol free, mix only *(Hodgson Mill)*	1/4 cup	120	5	23	170	1	0.0	0
sandwich, gluten-free, 'Favorite' *(Gluten Free Pantry)*	1 slice	110	3	24	170	1	0.0	0
tapioca, gluten-free *(Gluten Free Pantry)*	1 serving	110	2	25	115	1	0.0	0
white, crusty, for bread machines *(Pillsbury)*	1/8 pkg	130	4	25	250	1	2.0	0
white, unbleached flour, mix only *(Hodgson Mill)*	1/4 cup	120	5	22	170	3	2.0	0
whole grain, stone ground, w/honey, mix only *(Hodgson Mill)*	1/4 cup	120	5	22	160	3	2.0	0
whole wheat, low-fat, cholesterol free, mix only *(Hodgson Mill)*	1/4 cup	120	5	22	160	3	2.0	na
whole wheat, 100% all natural, stone ground *(Bob's Red Mill)*	1.5 oz	152	7	28	245	2	2.0	0
BREAD PUDDING								
w/apples, frozen, food service product *(Stouffer's)*	1 oz	42	2	5	77	1	1.6	30
BREADFRUIT								
Fresh, raw, whole, small fruit	1/4 fruit	99	1	26	2	5	0.2	0
Frozen, unthawed	1 cup	227	2	60	4	11	0.5	0
BREADFRUIT SEEDS								
boiled	1 oz	48	2	9	7	1	0.7	0
raw	1 oz	54	2	8	7	1	1.6	0
roasted	1 oz	59	2	11	8	2	0.8	0
BREADNUT TREE SEEDS/Jamaican breadnut								
dried	1 cup	587	14	127	85	24	2.7	0
dried	1 oz	104	2	23	15	4	0.5	0
raw, 8–14 seeds	1 oz	62	2	13	9	na	0.3	0
BREADSTICK								
garlic, frozen *(Cole's)*	1.9 oz	170	4	27	290	1	5.0	1
garlic, Italian style *(Barbara's Bakery)*	1 oz	120	4	18	170	0	3.0	0
garlic and sesame *(Angonoa's)*	7 pieces	120	4	19	120	1	3.0	0
onion *(Stella D'oro)*	1 piece	40	1	6	0	0	1.3	0
pizza *(Fattorie & Pandea)*	3 pieces	59	2	10	100	0	1.0	0
pizza *(Stella D'oro)*	1 piece	43	1	7	0	0	1.2	0
plain *(Angonoa's)*	6 pieces	120	4	20	280	1	2.5	0
plain *(Stella D'oro)*	1 piece	41	1	7	0	0	1.2	0
plain, 4.25-inch length	1 breadstick	21	1	3	33	0	0.5	0
plain, 7-5/8 x 5/8 inch	1 breadstick	41	1	7	66	0	0.9	0
plain, 9-1/4 x 3/8 inch	1 breadstick	25	1	4	39	0	0.6	0
plain, dietetic *(Stella D'oro)*	1 piece	46	1	7	10	0	1.4	0
plain, regular *(Barbara's Bakery)*	1 oz	120	4	18	170	0	3.0	0
sesame, dietetic *(Stella D'oro)*	1 piece	49	1	6	10	0	2.1	0
soft *(Pillsbury)*	1 serving	110	3	18	290	1	2.5	0
sesame *(Fattorie & Pandea)*	3 pieces	65	2	10	100	0	2.0	0
sesame *(Stella D'oro)*	1 piece	51	1	6	0	0	2.2	0
sesame, Italian style *(Barbara's Bakery)*	1 oz	120	4	18	170	0	3.0	0
soft, refrigerated ready-to-bake *(Mrs. Wright's)*	1 stick	100	3	17	300	1	2.5	0

Food Name	Serv. Size	Total Cal.	Prot. gms	Carbs gms	Sod. mgs	Fiber gms	Fat gms	Chol. mgs
soft, refrigerated *(Roman Meal)*	1 piece	117	3	17	274	1	3.9	0
wheat *(Stella D'oro)*	1 piece	42	1	6	0	0	1.4	0
whole wheat, w/sesame *(Angonoa's)*	5 pieces	130	4	19	220	3	4.0	0
whole wheat *(Fattorie & Pandea)*	3 pieces	57	2	10	100	0	1.0	0
BREAKFAST BAR								
(Carnation)								
chocolate chip	1 bar	200	6	20	180	1	11.0	1
chocolate crunch	1 bar	190	6	20	150	1	10.0	1
peanut butter chocolate chip	1 bar	200	6	20	170	1	11.0	1
peanut butter crunch	1 bar	190	6	20	180	1	10.0	1
BREAKFAST BURRITO. See under BURRITO.								
BREAKFAST DRINK MIX								
(Carnation)								
regular, prepared w/8 fl oz 2% milk	9 oz	250	12	39	220	na	5.0	na
sugarless, prepared w/8 fl oz 2% milk	9 oz	190	12	24	220	na	5.0	na
(Ovaltine) traditional flavor, 'Classic'	4 tbsp	80	2	17	65	0	0.0	0
(Pillsbury)								
chocolate, variety pack, dry mix, 'Instant Breakfast'	1/10 pkg	130	6	25	135	0	0.0	0
BREAKFAST SANDWICH								
(Great Starts)								
egg, beefsteak, and cheese	4.9 oz	360	17	27	730	0	20.0	0
egg, Canadian bacon, cheese	5.2 oz	420	16	37	1845	0	22.0	0
muffin w/egg, Canadian style bacon, cheese	1 pkg	290	14	25	750	2	15.0	95
muffin w/egg, sausage, cheese	1 pkg	490	18	36	1110	3	30.0	145
sausage, egg, and cheese biscuit	1 entrée	460	16	37	1060	3	28.0	115
(Jimmy Dean)								
biscuit w/egg, bacon, cheese	1 biscuit	300	11	28	890	2	16.0	95
biscuit w/egg, ham, cheese	1 biscuit	240	13	26	720	1	10.0	100
biscuit w/egg, sausage, cheese	1 biscuit	390	14	28	1040	2	27.0	115
biscuit w/sausage, frozen	1 pkg	385	10	23	881	1	28.2	31
biscuit w/sausage, frozen	1 sandwich	192	5	12	441	1	14.1	16
biscuit w/sausage, frozen	1 serving	385	10	23	881	1	28.2	31
biscuit w/sausage, microwaveable	2 sandwiches	310	9	23	850	1	20.0	30
sausage, refrigerated, microwave	1 sandwich	160	5	10	360	0	11.0	0
(La Choy) ham, egg, and cheese breakfast roll,								
food service product	1 serving	237	10	22	463	2	12.6	91
(Morningstar Farms)								
vegetarian, 'Breakfast Sandwich' w/muffin, patty,								
cheese, and Scramblers	1 sandwich	280	28	35	1000	5	3.0	10
vegetarian, Scramblers patty sandwich	1 serving	300	18	29	590	na	12.0	na
(Owens)								
sausage, biscuit, refrigerated, 'Border Breakfasts'	2 oz	210	6	14	400	0	14.0	0
sausage, egg, and cheese, biscuit, refrigerated,								
'Border Breakfasts'	2.5 oz	250	8	15	500	0	15.0	0
sausage, smoked, biscuit, refrigerated,								
'Border Breakfasts'	2 oz	200	4	15	786	0	6.0	0
(Red Baron)								
bacon scramble, 'Sunrise Singles'	1 unit	420	16	34	830	2	24.0	65
(Pierre)								
ham and cheese, wrapped, product 1295, 'Ham n Go'	1 piece	236	11	26	677	1	10.6	26
ham, wrapped, product 1293, 'Ham-n-Go'	1 piece	223	11	26	660	1	8.9	26
wrapped, 'Link-N-Dog' 'Dine'n w/Pierre'	1 piece	203	11	20	364	2	9.1	22
wrapped, 'Saus-A-Rage' 'Dine'n w/Pierre'	1 piece	263	11	26	495	2	13.2	22
(Quick Meal)								
sausage, biscuit	3.7 oz	350	10	29	870	0	22.0	40
sausage, w/cheese, biscuit	4.3 oz	420	13	31	1060	0	27.0	60
sausage, w/egg and cheese, muffin	5.1 oz	76	3	5	143	0	4.0	26

Food Name	Serv. Size	Total Cal.	Prot. gms	Carbs gms	Sod. mgs	Fiber gms	Fat gms	Chol. mgs
sausage, w/egg, biscuit	4.5 oz	350	11	30	780	0	21.0	110
(Red Baron)								
ham scramble, 'Sunrise Singles'	1 unit	370	15	34	770	2	19.0	65
(Sunny Fresh)								
biscuit w/ham and cheese, pre-cooked, frozen	1 pkg	29206	1470	3028	87040	14	1165.4	13736
biscuit w/ham and cheese, pre-cooked, frozen	1 serving	243	12	25	725	0	9.7	114
egg and cheese biscuit, pre-cooked, frozen	1 pkg	26910	1187	2957	67751	0	1066.9	13336
egg and cheese biscuit, pre-cooked, frozen	1 serving	224	10	25	565	0	8.9	111
egg and cheese pocket sandwich, pre-cooked, frozen, 'Breakfast Stuff-Its'	1 pkg	17605	814	1760	27862	115	913.9	11176
egg and cheese pocket sandwich, pre-cooked, frozen, 'Breakfast Stuff-Its'	1 serving	147	7	15	232	1	7.6	93
(Red Baron) sausage scramble 'Sunrise Singles'	1 unit	380	15	34	730	2	21.0	65
(Swanson) egg, sausage & cheese 'Great Starts'	5.5 oz	460	18	35	1310	0	28.0	0
(Weight Watchers) sausage, biscuit	1 biscuit	230	11	20	660	2	11.0	25

BREAKFAST STRIPS. See under BACON SUBSTITUTE.
BREWER'S YEAST. See under YEAST.
BROAD BEAN. See BEAN, FAVA.
BROCCOLI
Fresh

Food Name	Serv. Size	Total Cal.	Prot. gms	Carbs gms	Sod. mgs	Fiber gms	Fat gms	Chol. mgs
boiled, drained, chopped	1/2 cup	22	2	4	20	2	0.3	0
boiled, drained, spears, large, 11-12 inches long	1 spear	78	8	14	73	8	1.0	0
boiled, drained, spears, medium, 7.5–8 inches long	1 spear	50	5	9	47	5	0.6	0
boiled, drained, spears, small, 5 inches long	1 spear	39	4	7	36	4	0.5	0
raw, bunch	1 medium	170	18	32	164	18	2.1	0
raw, chopped	1 cup	25	3	5	24	3	0.3	0
raw, chopped or diced	1/2 cup	12	1	2	12	1	0.2	0
raw, florets	1 cup	20	2	4	19	na	0.2	0
raw, florets	1 medium	3	0	1	3	na	0.0	0
raw, spears, medium *(Dole)*	1 spear	40	5	4	75	5	1.0	0
raw, spears, medium, 7.5–8 inches long	1 spear	42	5	8	41	5	0.5	0
raw, spears, small, 5 inches long	1 spear	9	1	2	8	1	0.1	0
Frozen								
(Flav-R-Pac)	1 cup	25	2	4	20	2	0.0	0
(Health Valley)	1/2 cup	26	3	5	24	3	0.0	0
chopped *(A&P)*	3.3 oz	25	3	5	25	0	1.0	0
chopped *(Birds Eye)*	3.3 oz	25	3	5	15	3	0.0	0
chopped *(Finast)*	3.3 oz	25	3	5	20	0	0.0	0
chopped *(Flav-R-Pac)*	3/4 cup	30	2	5	5	3	0.0	0
chopped *(Frosty Acres)*	3.3 oz	25	3	5	18	1	0.0	0
chopped *(Seabrook)*	3.3 oz	25	3	5	18	1	0.0	0
chopped *(Southern)*	3.5 oz	28	3	4	25	0	0.3	0
chopped, drained	1 cup	52	6	10	478	6	0.2	0
chopped, no salt added, drained	1 cup	52	6	10	44	6	0.2	0
chopped, 'Plain Polybag' *(Green Giant)*	3/4 cup	25	2	4	25	2	0.0	0
chopped, unprepared	1 cup	41	4	7	37	5	0.5	0
chopped, unprepared	10-oz pkg	74	8	14	68	9	0.8	0
cuts *(A&P)*	3.3 oz	25	3	5	25	0	1.0	0
cuts *(Birds Eye)*	3.2 oz	25	3	5	25	3	0.0	0
cuts *(Flav-R-Pac)*	1 cup	25	2	4	20	2	0.0	0
cuts *(Frosty Acres)*	3.3 oz	25	3	5	50	1	0.0	0
cuts *(Pictsweet)*	1 cup	25	2	4	20	2	0.0	0
cuts *(Seabrook)*	3.3 oz	25	3	5	50	1	0.0	0
cuts, 'Plain Polybag' *(Green Giant)*	1/2 cup	18	2	5	25	4	0.0	0
cuts, 'Portion Pack' *(Birds Eye)*	3 oz	20	3	4	20	2	0.0	0
cuts, 'Singles' *(Stokely)*	3 oz	25	3	5	15	0	1.0	0
drained	1/2 cup	26	3	5	239	3	0.1	0

Food Name	Serv. Size	Total Cal.	Prot. gms	Carbs gms	Sod. mgs	Fiber gms	Fat gms	Chol. mgs
drained	10-oz pkg	70	8	13	650	8	0.3	0
florets *(C&W)*	3.3 oz	25	3	5	20	0	0.0	0
florets *(Frosty Acres)*	3.3 oz	30	3	5	14	1	0.0	0
florets, 'Deluxe' *(Birds Eye)*	3.3 oz	25	3	5	20	3	0.0	0
florets, 'Select Polybag' *(Green Giant)*	1 1/3 cup	25	2	4	25	2	0.0	0
Normandy *(Flav-R-Pac)*	3/4 cup	25	2	4	30	2	0.0	0
Normandy, w/buttery sauce *(Flav-R-Pac)*	1/2 cup	45	2	7	490	3	2.5	0
spears *(A&P)*	3.3 oz	25	3	5	20	0	1.0	0
spears *(Birds Eye)*	3.3 oz	25	3	5	20	3	0.0	0
spears *(Frosty Acres)*	3.3 oz	25	3	5	20	1	0.0	0
spears *(Seabrook)*	3.3 oz	25	3	5	20	1	0.0	0
spears *(Southern)*	3.5 oz	30	3	5	30	0	0.2	0
spears and florets, 'Deluxe' *(Birds Eye)*	3.3 oz	25	3	5	20	3	0.0	0
spears, 'Select Polybag' *(Green Giant)*	3 oz	25	2	4	25	2	0.0	0
spears, baby *(Seabrook)*	3.3 oz	30	3	5	14	1	0.0	0
spears, baby, 'Deluxe' *(Birds Eye)*	3.3 oz	30	3	5	15	3	0.0	0
spears, mini, *(Green Giant)*	1/5 pkg	18	2	5	25	3	0.0	0
spears, no salt added, drained	10-oz pkg	70	8	13	60	8	0.3	0
spears, no salt added, drained	1/2 cup	26	3	5	22	3	0.1	0
spears, whole, 'Farm Fresh' *(Birds Eye)*	4 oz	30	4	6	25	3	0.0	0
unprepared	2-lb pkg	263	28	49	154	27	3.1	0
unprepared	10-oz pkg	82	9	15	48	9	1.0	0
BROCCOLI, CHINESE, cooked	1 cup	19	1	3	6	2	0.6	0
BROCCOLI DISH/ENTRÉE								
(A&P) w/cauliflower, frozen	3.2 oz	25	2	4	20	0	1.0	0
(Amy's Kitchen)								
pie, w/cheddar cheese, organic	8-oz pie	390	10	46	500	3	18.0	0
pot pie	1 serving	430	11	46	630	4	22.0	45
(Birds Eye)								
stir-fry, 'Farm Fresh Mixtures'	1 cup	30	2	5	30	2	0.0	0
w/baby carrots and water chestnuts, 'Farm Fresh'	4 oz	45	2	10	35	3	0.0	0
(Flav-R-Pac) cheddar broccoli Normandy, frozen,								
'Grande Classics'	1/2 cup	45	3	6	210	2	2.0	5
(Frosty Acres) w/cauliflower, 'Swiss Mix'	3 oz	25	2	5	36	1	0.0	0
(Green Giant)								
'Broccoli Fanfare' 'Valley Combinations'	1/2 cup	80	3	14	340	3	2.0	0
in cheese flavored sauce	1 pkg	188	6	25	1344	na	7.0	na
in cheese flavored sauce	1 cup	113	4	15	806	na	4.2	na
in cheese flavored sauce	1 serving	75	3	10	538	na	2.8	na
w/cauliflower, 'Valley Combinations'	1/2 cup	60	2	9	340	3	2.0	0
w/red peppers, 'Select'	1/2 cup	25	2	4	15	2	0.0	0
(Nancy's) broccoli-cheddar quiche, frozen, microwave,								
'French Baked'	1 quiche	490	17	33	750	2	33.0	165
(Pepperidge Farm) w/cheese, in pastry, frozen	1 piece	230	5	18	380	0	16.0	0
(Stokely)								
w/cauliflower 'Singles'	3 oz	20	2	4	15	0	1.0	0
w/whole baby carrots, and water chestnuts, 'Singles'	3 oz	30	2	6	22	0	1.0	0
(Stouffer's)								
and cheese soufflé, frozen, food service product	1 oz	35	2	2	129	0	2.1	32
au gratin, frozen, food service product	1 oz	27	1	3	105	0	1.3	3
BROCCOLI DISH/ENTRÉE MIX								
(Pasta Roni) and mushroom noodles entrée,								
'Tenderthin'	1 serving	260	7	28	644	1	13.6	3
(Rice A Roni)								
and cheese rice, 'Fast Cook'	2.5 oz	169	4	23	412	1	6.8	3
au gratin	2.5 oz	209	4	27	500	1	9.6	3
au gratin, w/rice, 1/3 less sodium	2.5 oz	181	4	28	333	1	6.2	3

Food Name	Serv. Size	Total Cal.	Prot. gms	Carbs gms	Sod. mgs	Fiber gms	Fat gms	Chol. mgs
BROTH. See under SOUP.								
BROWN RICE. See under RICE.								
BROWNIE. See under CAKE, SNACK.								
BRUSSELS SPROUTS								
Fresh								
boiled, drained	1/2 cup	30	2	7	16	2	0.4	0
boiled, drained, whole	1 medium	8	1	2	4	1	0.1	0
raw	1 cup	38	3	8	22	3	0.3	0
raw	1 medium	8	1	2	5	1	0.1	0
raw *(Dole)*	1/2 cup	19	1	4	11	2	0.1	0
Frozen								
(A&P)	3.3 oz	35	3	7	15	0	1.0	0
(Birds Eye)	3.3 oz	35	3	7	15	3	0.0	0
(Flav-R-Pac)	6 medium	35	3	5	25	3	0.0	0
(Frosty Acres)	3.3 oz	35	3	7	12	1	0.0	0
(Pictsweet)	85 grams	35	3	5	25	3	0.0	0
(Seabrook)	3.3 oz	35	3	7	12	1	0.0	0
(Southern)	3.5 oz	37	3	8	20	0	0.0	0
baby *(Seabrook)*	3.3 oz	40	4	7	5	1	0.0	0
no salt, drained	1 cup	65	6	13	36	6	0.6	0
petite *(C&W)*	3.2 oz	30	3	5	25	3	0.0	0
'Plain Polybag' *(Green Giant)*	1/2 cup	25	2	6	10	2	0.0	0
'Singles' *(Stokely)*	3 oz	35	4	7	10	0	0.0	0
unprepared	2-lb pkg	372	34	71	91	34	3.7	0
unprepared	10-oz pkg	116	11	22	28	11	1.2	0
w/salt, drained	1 cup	65	6	13	401	6	0.6	0
BUBBLE GUM. See under CANDY, GUM.								
BUCKWHEAT	1 cup	583	23	122	2	17	5.8	0
BUCKWHEAT FLOUR. See under FLOUR.								
BUCKWHEAT GROATS, ROASTED/kasha								
cooked	1 cup	155	6	33	7	5	1.0	0
dry	1 cup	567	19	123	18	17	4.4	0
(Wolff's Kasha)	3/4 cup	150	4	35	2	4	0.0	0
BUFFALO. See BISON.								
BULGUR. See also CEREAL, HOT.								
cooked	1 cup	151	6	34	9	8	0.4	0
cooked	1 tbsp	7	0	2	0	0	0.0	0
dry	1 cup	479	17	106	24	26	1.9	0
BULGUR DISH/ENTRÉE MIX								
(Casbah)								
pilaf mix, dry	1 oz	100	3	21	270	2	0.0	0
tabbouleh, seasoned, prepared	2/3 cup	120	6	24	410	1	0.5	0
(Fantastic Foods) tabbouleh, seasoned	1/4 cup	120	4	26	450	6	0.5	0
BULLOCK'S HEART. See CUSTARD APPLE.								
BUN. See also BISCUIT; BUN, FRANKFURTER; BUN, HAMBURGER; BUN, SWEET; CROISSANT; ENGLISH MUFFIN; ROLL.								
hoagie, deli *(Wonder)*	1 serving	260	8	49	500	2	3.5	0
'Sof-Buns' *(Holsum)*	1 bun	120	3	23	190	0	2.0	0
spelt, yeast-free, organic *(French Meadow)*	1 bun	160	9	33	155	5	1.4	0
w/sesame seeds, 'Big BBQ Buns' *(Holsum)*	1 bun	200	5	38	320	0	3.0	0
BUN, FRANKFURTER								
	1 oz	81	2	14	159	1	1.4	0
(Arnold)								
	1 bun	100	3	20	162	1	1.8	0
'New England Style'	1 bun	108	4	21	178	1	2.0	0
oat bran	1 bun	110	4	20	210	1	2.0	0
(Aunt Hattie's) potato	1 bun	150	5	23	260	0	4.0	0

Food Name	Serv. Size	Total Cal.	Prot. gms	Carbs gms	Sod. mgs	Fiber gms	Fat gms	Chol. mgs
(Country Grain)	1 bun	100	4	18	230	1	1.0	0
(Mrs. Wright's)								
crushed wheat	1 bun	110	4	20	230	1	1.5	0
enriched	1 bun	100	3	19	190	1	1.5	0
(Pepperidge Farm)								
	1 bun	140	5	24	270	1	3.0	0
Dijon	1 bun	160	5	23	230	2	5.0	0
(Roman Meal)								
'Original'	1 bun	104	4	20	210	2	1.9	0
whole-grain	1 bun	120	4	19	210	0	3.0	0
(Wonder)								
	1 bun	110	3	21	220	0	1.5	0
footlong Coney	1 bun	220	7	42	430	1	3.0	0
'Light'	1 bun	80	5	13	210	4	1.0	0
BUN, HAMBURGER								
	1 oz	81	2	14	159	1	1.4	0
(Arnold)	1 bun	115	4	22	223	2	2.2	0
(Aunt Hattie's) potato	1 bun	150	5	23	260	0	4.0	0
(Mrs. Wright's)								
crushed wheat	1 bun	110	3	21	240	1	1.5	0
enriched	1 bun	110	3	21	190	1	1.5	0
enriched, w/sesame	1 bun	110	4	21	190	1	1.5	0
(Pepperidge Farm)	1 bun	130	5	22	240	1	2.0	0
(Roman Meal)								
'Original'	1 bun	113	5	21	228	2	1.9	0
whole grain	1 bun	130	4	20	230	0	3.0	0
(Wonder)								
	1 bun	110	3	21	220	0	1.5	0
4-inch diam *(Wonder)*	1 bun	110	3	21	220	1	1.5	0
'Light'	1 bun	80	5	13	210	4	1.0	0
BUN, SWEET. See also PASTRY; ROLL, SWEET.								
(Aunt Fanny's)								
honey	3 oz	360	4	42	150	0	30.0	10
honey, apple bear	4 oz	460	6	50	220	0	26.0	5
honey, applesauce-filled	1 bun	330	6	43	300	4	17.0	0
honey, banana creme–filled	1 bun	350	5	32	290	2	18.0	0
honey, birdie, jelly-filled	4 oz	450	6	53	210	0	24.0	5
honey, bogie, creme-filled	4 oz	460	6	49	200	0	27.0	10
honey, chocolate creme–filled	1 bun	350	5	32	290	2	18.0	0
honey, iced	1 bun	350	5	32	290	2	18.0	0
honey, lemon bear	4 oz	440	5	52	200	0	23.0	5
honey, raspberry-filled	1 bun	350	5	45	290	2	17.0	0
honey, regular	1 bun	360	5	41	300	2	20.0	0
honey, snow bear	4 oz	480	6	60	220	0	24.0	5
honey, vanilla creme–filled	1 bun	350	5	32	290	2	18.0	0
(Break Cake)								
apple honey, multi pak, 1.5 oz	1 bun	170	2	20	90	0	10.0	0
honey, 3 oz	1 bun	420	4	38	160	0	28.0	0
honey, multi pak, 2.75 oz	1 bun	380	3	34	150	0	24.0	0
(Entenmann's)								
blueberry cheese, nonfat, no cholesterol	1 serving	140	4	31	150	1	0.0	0
cheese-topped	1 bun	240	5	29	240	0	12.0	0
cinnamon	1 bun	230	4	31	200	0	10.0	0
pineapple cheese, nonfat, no cholesterol	1 serving	140	4	30	150	1	0.0	0
raspberry cheese, nonfat, no cholesterol	1 serving	160	4	36	135	1	0.0	0
(Hostess)								
honey glazed, 'Breakfast Bake Shop'	1 piece	360	5	38	230	1	21.0	15
honey iced, 'Breakfast Bake Shop'	1 piece	430	5	55	240	2	22.0	20

Food Name	Serv. Size	Total Cal.	Prot. gms	Carbs gms	Sod. mgs	Fiber gms	Fat gms	Chol. mgs
(Morton) honey, microwave	1 bun	250	3	35	160	2	10.0	0
(Pepperidge Farm) cinnamon, frozen, '2/pkg.'	1 piece	280	4	34	190	0	14.0	0
(Rich's)								
cinnamon, frozen, 2.5 oz, 'Ever Fresh'	1 bun	293	4	38	0	0	14.6	0
honey, frozen, mini, 'Ever Fresh'	1.36 oz	133	2	18	0	0	6.6	0
(Tastykake)								
honey glazed	3.25 oz	362	6	42	219	4	20.4	2
honey iced	3.25 oz	348	5	50	254	2	14.9	2
(Weight Watchers)								
cheese bun, frozen, 'Microwave'	1/2 pkg	180	5	32	5	0	4.0	210
BURBOT								
baked, broiled, grilled, or microwaved	3 oz	98	21	0	105	0	0.9	65
raw	3 oz	77	16	0	82	0	0.7	51
BURDOCK ROOT/gobo								
boiled, drained, sliced, 1-inch pieces	1 cup	110	3	26	5	2	0.2	0
boiled, drained, whole	1 med root	146	3	35	7	3	0.2	0
raw, sliced, 1-inch pieces	1 cup	85	2	20	6	4	0.2	0
raw, whole	1 med root	112	2	27	8	5	0.2	0

BURGER. See under BEEF DINNER/ENTRÉE; BEEF SUBSTITUTE DINNER/ENTRÉE; and individual ground meat listings.

BURGUNDY. See under WINE.

Food Name	Serv. Size	Total Cal.	Prot. gms	Carbs gms	Sod. mgs	Fiber gms	Fat gms	Chol. mgs
BURRITO								
(Amy's Kitchen)								
bean and cheese burrito	1 burrito	280	10	43	460	6	8.0	10
bean and rice burrito	1 burrito	250	9	44	450	6	5.0	0
bean burrito, w/rice and cheese, organic, frozen, 6 oz	1 burrito	280	10	43	460	6	8.0	10
breakfast burrito	1 serving	230	9	38	480	5	5.0	0
(Don Miguel)								
beef, cheese, and green chili	1 burrito	390	20	53	910	3	11.0	40
chicken, cheese, no beans	1 burrito	410	18	52	950	3	14.0	45
(Great Starts)								
breakfast burrito, hot and spicy	1 pkg	220	9	30	490	3	7.0	55
breakfast burrito, w/cheese and chili peppers, 'Original'	1 pkg	200	8	25	510	2	8.0	60
breakfast burrito, w/eggs, bacon, cheese	1 pkg	250	10	27	540	0	11.0	90
breakfast, burrito, w/eggs, ham, cheese	1 pkg	210	9	29	350	0	6.0	60
breakfast, burrito, w/eggs, pepperoni, cheese w/pizza sauce	1 pkg	240	9	28	410	0	9.0	60
(Healthy Choice)								
beef and bean, 'Quick Meals'	5.2 oz	270	12	42	520	0	7.0	15
chicken con queso, frozen, 'Quick Meals'	5.4 oz	280	15	40	500	0	8.0	20
chicken con queso entrée	1 entrée	350	14	60	590	6	6.0	35
(Homestyle Kitchens) black bean, organic, frozen	1 burrito	190	8	36	240	7	1.5	0
(Hormel)								
beef, frozen	1 piece	205	9	31	780	0	8.0	0
cheese, frozen	1 piece	210	9	32	792	0	5.0	0
chicken and rice, frozen	1 piece	200	9	32	594	0	4.0	0
chili, hot, frozen	1 piece	240	9	33	619	0	8.0	0
(Las Campanas)								
bean and cheese, no lard	1 burrito	272	10	42	480	6	7.0	3
beef and bean, frozen	1 pkg	2964	87	382	5791	8	120.8	125
beef and bean, frozen	1 serving	296	9	38	579	1	12.1	13
beef and bean, no lard	1 burrito	304	10	39	504	5	12.0	12
(Maria's)								
bean and cheese, jalapeño	1 burrito	360	12	54	620	8	11.0	10
beef and bean	1 burrito	420	13	49	660	5	19.0	25
(Marquez Pimera)								
beef, green chili, and cheese, 'Primera'	1 burrito	330	14	43	950	2	11.0	30

Food Name	Serv. Size	Total Cal.	Prot. gms	Carbs gms	Sod. mgs	Fiber gms	Fat gms	Chol. mgs
beef, green chili, and Monterey Jack cheese, frozen ..... 1 pkg		324	15	40	768	na	11.6	27
(Old El Paso)								
bean and cheese, frozen .... 1 burrito		330	14	45	740	0	11.0	0
beef and bean, frozen, 'Festive Dinners' .... 11 oz		470	23	72	1180	0	9.0	0
beef and bean, hot, frozen .... 1 burrito		310	12	41	710	0	11.0	0
beef and bean, medium, frozen .... 1 burrito		330	13	41	630	0	13.0	29
beef and bean, mild, frozen .... 1 burrito		320	13	42	500	0	11.0	0
packaged, prepared, w/filling .... 1 burrito		299	11	36	430	4	13.0	23
(Patio)								
beef and bean, frozen .... 5 oz		370	11	43	830	0	16.0	0
beef and bean, frozen, 'Britos' .... 3.63 oz		250	6	33	340	0	10.0	15
beef and bean, green chili, frozen .... 5 oz		330	12	43	770	0	12.0	0
beef and bean, nacho, frozen, 'Britos' .... 3.63 oz		270	9	30	420	0	13.0	25
beef and bean, red chili, frozen .... 5 oz		340	11	44	810	0	13.0	0
beef and bean, w/green chili, mild .... 1 pkg		325	10	44	879	4	11.9	20
beef and bean, w/green chili, mild .... 1 serving		325	10	44	879	4	11.9	20
chicken, spicy, frozen, 'Britos' .... 3.63 oz		250	6	33	330	0	10.0	25
frozen .... 12 oz		517	18	74	1643	0	16.0	0
green chili, frozen, 'Britos' .... 3.63 oz		250	6	33	420	0	10.0	15
nacho cheese, frozen, 'Britos' .... 3.63 oz		250	7	32	330	0	10.0	20
red chili, frozen, 'Britos' .... 3.63 oz		240	6	31	370	0	10.0	15
red hot, frozen, 'Britos' .... 5 oz		360	12	43	800	0	15.0	0
(Ruiz)								
beefsteak fajita, 'Supreme' .... 1 burrito		290	11	42	240	1	9.0	5
chicken fajita, 'Supreme' .... 1 burrito		260	12	50	500	10	1.0	5
BURRITO FILLING								
beans *(Del Monte)* .... 1/2 cup		110	6	20	900	0	1.0	0
'Manwich' *(Hunt's)* .... 1/4 cup		25	1	6	559	4	0.2	0
BURRITO SEASONING. See under SEASONING MIX.								
BUSH NUT. See MACADAMIA NUT.								
BUTTER								
light, salted, stick *(Land O'Lakes)* stick .... 1 tbsp		50	0	0	70	0	6.0	20
light, salted, whipped *(Land O'Lakes)* whipped .... 1 tbsp		35	0	0	45	0	4.0	10
light, unsalted, stick *(Land O'Lakes)* .... 1 tbsp		50	0	0	5	0	6.0	15
lightly salted *(Darigold)* .... 1 tsp		25	0	0	25	0	3.0	7
lightly salted *(Hotel Bar)* .... 1 tsp		35	0	0	35	0	4.0	0
lightly salted *(Kellers)* .... 1 tsp		35	0	0	35	0	4.0	0
lightly salted, stick *(Breakstone's)* .... 1 tbsp		100	0	0	90	0	11.0	35
lightly salted, whipped *(Breakstone's)* .... 1 tbsp		70	0	0	65	0	7.0	20
lightly salted, whipped *(Breakstone's)* .... 1 tbsp		70	0	0	65	0	7.0	20
'Quarters' *(Darigold)* .... 1 tsp		35	0	0	2	0	4.0	11
salted .... 1 cup		1628	2	0	1875	0	184.1	497
salted .... 1 pat		36	0	0	41	0	4.1	11
salted .... 1 stick		813	1	0	937	0	92.0	248
salted .... 1 tbsp		102	0	0	117	0	11.5	31
salted *(Hotel Bar)* .... 1 tsp		35	0	0	35	0	4.0	0
salted *(Kellers)* .... 1 tsp		35	0	0	35	0	4.0	0
salted, 'Quarters' *(Darigold)* .... 1 tsp		35	0	0	40	0	4.0	11
salted, stick *(Land O'Lakes)* .... 1 tbsp		100	0	0	85	0	11.0	30
salted, whipped *(Land O'Lakes)* .... 1 tsp		25	0	0	25	0	3.0	5
salted, whipped .... 1 cup		1082	1	0	1248	0	122.5	331
salted, whipped .... 1 pat		27	0	0	31	0	3.1	8
salted, whipped .... 1 stick		542	1	0	625	0	61.3	165
salted, whipped .... 1 tbsp		67	0	0	78	0	7.6	21
unsalted .... 1 pat		36	0	0	1	0	4.1	11
unsalted .... 1 cup		1628	2	0	25	0	184.1	497
unsalted .... 1 stick		813	1	0	12	0	92.0	248

Food Name	Serv. Size	Total Cal.	Prot. gms	Carbs gms	Sod. mgs	Fiber gms	Fat gms	Chol. mgs
unsalted	1 tbsp	102	0	0	2	0	11.5	31
unsalted *(Land O'Lakes)*	1 tsp	35	0	0	0	0	4.0	10
unsalted, sweet, stick *(Breakstone's)*	1 tbsp	100	0	0	0	0	11.0	35
unsalted, sweet, whipped *(Breakstone's)*	1 tbsp	70	0	0	0	0	7.0	20
unsalted, whipped *(Darigold)*	1 tsp	25	0	0	2	0	3.0	7
unsalted, whipped *(Land O'Lakes)*	1 tsp	25	0	0	0	0	3.0	5
whipped *(Breakstone's)*	1 tbsp	70	0	0	0	0	7.0	0
whipped *(Darigold)*	1 tsp	25	0	0	2	0	3.0	7
whipped *(Land O'Lakes)*	1 tsp	25	0	0	0	0	3.0	5
BUTTER ALTERNATIVE								
(Canola Harvest) canola oil spread	1 tbsp	100	0	0	110	0	11.0	0
(Fleischmann's) corn oil spread, 60% oil, 'Light'	1 tbsp	80	0	0	70	0	8.0	0
(I Can't Believe It's Not Butter!)								
buttermilk, no salt	1 tbsp	90	0	0	0	0	10.0	0
buttermilk, stick	1 tbsp	90	0	0	95	0	10.0	0
cream, buttermilk, squeezable	1 tbsp	90	0	0	90	0	10.0	0
light spread, 40% vegetable oil, stick	1 tbsp	50	0	0	90	0	6.0	0
soft, 70% vegetable oil	1 tbsp	90	0	0	95	0	10.0	0
whipped	1 tbsp	60	0	0	70	0	7.0	0
(Land O'Lakes)								
stick, no salt	1 tbsp	90	na	na	0	0	10.0	0
tub	1 tbsp	80	na	na	70	0	8.0	0
w/sweet cream, salted, stick	1 tbsp	90	na	na	95	0	10.0	0
(Mazola) corn oil spread, 40% corn oil, light	1 tbsp	50	0	0	100	0	6.0	0
(Spectrum Naturals) canola oil spread, 100% dairy-free, nonhydrogenated	1 tbsp	94	0	0	84	0	11.0	0
BUTTER FLAVORING								
(Butter Buds) fat-free, sprinkles	1 tsp	5	0	2	120	na	0.0	0
(Fry's)	1/2 tsp	4	0	0	70	0	0.0	0
(Molly McButter) fat-free, natural butter flavor, sprinkles	1 tsp	5	0	1	180	na	0.0	0
(Schilling) naturally flavored, 'Best 'O Butter'	1/2 tsp	4	1	1	65	0	1.0	0
BUTTER OIL								
anhydrous	1 cup	1796	1	0	3	0	203.9	525
anhydrous	1 tbsp	112	0	0	0	0	12.7	33
BUTTERBEAN. See BEAN, LIMA.								
BUTTERBUR/fuki								
Canned								
chopped	1 cup	4	0	0	5	na	0.2	0
stalks, whole	3 medium	1	0	0	2	na	0.1	0
Fresh								
raw, chopped	1 cup	13	0	3	7	na	0.0	0
raw, petioles, whole	1 medium	1	0	0	0	na	0.0	0
BUTTERFISH								
baked, broiled, grilled, or microwaved	3 oz	159	19	0	97	0	8.7	71
raw	3 oz	124	15	0	76	0	6.8	55
BUTTERHEAD LETTUCE. See under LETTUCE.								
BUTTERMILK								
cultured *(A&P)*	1 cup	90	8	12	260	0	1.0	0
cultured *(Crowley)*	1 cup	110	9	12	390	0	4.0	15
cultured, low-fat	1 quart	396	32	47	1028	0	8.6	34
cultured, low-fat	1 cup	99	8	12	257	0	2.2	9
cultured, low-fat	1 fl oz	12	1	1	32	0	0.3	1
cultured, 1.5%, 'Golden Churn' *(Borden)*	1 cup	120	8	11	250	0	4.0	0
cultured, 1.5%, 'Unsalted' *(Friendship)*	1 cup	120	9	12	125	0	4.0	14
cultured, 2%, *(Knudsen)*	1 cup	120	8	12	140	0	5.0	0
cultured, 'Unsalted' *(Crowley)*	1 cup	110	9	12	130	0	4.0	15
cultured, 'Unsalted' (Friendship)	1 cup	120	9	12	125	0	4.0	14

Food Name	Serv. Size	Total Cal.	Prot. gms	Carbs gms	Sod. mgs	Fiber gms	Fat gms	Chol. mgs
dry	1 cup	464	41	59	621	0	6.9	83
dry	1 tbsp	25	2	3	34	0	0.4	5
dry, blend, cultured *(Saco Foods)*	3.5 tbsp	79	8	11	168	0	0.7	0
BUTTERNUT								
dried	1 cup	734	30	14	1	6	68.4	0
dried	1 oz	174	7	3	0	1	16.2	0
dried	1 nutmeat	18	1	0	0	0	1.7	0
BUTTERNUT SQUASH. See under SQUASH.								
BUTTERSCOTCH. See under CANDY.								
BUTTERSCOTCH TOPPING								
(Kraft)	1 tbsp	60	0	13	70	0	1.0	0
(Smucker's)	2 tbsp	140	0	33	75	0	1.0	0
BUTTON MUSHROOM. See MUSHROOM, WHITE.								

C

Food Name	Serv. Size	Total Cal.	Prot. gms	Carbs gms	Sod. mgs	Fiber gms	Fat gms	Chol. mgs
CABBAGE, COMMON								
boiled, drained, shredded	1/2 cup	17	1	3	6	2	0.3	0
boiled, drained, whole, medium, approx 5.75-inch diam	1 head	278	13	56	101	29	5.4	0
raw, chopped	1 cup	22	1	5	16	2	0.2	0
raw, leaf, large leaf	1 leaf	8	0	2	6	1	0.1	0
raw, leaf, medium leaf	1 leaf	6	0	1	4	1	0.1	0
raw, leaf, small leaf	1 leaf	4	0	1	3	0	0.0	0
raw, shredded	1 cup	18	1	4	13	2	0.2	0
raw, whole, large, approx 7-inch diam	1 head	312	18	68	225	29	3.4	0
raw, whole, medium head, approx 5.75-inch diam	1 head	227	13	49	163	21	2.5	0
raw, whole, small head, approx 4.5-inch diam	1 head	179	10	39	129	16	1.9	0
CABBAGE, DANISH								
raw, shredded	1/2 cup	8	0	2	6	1	0.1	0
raw, whole, medium	1 head	218	11	49	163	21	1.6	0
CABBAGE, NAPA. See BOK CHOY.								
CABBAGE, RED								
Canned or jarred								
sweet and sour *(Green Giant)*	1/2 cup	90	1	21	640	2	0.0	0
sweet and sour *(S&W)*	2 tbsp	15	0	3	160	0	0.0	0
Fresh								
boiled, drained, leaf	1 leaf	5	0	1	2	0	0.0	0
boiled, drained, shredded	1/2 cup	16	1	3	6	2	0.1	0
raw, chopped	1 cup	24	1	5	10	2	0.2	0
raw, leaf, medium	1 leaf	6	0	1	3	0	0.1	0
raw, shredded	1 cup	19	1	4	8	1	0.2	0
raw, whole, large, approx 5.5-inch diam	1 head	306	16	69	125	23	2.9	0
raw, whole, medium, approx 5-inch diam	1 head	227	12	51	92	17	2.2	0
raw, whole, small, approx 4-inch diam	1 head	153	8	35	62	11	1.5	0
CABBAGE, SAVOY								
boiled, drained, shredded	1 cup	35	3	8	35	4	0.1	0
raw, shredded	1 cup	19	1	4	20	2	0.1	0
CABBAGE, SKUNK/swamp cabbage/water convolvulus								
boiled, drained, chopped	1 cup	20	2	4	120	2	0.2	0
raw, chopped	1 cup	11	1	2	63	1	0.1	0
raw, medium shoot	1 shoot	2	0	0	15	0	0.0	0
CABBAGE DISH/ENTRÉE								
(Lean Cuisine)								
stuffed cabbage, w/whipped potatoes	1 entrée	220	11	27	460	5	7.0	25

Food Name	Serv. Size	Total Cal.	Prot. gms	Carbs gms	Sod. mgs	Fiber gms	Fat gms	Chol. mgs
stuffed cabbage w/meat and tomato sauce, potato ...... 1 pkg		199	12	26	412	6	5.6	24
(Efficienc)								
stuffed cabbage roll entrée, food service product ..... 1 serving		168	11	17	1026	na	6.0	na
(Stouffer's)								
stuffed cabbage, w/o sauce, frozen, food service product ... 1 oz		36	2	3	136	1	1.9	6
stuffed cabbage, w/sauce, frozen, food service product .... 1 oz		27	1	3	128	0	1.2	3

CABBAGE TURNIP. See KOHLRABI.
CAJUN SEASONING. See under MARINADE MIX; SEASONING MIX; SEASONING AND COATING MIX.
CAKE. See also BREAD, QUICK; CAKE, SNACK; CAKE MIX.

Food Name	Serv. Size	Total Cal.	Prot. gms	Carbs gms	Sod. mgs	Fiber gms	Fat gms	Chol. mgs
(Awrey's)								
'Best Wishes' 6-inch diam .... 1/4 cake		150	1	18	170	0	9.0	25
'Four-in-One Occasion' .... 1.3 oz		150	1	18	170	0	8.0	25
BANANA								
(Entenmann's)								
crunch, fat-free, cholesterol-free .... 1 slice		140	2	33	150	2	0.0	0
loaf, fat-free, cholesterol-free .... 1 slice		150	2	34	190	1	0.0	0
(Sara Lee) single layer, iced .... 1/8 cake		170	1	28	160	0	6.0	0
BLACK FOREST								
(Awrey's) torte .... 1/14 cake		350	3	38	330	1	21.0	50
(Sara Lee) two-layer, frozen .... 1/8 cake		190	2	28	100	0	8.0	0
BLUEBERRY								
(Entenmann's) crunch, fat-free, cholesterol-free .... 1 slice		140	2	32	200	2	0.0	0
BOSTON CREAM PIE								
(Pepperidge Farm) .... 1 slice		260	3	42	120	1	9.0	45
(Weight Watchers) frozen, approx 1/2 pkg .... 3 oz		160	3	34	260	0	4.0	5
CARAMEL FUDGE *(Weight Watchers)* à la mode ...... 1 serving		160	4	29	180	0	3.0	5
CARROT								
(Awrey's) cream cheese iced, three-layer .... 1/12 cake		390	5	44	310	1	23.0	45
(Entenmann's) fat-free, cholesterol-free .... 1 slice		170	3	40	230	1	0.0	0
(Pepperidge Farm)								
cream cheese iced, frozen, 'Old Fashioned' .... 1.5 oz		150	1	19	160	0	9.0	15
'Deluxe' .... 1 slice		310	2	39	320	1	16.0	40
(Sara Lee) single layer, iced, frozen .... 1/8 cake		250	3	30	240	0	13.0	25
(Stilwell) frozen, 'Oregon Farms' .... 1/6 cake		280	4	38	370	3	15.0	30
(Weight Watchers) frozen, 1/2 pkg .... 3 oz		170	4	27	280	0	5.0	5
CHEESECAKE								
(Sara Lee)								
cream strawberry, frozen .... 1/6 cake		222	4	34	171	0	8.0	0
cream, cherry, frozen .... 1/6 cake		243	4	35	184	0	8.0	0
cream, plain, frozen .... 1/6 cake		230	5	27	153	0	11.0	0
French, frozen, 'Classics' .... 1/8 cake		250	4	23	120	0	16.0	20
strawberry, French, frozen, 'Classics' .... 1/8 cake		240	3	28	125	0	13.0	20
(Tofutti) nondairy, frozen, 'Better than Cheesecake' .... 1/10 cake		160	2	16	110	0	10.0	0
(Weight Watchers)								
brownie .... 1 serving		200	9	33	220	4	6.0	5
frozen .... 3.9 oz		210	10	29	230	0	7.0	20
New York style .... 1 serving		150	6	21	140	0	5.0	10
strawberry, frozen, 'Sweet Celebrations' .... 3.9 oz		180	7	28	210	0	4.0	20
triple chocolate .... 1 serving		200	7	32	200	1	5.0	10
triple chocolate, frozen, 'Sweet Celebrations' .... 1 cake		190	8	30	220	0	4.0	5
CHERRY *(Weight Watchers)* cherries and cream, frozen ..... 3 oz		190	3	32	200	0	6.0	5
CHOCOLATE								
(Awrey's)								
double chocolate torte .... 1/14 cake		340	3	51	300	2	15.0	35
double chocolate, three-layer .... 1/12 cake		310	3	48	290	2	14.0	35
double chocolate, two-layer .... 1/12 cake		250	3	38	260	1	11.0	35
German, iced, 2 x 2-inch piece .... 1 piece		160	2	19	150	0	9.0	20

Food Name	Serv. Size	Total Cal.	Prot. gms	Carbs gms	Sod. mgs	Fiber gms	Fat gms	Chol. mgs
German chocolate, three-layer	1/12 cake	350	3	46	300	1	18.0	40
'Happy Birthday'	1.4 oz	150	1	18	150	1	8.0	25
milk chocolate, yellow, two-layer	1/12 cake	290	3	33	320	0	17.0	50
white iced, two-layer	1/12 cake	270	3	34	290	1	15.0	40
(Entenmann's)								
crunch, fat-free, cholesterol-free	1 slice	130	2	32	170	2	0.0	0
devil's food, fudge iced	1.2 oz	130	2	19	120	0	5.0	0
fudge iced, fat-free, cholesterol-free	1 slice	210	3	51	270	2	0.0	0
loaf, fat-free, cholesterol-free	1 slice	130	3	30	250	1	0.0	0
(Pepperidge Farm)								
chocolate mousse	1 slice	250	2	35	120	2	10.0	25
devil's food, layer	1 slice	290	2	40	220	2	14.0	35
frozen, 'Supreme'	2 7/8 oz	300	3	37	140	0	16.0	25
fudge layer cake	1 slice	300	2	38	230	2	16.0	35
fudge stripe layer cake	1 slice	290	2	38	150	2	14.0	35
German chocolate, layer	1 slice	300	2	37	280	2	16.0	35
(Sara Lee)								
chocolate mousse, frozen, 'Classics'	1/8 cake	260	3	23	100	0	17.0	20
double chocolate, three layer, frozen	1/8 cake	220	3	26	130	0	11.0	20
frozen, 'Free & Light'	1/8 cake	110	2	26	140	0	0.0	0
(Stilwell) bar cake, frozen	1/6 cake	260	3	43	410	2	9.0	40
(Weight Watchers)								
devil's food, 'Sweet Rewards'	1 serving	160	2	36	370	1	1.5	0
double fudge	1 serving	190	4	36	200	2	4.5	0
frozen	2.5 oz	180	5	31	250	0	5.0	5
German chocolate, frozen	2.5 oz	200	4	31	220	0	7.0	5
CHOCOLATE VANILLA ROLL								
(Ener-G Foods) gluten-free	2 oz	168	0	28	59	0	4.0	102
CINNAMON *(Pillsbury)* swirl, refrigerated	1/8 pkg	180	2	22	170	0	9.0	0
CINNAMON APPLE								
(Entenmann's) twist, fat-free, cholesterol-free	1 slice	150	3	35	110	1	0.0	0
COCONUT								
(Pepperidge Farm) layer	1 slice	300	2	41	200	1	14.0	40
(Awrey's) yellow, three-layer	1/12 cake	350	3	40	340	0	21.0	50
COFFEECAKE								
(Awrey's)								
caramel nut	1/12 cake	140	2	15	150	0	8.0	5
'Long John'	1/12 cake	160	2	19	130	0	8.0	10
(Entenmann's)								
cheese	1.6 oz	150	3	20	140	0	7.0	0
cinnamon apple, fat-free, cholesterol-free	1 slice	130	2	29	110	2	0.0	0
crumb	1.3 oz	160	3	21	160	0	7.0	0
crumb, cheese-filled	1.4 oz	130	3	18	140	0	6.0	0
(Pillsbury)								
cinnamon swirl, w/icing	1 serving	230	3	29	240	0	11.0	0
pecan crumb, w/icing	1 serving	230	3	29	240	0	12.0	0
(Sara Lee)								
cheese, all butter, frozen	1/8 cake	210	4	25	220	0	11.0	0
pecan, all butter, frozen	1/8 cake	160	3	19	180	0	8.0	0
streusel, all butter, frozen	1/8 cake	160	3	20	160	0	7.0	0
CRUMB								
(Entenmann's)								
apple spice, fat-free, cholesterol-free	1 slice	138	2	32	148	2	0.0	0
French, all butter	1.6 oz	180	2	26	220	0	8.0	0
golden, French, fat-free, cholesterol-free	1 slice	140	2	35	150	2	0.0	0
FRUIT *(Ener-G Foods)* loaf, gluten-free	1 slice	118	3	22	130	7	2.2	13
FUNNEL *(Funnel Cake Factory)* 5-inch	1 serving	270	4	31	230	1	14.0	30

Food Name	Serv. Size	Total Cal.	Prot. gms	Carbs gms	Sod. mgs	Fiber gms	Fat gms	Chol. mgs
GOLDEN								
(Entenmann's)								
fudge iced, fat-free, cholesterol-free	1 slice	220	3	52	200	2	0.0	0
thick fudge	1.2 oz	130	2	20	120	0	6.0	0
(Pepperidge Farm) layer	1 slice	290	3	38	230	1	14.0	50
LEMON								
(Awrey's)								
three-layer	1/12 cake	320	2	38	310	0	19.0	45
yellow, two-layer	1/12 cake	290	2	33	310	0	17.0	45
(Pepperidge Farm)								
lemon coconut, frozen, 'Supreme'	3 oz	280	3	38	220	0	13.0	30
lemon cream, frozen, 'Supreme'	1 5/8 oz	170	2	21	120	0	9.0	20
LOUISIANA CRUNCH								
(Entenmann's)								
	1.7 oz	180	2	27	180	0	8.0	0
fat-free, cholesterol-free	1 slice	220	3	51	220	1	0.0	0
MARBLE *(Entenmann's)* loaf, fat-free, cholesterol-free	1 slice	130	2	29	190	1	0.0	0
NEAPOLITAN *(Awrey's)* torte	1/14 cake	380	3	43	370	0	22.0	55
ORANGE *(Awrey's)* three-layer	1/12 cake	320	2	40	320	0	17.0	35
PEANUT BUTTER *(Awrey's)* torte	1/14 cake	380	7	44	340	1	22.0	40
PECAN STREUSEL *(Pillsbury)* refrigerated	1/8 pkg	180	2	21	170	0	9.0	0
PINEAPPLE								
(Entenmann's) crunch	1 oz slice	70	1	16	85	0	0.0	0
(Pepperidge Farm) pineapple cream, frozen, 'Supreme'	2 oz	190	2	28	130	0	7.0	20
PISTACHIO *(Awrey's)* torte	1/12 cake	370	3	41	370	1	22.0	35
POUND								
(Awrey's) golden	1/14 loaf	130	2	19	150	0	5.0	20
(Ener-G Foods) gluten-free	1 serving	236	4	32	576	3	9.9	9
(Entenmann's)								
all butter, loaf	1 oz	110	2	15	150	0	5.0	0
sour cream, loaf	1 oz	120	1	14	90	0	7.0	0
(Pepperidge Farm) frozen, 'Old Fashioned								
Cholesterol-Free'	1 oz	110	1	13	85	0	6.0	0
(Sara Lee)								
all butter, frozen, 'Family Size Original'	1/15 cake	130	2	14	85	0	7.0	0
all butter, frozen, 'Original'	1/10 cake	130	2	14	85	0	7.0	0
all butter, frozen, 1.6 oz	1 piece	200	2	23	190	0	11.0	0
frozen, 'Free & Light'	1/10 cake	70	1	17	105	0	0.0	0
RASPBERRY								
(Awrey's) nut	1/16 cake	310	3	39	220	0	16.0	30
(Entenmann's) twist, fat-free, cholesterol-free	1 slice	140	3	33	125	2	0.0	0
(Great Cakes) bar, all natural	3 oz	175	7	35	4	16	2.0	0
SHORTCAKE *(Sara Lee)* strawberry, frozen	1/8 cake	190	2	26	90	0	8.0	0
SPONGE *(Awrey's)* 2 x 2-inch piece	1 piece	80	1	11	125	0	3.0	15
STRAWBERRY								
(Awrey's) strawberry supreme torte	1/14 cake	270	3	38	310	1	12.0	45
(Pepperidge Farm)								
strawberry cream, frozen, 'Supreme'	2 oz	190	1	30	120	0	7.0	20
strawberry stripe, layer	1 slice	310	2	47	150	1	13.0	65
VANILLA *(Pepperidge Farm)* layer	1 slice	290	2	41	190	1	13.0	45
WALNUT *(Awrey's)* torte	1/14 cake	320	2	38	290	0	19.0	30
YELLOW *(Awrey's)* white iced, 2 x 2-inch piece	1 piece	150	1	18	180	0	9.0	25
CAKE, SNACK								
(Awrey's) 'Best Wishes, Miniature'	3 oz	320	5	33	280	0	22.0	0
(Break Cake)								
filled twins, 3 oz	2 cakes	310	2	53	260	0	10.0	15
filled twins, multi-pak, 1.5 oz	1 cake	150	1	26	130	0	5.0	5

Food Name	Serv. Size	Total Cal.	Prot. gms	Carbs gms	Sod. mgs	Fiber gms	Fat gms	Chol. mgs
(Drake's)								
cream filled, 'Sunny Doodle'	1 piece	100	1	16	100	0	3.0	10
cream filled, 'Ring Ding'	1 piece	100	1	16	110	0	4.0	0
'Funny Bone'	1.25 oz	150	3	18	110	0	8.0	0
'Zoinks'	1.25 oz	130	1	20	130	0	5.0	10
(Erewhon) 'Poppets'	1 oz	110	2	24	10	1	1.0	0
(Hostess)								
dessert cup	1 piece	90	2	18	170	0	2.0	15
'Lil' Angels'	1 piece	90	1	14	95	0	2.0	2
'Snowballs'	1 serving	180	1	31	190	1	5.0	5
'Suzy Q's'	1 serving	230	2	35	270	1	9.0	10
'Tiger Tail'	1 piece	240	4	38	290	1	8.0	25
'Twinkie'	1 serving	150	1	25	200	0	5.0	20
(Little Debbie)								
'Be My Valentine'	2.5 oz	330	2	44	125	0	17.0	1
'Caravella'	1.2 oz	200	2	26	95	0	9.0	1
Christmas tree	1 cake	190	1	26	100	0	10.0	0
dessert cup	0.79 oz	80	1	4	170	0	1.0	1
'Doodle Dandies'	2.5 oz	320	2	44	140	0	16.0	1
'Easter Bunny'	2.5 oz	320	2	45	135	0	15.0	1
'Tiger Cake'	1 cake	310	2	44	190	1	15.0	0
(Sunbelt) bar, baked	1.31 oz	130	1	28	130	0	2.0	1
(Tastykake) 'Tasty Twist'	1 piece	18	0	3	0	0	0.6	0
ANGEL FOOD *(Break Cake)*	1 oz	70	1	16	100	0	0.0	0
APPLE								
(Aunt Fanny's) applesauce	2.5 oz	234	3	40	230	0	7.0	0
(Awrey's) apple streusel	1 piece	160	2	18	120	0	9.0	15
(Erewhon) 'Apple Stroodles'	1 oz	90	3	23	15	3	0.0	0
(Hostess) 'Light'	1 piece	130	2	29	150	1	1.0	0
(Little Debbie)								
'Apple Delight'	1.25 oz	140	2	24	95	0	4.0	1
apple spice, 2.2 oz	1 piece	270	2	41	180	0	11.0	1
(Pepperidge Farm)								
apple spice, frozen, 'Dessert Lights' 4.25 oz	1 piece	170	2	37	105	0	2.0	10
(Sara Lee) frozen, apple crisp 'Lights' 3 oz	1 piece	150	1	31	130	0	2.0	5
(Weight Watchers) apple raisin bar	1 bar	70	1	14	60	2	2.0	0
BANANA								
(Awrey's) iced	1 piece	140	1	17	120	0	8.0	20
(Break Cake) banana marshmallow pie	1 pie	150	1	25	80	0	5.0	0
(Hostess) 'Suzy Q's'	1 piece	240	2	4	200	0	9.0	20
(Little Debbie) banana slices	3 oz	340	3	54	260	0	12.0	1
(Tastykake) 'Creamie'	1.5 oz	185	2	25	91	1	7.1	8
BLACK FOREST *(Sara Lee)* frozen, 3.6 oz, 'Lights'	1 piece	170	3	34	85	0	5.0	10
BOSTON CREAM *(Pepperidge Farm)* frozen, 'Hyannis'	1 piece	230	4	34	125	2	10.0	70
BROWN RICE TREAT								
(Glenny's)								
98% fat-free, 100% natural	1 pkg	120	1	28	25	1	3.0	0
caramel, 100% natural	1.25 oz	120	1	29	70	1	0.0	0
chocolate, 100% natural,	1.25 oz	120	1	28	10	2	0.0	0
BROWNIE								
(Auburn Farms)								
butterscotch, nonfat, 'Jammers'	1 brownie	100	2	22	65	2	0.0	0
cappuccino fudge, nonfat, 'Jammers'	1 brownie	100	2	22	90	2	0.0	0
chocolate fudge, nonfat, 'Jammers'	1 brownie	90	2	22	95	2	0.0	0
raspberry fudge, nonfat, 'Jammers'	1 brownie	90	2	22	95	2	0.0	0
whole wheat fudge	1 serving	90	2	22	35	2	0.0	0

Food Name	Serv. Size	Total Cal.	Prot. gms	Carbs gms	Sod. mgs	Fiber gms	Fat gms	Chol. mgs
(Awroy's)								
Dutch chocolate, 'Cake'	1/16 cake	340	3	40	260	1	20.0	35
fudge nut, iced, 'Sheet Cake' 2.5 oz	1 brownie	300	3	36	210	1	17.0	40
fudge nut, 'Sheet Cake' 1.25 oz	1 brownie	150	2	16	115	1	9.0	25
(Break Cake)								
chocolate nut, mini, 0.5 oz	1 brownie	70	1	9	60	0	4.0	0
fudge, 2.8 oz	1 brownie	370	4	47	260	0	18.0	35
(Ener-G Foods) gluten free	1 serving	108	2	16	178	2	4.1	10
(Entenmann's) fudge, cholesterol-free	1 piece	110	2	27	140	1	0.0	0
(Frito-Lay's) fudge nut, 3 oz	1 brownie	360	3	56	225	0	14.0	8
(Health Valley) fudge brownie bar, nonfat	1 bar	110	3	26	30	4	0.0	0
(Hostess) fudge, chocolate iced, lowfat, 'Lights'	1 brownie	140	2	29	95	1	2.6	10
(Little Debbie)								
fudge	1 brownie	270	2	39	170	1	13.0	15
low-fat	1 serving	190	3	39	200	1	3.0	0
twin wrapped	1 pkg	247	3	39	190	1	9.9	10
(Nestlé)								
chocolate chip, frozen, 'Toll House Ready to Bake'	1.4 oz	150	2	19	60	0	7.0	0
(Pepperidge Farm) hot fudge, 'Newport'	1 ramekin	400	4	50	160	0	20.0	80
(Tastykake) fudge walnut, 3 oz	1 brownie	335	4	53	222	5	14.2	22
(Weight Watchers)								
brownie à la mode	1 serving	190	5	34	170	2	4.0	5
chocolate, frosted	1 serving	100	2	22	135	3	2.5	0
chocolate, frozen, 'Sweet Celebrations'	1/3 pkg	100	3	16	150	0	3.0	5
mint frosted 'Sweet Celebrations'	1.23 oz	100	2	18	130	0	2.0	5
peanut butter fudge	1 serving	110	2	21	140	3	2.5	0
Swiss mocha fudge, 'Sweet Celebrations'	1.23 oz	90	2	18	140	0	2.0	5
BUTTERSCOTCH *(Tastykake)* 'Krimpets'	1 oz	103	1	19	83	0	2.6	22
CARAMEL *(Little Debbie)* peanut filled, chocolate coated	1 piece	230	3	28	120	0	12.0	1
CARROT								
(Break Cake)								
multi pak, 1.2 oz	1 cake	120	1	20	115	0	4.0	5
3.5 oz	2 cakes	370	3	64	380	0	12.0	20
(Pepperidge Farm) frozen 'Classic' 2.5 oz	1 piece	260	2	32	280	0	16.0	50
(Sara Lee)								
frozen, 1.8 oz, 'Deluxe'	1 piece	180	3	26	200	0	7.0	0
frozen, 2.5 oz, 'Lights'	1 piece	170	4	30	75	0	4.0	5
CHEESECAKE								
(Pepperidge Farm) strawberry, frozen, 'Manhattan'	1 piece	300	6	49	250	0	9.0	150
(Sara Lee)								
classic, 2 oz	1 piece	200	4	16	150	0	14.0	0
French, frozen, 3.2 oz, 'Lights'	1 piece	150	5	24	90	0	4.0	15
French, strawberry, frozen, 3.5 oz, 'Lights'	1 piece	150	3	29	65	0	2.0	5
(Weight Watchers)								
brownie, 'Sweet Celebrations'	3.5 oz	200	9	34	260	0	5.0	10
strawberry, 'Sweet Celebrations'	3.9 oz	180	7	28	210	0	4.0	20
CHERRY *(Pepperidge Farm)* frozen, supreme, 3.25 oz, 'Dessert Lights'	1 piece	170	0	38	35	0	2.0	80
CHOCOLATE								
(Aunt Fanny's)								
chocolate fudge	2.5 oz	222	4	39	402	0	6.0	0
fingers, devil's food	3 oz	288	4	49	438	0	9.0	0
(Awrey's) one piece	0.8 oz	70	1	11	110	0	3.0	15
(Break Cake)								
chocolate marshmallow pie	1 pie	150	1	24	70	0	5.0	0
chocolate marshmallow pie, double-decker	1 pie	360	3	61	170	0	11.0	0

Food Name	Serv. Size	Total Cal.	Prot. gms	Carbs gms	Sod. mgs	Fiber gms	Fat gms	Chol. mgs
devil's food marshmallow pie .... 1 pie		140	1	25	85	0	4.0	0
rounds, multi pak, 1.3 oz .... 1 cake		160	1	24	125	0	7.0	0
rounds, 3.25 oz .... 2 cakes		390	3	58	300	0	16.0	0
(Drake's)								
Swiss chocolate roll, cream filled .... 1.4 oz		170	2	22	140	0	8.0	15
chocolate mint, cream filled 'Ring Ding' .... 1.5 oz		190	2	22	115	0	11.0	0
chocolate roll, cream filled, 'Yodel' .... 1.1 oz		150	2	16	65	0	9.0	5
cream filled, 'Devil Dog' .... 1.5 oz		160	2	24	135	0	6.0	0
cream filled, 'Ring Ding' .... 1.5 oz		180	2	23	115	0	10.0	0
(Hostess)								
'Choco Bliss' .... 1 piece		200	2	29	210	1	9.0	5
'Chocodiles' .... 1 serving		240	2	33	180	1	11.0	20
'Chocolicious' .... 1 serving		190	1	30	210	1	7.0	10
creme filled, 'Ding Dongs' .... 1 serving		368	3	45	241	2	19.4	14
vanilla pudding filled, 'Light' .... 1 piece		130	2	28	180	1	1.0	0
(Little Debbie)								
.... 2.5 oz		320	2	45	135	0	14.0	1
'Be My Valentine' .... 1 cake		270	2	39	160	1	13.0	0
'Choco-Cake' .... 2.17 oz		270	2	37	220	0	13.0	1
'Choco-Jel' .... 1.16 oz		150	1	21	80	0	7.0	1
chocolate fudge, crispy .... 2.1 oz		260	2	48	90	0	7.0	1
chocolate fudge, round .... 2.75 oz		330	3	55	180	0	12.0	1
chocolate slices .... 3 oz		320	3	56	280	0	9.0	1
chocolate twins .... 2.2 oz		240	2	41	200	0	7.0	1
(Pepperidge Farm)								
chocolate fudge, frozen, 1.6 oz cake .... 1 piece		190	2	24	125	0	10.0	0
double chocolate, frozen, 2.25 oz, 'Classic' .... 1 piece		250	2	31	180	0	13.0	35
double chocolate, frozen, 2.5 oz, 'Lights' .... 1 piece		150	4	23	85	0	5.0	10
German chocolate, frozen, 2.25 oz, 'Classic' .... 1 piece		250	2	29	230	0	13.0	45
mousse, frozen, 1.5 oz, 'Dessert Lights' .... 1 piece		190	3	25	260	0	9.0	5
mousse, frozen, 3 oz serving .... 1 piece		180	5	20	125	0	9.0	15
mousse, frozen, 3 oz, 'Lights' .... 1 piece		170	4	20	60	0	8.0	10
(Snackwell's)								
devil's food cookie cake, nonfat .... 1 cookie		50	1	13	25	1	0.0	0
double fudge cookie cake, nonfat .... 1 serving		50	1	12	70	1	0.0	0
frosted fudge cake .... 1 cake		180	1	25	130	1	10.0	5
(Tastykake)								
cream filled, 'Krimpets' .... 1 piece		124	1	20	113	0	4.3	6
'Creamie' .... 1.5 oz		168	2	24	126	1	7.6	12
'Juniors' .... 3.3 oz		341	4	57	223	4	12.3	60
'Kandy Kakes' .... 0.7 oz		78	1	13	35	1	3.1	0
CHOCOLATE CHIP *(Little Debbie)* .... 1 cake		290	2	42	210	1	14.0	0
CINNAMON *(Aunt Fanny's)* twirl .... 1 oz		110	2	16	85	0	4.0	0
COCONUT								
(Little Debbie)								
coconut creme cake .... 1 cake		210	1	30	140	0	10.0	0
coconut crunch .... 2 oz		320	2	35	80	0	19.0	2
(Pepperidge Farm) frozen, 2.25 oz, 'Classic' .... 1 piece		230	2	31	160	0	11.0	20
(Tastykake) 'Juniors' .... 3.3 oz		296	4	60	304	4	6.0	49
COFFEECAKE								
(Drake's)								
cinnamon crumb .... 1.33 oz		150	2	22	110	0	6.0	10
'Jr.' .... 1.1 oz		140	2	18	90	0	6.0	10
'Small' .... 2 oz		220	3	33	160	0	9.0	15
(Hostess Snack Cake) .... 1 serving		130	1	19	110	0	5.0	10

Food Name	Serv. Size	Total Cal.	Prot. gms	Carbs gms	Sod. mgs	Fiber gms	Fat gms	Chol. mgs
(Little Debbie)								
....	2.1 oz	250	3	39	210	0	9.0	1
apple streusel	1 cake	230	2	39	190	1	7.0	10
(Sara Lee)								
apple cinnamon, individually wrapped	1 piece	290	4	40	270	0	13.0	0
butter streusel, individually wrapped	1 piece	230	4	27	270	0	12.0	0
pecan, individually wrapped	1 piece	280	5	30	270	0	16.0	0
(Tastykake)								
cream filled, 'Koffee Kake'	1 oz	110	1	18	81	0	4.0	16
'Koffee Kake Juniors'	2.5 oz	261	3	44	212	1	8.5	410
(Weight Watchers) cinnamon streusel, 'Microwave'	1/2 pkg	190	3	28	250	0	7.0	5
CRUMB *(Hostess)*	1 serving	90	1	19	100	0	0.5	0
CUPCAKE								
(Aunt Fanny's) orange	3 oz	334	3	54	363	0	12.0	0
(Break Cake)								
chocolate, 3.5 oz	2 cupcakes	350	3	64	350	0	9.0	0
chocolate, multi-pak, 1.3 oz	1 cupcake	130	1	24	135	0	4.0	0
white, 1.3 oz	1 cupcake	130	1	24	115	0	3.0	0
(Hostess)								
chocolate	1 cupcake	180	2	30	290	1	6.0	5
chocolate, creme-filled, 'Light'	1 cupcake	120	2	25	160	0	2.0	0
orange	1 serving	160	1	27	160	0	5.0	10
(Tastykake)								
butter cream, cream filled, 1.1 oz	1 cupcake	118	1	20	120	1	4.2	6
chocolate, 'Royale'	1 cupcake	171	2	28	130	2	6.6	7
chocolate, cream filled, 1.1 oz	1 cupcake	118	1	19	119	1	4.2	4
chocolate, cream filled, 1.1 oz, 'Tastylite'	1 cupcake	100	1	22	116	1	1.3	0
'Kreme Kup'	0.9 oz	86	1	15	113	1	2.8	4
vanilla, cream filled, 'Tastylite'	1 cupcake	100	1	21	121	1	1.5	0
FRUIT *(Hostess)* 'Fruit Loaf'	1 piece	400	4	77	520	0	9.0	7
GOLDEN *(Hostess)* creme-filled, 'Twinkies'	1 piece	150	2	27	200	1	5.0	20
JELLY								
(Little Debbie) jelly roll	2.2 oz	250	1	43	160	0	9.0	1
(Tastykake) 'Krimpets'	1 oz	85	1	19	82	1	1.0	21
LEMON								
(Little Debbie) lemon stix	1.5 oz	220	2	29	55	0	10.0	1
(Pepperidge Farm) frozen, supreme 'Dessert Lights'	1 piece	170	4	26	100	0	5.0	50
(Sara Lee) frozen, lemon cream 'Lights'	1 piece	180	3	29	60	0	6.0	10
(Tastykake) 'Juniors'	3.3 oz	306	3	64	255	0	4.0	0
ORANGE *(Tastykake)* 'Juniors'	3.3 oz	337	3	61	236	1	9.2	5
PEANUT BUTTER								
(Little Debbie) wafer, 'Peanut Butter Naturals'	1.25 oz	170	5	19	90	0	10.0	1
(Tastykake) 'Kandy Kakes'	0.7 oz	87	2	11	38	1	4.2	5
PECAN								
(Aunt Fanny's) twirls	2 twirls	210	2	33	160	2	8.0	5
(Little Debbie) twins	2 oz	220	3	34	170	0	10.0	1
(Tastykake) twirls	1 oz	109	1	17	74	0	4.9	0
POUND								
(Aunt Fanny's)	2.5 oz	260	3	41	253	0	9.0	0
(Drake's) approx. 1.1 oz	1/10 cake	110	2	16	70	0	5.0	25
(Sara Lee) frozen, all butter, 1.6 oz	1 piece	200	2	23	190	0	11.0	0
PUDDING *(Hostess)*	1 piece	170	2	32	200	0	4.0	8
RASPBERRY								
(Aunt Fanny's) fingers	3 oz	303	3	53	337	0	9.0	0
(Little Debbie) raspberry angel cake	1 cake	120	2	28	100	1	1.5	0
(Pepperidge Farm) vanilla swirl, frozen, 'Dessert Lights' ...	1 piece	160	4	25	140	0	5.0	15
SHORTCAKE								
(Pepperidge Farm) strawberry, frozen, 'Dessert Lights' ...	1 piece	170	2	30	50	1	5.0	70

Food Name	Serv. Size	Total Cal.	Prot. gms	Carbs gms	Sod. mgs	Fiber gms	Fat gms	Chol. mgs
(Weight Watchers) strawberry à la mode .... 1 serving		170	3	33	150	0	2.0	5
SPICE								
(Aunt Fanny's) fingers .... 3 oz		290	3	49	433	0	9.0	0
(Little Debbie) .... 1 cake		300	2	44	230	0	14.0	10
STRAWBERRY *(Hostess)* 'Twinkies Fruit 'N Creme' ...... 1.75 oz		160	2	32	210	1	3.0	20
VANILLA								
(Aunt Fanny's) fingers .... 3 oz		250	3	50	380	0	9.0	25
(Little Debbie) .... 2.6 oz		330	2	46	135	0	16.0	1
(Pepperidge Farm) fudge swirl, frozen, 'Classic' .... 1 piece		250	2	33	160	0	11.0	35
(Tastykake)								
cream filled 'Krimpets' .... 1.1 oz		116	1	19	77	1	4.1	19
'Creamie' .... 1.5 oz		184	1	25	117	1	9.0	26
YELLOW *(Awrey's)* one piece .... 0.9 oz		80	1	12	135	0	3.0	20
CAKE, SNACK, MIX								
APPLE								
(Pillsbury)								
apple streusel bar, deluxe, mix only .... 1/24 pkg		130	1	22	40	1	4.5	0
apple streusel bar, deluxe, prepared .... 1/24 pkg		150	1	23	55	1	6.0	0
BROWNIE								
regular, mix only .... 1 oz		123	1	22	86	na	4.2	0
regular, mix only .... 21.5-oz pkg		2647	24	467	1848	na	90.9	0
(Betty Crocker)								
caramel, 'Supreme' prepared .... 1 brownie		110	1	21	110	0	2.0	0
caramel, 'Supreme' prepared w/1/4 cup oil, 1 egg .... 1 brownie		120	1	21	115	0	4.0	10
chocolate chip, 'Supreme' prepared .... 1 brownie		110	1	20	85	0	3.0	0
chocoplate chip, 'Supreme' prepared w/1/4 cup oil,								
1 egg .... 1 brownie		130	1	20	90	0	5.0	10
frosted, 'Supreme' prepared .... 1 brownie		140	1	26	100	0	3.0	0
frosted, 'Supreme' prepared w/1/4 cup oil, 1 egg ..... 1 brownie		160	1	26	105	0	6.0	10
German chocolate, prepared w/oil, margarine, egg,								
2% milk .... 1 brownie		160	1	24	120	0	7.0	10
original, 'Supreme' prepared w/1/4 cup oil, 2 eggs ... 1 brownie		140	1	22	95	0	5.0	20
party, 'Supreme' prepared .... 1 brownie		140	1	26	100	0	3.0	0
party, 'Supreme' prepared w/1/4 cup oil, 1 egg ...... 1 brownie		160	1	26	105	0	6.0	10
peanut butter candies 'Supreme' mix only .... 1/24 pkg		120	2	21	80	0	3.0	0
peanut butter candies 'Supreme' prepared .... 1/24 pkg		140	2	21	85	0	5.0	0
(Duncan Hines)								
blonde, prepared .... 1 piece		160	2	22	100	0	8.0	10
'Dark 'n Fudgy' prepared .... 1 piece		170	2	25	110	1	8.0	15
double fudge, 'Brownies Plus' mix only .... 1 brownie		120	1	22	100	0	3.0	0
double fudge, 'Brownies Plus' prepared .... 1 brownie		150	2	22	105	0	6.0	0
double fudge, prepared .... 1 piece		170	2	29	130	1	7.0	20
fudge, chewy, prepared .... 1 piece		160	2	25	120	1	7.0	10
fudge, prepared .... 1 brownie		130	1	18	90	0	5.0	0
fudge, mix only .... 1 brownie		100	1	18	85	0	18.0	0
'Gourmet Turtle' mix only .... 1 brownie		160	2	27	120	0	5.0	0
'Gourmet Turtle' prepared .... 1 brownie		200	2	27	125	0	9.0	0
milk chocolate, 'Brownies Plus' prepared .... 1 brownie		160	1	20	95	0	8.0	0
milk chocolate, 'Brownies Plus' mix only .... 1 brownie		120	1	20	90	0	4.0	0
milk chocolate chunk, prepared .... 1 piece		170	2	26	120	1	7.0	20
Mississippi mud, prepared .... 1 piece		160	1	26	100	0	6.0	10
peanut butter, 'Brownies Plus' .... 1 brownie		150	3	16	105	0	8.0	0
peanut butter, 'Brownies Plus' mix only .... 1 brownie		120	3	16	100	0	5.0	0
peanut butter, prepared .... 1 piece		160	2	23	120	1	8.0	10
w/walnuts, 'Brownies Plus' .... 1 brownie		150	1	19	90	0	7.0	0
w/walnuts 'Brownies Plus' mix only .... 1 brownie		120	1	19	85	0	4.0	0
turtle, prepared .... 1 piece		160	2	26	110	1	6.0	10

Food Name	Serv. Size	Total Cal.	Prot. gms	Carbs gms	Sod. mgs	Fiber gms	Fat gms	Chol. mgs
walnut, prepared	1 piece	170	2	24	105	0	8.0	10
(Estee) prepared, 2-inch square	1 brownie	50	1	11	0	0	2.0	0
(Finast)								
fudge, 'Ultra Moist'	1/16 pkg	130	2	20	120	0	5.0	0
w/walnuts, 'Ultra Moist'	11/16 pkg	130	1	19	110	0	6.0	0
(General Mills)								
caramel 'Supreme' prepared	1 brownie	110	1	21	110	0	2.0	0
caramel 'Supreme' prepared w/1/4 cup oil, 1 egg	1 brownie	120	1	21	115	0	4.0	10
chocolate chip, 'Supreme' prepared	1 brownie	110	1	20	85	0	3.0	0
chocolate chip, 'Supreme' prepared w/1/4 cup oil, 1 egg	1 brownie	130	1	20	90	0	5.0	10
frosted, 'Supreme' prepared	1 brownie	140	1	26	100	0	3.0	0
frosted, 'Supreme' prepared w/1/4 cup oil, 1 egg	1 brownie	160	1	26	105	0	6.0	10
fudge, 'Family Size' prepared as directed	1 brownie	110	1	22	95	0	2.0	0
fudge, 'Family Size' prepared w/1/4 cup oil, 1 egg	1 brownie	140	1	22	100	0	5.0	10
fudge, 'Light' prepared	1 brownie	100	1	21	90	0	1.0	0
fudge, 'Regular Size' prepared	1 brownie	110	1	23	100	0	2.0	0
fudge, 'Regular Size' prepared w/1/4 cup oil, 1 egg	1 brownie	150	1	23	105	0	6.0	15
German chocolate, 'Supreme' prepared	1 brownie	130	1	24	105	0	3.0	0
German chocolate, prepared w/oil, margarine, egg, 2% milk	1 brownie	160	1	24	120	0	7.0	10
original, 'Supreme' prepared	1 brownie	120	1	22	90	0	3.0	0
original, 'Supreme' prepared w/1/4 cup oil, 2 eggs	1 brownie	140	1	22	95	0	5.0	20
party, 'Supreme' prepared	1 brownie	140	1	26	100	0	3.0	0
party, 'Supreme' prepared w/1/4 cup oil, 1 egg	1 brownie	160	1	26	105	0	6.0	10
walnut, 'Supreme' prepared	1 brownie	110	1	18	85	0	4.0	0
walnut, 'Supreme' prepared w/1/4 cup oil, 1 egg	1 brownie	130	1	18	85	0	6.0	10
(Gluten Free Pantry) chocolate truffle, gluten-free	1 serving	150	1	30	65	2	2.5	0
(Gold Medal)								
fudge, prepared	1 brownie	120	2	24	100	1	2.0	0
fudge, 'Pouch Mix'	1/16 pkg	100	1	16	85	0	4.0	0
(Great Additions)								
double chocolate, mix only	1/24 pkg	110	1	19	70	0	3.0	0
double chocolate, prepared w/1/3 cup oil, 1 egg, 2-inch square	1 brownie	140	1	19	75	0	6.0	10
double chocolate, prepared w/1/3 cup oil, 2 egg whites, 2-inch square	1 brownie	130	1	19	75	0	6.0	0
frosted, 'Funfetti Frosted' mix only	1/24 pkg	100	1	18	80	0	2.0	0
frosted, 'Funfetti' prepared w/1/3 cup oil, 1 egg, 2-inch square	1 brownie	160	1	23	100	0	7.0	10
frosted, 'Funfetti' prepared w/1/3 cup oil, 1 egg white, 2-inch square	1 brownie	150	1	23	100	0	6.0	0
walnut, mix only	1/24 pkg	110	1	16	70	0	4.0	0
walnut, prepared w/water, 1/3 cup oil 2 egg whites, 2-inch square	1 brownie	130	2	16	75	0	7.0	0
walnut, prepared w/water, 1/3 cup oil 1 egg, 2-inch square	1 brownie	140	2	16	70	0	8.0	10
(Krusteaz) fudge, prepared	1.5 oz mix	190	1	28	135	0	8.0	19
(Lovin' Lites)								
fudge, mix only	1/24 pkg	100	1	19	80	0	2.0	0
fudge, prepared w/water, 1 egg	1/24 pkg	100	1	19	80	0	2.0	10
fudge, prepared w/water, 2 egg whites	1/24 pkg	100	1	19	85	0	2.0	0
(Martha White) mix only	1 serving	114	1	23	138	na	1.8	na
(MicroRave)								
frosted	1 brownie	180	2	27	130	0	7.0	0
'Singles' prepared	1 brownie	250	4	39	230	0	9.0	0
walnut, 1.1 oz	1 brownie	160	2	21	95	0	7.0	0

Food Name	Serv. Size	Total Cal.	Prot. gms	Carbs gms	Sod. mgs	Fiber gms	Fat gms	Chol. mgs
w/hot fudge topping, 'Singles'	1 brownie	340	5	54	270	0	12.0	0
(Mixed Company) organic, chewy	1/4 cup	150	3	31	10	1	2.0	0
(Pillsbury)								
caramel fudge chunk, prepared, 2-inch square	1 brownie	170	2	25	105	0	7.0	0
chocolate chip, deluxe, mix only	1/20 pkg	140	1	28	110	1	3.0	0
chocolate chip, deluxe, prepared	1/20 pkg	180	2	28	110	1	7.0	10
cream cheese swirl, mix only	1/20 pkg	140	1	22	90	1	5.0	5
cream cheese swirl, prepared	1/20 pkg	180	2	22	95	1	9.0	25
double fudge, 2-inch square	1 brownie	160	2	24	105	0	6.0	0
fudge, deluxe 'Lovin' Bites'	1 piece	160	2	29	125	0	3.5	15
fudge, 15-oz pkg, mix only	1/16 pkg	110	1	21	90	0	2.0	0
fudge, 15-oz, prep	1/16 pkg	150	1	22	95	1	6.0	15
fudge, mix only	1/9 pkg	130	2	25	110	0	3.0	0
fudge, prepared	1 brownie	190	2	25	105	0	9.0	0
fudge, prepared w/1/4 cup oil	1/9 pkg	190	2	25	110	0	9.0	0
fudge, prepared w/1/2 cup oil, 2 egg whites, 2-inch square	1 brownie	150	1	20	90	0	7.0	0
fudge, prepared w/water, 1/4 cup oil, 1 egg, 2-inch square	1 brownie	140	2	21	95	0	6.0	15
fudge, prepared w/water, 1/4 cup oil, 1 egg white, 2-inch square	1 brownie	140	1	21	95	0	6.0	0
fudge, 21.5-oz pkg, mix only	1/24 pkg	100	1	20	85	0	2.0	0
fudge, 21.5-oz, prepared	1/20 pkg	180	2	25	105	1	8.0	10
fudge, w/fudge frosting, 'Microwave Mix'	1/9 pkg	50	0	7	30	0	2.0	0
fudge, w/fudge frosting, mix only	1/9 pkg	130	2	25	110	0	3.0	0
fudge, w/fudge frosting, prepared w/1/4 cup oil, frosting	1/9 pkg	240	2	32	140	0	11.0	0
fudge deluxe, 'Family Size' 2-inch square	1 brownie	150	1	20	95	0	7.0	0
fudge deluxe, 2-inch square	1 brownie	150	2	21	100	0	6.0	0
fudge deluxe, w/walnuts, 2-inch square	1 brownie	150	2	19	90	0	8.0	0
fudge swirl cookie bar, deluxe, mix only	1/20 pkg	150	1	25	105	1	5.0	0
fudge swirl cookie bar, deluxe, prepared	1/20 pkg	180	1	25	110	1	8.0	10
hot fudge, mix	1/24 pkg	130	1	24	100	1	3.5	0
hot fudge, prepared	1/24 pkg	160	1	24	100	1	7.0	10
rocky road, fudge, 2-inch square	1 brownie	170	2	24	95	0	8.0	0
walnut, mix only	1/18 pkg	140	2	22	90	1	5.0	0
walnut, prepared	1/18 pkg	180	2	22	90	1	9.0	10
traditional, mix only	1 serving	132	1	23	88	na	3.6	na
triple fudge, chunky, 2-inch square	1 brownie	170	2	25	105	0	7.0	0
(Robin Hood) fudge, 'Pouch Mix'	1/16 pkg	100	1	16	85	0	4.0	0
(Weight Watchers) fudge, low-fat, 'Sweet Rewards'	1 serving	130	2	27	115	1	2.5	0
CHEESECAKE								
(Pillsbury)								
lemon, bar, mix only	1/24 pkg	170	1	20	45	0	9.0	10
lemon, bar, prepared	1/24 pkg	180	2	20	50	0	10.0	25
CHOCOLATE								
(Pillsbury)								
Oreo bar, deluxe, mix only	1/24 pkg	130	1	22	125	1	4.0	0
Oreo bar, deluxe, prepared	1/24 pkg	150	1	22	130	1	6.0	10
CUPCAKE								
(Funfetti)								
chocolate, microwave, mix only	1/9 pkg	100	1	14	160	0	4.0	10
chocolate, microwave, w/chocolate fudge frosting, prepared	1/9 pkg	160	1	24	190	0	7.0	10
yellow, microwave, mix only	1/9 pkg	110	1	17	135	0	5.0	10
yellow, microwave, w/vanilla frosting, prepared	1/9 pkg	180	1	28	160	0	7.0	10

Food Name	Serv. Size	Total Cal.	Prot. gms	Carbs gms	Sod. mgs	Fiber gms	Fat gms	Chol. mgs
GINGERBREAD								
(Betty Crocker)								
'Classic' cholesterol-free recipe, prepared .... 1/9 pkg		210	3	35	330	0	6.0	0
'Classic' prepared w/1 egg .... 1/9 pkg		220	3	35	330	0	7.0	30
(Dromedary) mix only .... 3 tbsp		100	1	19	190	0	2.0	0
(Hodgson Mill) whole wheat, mix only .... 1/4 cup		110	2	24	260	2	0.0	0
(Pillsbury)								
.... 1 serving		220	3	40	340	1	5.0	0
prepared, 3-inch square .... 1 piece		190	2	36	310	0	4.0	0
prepared w/water .... 1/9 pkg		180	2	32	300	0	5.0	0
(Sweet 'n Low) w/'Sweet 'n Low' mix only .... 1/6 cake		150	2	30	30	1	3.0	0
NUT								
(Pillsbury)								
Nutter Butter bar, deluxe, mix only .... 1/18 pkg		150	2	26	140	0	4.0	0
Nutter Butter bar, deluxe, prepared .... 1/18 pkg		180	3	26	170	0	7.0	15
CAKE DECORATION. See also under FROSTING; TOPPING.								
candies, rainbow mix *(Dec-a-Cake)* .... 1 tsp		15	0	3	5	0	0.5	0
candies, sugar crystals *(Dec-a-Cake)* .... 1 tsp		15	0	3	0	0	0.0	0
CAKE MIX								
ANGEL FOOD								
(Betty Crocker)								
confetti, 'SuperMoist' .... 1/12 cake		150	3	34	320	0	0.0	0
one-step white, SuperMoist' prepared .... 1/12 cake		140	3	32	320	0	0.0	0
'Traditional' mix only .... 1/12 mix		130	3	30	170	0	0.0	0
'Traditional' 'SuperMoist' prepared .... 1/12 cake		130	3	30	150	0	0.0	0
(Duncan Hines)								
mix only .... 1/12 mix		140	3	30	130	0	0.0	0
prepared .... 1/12 cake		130	3	30	320	0	0.0	0
(General Mills)								
chocolate, mix only .... 1/12 mix		150	3	34	300	0	0.0	0
confetti, mix only .... 1/12 mix		150	3	34	300	0	0.0	0
lemon custard, mix only .... 1/12 mix		150	3	34	300	0	0.0	0
lemon pudding, mix only .... 1/12 mix		150	3	34	300	0	0.0	0
strawberry, mix only .... 1/12 mix		150	3	35	260	0	0.0	0
white, one-step, mix only .... 1/12 mix		150	3	34	300	0	0.0	0
(Gluten Free Pantry) gluten-free .... 1 serving		140	4	32	90	0	0.0	0
(Lovin' Loaf)								
mix only .... 1/8 pkg		90	2	20	210	0	0.0	0
prepared w/water .... 1/8 pkg		90	2	20	210	0	0.0	0
(Pillsbury)								
'Moist Supreme' mix only .... 1/12 pkg		140	3	31	330	0	0.0	0
prepared .... 1/12 cake		150	3	34	360	0	0.0	0
APPLE								
(Betty Crocker)								
apple cinnamon, 'SuperMoist' prepared .... 1/12 cake		250	3	36	280	0	10.0	55
apple cinnamon, 'SuperMoist' prepared,								
cholesterol-free recipe .... 1/12 cake		210	3	36	280	0	6.0	0
(Gold Medal) applesauce raisin, mix only .... 1/9 mix		140	1	28	160	0	3.0	0
(MicroRave)								
apple streusel, prepared .... 1/12 cake		240	2	33	190	0	11.0	45
apple streusel, prepared w/cholesterol-free								
egg product .... 1/12 cake		210	2	33	200	0	8.0	0
(Robin Hood) applesauce raisin, mix only .... 1/9 mix		140	1	28	160	0	3.0	0
BANANA								
(Duncan Hines)								
'Banana Supreme' prepared .... 1/12 cake		250	3	36	270	0	11.0	45
cholesterol-free recipe, prepared .... 1/12 cake		250	3	36	285	0	10.0	0
mix only .... 1/12 pkg		190	2	36	280	0	4.0	0

Food Name	Serv. Size	Total Cal.	Prot. gms	Carbs gms	Sod. mgs	Fiber gms	Fat gms	Chol. mgs
(Gold Medal) banana walnut, mix only	1/9 mix	150	1	27	200	0	4.0	0
(Pillsbury)								
microwave, mix only	1/9 pkg	110	1	17	140	0	5.0	10
'Moist Supreme' mix only	1/12 pkg	180	2	35	260	0	4.0	0
'Moist Supreme' prepared	1/12 pkg	260	3	36	280	0	11.0	55
'Pillsbury Plus' prepared	1/12 cake	260	3	36	280	0	11.0	55
'Pillsbury Plus' prepared w/water, 1/3 cup oil, 3 eggs ...	1/12 pkg	250	3	35	280	0	11.0	55
'Pillsbury Plus' prepared w/water, 3 egg whites, 2 tbsp flour	1/12 pkg	190	3	36	280	0	4.0	0
w/vanilla frosting, microwave, 'Snack' prepared	1/9 pkg	170	1	26	160	0	7.0	10
(Robin Hood) banana walnut, mix only	1/9 mix	150	1	27	200	0	4.0	0
(Sweet 'n Low) mix only	1/6 cake	150	2	30	30	1	3.0	0
BLACK FOREST								
(Duncan Hines) mousse, 'Tiarra'	1/12 cake	260	3	33	270	0	13.0	0
(Pillsbury)								
cherry 'Bundt Ring Cake' mix only	1/16 pkg	200	2	40	310	0	4.0	0
cherry, 'Bundt' prepared	1/16 cake	240	3	38	310	0	8.0	0
cherry, prepared w/1/2 cup oil, 3 egg whites	1/16 pkg	270	3	41	320	0	12.0	40
cherry, prepared w/1/2 cup oil, 4 egg whites	1/16 pkg	260	3	41	320	0	11.0	0
BLUEBERRY								
(Streusel Swirl)								
streusel, mix only	1/16 pkg	210	2	39	190	0	5.0	0
streusel, prepared w/1/3 cup oil, 3 eggs	1/16 pkg	260	3	39	200	0	11.0	40
streusel, prepared w/1/3 cup oil, 4 egg whites	1/16 pkg	250	3	39	200	0	10.0	0
BOSTON CREAM								
(Betty Crocker)								
'Classic' mix only	1/8 pkg	230	1	48	370	0	4.0	0
'Classic' prepared w/egg, 2% milk	1/8 pkg	270	4	50	390	0	6.0	30
(Pillsbury)								
'Bundt' prepared	1/16 cake	270	3	43	310	0	10.0	0
chocolate éclair, 'Bundt Ring' mix only	1/16 pkg	210	1	42	280	0	4.0	0
chocolate éclair, prepared w/1/2 cup oil, 4 egg whites .	1/16 cake	250	2	42	300	0	9.0	0
chocolate éclair, prepared w/1/3 cup oil, 3 eggs	1/16 pkg	260	3	42	290	0	10.0	40
BUTTER BRICKLE								
(Betty Crocker)								
'SuperMoist' prepared	1/12 cake	250	3	38	280	0	10.0	55
'SuperMoist' prepared w/cholesterol-free egg product	1/12 cake	220	3	38	280	0	6.0	0
BUTTER PECAN								
(Betty Crocker)								
'SuperMoist' mix only	1/12 mix	180	1	35	300	0	4.0	0
'SuperMoist' prepared w/3 eggs, 1/3 cup oil	1/12 cake	250	3	35	320	0	11.0	55
'SuperMoist' prepared w/oil, cholesterol-free egg product	1/12 cake	220	3	35	320	0	7.0	0
CARAMEL *(Duncan Hines)* prepared	1/12 cake	250	3	36	270	0	11.0	45
CARROT								
(Betty Crocker)								
'SuperMoist' mix only	1/12 mix	180	1	36	280	0	3.0	0
'SuperMoist' prepared	1/12 cake	200	2	42	320	0	3.0	0
'SuperMoist' prepared w/1/3 cup oil, 3 eggs	1/12 cake	250	3	36	300	0	10.0	55
'SuperMoist' prepared w/1/3 cup oil, egg substitute ...	1/12 cake	210	3	36	300	0	6.0	0
(Dromedary) prepared	1/12 cake	232	3	23	292	0	15.0	0
(Estee) prepared	1/10 cake	100	1	18	65	0	2.0	0
(Pillsbury)								
carrot 'n spice, 'Pillsbury Plus' prepared	1/12 cake	260	3	36	330	0	11.0	0
microwave, mix only	1/9 pkg	110	1	17	170	0	5.0	10
'Moist Supreme' mix only	1/12 pkg	180	2	35	280	1	4.0	0

Food Name	Serv. Size	Total Cal.	Prot. gms	Carbs gms	Sod. mgs	Fiber gms	Fat gms	Chol. mgs
'Moist Supreme' prepared	1/12 pkg	260	3	35	290	1	12.0	55
'Pillsbury Plus' prepared w/1/3 cup oil, 3 eggs	1/12 pkg	260	3	34	300	0	12.0	55
'Pillsbury Plus' prepared w/water, 3 egg whites, 2 tbsp flour	1/12 pkg	190	3	35	300	0	5.0	0
'Quick Bread Mix' mix only	1/12 pkg	110	2	22	150	1	1.0	0
'Quick Bread Mix' prepared	1/12 pkg	140	2	22	150	1	5.0	25
w/cream cheese frosting, microwave, prepared	1/9 pkg	170	1	25	200	0	7.0	10
CHEESECAKE								
(Jell-O)								
lemon, no bake, mix only	1 pkg	170	4	31	300	0	3.0	0
lemon, no bake, prepared, 8-inch cake	1/8 cake	270	5	36	400	0	13.0	25
New York style, no bake, mix only	1 pkg	180	4	33	320	0	3.0	0
New York style, no bake, prepared, 8-inch cake	1/8 cake	280	6	38	420	0	12.0	30
strawberry, no bake, prepared	1/12 cake	340	5	52	400	1	12.0	5
(Royal)								
lite, 'No-Bake'	1/8 cake	210	5	23	380	0	10.0	0
real, 'No-Bake'	1/8 cake	280	5	31	370	0	9.0	0
CHERRY								
(Betty Crocker)								
cherry chip, 'SuperMoist' mix only	1/12 mix	180	2	37	250	0	3.0	0
cherry chip, 'SuperMoist' prepared w/3 egg whites	1/12 mix	190	3	37	270	0	3.0	0
(Duncan Hines)								
cherries and cream 'Tiarra'	1/12 cake	250	4	34	265	0	11.0	0
cherry vanilla, prepared	1/12 cake	250	3	36	270	0	11.0	45
CHOCOLATE								
(Betty Crocker)								
butter recipe, 'SuperMoist' mix only	1/12 mix	190	2	35	300	0	5.0	0
butter recipe, 'SuperMoist' prepared w/1/2 cup butter, 3 eggs	1/12 mix	280	4	35	400	0	14.0	75
chocolate chocolate chip, 'SuperMoist' prepared w/1/3 cup oil, 3 eggs	1/12 mix	260	3	34	400	0	12.0	55
chocolate chocolate chip, 'SuperMoist' mix only	1/12 mix	190	2	34	380	0	5.0	0
chocolate fudge, 'SuperMoist' mix only	1/12 mix	180	2	35	430	0	4.0	0
chocolate fudge, 'SuperMoist' prepared w/1/3 cup oil, 3 eggs	1/12 mix	260	3	35	450	0	12.0	55
chocolate pudding, 'Classic Dessert' mix only	1/6 pkg	220	2	44	240	0	4.0	0
chocolate pudding, 'Classic Dessert' prepared w/1 egg	1/6 pkg	230	3	44	250	0	5.0	35
devil's food 'SuperMoist' 'Light' cholesterol-free recipe, prepared	1/12 mix	180	3	36	370	0	3.0	0
devil's food 'SuperMoist' 'Light' mix only	1/12 mix	180	2	36	330	0	3.0	0
devil's food 'SuperMoist' 'Light' prepared w/3 eggs	1/12 mix	200	4	36	340	0	4.0	55
devil's food, 'SuperMoist' mix only	1/12 mix	190	2	35	410	0	5.0	0
devil's food, 'SuperMoist' prepared w/1/3 cup oil, 3 eggs	1/12 mix	260	4	35	430	0	12.0	55
devil's food, 'SuperMoist' prepared w/oil, cholesterol-free egg product	1/12 mix	220	3	35	430	0	7.0	0
fudge marble, 'SuperMoist' mix only	1/12 mix	180	1	36	270	0	4.0	0
fudge marble, 'SuperMoist' prepared w/1/3 cup oil, 3 eggs	1/12 mix	260	3	36	290	0	11.0	55
fudge marble, 'SuperMoist' prepared w/oil, cholesterol-free egg substitute	1/12 mix	220	3	36	290	0	7.0	0
German chocolate, 'SuperMoist' cholesterol-free recipe, prepared	1/12 mix	220	3	35	420	0	8.0	0
German chocolate, 'SuperMoist' mix only	1/12 mix	180	2	35	400	0	4.0	0
German chocolate, 'SuperMoist' prepared w/1/3 cup oil, 3 eggs	1/12 mix	260	3	35	420	0	12.0	55

Food Name	Serv. Size	Total Cal.	Prot. gms	Carbs gms	Sod. mgs	Fiber gms	Fat gms	Chol. mgs
milk chocolate, 'SuperMoist' cholesterol-free recipe, prepared	1/12 mix	210	3	34	340	0	7.0	0
milk chocolate, 'SuperMoist' mix only	1/12 mix	190	2	34	320	0	5.0	0
milk chocolate, 'SuperMoist' prepared w/1/3 cup oil, 3 eggs	1/12 mix	260	4	34	340	0	12.0	55
sour cream, 'SuperMoist' mix only	1/12 mix	180	2	35	410	0	4.0	0
sour cream, 'SuperMoist' prepared w/egg substitute	1/12 mix	220	3	35	430	0	8.0	0
sour cream, 'SuperMoist' prepared w/1/3 cup oil, 3 eggs	1/12 mix	260	3	35	430	0	12.0	55
(Duncan Hines)								
chocolate mousse, Amaretto, 'Tiarra' prepared	1/12 cake	270	3	29	230	0	16.0	0
chocolate mousse, 'Tiarra' prepared	1/12 cake	270	3	29	235	0	16.0	0
dark Dutch fudge, prepared	1/12 cake	280	4	33	470	0	15.0	65
dark Dutch fudge, cholesterol-free recipe, prepared	1/12 cake	270	4	33	380	0	14.0	0
dark Dutch fudge, mix only	1/12 cake	190	2	33	455	0	5.0	0
devil's food, cholesterol-free recipe, prepared	1/12 cake	270	4	33	380	0	14.0	0
devil's food, mix only	1/12 pkg	190	2	33	360	0	5.0	0
devil's food, prepared	1/12 cake	280	4	33	375	0	15.0	65
fudge, butter recipe, mix only	1/12 cake	190	2	34	240	0	4.0	0
fudge, butter recipe, prepared	1/12 cake	320	3	40	300	2	17.0	80
fudge, butter recipe, prepared w/stick margarine	1/12 cake	270	3	34	350	0	13.0	65
fudge marble, cholesterol-free recipe, prepared	1/12 cake	250	3	36	285	0	10.0	0
fudge marble, mix only	1/12 cake	190	2	36	280	0	4.0	0
fudge marble, prepared	1/12 cake	260	3	36	295	0	11.0	65
Swiss chocolate, cholesterol-free recipe, prepared	1/12 cake	270	4	33	380	0	14.0	0
Swiss chocolate, mix only	1/12 pkg	190	2	33	360	0	5.0	0
Swiss chocolate, prepared	1/12 cake	280	4	33	375	0	15.0	65
(Estee) prepared	1/10 cake	100	1	18	100	0	2.0	0
(Finast) devil's food, 'Ultra Moist' prepared	1/12 cake	250	3	33	360	0	11.0	0
(Gold Medal) mix, chocolate chip fudge, mix only	1/9 mix	150	2	25	210	0	5.0	0
(Krusteaz) devil's food, 8-inch double cake, prepared	1/12 cake	190	4	37	330	0	2.0	25
(MicroRave)								
chocolate fudge, w/vanilla frosting, prepared	1/6 cake	310	3	40	300	0	15.0	35
devil's food, 'Lovin' Lites' mix only	1/12 pkg	160	3	32	370	0	2.0	0
devil's food, 'Lovin' Lites' prepared w/water, 2 eggs	1/12 pkg	170	4	32	380	0	3.0	35
devil's food, 'Lovin' Lites' prepared w/water, 3 egg whites	1/12 pkg	160	4	32	380	0	2.0	0
devil's food, microwave, 'Singles' mix only	1 cake	250	5	35	450	0	10.0	50
devil's food, w/chocolate frosting, microwave, mix only	1/6 pkg	210	2	35	240	0	7.0	0
devil's food, w/chocolate frosting, microwave, prepared	1/6 pkg	310	3	36	250	0	17.0	35
devil's food, w/chocolate frosting, microwave, prepared w/egg substitute	1/6 pkg	240	3	36	250	0	9.0	0
devil's food, w/chocolate frosting, microwave, 'Singles' prepared	1 cake	450	5	65	520	0	19.0	50
German chocolate, w/frosting, microwave, mix only	1/6 pkg	230	2	37	240	0	8.0	0
German chocolate, w/frosting, microwave, prepared	1/6 pkg	320	3	37	350	0	18.0	35
(Pillsbury)								
butter recipe, 'Moist Supreme' mix only	1/12 pkg	180	2	33	330	1	4.0	0
butter recipe, 'Moist Supreme' mix only	1/12 pkg	270	4	33	420	1	13.0	75
butter recipe, 'Pillsbury Plus' mix only	1/12 pkg	170	2	32	330	0	4.0	0
butter recipe, 'Pillsbury Plus' prepared	1/12 pkg	270	4	33	430	2	13.0	75
butter recipe, 'Pillsbury Plus' prepared w/1/2 cup margarine, 4 egg whites	1/12 cake	240	3	32	420	0	12.0	0
caramel nut, 'Bundt Ring Cake' mix	1/16 pkg	180	2	28	200	1	7.0	0
caramel nut, 'Bundt Ring Cake' prepared	1/16 cake	290	3	28	210	1	18.0	40

Food Name	Serv. Size	Total Cal.	Prot. gms	Carbs gms	Sod. mgs	Fiber gms	Fat gms	Chol. mgs
caramel, 'Bundt Ring Cake' mix only .... 1/16 pkg		220	2	43	350	0	5.0	5
caramel, prepared w/1/3 cup oil, 4 egg whites .... 1/16 cake		280	3	43	370	0	12.0	5
caramel, prepared w/water, 1/2 cup oil, 3 eggs ...... 1/16 cake		290	3	43	370	0	13.0	45
chocolate macaroon, prepared w/1/2 cup oil, 4 egg whites .... 1/16 cake		270	3	37	340	0	14.0	0
chocolate macaroon, 'Bundt Ring Cake' mix only ..... 1/16 pkg		210	2	37	330	0	7.0	0
chocolate macaroon, prepared w/1/2 cup oil, 3 eggs .... 1/16 cake		280	3	37	340	0	14.0	40
chocolate mousse, 'Bundt Ring Cake' mix only .... 1/16 pkg		180	2	37	300	0	4.0	0
chocolate mousse, prepared w/1/2 cup oil, 3 eggs .... 1/16 cake		260	3	37	310	0	12.0	40
chocolate mousse, prepared w/1/2 cup oil, 4 egg whites .... 1/16 cake		250	3	37	320	0	11.0	0
dark chocolate, 'Moist Supreme' mix only .... 1/12 pkg		180	2	34	320	1	4.0	0
dark chocolate, 'Moist Supreme' prepared .... 1/12 cake		250	3	34	340	1	11.0	55
dark chocolate, 'Pillsbury Plus' prepared w/3 egg whites, 2 tbsp flour .... 1/12 cake		180	3	33	340	0	5.0	0
dark chocolate, 'Pillsbury Plus' prepared w/water, 1/3 cup oil, 3 eggs .... 1/12 cake		250	3	32	340	0	12.0	55
devil's food, 'Lovin Lites' prepared .... 1/10 cake		230	4	41	420	2	5.0	45
devil's food, 'Lovin' Lites' mix only .... 1/10 pkg		210	2	41	410	2	4.5	0
devil's food, 'Moist Supreme' mix only .... 1/12 pkg		180	2	33	330	1	4.0	0
devil's food, 'Moist Supreme' prepared .... 1/12 cake		270	4	33	340	1	14.0	55
devil's food, 'Pillsbury Plus' prepared w/water, 3 egg whites, 2 tbsp flour .... 1/12 cake		180	3	33	340	0	4.0	0
double hot fudge, Bundt, prepared .... 1/12 cake		280	3	32	220	1	16.0	40
double supreme, microwave, prepared .... 1/8 cake		330	3	39	340	0	19.0	0
fudge, 'Tunnel of Fudge' mix only .... 1/16 pkg		210	2	42	330	0	4.0	0
fudge, 'Tunnel of Fudge' prepared w/3/4 cup oil, 4 egg whites .... 1/16 pkg		300	3	42	340	0	15.0	0
fudge, 'Tunnel of Fudge' prepared w/3/4 cup oil, 3 eggs .... 1/16 cake		310	3	42	340	0	16.0	40
fudge swirl, 'Moist Supreme' mix only .... 1/12 pkg		200	2	37	280	1	4.5	0
fudge swirl, 'Moist Supreme' prepared .... 1/12 cake		250	3	37	290	1	10.0	55
fudge swirl, 'Pillsbury Plus' prepared w/1/3 cup oil, 3 eggs .... 1/12 cake		270	3	36	300	0	12.0	55
fudge swirl, 'Pillsbury Plus' prepared w/water, 3 egg whites, 2 tbsp flour .... 1/12 cake		200	3	37	290	0	5.0	0
German chocolate, 'Moist Supreme' mix only .... 1/12 pkg		180	2	34	270	1	4.0	0
German chocolate, 'Moist Supreme' prepared .... 1/12 cake		250	3	34	280	1	11.0	35
German chocolate, 'Pillsbury Plus' prepared w/1/3 cup oil, 3 eggs .... 1/12 cake		250	3	34	280	0	11.0	55
German chocolate, 'Pillsbury Plus' prepared w/3 egg whites, 2 tbsp flour .... 1/12 cake		180	3	34	280	0	4.0	0
microwave, mix only .... 1/9 pkg		110	1	16	180	0	5.0	10
microwave, prepared .... 1/8 cake		210	2	23	260	0	13.0	0
'Pillsbury Plus' prepared .... 1/12 cake		260	3	34	330	1	12.0	55
'Pillsbury Plus' prepared w/1/2 cup butter, 3 eggs ..... 1/12 pkg		250	4	32	420	0	13.0	75
w/chocolate frosting, microwave, prepared .... 1/8 cake		300	2	35	310	0	17.0	0
w/chocolate fudge frosting, prepared .... 1/9 cake		160	2	24	210	0	7.0	10
w/vanilla frosting, microwave, prepared .... 1/8 cake		300	2	36	300	0	17.0	0
(Robin Hood) mix, chocolate chip fudge, mix only .... 1/9 mix		150	2	25	210	0	5.0	0
(Sweet 'n Low)								
low-fat, low-sodium, low-cholesterol, microwave, prepared1/10 cake 90		2	16	40	1	2.0	0.0	20%
mix only .... 1/6 cake		150	2	30	30	1	3.0	0

Food Name	Serv. Size	Total Cal.	Prot. gms	Carbs gms	Sod. mgs	Fiber gms	Fat gms	Chol. mgs
CHOCOLATE CHIP								
(Betty Crocker)								
'SuperMoist' mix only	1/12 mix	180	2	35	280	0	4.0	0
'SuperMoist' prepared w/oil, cholesterol-free								
egg substitute	1/12 mix	220	3	35	300	0	8.0	0
'SuperMoist' prepared w/1/2 cup oil, 3 eggs	1/12 mix	290	3	35	300	0	15.0	55
(Gold Medal) golden, mix only	1/9 mix	140	1	26	190	0	4.0	0
(Pillsbury)								
'Moist Supreme' mix only	1/12 pkg	190	2	35	270	1	5.0	0
'Moist Supreme' prepared	1/12 cake	240	3	35	280	1	10.0	35
'Pillsbury Plus' prepared w/1/4 cup oil, 2 eggs	1/12 cake	240	3	34	280	0	10.0	35
'Pillsbury Plus' w/2 egg whites, 2 tbsp flour	1/12 cake	190	3	35	280	0	5.0	0
(Robin Hood) golden, mix only	1/9 mix	140	1	26	190	0	4.0	0
CINNAMON								
(MicroRave)								
pecan, microwave	1/6 cake	290	3	39	210	0	13.0	45
pecan, microwave, prepared w/cholesterol-free								
egg product	1/6 cake	240	3	39	220	0	8.0	0
(Pillsbury)								
streusel, microwave, 'Streusel Swirl' prepared	1/8 cake	240	2	33	180	0	11.0	0
streusel, 'Streusel Swirl' mix only	1/16 pkg	210	2	38	210	0	5.0	0
streusel, 'Streusel Swirl' prepared	1/16 cake	260	3	38	200	0	11.0	0
streusel, 'Streusel Swirl' prepared w/1/3 cup oil,								
4 egg whites	1/16 pkg	250	2	38	200	0	10.0	0
streusel, 'Streusel Swirl' prepared w/water,								
1/3 cup oil, 3 eggs	1/16 pkg	260	3	38	200	0	11.0	40
COFFEECAKE								
(Aunt Jemima) 'easy'	1/3 cup	170	2	30	240	1	5.0	0
(Pillsbury) apple cinnamon	1/8 cake	240	3	40	150	0	7.0	0
FRUIT								
(Duncan Hines) tropical fruit, prepared	1/12 cake	250	3	36	270	0	11.0	45
GOLDEN								
(Betty Crocker) vanilla, 'SuperMoist' prepared	1/12 cake	170	1	35	270	0	3.0	0
(Duncan Hines)								
golden, butter recipe, mix only	1/12 pkg	190	2	36	160	0	4.0	0
golden, butter recipe, prepared	1/12 cake	320	3	42	190	2	16.0	80
golden, butter recipe, prepared w/stick margarine	1/12 cake	270	3	36	270	0	13.0	65
KEY LIME *(Duncan Hines)* prepared	1/12 cake	250	3	36	270	0	11.0	45
LEMON								
(Betty Crocker)								
'SuperMoist' mix only	1/12 mix	180	1	36	260	0	4.0	0
'SuperMoist' prepared w/1/3 cup oil, 3 eggs	1/12 mix	260	3	37	280	0	11.0	55
'SuperMoist' prepared w/3 tbsp oil, egg substitute	1/12 mix	220	3	37	280	0	7.0	0
lemon chiffon, 'Classic Dessert' mix only	1/12 pkg	190	3	36	190	0	4.0	0
lemon chiffon, 'Classic Dessert' w/2 eggs	1/12 pkg	200	4	36	200	0	5.0	35
lemon pudding, 'Classic Dessert' mix only	1/6 pkg	220	1	45	260	0	4.0	0
lemon pudding, 'Classic Dessert' prepared w/1 egg	1/6 pkg	230	2	45	270	0	5.0	35
(Duncan Hines)								
lemon supreme	1/12 cake	260	3	36	295	0	11.0	65
lemon supreme, cholesterol-free recipe, prepared . . .	1/12 cake	250	3	36	285	0	10.0	0
lemon supreme, mix only	1/12 cake	190	2	36	280	0	4.0	0
(Estee)	1/10 cake	100	1	18	68	0	2.0	0
(MicroRave) w/lemon frosting	1/6 cake	300	2	37	250	0	16.0	45
(Pillsbury)								
'Moist Supreme' mix only	1/10 pkg	210	2	42	330	1	4.0	0
'Moist Supreme' prepared	1/10 pkg	300	4	42	350	1	13.0	65
'Pillsbury Plus' prepared w/1/3 cup oil, 3 eggs	1/12 pkg	240	3	34	280	0	10.0	55

Food Name	Serv. Size	Total Cal.	Prot. gms	Carbs gms	Sod. mgs	Fiber gms	Fat gms	Chol. mgs
'Pillsbury Plus' prepared w/water, 3 egg whites, 2 tbsp flour	1/12 pkg	180	3	35	280	0	3.0	0
'Pillsbury Plus' prepared	1/12 cake	310	4	43	340	1	13.0	65
Bundt, 'Tunnel of Lemon' mix only	1/16 pkg	210	1	44	270	0	4.0	0
Bundt, 'Tunnel of Lemon' prepared	1/16 cake	270	2	45	300	0	9.0	0
Bundt, 'Tunnel of Lemon' prepared w/1/3 cup oil, 3 eggs	1/16 pkg	270	2	44	280	0	9.0	40
Bundt, 'Tunnel of Lemon' prepared w/1/3 cup oil, 4 egg whites	1/16 pkg	260	2	44	280	0	8.0	0
double supreme, microwave, prepared	1/8 cake	300	2	40	210	0	15.0	0
microwave, prepared	1/8 cake	220	2	23	180	0	13.0	0
w/lemon frosting, microwave, prepared	1/8 cake	300	2	37	220	0	17.0	0
(Streusel Swirl)								
lemon supreme, mix only	1/16 pkg	200	2	37	290	0	6.0	0
lemon supreme, prepared	1/16 cake	270	3	39	340	0	11.0	0
lemon supreme, prepared w/water, 1/3 cup oil, 3 eggs	1/16 pkg	260	3	37	300	0	11.0	40
lemon supreme, prepared w/water, 1/3c oil, 4 egg whites	1/16 pkg	250	3	37	300	0	10.0	0
(Sweet 'n Low) mix only	1/6 cake	150	2	30	30	1	3.0	0
ORANGE								
(Duncan Hines)								
orange supreme, cholesterol-free recipe, prepared	1/12 cake	250	3	36	285	0	10.0	0
orange supreme, mix only	1/12 cake	190	2	36	280	0	4.0	0
orange supreme, prepared	1/12 cake	260	3	36	295	0	11.0	65
PEACH (Duncan Hines) prepared	1/12 cake	250	3	36	270	0	11.0	45
PINEAPPLE								
(Betty Crocker)								
upside down, prepared w/egg substitute	1/9 cake	270	2	43	240	0	10.0	0
upside down, prepared w/eggs, margarine	1/9 cake	270	2	43	240	0	10.0	25
supreme, cholesterol-free recipe, prepared	1/12 cake	250	3	36	285	0	10.0	0
supreme, mix only	1/12 cake	190	2	36	280	0	4.0	0
supreme, prepared	1/12 cake	260	3	36	295	0	11.0	65
(Pillsbury)								
crème, Bundt, mix only	1/16 pkg	200	1	42	270	0	3.0	0
crème, Bundt, prepared	1/16 cake	260	2	41	300	0	9.0	0
crème, prepared w/water, 1/2 cup oil, 4 egg whites	1/16 pkg	270	2	42	280	0	10.0	0
crème, prepared w/water, 1/3 cup oil, 3 eggs	1/16 pkg	280	2	42	280	0	11.0	40
POUND								
(Betty Crocker) golden 'Classic Dessert' mix only	1/12 pkg	190	1	28	150	0	8.0	0
(Dromedary)								
mix only	5 tbsp	130	1	20	140	0	5.0	0
prepared	1 slice (1/2")	150	2	21	160	0	6.0	0
(Estee) prepared	1/8 cake	120	2	23	85	0	2.5	0
(Martha White) prepared	1/10 cake	120	2	19	110	0	4.0	20
RAINBOW CHIP								
(Betty Crocker)								
party cake, 'SuperMoist' mix only	1/12 mix	180	2	35	300	0	4.0	0
party cake, 'SuperMoist' prepared	1/12 cake	220	2	41	340	0	5.0	0
party cake, 'SuperMoist' prepared w/1/3 cup oil, 3 eggs	1/12 cake	250	3	35	320	0	11.0	55
RASPBERRY (Duncan Hines) prepared	1/12 cake	250	3	36	270	0	11.0	45
SPICE								
(Betty Crocker)								
'SuperMoist' mix only	1/12 mix	180	1	36	300	0	4.0	0
'SuperMoist' prepared w/1/3 cup oil, 3 eggs	1/12 cake	260	3	36	320	0	11.0	55

Food Name	Serv. Size	Total Cal.	Prot. gms	Carbs gms	Sod. mgs	Fiber gms	Fat gms	Chol. mgs
'SuperMoist' prepared w/3 tbsp oil, cholesterol-free egg product	1/12 cake	220	3	36	320	0	7.0	0
(Duncan Hines)								
cholesterol-free recipe, prepared	1/12 cake	250	3	36	285	0	10.0	0
mix only	1/12 cake	190	2	36	280	0	4.0	0
prepared	1/12 cake	260	3	36	295	0	11.0	65
(Estee)	1/8 cake	120	1	23	80	0	3.0	0
(Gluten Free Pantry) gluten-free	1 serving	110	1	26	170	0	0.0	0
STRAWBERRY								
(Duncan Hines)								
supreme, mix only	1/12 pkge	190	2	36	280	0	4.0	0
supreme, prepared	1/12 cake	260	3	36	295	0	11.0	65
supreme, prepared, cholesterol-free recipe	1/12 cake	250	3	36	285	0	10.0	0
(Pillsbury)								
'Moist Supreme' mix only	1/12 pkg	180	1	36	280	1	4.0	0
'Moist Supreme' prepared	1/12 cake	260	3	36	300	1	11.0	55
cream cheese, 'Bundt Ring Cake' mix only	1/16 pkg	190	1	34	180	0	5.0	5
cream cheese, 'Bundt Ring Cake' prepared	1/16 cake	300	3	34	200	0	17.0	60
'Pillsbury Plus' prepared	1/12 cake	260	3	36	310	0	11.0	55
'Pillsbury Plus' prepared w/1/3 cup oil & 3 eggs	1/12 pkg	190	3	36	310	0	4.0	0
SWIRL								
(Betty Crocker)								
party cake, 'SuperMoist' mix only	1/12 mix	190	2	36	270	0	4.0	0
party cake, 'SuperMoist' prepared, cholesterol-free recipe	1/12 cake	220	3	36	290	0	7.0	0
party cake, 'SuperMoist' prepared w/1/3 cup oil, 3 eggs	1/12 cake	260	3	36	280	0	11.0	55
(Pillsbury)								
white and fudge, 'Moist Supreme' mix only	1/12 pkg	200	2	37	280	1	4.5	0
white and fudge, 'Moist Supreme' prepared	1/12 pkg	250	3	37	290	1	10.0	35
white and fudge, 'Pillsbury Plus' mix only	1/12 pkg	190	2	36	280	0	4.0	0
white and fudge, 'Pillsbury Plus' prepared	1/12 pkg	250	3	36	290	0	10.0	35
white and fudge, 'Pillsbury Plus' prepared, cholesterol-free recipe	1/12 pkg	200	3	37	290	0	4.0	0
VANILLA								
(Betty Crocker)								
golden, 'SuperMoist' mix only	1/12 mix	180	1	36	250	0	4.0	0
golden, 'SuperMoist' prepared w/1/2 cup oil, 3 eggs	1/12 mix	280	3	36	270	0	14.0	55
golden, 'SuperMoist' prepared w/oil, egg substitute	1/12 mix	220	3	36	270	0	7.0	0
(Duncan Hines)								
French, mix only	1/12 cake	190	2	36	280	0	4.0	0
French, prepared	1/12 cake	260	3	36	295	0	11.0	65
French, prepared, cholesterol-free recipe	1/12 cake	250	3	36	285	0	10.0	0
(MicroRave) golden	1/6 cake	320	2	40	230	0	17.0	35
(Pillsbury)								
French, 'Moist Supreme' mix only	1/10 pkg	220	2	42	330	1	5.0	0
French, 'Moist Supreme' prepared	1/10 cake	300	3	42	350	1	13.0	45
French, 'Pillsbury Plus' mix only	1/10 pkg	230	2	41	340	1	6.0	0
French, 'Pillsbury Plus' prepared	1/10 pkg	320	4	41	360	1	15.0	65
sunshine, 'Moist Supreme' mix only	1/12 pkg	190	1	34	280	1	5.0	0
sunshine, 'Moist Supreme' prepared	1/12 cake	260	3	34	300	1	12.0	55
sunshine, 'Pillsbury Plus' prepared w/3 egg white, 2 tbsp flour	1/12 pkg	190	3	35	300	0	5.0	0
WHITE								
(Betty Crocker)								
'Light' prepared	1/12 mix	180	1	37	320	0	3.0	0
'Light' mix only	1/12 mix	180	2	34	300	0	4.0	0

Food Name	Serv. Size	Total Cal.	Prot. gms	Carbs gms	Sod. mgs	Fiber gms	Fat gms	Chol. mgs
'Light' prepared w/3 egg whites . . . . 1/12 mix		180	2	37	330	0	3.0	0
sour cream, 'SuperMoist' mix only . . . . 1/12 mix		180	2	36	280	0	3.0	0
sour cream, 'SuperMoist' prepared . . . . 1/12 cake		210	2	41	370	0	4.5	0
sour cream, 'SuperMoist' prepared w/3 egg whites . . . . 1/12 mix		180	3	36	290	0	3.0	0
'SuperMoist' prepared w/1/3 cup oil, 3 eggs . . . . 1/12 mix		230	2	34	320	0	10.0	0
(Duncan Hines)								
cholesterol-free recipe, prepared . . . . 1/12 cake		240	3	36	270	0	10.0	0
mix only . . . . 1/12 cake		190	2	36	250	0	4.0	0
prepared . . . . 1/12 cake		240	2	35	220	0	10.0	0
(Estee) . . . . 1/10 cake		100	1	18	68	0	2.0	0
(Krusteaz) prepared, 8-inch double cake . . . . 1/12 cake		190	3	37	280	0	3.0	2
(Pillsbury)								
'Lovin Lites' mix only . . . . 1/10 pkg		210	2	42	340	1	4.0	0
'Lovin Lites' prepared . . . . 1/10 cake		230	3	42	350	1	5.0	45
'Moist Supreme' mix only . . . . 1/10 pkg		220	2	41	330	1	5.0	0
'Moist Supreme' prepared . . . . 1/10 cake		280	3	41	350	1	11.0	0
'Pillsbury Plus' mix only . . . . 1/12 pkg		170	2	35	300	0	2.0	0
'Pillsbury Plus' prepared w/water, egg whites . . . . 1/12 cake		170	3	35	310	0	2.0	0
'Pillsbury Plus' prepared w/water, eggs . . . . 1/12 cake		180	3	35	310	0	3.0	35
'Pillsbury Plus' prepared w/1/4 cup oil, 3 egg whites . . . 1/12 cake		220	3	34	290	0	9.0	0
'Pillsbury Plus' prepared w/water, 3 egg whites, 2 tbsp flour . . . . 1/12 cake		190	3	35	290	0	4.0	0
(Lovin' Loaf)								
mix only . . . . 1/12 pkg		170	2	35	300	0	2.0	0
prepared w/water, 2 eggs . . . . 1/12 cake		180	3	35	310	0	3.0	35
prepared w/water, 3 egg whites . . . . 1/12 cake		170	3	35	310	0	2.0	0
(Sweet 'n Low) lowfat, mix only . . . . 1/6 pkg		140	2	30	30	1	3.0	0
(Weight Watchers) low-fat, 'Sweet Rewards' . . . . 1 serving		170	2	36	300	0	2.0	0
YELLOW								
(Betty Crocker)								
'SuperMoist' 'Light' prepared . . . . 1/12 cake		180	1	37	290	0	3.0	0
'SuperMoist' 'Light' prepared w/3 eggs . . . . 1/12 cake		200	3	37	310	0	4.0	55
'SuperMoist' 'Light' prepared w/egg substitute . . . . 1/12 cake		190	3	37	330	0	3.0	0
'SuperMoist' mix only . . . . 1/12 mix		180	1	36	280	0	4.0	0
'SuperMoist' prepared w/1/3 cup oil, 3 eggs . . . . 1/12 cake		260	3	36	300	0	11.0	55
'SuperMoist' prepared w/3 tbsp oil, egg substitute . . . . 1/12 cake		220	3	36	300	0	7.0	0
(Duncan Hines)								
cholesterol-free recipe, prepared . . . . 1/12 cake		250	3	36	285	0	10.0	0
mix only . . . . 1/12 pkg		190	2	36	280	0	4.0	0
prepared . . . . 1/12 cake		260	3	36	295	0	11.0	65
(Finast) 'Ultra Moist' prepared . . . . 1/12 cake		240	3	34	280	0	10.0	0
(Krusteaz) prepared, 8-inch double cake . . . . 1/12 cake		200	3	36	330	1	5.0	0
(Lovin' Loaf)								
prepared w/water, 2 eggs . . . . 1/12 pkg		180	3	35	300	0	3.0	35
prepared w/water, 3 egg whites . . . . 1/12 pkg		170	3	35	310	0	2.0	0
(MicroRave)								
microwave, 'Singles' prepared . . . . 1 cake		260	3	36	450	0	11.0	50
w/chocolate frosting, microwave, mix only . . . . 1/6 pkg		210	1	36	210	0	7.0	0
w/chocolate frosting, microwave, 'Singles' prepared . . . . . 1 cake		460	4	65	510	0	20.0	50
w/chocolate frosting, microwave, prepared w/1 tbsp oil, egg substitute . . . . 1/6 pkg		230	2	36	230	0	9.0	0
yellow, w/chocolate frosting, microwave, prepared w/1/4 cup oil, 1 egg . . . . 1/6 pkg		300	2	36	220	0	17.0	35
(Pillsbury)								
butter recipe, 'Moist Supreme' mix only . . . . 1/12 pkg		170	1	35	270	0	3.0	0
butter recipe, 'Pillsbury Plus' prepared . . . . 1/12 cake		260	3	36	370	0	12.0	75

Food Name	Serv. Size	Total Cal.	Prot. gms	Carbs gms	Sod. mgs	Fiber gms	Fat gms	Chol. mgs
butter recipe, 'Pillsbury Plus' prepared								
w/1/2 cup butter, 3 eggs	1/12 cake	260	3	35	370	0	12.0	75
butter recipe, 'Pillsbury Plus' prepared w/1/2 cup								
margarine, 4 egg whites	1/12 cake	250	3	35	360	0	11.0	0
butter recipe, 'SuperMoist' mix only	1/12 mix	170	1	37	250	0	2.0	0
butter recipe, 'SuperMoist' prepared w/1/2 cup butter,								
3 eggs	1/12 mix	260	3	37	340	0	11.0	75
'Lovin' Lites' mix only	1/10 pkg	220	2	43	370	1	4.0	0
'Lovin' Lites' prepared	1/10 cake	230	3	43	380	1	5.0	45
microwave, prepared	1/8 cake	220	2	23	170	0	13.0	0
'Moist Supreme' mix only	1/12 pkg	180	2	35	280	1	4.0	0
'Moist Supreme' prepared	1/12 cake	240	3	35	290	1	10.0	55
'Pillsbury Plus' prepared w/1/3 cup oil, 3 eggs	1/12 cake	260	3	34	300	0	12.0	55
'Pillsbury Plus' prepared w/water, 3 egg whites,								
2 tbsp flour	1/12 cake	190	3	35	300	0	5.0	0
w/chocolate frosting, microwave, prepared	1/8 cake	300	2	36	220	0	17.0	0
(Sweet 'n Low)								
low-fat, low-sodium, low-cholesterol,								
microwave, prepared	1/10 cake	90	2	16	40	1	2.0	5
mix only	1/6 pkg	150	2	30	30	1	3.0	0
(Weight Watchers) less fat 'Sweet Rewards'	1 serving	160	2	37	280	0	1.0	0

CALABASH GOURD. See GOURD, BOTTLE.
CALAMARI. See SQUID.
CALICO BASS. See SUNFISH.
CALZONE. See under SANDWICH.
CANADIAN BACON. See BACON, CANADIAN STYLE.
CANARY TREE. See PILI NUT.
CANDY. See also CANDY COATING.

Food Name	Serv. Size	Total Cal.	Prot. gms	Carbs gms	Sod. mgs	Fiber gms	Fat gms	Chol. mgs
(Boyer) 'Smoothie'	1.6 oz	250	5	24	0	0	15.0	0
(Brach's) 'Bridge Mix'	1 oz	140	2	17	30	0	7.0	0
(Estee) 'Estee-ets'	5 pieces	35	1	4	10	0	2.0	1
(Nestlé) 'Butterfinger' round 'BBs'	10 pieces	125	3	17	51	1	4.9	0
(Russell Stover) 'Home Fashioned Favorites'	1.4 oz	170	1	27	60	1	7.0	5
ALMOND								
(Brach's) candy-coated, 'Jordan Almonds'	1 oz	120	2	23	0	0	2.0	0
(Estee) chocolate covered	2 squares	60	1	5	10	0	4.5	2
(Featherweight) chocolate covered	1 section	90	1	6	20	0	7.0	0
(Hershey's) chocolate covered, solitaires,								
'Hershey's Golden Collection' 2.8-oz pieces	1 piece	444	9	37	44	3	28.9	10
(M&M Mars) candy-coated, 'M&M's'	1 oz	150	2	17	30	0	8.0	0
(Russell Stover) 'Almond Delights'	1.4 oz	210	3	22	55	1	12.0	10
BUTTERSCOTCH *(Russell Stover)* squares	1.4 oz	180	1	29	65	1	6.5	5
CANDY BAR								
(Barat)								
chocolate tofu, w/almonds	1 oz	170	3	13	10	0	11.0	0
chocolate tofu, w/almonds and raisins	1 oz	160	3	14	10	0	11.0	0
chocolate tofu truffle, w/pralines	1 oz	170	4	12	10	0	11.0	0
(Cadbury)								
chocolate, w/crisps and honey	1 oz	150	2	18	40	0	7.0	0
chocolate, w/fruit and nuts	1 oz	150	2	17	40	0	8.0	0
chocolate, w/roasted almonds	1 oz	150	3	15	40	0	9.0	0
'Dairy Milk'	1 oz	150	2	17	45	0	8.0	0
(Carafection)								
'Almond Crunch' date sweetened carob	1 oz	139	2	17	26	0	7.0	0
'Cashew Coconut Crunch' carob	1 oz	139	2	17	26	0	7.0	0
'Crispy Crunch' date sweetened carob	1 oz	139	2	17	26	0	7.0	0
'Mint Honey Graham' carob coated	1 oz	139	2	17	26	0	7.0	0

Food Name	Serv. Size	Total Cal.	Prot. gms	Carbs gms	Sod. mgs	Fiber gms	Fat gms	Chol. mgs
'Mint' date sweetened carob	1 oz	139	2	17	26	0	7.0	0
'Original Honey Graham' carob coated	1 oz	139	2	17	26	0	7.0	0
'Peanut Crunch' date sweetened, carob	1 oz	139	2	17	26	0	7.0	0
plain, date sweetened, carob	1 oz	139	2	17	26	0	7.0	0
(Caroby) carob	4 sections	150	4	13	55	0	9.0	0
(Cocofection) original	1 oz	155	2	15	23	0	10.0	0
(Estee)								
chocolate, coconut	2 squares	60	1	5	15	0	4.0	5
chocolate, dark, deluxe	2 squares	50	1	6	0	0	3.0	0
chocolate, fruit and nut	2 squares	60	1	5	10	0	4.5	2
chocolate, milk	2 squares	60	1	5	15	0	4.0	5
crunch	2 squares	45	1	4	10	0	3.0	2
mint	2 squares	50	1	6	0	0	3.0	0
(Fantastic Foods) 'Halvah'	1.5 oz	232	8	17	0	0	10.0	0
(Fifty 50)								
chocolate, milk, extra thick, w/o sugar	1 section	80	1	6	25	0	6.0	0
chocolate, milk, mini	4 pieces	90	2	6	20	0	6.0	0
chocolate, w/almonds, extra thick, w/o sugar	1 section	90	2	6	20	0	6.0	0
crunch, chocolate, extra thick, w/o sugar	1 section	70	1	6	20	0	5.0	0
fruit and nut, chocolate, extra thick, w/o sugar	1 section	80	1	6	20	0	5.0	0
(Ghirardelli)								
chocolate, dark, 'Premier Bar'	1 bar	428	4	51	5	5	28.6	0
chocolate, dark, w/almonds, 'Premier Bar'	1 bar	442	6	45	6	6	31.6	0
chocolate, dark, w/raspberries, 'Premier Bar'	1 bar	423	4	52	4	5	27.6	0
(Heath) 'Soft'n Crunchy Bar' 2 pieces	1.19 oz serving	190	1	19	85	0	12.0	0
(Hershey's)								
'Almond Joy' 1.7-oz bar	1 bar	229	2	29	72	2	13.1	2
'Almond Joy' snack size, 0.7 oz	1 bar	93	1	12	29	1	5.4	1
'Caramello' 5-oz bar	1 bar	673	9	90	195	2	30.8	38
'Caramello' 1.6-oz bar	1 bar	213	3	29	62	1	9.8	12
chocolate, 'Hershey's Milk Chocolate Bar'	1.55 oz	240	4	25	40	0	14.0	10
chocolate, snack size, 0.7-oz bar	1 bar	91	1	11	28	1	4.8	0
chocolate, w/almonds, 'Hershey's Milk Chocolate Bar w/Almonds'	1.45 oz	230	5	20	55	0	14.0	10
chocolate almond, 'Golden Collection'	2.8 oz	448	10	36	52	4	29.7	12
'Cookies 'N' Mint'	1 bar	220	3	26	75	0	12.0	0
'5th Avenue' 2-oz bar	1 bar	280	5	38	94	1	12.1	3
'5th Avenue' snack size, 0.6 oz	1 bar	79	1	11	26	0	3.4	1
'Kit Kat' 3.375-oz bar	1 bar	493	7	61	72	2	24.5	6
'Kit Kat' 2.8-oz bar	1 bar	401	6	50	59	1	19.9	5
'Kit Kat' 1.62-oz bar	1 bar	236	3	29	35	1	11.7	3
'Kit Kat' 1.5-oz bar	1 bar	216	3	27	32	1	10.7	3
'Kit Kat' mini, 0.35-oz bar	1 bar	51	1	6	8	0	2.5	1
'Krackel' 7-oz pkg	1 pkg	982	12	114	255	4	53.1	35
'Krackel' 2.2-oz bar	1 bar	329	4	38	86	1	17.8	12
'Krackel' 1.5-oz bar	1 bar	218	3	25	57	1	11.8	8
'Mounds' 1.9-oz bar	1 bar	253	2	31	79	3	13.3	1
'Mr. Goodbar' 2.6-oz bar	1 bar	398	8	38	109	3	25.5	6
'Mr. Goodbar' 1.75-oz bar	1 bar	267	5	25	73	2	17.1	4
'Skor' 1.4-oz bar	1 bar	217	2	23	108	1	13.3	20
'Special Dark' extra large, 8 oz	1 bar	1253	11	138	16	11	73.5	2
'Special Dark' large, 4-oz bar	1 bar	624	6	68	8	6	36.6	1
'Special Dark' 2.8-oz bar	1 bar	436	4	48	6	4	25.6	1
'Special Dark' 2.2-oz bar	1 bar	342	3	38	4	3	20.1	1
'Special Dark' 1.45-oz bar	1 bar	226	2	25	3	2	13.3	0
'Symphony' 1.5-oz bar	1 bar	232	3	24	39	1	13.8	9
'Symphony' 2.4-oz bar	1 bar	371	5	39	62	1	22.0	15

Food Name	Serv. Size	Total Cal.	Prot. gms	Carbs gms	Sod. mgs	Fiber gms	Fat gms	Chol. mgs
'Whatchamacallit' 1.7-oz bar	1 bar	214	4	29	99	1	9.3	5
(M&M Mars)								
'Bounty' milk chocolate	1 oz	140	1	17	30	0	7.0	0
'Dove' dark chocolate	1 bar	200	2	22	0	2	12.0	5
'Dove' dark chocolate, miniatures	4 pieces	130	1	14	0	0	8.0	0
'Dove' milk chocolate	1 bar	200	2	22	25	1	12.0	5
'Dove' milk chocolate, miniatures	4 pieces	130	1	14	20	0	8.0	0
'Mars' almond, 1.76-oz bar	1 bar	234	4	31	85	1	11.5	9
'Milky Way' 2.15-oz bar	1 bar	258	3	44	146	1	9.8	9
'Milky Way' 2.1-oz bar	1 bar	254	3	43	144	1	9.7	8
'Milky Way' 2.05-oz bar	1 bar	245	3	42	139	1	9.3	8
'Milky Way' 1.9-oz bar	1 bar	228	2	39	130	1	8.7	8
'Milky Way' 0.8-oz bar	1 bar	97	1	16	55	0	3.7	3
'Milky Way' fun size	1 bar	76	1	13	43	0	2.9	3
'Munch'	1.42 oz	220	6	19	110	0	14.0	0
'Snickers' king size, 4-oz bar	1 bar	541	9	67	301	3	27.8	15
'Snickers' 2-oz bar	1 bar	273	5	34	152	1	14.0	7
'Snickers' fun size	1 bar	72	1	9	40	0	3.7	2
'3 Musketeers' 2.13-oz bar	1 bar	250	2	46	116	1	7.7	7
'3 Musketeers' 1.813-oz bar	1 bar	212	2	39	99	1	6.6	6
'3 Musketeers' 0.8-oz bar	1 bar	96	1	18	45	0	3.0	3
'3 Musketeers' fun size	1 bar	69	1	13	32	0	2.1	2
'Twix' 11-oz pkg	1 pkg	1557	14	205	602	3	76.1	16
'Twix' 3.35-oz bar	4 bars	474	4	62	183	1	23.2	5
'Twix' 2.06-oz bar	2 bars	289	3	38	112	1	14.1	3
'Twix' 2-oz pkg	1 pkg	284	3	37	110	1	13.9	3
'Twix' peanut, 9.43-oz pkg	1 pkg	1415	27	141	726	9	85.9	13
'Twix' peanut, 2.06-oz pkg	1 pkg	307	6	31	158	2	18.7	3
'Twix' peanut, 1.89-oz pkg	1 pkg	286	5	28	147	2	17.4	3
'Twix' peanut, 1.77-oz pkg	1 pkg	265	5	26	136	2	16.1	3
(Nature's Warehouse)								
'A-Ok' fruit juice sweetened	1 oz	130	3	17	32	0	6.2	0
'My O My' fruit juice sweetened	1 oz	103	2	21	42	0	1.4	0
'No How' peanut butter, fruit juice sweetened	1 oz	140	6	11	48	0	10.0	0
'Non Stop' fruit juice sweetened	1 oz	122	2	18	48	0	5.0	0
'Nut Wit' carob caramel and peanuts	1 oz	135	3	17	32	0	6.3	0
(Necco) 'Sky Bar'	1.5 oz	196	2	32	57	0	7.1	0
(Nestlé)								
'100 Grand' 1.5-oz bar	1 bar	200	2	30	89	1	7.8	8
'100 Grand' miniature	1 bar	98	1	15	43	0	3.8	4
'Aero' regular size	1 bar	210	0	20	20	0	12.0	0
'Aero' bite size	2 bars	85	0	10	0	0	5.0	10
'Baby Ruth' 2.28-oz bar	1 bar	313	5	42	147	2	13.8	3
'Baby Ruth' 2.1-oz bar	1 bar	289	4	39	136	2	12.7	2
'Baby Ruth' 1.2-oz bar	1 bar	164	3	22	77	1	7.2	1
'Baby Ruth' miniature	1 bar	101	2	14	47	1	4.4	1
'Baby Ruth' fun size	1 bar	67	1	9	32	0	3.0	1
'Butterfinger' king size	1 bar	518	13	71	214	3	20.2	1
'Butterfinger' 2.16-oz bar	1 bar	293	8	40	121	1	11.4	1
'Butterfinger' 1.6-oz bar	1 bar	216	6	30	89	1	8.4	0
'Butterfinger' fun size	1 bar	101	3	14	42	1	3.9	0
'Butterfinger' bite size	1 bar	34	1	5	14	0	1.3	0
'Chunky' 1.4-oz bar	1 bar	198	4	23	21	2	11.7	4
'Chunky' 1.25-oz bar	1 bar	173	3	20	19	2	10.2	4
'Crunch' 1.55-oz bar	1 bar	230	3	29	59	1	11.6	6
'Crunch' 1.4-oz bar	1 bar	209	2	26	53	1	10.5	5
'Crunch' miniature	1 bar	52	1	7	13	0	2.6	1

Food Name	Serv. Size	Total Cal.	Prot. gms	Carbs gms	Sod. mgs	Fiber gms	Fat gms	Chol. mgs
'Oh Henry!' 2-oz bar .... 1 bar	246	6	37	135	2	9.6	5
(Pay Day) 'Pay Day' .... 1.85 oz	250	9	28	200	0	12.0	0
(Russell Stover)							
French chocolate .... 1 bar	200	3	20	30	1	13.0	10
mint, French chocolate .... 1 bar	230	3	20	25	2	15.5	10
peanut butter .... 1 bar	290	7	22	130	3	19.0	5
(Weight Watchers)							
caramel nut .... 1 bar	130	2	14	25	0	8.0	5
English toffee crunch .... 1 bar	120	2	12	25	0	7.0	5
(Yogafection)							
'Brazil Nut Crunch' .... 1 oz	180	2	17	70	0	10.0	5
'Cashew Nut Crunch' .... 1 oz	180	2	17	70	0	10.0	5
CARAMEL							
(Allen Wertz)							
.... 1 piece	37	0	6	2	0	2.0	1
nougat swirl .... 1 piece	32	0	6	2	0	1.0	1
(Brach's) chocolate, 'Milk Maid' .... 1 oz	110	1	20	55	0	3.0	0
(Estee)							
chocolate .... 2 pieces	50	1	9	25	0	2.0	0
vanilla .... 2 pieces	50	1	9	25	0	2.0	0
(Featherweight) .... 1 piece	30	0	5	10	0	1.0	0
(Hershey's)							
in milk chocolate, 1.91-oz pkg 'Rolo' .... 1 pkg	218	3	28	93	0	10.6	10
in milk chocolate, 1.74-oz roll 'Rolo' .... 1 roll	202	2	26	86	0	9.8	9
in milk chocolate, 0.2-oz pieces 'Rolo' .... 1 piece	12	0	2	5	0	0.6	1
(Kraft) .... 1 piece	30	0	6	25	0	1.0	0
(Pom Poms) chocolate coated .... 1 oz	100	1	15	70	0	3.0	0
(Russell Stover)							
butter cream, squares .... 1.4 oz	170	1	26	95	1	7.5	10
marshmallow, milk chocolate, soft-chewy, squares ...... 1.4 oz	190	2	25	85	5	10.0	0
CHERRY							
(Brach's)							
chocolate cream .... 1 oz	110	1	21	20	0	2.0	0
dark chocolate coated .... 1 oz	110	1	22	20	0	2.0	0
milk chocolate covered, 'Villa' .... 1 oz	110	1	22	20	0	2.0	0
(Russell Stover)							
'Cherry Cordials' .... 1.4 oz	170	1	25	25	2	7.5	5
squares .... 1.4 oz	160	1	28	40	1	5.5	0
CHOCOLATE							
(Allen Wertz) assortment, 'Gourmet' .... 11.9 grams	55	1	9	13	0	2.0	1
(Barat)							
tofu, 'Passionettes' .... 1 piece	70	1	6	5	0	5.0	0
tofu pastilles 'Bits' .... 0.75 oz	120	2	11	10	0	8.0	0
(Brach's)							
assorted, wrapped .... 1 oz	110	0	24	20	0	2.0	0
'Jots' .... 1 oz	130	1	21	30	0	5.0	0
milk, 'Stars' .... 1 oz	150	2	17	30	0	8.0	0
milk chocolate coated, 'Malted Milk Balls' .... 1 oz	130	1	21	40	0	5.0	0
(Callard and Bowser) cream .... 1 oz	120	0	22	0	0	3.7	0
(Cocofection) trail mix, premium .... 1 oz	130	4	13	14	0	9.0	0
(Featherweight)							
crunch .... 1 section	80	1	7	20	0	6.0	0
milk .... 1 section	80	1	7	20	0	6.0	0
(Great Cakes) amaretto, confection, 'Buffalo Ball' .... 1 ball	105	3	27	15	6	3.5	0
(Hershey's)							
milk, 'Kisses' .... 6 pieces	150	2	16	25	0	9.0	5
milk, creamy, w/almonds and toffee chips .... 0.75 oz	280	5	26	50	0	17.0	0

Food Name	Serv. Size	Total Cal.	Prot. gms	Carbs gms	Sod. mgs	Fiber gms	Fat gms	Chol. mgs
w/almonds, 'Kisses w/Almonds' .... 6 pieces	160	3	14	25	0	10.0	0
(M&M Mars)								
'M&M's' mini, 5-oz pkg .... 1 pkg	707	7	95	97	4	33.1	21
'M&Ms' plain .... 1 cup	1023	9	148	127	5	44.0	29
'M&Ms' plain .... 10 pieces	34	0	5	4	0	1.5	1
'M&Ms' plain, 1.69-oz pkg .... 1 pkg	236	2	34	29	1	10.1	7
'M&Ms' plain, 1.48-oz box .... 1 box	207	2	30	26	1	8.9	6
(Nabisco) milk, 'Stars' approx 13 pieces .... 1 oz	160	2	19	35	0	8.0	0
(Russell Stover)								
dark and milk mix, 'The Gift Box' .... 1.4 oz	180	2	26	45	0	8.5	5
milk, assortment .... 1.4 oz	190	2	27	50	0	8.5	5
(Saco Foods)								
'Choc'Oh's' .... 1.5 oz	111	1	14	14	0	6.6	0
chunks .... 3.5 oz	466	4	67	26	0	26.4	0
(Spangler)								
coated, creme center .... 1 piece	80	1	15	40	0	2.0	0
coated, creme center caramel, w/nuts .... 1 piece	100	2	11	30	0	6.0	0
coated, creme center cherry, w/nuts .... 1 piece	110	2	12	20	0	5.0	0
coated, creme center fudge, w/nuts .... 1 piece	140	2	17	25	0	6.0	0
coated, creme center fudge, w/pecans .... 1 piece	140	1	18	40	0	7.0	0
coated, creme center maple, w/nuts .... 1 piece	110	2	12	15	0	5.0	0
coated, creme center vanilla, w/nuts .... 1 piece	110	2	13	20	0	5.0	0
(Tootsie Roll) chewy roll .... 1 oz	112	0	23	6	0	2.5	0
(Whoppers) milk chocolate coated, malted milk balls .... 1 oz	136	1	20	0	0	6.0	0
COCONUT								
(Brach's) Neapolitan .... 1 oz	120	1	24	40	0	2.0	0
(Sunbelt) chocolate coated 'Macaroo' .... 2 oz	288	3	33	75	0	16.0	1
COFFEE								
(Allen Wertz)								
'Coffee Time' .... 1 piece	20	0	4	2	0	1.0	1
'Coffee Time' assorted .... 1 piece	28	0	5	2	0	1.0	1
'Coffee Time' decaffeinated .... 1 piece	20	0	4	2	0	1.0	1
(Brach's) .... 1 oz	120	0	25	35	0	2.0	0
FRUIT								
(Bonkers!) chews, all flavors .... 1 piece	20	0	5	0	0	0.0	0
(Featherweight)								
berry patch .... 1 piece	12	0	3	0	0	0.0	0
drops, all flavors .... 0.33 oz	30	0	8	15	0	0.0	0
orchard .... 1 piece	12	0	3	0	0	0.0	0
tropical blend .... 1 piece	12	0	3	0	0	0.0	0
(Glenny's)								
black cherry, 'Drops' .... 1 drop	6	1	1	1	0	1.0	0
lemon, twist of, 'Drops' .... 1 drop	6	1	1	1	0	1.0	0
mandarin orange, 'Drops' .... 1 drop	6	1	1	1	0	1.0	0
mixed fruit, 'Drops' .... 1 drop	6	1	1	1	0	1.0	0
(Hershey's) 'Jujyfruits' .... 11 pieces	100	1	25	0	0	1.0	0
(M&M Mars)								
'Skittles' original, bite size .... 1 cup	830	0	186	33	0	9.0	0
'Skittles' original, bite size, 4-oz pkg .... 1 pkg	458	0	102	18	0	4.9	0
'Skittles' original, bite size, 2.3-oz pkg .... 1 pkg	263	0	59	10	0	2.8	0
'Skittles' original, bite size, 2.17-oz pkg .... 1 pkg	251	0	56	10	0	2.7	0
'Skittles' original, bite size, 2-oz pkg .... 1 pkg	231	0	52	9	0	2.5	0
'Skittles' original, bite size .... 10 pieces	43	0	10	2	0	0.5	0
chews, 'Starburst' .... 1 piece	20	0	4	3	0	0.4	0
chews, 'Starburst' 2.07-oz pkg .... 1 pkg	234	0	50	33	0	4.9	0
chews, 'Starburst' fun size .... 1 pkg	166	0	35	24	0	3.5	0
(Rascals) chews, all flavors .... 1 piece	4	0	1	0	0	0.0	0

Food Name	Serv. Size	Total Cal.	Prot. gms	Carbs gms	Sod. mgs	Fiber gms	Fat gms	Chol. mgs
(SweeTARTS) chewy	1 oz	113	0	25	0	0	1.0	0
FUDGE								
(Kraft) 'Fudgies'	1 piece	35	0	6	25	0	1.0	0
(Woody's)								
cheese, w/walnuts	1 oz	120	2	18	25	0	4.0	5
chocolate, w/walnuts	1 oz	120	2	18	25	0	4.0	5
maple walnut	1 oz	120	1	19	25	0	4.0	5
mint, w/walnuts	1 oz	120	2	18	25	0	4.0	5
GUM								
(Beech-Nut)								
candy-coated, 'Beechies'	1 piece	6	0	2	0	0	0.0	0
cinnamon	1 piece	10	0	2	0	0	0.0	0
fruit	1 piece	10	0	2	0	0	0.0	0
peppermint	1 piece	10	0	2	0	0	0.0	0
spearmint	1 piece	10	0	2	0	0	0.0	0
(Brach's) balls, 'Gumdinger' all flavors,	1 oz	110	0	24	5	0	2.0	0
(Bubble Yum)								
bananaberry split	1 piece	25	0	7	0	0	0.0	0
checkermint	1 piece	25	0	7	0	0	0.0	0
cherry	1 piece	25	0	7	0	0	0.0	0
fruit	1 piece	25	0	7	0	0	0.0	0
fruit, sugarless	1 piece	20	0	5	0	0	0.0	0
grape	1 piece	25	0	7	0	0	0.0	0
grape, sugarless	1 piece	20	0	5	0	0	0.0	0
Hawaiian punch	1 piece	25	0	7	0	0	0.0	0
lime, luscious	1 piece	25	0	7	0	0	0.0	0
peppermint, sugarless	1 piece	20	0	5	0	0	0.0	0
strawberry stripe	1 piece	25	0	7	0	0	0.0	0
strawberry, sugarless	1 piece	20	0	5	0	0	0.0	0
3-flavor, grape, cherry, and fruit	1 piece	25	0	7	0	0	0.0	0
watermelon, wet 'n wild	1 piece	25	0	7	0	0	0.0	0
(Bubblicious)								
original	1 piece	25	0	6	0	0	0.0	0
sugarless	1 piece	5	0	1	0	0	0.0	0
(Care Free)								
bubble, fruit, sugarless	1 piece	10	0	2	0	0	0.0	0
bubble, wild cherry, sugarless	1 piece	10	0	2	0	0	0.0	0
bubble, wintergreen, sugarless	1 piece	10	0	2	0	0	0.0	0
cinnamon, sugarless	1 piece	8	0	2	0	0	0.0	0
peppermint, sugarless	1 piece	8	0	2	0	0	0.0	0
spearmint, sugarless	1 piece	8	0	2	0	0	0.0	0
(Chewels) all flavors	1 piece	8	0	2	0	0	0.0	0
(Chiclets)								
	10 pieces	55	0	15	1	0	0.0	0
candy-coated	1 piece	6	0	2	0	0	0.0	0
candy-coated, 'Tiny'	1 pkg	8	0	0	0	0	0.0	0
(Clorets) stick, all flavors	1 piece	9	0	2	0	0	0.0	0
(Dentyne)								
all flavors	1 piece	6	0	2	0	0	0.0	0
all flavors, sugarless	1 piece	5	0	1	0	0	0.0	0
(Extra)								
bubble, classic	1 piece	6	0	0	0	0	0.0	0
bubble, original	1 piece	7	0	0	0	0	0.0	0
cinnamon	1 stick	8	0	0	0	0	0.0	0
peppermint	1 stick	8	0	0	0	0	0.0	0
spearmint	1 stick	8	0	0	0	0	0.0	0
winter fresh	1 stick	8	0	0	0	0	0.0	0

Food Name	Serv. Size	Total Cal.	Prot. gms	Carbs gms	Sod. mgs	Fiber gms	Fat gms	Chol. mgs
(Freedent)								
cinnamon	1 stick	10	0	2	0	0	0.0	0
peppermint	1 stick	10	0	2	0	0	0.0	0
spearmint	1 stick	10	0	2	0	0	0.0	0
(Freshen-Up) all flavors	1 piece	13	0	3	0	0	0.0	0
(Fruit Stripe)								
bubble, cherry	1 piece	8	0	2	0	0	0.0	0
bubble, fruit	1 piece	8	0	2	0	0	0.0	0
bubble, grape	1 piece	8	0	2	0	0	0.0	0
bubble, lemon	1 piece	8	0	2	0	0	0.0	0
cherry	1 piece	10	0	2	0	0	0.0	0
lemon	1 piece	10	0	2	0	0	0.0	0
lime	1 piece	10	0	2	0	0	0.0	0
orange	1 piece	10	0	2	0	0	0.0	0
(Hubba Bubba)								
all flavors except cola and grape	1 piece	23	0	6	0	0	0.0	0
cola	1 piece	23	0	5	0	0	0.0	0
grape, sugar-free	1 piece	13	0	0	0	0	0.0	0
original, sugar-free	1 piece	14	0	0	0	0	0.0	0
(Wrigley's)								
	1 serving	10	0	2	0	0	0.0	0
'Big Red'	1 piece	10	0	2	0	0	0.0	0
'Doublemint'	1 piece	10	0	2	0	0	0.0	0
'Juicy Fruit'	1 piece	10	0	2	0	0	0.0	0
'Spearmint'	1 piece	10	0	2	0	0	0.0	0
GUMDROP								
1-inch diam	1 gumdrop	45	0	11	5	0	0.0	0
3/4-inch diam	1 gumdrop	16	0	4	2	0	0.0	0
(Estee)	4 pieces	25	0	6	0	0	0.0	0
HARD CANDY								
(Brach's)								
butterscotch, 'Disks'	1 oz	110	0	27	220	0	0.0	0
cinnamon, 'Disks'	1 oz	110	0	27	15	0	0.0	0
cinnamon, 'Imperials'	1 oz	110	0	27	5	0	0.0	0
'Cut Rock'	1 oz	110	0	27	10	0	0.0	0
filled, assorted	1 oz	110	0	27	15	0	0.0	0
lemon drops	1 oz	110	0	27	5	0	0.0	0
raspberry filled	1 oz	110	0	27	15	0	0.0	0
ribbon, crimp	1 oz	110	0	27	15	0	0.0	0
'Royals'	1 oz	100	1	20	60	0	2.0	0
'Spicettes'	1 oz	100	0	26	15	0	0.0	0
sour balls	1 oz	110	0	27	15	0	0.0	0
(Breath Savers)								
mint-cinnamon	1 piece	8	0	2	0	0	0.0	0
mint-cinnamon, cores	1 piece	2	0	1	0	0	0.0	0
peppermint	1 piece	8	0	2	0	0	0.0	0
peppermint, cores	1 piece	2	0	1	0	0	0.0	0
spearmint	1 piece	8	0	2	0	0	0.0	0
spearmint, cores	1 piece	2	0	1	0	0	0.0	0
wintergreen	1 piece	8	0	2	0	0	0.0	0
wintergreen, cores	1 piece	2	0	1	0	0	0.0	0
(Callard and Bowser) butterscotch	1 oz	115	0	25	0	0	1.9	0
(Ce De) 'Smarties'	1 roll	25	0	6	0	0	0.0	0
(Certs)								
mini, sugar-free	1 piece	1	0	0	0	0	0.0	0
mints, sugar-free	1 piece	6	0	2	0	0	0.0	0

Food Name	Serv. Size	Total Cal.	Prot. gms	Carbs gms	Sod. mgs	Fiber gms	Fat gms	Chol. mgs
(Clorets)								
clear mint	1 piece	8	0	2	0	0	0.0	0
pressed mints	1 piece	6	0	2	0	0	0.0	0
(Estee)	2 pieces	25	0	6	0	0	0.0	0
(Featherweight)								
butterscotch	1 piece	25	0	6	25	0	0.0	0
tropical blend, 'Sweet Pretenders'	1 piece	12	0	3	0	0	0.0	0
(Fruit Juicers)								
citrus fruits	1 piece	8	0	2	0	0	0.0	0
fruit punch	1 piece	8	0	2	0	0	0.0	0
grape	1 piece	8	0	2	0	0	0.0	0
mixed berries	1 piece	8	0	2	0	0	0.0	0
strawberry	1 piece	8	0	2	0	0	0.0	0
(Glenny's)								
fruit	1 piece	19	1	4	1	0	1.0	0
peppermint	1 piece	19	1	4	1	0	1.0	0
(Jolly Joes)	1 piece	9	0	2	1	0	0.0	0
(Jolly Rancher)								
apple	1 piece	23	0	6	5	0	0.0	0
butterscotch	1 piece	25	0	6	37	0	1.0	0
cherry	1 piece	23	0	6	3	0	0.0	0
fire cinnamon	1 piece	23	0	6	5	0	0.0	0
fruit punch	1 piece	23	0	6	5	0	0.0	0
grape	1 piece	23	0	6	5	0	0.0	0
lemon	1 piece	23	0	6	5	0	0.0	0
orange	1 piece	23	0	6	4	0	0.0	0
peach	1 piece	23	0	6	3	0	0.0	0
peppermint	1 piece	23	0	6	3	0	0.0	0
pink lemonade	1 piece	23	0	6	5	0	0.0	0
raspberry	1 piece	23	0	6	5	0	0.0	0
strawberry	1 piece	23	0	6	3	0	0.0	0
watermelon	1 piece	23	0	6	5	0	0.0	0
(Jurassic Park)								
jawbreakers, tropical flavors								
jawbreakers, wild cherry, 'Raptor Bites'	13 pieces	60	0	15	0	0	0.0	0
(Life Savers)								
butter creme mint	1 piece	8	0	2	5	0	0.0	0
butter rum	1 piece	8	0	2	10	0	0.0	0
butter rum, 'Holes'	1 piece	2	0	1	0	0	0.0	0
butterscotch	1 piece	8	0	2	10	0	0.0	0
'Cin-O-Mon'	1 piece	8	0	2	0	0	0.0	0
'Cryst-O-Mint'	1 piece	8	0	2	0	0	0.0	0
fancy fruits	1 piece	8	0	2	0	0	0.0	0
five flavor	1 piece	8	0	2	0	0	0.0	0
five flavor, 'Holes'	1 piece	2	0	1	0	0	0.0	0
'Pep-O-Mint'	1 piece	8	0	2	0	0	0.0	0
'Pep-O-Mint,' 'Holes'	1 piece	2	0	1	0	0	0.0	0
root beer flavor	1 piece	8	0	2	0	0	0.0	0
'Spear-O-Mint'	1 piece	8	0	2	0	0	0.0	0
sunshine fruits	1 piece	8	0	2	0	0	0.0	0
sunshine fruits, 'Holes'	1 piece	2	0	1	0	0	0.0	0
tangerine, 'Holes'	1 piece	2	0	1	0	0	0.0	0
tropical fruits	1 piece	8	0	2	0	0	0.0	0
wild cherry	1 piece	8	0	2	0	0	0.0	0
'Wint-O-Green'	1 piece	8	0	2	0	0	0.0	0
'Wint-O-Green,' 'Holes'	1 piece	2	0	1	0	0	0.0	0
(Mike and Ike)	1 piece	9	0	2	1	0	0.0	0

Food Name	Serv. Size	Total Cal.	Prot. gms	Carbs gms	Sod. mgs	Fiber gms	Fat gms	Chol. mgs
(Russell Stover) mixed, sugar-free .... 3 pieces		70	0	18	5	0	0.0	0
'Spitters' .... 13 pieces		60	0	15	0	0	0.0	0
(Spree) fruit .... 1 oz		110	0	26	0	0	0.0	0
(SweeTARTS) fruit .... 1 oz		110	0	26	0	0	0.0	0
(Sunmark) jawbreakers, 'Willy Wonka's Everlasting Gobstoppers' .... 6 pieces		59	0	15	1	na	0.0	na
HOLIDAY								
(Brach's) holiday mints .... 1 oz		110	0	26	0	0	1.0	0
Christmas								
(Brach's)								
bell, chocolate, in foil .... 1 oz		150	2	17	25	0	8.0	0
candy cane .... 1 oz		110	0	27	10	0	0.0	0
chocolate, assorted .... 1 oz		110	0	23	25	0	2.0	0
jellies .... 1 oz		100	0	24	10	0	0.0	0
jellies, snowbase .... 1 oz		100	0	24	5	0	0.0	0
'Jots' .... 1 oz		130	1	21	30	0	5.0	0
mint 'Pearls' .... 1 oz		110	0	25	5	0	1.0	0
mint 'Starlight' .... 1 oz		110	0	27	15	0	0.0	0
nougat .... 1 oz		110	0	24	20	0	2.0	0
ornaments .... 1 oz		150	2	17	50	0	8.0	0
'Perkys' .... 1 oz		90	0	23	20	0	0.0	0
Santa, chocolate, in foil .... 1 oz		140	2	18	40	0	7.0	0
Santa, marshmallow .... 1 oz		120	1	23	35	0	3.0	0
(Just Born)								
snowman, marshmallow, large .... 1 piece		111	1	27	8	0	0.1	0
snowman, marshmallow, small .... 1 piece		37	0	9	3	0	0.1	0
tree, marshmallow, large .... 1 piece		111	1	27	8	0	0.1	0
tree, marshmallow, small .... 1 piccc		37	0	9	3	0	0.1	0
(Spangler) candy cane .... 1 piece		60	1	14	0	0	1.0	0
Easter								
(Brach's)								
assorted, 'Chicks and Rabbits' .... 1 oz		100	0	26	10	0	0.0	0
assorted, 'Easter Fun' .... 1 oz		100	0	26	10	0	0.0	0
corn .... 1 oz		100	0	26	66	0	0.0	0
eggs, 'Hide'n Seek' .... 1 oz		110	0	27	5	0	0.0	0
eggs, chocolate malted milk .... 1 oz		130	1	21	40	0	5.0	0
eggs, chocolate, in foil .... 1 oz		150	2	17	25	0	8.0	0
eggs, creme, chocolate coated buttercream .... 1 oz		120	1	22	50	0	3.0	0
eggs, creme, chocolate coated cherry .... 1 oz		110	1	23	20	0	2.0	0
eggs, creme, chocolate coated coconut .... 1 oz		110	0	22	40	0	3.0	0
eggs, creme, chocolate coated fruit and nut .... 1 oz		110	0	23	35	0	2.0	0
eggs, creme, chocolate coated maple .... 1 oz		110	0	23	30	0	2.0	0
eggs, creme, chocolate coated vanilla .... 1 oz		110	0	23	25	0	2.0	0
eggs, jelly .... 1 oz		100	0	24	15	0	0.0	0
eggs, jelly, 'Tiny' .... 1 oz		100	0	26	10	0	0.0	0
eggs, jelly, speckled .... 1 oz		110	0	27	40	0	0.0	0
eggs, jelly, spiced .... 1 oz		90	0	22	10	0	0.0	0
eggs, marshmallow .... 1 oz		100	0	25	5	0	0.0	0
eggs, pastel 'Fiesta' .... 1 oz		120	1	23	25	0	3.0	0
lollipop, pastels, 'Easter' .... 1 lollipop		40	0	10	0	0	0.0	0
mint, 'Starlight' .... 1 oz		110	0	27	15	0	0.0	0
nougats .... 1 oz		100	0	24	25	0	1.0	0
rabbits, jel, 'Jube' .... 1 oz		100	0	24	15	0	0.0	0
rabbits, marshmallow .... 1 oz		120	1	22	55	0	3.0	0
'Robin's Eggs' .... 1 oz		140	1	20	30	0	6.0	0
(Cadbury)								
eggs, creme .... 1.37 oz		190	2	26	0	0	8.0	0
eggs, creme, mini .... 1 oz		140	2	20	0	0	7.0	0

Food Name	Serv. Size	Total Cal.	Prot. gms	Carbs gms	Sod. mgs	Fiber gms	Fat gms	Chol. mgs
(Just Born) peeps, marshmallow	1 piece	27	0	7	2	0	0.1	0
Halloween								
(Brach's)								
corn, Indian	1 oz	100	0	26	75	0	0.0	0
corn, three color	1 oz	100	0	26	95	0	0.0	0
jelly beans	1 oz	100	0	26	15	0	0.0	0
lollipops 'Picture Pops'	1 oz	110	0	27	10	0	0.0	0
'Mellowcremes'	1 oz	100	0	26	40	0	0.0	0
pumpkin heads, crazy	1 oz	100	0	24	15	0	1.0	0
pumpkins	1 oz	100	0	26	65	0	0.0	0
'Scary Cats'	1 oz	100	0	26	85	0	0.0	0
'Trick or Treat Party Pack'	1 oz	110	0	27	20	0	0.0	0
witches' teeth	1 oz	100	0	26	75	0	0.0	0
(Just Born)								
cats, marshmallow	1 piece	28	0	7	2	0	0.1	0
pumpkins, marshmallow, large	1 piece	111	1	27	8	0	0.1	0
pumpkins, marshmallow, small	1 piece	14	0	3	1	0	0.1	0
Valentine's Day								
(Brach's)								
chocolate, 'I Luv U'	1 oz	150	2	17	25	0	8.0	0
'Heart Box' 1/2-lb box	1 oz	110	1	23	35	0	2.0	0
hearts	1 oz	110	1	23	30	0	2.0	0
hearts, cherry jel 'Jube'	1 oz	100	0	26	20	0	0.0	0
hearts, cinnamon 'Imperial'	1 oz	110	0	27	5	0	0.0	0
hearts, 'Conversation' large	1 oz	110	0	27	5	0	0.0	0
hearts, 'Conversation' small	1 oz	110	0	27	0	0	0.0	0
hearts, fruity	1 oz	100	0	24	5	0	0.0	0
hearts, jelly, red	1 oz	100	0	24	10	0	0.0	0
hearts, 'Sassy Hearts'	1 oz	100	0	25	0	0	0.0	0
kisses, nougat	1 oz	110	0	24	15	0	2.0	0
'Love'	1 oz	150	2	17	25	0	8.0	0
'Mellowcremes'	1 oz	100	0	26	75	0	0.0	0
'Valentine Heart' 1/3-lb box	1 oz	110	1	23	25	0	2.0	0
'Valentine Heart' 1-lb box	1 oz	110	1	23	30	0	2.0	0
JELLIED AND GUMMED								
jellybeans, large	10 pieces	104	0	26	7	0	0.1	0
jellybeans, small	10 pieces	40	0	10	3	0	0.1	0
(Brach's)								
cinnamon bears	1 oz	80	0	21	10	0	0.0	0
'Fruit Bunch'	1 oz	100	0	24	10	0	0.0	0
gummi bears	1 oz	100	2	22	15	0	0.0	0
gummi worms	1 oz	100	2	22	15	0	0.0	0
jelly beans	1 oz	100	0	26	5	0	0.0	0
jelly nougat	1 oz	100	0	24	35	0	1.0	0
'Jels' sour cherry	1 oz	100	0	26	10	0	0.0	0
'Jube'	1 oz	100	0	24	10	0	0.0	0
jube jels	1 oz	100	0	24	10	0	0.0	0
mint, assorted	1 oz	100	0	26	0	0	0.0	0
'Rainbow Bears'	1 oz	100	0	24	10	0	0.0	0
'Spearmint Leaves'	1 oz	100	0	24	5	0	0.0	0
spicettes	1 oz	100	0	26	15	0	0.0	0
(Callard and Bowser) juicy	1 oz	90	0	23	0	0	0.0	0
(Estee)								
gummi bears	4 pieces	20	1	4	0	0	0.0	0
ring, 1.25-inch diam	1 piece	39	0	10	4	0	0.0	0
(Hershey's)								
gummi bears, 'Amazin Fruit' 12 pieces	1 oz	90	2	21	20	0	1.0	0

Food Name	Serv. Size	Total Cal.	Prot. gms	Carbs gms	Sod. mgs	Fiber gms	Fat gms	Chol. mgs
gummi bears, tropical, 'Amazin Fruit'	1 oz	90	2	21	20	0	1.0	0
(Hot Tamales) cinnamon, hot	1 piece	9	0	2	1	0	0.0	0
(Jurassic Park) gummi dinosaurs, tropical	15 pieces	140	3	31	0	0	0.0	0
(Just Born)								
eggs, 'Petite'	1 piece	4	0	1	1	0	0.0	0
'Teenee Beanee Gourmet'	1 piece	4	0	1	1	0	0.0	0
(Life Savers) 'Gummi Savers'	1 piece	12	0	3	0	0	0.0	0
(Rodda) eggs	1 piece	7	0	2	1	0	0.0	0
LEMON *(Russell Stover)* squares	1.4 oz	160	1	27	35	2	5.5	0
LICORICE								
(Brach's)								
'Red Laces'	1 oz	100	2	22	10	0	0.0	0
'Twin Twists'	1 oz	100	2	22	10	0	0.0	0
'Twists'	1 oz	100	2	22	50	0	1.0	0
(Good and Fruity) candy-coated	1 oz	106	1	26	8	0	0.1	0
(Hershey's)								
cherry bits, 'Twizzlers'	5 oz pkg	474	5	110	351	2	2.3	0
cherry bits, 'Twizzlers' 4-oz bag	22 pieces	139	1	31	85	1	1.0	0
strawberry bits, 'Twizzlers' 2.5-oz pkg	1 pkg	237	2	55	175	1	1.1	0
LOLLIPOP								
(Brach's) all flavors, 'Pops'	1 oz	110	0	27	10	0	0.0	0
(Estee) all flavors	1 lollipop	30	0	7	0	0	0.0	0
(Fruit Juicers)								
black raspberry	1 lollipop	40	0	10	0	0	0.0	0
fruit punch	1 lollipop	40	0	10	0	0	0.0	0
pineapple	1 lollipop	40	0	10	0	0	0.0	0
strawberry	1 lollipop	40	0	10	0	0	0.0	0
(Glenny's)								
fruit	1 lollipop	21	1	5	1	0	1.0	0
Vit-C	1 lollipop	35	1	8	1	0	1.0	0
(Life Savers)								
assorted	1 lollipop	45	0	11	10	0	0.0	0
swirled	1 lollipop	45	0	11	10	0	0.0	0
(Sorbee) assorted fruit flavors	1 lollipop	22	0	5	0	0	0.0	0
(Spangler)								
all flavors, 'Dum Dums'	1 lollipop	25	1	6	0	0	1.0	0
all flavors, 'Saf-T-Pops'	1 lollipop	45	1	11	0	0	1.0	0
bubble gum center, all flavors	1 lollipop	57	1	14	5	0	1.0	0
(Tootsie Pop)								
all flavors except chocolate	1 oz	111	0	26	1	0	0.6	0
chocolate	1 oz	110	0	26	2	0	0.6	0
MARSHMALLOW								
(Boyer) 'Mallow Cup'	2 pieces	224	2	30	0	0	11.0	0
(Brach's) 'Perky's Circus Peanuts'	1 oz	100	0	26	10	0	0.0	0
(Campfire) large	2 pieces	40	0	10	10	0	0.0	0
(FunMallows)								
	1 piece	30	0	7	15	0	0.0	0
miniature	10 pieces	18	0	5	5	0	0.0	0
(Just Born) coconut, toasted	1 piece	30	0	6	6	1	0.6	0
(Spangler) 'Circus Peanuts'	4 pieces	110	1	26	5	0	1.0	0
MINT								
(Andes) chocolate mint thins, 'Creme de Menthe'	6 pieces	150	2	16	20	0	9.0	0
(Barat)								
chocolate tofu, 'Bits'	0.75 oz	120	2	11	15	0	8.0	0
chocolate tofu, after dinner	1 piece	40	1	4	0	0	2.0	0
(Brach's)								
'Kentucky Mints'	1 oz	110	0	27	0	0	0.0	0

Food Name	Serv. Size	Total Cal.	Prot. gms	Carbs gms	Sod. mgs	Fiber gms	Fat gms	Chol. mgs
chocolate covered, thin	1 oz	110	0	24	10	0	2.0	0
'Coolers/Starlight'	1 oz	110	0	27	15	0	0.0	0
creme, chocolate covered, regular	1 oz	110	0	24	10	0	2.0	0
'Creme de Menthe'	1 oz	150	2	16	20	0	9.0	0
'Dessert Mints' assorted	1 oz	110	0	27	0	0	0.0	0
'Jots/Pearls'	1 oz	120	0	25	10	0	2.0	0
parfait	1 oz	150	2	16	35	0	9.0	0
peppermint, 'Star Brites'	3 pieces	59	0	15	6	na	0.0	na
peppermint kisses	1 oz	100	0	24	25	0	1.0	0
straws, filled	1 oz	110	0	26	10	0	1.0	0
(Featherweight)								
'Cool Blue'	1 piece	25	0	6	0	0	0.0	0
peppermint swirls	1 piece	20	0	5	0	0	0.0	0
(Glenny's) gentle, 'Drops'	1 piece	6	1	1	1	0	1.0	0
(Hershey's)								
'Peppermnt Pattie' large, 1.5 oz	1 piece	165	1	34	10	1	3.0	0
'Peppermint Pattie' 0.6 oz	1 patty	67	0	14	4	0	1.2	0
'Peppermint Pattie' 0.5 oz	1 patty	55	0	11	3	0	1.0	0
(Kraft)								
butter	1 piece	8	0	2	0	0	0.0	0
party	1 piece	8	0	2	0	0	0.0	0
(Mint) 'Meltaway'	1 piece	50	0	5	10	0	3.0	0
(Nestlé)								
'After Eight'	5 pieces	147	1	31	5	1	5.6	0
'After Eight'	1 piece	29	0	6	1	0	1.1	0
(Rowntree) dark chocolate, wafer thin, 'After Eight'	1 piece	35	0	6	0	0	1.0	0
(Russell Stover) squares	1.4 oz	160	1	28	35	1	5.0	0
(Saco Foods) 'Mint'Oh's'	1.5 oz	111	1	14	14	0	6.6	0
(Spangler) dark chocolate coated	1 piece	80	1	14	25	0	2.0	0
(Velamints)								
all flavors except cocoamint	1 piece	7	0	2	0	0	0.0	0
cocoamint	1 piece	7	5	2	0	0	0.3	0
NONPAREILS								
(Brach's) dark chocolate	1 oz	140	1	20	20	0	6.0	0
(Nestlé) 'Sno-Caps'	1 oz	140	1	21	0	0	6.0	0
ORANGE								
(Brach's)								
'Orangettes'	1 oz	100	0	24	20	0	0.0	0
sticks, chocolate coated	1 oz	110	1	23	25	0	2.0	0
PEANUT								
(Barat) chocolate tofu, dipped, 'Bits'	1 oz	120	4	8	15	0	8.0	0
(Brach's)								
caramel cluster	1 oz	150	4	15	50	0	8.0	0
chocolate covered 'Small'	1 oz	140	4	15	40	0	7.0	0
filled	1 oz	110	1	25	20	0	1.0	0
French, burnt	1 oz	130	4	18	5	0	5.0	0
'Jots'	1 oz	140	3	18	25	0	6.0	0
milk chocolate coated	1 oz	150	3	15	30	0	9.0	0
milk chocolate, 'Peanut Clusters'	1 oz	150	3	15	25	0	9.0	0
'Nut Goodies'	1 oz	130	2	21	10	0	4.0	0
parfait	1 oz	160	3	14	60	0	10.0	0
(Cocofection) enrobed in chocolate	1 oz	140	5	10	12	0	12.0	0
(Estee)								
candy-coated	10 pieces	70	2	8	10	0	4.0	0
chocolate-covered	2 squares	60	1	5	10	0	4.5	2
(M&M Mars)								
chocolate, candy-coated, 'M&Ms'	1 cup	877	16	103	82	6	44.6	15
chocolate, candy-coated, 'M&Ms' 1.74-oz pkg	1 pkg	253	5	30	24	2	12.9	4

Food Name	Serv. Size	Total Cal.	Prot. gms	Carbs gms	Sod. mgs	Fiber gms	Fat gms	Chol. mgs
chocolate, candy-coated, 'M&Ms' 1.67-oz pkg . . . . 1 pkg		243	4	28	23	2	12.3	4
chocolate, candy-coated, 'M&Ms' fun size pkg . . . . 1 pkg		108	2	13	10	1	5.5	2
chocolate, candy-coated, 'M&Ms' . . . . 10 pieces		103	2	12	10	1	5.2	2
(Nabisco) chocolate covered, approx 14 pieces . . . . 1 oz		160	4	14	15	0	9.0	0
(Nestlé)								
chocolate-covered, 'Goobers' 7-oz pkg . . . . 1 pkg		1016	27	96	81	12	66.3	18
chocolate-covered, 'Goobers' . . . . 1/4 cup		210	6	20	17	3	13.7	4
chocolate-covered, 'Goobers' 1.375-oz pkg . . . . 1 pkg		200	5	19	16	2	13.1	4
chocolate-covered, 'Goobers' . . . . 10 pieces		51	1	5	4	1	3.4	1
(Russell Stover) 'Peanut Delights' . . . . 1.4 oz		210	4	22	130	1	12.0	10
PEANUT BRITTLE								
(Estee) . . . . 0.5 oz		60	1	10	20	0	2.0	0
(Kraft) . . . . 1 oz		130	3	20	135	0	5.0	0
(Sophie Mae) . . . . 1.4 oz		170	4	30	130	1	5.0	0
PEANUT BUTTER								
(Boyer)								
cup . . . . 1.6 oz		250	5	23	0	0	15.0	0
cup, 0.5 oz . . . . 1 piece		75	3	12	0	0	7.5	0
(Brach's) kisses . . . . 1 oz		110	1	22	135	0	2.0	0
(Estee) cup . . . . 1 piece		40	1	3	20	0	3.0	1
(Hershey's)								
'Reese's Crunchy Peanut Butter Cup' . . . . 1.8 oz		280	7	24	130	0	18.0	5
'Reese's Peanut Butter Cup' individual, 0.6 oz . . . . 1 piece		92	2	9	54	1	5.3	1
'Reese's Peanut Butter Cup' miniature . . . . 5 pieces		211	4	21	124	1	12.2	2
'Reese's Peanut Butter Cup' miniature . . . . 1 piece		38	1	4	22	0	2.2	0
'Reese's Peanut Butter Cup' 2-pack, 1.6 oz . . . . 1 pkg		243	5	25	143	1	14.1	2
'Reese's Pieces' . . . . 1/4 cup		231	6	29	69	1	9.9	1
'Reese's Pieces' . . . . 1.6-oz pkg		226	6	28	68	1	9.7	1
'Reese's Pieces' . . . . 50 pieces		191	5	24	57	1	8.2	1
'Reese's Pieces' . . . . 10 pieces		39	1	5	12	0	1.7	0
(M&M Mars)								
chocolate-covered, 'Kudos' . . . . 1.3 oz		200	4	19	80	0	12.0	0
chocolate-covered cookie, 'PB Max' . . . . 1 piece		240	5	20	150	0	15.0	0
PECAN								
(Russell Stover)								
'Pecan Crowns' . . . . 1.4 oz		200	2	19	60	1	13.0	5
'Pecan Delights' . . . . 1.4 oz		220	2	19	55	1	14.5	5
(Demet's)								
turtles . . . . 6-oz pkg		825	11	99	160	4	47.3	37
turtles . . . . 1 piece		82	1	10	16	0	4.7	4
POWDER CANDY								
(Lik-m-aid Fun Dip) . . . . 1 oz		110	0	26	0	0	0.0	0
(Pixy Stix) . . . . 1 oz		100	0	26	0	0	0.0	0
RAISIN								
(Barat) chocolate tofu, 'Bits' . . . . 1 oz		120	1	14	10	0	7.0	0
(Brach's) chocolate-coated . . . . 1 oz		130	1	20	30	0	5.0	0
(Cocofection) enrobed in chocolate . . . . 1 oz		120	1	20	14	0	5.0	0
(Estee) chocolate-coated . . . . 8 pieces		30	1	5	5	0	1.0	0
(Fruit Source) yogurt-coated, made w/real fruit juice . . . . 9 pieces		170	3	27	35	1	7.0	0
(Harmony) chocolate-coated . . . . 44 pieces		160	2	29	15	1	5.0	5
(Nabisco) chocolate-coated, approx 29 pieces . . . . 1 oz		130	1	21	15	0	5.0	1
(Nestlé)								
chocolate-covered, 'Raisinets' . . . . 1.58-oz pkg		185	2	32	16	2	7.2	2
chocolate-covered, 'Raisinets' . . . . 10 pieces		41	0	7	4	1	1.6	0
TAFFY								
(Beich's)								
all flavors, 'Salt Water Taffy' . . . . 1 oz		100	0	24	30	0	1.0	0

Food Name	Serv. Size	Total Cal.	Prot. gms	Carbs gms	Sod. mgs	Fiber gms	Fat gms	Chol. mgs
apple flavor chews, 'Laffy Taffy'	2 pieces	110	0	26	55	0	1.0	0
banana flavor chews, 'Laffy Taffy'	2 pieces	120	0	26	55	0	1.0	0
cherry flavor chews, 'Laffy Taffy'	2 pieces	110	0	26	55	0	1.0	0
grape flavor chews, 'Laffy Taffy'	2 pieces	110	0	26	60	0	1.0	0
passion punch flavor, 'Laffy Taffy'	2 pieces	120	0	26	50	0	1.0	0
strawberry flavor chews, 'Laffy Taffy'	2 pieces	110	0	26	55	0	1.0	0
watermelon flavor chews, 'Laffy Taffy'	2 pieces	110	0	26	55	0	1.0	0
TOFFEE								
(Brach's)	1 oz	110	1	23	80	0	2.0	0
(Callard and Bowser)	1 oz	135	1	19	0	0	6.5	0
(Flavor House) peanut butter	1 oz	150	4	17	90	0	7.0	0
(Heath)								
'Bits O'Brickle'	3 oz	448	1	50	472	0	28.0	0
English, 'Bits O'Heath'	3.5 oz	520	3	62	390	0	31.0	0
English, 'Heath Bar'	2 pieces	180	1	20	130	0	11.0	0
CANDY COATING								
bars, butterscotch, confectioner's coating	1 oz	153	1	19	25	0	8.2	0
bars, white, confectioner's coating	3 oz	458	5	50	77	0	27.3	18
chips, butterscotch, confectioner's coating	1 cup	916	4	114	151	0	49.4	0
chip, white, confectioner's coating	1 cup	916	10	101	153	0	54.6	36
CANNELLINI BEAN. See BEAN, CANNELLINI, CANNED.								
CANOLA OIL								
	1 cup	1927	0	0	0	0	218.0	0
	1 tbsp	124	0	0	0	0	14.0	0
(Hain)	1 tbsp	120	0	0	0	0	14.0	0
(Kroger)	1 tbsp	122	0	0	0	0	13.6	0
(Smart Beat)	1 tbsp	117	0	0	0	0	13.6	0
(Wesson)	1 tbsp	122	0	0	0	0	13.6	0
(Westbrae Naturals)	1 tbsp	100	0	0	90	0	11.0	5
cholesterol-free, no sodium (Country Pure)	1 tbsp	120	0	0	0	0	14.0	0
'Food Service' (Wesson)	1 tbsp	122	0	0	0	0	13.6	0
'Heart Beat' (Nucoa)	1 tbsp	120	0	0	0	0	14.0	0
100% pure pressed (Loriva')	1 tbsp	120	0	0	0	0	14.0	0
pure pressed, organic, lowest in saturated fat (Spectrum Naturals)	1 tbsp	120	0	0	0	0	14.0	0
CANTALOUPE. See MELON, CANTALOUPE.								
CAPERS								
canned, drained	1 tbsp	2	0	0	255	0	0.1	0
canned, drained (Progresso)	1 tsp	0	0	0	105	0	0.0	0
canned, non-pareilles (Reese)	1 tsp	0	0	0	105	0	0.0	0
CAPPUCCINO. See under COFFEE, FLAVORED.								
CARAMBOLA. See STAR FRUIT.								
CARAMEL. See under CANDY.								
CARAMEL TOPPING								
(Kraft)	2 tbsp	120	2	28	90	0	0.0	0
(Mrs. Richardson's)								
	2 tbsp	130	1	28	90	0	2.0	5
nonfat	2 tbsp	130	1	31	55	0	0.0	0
(Smucker's)								
hot	2 tbsp	150	1	28	75	0	4.0	0
'Special Recipe'	2 tbsp	160	1	33	40	0	3.0	0
CARAWAY SEED								
	1 tbsp	22	1	3	1	3	1.0	0
	1 tsp	7	0	1	0	1	0.3	0
(Spice Islands)	1 tsp	8	0	1	1	0	0.4	0
(Tone's)	1 tsp	7	0	1	1	1	0.3	0
dried (McCormick/Schilling)	1 tsp	14	1	1	0	1	0.8	0

Food Name	Serv. Size	Total Cal.	Prot. gms	Carbs gms	Sod. mgs	Fiber gms	Fat gms	Chol. mgs
whole seeds *(Durkee)*	1 tsp	9	0	0	0	0	0.0	0
whole seeds *(Laurel Leaf)* whole seeds	1 tsp	9	0	0	0	0	0.0	0
CARDAMOM								
ground	1 tbsp	18	1	4	1	2	0.4	0
ground	1 tsp	6	0	1	0	1	0.1	0
ground *(Tone's)*	1 tsp	6	0	1	1	0	0.1	0
ground, fresh *(Durkee)*	1 tsp	7	0	0	0	0	0.0	0
ground, fresh *(Laurel Leaf)*	1 tsp	7	0	0	0	0	0.0	0
whole *(McCormick/Schilling)*	1 tsp	7	0	2	0	1	0.0	0
whole *(Spice Islands)*	1 tsp	6	0	1	0	0	0.1	0
CARDONI. See CARDOON.								
CARDOON/cardoni								
boiled, drained	4 oz	25	0.9	6.0	200	2.1	0.1	0
raw, shredded	1 cup	36	1.0	9.0	303	3.0	0.2	0
CARIBOU								
raw	1 oz	36	6	0	16	0	1.0	24
roasted	3 oz	142	25	0	51	0	3.8	93
CARISSA/Natal plum								
Fresh								
raw, sliced	1 cup	93	1	20	5	na	1.9	0
raw, whole, peeled and seeded	1 fruit	12	0	3	1	na	0.3	0
CAROB CHIPS, unsweetened *(Sunspire)*	1 oz	133	4	15	123	0	6.0	2
CAROB FLAVOR DRINK								
mix, powder	1 tbsp	45	0	11	12	1	0.0	0
mix, powder, prepared w/milk	8 fl oz	195	8	23	133	1	8.2	33
CAROB FLOUR. See under FLOUR.								
CARP								
baked, broiled, grilled, or microwaved	3 oz	138	19	0	54	0	6.1	71
raw	3 oz	108	15	0	42	0	4.8	56
CARROT								
Canned								
(A&P)	1/2 cup	30	1	6	300	0	1.0	0
(Stokely)	1/2 cup	35	1	7	300	0	0.0	0
baby, petite, whole *(Stokely)*	4.5 oz	30	0	5	390	2	0.0	0
baby, whole *(Allens)*	1/2 cup	30	1	6	240	0	1.0	0
baby, whole, 'LeSueur' *(Green Giant)*	1/2 cup	35	1	8	410	3	0.0	0
crinkle sliced *(Freshlike)*	1/2 cup	30	1	6	300	0	0.0	0
crinkle sliced *(Stokely)*	1/2 cup	35	1	7	300	na	0.0	na
crinkle sliced *(Veg-All)*	1/2 cup	30	1	6	300	0	0.0	0
diced *(Allens)*	1/2 cup	30	1	5	190	0	1.0	0
diced, 'Fancy' *(S&W)*	1/2 cup	30	1	7	240	0	0.0	0
diced, w/liquid *(Del Monte)*	1/2 cup	30	0	7	265	0	0.0	0
mashed, no salt added, drained	1 cup	57	1	13	96	3	0.4	0
no salt added *(A&P)*	1/2 cup	25	1	6	40	0	1.0	0
no salt or sugar added *(Stokely)*	1/2 cup	35	1	7	35	0	0.0	0
regular pack, mashed, drained	1 cup	57	1	13	552	3	0.4	0
regular pack, sliced, drained	1 cup	37	1	8	353	2	0.3	0
regular pack, sliced, drained	1 slice	1	0	0	7	0	0.0	0
regular pack, sliced, w//liquid	1/2 cup	28	1	7	295	2	0.2	0
sliced *(Featherweight)*	1/2 cup	30	1	6	30	0	0.0	0
sliced *(Finast)*	1/2 cup	35	1	8	370	0	0.0	0
sliced *(Green Giant)*	1/2 cup	25	1	6	380	2	0.0	0
sliced *(IGA)*	1/2 cup	30	1	6	300	0	0.0	0
sliced *(Pathmark)*	1/2 cup	35	1	7	310	0	0.0	0
sliced, no salt added, drained	1 cup	37	1	8	61	2	0.3	0
sliced, no salt added, drained	1 slice	1	0	0	1	0	0.0	0
sliced, no salt added, w/liquid	1/2 cup	28	1	7	42	2	0.2	0

Food Name	Serv. Size	Total Cal.	Prot. gms	Carbs gms	Sod. mgs	Fiber gms	Fat gms	Chol. mgs
sliced, large *(Allens)*	1/2 cup	30	1	7	250	0	1.0	0
sliced, medium *(Allens)*	1/2 cup	30	1	7	250	0	1.0	0
sliced, Nutradiet *(S&W)*	1/2 cup	30	0	7	50	0	0.0	0
sliced, small *(Allens)*	1/2 cup	30	1	7	250	0	1.0	0
sliced no salt added *(Finast)*	1/2 cup	35	1	8	30	0	0.0	0
sliced no salt added *(Pathmark)*	1/2 cup	35	1	8	35	0	0.0	0
sliced, water packed, no salt *(Freshlike)*	1/2 cup	30	1	6	40	0	0.0	0
Fresh								
baby, raw, large	1 carrot	6	0	1	5	0	0.1	0
baby, raw, medium	1 carrot	4	0	1	4	0	0.1	0
boiled, drained, sliced	1/2 cup	35	1	8	51	3	0.1	0
boiled, drained, whole, medium	1 carrot	21	1	5	30	2	0.1	0
raw, chopped	1 cup	55	1	13	45	4	0.2	0
raw, cut, 3-inch strips	1 strip	3	0	1	2	0	0.0	0
raw, cut, strips or slices	1 cup	52	1	12	43	4	0.2	0
raw, grated	1 cup	47	1	11	39	3	0.2	0
raw, shredded	1/2 cup	24	0.6	5.6	19	1.7	0.1	0
raw, whole, medium *(Dole)*	1 carrot	40	1.0	8.0	40	1.0	1.0	na
raw, whole, large, 7.25–8.5-inch long	1 carrot	31	1	7	25	2	0.1	0
raw, whole, small, 5.5-inch long	1 carrot	22	1	5	18	2	0.1	0
Frozen								
(A&P)	3.3 oz	40	1	9	45	0	1.0	0
(Seabrook)	3.3 oz	40	1	9	44	1	0.0	0
baby, cut, 'Select Polybag' *(Green Giant)*	3/4 cup	30	1	7	40	3	0.0	0
baby, whole *(C&W)*	2/3 cup	35	1	7	60	3	0.0	0
baby, whole *(Flav-R-Pac)*	2/3 cup	35	1	6	45	2	0.0	0
baby, whole, 'Deluxe' *(Birds Eye)*	3.3 oz	40	1	9	45	2	0.0	0
baby, whole, 'Harvest Fresh' *(Green Giant)*	1/2 cup	18	1	5	75	2	0.0	0
baby, whole, 'Select' *(Green Giant)*	1/2 cup	20	1	7	35	2	0.0	0
baby, whole, 'Singles' *(Stokely)*	3 oz	35	1	8	50	0	0.0	0
Parisienne, 'Deluxe' *(Birds Eye)*	2.6 oz	30	1	7	35	2	0.0	0
sliced *(Birds Eye)*	3.2 oz	35	1	8	40	1	0.0	0
sliced *(Flav-R-Pac)*	2/3 cup	35	1	6	45	2	0.0	0
sliced *(Frosty Acres)*	3.3 oz	40	1	9	44	1	0.0	0
sliced, drained	1 cup	53	2	12	431	5	0.2	0
sliced, no salt, drained	1 cup	53	2	12	86	5	0.2	0
sliced, unprepared	10-oz pkg	111	3	26	168	9	0.6	0
sliced, unprepared	1/2 cup	25	1	6	38	2	0.1	0
small, round, European style, 'Parisienne' *(C&W)*	2/3 cup	40	0	10	50	3	0.0	0
whole *(Southern)*	3.5 oz	42	1	9	60	0	0.2	0
CARROT CHIPS								
(Hain)								
	1 oz	150	2	16	160	0	9.0	0
barbecue	1 oz	140	2	16	160	0	8.0	0
no salt added	1 oz	150	2	16	30	0	7.0	0
CARROT DISH								
(Birds Eye)								
w/sweet peas, pearl onions, 'Deluxe'	3.3 oz	50	2	10	60	2	0.0	0
(Flav-R-Pac)								
baby, orange glazed, 'Grande Classics'	1/2 cup	60	1	14	85	3	1.5	0
baby, whole, w/buttery sauce	1/2 cup	45	1	9	420	3	2.0	0
shoestring, frozen	1 cup	35	1	6	45	2	0.0	0
CARROT JUICE								
Canned or bottled								
	1 cup	94	2	22	68	2	0.4	0
	1 fl oz	12	0	3	9	0	0.0	0
(Biotta)	6 fl oz	51	2	11	158	0	0.1	0

Food Name	Serv. Size	Total Cal.	Prot. gms	Carbs gms	Sod. mgs	Fiber gms	Fat gms	Chol. mgs
(Hain)	6 fl oz	80	1	17	170	0	0.0	0
(Hollywood)	6 fl oz	80	1	17	170	2	0.0	0

CASABA MELON. See MELON, CASABA.

CASHEW/heart nut

(Beer Nuts)	1 oz	170	5	8	65	0	13.0	0
(Frito-Lay's)	1 oz	170	4	9	115	0	14.0	0
halves *(Fisher)*	1 oz	160	5	8	0	0	13.0	0
halves, lightly salted *(Eagle)*	1 oz	180	5	8	65	1	14.0	0
lightly salted *(Eagle)*	1 oz	190	5	8	65	1	14.0	0
pieces *(Fisher)*	1 oz	170	5	8	135	0	14.0	0
salted, whole *(Guy's)*	1 oz	170	5	5	140	0	14.0	0
salted *(Pathmark)*	1 oz	170	4	9	150	0	13.0	0
salted, 'No Frills' *(Pathmark)*	1 oz	170	5	8	220	0	13.0	0
salted *(Planters)*	1 oz	160	5	9	230	0	13.0	0
unsalted, natural *(Flanigan Farms)*	1/4 cup	160	4	9	0	2	13.0	0
whole *(Fisher)*	1 oz	160	5	8	100	0	13.0	0

Dry roasted

halves and whole, salted	1 cup	786	21	45	877	4	63.5	0
halves and whole, unsalted	1 cup	786	21	45	22	4	63.5	0
lightly salted *(Planters)*	1 oz	160	5	9	0	0	13.0	0
salted	1 oz	163	4	9	181	1	13.1	0
unsalted	1 oz	163	4	9	5	1	13.1	0
unsalted	1 tbsp	49	1	3	1	0	4.0	0
unsalted *(Planters)*	1 oz	160	5	9	0	0	13.0	0

Honey roasted

(Eagle)	1 oz	180	4	9	130	1	14.0	0
(Planters)	1 oz	170	4	11	170	0	12.0	0
halves *(Eagle)*	1 oz	180	4	9	130	1	14.0	0
halves *(Fisher)*	1 oz	150	4	7	0	0	13.0	0
whole *(Fisher)*	1 oz	150	4	7	90	0	13.0	0
w/peanuts *(Planters)*	1 oz	170	5	9	170	0	12.0	0

Oil roasted

halves, salted *(Fisher)*	1/4 cup	170	5	8	160	1	15.0	0
halves, salted *(Planters)*	1 oz	170	5	8	135	0	14.0	0
halves, salted *(Planters)*	1 oz	170	5	8	135	0	14.0	0
halves, unsalted *(Planters)*	1 oz	170	5	8	0	0	14.0	0
halves and whole, salted	1 cup	749	21	37	814	5	62.7	0
halves and whole, unsalted	1 cup	749	21	37	22	5	62.7	0
lightly salted *(Planters)*	1 oz	160	5	8	80	0	14.0	0
salted *(Flavor House)*	1 oz	180	7	3	125	0	16.0	0
salted *(Pathmark)*	1 oz	170	5	8	150	0	14.0	0
salted, approx 18 kernels	1 oz	163	5	8	177	1	13.7	0
salted, 'Fancy' *(Planters)*	1 oz	170	5	8	135	0	14.0	0
salted, 'No Frills' *(Pathmark)*	1 oz	170	5	8	150	0	14.0	0
unsalted, approx 18 kernels	1 oz	163	5	8	5	1	13.7	0
w/almonds *(Fisher)*	1 oz	170	5	6	95	0	15.0	0
whole *(Fisher)*	1/4 cup	170	5	8	130	1	15.0	0

CASHEW BUTTER

creamy, roasted fresh, no salt added *(Roaster Fresh)*	1 oz	165	4	9	4	0	14.0	0
gourmet *(Roaster Fresh)*	1 oz	165	4	9	4	0	14.0	0
peanut date *(Maranatha Natural)*	2 tbsp	190	8	8	8	0	14.0	0
peanut date, 'Natural' *(Westbrae)*	2 tbsp	200	6	8	2	0	15.0	0
raw *(Hain)*	2 tbsp	190	6	8	0	0	15.0	0
raw, 'Natural' *(Westbrae)*	2 tbsp	300	6	8	0	0	28.0	0
raw, unsalted *(Hain)*	2 tbsp	210	5	8	10	0	19.0	0
roasted *(Maranatha Natural)*	2 tbsp	190	6	10	5	0	14.0	0
roasted, 'Natural' *(Westbrae)*	2 tbsp	190	6	8	0	0	17.0	0

Food Name	Serv. Size	Total Cal.	Prot. gms	Carbs gms	Sod. mgs	Fiber gms	Fat gms	Chol. mgs
roasted, organic *(Maranatha Natural)*	2 tbsp	210	8	8	9	6	16.0	0
salted	1 oz	166	5	8	174	1	14.0	0
salted	1 tbsp	94	3	4	98	0	7.9	0
toasted *(Hain)*	2 tbsp	210	7	7	15	0	17.0	0
unsalted	1 oz	166	5	8	4	1	14.0	0
unsalted	1 tbsp	94	3	4	2	0	7.9	0
unsalted, 'Fancy' *(Planters)*	1 oz	170	5	8	0	0	14.0	0
CASSAVA/manioc/yuca								
raw, chopped or sliced	1 cup	330	3	78	29	4	0.6	0
raw, whole	1 root	653	6	155	57	7	1.1	0
CATFISH, CHANNEL								
Fresh								
breaded, fried	3 oz	195	15	7	238	1	11.3	69
farmed, baked, broiled, grilled, or microwaved	3 oz	129	16	0	68	0	6.8	54
farmed, raw	3 oz	115	13	0	45	0	6.5	40
wild, baked, broiled, grilled, or microwaved	3 oz	89	16	0	43	0	2.4	61
wild, raw	3 oz	81	14	0	37	0	2.4	49
Frozen, fillets *(Delta Pride)*	4 oz	132	18	5	1	0	4.9	62
CATFISH, OCEAN. See WOLF FISH.								
CATSUP/ketchup								
	1 cup	250	4	65	2846	3	0.9	0
	1 tbsp	16	0	4	178	0	0.1	0
	1 pkt	6	0	2	71	0	0.0	0
low-salt	1 cup	250	4	65	48	3	0.9	0
low-salt	1 tbsp	16	0	4	3	0	0.1	0
low-salt	1 pkt	6	0	2	1	0	0.0	0
(Del Monte)								
	1/4 cup	60	1	16	675	0	0.0	0
	1 tbsp	15	0	4	190	0	0.0	0
'No Salt Added'	1/4 cup	60	1	16	25	0	0.0	0
(Estee)	1 tbsp	6	0	0	20	0	0.0	0
(Featherweight)	1 tbsp	6	0	1	5	0	0.0	0
(Hain)								
'Natural'	1 tbsp	16	0	4	155	0	0.0	0
'Natural No Salt Added'	1 tbsp	16	0	4	5	0	0.0	0
(Healthy Choice)	0.5 oz	9	0	2	97	0	0.1	0
(Heinz)								
hot	1 tbsp	16	0	4	195	0	0.0	0
light	1 tbsp	10	0	3	95	0	0.0	0
regular	1 tbsp	16	0	4	213	0	0.0	0
w/onions	1 tbsp	19	5	0	289	0	0.0	0
(Hunt's)								
	1 tbsp	16	0	4	158	0	0.1	0
bulk packaged, food service product	1 tbsp	16	0	4	197	0	0.1	0
no salt added	1 tbsp	16	0	3	6	0	0.1	0
packets, food service product	1 pkt	10	0	2	96	0	0.1	0
(Life) 'All Natural'	1 tbsp	17	0	4	10	0	0.0	0
(Millina's Finest)								
organic	1 oz	17	1	4	143	0	0.1	0
organic, fruit juice sweetened	1 tbsp	25	0	6	143	0	0.0	0
(Smucker's)	1 tsp	8	0	2	45	0	0.0	0
(Snider's)	1 tbsp	16	0	4	158	0	0.1	0
(Stokely)	1 tbsp	20	0	5	190	0	0.0	0
(Weight Watchers)	2 tsp	8	0	2	110	0	0.0	0
(Westbrae)								
fruit sweetened	1 tbsp	12	0	2	110	0	0.0	0
fruit sweetened, no salt	1 tbsp	12	0	2	10	0	0.0	0

Food Name	Serv. Size	Total Cal.	Prot. gms	Carbs gms	Sod. mgs	Fiber gms	Fat gms	Chol. mgs
unsweetened	1 tbsp	5	0	1	60	0	0.0	0
unsweetened 'Unketchup'	1 tbsp	8	0	1	105	0	0.0	0
CAULIFLOWER								
Canned or jarred								
pickled, 'Hot & Spicy' *(Vlasic)*	1 oz	4	0	1	435	0	0.0	0
sweet *(Vlasic)*	1 oz	35	0	9	225	0	0.0	0
Fresh								
green, cooked	1/5 head	29	3	6	21	3	0.3	0
green, raw, chopped	1 cup	20	2	4	15	2	0.2	0
green, raw, florets	1 floret	8	1	2	6	1	0.1	0
green, raw, whole, large, approx 6-7-inch diam	1 head	158	15	31	118	16	1.5	0
green, raw, whole, medium, approx 5-6-inch diam	1 head	134	13	26	99	14	1.3	0
green, raw, whole, small, approx 4-inch diam	1 head	101	10	20	75	10	1.0	0
white, boiled, drained, florets	3 florets	12	1	2	8	1	0.2	0
white, boiled, drained, 1-inch pieces	1/2 cup	14	1	3	9	2	0.3	0
white, raw, chopped	1 cup	25	2	5	30	3	0.2	0
white, raw, florets	1 floret	3	0	1	4	0	0.0	0
white, raw, whole, large, approx 6-7-inch diam	1 head	210	17	44	252	21	1.8	0
white, raw, whole, medium, approx 5-6-inch diam	1 head	144	11	30	173	14	1.2	0
white, raw, whole, small, approx 4-inch diam	1 head	66	5	14	80	7	0.6	0
Frozen								
(A&P)	3.3 oz	25	2	5	20	0	1.0	0
(Birds Eye)	3.3 oz	25	2	5	20	2	0.0	0
(Finast)	3.3 oz	25	2	5	15	0	0.0	0
(Flav-R-Pac)	4 pieces	20	2	3	25	2	0.0	0
(Frosty Acres)	3.3 oz	25	2	5	16	1	0.0	0
(Kohl's)	3 oz	20	2	4	15	0	1.0	0
(Seabrook)	3.3 oz	25	2	5	16	1	0.0	0
(Southern)	3.5 oz	26	2	5	30	0	0.2	0
cuts *(Green Giant)*	1/2 cup	12	1	3	25	1	0.0	0
cuts, no salt, drained, 1-inch pieces	1 cup	34	3	7	32	5	0.4	0
cuts, unprepared, 1-inch pieces	1/2 cup	16	1	3	16	2	0.2	0
cuts, w/salt, drained, 1-inch pieces	1 cup	34	3	7	457	5	0.4	0
florets, 'Plain Polybag' *(Green Giant)*	1/2 cup	12	1	3	25	2	0.0	0
'Singles' *(Stokely)*	3 oz	20	2	4	20	0	0.0	0
unprepared	10-oz pkg	68	6	13	68	7	0.8	0
CAULIFLOWER DISH								
(Green Giant) w/cheese flavored sauce	1/2 cup	60	2	8	510	2	2.5	3
CAVATELLI. See under PASTA DISH/ENTRÉE.								
CAVIAR								
black or red, granular	1 oz	71	7	1	425	0	5.1	167
black or red, granular	1 tbsp	40	4	1	240	0	2.9	94
CAYENNE. See under PEPPER, GROUND.								
CECI. See CHICKPEA.								
CELERIAC								
boiled, drained, chopped	1 cup	42	1	9	95	2	0.3	0
raw, chopped	1 cup	66	2	14	156	3	0.5	0
CELERY								
boiled, drained, diced	1 cup	27	1	6	137	2	0.2	0
boiled, drained, whole	2 stalks	14	1	3	68	1	0.1	0
raw, cut, approx 4-inch strips	1 cup	20	1	5	108	2	0.2	0
raw, cut, approx 4-inch strips	1 strip	1	0	0	3	0	0.0	0
raw, diced	1 cup	19	1	4	104	2	0.2	0
raw, diced	1 tbsp	1	0	0	7	0	0.0	0
raw, whole, large, 11-12 inches long	1 stalk	10	0	2	56	1	0.1	0
raw, whole, medium, 7.5–8 inches long	1 stalk	6	0	1	35	1	0.1	0
raw, whole, small, approx 5 inches long	1 stalk	3	0	1	15	0	0.0	0

Food Name	Serv. Size	Total Cal.	Prot. gms	Carbs gms	Sod. mgs	Fiber gms	Fat gms	Chol. mgs
CELERY FLAKES *(Tone's)*	1 tsp	9	0	1	4	0	0.5	0
CELERY ROOT JUICE, bottled *(Biotta)*	6 fl oz	67	3	13	195	0	0.2	0
CELERY SALT *(Tone's)*	1 tsp	6	0	1	1584	0	0.4	0
CELERY SEED								
	1 tbsp	25	1	3	10	1	1.6	0
	1 tsp	8	0	1	3	0	0.5	0
(McCormick/Schilling)	1 tsp	7	0	1	3	1	0.4	0
(Spice Islands)	1 tsp	11	0	1	4	0	0.5	0
(Tone's)	1 tsp	9	0	1	4	0	0.5	0
whole seeds *(Durkee)*	1 tsp	9	0	0	0	0	0.0	0
whole seeds *(Laurel Leaf)*	1 tsp	9	0	0	0	0	0.0	0
CELLOPHANE NOODLES. See under NOODLE.								
CELTUCE, fresh, raw	1 med leaf	1	0	0	1	0	0.0	0
CEREAL, HOT								
(Krusteaz)								
'Ala'	1/4 cup	150	4	33	0	7	0.0	0
'Zoom'	1/3 cup	120	5	24	0	4	0.0	0
(Malt-O-Meal)								
'Maple Brown Sugar' 30% formulation, prepared, w/2% milk	1 oz	160	7	28	60	1	3.0	10
'Maple Brown Sugar' 30% formulation, unprepared	1 oz	100	3	22	0	1	0.0	0
(Quaker) plus fiber, prepared w/1/2 cup nonfat milk	1/2 cup	170	10	27	66	6	2.5	0
BARLEY								
(Erewhon) organic	1 oz	110	3	22	0	1	1.0	0
(Quaker) Scotch, quick	1/3 cup	170	5	37	0	5	1.0	0
BRAN								
(Breadshop) oat, rice, corn, 'Triple Bran' unprepared	1 oz	100	6	15	5	6	2.0	0
(H-O Brand) 'Super Bran' unprepared	1/3 cup	110	4	18	0	8	2.0	0
BULGUR								
(Arrowhead Mills)	2 oz	200	6	43	0	5	1.0	0
(Hodgson Mill) w/soy grits, unprepared	1/4 cup	120	6	24	0	1	1.0	0
CORN GRITS. See GRITS.								
FARINA								
(H-O Brand) instant, unprepared	1 pkt	110	3	22	235	3	0.0	0
(Krusteaz)	1 oz	100	3	22	1	1	0.0	0
(Pillsbury)								
unprepared	1/12 pkg	80	3	18	0	0	0.0	0
prepared w/water, 1/8 tsp salt	2/3 cup	80	3	18	270	0	0.0	0
(Quaker)	1/4 cup	154	5	33	1	1	0.4	0
GRANOLA								
(Breadshop)								
almond raisin, nectarsweet	1 oz	120	4	18	2	3	4.0	0
'Blueberry 'N Cream' nectarsweet	1 oz	115	4	19	2	3	3.0	0
'California Orange Crunch' honeysweet	1 oz	130	4	18	1	2	5.0	0
'Cinnapple Spice' honeysweet	1 oz	125	3	19	2	2	4.5	0
'Crunchy Oat Bran' nectarsweet	1 oz	120	3	18	2	3	5.0	0
'Golden Maple Nut' honeysweet	1 oz	130	4	17	2	2	5.0	0
'Golden Maple Nut'	1/2 cup	230	6	32	0	4	9.5	0
'Gone Nuts!' nectarsweet	1 oz	125	4	17	2	3	5.0	0
honey apple blueberry, honeysweet	1 oz	125	4	18	1	3	5.0	0
'Honey Gone Nuts!' honeysweet	1 oz	130	4	18	2	3	5.5	0
'New England Supernatural'	1/2 cup	220	5	31	0	3	9.0	0
orange almond	1/2 cup	240	7	35	0	5	8.5	0
orange almond, nectarsweet	1 oz	120	4	18	2	3	4.0	0
'Oregon Blueberry Crunch' honeysweet	1 oz	125	4	18	2	3	5.0	0
'Peaches 'N Cream' nectarsweet	1 oz	115	4	19	2	3	3.0	0
raspberries and cream, w/organic oats	1/2 cup	220	6	34	0	4	7.5	0

Food Name	Serv. Size	Total Cal.	Prot. gms	Carbs gms	Sod. mgs	Fiber gms	Fat gms	Chol. mgs
'Raspberry 'N Cream' nectarsweet	1 oz	115	4	19	2	3	3.0	0
'Strawberry 'N Cream' nectarsweet	1 oz	110	3	16	5	3	4.0	0
'Supernatural New England' honeysweet	1 oz	130	3	18	2	2	5.0	0
'Supernatural' honeysweet	1 oz	100	4	18	2	4	5.0	0
(Ener-G Foods) gluten-free	1 cup	436	9	47	178	7	26.8	0
(Erewhon)								
apple, spiced	1 oz	130	3	17	55	0	6.0	0
honey almond	1 oz	130	3	17	65	0	6.0	0
maple	1 oz	130	3	17	55	0	5.0	0
'Sunflower Crunch'	1 oz	130	3	18	60	0	4.0	0
w/bran, '#9'	1 oz	130	3	17	10	4	6.0	0
w/dates and nuts	1 oz	130	3	17	45	0	6.0	0
(Golden Temple)								
apple cinnamon, low-fat	1/2 cup	190	6	39	5	4	2.0	0
blueberry	1 oz	132	4	19	6	2	5.0	0
blueberry, coconut-free	1 oz	131	4	19	3	2	4.5	0
blueberry, wild	1/2 cup	230	6	33	5	4	9.0	0
cashew almond	1 oz	129	4	19	3	4	3.5	0
cinnamon apple raisin	1 oz	125	3	20	3	2	3.5	0
coconut almond	1 oz	145	4	18	3	2	3.5	0
fruit and nut	1 oz	129	3	19	26	2	4.5	0
golden	1 oz	138	4	19	25	2	6.0	0
Hawaiian	1 oz	126	4	19	3	2	4.0	0
high-protein	1 oz	124	4	19	6	2	3.5	0
honey almond	1 oz	130	4	20	25	3	3.5	0
honey blueberry apple	1 oz	128	4	20	2	2	3.5	0
'Lite & Crunchy'	1/2 cup	220	6	33	5	4	8.0	0
maple almond	1 oz	129	4	20	25	2	3.5	0
'Natural Delite'	1 oz	128	3	20	26	2	3.5	0
oat bran, w/berries	1 oz	120	4	20	3	3	3.5	0
oat bran, w/raisins and almonds	1 oz	119	3	19	3	3	3.5	0
orange almond	1 oz	133	4	19	25	2	4.0	0
'Rainforest Granola'	1/2 cup	240	7	33	0	4	10.0	0
raisin apricot date	1 oz	127	3	20	25	2	3.5	0
'Super Nutty'	1 oz	135	4	19	25	3	5.0	0
'Super Nutty'	1/2 cup	230	6	33	45	4	9.0	0
'Sweet Home Farm' low-fat	1 oz	110	3	22	65	2	2.0	0
(Health Valley)								
date and almond, nonfat	1 oz	90	2	21	20	3	0.0	0
raisin cinnamon, nonfat	1 oz	90	2	21	20	3	0.0	0
raspberry, nonfat	1 bar	140	2	35	5	3	0.0	0
tropical fruit, nonfat	1 oz	90	2	21	20	3	0.0	0
(Stone-Buhr) apple, no preservatives, no added sugar	1/3 cup	130	5	31	0	5	1.0	0
GRITS. See GRITS.								
MULTIGRAIN								
(Arrowhead Mills)								
four grain, unprepared	1 oz	94	4	18	1	7	1.0	0
seven grain, unprepared	1 oz	100	4	17	1	4	1.0	0
(Pritikin) hearty, microwave, prepared	1 pkt	190	9	38	65	0	2.0	0
(Quaker)								
unprepared	1/2 cup	133	5	29	1	5	1.0	0
prepared w/1/2 cup nonfat milk	1/2 cup	170	9	30	65	5	1.5	0
(Roman Meal)								
oats, wheat, and other grains, prepared w/water	1 cup	170	7	34	540	8	1.9	0
oats, wheat, and other grains, prepared w/water	3/4 cup	128	5	26	405	6	1.4	0
oats, wheat, and other grains, unprepared	1 cup	340	15	69	20	na	4.0	0
oats, wheat, and other grains, unprepared	1/4 cup	85	4	17	5	na	1.0	0

Food Name	Serv. Size	Total Cal.	Prot. gms	Carbs gms	Sod. mgs	Fiber gms	Fat gms	Chol. mgs
wheat w/other grains, plain, prepared w/water	1 cup	147	7	33	198	8	1.0	0
wheat w/other grains, plain, prepared w/water	3/4 cup	110	5	25	148	6	0.7	0
wheat w/other grains, unprepared	1 cup	299	13	67	6	17	2.0	0
wheat w/other grains, unprepared	1/3 cup	100	4	22	2	6	0.7	0
wheat w/other grains, unprepared	1 tbsp	19	1	4	0	1	0.1	0
w/apple cinnamon, prepared	2/3 cup	112	4	24	14	6	2.8	1
OAT BRAN								
(Arrowhead Mills) unprepared	1 oz	110	6	17	1	5	1.0	0
(Breadshop)								
'Oat Bran Muesli' unprepared	1 oz	100	4	20	5	3	2.0	0
100% pure 'Oat Bran' unprepared	1 oz	100	6	17	5	4	2.0	0
(Erewhon) w/toasted wheat germ *(Erewhon)*	1 oz	115	5	18	15	3	2.0	0
(Health Valley)								
apple/cinnamon, 'Natural' unprepared	1/4 cup	100	3	19	10	4	1.0	0
raisin, nonfat	1 oz	100	3	19	10	4	1.0	0
(Hodgson Mill) low-fat, cholesterol-free, unprepared	1/4 cup	120	6	23	3	6	3.0	0
(Malt-O-Meal)								
'Plus 40% Oat Bran' prepared, w/1/2 cup nonfat milk	1.3 oz	170	10	31	65	3	2.0	0
'Plus 40% Oat Bran' prepared, w/1/2 cup 2% milk	1.3 oz	190	10	31	65	3	4.0	10
'Plus 40% Oat Bran' unprepared	1.3 oz	130	6	25	0	3	2.0	0
(Mother's)								
prepared w/o salt	2/3 cup	92	6	17	1	4	2.0	0
prepared w/1/2 cup whole milk, w/o salt	1 oz	180	10	22	60	1	7.0	15
unprepared	1/3 cup	92	6	17	1	4	2.1	0
(Quaker) 'Mother's' unprepared	1/2 cup	146	7	25	2	6	3.2	0
(3-Minute Brand)								
'Quick' unprepared	1 oz	100	5	18	0	3	2.0	0
'Regular' unprepared	1 oz	90	6	17	0	4	2.0	0
(Wholesome 'N Hearty)								
apple cinnamon, unprepared	1 pkt	130	3	30	160	5	2.0	0
honey, unprepared	1 pkt	110	3	26	160	5	2.0	0
regular, unprepared	1 oz	100	4	18	0	5	2.0	0
OATMEAL AND OATS								
(Arrowhead Mills)								
apple, date, and almond, unprepared	1 oz	130	5	23	3	4	3.0	0
apple spice, unprepared	1 oz	130	5	23	1	3	2.0	0
cinnamon, raisin, almond, unprepared	1 oz	140	6	23	3	4	3.0	0
instant, unprepared	1 oz	100	6	18	0	4	2.0	0
(Erewhon)								
apple cinnamon, instant	1.25 oz	145	4	25	100	0	3.0	0
apple cinnamon, 100% natural, instant	1 pkt	130	5	24	100	3	2.0	0
apple raisin, instant	1.3 oz	150	4	27	100	0	3.0	0
apple raisin, 100% natural, instant	1 pkt	150	4	27	100	0	3.0	0
maple spice, instant	1.2 oz	140	4	24	100	0	3.0	0
maple spice, 100% natural, instant	1 pkt	130	2	25	100	3	2.0	0
w/oat bran, instant	1.25 oz	125	6	23	0	4	3.0	0
w/raisins, dates, and walnuts, instant	1.2 oz	130	3	24	60	3	3.0	0
(General Mills)								
apple and cinnamon, instant, unprepared	1.5 oz	150	4	32	105	3	2.0	0
cinnamon raisin, unprepared	1.8 oz	170	4	38	130	3	2.0	0
(H-O Brand)								
apple and bran w/fiber, instant, unprepared	1 pkt	130	3	26	140	3	2.0	0
apple and cinnamon, instant, unprepared	1 pkt	130	3	26	220	3	2.0	0
'Gourmet' unprepared	1/3 cup	100	5	18	0	3	2.0	0
instant, unprepared	1 pkt	110	4	18	230	3	2.0	0
instant, unprepared	1/2 cup	130	5	22	5	3	2.0	0
maple brown sugar, unprepared	1 pkt	160	4	32	285	3	2.0	0

Food Name	Serv. Size	Total Cal.	Prot. gms	Carbs gms	Sod. mgs	Fiber gms	Fat gms	Chol. mgs
'Quick' unprepared	1/2 cup	130	5	23	5	3	2.0	0
raisin and bran, w/fiber, instant, unprepared	1 pkt	150	4	32	140	3	2.0	0
raisins and spice, instant, unprepared	1 pkt	150	4	32	240	3	2.0	0
sweet'n mellow, instant, unprepared	1 pkt	150	5	30	270	3	2.0	0
w/fiber, instant, unprepared	1 pkt	110	5	18	140	3	2.0	0
w/fiber, instant, unprepared	1/3 cup	100	5	15	5	3	2.0	0
(Maypo)								
maple flavored, 'Vermont Style' unprepared	1 oz	105	4	20	0	2	1.0	0
'Maypo' prepared w/water, salt	1 cup	170	6	32	259	6	2.4	0
'Maypo' prepared w/water, salt	3/4 cup	128	4	24	194	4	1.8	0
'Maypo' prepared w/water, no salt added	1 cup	170	6	32	10	6	2.4	0
'Maypo' prepared w/water, no salt added	3/4 cup	128	4	24	7	4	1.8	0
'Maypo' prepared w/water, no salt added	1 tbsp	11	0	2	1	0	0.1	0
'Maypo' '30 Second' unprepared	1 oz	100	4	19	0	2	1.0	0
'Maypo' unprepared	1 cup	362	12	68	18	10	5.0	0
'Maypo' unprepared	1/2 cup	181	6	34	9	5	2.5	0
(Mother's)								
instant, prepared w/1/2 cup whole milk	1 oz	190	9	24	60	0	6.0	15
instant, unprepared	1 oz	110	5	18	0	0	2.0	0
(Oatmeal Swirlers)								
cherry, unprepared	1.7 oz	150	3	33	130	2	2.0	0
cinnamon spice, unprepared	1.6 oz	160	3	35	100	2	2.0	0
maple brown sugar, unprepared	1.6 oz	160	3	35	100	2	2.0	0
milk chocolate, unprepared	1.7 oz	170	3	37	100	2	2.0	0
apple and cinnamon, instant, unprepared	1.7 oz	160	3	34	120	2	2.0	0
strawberry, unprepared	1.6 oz	150	3	32	120	2	2.0	0
(Quaker)								
apple spice, microwave, 'Quick 'n Hearty'	1 pkt	166	4	35	306	3	2.0	0
apples and cinnamon, instant, unprepared	1 pkt	130	4	26	105	3	1.5	0
apples and spice, instant, 'Extra' unprepared	1 pkt	133	4	27	191	3	1.9	0
brown sugar cinnamon, microwave, 'Quick 'n Hearty'	1 pkt	155	4	31	255	3	2.2	0
cinnamon and spice, instant, unprepared	1 pkt	164	5	35	322	3	2.1	0
cinnamon double raisin, microwave, 'Quick 'n Hearty'	1 pkt	169	4	35	275	3	2.2	0
cinnamon graham, instant, 'Kids' Choice' unprepared	1 pkt	140	4	29	170	3	2.0	0
cinnamon graham cookie, instant, 'Kids Choice'	1 pkt	190	8	35	230	3	2.0	0
cinnamon toast, instant, unprepared	1 pkt	130	3	27	160	2	2.0	0
'Cinnamagic' instant, unprepared	1 pkt	144	4	30	165	3	2.0	0
'Extra' unprepared	1 pkt	95	4	18	219	3	2.0	0
fruit punch flavor, instant, 'Power Rangers' unprepared	1 pkt	149	4	31	165	3	2.0	0
fruit and cream, instant, unprepared	1 pkt	135	3	26	169	2	2.5	0
fruit and cream blueberry, instant, unprepared	1 pkt	130	3	27	140	2	2.5	0
honey bran, microwave, 'Quick 'n Hearty'	1 pkt	151	4	31	253	3	2.1	0
honey nut, instant, unprepared	1 pkt	130	3	25	210	2	3.0	0
instant, unprepared	1 pkt	94	4	18	270	3	2.0	0
low-salt, instant, unprepared	1 pkt	103	4	19	78	3	2.0	0
maple and brown sugar, instant, prepared w/water	1 pkt	153	4	31	234	3	1.8	0
maple and brown sugar, instant, 'Kids' Choice' unprepared	1 pkt	140	4	31	240	3	2.0	0
maple and brown sugar, instant, unprepared	1 pkt	152	5	32	320	3	2.1	0
'Old Fashioned' prepared	2/3 cup	99	4	19	1	3	2.0	0
'Old Fashioned' unprepared	1/3 cup	99	4	19	1	3	2.0	0
peaches and cream, instant, unprepared	1 pkt	129	3	26	179	2	2.2	0
plus fiber, instant, unprepared	1/2 cup	130	6	21	0	6	2.5	0
'Quick' prepared	2/3 cup	99	4	19	1	3	2.0	0
'Quick' unprepared	1/3 cup	99	4	19	1	3	2.0	0
radical raspberry, instant, 'Kids' Choice' unprepared	1 pkt	150	4	28	170	3	3.0	0
raisin bran, plus fiber, instant, unprepared	1 pkt	190	9	34	125	6	2.0	0

Food Name	Serv. Size	Total Cal.	Prot. gms	Carbs gms	Sod. mgs	Fiber gms	Fat gms	Chol. mgs
raisins and cinnamon, instant, 'Extra' unprepared .... 1 pkt		129	4	27	119	3	1.9	0
raisins and spice, instant, unprepared .... 1 pkt		149	4	32	266	3	2.0	0
raisins, dates, and walnuts, instant, unprepared .... 1 pkt		141	4	25	216	2	3.8	0
regular flavor, instant .... 1 pkt		94	4	18	270	3	2.0	0
regular flavor, microwave, 'Quick 'n Hearty' .... 1 pkt		106	4	19	153	2	2.1	0
strawberries and cream, instant, unprepared .... 1 pkt		129	3	27	204	2	2.0	0
strawberries and stuff, instant, 'Kids' Choice' unprepared ... 1 pkt		140	4	30	170	3	2.0	0
unprepared .... 1/3 cup		99	4	19	1	3	2.0	0
w/apples and cinnamon, instant, prepared w/water .... 1 pkt		125	3	26	121	3	1.4	0
w/apples and cinnamon, instant, unprepared .... 1 pkt		128	3	27	121	3	1.5	0
(Ralston)								
prepared w/water, salt .... 1 cup		134	6	28	476	6	0.8	0
prepared w/water, salt .... 3/4 cup		101	4	21	357	5	0.6	0
(3-Minute Brand)								
'Old Fashioned' unprepared .... 1 oz		100	5	18	0	3	2.0	0
'Quick' unprepared .... 1 oz		100	5	18	0	3	2.0	0
raisin, unprepared .... 1 oz		100	5	18	0	3	2.0	0
raisin, w/oat bran, unprepared .... 1 oz		100	4	18	0	3	2.0	0
(Total)								
instant, unprepared .... 1.2 oz		110	4	22	220	3	2.0	0
maple brown sugar, unprepared .... 1.6 oz		160	4	34	150	3	2.0	0
'Quick' unprepared .... 1 oz		90	4	18	0	3	2.0	0
(Under Cover Bears) plain, instant, prepared w/water ...... 1 pkt		71	3	12	195	2	1.2	0
RICE								
(Arrowhead Mills)								
brown, 'Rise and Shine' unprepared .... 1.5 oz		160	3	35	1	2	1.0	0
(Cream of Rice)								
cream of, prepared w/water, no salt .... 1 cup		127	2	28	2	0	0.2	0
cream of, prepared w/water, no salt .... 3/4 cup		95	2	21	2	0	0.2	0
cream of, prepared w/water, no salt .... 1 tbsp		8	0	2	0	0	0.0	0
cream of, prepared w/water, salt .... 1 cup		127	2	28	422	0	0.2	0
cream of, prepared w/water, salt .... 3/4 cup		95	2	21	317	0	0.2	0
cream of, unprepared .... 1 cup		640	11	143	10	1	0.9	0
cream of, unprepared .... 1 tbsp		38	1	8	1	0	0.1	0
(Erewhon)								
brown, cream of, organic .... 1 oz		110	3	23	20	0	1.0	0
(Lundberg Family)								
almond-date, 'Hot'n Creamy' prepared .... 1 oz		110	2	24	25	0	1.0	0
organic, 'Hot'n Creamy' prepared .... 1 oz		110	3	23	20	0	1.0	0
RYE								
(Breadshop) 'Rye Date Muesli' unprepared .... 1 oz		100	3	19	5	4	2.0	0
(Roman Meal) cream of, unprepared .... 1/3 cup		110	4	27	0	5	1.0	0
WHEAT								
(Ancient Harvest) whole-grain, steam rolled .... 1/3 cup		105	3	23	5	3	1.0	0
(Arrowhead Mills)								
'Bear Mush' unprepared .... 1 oz		100	3	21	1	1	0.0	0
cracked wheat, unprepared .... 2 oz		180	7	40	1	2	1.0	0
(Cream of Wheat)								
cream of, apple, banana and maple flavored, instant, 'Mix 'N Eat' prepared .... 1 pkt		132	2	29	242	0	0.5	0
cream of, apple, banana and maple flavored, instant, 'Mix 'N Eat' unprepared .... 1 pkt		132	2	29	241	1	0.4	0
cream of, apple and cinnamon, 'Mix'n Eat' unprepared .... 1 oz		130	2	29	250	1	0.0	0
cream of, brown sugar cinnamon, 'Mix'n Eat' unprepared ... 1 oz		130	2	29	230	1	0.0	0
cream of, instant, prepared w/water, no salt .... 1 cup		121	4	26	1	1	0.2	0
cream of, instant, prepared w/water, no salt .... 3/4 cup		116	3	24	5	2	0.4	0
cream of, instant, prepared w/water, salt .... 1 serving		96	3	20	160	1	0.2	0

Food Name	Serv. Size	Total Cal.	Prot. gms	Carbs gms	Sod. mgs	Fiber gms	Fat gms	Chol. mgs
cream of, instant, prepared w/water, salt	1 cup	154	4	32	364	3	0.5	0
cream of, instant, prepared w/water, salt	3/4 cup	116	3	24	273	2	0.4	0
cream of, instant, prepared w/water, salt	1 tbsp	10	0	2	0	0	0.0	0
cream of, instant, unprepared	1 cup	651	19	134	27	6	2.5	0
cream of, instant, unprepared	1 tbsp	42	1	9	2	0	0.2	0
cream of, maple brown sugar, 'Mix'n Eat' unprepared	1 oz	130	2	29	180	1	0.0	0
cream of, original, 'Mix'n Eat' unprepared	1 oz	100	3	21	170	1	0.0	0
cream of, plain, instant, 'Mix 'N Eat' prepared	1 pkt	102	3	21	241	0	0.3	0
cream of, plain, instant, 'Mix 'N Eat' unprepared	1 pkt	102	3	21	241	1	0.3	0
cream of, quick, prepared w/water	1 cup	129	4	27	139	1	0.5	0
cream of, quick, prepared w/water	3/4 cup	97	3	20	104	1	0.4	0
cream of, quick, prepared w/water	1 tbsp	8	0	2	9	0	0.0	0
cream of, quick, prepared w/water, salt	1 cup	129	4	27	464	1	0.5	0
cream of, quick, prepared w/water, salt	3/4 cup	97	3	20	347	1	0.4	0
cream of, quick, unprepared	1 cup	635	18	132	688	5	2.3	0
cream of, quick, unprepared	1 tbsp	40	1	8	43	0	0.1	0
cream of, regular, prepared w/water, no salt	1 cup	133	4	28	3	2	0.5	0
cream of, regular, prepared w/water, no salt	3/4 cup	100	3	21	2	1	0.4	0
cream of, regular, prepared w/water, no salt	1 tbsp	8	0	2	0	0	0.0	0
cream of, regular, prepared w/water, salt	1 cup	133	4	28	336	2	0.5	0
cream of, regular, prepared w/water, salt	3/4 cup	100	3	21	252	1	0.4	0
cream of, regular, unprepared	1 cup	640	18	132	12	7	2.6	0
cream of, regular, unprepared	1 tbsp	39	1	8	1	0	0.2	0
(General Mills)								
'Wheat Hearts' prepared, w/3/4 cup nonfat milk	3/4 cup	170	10	29	95	1	1.0	0
'Wheat Hearts' unprepared	1 oz	110	4	21	0	0	1.0	0
(Wheat Hearts) unprepared	1 oz	110	4	21	0	0	1.0	0
(H-O Brand) wheat farina, cream of, unprepared	3 tbsp	120	3	26	0	3	0.0	0
(Hodgson Mill) cracked, coarse milled, unprepared	1/4 cup	110	4	26	0	8	1.0	0
(Malt-O-Meal)								
and barley, chocolate, prepared, w/1/2 cup 2% milk	1 oz	160	7	28	60	1	3.0	10
and barley, chocolate, unprepared	1 cup	607	17	128	17	na	1.5	0
and barley, chocolate, unprepared	1 oz	100	3	22	0	1	0.0	0
and barley, plain or chocolate, prepared w/water	1 cup	122	4	26	2	1	0.2	0
and barley, plain or chocolate, prepared w/water	3/4 cup	92	3	19	2	1	0.2	0
and barley, plain or chocolate, prepared w/water	1 tbsp	8	0	2	0	0	0.0	0
and barley, plain or chocolate, prepared w/water, salt	1 cup	122	4	26	324	1	0.2	0
and barley, plain or chocolate, prepared w/water, salt	3/4 cup	92	3	19	243	1	0.2	0
and barley, plain, unprepared	1 cup	607	17	128	12	na	1.5	0
and barley, plain, unprepared	1 tbsp	38	1	8	1	na	0.1	0
(Maltex)								
and barley, unprepared	1 oz	105	3	21	0	3	1.0	0
'Maltex' prepared w/water, no salt	1 cup	179	6	40	10	3	1.0	0
'Maltex' prepared w/water, no salt	3/4 cup	135	4	30	7	2	0.7	0
'Maltex' prepared w/water, no salt	1 tbsp	11	0	2	1	0	0.1	0
'Maltex' prepared w/water, salt	1 cup	179	6	40	189	3	1.0	0
'Maltex' prepared w/water, salt	3/4 cup	135	4	30	142	2	0.7	0
'Maltex' unprepared	1 cup	532	17	117	26	6	3.2	0
'Maltex' unprepared	1/4 cup	134	4	29	6	2	0.8	0
(Mother's)								
whole wheat, prepared, w/1/2 cup whole milk	1 oz	180	8	26	60	1	5.0	0
whole wheat, unprepared	1/3 cup	92	3	21	1	2	0.6	0
(Nabisco)								
cream of, apple cinnamon, prepared	1 serving	114	2	25	202	1	0.3	0
cream of, apple cinnamon, unprepreed	1 oz	108	2	24	192	1	0.3	0
cream of, enriched w/iron, quick, prepared	1 cup	78	3	16	59	1	0.3	0
cream of, enriched w/iron, quick, unprepared	1 cup	629	21	127	474	8	2.1	0

Food Name	Serv. Size	Total Cal.	Prot. gms	Carbs gms	Sod. mgs	Fiber gms	Fat gms	Chol. mgs
cream of, enriched w/iron, unprepared	1 oz	105	3	21	233	1	0.4	0
(Ralston)								
100% wheat, prepared	1/2 cup	160	5	31	0	5	1.0	0
'Ralston' prepared w/water, no salt	1 cup	134	6	28	5	6	0.8	0
'Ralston' prepared w/water, no salt	3/4 cup	101	4	21	4	5	0.6	0
'Ralston' prepared w/water, no salt	1 tbsp	8	0	2	0	0	0.0	0
'Ralston' unprepared	1 cup	402	17	85	13	16	2.5	0
'Ralston' unprepared	1/4 cup	102	4	22	3	4	0.6	0
(Roman Meal)								
w/dates, raisins, almonds, unprepared	1/3 cup	140	4	26	0	3	3.0	0
w/honey, coconut, almond	1/3 cup	150	5	21	5	3	6.0	0
w/rye, bran, flax, unprepared	1/3 cup	116	5	25	5	5	1.7	0
(Wheatena)								
wheat, unprepared	1 oz	100	3	21	0	4	1.0	0
'Wheatena' prepared w/water, no salt	1 cup	136	5	29	5	7	1.2	0
'Wheatena' prepared w/water, no salt	3/4 cup	102	4	21	4	5	0.9	0
'Wheatena' prepared w/water, salt	1 cup	136	5	29	578	7	1.2	0
'Wheatena' prepared w/water, salt	3/4 cup	102	4	21	433	5	0.9	0
'Wheatena' unprepared	1 cup	503	18	107	18	18	4.1	0
'Wheatena' unprepared	1/4 cup	125	5	26	5	4	1.0	0
CEREAL, READY-TO-EAT								
(Arrowhead Mills)								
bran flakes	1 oz	100	5	21	100	4	1.0	0
buckwheat groats, brown	2 oz	190	7	41	1	7	1.0	0
buckwheat groats, white	2 oz	190	7	41	1	7	1.0	0
corn flakes	1 oz	100	2	25	100	2	0.0	0
corn flakes, organic	1 cup	130	3	30	65	2	0.0	0
'Maple Corns'	1 oz	100	3	23	75	3	1.0	0
'Maple Corns' organic	1 cup	190	5	43	140	6	3.0	0
multigrain, organic	1 cup	140	3	29	130	3	1.5	0
'Nature-O's' organic	1 cup	130	5	24	5	3	2.0	0
oat bran flakes	1 oz	100	5	19	100	3	2.0	0
oat flakes	2 oz	220	10	39	1	8	4.0	0
oat groats	2 oz	220	8	38	1	6	4.0	0
puffed corn	0.5 oz	50	3	11	1	3	0.0	0
puffed rice	0.5 oz	50	1	12	1	3	0.0	0
puffed wheat	0.5 oz	50	2	11	1	6	0.0	0
wheat flakes	2 oz	210	8	42	1	7	1.0	0
(Barbara's Bakery)								
raisin bran	1 oz	170	3	36	80	0	1.0	0
'Shredded Spoonfuls' natural, 97% fat-free	3/4 cup	120	5	23	200	4	1.5	0
'Shredded Wheat'	2 biscuits	140	4	31	0	5	1.0	0
(Breadshop)								
'Almond Raisin' nectarsweet premium	1 oz	120	4	18	2	3	4.0	0
'Blueberry 'N Cream' nectarsweet gourmet	1 oz	115	4	19	2	3	3.0	0
'California Orange Crunch' honeysweet premium	1 oz	130	4	18	1	2	5.0	0
'Cinnapple Spice' honeysweet premium	1 oz	125	3	19	2	2	4.5	0
'Crunchy Oat Bran' nectarsweet gourmet	1 oz	120	3	18	2	3	5.0	0
'Golden Maple Nut' honeysweet premium	1 oz	130	4	17	2	2	5.0	0
'Gone Nuts!' nectarsweet premium	1 oz	125	4	17	2	3	5.0	0
'Honey Apple Blueberry' honeysweet premium	1 oz	125	4	18	1	3	5.0	0
'Honey Gone Nuts!' honeysweet premium	1 oz	130	4	18	2	3	5.5	0
'Orange Almond' nectarsweet premium	1 oz	120	4	18	2	3	4.0	0
'Oregon Blueberry Crunch' honeysweet gourmet	1 oz	125	4	18	2	3	5.0	0
'Peaches 'N Cream' nectarsweet gourmet	1 oz	115	4	19	2	3	3.0	0
'Raspberry 'N Cream' nectarsweet gourmet	1 oz	115	4	19	2	3	3.0	0
'Strawberry 'N Cream' nectarsweet gourmet	1 oz	110	3	16	5	3	4.0	0

Food Name	Serv. Size	Total Cal.	Prot. gms	Carbs gms	Sod. mgs	Fiber gms	Fat gms	Chol. mgs
'Supernatural' honeysweet gourmet	1 oz	100	4	18	2	4	5.0	0
'Supernatural New England' honeysweet gourmet	1 oz	130	3	18	2	2	5.0	0
(Eden Foods) 'Puffed Rice' five-flavor	30 puffs	110	3	24	160	2	0.0	0
(Erewhon)								
'Aztec' natural, nonfat	1 cup	110	2	26	70	1	0.0	0
'Banana-O's' organic, natural	3/4 cup	110	2	26	15	2	0.0	0
'Brown Rice' crispy	1 oz	110	2	24	185	4	1.0	0
brown rice, crispy, low-sodium	1 oz	110	2	24	5	4	1.0	0
brown rice, crispy, nonfat	1 cup	110	2	25	180	1	0.0	0
corn flakes, natural, no sweeteners	3/4 cup	100	2	22	50	1	1.0	0
'Crisp Rice' brown, natural	1 cup	110	2	25	180	1	0.0	0
'Fruit 'N Wheat'	1 oz	100	2	21	75	3	1.0	0
'Galaxy Grahams' natural, organic	3/4 cup	100	3	23	60	2	0.5	0
kamut flakes	3/4 cup	90	4	18	60	0	0.0	0
'Poppets' natural, organic	1 cup	120	2	25	10	0	1.0	0
raisin bran	1 oz	100	3	22	80	3	0.0	0
raisin bran, high-fiber, low-fat, low-sodium	1 cup	170	5	40	100	6	1.0	0
'Raisin Grahams' natural, nonfat, low-sodium	3/4 cup	100	4	23	55	3	0.0	0
'Right Start'	1 oz	90	3	24	80	5	0.0	0
'Right Start w/Raisins'	1 oz	90	3	22	80	5	0.0	0
'Wheat Flakes'	1 oz	110	3	22	75	4	0.0	0
'Super O's'	1 oz	110	3	24	5	4	0.0	0
(General Mills)								
'Addam's Family'	1 oz	110	1	25	65	0	1.0	0
'Basic 4'	1 cup	201	4	42	323	3	2.8	0
'Batman Returns'	1 oz	110	1	26	190	0	0.0	0
'Berry Berry Kix'	3/4 cup	120	1	26	185	0	1.2	0
'Body Buddies'	1 cup	115	2	26	288	1	0.9	0
'Boo Berry'	1 cup	116	1	27	214	0	0.5	0
'Bunuelitos'	1 oz	120	1	25	120	0	2.0	0
'Cheerios'	1 cup	110	3	23	284	3	1.8	0
'Cheerios' apple cinnamon	3/4 cup	118	2	25	150	2	1.6	0
'Cheerios' apple cinnamon, breakfast pack	1-oz box	120	2	24	200	2	2.0	0
'Cheerios' honey nut	1 cup	115	3	24	259	2	1.2	0
'Cheerios' multigrain	1 cup	112	3	24	254	2	1.1	0
'Cheerios Plus' multigrain	1 cup	108	3	24	201	3	1.1	0
'Cheerios-To-Go' apple cinnamon	1 pouch	110	2	22	180	2	2.0	0
'Cheerios-To-Go' honey nut	1 pouch	110	3	23	250	2	1.0	0
'Cheerios-To-Go'	1 pouch	80	3	15	220	2	2.0	0
'Chex' corn	1 cup	113	2	26	289	1	0.4	0
'Chex' honey nut	3/4 cup	117	2	26	224	0	0.7	0
'Chex' multi-bran	1 cup	165	4	41	325	6	1.2	0
'Chex' rice	1.25 cup	117	2	27	291	0	0.2	0
'Chex' wheat	1 cup	104	3	24	269	3	0.7	0
'Cinnamon Streusel' Betty Crocker	3/4 cup	120	2	25	167	1	1.3	0
'Cinnamon Toast Crunch'	3/4 cup	124	2	24	210	2	3.0	0
'Cocoa Puffs'	1 cup	119	1	27	181	0	0.9	0
'Cookie-Crisp'	1 cup	120	2	26	207	0	1.1	0
'Corn Flakes'	1 cup	98	2	22	239	0	0.1	0
'Count Chocula'	1 cup	117	1	26	209	0	0.9	0
'Country Corn Flakes'	1 cup	114	2	26	284	0	0.5	0
'Crispy Wheats 'N Raisins'	1 cup	191	4	44	285	3	0.8	0
'Crunchy Bran'	3/4 cup	90	2	23	253	5	0.9	0
'Dutch Apple' Betty Crocker	1 cup	219	4	46	309	2	2.0	0
'Fiber One'	1/2 cup	62	3	24	143	14	0.8	0
'Fingos' cinnamon	1 oz	110	1	22	170	2	3.0	0
'Fingos' honey toasted oat	1 oz	110	2	21	210	2	3.0	0

Food Name	Serv. Size	Total Cal.	Prot. gms	Carbs gms	Sod. mgs	Fiber gms	Fat gms	Chol. mgs
'40% Bran Flakes'	1 cup	159	6	39	456	7	0.7	0
'Frankenberry'	1 cup	117	1	27	209	0	0.5	0
'Golden Grahams'	3/4 cup	116	2	26	275	1	1.1	0
'Hidden Treasures' fruit juice added	3/4 cup	120	1	25	140	0	2.0	0
'Honey Almond Delight'	1 oz	110	2	23	200	1	2.0	0
'Honey Frosted Wheaties'	3/4 cup	110	2	26	211	2	0.3	0
'Honey Nut Clusters'	1 cup	213	5	43	239	4	3.5	0
'Kaboom'	1.25 cup	118	3	24	275	2	1.1	0
'Kix'	1 1/3 cup	114	2	26	263	1	0.6	0
'Lucky Charms'	1 cup	116	2	25	203	1	1.1	0
'Muesli' apple almond	1.45 oz	150	4	31	140	3	2.0	0
'Muesli' banana walnut	1.45 oz	150	4	30	150	3	3.0	0
'Muesli' cranberry walnut	1.45 oz	150	4	30	95	3	3.0	0
'Muesli' date almond	1.45 oz	140	4	32	95	3	2.0	0
'Muesli' peach pecan	1.45 oz	150	4	30	150	3	3.0	0
'Muesli' raspberry almond	1.45 oz	150	4	30	140	3	3.0	0
'Nature Valley Granola' cinnamon and raisin	3/4 cup	235	5	38	88	3	7.7	0
'Nature Valley Granola' fruit, low-fat	2/3 cup	212	5	44	205	3	3.0	0
'Nature Valley Granola' fruit and nut	2/3 cup	253	6	34	77	3	11.2	0
'Nature Valley Granola' fruit and nut	1/3 cup	130	2	19	45	1	5.0	0
'Nature Valley Granola' toasted oats	3/4 cup	248	6	36	89	4	9.7	0
'Nature Valley Granola' toasted oats	1/3 cup	130	2	20	50	1	5.0	0
'Oatmeal Crisp w/Almonds'	1 cup	219	6	42	250	4	4.6	0
'Oatmeal Crisp w/Apples'	1 cup	205	4	46	282	4	1.8	0
'Oatmeal Raisin Crisp'	1 cup	204	4	44	224	4	2.4	0
'Raisin Bran'	1 cup	178	4	46	486	8	0.3	0
'Raisin Bran'	1 1/3 oz box	120	3	31	328	5	0.2	0
'Raisin Nut Bran'	1 cup	209	5	41	246	5	4.4	0
'Reese's Peanut Butter Puffs'	3/4 cup	129	3	23	177	0	3.2	0
'Ripple Crisp'	1 oz	110	1	24	280	1	1.0	0
'Ripple Crisp' honey bran	1 oz	100	2	24	210	3	1.0	0
'S'Mores Grahams'	3/4 cup	117	2	26	212	1	1.2	0
'Sprinkle Spangles' corn puffs w/sprinkles	1 oz	110	1	25	130	0	1.0	0
'Sugar Frosted Flakes'	1 cup	149	2	34	247	1	0.5	0
'Sun Crunchers'	1 cup	216	5	44	380	2	3.2	0
'Sunflakes' multigrain	1 oz	100	2	24	240	0	1.0	0
'Team Cheerios'	1 cup	113	2	25	224	2	1.1	na
'Teenage Mutant Ninja Turtles'	1 oz	110	1	26	190	0	0.0	0
'Total'	3/4 cup	105	3	24	199	3	0.7	0
'Total Corn Flakes'	1 1/3 cup	112	2	26	203	1	0.5	0
'Total Raisin Bran'	1 cup	178	4	43	240	5	1.0	0
'Triples'	1 cup	116	2	25	191	1	1.0	0
'Trix'	1 cup	122	1	26	197	1	1.7	0
'Urkel-O's'	1 oz	110	1	25	160	0	1.0	0
'Wheaties'	1 cup	110	3	24	222	2	0.9	0
'Wheaties' honey gold'	3/4 cup	100	2	25	200	1	1.0	0
(Glenny's)								
'Maple Frosted Corn' mini puffs	1 oz	109	4	20	50	0	0.5	0
'Oat Mini Puffs'	1 oz	108	5	22	30	0	0.5	0
'Oat Mini Puffs' no salt, no sugar	1 oz	108	5	22	7	0	0.5	0
'Rice Mini Puffs'	1 oz	109	4	20	30	0	0.5	0
(Golden Temple)								
'Almond Raisin' low-fat	1 oz	110	2	22	57	2	1.5	0
'Apple Cinnamon' low-fat	1 oz	110	2	22	59	2	1.5	0
'Cashew Almond Granola'	1 oz	129	4	19	3	4	3.5	0
'Cinnamon & Spice Crunch' psyllium and chia seed	1 oz	132	3	20	26	2	4.5	0
'Cinnamon Granola' apple and raisin	1 oz	125	3	20	3	2	3.5	0

Food Name	Serv. Size	Total Cal.	Prot. gms	Carbs gms	Sod. mgs	Fiber gms	Fat gms	Chol. mgs
'Coconut Almond Granola'	1 oz	145	4	18	26	3	7.0	0
'Fruit 'N Nut Granola'	1 oz	129	3	19	26	2	4.5	0
'Golden Granola'	1 oz	138	4	19	25	2	6.0	0
'Hawaiian Granola'	1 oz	126	4	19	3	2	4.0	0
'Hazelnut Boysenberry' organic oats	1 oz	135	4	19	2	3	5.5	0
'High-Protein Granola'	1 oz	124	4	19	6	2	3.5	0
'Honey Almond Granola'	1 oz	130	4	20	25	3	3.5	0
'Honey Blueberry Granola' apple	1 oz	128	4	20	2	2	3.5	0
'Lite 'N Crunchy Granola'	1 oz	129	4	19	9	2	4.5	0
'Lite Muesli'	1 oz	102	3	20	60	2	1.0	0
'Maple Almond Granola'	1 oz	129	4	20	25	2	3.5	0
'Natural Blueberry Granola'	1 oz	132	4	19	3	2	5.0	0
'Natural Blueberry Granola' coconut-free	1 oz	131	4	19	3	2	4.5	0
'Natural Delite Granola'	1 oz	128	3	20	26	2	3.5	0
'Natural Foods' almond and raisin, lowfat	1 oz	110	3	22	3	2	1.0	0
'Natural Foods' apple and cinnamon, lowfat	1 oz	110	3	22	3	2	1.0	0
'Natural Foods' strawberry and raspberry, lowfat	1 oz	111	3	22	3	2	1.0	0
'Oat Bran Almond'	1 oz	120	4	20	3	3	3.5	0
'Oat Bran Apple'	1 oz	112	4	19	3	3	3.5	0
'Oat Bran Granola' berries	1 oz	120	4	20	3	3	3.5	0
'Oat Bran Granola' raisins and almonds	1 oz	119	3	19	3	3	3.5	0
'Oat Bran Muesli' dates and almonds	1 oz	108	3	21	79	2	1.5	0
'Oat Bran Muesli' raisins and hazelnut	1 oz	102	3	20	59	3	1.5	0
'Oat Bran Oregonberry'	1 oz	116	4	20	3	3	3.5	0
'100% Natural Almond'	1 oz	123	3	18	15	2	4.0	0
'100% Natural Apple/Cinnamon'	1 oz	120	3	18	14	2	4.0	0
'100% Natural Oat Bran'	1 oz	70	5	19	1	5	2.5	0
'100% Natural Raisin/Almond'	1 oz	120	3	19	7	2	4.0	0
'Orange Almond Granola'	1 oz	133	4	19	25	2	4.0	0
'Raisin Granola' apricot and dates	1 oz	127	3	20	25	2	3.5	0
'Six-Grain Crisp' fruit and flaxseed	1 oz	118	3	20	73	2	3.5	0
'Super Nutty Granola'	1 oz	135	4	19	25	3	5.0	0
'Sweet Home Farm Almond'	1 oz	123	3	18	14	2	4.0	0
'Sweet Home Farm Granola' lowfat	1 oz	110	3	22	65	2	2.0	0
'Sweet Home Farm Muesli' crunchy, lowfat	1 oz	105	3	21	98	2	2.0	0
'Sweet Home Farm Raisin'	1 oz	120	3	19	13	2	4.0	0
'Swiss Style Muesli'	1 oz	105	3	19	15	3	1.5	0
'35% Fruit Muesli'	1 oz	97	3	19	16	3	1.0	0
(Health Valley)								
'Almond Flavor O's' fat-free	1 oz	90	3	19	5	5	0.0	0
granola, date and almond flavor, nonfat	1 oz	90	2	21	20	3	0.0	0
granola, raisin cinnamon, nonfat	1 oz	90	2	21	20	3	0.0	0
granola, tropical fruit, nonfat	1 oz	90	2	21	20	3	0.0	0
'High-Fiber O's, nonfat'	1 oz	90	3	19	5	5	0.0	0
'100% Organic Blue Corn Flakes'	1 oz	90	3	19	10	3	1.0	0
'Organic Amaranth Flakes'	1 oz	90	3	20	10	3	0.0	0
'Sprouts 7' bananas and Hawaiian fruit, nonfat	1 oz	90	3	16	0	4	0.0	0
'Sprouts 7' raisins, nonfat	1 oz	90	4	16	0	5	0.0	0
(Heartland)								
'Heartland Natural' plain	1 cup	499	12	79	293	7	17.7	0
'Heartland Natural, plain	1 oz	123	3	19	72	2	4.4	0
'Heartland Natural' w/coconut	1 cup	463	11	71	213	7	17.1	0
'Heartland Natural' w/coconut	1 oz	125	3	19	58	2	4.6	0
'Heartland Natural' w/raisins	1 cup	468	11	76	226	6	15.6	0
(Honeybran)								
'Honeybran'	1 cup	119	3	29	202	4	0.7	0
'Honeybran'	1 oz	97	2	23	164	3	0.6	0

Food Name	Serv. Size	Total Cal.	Prot. gms	Carbs gms	Sod. mgs	Fiber gms	Fat gms	Chol. mgs
(Kashi)								
'Multigrain' medley	1 oz	100	4	20	50	2	1.0	0
'Puffed' honey, no refined sugars, no added oils	2 oz	120	3	25	6	2	1.0	0
'Puffed' sodium-free	2 oz	70	3	19	0	2	1.0	0
(Kellogg's)								
'All-Bran'	1/2 cup	79	4	23	61	10	0.9	0
'All-Bran Bran Buds'	1/3 cup	83	3	24	200	12	0.7	0
'All-Bran' w/extra fiber	1/2 cup	53	4	23	127	15	0.9	0
'Apple Jacks'	1 cup	116	1	27	134	1	0.4	0
'Apple Raisin Crisp'	1 cup	185	3	47	373	4	0.5	0
'Bran Flakes'	3/4 cup	95	3	23	226	5	0.6	0
'Cinnamon Mini Buns'	3/4 cup	115	1	27	208	1	0.6	0
'Cocoa Frosted Flakes'	3/4 cup	120	1	28	208	0	0.5	0
'Cocoa Krispies'	3/4 cup	120	2	27	210	0	0.8	0
'Common Sense Oat Bran Flakes'	3/4 cup	109	4	23	270	4	1.2	0
'Corn Flakes'	1 cup	102	2	24	298	1	0.2	0
'Corn Pops'	1 cup	118	1	28	123	0	0.2	0
'Cracklin' Oat Bran'	3/4 cup	225	5	40	195	7	7.0	0
'Crispix'	1 cup	108	2	25	240	1	0.3	0
'Double Dip Crunch'	3/4 cup	115	1	27	176	0	0.1	0
'Fiberwise'	1 oz	90	3	23	140	5	1.0	0
'Froot Loops'	1 cup	117	1	26	141	1	0.9	0
'Frosted Bran'	3/4 cup	101	2	25	206	3	0.3	0
'Frosted Flakes'	3/4 cup	119	1	28	200	1	0.2	0
'Frosted Krispies'	3/4 cup	113	1	27	219	0	0.2	0
'Frosted Mini-Wheats' bite size	1 cup	187	5	45	2	6	0.9	0
'Frosted Mini-Wheats' regular	1 cup	173	5	42	2	5	0.8	0
'Fruity Marshmallow Krispies'	3/4 cup	113	1	27	179	0	0.1	0
granola, w/o raisins, low-fat	1/2 cup	213	5	44	135	3	3.2	0
granola, w/raisins, low-fat	2/3 cup	202	5	44	124	3	2.8	0
'Healthy Choice Almond Crunch with Raisins'	1 cup	198	5	43	215	5	2.6	0
'Healthy Choice Multigrain' clusters w/raisins and almonds	1 1/4 cup	200	4	44	240	4	2.0	0
'Healthy Choice Multigrain' flakes w/brown sugar	1 cup	110	3	26	210	3	0.0	0
'Healthy Choice Multigrain' flakes	1 cup	104	3	25	174	3	0.4	0
'Healthy Choice Multigrain' squares w/honey	1 1/4 cup	190	5	45	0	6	1.0	0
'Healthy Choice Toasted Brown Sugar Squares'	1.25 cup	189	5	45	2	5	1.0	0
'Honey Crunch Corn Flakes'	3/4 cup	115	2	26	216	1	0.9	0
'Just Right' fruit and nut	1 cup	193	4	44	266	3	1.6	0
'Just Right' w/crunchy nuggets	1 cup	204	4	46	338	3	1.5	0
'Kenmei Rice Bran'	3/4 cup	110	2	24	230	1	1.0	0
'Mini-Wheats' apple cinnamon	3/4 cup	182	4	44	20	5	1.0	0
'Mini-Wheats' blueberry	3/4 cup	182	4	44	20	5	1.0	0
'Mini-Wheats' raisin	3/4 cup	187	4	43	3	5	1.5	0
'Mini-Wheats' strawberry	1 cup	187	4	43	17	5	1.3	0
'Mueslix' apple and orange crunch	3/4 cup	211	5	41	270	5	5.0	0
'Mueslix' raisin and almond crunch, w/dates	2/3 cup	200	4	40	160	4	3.2	0
'Nut & Honey Crunch'	1.25 cup	223	4	46	370	1	2.5	0
'Nutri-Grain Raisin Bran'	1 cup	130	4	31	200	5	1.0	0
'Nutri-Grain Wheat'	3/4 cup	101	3	24	221	4	1.0	0
'Oatbake Honey Bran'	1/3 cup	110	2	21	190	3	3.0	0
'Oatbake Raisin Nut'	1 oz	110	2	21	190	3	3.0	0
'Pop Tarts Crunch' cinnamon, brown sugar, frosted	3/4 cup	120	1	26	160	1	1.0	0
'Pop-Tarts Crunch' strawberry, frosted	3/4 cup	118	1	27	114	0	0.8	0
'Product 19'	1 cup	110	3	25	216	1	0.4	0
'Raisin Bran'	1 cup	186	6	47	354	8	1.5	0
'Razzle Dazzle Rice Krispies'	3/4 cup	108	1	25	166	0	0.3	0

Food Name	Serv. Size	Total Cal.	Prot. gms	Carbs gms	Sod. mgs	Fiber gms	Fat gms	Chol. mgs
'Rice Krispies'	1.25 cup	124	2	29	354	0	0.4	0
'Rice Krispies' apple cinnamon	3/4 cup	112	2	27	223	0	0.1	0
'Rice Krispies Treats'	3/4 cup	120	1	26	190	0	1.6	0
'Smacks'	3/4 cup	103	2	24	51	1	0.5	0
'Smart Start'	1 cup	183	3	43	313	2	0.7	0
'Special K'	1 cup	115	6	22	250	1	0.3	0
'Temptations' French vanilla almond	3/4 cup	119	2	25	207	1	1.6	0
'Temptations' honey roasted pecan	1 cup	122	2	24	248	1	2.3	0
'Whole Grain Shredded Wheat'	1 oz	90	3	23	0	4	0.0	0
(Kolln) 'Oat Bran Crunch'	1 oz	100	5	20	0	0	2.0	0
(Krusteaz)								
'Corn Flakes'	1 oz	110	2	24	280	1	1.0	0
'Crisp Rice'	1 oz	110	2	25	270	1	0.0	0
'Fruit Whirls'	1 oz	110	1	25	120	1	1.0	0
'Honey Nut O's'	1 oz	110	3	23	190	2	1.0	0
'Raisin Bran'	3/4 cup	120	3	30	210	4	1.0	0
'Sugar Frosted Flakes'	1 oz	110	1	26	230	1	0.0	0
'Toasted Oats'	1 oz	110	4	22	290	2	1.0	0
(Lundberg Family) 'Crunchies' brown rice	1 cup	171	3	38	7	0	0.8	0
(Malt-O-Meal)								
'Apple & Cinnamon Toasted Oat'	1 oz	110	2	22	180	1	2.0	0
'Berry Colossal Crunch'	3/4 cup	120	1	26	220	1	1.7	0
'Bran Flakes'	1 oz	90	3	23	210	5	1.0	0
'Colossal Crunch'	3/4 cup	120	1	26	230	1	1.7	0
'Corn Bursts'	1 cup	118	1	29	122	0	0.1	0
'Corn Flakes'	1 oz	110	2	25	290	1	0.0	0
'Crisp 'N' Crackling Rice'	1 oz	110	2	25	240	0	0.0	0
'Crispy Rice'	1 cup	125	2	29	320	0	0.4	0
'Fruit & Frosted O's' multigrain	1 oz	110	2	25	120	1	1.0	0
'Honey & Nut Toasted Oat'	1 oz	110	3	23	190	2	1.0	0
'Marshmallow Mateys'	1 cup	115	2	25	211	1	1.0	0
'Puffed Rice'	0.5 oz	50	1	12	0	0	0.0	0
'Puffed Wheat'	0.5 oz	50	2	10	0	1	0.0	0
'Raisin Bran Flakes'	1.4 oz	130	3	30	200	5	2.0	0
'Sugar Frosted Flakes'	1 oz	110	1	26	170	1	0.0	0
'Sugar Puffs'	1 oz	110	2	25	25	0	0.0	0
'Sweetened Puffed Wheat'	1 oz	110	2	25	25	1	0.0	0
'Toasted Oats'	1 oz	110	4	20	240	2	2.0	0
'Toasty O's'	1 cup	112	3	22	284	3	1.8	0
'Tootie Fruities'	1 cup	125	2	28	149	1	1.0	0
(Nabisco)								
'Fruit Wheats' apple	1 oz	90	2	23	15	3	0.0	0
'Team Flakes'	1 oz	110	2	24	180	0	1.0	0
(Nature Valley) See under General Mills.								
(Nature's Path) 'Heritage O's'	1 cup	165	5	34	140	5	1.0	0
(Perky's) 'Rice' nutty	1/2 cup	210	4	47	110	2	1.5	0
(Post)								
'Alpha-Bits' w/marshmallows	1 cup	115	2	25	206	0	1.0	0
'Banana Nut Crunch'	1 cup	249	5	44	253	4	6.1	0
'Blueberry Morning'	1.25 cup	211	4	43	266	2	2.5	0
'Bran Flakes'	3/4 cup	96	3	24	220	5	0.7	0
'C.W. Post Hearty Granola'	1 oz	130	2	21	80	2	4.0	0
'Cocoa Pebbles'	3/4 cup	115	1	25	157	0	1.2	0
'Dino Pebbles'	1 oz	110	1	25	150	0	1.0	0
'Frosted Alpha-Bits'	1 cup	130	3	27	212	1	1.3	0
'Frosted Shredded Wheat' bite size	1 cup	183	4	44	10	5	1.0	0
'Fruit & Fibre' tropical fruit	1.25 oz	120	3	27	170	5	3.0	0

Food Name	Serv. Size	Total Cal.	Prot. gms	Carbs gms	Sod. mgs	Fiber gms	Fat gms	Chol. mgs
'Fruit & Fibre' w/dates, raisins and walnuts	1 cup	212	4	42	280	5	3.1	0
'Fruity Pebbles'	3/4 cup	108	1	24	158	0	1.1	0
'Golden Crisp'	3/4 cup	107	1	25	41	0	0.4	0
'Grape-Nuts'	1/2 cup	208	6	47	354	5	1.1	0
'Grape-Nuts Flakes'	3/4 cup	106	3	24	140	3	0.8	0
'Great Grains' crunchy pecan	2/3 cup	216	5	38	214	4	6.3	0
'Great Grains' double pecan	1 oz	120	3	20	60	3	3.0	0
'Great Grains' raisin, date, and pecan	2/3 cup	204	4	40	156	4	4.5	0
'Honey Bunches Of Oats'	3/4 cup	118	2	25	193	1	1.6	0
'Honey Bunches Of Oats' w/almonds	3/4 cup	126	2	24	187	1	2.6	0
'Honeycomb'	1 1/3 cup	115	2	26	215	1	0.6	0
'Oat Flakes'	1 oz	110	4	21	130	2	1.0	0
'100% Bran'	1/3 cup	83	4	23	121	8	0.6	0
'Oreo O's'	3/4 cup	112	1	22	128	1	2.4	0
'Raisin Bran'	1 cup	187	5	46	360	8	1.1	0
'Raisin Grape-Nuts'	1 oz	100	3	23	140	2	0.0	0
'Shredded Wheat' original	2 biscuits	156	5	38	3	5	0.6	0
'Shredded Wheat' spoon size	1 cup	167	5	41	3	6	0.5	0
'Shredded Wheat 'N Bran' original	1.25 cup	197	7	47	3	8	0.8	0
'Smurf-Magic Berries'	1 oz	120	2	26	60	0	1.0	0
'Toasties' corn flakes	1 cup	101	2	24	266	1	0.0	0
'Waffle Crisp'	1 cup	129	2	24	130	1	2.9	0
(Quaker)								
'Apple Zaps'	3/4 cup	118	1	27	132	1	1.0	0
'Cap'n Crunch'	3/4 cup	107	1	23	208	1	1.4	0
'Cap'n Crunch's Crunchberries'	3/4 cup	104	1	22	190	1	1.3	0
'Cap'n Crunch's Peanut Butter Crunch'	3/4 cup	112	2	22	204	1	2.3	0
'Cinnamon Life'	1 cup	190	4	40	220	3	1.7	0
'Cinnamon Oatmeal Squares'	1 cup	232	8	47	266	5	2.6	0
'Cocoa Blasts'	1 cup	129	1	29	133	1	1.2	0
'Corn Blasts'	1 cup	133	1	28	240	1	1.9	0
'Frosted Flakers'	3/4 cup	117	1	28	281	1	0.2	0
'Fruitangy Oh!s'	1 cup	122	2	27	152	1	1.1	0
'Honey Graham Oh!'	3/4 cup	112	1	23	178	1	1.9	0
'King Vitaman'	1.25 cup	120	2	26	260	1	1.1	0
'Kretschmer Honey Crunch Wheat Germ'	1 2/3 tbsp	52	4	8	2	1	1.1	0
'Marshmallow Safari'	3/4 cup	119	2	25	192	1	1.5	0
'Oat Bran'	1.25 cup	213	9	41	205	6	2.9	0
'Oat Life, Plain'	3/4 cup	121	3	25	174	2	1.3	0
'Oatmeal Squares'	1 cup	216	7	43	263	4	2.6	0
'100% Natural,' oats, honey, and raisins	1/2 cup	218	5	36	11	4	7.3	1
'100% Natural,' oats and honey	1/2 cup	213	5	33	13	4	7.9	0
'100% Natural,' whole grain w/raisins, lowfat	1/2 cup	195	4	40	129	3	2.7	1
'Puffed Rice'	1 cup	54	1	12	1	0	0.1	0
'Puffed Wheat'	1.25 cup	55	2	11	1	1	0.3	0
'Quisp'	1 cup	109	1	23	194	1	1.5	0
'Sun Country Granola' w/almonds	1/2 cup	266	7	38	19	3	10.3	0
'Sun Country Granola' w/raisins and dates	1/2 cup	135	3	22	8	2	4.2	0
'Toasted Oatmeal' honey nut	1 cup	191	5	39	166	3	2.7	0
'Toasted Oatmeal' original	1 oz	100	3	22	160	2	1.0	0
(Rainforest Flake)								
flakes w/cashews, Brazil nuts, and raisins	4 oz	230	7	35	40	5	8.0	0
'Honey Nut Clusters' lowfat	4 oz	210	4	45	200	4	1.5	0
(Ralston Purina) See under *(General Mills)*.								
(Rice Krinkles)								
'Frosted Rice Krinkles'	1 cup	173	2	41	284	0	0.1	0
'Frosted Rice Krinkles' single serving box	0.75 oz	82	1	19	134	0	0.0	0

Food Name	Serv. Size	Total Cal.	Prot. gms	Carbs gms	Sod. mgs	Fiber gms	Fat gms	Chol. mgs
(Stone-Buhr)								
'Cereal Mates' 4-grain	1/3 cup	140	6	31	0	5	1.5	0
'Cereal Mates' 7-grain	1/3 cup	140	6	31	0	7	2.0	0
(Sunbelt)								
granola, banana almond	1 oz	130	3	20	25	0	4.0	2
granola, fruit and nut	1 oz	120	3	19	20	0	5.0	0
(US Mills) 'Uncle Sam'	1 oz	110	4	20	65	7	1.0	0
(Wonder)								
'Apple Cinnamon Corn Flakes'	1 oz	110	2	25	200	0	0.0	0
'Crunch Graham Oat Rings'	1 oz	110	2	24	125	0	1.0	0
'Honey Nut Crispy Rice'	1 oz	110	2	25	205	0	1.0	0

CEREAL BAR. See GRANOLA/CEREAL BAR.
CEREAL GRAIN BEVERAGE. See COFFEE SUBSTITUTE.
CEREAL SNACK. See also GRANOLA/CEREAL BAR.

Food Name	Serv. Size	Total Cal.	Prot. gms	Carbs gms	Sod. mgs	Fiber gms	Fat gms	Chol. mgs
(Barbara's Bakery)								
chocolate chip, 'Grrr-nola Treat'	1 serving	80	1	15	5	1	2.0	0
peanut butter and jelly, 'Grrr-nola Treat'	1 serving	80	1	14	5	1	3.0	0
(General Mills)								
'Cheerios-to-Go' apple cinnamon	1 pouch	110	2	22	180	2	2.0	0
'Cheerios-to-Go' honey nut	1 pouch	110	3	23	250	2	1.0	0
'Cheerios-to-Go' plain	1 pouch	80	3	15	220	2	2.0	0
'Fingos' cinnamon	1 oz	110	1	22	170	2	3.0	0
'Fingos' honey toasted oat	1 oz	110	2	21	210	2	3.0	0
(Natural Nectar)								
granola, almond butter crunch 'Nectar Nuggets'	1 cup	120	3	11	30	5	7.0	0
granola, almond cappuccino crunch 'Nectar Nuggets'	1 cup	110	2	14	30	5	5.0	0
granola, coconut almond crunch, 'Nectar Nuggets'	1 cup	110	2	15	20	4	5.0	0
granola, peanut butter crunch, 'Nectar Nuggets'	1 cup	120	4	11	30	5	7.0	0
(Nature Valley)								
granola, apple-cinnamon, 'Granola Bites'	1 pouch	170	3	25	100	2	7.0	0
granola, honey nut, 'Granola Bites'	1 pkg	170	3	24	120	2	8.0	0
granola, variety pack, 'Granola Bites'	1 pkg	170	3	24	120	2	8.0	0
(Nature's Choice)								
granola, chocolate chip, 'Grrr-Nola Treats'	0.75 oz	80	1	15	5	0	2.0	0
granola, cinnamon toast, 'Grrr-Nola Treats'	0.75 oz	80	1	15	5	0	2.0	0
granola, peanut butter and jelly, 'Grrr-Nola Treats'	0.75 oz	80	1	14	5	0	3.0	0
granola, tutti-frutti, 'Grrr-Nola Treats'	0.75 oz	75	1	15	5	0	2.0	0

CHARD. See SWISS CHARD.
CHAYOTE
Fresh

Food Name	Serv. Size	Total Cal.	Prot. gms	Carbs gms	Sod. mgs	Fiber gms	Fat gms	Chol. mgs
boiled, drained, chopped, 1-inch pieces	1 cup	38	1	8	2	4	0.8	0
raw, chopped, 1-inch pieces	1 cup	25	1	6	3	2	0.2	0
raw, whole, 5.75-inches	1 chayote	39	2	9	4	3	0.3	0

CHEDDARWURST. See under SAUSAGE.
CHEESE. See also CHEESE FOOD; CHEESE PRODUCT; CHEESE SPREAD; CHEESE SUBSTITUTE.
AMERICAN

Food Name	Serv. Size	Total Cal.	Prot. gms	Carbs gms	Sod. mgs	Fiber gms	Fat gms	Chol. mgs
pasteurized, process	1 oz	106	6	0	184	0	8.9	27
pasteurized process, w/disodium phosphate added	1 oz	106	6	0	406	0	8.9	27
(Borden)								
processed, 'Light'	1 1/3 slices	70	6	1	420	0	4.0	15
processed, 'Loaf'	1 oz	110	6	1	40	0	9.0	0
processed, nonfat, low-cholesterol	1 oz	40	6	4	380	0	0.0	5
processed, 'Slices'	1 oz	110	6	1	40	0	9.0	0
processed, slices, 'Premium'	1 oz	110	6	1	460	0	9.0	0
(Dorman's)								
processed	1 oz	110	6	1	440	0	9.0	0
processed, low-sodium, 'Loaf'	1 oz	110	6	1	140	0	9.0	0

Food Name	Serv. Size	Total Cal.	Prot. gms	Carbs gms	Sod. mgs	Fiber gms	Fat gms	Chol. mgs
(Healthy Choice)								
white, singles	1 slice	40	5	2	200	0	1.0	5
yellow, singles	1 slice	40	5	2	200	0	1.0	5
(Healthy Favorites) processed	2/3 oz	45	4	2	260	0	2.0	10
(Hoffman's) processed	1 oz	110	6	1	400	0	9.0	0
(Kraft)								
processed, 'Deluxe Loaf'	1 oz	110	6	1	430	0	9.0	25
processed, 'Deluxe Slices'	1 oz	110	6	1	450	0	9.0	25
(Land O'Lakes)								
processed	1 oz	110	6	1	405	0	9.0	25
processed, sharp	1 oz	100	6	1	360	0	9.0	30
(Old English)								
processed, sharp, 'Loaf'	1 oz	110	6	1	400	0	9.0	30
processed, sharp, 'Slices'	1 oz	110	6	1	440	0	9.0	30
(Sargento) hot pepper, pasteurized process	1 oz	106	6	0	406	0	8.9	27
(Smart Beat) fat-free	1 slice	25	4	3	180	0	0.0	0
(Weight Watchers) low-fat	1 slice	30	5	2	151	0	0.0	0
ASIAGO *(Frigo)* natural, wheel	1 oz	110	7	1	400	0	9.0	0
BABYBEL								
(Laughing Cow)								
natural	1 oz	91	7	0	227	0	7.0	22
natural, mini	3/4 oz	74	5	0	170	0	6.0	18
BEL PAESE								
(Bel Paese)								
'Domestic Traditional'	1 oz	101	6	1	145	0	8.0	20
'Imported'	1 oz	90	6	0	196	0	7.4	22
'Lite'	1 oz	76	7	1	155	0	5.0	16
primavera, 'Lite'	1 oz	68	6	2	165	0	4.0	14
BLUE								
	1 oz	100	6	1	396	0	8.1	21
(Dorman's)								
natural, 'Castello 70%'	1 oz	134	4	0	286	0	12.3	29
natural, 'Danablu 50%'	1 oz	100	6	0	200	0	8.2	23
natural, 'Danablu 60%'	1 oz	108	5	0	200	0	9.7	31
natural, 'Saga 70%'	1 oz	134	4	0	286	0	12.3	29
(Frigo) natural	1 oz	100	6	1	400	0	8.0	0
(Hickory Farms) natural, 'Domestic'	1 oz	101	6	1	396	0	8.3	21
(Kraft) natural	1 oz	100	6	1	330	0	9.0	30
(Sargento)								
crumbled	1/4 cup	100	6	1	380	0	8.0	20
natural	1 oz	100	6	1	400	0	8.0	21
BONBEL								
(Laughing Cow)								
mini	3/4 oz	74	5	0	170	0	6.0	18
natural	1 oz	100	6	0	227	0	8.0	24
BONBINO *(Laughing Cow)* natural	1 oz	103	7	0	227	0	9.0	27
BRICK								
	1 oz	105	7	1	159	0	8.4	27
(Dorman's) natural	1 oz	110	7	1	180	0	8.0	0
(Kraft) natural	1 oz	110	7	0	180	0	9.0	30
(Land O'Lakes) natural	1 oz	110	7	1	160	0	8.0	25
BRIE								
	1 oz	95	6	0	178	0	7.8	28
(Dorman's) natural	1 oz	81	5	0	229	0	6.6	20
(Sargento) natural	1 oz	100	6	0	180	0	8.0	28
BURGER *(Sargento)* natural	1 oz	110	6	1	410	0	9.0	27
BUTTERNIP *(Hickory Farms)* natural	1 oz	110	5	1	82	0	9.4	25

Food Name	Serv. Size	Total Cal.	Prot. gms	Carbs gms	Sod. mgs	Fiber gms	Fat gms	Chol. mgs
CAJUN *(Sargento)*	1 oz	110	7	0	165	0	9.0	28
CALJACK *(Churny)*	1 oz	100	6	1	0	0	8.0	0
CAMEMBERT								
....	1 cup	737	49	1	2071	0	59.7	177
(Dorman's)								
'45%'	1 oz	82	6	0	226	0	6.3	17
'50%'	1 oz	89	6	0	285	0	7.3	23
(Hickory Farms)	1 oz	90	6	0	239	0	7.0	26
(Sargento)	1 oz	90	6	0	240	0	7.0	20
CHEDDAR								
....	1 oz	114	7	0	176	0	9.4	30
low-fat	1 oz	49	7	1	174	0	2.0	6
low-salt	1 oz	113	7	1	6	0	9.2	28
(Alpine Lace)								
'Cheddar Flavored'	1 oz	100	7	1	95	0	8.0	25
milk, natural, shredded, 'Ched-R-Lo'	1 oz	80	7	1	95	0	5.0	20
(Alta Dena)								
mild, natural	1 oz	110	7	1	200	0	9.0	0
sharp, natural	1 oz	110	7	1	200	0	9.0	0
(Axelrod)								
extra sharp	1 oz	110	7	1	200	0	9.0	30
sharp...	1 oz	110	7	1	200	0	9.0	30
(Boar's Head) sharp sliced	1 oz	110	7	1	100	0	9.0	18
(Darigold)	1 oz	110	7	1	170	0	9.0	29
(Dorman's)								
....	1 oz	110	7	1	200	0	9.0	0
'Chedda-Delite'	1 oz	90	7	1	100	0	7.0	0
cheddar Jack, low-salt	1 oz	80	8	1	140	0	5.0	19
less fat, 'Low Sodium'	1 oz	80	8	1	100	0	5.0	20
low-salt, low-fat	1 oz	80	8	1	140	0	5.0	20
w/Monterey Jack, 'Chedda-Jack'	1 oz	90	7	1	100	0	7.0	0
(Featherweight) 'Low Sodium'	1 oz	110	7	1	5	0	9.0	0
(Frigo)								
....	1 oz	110	7	1	200	0	9.0	0
low-fat	1 oz	20	3	1	20	0	1.0	5
(Golden Balance)								
mild, natural, shredded 'Natural Shreds'	1 oz	90	8	1	150	0	6.0	20
sharp, natural, shredded 'Natural Shreds'	1 oz	90	8	1	130	0	6.0	20
(Healthy Choice)								
low-fat, 'Fancy Shreds'	1/4 cup	50	8	1	220	1	1.5	3
mild, natural, 'Fancy Shreds'	1 oz	70	8	0	220	0	4.0	15
(Hickory Farms)								
....	1 oz	110	7	1	176	0	9.0	30
raw milk, 'Light Choice Low Sodium'	1 oz	114	6	0	100	0	8.0	30
(Hoffman's) super sharp, processed	1 oz	110	6	2	390	0	8.0	0
(Kraft)								
mild, natural	1 oz	110	7	1	180	0	9.0	30
mild, natural, low-fat, made w/2% milk	1 oz	90	7	1	240	0	6.0	20
mild, natural, shredded 'Light Naturals'	1 oz	80	8	1	220	0	5.0	20
sharp, less fat, 'Light Naturals'	1 oz	80	9	1	220	0	5.0	20
sharp, low-fat, natural, made w/2% milk	1 oz	90	7	1	240	0	6.0	20
sharp, natural, made w/2% milk, 'Cracker Barrel'	1 oz	90	7	1	240	0	6.0	20
sharp, white, light, 'Cracker Barrel'	1 oz	80	9	1	220	0	5.0	20
(Land O'Lakes)								
natural......................................	1 oz	110	7	1	175	0	9.0	30
natural, 'Chedarella'	1 oz	100	7	1	180	0	8.0	25

Food Name	Serv. Size	Total Cal.	Prot. gms	Carbs gms	Sod. mgs	Fiber gms	Fat gms	Chol. mgs
(Laughing Cow)								
....	1 oz	110	7	0	227	0	9.0	28
'Reduced Mini'	3/4 oz	45	6	0	170	0	2.5	8
(Sargento)								
....	1 oz	110	7	0	176	0	9.0	30
mild, fancy, shredded, 'Preferred Light'	1/4 cup	70	8	1	200	0	4.5	10
mild, light, 'Mootown Snackers'	1 piece	60	7	1	170	0	4.0	10
mild, shredded, 'Classic Supreme'	1/4 cup	110	6	1	160	0	9.0	30
mild or sharp, 'Mootown Snackers'	1 piece	100	5	1	130	0	8.0	25
'New York'	1 oz	110	7	0	180	0	9.0	30
sliced	1 slice	110	6	1	160	0	9.0	30
(Smart Beat) sharp, nonfat	1 slice	25	4	3	230	0	0.0	0
(Stilwell) cheddar, frozen 'Bumpers'	1 piece	60	1	6	230	1	3.0	5
(Weight Watchers)								
mild, 'Natural'	1 oz	80	8	1	150	0	5.0	15
mild, shredded, 'Natural'	1 oz	80	8	1	150	0	5.0	15
sharp, 'Natural'	1 oz	80	8	1	150	0	5.0	15
CHESHIRE	1 oz	110	7	1	198	0	8.7	29
CHUTTER *(Hickory Farms)* 'Cold Pack'	1 oz	87	6	3	213	0	5.8	46
COLBY								
....	1 oz	112	7	1	171	0	9.1	27
low-fat	1 oz	49	7	1	174	0	2.0	6
low-salt	1 oz	113	7	1	6	0	9.2	28
(Alpine Lace) 'Colby-Lo'	1 oz	80	7	1	85	0	5.0	20
(Dorman's)	1 oz	110	7	1	190	0	9.0	0
(Hickory Farms)								
'Light Choice Low Sodium'	1 oz	100	8	1	4	0	6.0	20
'Longhorn'	1 oz	112	7	1	171	0	8.6	27
low-fat, calcium-enriched 'Light Choice'	1 oz	100	7	1	180	0	8.0	0
(Kraft)								
....	1 oz	110	7	1	180	0	9.0	30
made w/2% milk, natural	1 oz	80	7	0	220	0	6.0	20
w/Monterey Jack, less fat, 'Light Naturals'	1 oz	80	8	1	220	0	5.0	20
w/Monterey Jack, natural, shredded, 'Light Naturals'	1 oz	80	8	1	220	0	5.0	20
(Land O'Lakes) natural	1 oz	110	7	1	170	0	9.0	25
(Sargento)								
....	1 oz	110	7	1	170	0	9.0	27
Jack	1 oz	110	7	1	160	0	9.0	27
Jack, 'Mootown Snackers'	1 piece	90	5	1	160	0	8.0	20
Jack, shredded, 'Fancy Supreme'	1/4 cup	110	6	1	190	0	9.0	25
sliced	1 slice	110	6	0	190	0	9.0	30
(Weight Watchers) 'Natural'	1 oz	80	8	1	130	0	5.0	15
COTTAGE CHEESE								
creamed, not packed	1 cup	217	26	6	850	0	9.5	31
dry, large or small curd, not packed	1 cup	123	25	3	19	0	0.6	10
nonfat, dry, large or small curd	4 oz	96	20	2	14	0	0.5	8
(Bison)								
chive, creamed	1/2 cup	120	14	4	420	0	5.0	20
creamed, low-fat, 1% milk fat	1/2 cup	90	14	4	350	0	2.0	5
creamed, 4% milk fat	1/2 cup	120	14	4	420	0	5.0	20
garden salad, creamed	1/2 cup	110	12	4	420	0	4.0	15
w/pineapple, creamed	1/2 cup	140	10	18	340	0	4.0	15
(Borden)								
creamed, 4% milk fat	1/2 cup	120	14	4	400	0	5.0	0
creamed, 4% milk fat, unsalted	1/2 cup	120	14	4	40	0	5.0	0
dry curd, unsalted	1/2 cup	80	18	3	20	0	1.0	0

Food Name	Serv. Size	Total Cal.	Prot. gms	Carbs gms	Sod. mgs	Fiber gms	Fat gms	Chol. mgs
(Breakstone's)								
creamed	4 oz	110	13	3	370	0	5.0	25
creamed, low-fat, 2% milk fat	4 oz	100	14	4	510	0	2.0	15
dry curd, nonfat, unsalted	4 oz	90	16	6	65	0	0.0	10
(Carnation)								
large curd, 4% milk fat	1/2 cup	115	14	4	440	0	5.0	0
low-fat, 1.5% milk fat, 'Slender'	1/2 cup	90	14	4	440	0	2.0	0
small curd, 4% milk fat	1/2 cup	115	14	4	440	0	5.0	0
w/pineapple, 4% milk fat,	1/2 cup	130	10	12	430	0	5.0	0
(Crowley)								
calcium-fortified, creamed, low-fat, 1% milk fat	1/2 cup	90	14	4	390	0	1.0	5
creamed, 4% milk fat	1/2 cup	120	14	4	390	0	5.0	15
creamed, low-fat, 1% milk fat	1/2 cup	90	14	4	390	0	1.0	5
no salt added, creamed, low-fat, 1% milk fat	1/2 cup	90	14	4	50	0	1.0	5
w/peaches, creamed, 4% milk fat	1/2 cup	140	10	17	340	0	3.0	10
w/pineapple, creamed, 4% milk fat	1/2 cup	140	11	15	330	0	4.0	15
w/pineapple, creamed, low-fat, 1% milk fat	1/2 cup	110	11	15	330	0	1.0	5
(Darigold)								
creamed, 4% milk fat	4 oz	120	14	4	510	0	4.2	17
dry curd, unsalted	4 oz	80	18	3	15	0	1.0	10
'Trim' creamed, low-fat, 2% milk fat	4 oz	100	14	4	510	0	3.2	17
(Friendship)								
'California Style' creamed, 4% milk fat	1/2 cup	120	14	4	380	0	5.0	17
creamed, low-fat, 1% milk fat	1/2 cup	90	14	4	350	0	1.0	5
lactose-reduced, creamed, low-fat, 1% milk fat	1/2 cup	90	14	4	350	0	1.0	5
no salt added, creamed, low-fat, 1% milk fat	1/2 cup	90	14	4	31	0	1.0	5
pot style, large curd, creamed, low-fat, 2% milk fat	1/2 cup	100	14	4	405	0	2.0	9
w/pineapple, creamed, 4% milk fat	1/2 cup	140	11	15	300	0	4.0	17
w/pineapple, creamed, low-fat, 1% milk fat	1/2 cup	110	11	15	300	0	1.0	5
(Knudsen)								
creamed, 4% milk fat	4 oz	120	14	4	340	0	5.0	20
low-fat, 2% milk fat	4 oz	100	14	4	370	0	2.0	15
nonfat	1/2 cup	80	14	4	380	0	0.0	0
nonfat	4 oz	70	15	3	420	0	0.0	5
small curd, creamed, 4% milk fat	4 oz	120	14	4	370	0	5.0	20
w/fruit cocktail low-fat, 2% milk fat	4 oz	130	11	16	330	0	2.0	10
w/mandarin orange, low-fat, 2% milk fat	4 oz	110	11	11	320	0	2.0	10
w/peach, low-fat, 2% milk fat	6 oz	170	16	19	270	0	2.0	15
w/pear, low-fat, 2% milk fat	4 oz	110	11	12	320	0	2.0	10
w/pineapple, creamed, 4% milk fat	4 oz	140	10	14	260	0	5.0	25
w/pineapple, low-fat, 2% milk fat	6 oz	170	16	18	300	0	2.0	15
w/spiced apple, low-fat, 2% milk fat	6 oz	180	16	20	280	0	2.0	15
w/strawberry, low-fat, 2% milk fat	6 oz	170	16	19	320	0	2.0	15
(Light n' Lively)								
garden salad, low-fat, 1% milk fat	4 oz	80	18	5	350	0	2.0	10
low-fat, 1% milk fat	4 oz	80	14	4	370	0	2.0	10
nonfat	4 oz	90	14	7	400	0	0.0	10
w/peach and pineapple, low-fat	4 oz	100	11	12	320	0	1.0	10
(Lite-Line) creamed, low-fat 1.5% milk fat	1/2 cup	90	14	4	400	0	2.0	0
(Lucerne)								
no added salt	1/2 cup	80	14	4	40	0	1.0	5
nonfat	1/2 cup	70	14	4	420	0	0.0	0
(Sealtest) low-fat, 2% milk fat	4 oz	100	14	4	340	0	2.0	15
(Weight Watchers)								
creamed, low-fat, 1% milk fat	1/2 cup	90	14	4	460	0	1.0	0
creamed, low-fat, 2% milk fat	1/2 cup	100	14	4	460	0	2.0	0

Food Name	Serv. Size	Total Cal.	Prot. gms	Carbs gms	Sod. mgs	Fiber gms	Fat gms	Chol. mgs
CREAM CHEESE								
.... 1 cup	1 cup	810	18	6	686	0	80.9	255
.... 3-oz pkg	3-oz pkg	297	6	2	251	0	29.6	93
.... 1 oz	1 oz	99	2	1	84	0	9.9	31
.... 1 tbsp	1 tbsp	51	1	0	43	0	5.1	16
whipped .... 1 tbsp	1 tbsp	35	1	0	30	0	3.5	11
(Alta Dena) pasteurized .... 1 oz	1 oz	100	2	2	110	0	10.0	0
(Crowley) .... 1 oz	1 oz	110	2	1	100	0	9.0	30
(Darigold) .... 1 oz	1 oz	99	2	1	84	0	9.9	31
(Dorman's)								
'65%' .... 1 oz	1 oz	90	3	1	200	0	8.4	26
'70%' .... 1 oz	1 oz	102	3	1	200	0	9.9	30
(Friendship) soft .... 1 oz	1 oz	103	2	1	70	0	10.0	31
(Healthy Choice) plain, nonfat .... 2 tbsp	2 tbsp	25	4	2	200	1	0.0	0
(Healthy Favorites) .... 1 oz	1 oz	60	3	2	110	0	5.0	15
(Philadelphia Brand)								
.... 1 oz	1 oz	100	2	1	90	0	10.0	30
brick .... 1 oz	1 oz	100	2	1	90	0	10.0	30
light, soft .... 2 tbsp	2 tbsp	70	3	2	150	0	5.0	15
nonfat, 'Free' .... 1 oz	1 oz	25	4	1	170	0	0.0	5
pasteurized process, 'Light' .... 1 oz	1 oz	60	3	2	160	0	5.0	10
soft .... 2 tbsp	2 tbsp	100	2	1	100	0	10.0	30
strawberry, soft .... 2 tbsp	2 tbsp	110	1	5	100	0	9.0	25
whipped .... 2 tbsp	2 tbsp	70	1	1	85	0	7.0	25
w/chives .... 1 oz	1 oz	90	2	1	125	0	9.0	30
w/chives, brick .... 1 oz	1 oz	90	2	1	135	0	9.0	25
w/chives, whipped .... 2 tbsp	2 tbsp	70	1	1	130	0	6.0	20
w/chives and onion, soft .... 2 tbsp	2 tbsp	110	1	2	135	0	10.0	30
w/herb and garlic, soft .... 1 oz	1 oz	100	1	2	160	0	9.0	25
w/olive and pimiento, nonfat .... 1 oz	1 oz	90	2	2	160	0	8.0	0
w/olive and pimiento, soft .... 1 oz	1 oz	90	2	2	160	0	8.0	25
w/onion, whipped .... 1 oz	1 oz	90	2	2	170	0	8.0	25
w/pimiento .... 1 oz	1 oz	90	2	1	150	0	9.0	30
w/pineapple, soft .... 2 tbsp	2 tbsp	100	1	4	100	0	9.0	25
w/salmon, soft .... 2 tbsp	2 tbsp	100	2	1	200	0	9.0	30
w/smoked salmon, whipped .... 2 tbsp	2 tbsp	70	2	1	140	0	6.0	20
(Stilwell) frozen, 'Bumpers' .... 1 piece	1 piece	60	2	5	210	0	3.0	5
(Temp-Tee) whipped .... 1 oz	1 oz	100	2	1	85	0	10.0	30
CREMA DANIA (Dorman's) 'Crema Dania 70%' .... 1 oz	1 oz	134	4	0	286	0	12.3	29
DANBO								
(Dorman's)								
45% .... 1 oz	1 oz	98	7	0	200	0	7.5	23
20% .... 1 oz	1 oz	62	9	0	200	0	2.8	9
EDAM								
.... 1 oz	1 oz	101	7	0	274	0	7.9	25
(Dorman's)								
.... 1 oz	1 oz	100	7	1	200	0	8.0	0
45% .... 1 oz	1 oz	91	7	0	200	0	7.0	21
(Hickory Farms) 'Domestic' .... 1 oz	1 oz	100	6	1	182	0	8.4	24
(Kaukauna) .... 1 oz	1 oz	100	7	1	275	0	8.0	25
(Kraft) .... 1 oz	1 oz	90	8	0	310	0	7.0	20
(Land O'Lakes) natural .... 1 oz	1 oz	100	7	1	275	0	8.0	25
(Laughing Cow) .... 1 oz	1 oz	100	6	0	227	0	8.0	26
(May-Bud) .... 1 oz	1 oz	100	7	0	275	0	8.0	0
(Sargento) .... 1 oz	1 oz	100	7	0	270	0	8.0	25
FARMER								
(Friendship)								
.... 1/2 cup	1/2 cup	160	16	4	356	0	12.0	40

Food Name	Serv. Size	Total Cal.	Prot. gms	Carbs gms	Sod. mgs	Fiber gms	Fat gms	Chol. mgs
'No Salt Added' .... 1/2 cup		160	16	4	8	0	12.0	40
(Hickory Farms)								
.... 1 oz		90	6	1	210	0	7.0	20
'Light Choice' .... 1 oz		90	6	1	150	0	7.0	20
(Kaukauna) .... 1 oz		100	7	1	0	0	8.0	25
(May-Bud) .... 1 oz		90	6	1	210	0	7.0	20
(Sargento) .... 1 oz		100	7	1	130	0	8.0	26
FETA								
.... 1 oz		75	4	1	316	0	6.0	25
(Churny) 'Natural' .... 1 oz		75	5	1	316	0	6.5	25
(Dorman's) 45% .... 1 oz		91	6	0	0	0	7.3	0
(Sargento) .... 1 oz		80	4	1	320	0	6.0	25
FONTINA								
.... 1 oz		110	7	0	227	0	8.8	33
(Sargento) .... 1 oz		110	7	0	0	0	9.0	33
GJETOST								
.... 1 oz		132	3	12	170	0	8.4	27
(Sargento) .... 1 oz		130	3	12	170	0	8.0	0
GOAT								
hard .... 1 oz		128	9	1	98	0	10.1	30
semisoft .... 1 oz		103	6	1	146	0	8.5	22
soft .... 1 oz		76	5	0	104	0	6.0	13
GOUDA								
.... 1 oz		101	7	1	232	0	7.8	32
(Dorman's) .... 1 oz		100	7	1	210	0	8.0	0
(Kaukauna)								
.... 1 oz		100	7	1	230	0	8.0	30
w/caraway seed .... 1 oz		100	7	1	230	0	8.0	30
w/hickory smoke flavor .... 1 oz		100	7	1	230	0	8.0	25
(Kraft) .... 1 oz		110	7	0	200	0	9.0	30
(Land O'Lakes) natural .... 1 oz		100	7	1	230	0	8.0	30
(Laughing Cow)								
.... 1 oz		110	7	0	227	0	9.0	28
mini .... 3/4 oz		80	5	0	170	0	6.4	21
(May-Bud) .... 1 oz		100	7	1	230	0	8.0	0
(Sargento) .... 1 oz		100	7	1	230	0	8.0	32
GRUYÈRE .... 1 oz		117	8	0	95	0	9.2	31
HAVARTI								
(Casino) .... 1 oz		120	6	0	140	0	11.0	35
(Dorman's)								
45% .... 1 oz		91	7	0	200	0	7.0	21
60% .... 1 oz		118	5	0	200	0	10.6	31
(Hickory Farms) 'Danish Special' .... 1 oz		117	5	0	198	0	10.5	31
(Sargento) .... 1 oz		120	5	0	200	0	11.0	31
HORSERADISH *(Kaukauna)* hearty, cold pack 'Cup' .... 1 oz		100	6	3	250	0	7.0	25
HOT PEPPER *(Hickory Farms)* .... 1 oz		106	6	1	406	0	8.9	27
ITALIAN STYLE								
(Sargento)								
grated .... 1 oz		110	8	1	105	0	8.0	26
6-cheese blend, 'Recipe Blend' .... 1/4 cup		90	7	0	180	0	7.0	20
JACK. See MONTEREY JACK.								
JARLSBERG								
(Hickory Farms) .... 1 oz		100	7	1	130	0	7.0	16
(Norseland) .... 1 oz		97	7	1	135	0	7.0	18
(Sargento) sliced .... 1 slice		120	9	1	160	0	9.0	20
LIMBURGER								
.... 1 cup		438	27	1	1072	0	36.5	121

Food Name	Serv. Size	Total Cal.	Prot. gms	Carbs gms	Sod. mgs	Fiber gms	Fat gms	Chol. mgs
(Mohawk Valley) natural 'Little Gem'	1 oz	90	6	0	250	0	8.0	25
(Sargento)	1 oz	90	6	0	230	0	8.0	26
MASCARPONE *(Galbani)* 'Imported'	1 oz	128	2	1	17	0	13.1	39
MEXICAN STYLE								
(Healthy Choice) fancy shreds	1/4 cup	50	8	1	220	1	1.5	3
(Sargento) 4-cheese blend, 'Recipe Blend'	1/4 cup	110	6	1	200	0	9.0	25
(Velveeta) mild, pasteurized process, shredded	1/4 cup	120	8	3	520	0	9.0	30
MONTEREY JACK								
	1 oz	106	7	0	152	0	8.6	25
(Alpine Lace)								
'Monti-Jack-Lo'	1 oz	80	7	1	75	0	5.0	15
natural, milk cheese 'Monti-Jack-Lo'	1 oz	80	7	1	75	0	5.0	15
(Alta Dena)								
natural	1 oz	100	7	1	180	0	8.0	0
natural, w/jalapeño peppers	1 oz	100	7	1	180	0	8.0	0
(Axelrod)								
	1 oz	100	6	1	150	0	8.0	30
w/jalapeño pepper	1 oz	100	6	1	220	0	8.0	30
(Darigold)	1 oz	110	7	1	150	0	8.0	25
(Dorman's)								
	1 oz	100	6	1	180	0	8.0	0
less fat, 'Low Sodium'	1 oz	80	8	1	90	0	5.0	18
low-salt	1 oz	80	8	1	140	0	5.0	18
'Slim Jack'	1 oz	90	6	1	90	0	7.0	0
(Hickory Farms) 'Light Choice Low Sodium'	1 oz	110	6	0	100	0	8.0	30
(Kaukauna)	1 oz	110	7	1	150	0	9.0	25
(Kraft)								
	1 oz	110	6	0	190	0	9.0	30
natural, low-fat, made w/2% milk	1 oz	80	7	1	240	0	6.0	20
natural, w/jalapeño peppers	1 oz	110	7	1	190	0	9.0	30
w/caraway	1 oz	100	7	1	180	0	8.0	30
w/peppers, less fat, 'Light Naturals'	1 oz	80	8	1	220	0	5.0	20
(Land O'Lakes)								
natural	1 oz	110	7	1	150	0	9.0	20
natural, hot pepper	1 oz	110	7	1	150	0	9.0	20
processed, 'Jalapeño Jack'	1 oz	90	5	1	430	0	8.0	20
(May-Bud)	1 oz	110	7	0	150	0	9.0	0
(Sargento)								
	1 oz	110	7	0	150	0	9.0	25
shredded	1/4 cup	100	6	0	190	0	9.0	30
sliced	1 slice	100	6	0	190	0	9.0	30
(Weight Watchers) 'Natural'	1 oz	80	8	1	120	0	5.0	15
MOZZARELLA								
part skim	1 oz	72	7	1	132	0	4.5	16
part skim, low-moisture	1 oz	79	8	1	150	0	4.9	15
part skim, low-moisture, diced	1 cup	370	36	4	697	0	22.6	71
part skim, low moisture, shredded	1 cup	316	31	4	596	0	19.3	61
whole milk	1 oz	80	6	1	106	0	6.1	22
whole milk, low moisture	1 oz	90	6	1	118	0	7.0	25
whole milk, low-moisture, shredded	1 cup	315	22	2	418	0	24.2	88
(Alpine Lace)								
natural, shredded	1 oz	70	7	1	75	0	5.0	15
natural, sliced	1 oz	70	7	1	75	0	5.0	15
part skim, low-moisture	1 oz	70	7	1	75	0	5.0	15
(Crowley)								
part skim	1 oz	70	8	1	240	0	4.0	15
whole milk	1 oz	90	5	1	240	0	7.0	25

Food Name	Serv. Size	Total Cal.	Prot. gms	Carbs gms	Sod. mgs	Fiber gms	Fat gms	Chol. mgs
(Dorman's)								
....	1 oz	90	7	1	190	0	6.0	0
less fat, 'Low Sodium'	1 oz	80	9	1	90	0	4.0	17
low-salt	1 oz	80	9	1	140	0	4.0	15
part skim, low-moisture, 'Low Sodium'	1 oz	80	8	1	90	0	5.0	15
(Frigo)								
part skim, low-moisture	1 oz	80	7	1	190	0	5.0	10
part skim, low-moisture, less fat	1 oz	60	8	1	150	0	3.0	10
whole milk, low-moisture...........................	1 oz	90	6	1	190	0	7.0	15
(Healthy Choice)								
ball	1 oz	45	10	1	200	1	0.0	0
fat-free, shredded	1 oz	40	9	1	200	0	0.0	5
low-fat, fancy, shredded	1/4 cup	50	8	1	220	0	1.5	3
natural, fat-free, chunk	1 oz	40	9	1	200	0	0.0	5
string	1 oz	50	8	1	220	0	1.5	3
(Hickory Farms)								
....	1 oz	72	7	1	132	0	4.5	16
low-salt, 'Light Choice Low Sodium'	1 oz	80	8	1	90	0	5.0	15
(Kraft)								
....	1 oz	90	6	1	190	0	7.0	20
less fat, 'Light Naturals'	1 oz	80	8	1	200	0	4.0	15
natural, low-fat, made w/2% milk	1/3 cup	80	9	1	210	0	5.0	15
part skim, low-moisture............................	1 oz	80	8	1	200	0	5.0	15
part skim, w/jalapeño pepper	1 oz	80	8	1	230	0	5.0	20
(Land O'Lakes) natural, low moisture, part skim	1 oz	80	8	1	150	0	5.0	15
(Polly-O)								
fresh 'Fior di Latte'	1 oz	80	5	1	20	0	6.0	20
grated	1 oz	130	11	1	530	0	10.0	25
'Lite'	1 oz	70	7	1	200	0	4.0	15
part skim	1 oz	80	6	1	280	0	5.0	15
whole milk......................................	1 oz	90	5	1	280	0	6.0	20
(Sargento)								
light, sliced, 'Preferred Light'	1 slice	90	11	0	230	0	5.0	15
part skim, low-moisture............................	1 oz	80	8	1	150	0	5.0	15
shredded, 'Classic Supreme'	1/4 cup	80	7	1	150	0	6.0	15
shredded, 'Preferred Light'	1/4 cup	70	8	1	140	0	3.0	10
sliced	1 slice	130	11	2	230	0	9.0	25
whole milk	1 oz	90	6	1	120	0	7.0	25
(Weight Watchers)								
'Natural'	1 oz	70	8	1	150	0	4.0	15
shredded, 'Natural'	1 oz	80	8	1	150	0	4.0	15
MUENSTER								
....	1 oz	104	7	0	178	0	8.5	27
(Alpine Lace)								
....	1 oz	100	7	1	85	0	8.0	30
low-salt, natural, sliced 'Low Sodium'	1 oz	100	7	1	85	0	9.0	25
(Dorman's)								
....	1 oz	110	7	0	190	0	9.0	0
50%	1 oz	100	6	0	200	0	8.2	24
less fat, 'Low Sodium'	1 oz	80	8	0	140	0	5.0	18
low-salt	1 oz	80	8	0	140	0	5.0	18
low-salt, 'Low Sodium'	1 oz	110	7	0	95	0	9.0	0
(Hickory Farms)								
....	1 oz	100	7	0	180	0	8.5	25
low-salt, 'Light Choice Low Sodium'	1 oz	110	7	0	95	0	9.0	27
(Kaukauna)	1 oz	110	7	1	180	0	9.0	25
(Land O'Lakes) natural	1 oz	100	7	1	180	0	9.0	25

Food Name	Serv. Size	Total Cal.	Prot. gms	Carbs gms	Sod. mgs	Fiber gms	Fat gms	Chol. mgs
(Sargento) sliced	1 slice	100	6	1	200	0	9.0	25
NACHO *(Sargento)* shredded, 'Fancy Supreme'	1/4 cup	110	6	1	240	0	9.0	25
NEUFCHATEL CHEESE								
. . . .	3-oz pkg	221	8	2	339	0	19.9	65
. . . .	1 oz	74	3	1	113	0	6.6	22
(Hickory Farms)								
chocolate	1 oz	110	2	8	90	0	8.0	33
date nut, rum	1 oz	100	2	4	80	0	8.0	31
orange	1 oz	100	2	4	75	0	8.0	45
peach	1 oz	90	2	3	85	0	8.0	39
pineapple	1 oz	90	2	2	60	0	8.0	33
strawberry	1 oz	90	2	3	70	0	8.0	32
(Kaukauna)								
garlic and herbs	1 oz	80	3	1	150	0	7.0	25
vegetable, garden	1 oz	80	3	1	200	0	7.0	25
(Philadelphia Brand)								
. . . .	1 oz	70	3	1	120	0	6.0	20
'Light'	1 oz	80	3	1	115	0	7.0	25
NEW HOLLAND								
(Hickory Farms) w/herbs, 'Light Choice'	1 oz	90	7	1	100	0	8.0	27
PARMESAN								
grated	1 cup	456	42	4	1862	0	30.0	79
grated	1 oz	129	12	1	528	0	8.5	22
grated	1 tbsp	23	2	0	93	0	1.5	4
hard	1 oz	111	10	1	454	0	7.3	19
shredded	1 tbsp	21	2	0	85	0	1.4	4
(Churny) 'Natural'	1 oz	110	10	1	455	0	7.0	20
(Frigo)								
fresh, grated	1 oz	110	10	1	350	0	7.0	0
grated	1 oz	130	12	1	510	0	9.0	0
wheel	1 oz	110	10	1	350	0	7.0	0
w/Romano cheese, grated	1 oz	130	12	1	510	0	9.0	0
(Hickory Farms)	1 oz	110	10	1	350	0	7.0	0
(Kraft)								
. . . .	1 oz	100	9	1	290	0	7.0	20
grated	1 oz	130	12	1	430	0	9.0	30
(Polly-O) grated	1 oz	130	11	1	530	0	9.0	20
(Progresso) grated	1 tbsp	23	2	1	95	0	2.0	4
(Sargento)								
fresh	1 oz	110	10	1	450	0	7.0	19
grated	1 oz	130	12	2	530	0	9.0	22
shredded, 'Fancy Supreme'	1/4 cup	110	9	1	300	0	7.0	25
w/Romano, grated	1 oz	110	10	1	400	0	7.0	24
w/Romano, shredded, 'Fancy Supreme'	1/4 cup	110	9	1	340	0	7.0	25
PARMESANO REGGIANO *(Galbani)* 'Imported'	1 oz	105	10	1	188	0	7.1	21
PIZZA								
(Frigo)								
low-fat, shredded	1 oz	65	9	1	150	0	3.0	10
shredded	1 oz	90	6	1	190	0	7.0	20
(Healthy Choice) low-fat, fancy, shredded	1/4 cup	50	8	1	220	1	1.5	5
(Precious) mozzarella cheddar, natural, shredded	1 oz	95	7	1	180	0	7.0	0
(Sargento)								
double cheese, shredded, 'Fancy Supreme'	1/4 cup	90	7	1	150	0	6.0	20
shredded, 'Classic Supreme'	1/4 cup	90	7	0	210	0	6.0	20
PORT DU SALUT	1 oz	100	7	0	151	0	8.0	35
PORT WINE *(Hickory Farms)* natural	1 oz	97	6	2	262	0	6.9	18
POT *(Sargento)*	1 oz	25	5	1	1	0	0.2	0

Food Name	Serv. Size	Total Cal.	Prot. gms	Carbs gms	Sod. mgs	Fiber gms	Fat gms	Chol. mgs
PROVOLONE
....	1 oz	100	7	1	248	0	7.5	20
(Alpine Lace) 'Provo-Lo'	1 oz	70	7	1	85	0	5.0	15
(Dorman's)
....	1 oz	90	7	1	290	0	7.0	0
low-salt	1 oz	80	9	1	140	0	4.0	17
(Frigo)
....	1 oz	100	7	1	230	0	7.0	0
smoked	1 oz	100	7	1	230	0	7.0	0
(Hickory Farms) low-salt, 'Light Choice Low Sodium'	1 oz	90	7	1	140	0	7.0	20
(Kraft)	1 oz	100	7	1	260	0	7.0	25
(Land O'Lakes) natural	1 oz	100	7	1	250	0	8.0	20
(Sargento) sliced	1 slice	100	7	0	190	0	8.0	25
PUB (Hickory Farms)	1 oz	94	6	2	237	0	6.9	18
QUESO ANEJO
Mexican	1 oz	106	6	1	321	0	8.5	30
Mexican, crumbled	1 cup	492	28	6	1493	0	39.6	139
QUESO ASEDERO
Mexican	1 oz	101	6	1	186	0	8.0	30
Mexican, diced	1 cup	470	30	4	865	0	37.3	139
Mexican, shredded	1 cup	402	26	3	740	0	31.9	119
QUESO BLANCO (Sargento)	1 oz	100	7	0	180	0	9.0	27
QUESO CHIHUAHUA
Mexican	1 oz	106	6	2	175	0	8.4	30
Mexican, diced	1 cup	494	28	7	814	0	39.2	139
Mexican, shredded	1 cup	423	24	6	697	0	33.5	119
QUESO DE PAPA (Sargento)	1 oz	110	7	0	180	0	9.0	30
QUESO DE TACO (Hickory Farms)	1 oz	106	6	1	450	0	8.9	27
RICOTTA
part skim	1 cup	340	28	13	307	0	19.5	76
part skim	1 oz	39	3	1	35	0	2.2	9
whole milk	1 cup	428	28	7	207	0	31.9	124
(Breakstone's) whole milk	4 oz	200	12	6	95	0	15.0	55
(Crowley)
part skim	2 oz	80	7	3	50	0	4.0	15
whole milk	2 oz	100	6	3	50	0	7.0	25
(Frigo)
low-fat	1/4 cup	64	9	3	98	0	1.9	11
nonfat	1/4 cup	48	8	2	122	0	0.4	6
nonfat, 'Truly Lite'	1 oz	20	4	2	15	0	0.0	3
part skim	1 oz	45	3	1	100	0	3.0	10
whole milk	1 oz	50	3	1	100	0	4.0	15
(Gardenia) low-fat	1/4 cup	65	8	2	159	0	2.8	14
(Polly-O)
light, 'Lite'	2 oz	80	7	3	65	0	4.0	15
part skim	2 oz	90	7	2	45	0	6.0	20
whole milk	2 oz	100	7	2	45	0	7.0	20
(Precious) low-fat, natural	1 oz	40	3	2	20	0	2.0	10
(Sargento)
....	1 oz	40	3	1	25	0	3.0	13
light	1/4 cup	60	5	3	55	0	2.5	15
old fashioned	1/4 cup	90	7	3	75	0	6.0	25
part skim	1/4 cup	80	7	2	75	0	5.0	20
ROMANO
....	1 oz	110	9	1	340	0	7.6	29
(Frigo)
grated	1 oz	130	12	1	510	0	9.0	0
wedge	1 oz	110	9	1	350	0	8.0	0

Food Name	Serv. Size	Total Cal.	Prot. gms	Carbs gms	Sod. mgs	Fiber gms	Fat gms	Chol. mgs
(Kraft) grated	1 oz	130	11	1	350	0	9.0	30
(Hickory Farms) loaf	1 oz	110	9	1	350	0	8.0	0
(Kraft) 'Natural'	1 oz	100	8	1	250	0	7.0	20
(Polly-O) grated	1 oz	130	11	1	530	0	10.0	30
(Progresso) grated	1 tbsp	23	2	1	70	0	2.0	6
(Sargento)	1 oz	110	9	1	340	0	8.0	29
ROQUEFORT	1 oz	105	6	1	513	0	8.7	26
SMOKED								
(Hickory Farms) 'Light Choice Smoky Lyte'	1 oz	80	7	1	449	0	6.0	5
(Hoffman's) sharp, processed	1 oz	110	6	1	440	0	9.0	0
(Sargento) 'Smokestick'	1 oz	100	7	1	390	0	7.0	24
SOY. See under CHEESE SUBSTITUTE.								
STRING								
(Frigo)	1 oz	80	7	1	190	0	5.0	0
(Kraft) low moisture	1 oz	80	8	1	230	0	5.0	20
(Polly-O)	1 oz slice	90	7	2	200	0	6.0	15
(Sargento)								
	1 oz	80	8	1	150	0	5.0	15
light, 'Mootown Snackers'	1 piece	60	7	1	200	0	3.0	10
smoked	1 oz	80	8	1	150	0	5.0	15
SWISS								
	1 oz	107	8	1	74	0	7.8	26
diced	1 cup	496	38	4	343	0	36.2	121
pasteurized process, w/disodium phosphate added	1 oz	95	7	1	388	0	7.1	24
shredded	1 cup	406	31	4	281	0	29.6	99
(Alpine Lace)								
light, 'Swiss-Lo'	1 oz	100	8	1	35	0	7.0	20
natural, milk, sliced, 'Swiss-Lo'	1 oz	90	8	1	35	0	6.0	20
(Boar's Head)								
'Domestic'	1 oz	110	7	1	75	0	8.0	25
no salt added	1 oz	100	8	1	12	0	8.0	26
(Borden)								
processed	1 oz	100	7	1	380	0	8.0	0
processed, fat-free, low cholesterol	1 oz	40	6	4	0	0	0.0	5
(Casino)	1 oz	110	8	1	35	0	8.0	30
(Dorman's)								
	1 oz	100	8	0	80	0	8.0	0
less fat	1 oz	90	10	0	80	0	5.0	17
low-fat, low-sodium	1 oz	90	10	0	60	0	5.0	17
no salt added	1 oz	100	8	0	8	0	8.0	0
no salt added, 'Deli Light'	1 oz	100	8	0	8	0	8.0	26
smoked	1 oz	100	7	1	390	0	7.0	0
(Healthy Favorites) less fat, natural, sliced	1 oz	80	9	1	70	0	4.0	15
(Hickory Farms)								
creamy, 'Cold Pack'	1 oz	92	6	3	237	0	7.2	24
'Domestic'	1 oz	110	8	1	75	0	7.8	25
light, 'Light Choice Lorraine'	1 oz	100	8	0	35	0	7.8	25
low-salt, 'Light Choice Low Sodium'	1 oz	100	8	0	8	0	8.0	26
(Hoffman's) w/cheddar, smoky	1 oz	110	7	1	410	0	8.0	0
(Kraft)								
	1 oz	110	8	1	40	0	8.0	25
aged	1 oz	110	8	1	45	0	8.0	25
light, 'Light Naturals'	1 oz	90	10	1	45	0	5.0	20
low-salt, '75% Very Low Sodium'	1 oz	110	8	1	10	0	8.0	25
natural, baby, 'Cracker Barrel'	1 oz	110	7	0	65	0	9.0	25
natural, less fat, 'Light Naturals'	1 oz	90	10	1	70	0	5.0	20
processed, 'Deluxe'	1 oz	90	7	1	420	0	7.0	25

Food Name	Serv. Size	Total Cal.	Prot. gms	Carbs gms	Sod. mgs	Fiber gms	Fat gms	Chol. mgs
processed, 'Light'	1 oz	70	6	2	350	0	3.0	15
(Land O'Lakes) natural	1 oz	110	8	1	75	0	8.0	25
(Sargento)								
'Finland'	1 oz	110	8	1	75	0	8.0	26
light, thin sliced, 'Preferred Light'	1 slice	80	9	1	50	0	4.0	15
mild, wafer thin sliced	1 slice	110	8	0	40	0	9.0	25
shredded, 'Fancy Supreme'	1/4 cup	110	8	0	40	0	8.0	30
sliced	1 slice	80	6	0	30	0	6.0	20
(Weight Watchers)								
'Natural'	1 oz	90	9	1	50	0	5.0	15
nonfat	1 slice	30	5	2	281	0	0.0	0
TACO								
(Frigo) shredded	1 oz	110	7	1	200	0	9.0	0
(Kraft) shredded	1 oz	110	7	1	190	0	9.0	30
(Sargento)								
	1 oz	110	7	1	160	0	9.0	27
shredded, 'Classic Supreme'	1/4 cup	110	6	1	220	0	9.0	25
shredded, 'Preferred Light'	1/4 cup	70	8	1	240	0	4.5	15
TALEGGIO (Tal-Fino) natural, 'Brand Imported'	1 oz	89	5	0	176	0	7.4	0
TILSIT								
	1 oz	96	7	1	213	0	7.4	29
(Sargento)	1 oz	100	7	1	210	0	7.0	29
TYBO								
(Dorman's) 45%	1 oz	98	7	0	200	0	7.5	23
(Sargento) red wax	1 oz	100	7	0	200	0	7.0	23
VERMONT (Churny)	1 oz	110	7	1	180	0	9.0	30
CHEESE-BALL								
cheddar, sharp, w/almonds (Kaukauna)	1 oz	100	6	3	250	0	7.0	25
cheddar, w/almonds and bacon (Kaukauna)	1 oz	100	6	3	250	0	7.0	25
green onion flavor, w/almonds (Kaukauna)	1 oz	100	6	3	250	0	7.0	25
Port wine, w/almonds (Kaukauna)	1 oz	100	6	3	250	0	7.0	25
CHEESE DISH/ENTRÉE								
(Snow's) Welsh rarebit, canned	1/2 cup	170	9	10	460	0	11.0	0
(Stouffer's)								
Swiss cheese strata, frozen, food service product	4 oz	176	8	10	376	1	11.2	119
Welsh rarebit	1/4 cup	120	5	5	280	0	9.0	20
CHEESE FLAVORED SEASONING								
(Molly McButter)	1/2 tsp	4	0	1	61	0	0.1	0
CHEESE FLAVORED SNACK								
(Barbara's Bakery)								
cheese flavored puffs, tangy triple cheese, 'Pinta Puffs'	1 oz	70	2	10	100	0	2.0	5
cheese puff bakes (Barbara's Bakery)	1 1/2 cup	160	2	13	190	0	11.0	0
(Bearitos)								
cheddar flavored puffs, light	1 oz	120	2	20	150	na	4.0	0
cheddar flavored puffs, original	1 oz	160	2	14	260	na	10.0	4
(Cheetos)								
cheddar valley	1 oz	160	2	16	240	1	9.0	0
cheese flavored puffs	1 oz	160	2	15	370	1	10.0	0
cheese flavored puffs, balls	1 oz	150	2	15	300	1	10.0	0
cheese flavored puffs, crunchy	1 oz	160	2	15	290	1	10.0	0
cheese flavored puffs, curls	1 oz	150	2	15	290	1	10.0	0
cheese flavored puffs, flamin' hot	1 oz	160	2	15	240	1	10.0	0
cheese flavored puffs, jumbo	1 oz	160	2	13	350	0	10.0	0
light, approx 38 pieces	1 oz	140	2	19	280	1	6.0	0
paws, approx 16 pieces	1 oz	160	1	15	310	1	10.0	0
(Eagle)								
cheese crunch, 'Cheegles'	1 cup	160	2	15	240	0	10.0	0

Food Name	Serv. Size	Total Cal.	Prot. gms	Carbs gms	Sod. mgs	Fiber gms	Fat gms	Chol. mgs
cheese flavored balls, 'Cheegles'	2 1/2 cups	160	2	15	260	0	10.0	0
cheese flavored balls, less fat, 'Cheegles'	2 1/2 cups	150	2	18	200	0	6.0	0
'Shamu Shapes'	1 cup	160	2	15	260	0	10.0	0
(Flavor Tree)								
cheese flavored sticks, cheddar	1/4 cup	129	3	12	335	0	8.1	0
(Health Valley)								
cheese flavored puffs, baked, w/organic corn, 'Cheddar Lite'	0.25 oz	40	1	4	35	0	2.0	0
cheese flavored puffs, nonfat	1 cup	73	2	15	173	1	0.0	0
cheese flavored puffs, w/chili, nonfat	1 oz	100	3	21	75	0	0.0	0
(Keebler)								
zesty cheddar, 'RC Ricers'	1 oz	140	2	17	200	0	8.0	0
(Planters)								
cheese flavored balls, 'Cheez Balls'	1 oz	160	2	14	270	0	11.0	5
cheese flavored balls, nacho, 'Cheez Balls'	1 oz	160	2	15	290	0	10.0	5
cheese flavored curls, 'Cheez Curls'	1 oz	160	2	14	290	0	11.0	5
cheese flavored curls, nacho, 'Cheez Curls'	1 oz	160	2	15	290	0	10.0	5
(Ralston)								
cheddar snacks, 'Stop & Shop'	18 crackers	150	2	20	240	2	7.0	na
(Weight Watchers)								
cheese curls	1 serving	70	1	10	85	0	2.5	0
(Wise)								
cheese flavored puffs, baked, 'Cheez Doodles'	1 oz	150	2	16	360	0	9.0	0
cheese flavored spirals, nacho cheese	1 oz	160	2	16	190	0	10.0	0
'Cheez Waffies'	1 oz	140	3	14	420	0	8.0	0
cheese flavored twists, nacho cheese, crispy	1 oz	160	2	16	190	0	10.0	0
fried, crunchy, 'Cheez Doodles'	1 oz	160	2	16	230	0	10.0	0
CHEESE FOOD. See also CHEESE PRODUCT.								
(Kraft)								
nonfat, processed, singles, 'Free'	1 oz	45	6	4	430	0	0.0	5
pasteurized process, shredded, 'Velveeta'	1/4 cup	130	8	3	500	0	9.0	30
shredded, 'Velveeta'	1 oz	100	6	3	410	0	7.0	20
(Land O'Lakes)								
processed	1 oz	90	5	2	350	0	6.0	20
processed, slices	3/4 oz	70	4	2	260	0	5.0	15
(Nippy)	1 oz	90	5	2	380	0	7.0	20
AMERICAN								
(Borden)								
processed, sharp, 'Singles'	1 oz	90	5	2	470	0	7.0	0
processed, 'Singles'	1 oz	90	5	3	350	0	7.0	0
processed, 'Slices'	1 oz	100	6	2	420	0	7.0	0
(Darigold) processed	1 oz	80	5	2	381	0	6.0	16
(Hoffman's) processed, colored	1 oz	100	5	3	490	0	7.0	0
(Kraft)								
processed, grated	1 oz	130	8	8	740	0	7.0	25
processed, 'Light'	1 oz	70	6	2	420	0	4.0	15
processed, 'Singles'	1 oz	90	5	2	390	0	7.0	25
processed, white, 'Singles'	1 oz	90	5	2	400	0	7.0	20
(Land O'Lakes) processed, w/Swiss cheese	1 oz	100	7	1	400	0	8.0	25
BACON								
(Hoffman's) 'Chees'N Bacon'	1 oz	90	6	3	540	0	6.0	0
(Kraft)								
'Chees'N Bacon'	1 oz	90	6	2	400	0	7.0	25
'Cracker Barrel'	1 oz	90	5	3	280	0	7.0	20
CARAWAY (Hoffman's) 'Swisson Rye'	1 oz	90	6	2	400	0	7.0	0
CHEDDAR								
(Alpine Lace) nonfat	1 oz	45	8	2	280	0	0.0	0

Food Name	Serv. Size	Total Cal.	Prot. gms	Carbs gms	Sod. mgs	Fiber gms	Fat gms	Chol. mgs
(Kaukauna)								
extra sharp, cold pack, 'Cup'	1 oz	100	6	3	250	0	7.0	25
nacho, processed, cold pack 'Cup'	1 oz	100	6	3	250	0	7.0	25
sharp, 'Lite'	1 oz	70	5	5	230	0	4.0	15
sharp, cold pack, 'Cup'	1 oz	100	6	3	250	0	7.0	25
sharp, cup, 'Lite 50'	1 oz	70	5	5	190	0	3.0	15
smoky, 'Lite'	1 oz	70	5	5	230	0	4.0	15
w/bacon and horseradish, cold pack, 'Cup'	1 oz	100	6	3	250	0	7.0	25
(Kraft)								
extra sharp, processed, 'Cracker Barrel'	1 oz	90	5	3	240	0	7.0	20
sharp, processed, 'Cracker Barrel'	1 oz	100	4	4	230	0	7.0	20
sharp, 'Singles'	1 oz	100	6	1	400	0	8.0	25
(Land O'Lakes)								
extra sharp, processed	1 oz	100	6	1	370	0	9.0	30
'La Chedda'	1 oz	90	6	2	335	0	7.0	20
processed, w/bacon	1 oz	110	6	1	350	0	9.0	25
(Wispride) sharp, cold pack	1 oz	100	5	2	210	0	7.0	25
GARLIC *(Kraft)* pasteurized process	1 oz	90	5	2	370	0	7.0	20
ITALIAN HERB *(Land O'Lakes)* processed	1 oz	90	6	2	430	0	7.0	20
JALAPEÑO								
(Hoffman's)	1 oz	90	5	2	580	0	7.0	0
(Kraft)								
pasteurized process	1 oz	90	5	2	370	0	7.0	20
'Singles'	1 oz	90	5	2	450	0	7.0	25
(Land O'Lakes)								
	1 oz	90	6	2	360	0	7.0	20
processed	1 oz	90	6	2	400	0	7.0	20
MEXICAN								
(Kraft)								
hot, pasteurized process, shredded, 'Velveeta'	1/4 cup	130	8	3	540	0	9.0	30
hot, shredded, 'Velveeta'	1 oz	100	6	3	430	0	7.0	25
mild, shredded, 'Velveeta'	1 oz	100	6	3	420	0	7.0	25
ONION								
(Hoffman's) 'Chees'N Onion'	1 oz	100	5	3	490	0	7.0	0
(Land O'Lakes) processed	1 oz	90	6	2	330	0	7.0	15
PEPPERONI *(Land O'Lakes)* processed	1 oz	90	6	1	395	0	7.0	20
PIMIENTO								
(Kraft)								
'Singles'	1 oz	90	5	2	390	0	7.0	25
processed, 'Deluxe'	1 oz	100	6	1	440	0	8.0	25
PORT WINE								
(Kaukauna)								
cold pack, 'Cup'	1 oz	100	6	3	250	0	7.0	25
cup, 'Lite 50'	1 oz	70	5	5	190	0	3.0	15
(Wispride) cold pack	1 oz	100	5	3	210	0	7.0	25
SALAMI								
(Hoffman's) 'Chees'N Salami'	1 oz	90	5	3	560	0	6.0	0
(Land O'Lakes) processed	1 oz	90	6	2	410	0	7.0	20
SMOKY *(Kaukauna)* cold pack 'Cup'	1 oz	100	6	3	250	0	7.0	25
SWISS								
(Borden) processed, slices 'Singles'	1 oz	100	6	2	420	0	7.0	0
(Kaukauna)								
almond, cup, 'Lite 50'	1 oz	70	5	5	180	0	3.0	15
country, cold pack 'Cup'	1 oz	100	6	3	250	0	7.0	25
country, 'Lite'	1 oz	70	6	5	200	0	4.0	15
(Kraft)								
fat-free, singles, 'Free'	1 oz	45	6	4	390	0	0.0	5

Food Name	Serv. Size	Total Cal.	Prot. gms	Carbs gms	Sod. mgs	Fiber gms	Fat gms	Chol. mgs
singles	1 oz	90	6	2	440	0	7.0	25
(Velveeta)	1 oz	100	6	3	410	0	7.0	20
CHEESE-LOG								
CHEDDAR								
(Kraft)								
sharp, w/almonds, 'Cracker Barrel'	1 oz	90	5	4	410	0	6.0	15
smoky, w/almonds, 'Cracker Barrel'	1 oz	90	5	4	410	0	6.0	15
(Kaukauna)								
white, sharp, w/green onion	1 oz	100	6	3	250	0	7.0	25
white, sharp hickory smoke	1 oz	100	6	3	250	0	7.0	25
(Sargento)								
Port wine	1 oz	100	6	3	250	0	7.0	18
sharp	1 oz	100	6	3	250	0	7.0	18
SWISS								
(Kaukauna) w/almonds	1 oz	100	6	3	250	0	7.0	25
(Sargento) w/almonds	1 oz	90	6	2	350	0	7.0	21
CHEESE NUGGET, mozzarella, breaded, frozen,								
'Cheese Hot Bites' (Banquet)	2.63 oz	240	14	16	530	0	13.0	0
CHEESE NUT								
(Kraft)								
cheddar, sharp, 'Cracker Barrel'	1 oz	100	5	4	250	0	7.0	20
Port wine, 'Cracker Barrel'	1 oz	90	5	4	260	0	6.0	15
(Kaukauna) sharp, w/bell and jalapeño peppers	1 oz	100	6	3	250	0	7.0	25
CHEESE PRODUCT								
(Borden) 'Singles' processed, slices, fat-free	1 oz	40	6	4	380	0	0.0	5
(Kraft)								
'Cheez Whiz' light, pasteurized process	2 tbsp	75	6	6	597	0	3.3	12
'Cheez Whiz' pasteurized process	2 tbsp	91	4	3	541	0	6.9	25
'Velveeta' less fat, pasteurized process	1 oz	62	5	3	444	0	3.0	12
(Lite-Line) slices, processed, fat-free	1 slice	25	4	3	250	0	0.0	5
(Lunch Wagon) sandwich slices, processed	1 oz	90	5	2	370	0	7.0	5
AMERICAN FLAVOR								
(Alpine Lace) processed	1 oz	90	6	2	200	0	7.0	20
(Borden) processed, 'Light'	1 oz	70	6	1	420	0	5.0	0
(Harvest Moon) processed	1 oz	70	6	2	420	0	4.0	15
(Kraft)								
pasteurized process	1 slice	31	5	2	273	0	0.2	3
processed, 'Light Singles'	1 oz	70	6	2	420	0	4.0	15
white, processed, 'Light Singles'	1 oz	70	6	2	410	0	4.0	15
(Light n' Lively) white, processed, 'Singles'	1 oz	70	6	2	410	0	4.0	15
(Lite-Line)								
processed	1 oz	50	7	1	410	0	2.0	0
processed, reduced sodium	1 oz	70	6	2	90	0	4.0	0
processed, 'Sodium Lite'	1 oz	70	6	2	200	0	4.0	0
CHEDDAR FLAVOR								
(Kraft)								
sharp, processed, 'Free'	1 oz	45	6	4	390	0	0.0	5
sharp, processed, 'Light'	1 oz	70	6	2	380	0	4.0	15
sharp, processed, 'Singles'	1 oz	100	6	1	400	0	8.0	25
(Light n' Lively) sharp, processed, 'Singles'	1 oz	70	6	2	380	0	4.0	15
(Lite-Line)								
mild, processed	1 oz	50	7	1	380	0	2.0	0
sharp, processed	1 oz	50	7	1	440	0	2.0	0
sharp, processed, slices	1 slice	35	4	1	300	0	2.0	5
(Spreadery)								
medium, processed	1 oz	70	5	3	250	0	4.0	15
sharp, processed	1 oz	70	5	3	240	0	4.0	15
Vermont white, processed	1 oz	70	5	3	230	0	4.0	15

Food Name	Serv. Size	Total Cal.	Prot. gms	Carbs gms	Sod. mgs	Fiber gms	Fat gms	Chol. mgs
CREAM CHEESE FLAVOR								
(Philadelphia Brand) processed, 'Light'	1 oz	60	3	2	160	0	5.0	10
MEXICAN FLAVOR								
(Spreadery) mild, w/jalapeños, processed	1 oz	70	5	3	260	0	4.0	15
MOZZARELLA FLAVOR								
(Alpine Lace) nonfat	1 oz	45	8	2	280	0	0.0	0
(Lite-Line) processed	1 oz	50	7	1	340	0	2.0	0
MUENSTER FLAVOR *(Lite-Line)* processed	1 oz	50	7	1	450	0	2.0	0
NACHO FLAVOR *(Spreadery)* processed	1 oz	70	5	3	240	0	4.0	15
NEUFCHATEL								
(Spreadery)								
French onion, processed	1 oz	70	2	2	135	0	6.0	20
garden vegetable, processed	1 oz	70	2	2	220	0	6.0	20
garlic and herb, processed	1 oz	70	2	1	140	0	6.0	20
ranch, classic, processed	1 oz	70	2	1	190	0	7.0	20
strawberry, processed	1 oz	70	2	1	270	0	5.0	15
PORT WINE FLAVOR *(Spreadery)* processed	1 oz	70	5	3	250	0	4.0	15
SWISS FLAVOR								
(Kraft) processed, slices, 'Free Singles'	1 oz	45	6	4	390	0	0.0	5
(Light n' Lively) processed, 'Singles'	1 oz	70	6	2	350	0	3.0	15
(Lite-Line) processed	1 oz	50	7	1	380	0	2.0	0
CHEESE SPREAD								
(Kraft)								
'Velveeta'	1 oz	80	5	3	430	0	6.0	20
'Velveeta' pasteurized process	1 oz	85	5	3	420	0	6.2	22
'Velveeta' slices	1 oz	90	5	3	400	0	6.0	20
(Land O'Lakes) processed, 'Golden Velvet'	1 oz	80	5	2	380	0	6.0	15
(Laughing Cow) 'Cheezbits'	1/6 oz	13	1	0	55	0	1.0	3
(Micro Melt)	1 oz	80	4	2	380	0	6.0	15
AMERICAN								
(Easy Cheese) pasteurized process	2 tbsp	100	6	2	400	0	7.0	25
(Kraft) processed	1 oz	80	4	2	470	0	6.0	15
(Nabisco) 'Easy Cheese American'	1 oz	80	4	2	350	0	6.0	0
(Sargento)								
sharp, processed, 'Cracker Snacks'	1 oz	110	6	1	410	0	9.0	27
w/pimento, processed, 'Cracker Snacks'	1 oz	110	6	1	410	0	9.0	27
BACON								
(Kraft)	1 oz	80	5	1	560	0	7.0	20
(Squeez-A-Snak)	1 oz	80	5	1	500	0	7.0	20
BLUE *(Roka)*	1 oz	70	3	2	270	0	6.0	20
BRICK 'Cracker Snacks' *(Sargento)*	1 oz	100	6	1	430	0	9.0	25
CHEDDAR								
(Kraft)								
extra sharp, 'Cracker Barrel'	2 tbsp	80	3	1	180	0	8.0	20
sharp, and cream cheese, 'Cracker Barrel'	2 tbsp	80	3	1	180	0	8.0	20
(Nabisco)								
'Easy Cheese Cheddar'	1 oz	80	4	2	370	0	6.0	0
'Easy Cheese Cheddar 'n Bacon'	1 oz	80	4	2	350	0	6.0	0
'Easy Cheese Sharp Cheddar'	1 oz	80	4	2	320	0	6.0	0
(Old English) sharp	1 oz	80	5	1	480	0	7.0	20
(Squeez-A-Snak) sharp	1 oz	80	5	1	440	0	7.0	20
(Weight Watchers) sharp, 'Cup'	1 oz	70	4	7	190	0	3.0	10
GARLIC *(Squeez-A-Snak)*	1 oz	80	5	1	430	0	7.0	20
HICKORY SMOKE *(Squeez-A-Snak)*	1 oz	80	5	1	440	0	7.0	20
JALAPEÑO								
(Kraft)								
	1 oz	70	2	3	95	0	5.0	15

Food Name	Serv. Size	Total Cal.	Prot. gms	Carbs gms	Sod. mgs	Fiber gms	Fat gms	Chol. mgs
loaf	1 oz	80	5	2	470	0	6.0	20
(Squeez-A-Snak)	1 oz	80	5	1	510	0	6.0	20
LIMBURGER (Mohawk Valley)	1 oz	70	4	0	420	0	6.0	20
MEXICAN (Velveeta) mild	1 oz	80	5	3	440	0	6.0	20
NACHO (Nabisco) 'Easy Cheese Nacho'	1 oz	80	4	2	340	0	6.0	0
OLIVE (Kraft) olives and pimiento	1 oz	60	2	2	160	0	5.0	15
PIMIENTO								
(Kraft)	1 oz	70	2	3	120	0	5.0	15
'Velveeta' (Kraft)	1 oz	80	5	3	400	0	6.0	20
PINEAPPLE (Kraft)	1 oz	70	2	4	15	0	5.0	75
PORT WINE 'Cup' (Weight Watchers)	1 oz	70	4	7	190	0	3.0	10
GARLIC								
(Alouette) and spices	1 oz	95	2	2	165	0	9.0	31
(Rondel) w/herbs, soft, 'Lite'	1 oz	70	3	2	170	0	6.0	15
HERB								
(Alouette) and garlic, soft, 'Light'	1 oz	60	3	2	130	0	4.5	15
(Rondel) soft, 'Fines Herbes'	1 oz	90	3	2	170	0	8.0	0
HORSERADISH (Alouette) and chive	1 oz	85	2	1	130	0	8.0	28
LIMBURGER (Mohawk Valley)	1 oz	70	4	0	420	0	6.0	20
MEXICAN								
(Kraft)								
hot, 'Velveeta'	1 oz	80	5	3	520	0	6.0	20
mild, 'Velveeta'	1 oz	80	5	3	440	0	6.0	20
ONION (Alouette) French	1 oz	95	2	2	205	0	9.0	31
PIMENTO								
(Kraft)								
	1 oz	70	2	3	120	0	5.0	15
'Velveeta'	1 oz	80	5	3	400	0	6.0	20
PINEAPPLE (Kraft)	1 oz	70	2	4	75	0	5.0	15
PORT WINE (Weight Watchers) 'Cup'	1 oz	70	4	7	190	0	3.0	10
SALMON (Alouette)	1 oz	70	2	2	140	0	6.0	20
SPINACH (Alouette) creamy	1 oz	90	2	2	125	0	8.0	0
SWISS (Sargento) 'Cracker Snacks'	1 oz	100	7	1	390	0	7.0	24
VEGETABLE								
(Alouette) spring, soft, 'Light'	1 oz	60	3	1	120	0	4.5	15
(Rondel) garden, soft	1 oz	90	3	3	160	0	8.0	0
CHEESE STICK								
CHEDDAR								
(Farm Rich) breaded, frozen	3 oz	300	11	19	740	0	21.0	0
(Flavor Tree) snack	1/4 cup	129	3	12	335	0	8.1	0
(Stilwell) battered, frozen	1 piece	80	4	8	40	1	4.0	10
PEPPER								
(Farm Rich) hot, breaded, frozen	3 oz	260	8	20	700	0	17.0	0
(Stilwell) jalapeño, breaded, frozen	1 piece	70	4	8	220	1	3.0	10
MOZZARELLA								
(Farm Rich) breaded, frozen	3 oz	240	10	19	570	0	13.0	0
(Frigo) string, natural, 'Truly Lite'	0.83 oz	50	8	1	116	0	2.0	7
(Stilwell)								
baby, battered, frozen	3 pieces	80	4	8	350	1	4.0	10
battered, frozen	1 piece	80	4	7	180	1	5.0	10
premium, battered, frozen	1 piece	100	5	9	180	0	5.0	15
PROVOLONE								
(Farm Rich) provolone, breaded, frozen	3 oz	270	10	22	820	0	16.0	0
CHEESE SUBSTITUTE. See also CHEESE FOOD; CHEESE PRODUCT.								
(Cheeztwin)	1 oz	90	5	3	400	0	6.0	0
(Fisher) 'Sandwich-Mate'	1 oz	90	5	3	400	0	6.0	0
(Lite-Line) low-cholesterol	1 oz	90	5	2	430	0	7.0	0
(Nucoa) 'Heart Beat'	1 1/2 slices	50	7	2	280	0	2.0	0

Food Name	Serv. Size	Total Cal.	Prot. gms	Carbs gms	Sod. mgs	Fiber gms	Fat gms	Chol. mgs
AMERICAN STYLE								
(Delicia)								
....	1 oz	80	6	1	300	0	6.0	3
hickory smoked	1 oz	80	6	0	470	0	6.0	1
w/caraway	1 oz	80	6	1	275	0	6.0	3
w/hot pepper	1 oz	80	6	1	300	0	6.0	3
w/salami	1 oz	80	6	1	370	0	6.0	3
(Formagg) lactose-free, singles	3/4 oz	70	5	1	280	0	5.0	0
(Golden Image)	1 oz	90	7	2	360	0	6.0	5
CHEDDAR STYLE								
(Fisher) shredded, 'Ched-O-Mate'	1 oz	90	6	1	330	0	7.0	0
(Formagg) fancy, shredded	1 oz	70	7	1	70	0	5.0	0
(Frigo)	1 oz	90	5	1	280	0	7.0	0
(Golden Image) mild	1 oz	110	7	0	190	0	9.0	5
(Nu Tofu)								
....	1 oz	70	6	1	190	0	4.0	0
low salt	1 oz	70	7	1	75	0	4.0	0
nonfat	1 oz	40	7	2	240	0	0.0	0
(Rella Good)								
California style, 'AlmondRella'	1 oz	50	7	1	170	0	1.4	0
California style, 'Zero-Fat Rella'	1 oz	45	8	3	170	0	0.0	0
mild, 'TofuRella'	1 oz	80	8	1	170	0	5.0	0
mild, slices, 'TofuRella'	0.75-oz slice	60	5	1	280	0	4.0	0
(Sargento)								
....	1 oz	90	7	1	350	0	6.0	2
shredded, 'Fancy Supreme'	1/4 cup	90	5	2	420	0	7.0	0
(Savoldi)	1 oz	90	6	1	400	0	6.0	0
(Soya Kaas)	1 oz	79	6	2	250	0	5.4	0
COLBY STYLE								
(Golden Image)	1 oz	110	7	1	190	0	9.0	5
(Delicia) Longhorn style	1 oz	80	6	1	550	0	6.0	3
(Dorman's) 'LoChol'	1 oz	90	7	1	140	0	6.0	1
CREAM CHEESE STYLE								
(Soya Kaas)	1 oz	90	2	0	60	0	9.4	0
(Tofutti) 'Better Than Cheese'	1 tbsp	40	1	1	68	na	4.0	0
(Weight Watchers)	1 oz	35	3	1	40	0	2.0	0
GARLIC HERB								
(Rella Good)								
'AlmondRella'	1 oz	60	5	3	250	1	3.0	0
'TofuRella'	1 oz	80	5	2	290	0	5.0	0
ITALIAN STYLE								
(Rella Good) 'VeganRella'	1 oz	60	1	7	130	1	3.0	0
(Weight Watchers) Italian topping, grated, nonfat	1 tbsp	20	2	2	60	0	0.0	0
JACK								
(Nu Tofu)								
....	1 oz	70	6	2	210	0	4.0	0
nonfat	1 oz	40	7	2	240	0	0.0	0
(Rella Good) 'TofuRella'	1 oz	80	5	2	290	0	5.0	0
JALAPEÑO								
(Rella Good)								
jack, 'Zero-FatRella'	1 oz	45	8	3	170	0	0.0	0
'TofuRella'	1 oz	80	5	2	290	0	5.0	0
'Zero-FatRella'	1 oz	40	7	3	250	0	0.0	0
(Soya Kaas) 'Jalapeno Mexi Kaas'	1 oz	77	7	0	160	0	5.3	0
MEXICAN *(Rella Good)* 'VeganRella'	1 oz	60	1	7	130	1	3.0	0
MOZZARELLA STYLE								
(Fisher) shredded, 'Pizza-Mate'	1 oz	90	6	1	310	0	7.0	0

Food Name	Serv. Size	Total Cal.	Prot. gms	Carbs gms	Sod. mgs	Fiber gms	Fat gms	Chol. mgs
(Frigo)	1 oz	90	6	1	240	0	7.0	0
(Nu Tofu)								
	1 oz	70	6	2	190	0	4.0	0
low sodium	1 oz	70	6	2	80	0	4.0	0
nonfat	1 oz	40	7	2	220	0	0.0	0
(Rella Good)								
'AlmondRella'	1 oz	60	5	3	250	1	3.0	0
slices	0.75-oz slice	60	5	1	280	0	4.0	0
'TofuRella'	1 oz	80	5	2	290	0	5.0	0
'Zero-Fat Rella'	1 oz	40	7	3	250	0	0.0	0
(Sargento)								
	1 oz	80	7	1	310	0	6.0	2
'Classic Supreme'	1/4 cup	80	6	1	320	0	6.0	0
(Savoldi)	1 oz	80	6	1	360	0	6.0	0
(Soya Kaas)	1 oz	78	7	2	155	0	5.6	0
MUENSTER STYLE 'LoChol' *(Dorman's)*	1 oz	100	7	1	140	0	7.0	1
PARMESAN STYLE *(Soyco)* grated	1 tbsp	23	3	1	120	0	0.8	0
SWISS STYLE								
(Dorman's) 'LoChol'	1 oz	100	7	1	140	0	7.0	1
(Formagg) lactose-free, singles	3/4 oz	70	5	1	280	0	5.0	0
CHEESE TOPPING *(Tone's)* cheddar, w/bacon	1 tsp	10	1	1	81	0	1.0	1
CHERIMOYA. See CUSTARD APPLE.								
CHERRY								
SOUR								
Canned								
red, in extra heavy syrup, w/liquid	1 cup	298	2	76	18	2	0.2	0
red, in heavy syrup, w/liquid	1 cup	233	2	60	18	3	0.3	0
red, in light syrup, w/liquid	1 cup	189	2	49	18	2	0.3	0
red, in water, w/liquid	1 cup	88	2	22	17	3	0.2	0
Fresh								
red, raw	1 cup	52	1	13	3	2	0.3	0
red, raw, pitted	1 cup	78	2	19	5	2	0.5	0
Frozen								
red, unsweetened	18-oz pkg	235	5	56	5	8	2.2	0
red, unsweetened, unthawed	1 cup	71	1	17	2	2	0.7	0
SWEET								
Canned								
pitted, in extra heavy syrup w/liquid	1 cup	266	2	68	8	4	0.4	0
pitted, in heavy syrup, w/liquid	1 cup	210	2	54	8	4	0.4	0
pitted, in juice, w/liquid	1 cup	135	2	35	8	4	0.1	0
pitted, in light syrup, w/liquid	1 cup	169	2	44	8	4	0.4	0
pitted, in water, w/liquid	1 cup	114	2	29	2	4	0.3	0
Fresh								
raw	1 cup	84	1	19	0	3	1.1	0
raw, medium	1 cherry	5	0	1	0	0	0.1	0
raw, pitted	1 cup	104	2	24	0	3	1.4	0
Frozen								
	10-oz pkg	253	3	64	3	6	0.4	0
thawed	1 cup	231	3	58	3	5	0.3	0
CHERRY JUICE. See also BLACK CHERRY JUICE; FRUIT DRINK; FRUIT JUICE DRINK; FRUIT DRINK MIX.								
Canned, bottled, or boxed								
(Dole) blend 'Pure & Light Mountain Cherry'	6 fl oz	87	0	22	8	0	0.1	0
(Juicy Juice)	6 fl oz	90	0	22	5	0	0.0	0
(Knudsen & Sons) tart	8 fl oz	125	1	30	0	0	0.0	0
(Mountain Sun) organic, 'Mountain Cherry'	8 fl oz	109	0	27	0	0	0.0	0
(Santa Cruz Natural) organic, 'Cruz'	8 fl oz	125	1	29	0	0	1.0	0
(Welch's) 'Orchard'	6 fl oz	180	0	45	10	0	0.0	0

Food Name	Serv. Size	Total Cal.	Prot. gms	Carbs gms	Sod. mgs	Fiber gms	Fat gms	Chol. mgs
Frozen								
(Welch's) concentrate, 'Welchade'	2 fl oz	130	0	31	15	0	0.0	0
CHERRY PEPPER. See PEPPER, CHERRY.								
CHERRY, SURINAM. See PITANGA.								
CHERVIL								
dried	1 tbsp	4	0	1	2	0	0.1	0
dried	1 tsp	1	0	0	0	0	0.0	0
dried *(McCormick/Schilling)*	1 tsp	2	0	0	1	0	0.0	0
dried *(Tone's)*	1 tsp	1	0	0	2	0	0.1	0
CHESTNUT, CHINESE								
boiled or steamed	1 oz	43	0.8	9.6	1	>0.3 c	0.2	0
dried	1 oz	103	1.9	22.6	1	>0.8 c	0.5	0
raw	1 oz	64	1.2	13.9	1	>0.5 c	0.3	0
raw, in shell	1 lb	852	16.0	187.0	13	>6.2 c	4.2	0
roasted	1 oz	68	1.3	14.9	1	>0.5 c	0.3	0
CHESTNUT, EUROPEAN/Italian chestnut/sweet chestnut								
boiled or steamed, shelled	1 oz	37	0.8	7.9	8	>.2 c	0.4	0
dried, in shell	1 lb	1357	23.2	280.5	135	>19.8 c	16.1	0
dried, shelled, peeled	1 oz	105	1.4	22.3	11	>1.4 c	1.1	0
dried, shelled, unpeeled	1 oz	106	1.8	22.0	11	3.3	1.3	0
raw, in shell	1 lb	714	8.1	152.8	9	33.3	7.6	0
raw, shelled, peeled	1 oz	56	0.5	12.5	1	>.3 c	0.4	0
raw, shelled, unpeeled	1 cup	309	3.5	66.0	4	11.7	3.3	0
raw, shelled, unpeeled	1 oz	60	0.7	12.9	1	2.3	0.6	0
roasted, in shell	1 lb	700	9.1	151.3	6	33.4	6.3	0
roasted, in shell	1 cup	350	4.5	75.7	3	18.4	3.2	0
roasted, in shell	1 oz	70	0.9	15.0	1	3.7	0.6	0
roasted, shelled	1 oz	70	0.9	15.0	1	3.3	0.6	0
roasted, shelled, approx 17 nuts	1 cup	350	4.3	75.7	3	16.7	3.2	0
CHESTNUT, ITALIAN. See CHESTNUT, EUROPEAN.								
CHESTNUT, JAPANESE								
boiled or steamed	1 oz	16	0.2	3.6	1	>.1 c	0.1	0
dried, in shell	1 lb	1078	15.7	243.7	101	>6.8 c	3.7	0
dried, shelled	1 oz	102	1.5	23.1	10	>.6 c	0.4	0
dried, shelled	1 cup	558	8.1	126.2	53	>3.5 c	1.9	0
raw, in shell	1 lb	462	6.7	104.5	43	>2.9 c	1.6	0
raw, shelled	1 oz	44	0.6	9.9	4	>.3 c	0.2	0
roasted	1 oz	57	0.8	12.8	5	>.3 c	0.2	0
CHESTNUT, SWEET. See CHESTNUT, EUROPEAN.								
CHESTNUT FLOUR. See under FLOUR.								
CHEWING GUM. See under CANDY, GUM.								
CHIA SEEDS, dried	1 oz	134	4.7	13.6	11	>7.2 c	7.4	0
CHICKEN								
AVERAGE OF ALL PARTS								
Fresh								
capon, meat and skin, raw	1 lb	1056	84.8	0.0	208	0	76.8	336
capon, meat and skin, raw	1 oz	66	5.3	0.0	13	0	4.8	21
capon, meat and skin, roasted	4 oz	260	32.8	0.0	56	0	13.2	98
roaster, meat and skin, raw	1 lb	976	78.4	0.0	304	0	72.0	336
roaster, meat and skin, raw	1 oz	61	4.9	0.0	19	0	4.5	21
roaster, meat and skin, roasted	4 oz	253	27.2	0.0	83	0	15.2	86
stewing, meat and skin, raw	1 oz	73	5.0	0.0	20	0	5.8	20
stewing, meat and skin, stewed	4 oz	323	30.5	0.0	83	0	21.4	90
BACK								
Fresh								
broiler/fryer, meat and skin, flour-coated, fried	4 oz	375	31.5	7.4	102	>.1 c	23.5	101
broiler/fryer, meat and skin, raw	1 oz	90	4.0	0.0	18	0	8.1	22

Food Name	Serv. Size	Total Cal.	Prot. gms	Carbs gms	Sod. mgs	Fiber gms	Fat gms	Chol. mgs
broiler/fryer, meat and skin, roasted	4 oz	340	29.4	0.0	99	0	23.8	100
broiler/fryer, meat and skin, stewed	4 oz	293	25.2	0.0	73	0	20.6	88
broiler/fryer, meat only, raw	1 lb	624	88.0	0.0	400	0	28.8	400
broiler/fryer, meat only, raw	1 oz	39	5.5	0.0	23	0	1.7	23
broiler/fryer, meat only, roasted	4 oz	271	32.0	0.0	109	0	14.9	102
broiler/fryer, meat only, stewed	4 oz	237	28.7	0.0	76	0	12.7	96
BREAST								
Canned								
chunk *(Hormel)*	6.75 oz	350	41	0	855	0	20.0	0
Fresh								
broiler/fryer, meat and skin, batter-dipped, fried	4 oz	295	28.2	10.2	312	0.4	15.0	96
broiler/fryer, meat and skin, flour-coated, fried	4 oz	252	36.1	1.9	86	>.1 c	10.1	101
broiler/fryer, meat and skin, raw	1 lb	784	94.4	0.0	288	0	41.6	288
broiler/fryer, meat and skin, raw	1 oz	49	5.9	0.0	18	0	2.6	18
broiler/fryer, meat and skin, roasted	4 oz	223	33.8	0.0	81	0	8.8	95
broiler/fryer, meat and skin, stewed	4 oz	209	31.1	0.0	70	0	8.4	85
broiler/fryer, meat only, raw	1 lb	496	104.0	0.0	288	0	6.4	256
broiler/fryer, meat only, raw	1 oz	31	6.5	0.0	18	0	0.4	16
broiler/fryer, meat only, roasted	4 oz	187	35.2	0.0	84	0	4.0	96
broiler/fryer, meat only, stewed	4 oz	171	32.9	0.0	71	0	3.4	87
Frozen or refrigerated								
Breast								
baked, 'Classic' *(Carving Board)*	1 slice	40	9	1	530	0	0.5	25
boneless, barbecue marinated, frozen *(Tyson)*	3.75 oz	120	22	5	400	0	3.0	0
boneless, butter garlic marinated *(Tyson)*	3.75 oz	160	21	3	320	0	7.0	0
boneless, Italian marinated, frozen *(Tyson)*	3.75 oz	130	22	6	320	0	2.0	0
boneless, teriyaki marinated, frozen *(Tyson)*	3.75 oz	130	22	6	290	0	2.0	0
broiler/fryer, baked *(Tyson)*	3 oz	116	24	0	63	0	1.5	72
fillet, barbecue, boneless, frozen *(Tyson)*	3 oz	110	14	6	310	0	3.0	35
fillet, boneless, grilled *(Tyson)*	2.75 oz	100	15	4	410	0	3.0	45
fillet, boneless, skinless, raw *(Delightful Farms)*	1 med breast	140	29	0	85	0	1.5	75
fillet, lemon-pepper breast, boneless, frozen *(Tyson)*	2.75 oz	100	14	4	380	0	3.0	40
grilled *(Carving Board)*	1 slice	40	9	1	530	0	0.5	25
half, roasted, w/skin *(Tyson)*	1 med piece	250	34	1	670	0	13.0	110
hickory smoked, nonfat *(Tyson)*	1 slice	35	7	1	450	0	0.0	0
honey flavor, nonfat *(Tyson)*	1 slice	35	7	2	450	0	0.0	0
mesquite flavor, roasted, nonfat *(Tyson)*	1 slice	35	7	1	440	0	0.0	0
peppered, roasted, nonfat *(Tyson)*	1 slice	35	7	1	480	0	0.0	0
roasted, nonfat *(Tyson)*	1 slice	35	7	1	460	0	0.0	0
split, skinless, raw *(Hudson)*	1 med breast	140	29	0	85	0	1.5	75
split, w/skin, raw *(Hudson)*	1 med breast	270	33	0	100	0	14.0	100
w/rib meat, boneless, skinless, raw *(Hudson)*	1 med breast	140	29	0	85	0	1.5	75
CHUNK								
Canned								
(Featherweight)	3 oz	90	16	0	60	0	3.0	65
(Swanson)	1 cup	360	64	8	800	0	12.0	140
DARK MEAT								
Canned, chunk *(Hormel)*	6.75 oz	327	42	0	933	0	18.0	0
Fresh								
broiler/fryer, meat and skin, batter-dipped, fried	4 oz	338	24.8	10.6	335	>.1 c	21.1	101
broiler/fryer, meat and skin, flour-coated, fried	4 oz	323	30.9	4.6	101	>.1 c	19.2	104
broiler/fryer, meat and skin, raw	1 oz	67	4.7	0.0	21	0	5.2	23
broiler/fryer, meat and skin, roasted	4 oz	287	29.4	0.0	99	0	17.9	103
broiler/fryer, meat and skin, stewed	4 oz	264	26.6	0.0	79	0	16.6	93
broiler/fryer, meat only, fried, chopped or diced	1 cup	335	40.6	3.6	136	0	16.3	134
broiler/fryer, meat only, raw	1 oz	35	6.0	0.0	24	0	1.2	23
broiler/fryer, meat only, roasted	1 cup	287	38.3	0.0	130	0	13.6	130

Food Name	Serv. Size	Total Cal.	Prot. gms	Carbs gms	Sod. mgs	Fiber gms	Fat gms	Chol. mgs
broiler/fryer, meat only, roasted	4 oz	232	31.0	0.0	105	0	11.0	105
broiler/fryer, meat only, roasted, chopped or diced	1 cup	286	38.3	0.0	130	0	13.6	130
broiler/fryer, meat only, stewed	1 cup	269	36.4	0.0	104	0	12.6	123
broiler/fryer, meat only, stewed	4 oz	218	29.4	0.0	84	0	10.2	100
broiler/fryer, meat only, stewed, chopped or diced	1 cup	269	36.4	0.0	104	0	12.6	123
roaster, meat only, raw	1 oz	32	5.3	0.0	27	0	1.0	20
roaster, meat only, roasted	4 oz	202	26.4	0.0	108	0	9.9	85
stewing, meat only, raw	1 oz	45	5.6	0.0	29	0	2.3	22
stewing, meat only, stewed	1 cup	361	39.4	0.0	133	0	21.4	133
stewing, meat only, stewed	4 oz	293	31.9	0.0	108	0	17.3	108
DRUMSTICK								
Fresh								
broiler/fryer, meat and skin, batter-dipped, fried	4 oz	304	24.9	9.4	305	>.1 c	17.9	98
broiler/fryer, meat and skin, flour-coated, fried	4 oz	278	30.6	1.8	101	>.1 c	15.6	102
broiler/fryer, meat and skin, raw	1 lb	736	88.0	0.0	384	0	40.0	368
broiler/fryer, meat and skin, raw	1 oz	46	5.5	0.0	24	0	2.5	23
broiler/fryer, meat and skin, roasted	4 oz	245	30.7	0.0	102	0	12.6	103
broiler/fryer, meat and skin, stewed	4 oz	231	28.7	0.0	86	0	12.1	94
broiler/fryer, meat only, raw	1 lb	544	92,8	0.0	400	0	16.0	352
broiler/fryer, meat only, raw	1 oz	34	5.8	0.0	25	0	1.0	22
broiler/fryer, meat only, roasted	4 oz	195	32.1	0.0	108	0	6.4	105
broiler/fryer, meat only, stewed	4 oz	192	31.2	0.0	91	0	6.5	100
DRUMSTICK AND WING								
Frozen								
drumette and wing portions, raw *(Delightful Farms)*	4 sections	150	13	0	310	0	10.0	70
GIBLETS								
Fresh								
all classes, fried	1 cup	402	47.2	6.3	164	0	19.5	647
all classes, simmered	1 cup	228	37.5	1.4	84	0	6.9	570
broiler/fryer, fried, chopped or diced	1 cup	402	47	6	164	0	19.5	647
broiler/fryer, raw	2.6 oz	93	13	1	58	0	3.4	197
broiler/fryer, simmered, chopped or diced	1 cup	228	37	1	84	0	6.9	570
capon, raw	1 lb	592	83.2	6.4	352	0	24.0	1328
capon, raw	1 oz	37	5.2	0.4	22	0	1.5	83
capon, simmered	1 cup	238	38.3	1.1	80	0	7.8	629
capon, simmered	4 oz	186	29.9	0.9	62	0	6.1	492
roaster, simmered	1 cup	239	38.8	1.3	87	0	7.6	518
stewing, raw	1 lb	560	81.6	8.0	352	0	20.8	1184
stewing, raw	1 oz	35	5.1	0.5	22	0	1.3	74
stewing, simmered	1 cup	281	37.3	0.2	81	0	13.5	515
GIZZARD								
Fresh								
all classes, simmered	1 cup	222	39.4	1.6	97	0	5.3	281
broiler-fryer, raw, approx 1.3 oz	1 medium	44	6.7	0.2	28	0	1.6	48
broiler-fryer, simmered, approx .8 oz	1 medium	34	6.0	0.3	15	0	0.8	43
roaster, raw	1 medium	44	7	0	28	0	1.6	48
roaster, simmered	1 medium	11	2	0	5	0	0.3	14
roaster, simmered, chopped or diced	1 cup	222	39	2	97	0	5.3	281
HEART								
Fresh								
all classes, simmered	1 cup	268	38.3	0.2	70	0	11.5	351
broiler-fryer, raw, 1 heart	2 oz	9	1.0	<.1	5	0	0.6	8
broiler-fryer, simmered	4 oz	210	29.9	0.1	54	0	9.0	275
roaster, raw	1 medium	9	1	0	5	0	0.6	8
roaster, simmered, chopped or diced	1 cup	268	38	0	70	0	11.5	351
LEG								
Fresh								
broiler/fryer, meat and skin, batter-dipped, fried	4 oz	310	24.7	9.9	316	>.1 c	18.3	102

Food Name	Serv. Size	Total Cal.	Prot. gms	Carbs gms	Sod. mgs	Fiber gms	Fat gms	Chol. mgs
broiler/fryer, meat and skin, flour-coated, fried .... 4 oz		285	30.1	2.8	99	>.1 c	16.2	105
broiler/fryer, meat and skin, raw .... 1 lb		848	81.6	0.0	352	0	54.4	384
broiler/fryer, meat and skin, raw .... 1 oz		53	5.1	0.0	22	0	3.4	24
broiler/fryer, stewed .... 4 oz		249	27.4	0.0	83	0	14.7	95
broiler/fryer, meat only, raw .... 1 lb		544	91.2	0.0	384	0	17.6	368
broiler/fryer, meat only, raw .... 1 oz		34	5.7	0.0	24	0	1.1	23
broiler/fryer, meat only, roasted .... 4 oz		217	30.7	0.0	103	0	9.6	107
broiler/fryer, meat only, stewed .... 4 oz		210	29.8	0.0	88	0	9.1	101
Frozen or refrigerated								
broiler/fryer, baked (Tyson) .... 3 oz		131	23	0	81	0	3.8	79
raw (Delightful Farms) .... 1 med drumstick		200	24	0	105	0	11.0	100
w/skin (Hudson) .... 2 med drumsticks		230	27	0	115	0	12.0	115
LIGHT MEAT								
Fresh								
broiler/fryer, meat and skin, batter-dipped, fried .... 4 oz		312	26.6	10.7	324	>.1 c	17.4	94
broiler/fryer, meat and skin, flour-coated, fried .... 4 oz		279	34.5	2.1	87	>.1 c	13.7	99
broiler/fryer, meat and skin, raw .... 1 oz		53	5.7	0.0	18	0	3.1	19
broiler/fryer, meat and skin, roasted .... 4 oz		252	32.9	0.0	85	0	12.3	95
broiler/fryer, meat and skin, stewed .... 4 oz		228	29.6	0.0	71	0	11.3	84
broiler/fryer, meat only, fried .... 8 oz		269	46.0	0.6	113	0	7.8	126
broiler/fryer, meat only, raw .... 1 oz		32	6.6	0.0	19	0	0.5	16
broiler/fryer, meat only, roasted .... 1 cup		242	43.3	0.0	108	0	6.3	119
broiler/fryer, meat only, roasted .... 4 oz		196	35.1	0.0	87	0	5.1	96
broiler/fryer, meat only, roasted, chopped or diced .... 1 cup		242	43.3	0.0	108	0	6.3	118
broiler/fryer, meat only, stewed, chopped or diced .... 1 cup		223	40.4	0.0	91	0	5.6	107
broiler/fryer, meat only, stewed .... 4 oz		180	32.7	0.0	74	0	4.5	87
roaster, meat only, raw .... 1 oz		31	6.3	0.0	14	0	0.5	16
roaster, meat only, roasted .... 4 oz		174	30.8	0.0	58	0	4.6	85
roaster, meat only, roasted, chopped or diced .... 1 cup		214	38.0	0.0	71	0	5.7	105
stewing, meat only, raw .... 1 oz		39	6.5	0.0	15	0	1.2	13
stewing, meat only, stewed .... 1 cup		298	46.3	0.0	81	0	11.2	98
stewing, meat only, stewed .... 4 oz		242	37.5	0.0	66	0	9.0	79
LIVER								
Fresh								
all classes, simmered .... 1 cup		220	34.1	1.2	71	0	7.6	883
broiler-fryer, chopped, simmered .... 1 cup		219	34.1	1.2	71	0	7.6	883
broiler-fryer, raw, approx 1.1 oz .... 1 liver		40	5.8	1.1	25	0	1.2	140
broiler-fryer, simmered .... 4 oz		178	27.6	1.0	58	0	6.2	716
NECK								
Fresh								
broiler/fryer, meat and skin, batter-dipped, fried .... 4 oz		374	22.5	9.9	313	>.1 c	26.7	103
broiler/fryer, meat and skin, flour-coated, fried .... 4 oz		376	27.2	4.8	93	>.1 c	26.8	107
broiler/fryer, meat and skin, raw .... 1 lb		1344	64.0	0.0	288	0	118.4	448
broiler/fryer, meat and skin, raw .... 1 oz		84	4.0	0.0	18	0	7.4	28
broiler/fryer, meat and skin, simmered .... 4 oz		280	22.2	0.0	59	0	20.5	79
broiler/fryer, meat only, raw .... 1 lb		704	80.0	0.0	368	0	40.0	384
broiler/fryer, meat only, raw .... 1 oz		44	5.0	0.0	23	0	2.5	24
broiler/fryer, meat only, simmered .... 4 oz		203	27.9	0.0	73	0	9.3	90
SKIN								
Fresh								
broiler/fryer, batter-dipped, fried .... 1 oz		112	2.9	6.6	165	>.1 c	8.2	21
broiler/fryer, roasted .... 1 oz		129	5.8	0.0	18	0	11.5	24
broiler/fryer, stewed .... 1 oz		103	4.3	0.0	16	0	9.4	18
THIGH								
Fresh								
broiler/fryer, meat and skin, batter-dipped, fried .... 4 oz		314	24.5	10.3	327	>.1 c	18.7	105
broiler/fryer, meat and skin, flour-coated, fried .... 4 oz		297	30.3	3.6	100	>.1 c	17.0	110

Food Name	Serv. Size	Total Cal.	Prot. gms	Carbs gms	Sod. mgs	Fiber gms	Fat gms	Chol. mgs
broiler/fryer, meat and skin, raw	1 lb	960	78.4	0.0	352	0	68.8	384
broiler/fryer, meat and skin, raw	1 oz	60	4.9	0.0	22	0	4.3	24
broiler/fryer, meat and skin, roasted	4 oz	280	28.4	0.0	95	0	17.6	105
broiler/fryer, meat and skin, stewed	4 oz	263	26.4	0.0	81	0	16.7	95
broiler/fryer, meat only, raw	1 lb	544	89.6	0.0	384	0	17.6	384
broiler/fryer, meat only, raw	1 oz	34	5.6	0.0	24	0	1.1	24
broiler/fryer, meat only, roasted	4 oz	237	29.4	0.0	100	0	12.3	108
broiler/fryer, meat only, stewed	4 oz	221	28.4	0.0	85	0	11.1	102
Frozen or refrigerated								
boneless, skinless, raw (Hudson)	1 med thigh	100	16	0	70	0	3.0	70
broiler/fryer, baked (Tyson)	3 oz	152	21	0	75	0	6.7	81
roasted, w/skin (Tyson)	1 med piece	270	22	1	490	0	19.0	140
w/skin, raw (Hudson)	1 med thigh	230	19	0	85	0	17.0	90
THIGH AND DRUMSTICK								
Frozen, 'Plump and Juicy' (Swanson)	3.25 oz	290	15	17	610	0	18.0	0
WHITE AND DARK MEAT								
Canned								
(Swanson)	2.5 oz	100	16	0	240	0	4.0	40
chunk (Hormel)	6.75 oz	340	39	0	857	0	20.0	0
chunk, unsalted (Hormel)	6.75 oz	330	42	0	75	0	18.0	0
cooked, in water, 96% fat-free (Valley Fresh)	2 oz	80	15	0	130	0	2.0	50
puréed (Bryan Foods)	1/3 cup	120	12	0	45	0	7.0	45
WHITE MEAT								
Canned								
(Swanson)	2.5 oz	100	15	0	235	0	4.0	35
chunk, cooked, in water, 98% fat-free (Valley Fresh)	2 oz	70	15	0	130	0	1.0	25
chunk, premium (Swanson)	3 oz	80	16	1	340	1	1.0	40
WHOLE								
Frozen or refrigerated								
barbecue (Empire Kosher)	5 oz	280	31	1	460	0	17.0	110
broiler/fryer, baked (Tyson)	3 oz	134	23	0	73	0	4.1	76
roasted, w/skin (Tyson)	3 oz	180	19	1	300	0	12.0	100
WING								
Fresh								
broiler/fryer, meat and skin, batter-dipped, fried	4 oz	367	22.5	12.4	363	>.1 c	24.7	90
broiler/fryer, meat and skin, flour-coated, fried	4 oz	364	29.6	2.7	87	>.1 c	25.1	92
broiler/fryer, meat and skin, raw	1 lb	1008	83.2	0.0	336	0	72.0	352
broiler/fryer, meat and skin, raw	1 oz	63	5.2	0.0	21	0	4.5	22
broiler/fryer, meat and skin, roasted	4 oz	329	30.5	0.0	93	0	22.1	95
broiler/fryer, meat and skin, stewed	4 oz	282	25.8	0.0	76	0	19.1	79
broiler/fryer, meat only, raw	1 lb	576	99.2	0.0	368	0	16.0	256
broiler/fryer, meat only, raw	1 oz	36	6.2	0.0	23	0	1.0	16
broiler/fryer, meat only, roasted	4 oz	230	34.5	0.0	104	0	9.2	96
broiler/fryer, meat only, stewed	4 oz	205	30.8	0.0	83	0	8.1	84
Frozen or refrigerated								
w/skin (Hudson)	3 med wings	280	23	0	90	0	20.0	95
broiler/fryer, baked (Tyson)	3 oz	147	23	0	78	0	5.6	72

CHICKEN DINNER/ENTRÉE. See also BURRITO; CHICKEN, CANNED; CHICKEN DINNER/ENTRÉE MIX; CHILI; CHIMICHANGA; ENCHILADA; FAJITA; LUNCH COMBINATION, PACKAGED; RAVIOLI DISH/ENTRÉE; SANDWICH; TORTELLINI DISH/ENTRÉE.

(Armour)

Food Name	Serv. Size	Total Cal.	Prot. gms	Carbs gms	Sod. mgs	Fiber gms	Fat gms	Chol. mgs
à la king, frozen, 'Classics Lite'	11.25 oz	290	19	38	630	0	7.0	55
Burgundy, frozen, 'Classics Lite'	10 oz	210	23	25	780	0	2.0	45
glazed, frozen, 'Classics'	10.75 oz	300	15	24	960	0	16.0	60
Marsala, frozen, 'Classics Lite'	10.5 oz	250	20	27	930	0	7.0	80
mesquite, frozen, 'Classics'	9.5 oz	370	15	42	660	0	16.0	55
Oriental, 'Classics Lite'	10 oz	180	18	24	660	0	1.0	35
parmigiana, frozen, 'Classics'	11.5 oz	370	22	27	1060	0	19.0	75

Food Name	Serv. Size	Total Cal.	Prot. gms	Carbs gms	Sod. mgs	Fiber gms	Fat gms	Chol. mgs
sweet and sour, frozen, 'Classics Lite'	11 oz	240	18	39	820	0	2.0	35
w/noodles, frozen, 'Classics'	11 oz	230	19	23	660	0	7.0	50
w/wine and mushroom sauce, frozen, 'Classics'	10.75 oz	280	22	24	900	0	11.0	50
(Banquet)								
à la king, frozen, 'Cookin' Bags'	4 oz	110	8	9	0	0	5.0	0
and dumplings, w/gravy	1 entrée	270	13	35	780	3	9.0	40
breast patty, fried, w/biscuit, frozen, 'Southern'	4 oz	320	12	37	980	0	14.0	0
chow mein, w/egg roll	1 entrée	210	9	28	850	3	7.0	30
drumsticks, frozen, 'Drumsnackers' 'Platters'	7 oz	430	20	49	690	0	19.0	0
fingers, barbecue	1 entrée	340	13	36	800	3	16.0	60
fried, 'Original'	1 entrée	470	21	35	1500	2	27.0	90
fried, white meat	1 entrée	480	18	40	1100	3	28.0	100
fried, white meat, frozen, 'Extra Helping'	16 oz	570	20	70	1470	0	28.0	0
fried, white meat, hot 'n spicy, frozen, 'Platter'	9 oz	430	38	21	0	0	22.0	105
fried, w/mashed potatoes and corn, seasoned sauce	1 entrée	470	21	35	1500	2	27.0	89
grilled	1 entrée	330	16	37	1210	3	13.0	50
hot'n spicy, frozen, 'Snack'n'	3.75 oz	140	6	8	480	0	9.0	0
nugget meal, frozen	1 meal	410	18	38	650	4	21.0	45
nuggets, fried	1 entrée	430	14	42	650	4	23.0	50
nuggets, hot'n spicy, w/barbecue sauce	4.5 oz	360	20	23	820	0	21.0	0
nuggets, sweet and sour, 'Extra Helping'	10 oz	650	28	64	0	0	34.0	0
nuggets, sweet and sour, w/sauce, 'Microwave'	4.5 oz	360	20	22	770	0	21.0	0
nuggets, w/BBQ sauce, 'Extra Helping'	10 oz	640	29	56	1390	0	36.0	0
nuggets, w/BBQ sauce, frozen, 'Southern'	4.5 oz	370	19	20	930	0	23.0	0
Oriental, w/egg rolls	1 entrée	260	10	36	790	3	9.0	40
parmigiana	1 entrée	320	10	29	900	3	18.0	50
patty, frozen, 'Platters'	7.5 oz	380	15	34	760	0	21.0	0
pie, frozen	7 oz	550	15	39	860	0	36.0	35
pie, frozen, 'Supreme Microwave'	7 oz	430	15	30	740	0	28.0	40
pot pie, frozen	1 serving	382	10	36	948	1	22.0	40
primavera, w/vegetable, frozen, 'Cookin' Bags'	4 oz	100	6	14	0	0	2.0	0
primavera, w/vegetable, frozen, 'Family Entrées'	7 oz	140	9	18	0	0	3.0	0
Southern fried	1 entrée	560	26	40	1540	3	33.0	100
sweet and sour, frozen, 'Cookin' Bags'	4 oz	130	5	22	0	0	2.0	0
w/dumplings, frozen	10 oz	430	17	34	940	0	24.0	45
(Barber Foods)								
cordon bleu, w/cheese and ham, frozen	1 pkg	697	52	30	1527	na	41.5	163
cordon bleu, w/cheese and ham, frozen	1 serving	344	26	15	754	na	20.5	81
w/broccoli and cheese stuffing, frozen	1 pkg	527	42	12	1054	na	34.7	126
w/broccoli and cheese stuffing, frozen	1 serving	260	21	6	521	na	17.1	62
(Budget Gourmet)								
and egg noodles, w/broccoli, frozen	10 oz	450	23	31	1110	0	26.0	130
au gratin, 'Light'	1 entrée	250	18	26	820	3	8.0	45
breast, herbed, frozen, 'Special Selections'	1 entrée	300	25	34	620	5	8.0	65
breast, honey mustard	1 entrée	310	19	45	620	3	6.0	35
breast, honey mustard, 'Light & Healthy'	1 dinner	310	20	46	540	6	6.0	50
breast, orange glazed	1 entrée	280	11	51	790	2	3.0	30
breast, orange glazed, 'Light'	1 entrée	300	15	56	920	1	2.0	30
cacciatore, frozen	11 oz	300	20	27	810	0	13.0	60
French, light, w/vegetables, potato, sauce	1 serving	179	23	9	864	6	5.6	26
French recipe, 'Light'	1 entrée	200	13	19	950	4	8.0	30
frozen, w/egg noodles, frozen	1 entrée	410	21	30	930	3	23.0	110
herbed, w/fettuccini	1 entrée	260	19	29	640	4	8.0	80
Italian style, frozen, 'Special Selections'	1 entrée	280	10	44	660	3	7.0	25
Mandarin, w/vegetables, frozen, 'Special Selections'	1 entrée	250	16	37	850	4	5.0	45
Marsala, frozen	10 oz	250	15	37	660	0	5.0	65
Mexican, frozen	12.8 oz	510	23	70	1210	0	15.0	40

Food Name	Serv. Size	Total Cal.	Prot. gms	Carbs gms	Sod. mgs	Fiber gms	Fat gms	Chol. mgs
Oriental, w/vegetables	1 entrée	290	11	43	730	3	8.0	25
Oriental, w/vegetables, 'Light & Healthy'	9 oz	280	19	44	690	0	6.0	20
Oriental, w/vegetables and rice, frozen, 'Special Selections'	1 entrée	290	11	42	720	4	9.0	15
roasted, frozen	11.2 oz	280	19	34	1110	0	7.0	40
roasted, w/herb gravy	1 entrée	260	14	34	610	4	8.0	45
sweet and sour, w/rice	10 oz	350	18	53	640	0	7.0	40
Szechuan, spicy, w/vegetable, frozen, 'Special Selections'	1 entrée	300	14	41	710	5	9.0	10
teriyaki, frozen	12 oz	360	20	44	610	0	12.0	55
teriyaki, w/Oriental style vegetables, frozen, 'Light and Healthy'	1 entrée	317	19	52	675	4	3.7	25
w/fettuccini	1 entrée	380	20	33	810	3	19.0	85
w/rigatoni, broccoli 'Special Selections'	1 entrée	310	17	46	670	5	6.0	15
white meat, w/Chinese style vegetables, rice	1 entrée	250	8	39	640	3	7.0	15
white meat, w/Italian style vegetables, rice	1 entrée	250	8	39	540	2	7.0	25
(Celentano)								
breaded, w/pasta marinara w/cheese	10 oz tray	390	19	36	1040	8	19.0	50
parmigiana, frozen	9 oz	330	32	15	560	0	20.0	0
primavera, frozen	11.5 oz	270	25	18	580	0	10.0	0
(Chicken By George)								
Cajun, boneless, skinless	1 med breast	120	20	2	650	0	4.0	55
Cajun, packaged	5 oz	180	25	4	890	0	8.0	80
Caribbean grill, packaged	5 oz	200	25	10	610	0	6.0	80
Italian bleu cheese, packaged	5 oz	180	26	2	890	0	8.0	85
lemon herb, boneless, skinless, raw	1 med breast	120	19	3	800	0	3.0	50
lemon herb, packaged	5 oz	170	24	6	870	0	6.0	70
lemon oregano, packaged	5 oz	160	26	4	580	0	4.0	75
mesquite barbecue, packaged	5 oz	170	25	6	790	0	6.0	70
mustard dill, packaged	5 oz	180	26	3	640	0	7.0	80
roasted, packaged	5 oz	150	26	2	710	0	4.0	70
teriyaki, breast, boneless, skinless, raw	1 med breast	130	20	6	650	0	3.0	50
tomato herb, w/basil, packaged,	5 oz	190	25	7	800	0	7.0	80
(Chun King)								
chow mein, frozen	13 oz	370	25	53	1560	0	6.0	0
imperial, frozen	13 oz	300	17	54	1540	0	1.0	0
sweet and sour, w/vegetables, fruit, and sauce, canned	1 pkg	802	28	154	2739	na	8.6	111
sweet and sour, w/vegetables, fruit, and sauce, canned	1 serving	165	6	32	564	na	1.8	23
walnut, crunchy, frozen	13 oz	310	16	49	1700	0	5.0	0
(Contadina) parmigiana, frozen, food service product	1 oz	43	2	3	130	0	2.3	7
(Country Pride) primavera, sticks, frozen	3 oz	240	10	16	400	0	15.0	0
(Dining Lite)								
à la king, frozen	9 oz	240	14	30	780	0	7.0	40
and noodles, frozen	9 oz	240	17	28	570	0	7.0	50
chow mein, frozen	9 oz	180	10	31	650	0	2.0	30
glazed, frozen	9 oz	220	17	30	680	0	4.0	45
(Dinty Moore)								
and dumplings, microwave cup	1 cup	100	6	12	940	1	3.0	35
stew, microwave cup	7.5 oz	260	11	15	850	0	18.0	80
w/dumplings, microwave cup	7.5 oz	166	12	17	683	0	5.0	19
w/gravy and mashed potatoes, packaged	1 bowl	220	22	24	1180	2	4.0	25
w/noodles, 'Micro Meal'	1 bowl	260	21	26	1150	2	8.0	80
(Empire Kosher)								
breast, battered and breaded, fried, kosher	3 oz	170	21	3	440	1	8.0	45
cutlets, battered and breaded, fried, kosher	1 med cutlet	200	18	11	320	2	9.0	25

Food Name	Serv. Size	Total Cal.	Prot. gms	Carbs gms	Sod. mgs	Fiber gms	Fat gms	Chol. mgs
nuggets, battered and breaded, fried, kosher	5 nuggets	200	13	9	650	1	13.0	30
nuggets, kosher	5 nuggets	180	13	12	370	1	9.0	15
pie, kosher	1 pie	440	23	41	960	11	21.0	30
(Featherweight)								
stew, w/wild rice, canned	7.5 oz	140	10	23	400	0	1.0	20
w/dumplings, canned	7.5 oz	160	12	18	115	0	5.0	0
(Freezer Queen)								
à la king, frozen, 'Cook-In-Pouch'	4 oz	70	9	6	460	0	1.0	0
à la king, w/rice, frozen, 'Single Serve'	9 oz	270	20	37	520	0	5.0	0
cacciatore, frozen, 'Single Serve'	9 oz	270	20	33	710	0	6.0	0
croquettes, breaded, 'Family Suppers'	7 oz	240	12	20	1000	0	12.0	0
nuggets, frozen, 'Deluxe Family Suppers'	3 oz	270	14	15	770	0	17.0	0
nuggets, platter, frozen	6 oz	410	14	36	950	0	23.0	0
patty, frozen, 'Platter'	7.5 oz	360	17	33	1160	0	17.0	0
primavera, sliced, w/gravy, 'Cook-In-Pouch'	5 oz	80	7	6	820	0	3.0	0
sweet and sour, w/rice, frozen, 'Single Serve'	9 oz	300	20	48	700	0	4.0	0
(Green Giant) and broccoli, frozen, 'Entrees'	9.5 oz	340	23	28	890	0	15.0	0
(Healthy Choice)								
à l'orange, frozen	9 oz	260	23	38	340	0	2.0	40
and broccoli, 'Hearty Handfuls'	1 entrée	320	17	51	580	5	5.0	20
and mushrooms, 'Hearty Handfuls'	1 entrée	310	17	49	590	4	5.0	20
broccoli Alfredo	1 entrée	300	25	34	530	2	7.0	50
cacciatore	1 entrée	340	21	52	590	6	5.0	20
cacciatore, in sauce, w/vegetables	1 serving	266	22	36	552	5	4.0	32
Cantonese	1 entrée	280	22	34	480	2	6.0	50
chow mein, lowfat, low-cholesterol, frozen	9 oz	240	20	29	530	0	5.0	45
country breaded	1 entrée	350	16	51	480	5	9.0	45
country glazed	1 entrée	230	17	30	480	3	4.0	45
country herb	1 entrée	320	18	44	540	3	8.0	45
Dijon	1 entrée	270	23	33	470	6	5.0	40
divan, w/pasta, frozen	11.5 oz	300	25	41	520	0	4.0	50
entree	1 entrée	250	17	31	470	3	6.0	50
Francesca	1 entrée	330	23	46	600	4	6.0	30
garlic, 'Hearty Handfuls'	1 entrée	330	20	53	600	6	5.0	25
glazed, frozen	8.5 oz	220	21	27	510	0	3.0	45
grilled, Sonoma	1 entrée	230	18	30	530	5	4.0	15
grilled, Southwestern	1 entrée	260	21	30	450	4	6.0	40
grilled, w/mashed potatoes	1 entrée	170	18	18	600	3	3.5	40
herb roasted, frozen	11 oz	380	26	56	470	0	7.0	60
honey mustard	1 entrée	290	21	38	520	1	6.0	40
Mandarin	1 entrée	280	20	44	520	4	2.5	35
Marsala, w/vegetables	1 entrée	240	20	32	440	3	4.0	30
mesquite barbecue	1 entrée	310	18	48	480	6	5.0	55
mesquite barbecue, w/rice, vegetable, apple raisin cobbler	1 serving	310	18	48	483	6	5.0	54
Mexican, low-fat, low-cholesterol, frozen	12.5 oz	340	25	51	550	0	5.0	60
Milano, garlic	1 entrée	260	18	34	510	3	6.0	35
Oriental, frozen	11.25 oz	200	19	32	440	0	1.0	35
parmigiana	1 entrée	330	19	46	490	3	8.0	40
picante	1 entrée	250	18	30	550	4	7.0	45
roasted	1 entrée	230	20	25	480	6	5.0	45
roasted, frozen	1 serving	290	25	39	430	0	4.0	50
'Salsa Chicken Dinner' frozen	1 serving	240	20	36	450	0	2.0	50
sesame	1 entrée	250	16	38	600	2	4.0	35
Shanghai, sesame	1 entrée	360	19	54	600	4	7.0	20
stir-fry, w/vermicelli, frozen, 'Extra Portion'	12 oz	300	23	42	550	0	5.0	30
sweet and sour	1 entrée	360	20	53	360	5	7.0	45

Food Name	Serv. Size	Total Cal.	Prot. gms	Carbs gms	Sod. mgs	Fiber gms	Fat gms	Chol. mgs
sweet and sour, frozen	11.5 oz	280	20	52	320	0	2.0	35
teriyaki	1 entrée	270	17	37	600	3	6.0	45
teriyaki, w/rice, vegetable, apple cherry compote	1 serving	268	17	37	602	3	5.6	44
(Heinz) stew, w/dumplings, canned	7.5 oz	210	9	22	850	0	9.0	0
(Hormel) loaf, canned	2 oz	130	7	0	608	0	10.0	0
(Hot Bites)								
breast tenders, boneless	2.25 oz	150	11	12	280	0	6.0	0
breast tenders, boneless, 'Microwave'	4 oz	260	19	24	560	0	10.0	0
drumsticks, frozen, 'Drumsnackers'	2.63 oz	220	10	13	530	0	15.0	0
nuggets, fried, frozen, 'Southern'	2.63 oz	220	10	13	530	0	14.0	0
nuggets, frozen	2.63 oz	210	11	11	550	0	14.0	0
nuggets, hot'n spicy, frozen	2.63 oz	250	10	10	380	0	19.0	0
nuggets, w/cheddar, frozen	2.63 oz	250	11	11	560	0	18.0	0
sticks, primavera, frozen	2.63 oz	220	10	11	350	0	15.0	0
(Kid Cuisine)								
fried, frozen 'Mega Meal'	10.8 oz	720	34	53	1400	0	41.0	0
fried, frozen	7.25 oz	420	15	41	1050	0	22.0	0
fried, white meat, w/potato, corn, chocolate pudding, frozen	1 meal	440	19	48	710	6	20.0	65
nuggets, frozen	6.25 oz	400	11	46	610	0	19.0	60
nuggets, frozen, 'Mega Meal'	8.4 oz	470	21	51	1010	0	20.0	0
nuggets, w/macaroni and cheese, corn, pudding, 'Cosmic'	1 serving	524	18	53	974	3	26.7	49
nuggets, w/macaroni, corn, chocolate pudding	1 meal	360	14	46	500	6	13.0	30
(La Choy)								
almond, w/rice, vegetable, 'Fresh and Lite'	9.75 oz	270	14	40	1092	3	8.0	42
chow mein, canned	1 cup	80	8	6	1352	3	3.5	9
chow mein, canned, 'Bi-Pack'	3/4 cup	80	7	8	980	1	3.0	18
chow mein, canned, food service product	1 cup	91	5	11	865	2	3.6	9
chow mein, frozen, food service product	1 cup	133	8	19	857	1	3.1	5
imperial, w/rice, frozen, 'Fresh and Lite'	11 oz	260	13	45	1269	3	6.0	46
Oriental, canned, 'Bi-Pack'	3/4 cup	240	9	47	1400	1	2.0	0
Oriental, spicy, frozen, 'Fresh and Lite'	9.75 oz	270	11	52	560	4	4.0	42
Oriental, w/noodles, canned, 'Bi-Pack'	9 oz	160	11	23	1163	4	3.8	13
sweet and sour, canned	3/4 cup	240	8	47	1420	1	2.0	19
sweet and sour, canned, 'Dinner Classics'	1/4 pkg	120	1	29	840	1	1.0	0
sweet and sour, packaged, 'Dinner Classics'	3/4 cup	310	32	30	860	1	6.0	50
sweet and sour, w/noodles, frozen	1 cup	256	7	49	697	9	3.1	10
sweet and sour, w/rice, vegetables, frozen 'Fresh & Lite'	10 oz	260	13	50	601	4	3.0	53
Szechwan, spicy, bi-pack	1 cup	98	8	11	857	1	2.6	19
(Le Menu)								
à la king, w/seasoned rice, frozen, 'LightStyle'	8.25 oz	240	19	29	670	0	5.0	30
breast, glazed, frozen, 'LightStyle'	10 oz	230	25	25	430	0	3.0	55
breast, roasted, w/herbs, rice, and vegetable	7.75 oz	260	22	29	500	0	6.0	45
cordon bleu, frozen	11 oz	460	23	47	850	0	20.0	0
Dijon, w/pasta and vegetables, 'LightStyle'	8.5 oz	240	22	21	500	0	7.0	40
herb roasted, frozen, 'LightStyle'	10 oz	240	27	18	400	0	7.0	70
in wine sauce, frozen	10 oz	280	26	27	680	0	7.0	0
Kiev, frozen	8 oz	530	20	24	780	0	39.0	0
Oriental, à la king, frozen	10.25 oz	330	23	29	830	0	13.0	0
parmigiana, frozen	11.75 oz	410	26	31	1030	0	20.0	0
sweet and sour, frozen	11.25 oz	400	19	41	1020	0	18.0	0
sweet and sour, frozen, 'LightStyle'	10 oz	250	18	29	530	0	7.0	2
(Lean Cuisine)								
'Fiesta' frozen	8.5 oz	240	19	30	560	0	5.0	40
à l'orange	1 entrée	260	19	40	260	1	2.5	40
à l'orange, in sauce, w/broccoli and rice	1 serving	268	24	39	360	na	1.8	46

Food Name	Serv. Size	Total Cal.	Prot. gms	Carbs gms	Sod. mgs	Fiber gms	Fat gms	Chol. mgs
and vegetables, w/vermicelli . . . . 1 pkg		252	19	32	582	5	5.6	24
and vegetables, w/vermicelli, frozen . . . . 11.75 oz		240	18	30	500	0	5.0	30
baked . . . . 1 entrée		230	18	31	520	5	4.0	35
baked, w/whipped potatoes . . . . 1 entrée		250	19	30	590	2	6.0	30
barbecue, w/rice pilaf, frozen . . . . 8.75 oz		260	20	32	500	0	6.0	50
barbecue, w/sauce, 'Hearty Portions' . . . . 1 entrée		380	23	58	790	7	6.0	45
breaded, baked, w/potato and vegetable, frozen . . . . 8 oz		200	17	21	480	0	5.0	35
cacciatore, w/vermicelli, frozen . . . . 10 7/8 oz		280	22	31	570	0	7.0	45
Calypso, frozen, 'Café Classics' . . . . 1 pkg		280	15	42	590	3	6.0	40
carbonara . . . . 1 entrée		280	18	33	580	2	8.0	30
chow mein . . . . 1 entrée		220	12	33	560	3	5.0	35
chow mein, w/rice, frozen . . . . 9 oz		240	14	34	530	0	5.0	30
classica, frozen, food service product . . . . 1 oz		23	2	2	85	0	0.8	5
fiesta, w/rice and vegetables . . . . 1 entrée		260	19	35	550	3	5.0	40
Florentine, 'Hearty Portions' . . . . 1 entrée		420	23	61	720	5	9.0	60
glazed . . . . 1 entrée		240	22	25	480	0	6.0	55
glazed, frozen, food service product . . . . 1 oz		26	3	1	101	0	1.1	9
glazed, w/vegetable rice, frozen . . . . 8.5 oz		250	21	24	590	0	7.0	50
grilled, and penne pasta, 'Hearty Portions' . . . . 1 entrée		380	25	52	750	7	8.0	45
grilled, w/salsa, frozen, 'Café Classics' . . . . 1 pkg		240	15	32	550	4	6.0	40
herb roasted . . . . 1 entrée		210	13	27	540	3	5.0	40
herb roasted, 'Café Classics' . . . . 1 entrée		210	17	25	430	4	5.0	40
honey mustard, 'Café Classics' . . . . 1 entrée		270	16	39	580	3	5.0	35
honey mustard, frozen . . . . 7.5 oz		230	18	30	540	0	4.0	40
honey roasted . . . . 1 entrée		290	14	46	590	5	6.0	25
in peanut sauce . . . . 1 entrée		290	23	35	550	4	6.0	30
Italienne, frozen, food service product . . . . 1 oz		20	2	1	122	0	0.9	7
medallions, w/creamy cheese sauce . . . . 1 entrée		260	16	31	590	4	8.0	50
Marsala, w/vegetables, frozen . . . . 8 1/8 oz		180	22	13	430	0	4.0	55
Mediterranean, frozen, 'Café Classics' . . . . 1 pkg		260	19	36	580	4	4.0	35
Mexicali style, frozen, food service product . . . . 1 oz		20	2	2	48	1	0.7	6
Oriental . . . . 1 entrée		250	19	30	530	4	6.0	35
Oriental, glazed, 'Hearty Portions' . . . . 1 entrée		410	19	69	790	4	6.0	50
Oriental, w/vermicelli, frozen . . . . 9 oz		280	22	31	480	0	7.0	35
Parmesan . . . . 1 entrée		220	18	27	560	4	5.0	50
Parmesan, 'Café Classics' . . . . 1 entrée		240	20	25	580	4	7.0	50
piccata . . . . 1 entrée		270	13	41	530	2	6.0	25
piccata, frozen, 'Café Classics' . . . . 1 pkg		290	15	45	540	1	6.0	30
pie . . . . 1 entrée		320	18	39	590	3	10.0	35
pie, 100% white meat, frozen . . . . 1 pkg		310	23	32	590	0	10.0	40
primavera, frozen, food service product . . . . 1 oz		16	1	1	82	0	0.7	5
roasted, w/herbs, frozen, 'Café Classics' . . . . 1 pkg		210	17	25	430	4	5.0	40
roasted, w/mushrooms, 'Hearty Portions' . . . . 1 entrée		380	21	57	790	4	7.0	35
sweet and sour, frozen, food service product . . . . 1 oz		22	2	3	40	0	0.5	4
sweet and sour, w/rice, frozen . . . . 9 oz		280	17	39	490	0	6.0	50
tenderloins, in herb sauce, frozen . . . . 9.5 oz		240	29	19	490	0	5.0	60
tenderloins, in peanut sauce, frozen . . . . 9 oz		290	23	33	530	0	7.0	45
w/bow tie pasta, frozen, 'Café Classics' . . . . 1 pkg		270	19	34	550	5	6.0	60
w/rice and vegetables . . . . 1 entrée		240	22	24	460	2	6.0	60
(Libby's)								
chow mein, microwave cup . . . . 7.75 oz		130	5	19	830	2	4.0	10
w/pasta spirals, microwave cup, 'Diner' . . . . 7.75 oz		120	8	16	910	2	3.0	15
(Lloyds) breast fillet, roasted, barbecue, w/sauce . . . . 1 fillet		140	16	12	930	1	3.0	60
(Luck's)								
and dumplings, microwave bowl . . . . 1 serving		150	16	21	1400	1	1.0	35
and rice, microwaveable bowl . . . . 1 serving		140	14	19	1180	1	1.0	30
Brunswick stew, microwave bowl . . . . 1 serving		130	9	23	910	3	0.0	0

Food Name	Serv. Size	Total Cal.	Prot. gms	Carbs gms	Sod. mgs	Fiber gms	Fat gms	Chol. mgs
thighs and wings, w/dumplings, in sauce	1 cup	340	24	23	810	2	20.0	140
w/dumplings, canned	7.25 oz	240	16	18	605	0	11.0	0
(Lunch Bucket)								
w/beans and rice, micro cup, 'Light'n Healthy'	7.5 oz	170	7	28	600	0	3.0	10
w/dumplings, microwave lunch cup	7.5 oz	140	4	25	880	0	2.0	0
(Lunch Express)								
Alfredo	1 entrée	373	19	33	588	4	18.5	57
chow mein	1 entrée	260	13	43	940	3	4.0	30
Mandarin	1 entrée	270	12	41	520	2	6.0	30
Oriental	1 entrée	370	11	55	910	3	12.0	28
stir-fry, w/rice and vegetables, frozen	1 entrée	270	12	40	632	6	7.4	26
w/vegetables and rice	1 entrée	340	15	45	750	2	11.0	30
(Manor House) fried, assorted pieces	3 oz	270	14	13	620	1	18.0	65
(Marie Callender's)								
and noodles	13 oz	520	21	42	1320	5	30.0	65
and noodles, escalloped, frozen	1 pkg	629	21	61	1597	na	33.6	na
and noodles, escalloped, frozen	1 cup	397	13	38	1007	na	21.2	na
and noodles, escalloped, frozen	1 serving	292	10	28	742	na	15.6	na
chicken and dumplings	1 cup	250	13	22	1030	3	12.0	80
cordon bleu	13 oz	590	33	58	1920	7	25.0	55
country fried, w/gravy	16 oz	620	24	63	2300	6	30.0	75
grilled, in mushroom sauce	14 oz	480	33	54	1030	7	15.0	65
grilled, w/rice pilaf	11.7 oz	360	20	38	1070	6	14.0	40
herb roasted, w/mashed potatoes	14 oz	670	43	32	2100	7	31.0	205
Marsala	14 oz	450	33	42	1260	6	17.0	70
parmigiana, breaded	16 oz	620	31	63	730	9	27.0	50
pot pie	1 pie	600	14	53	1070	4	37.0	15
pot pie, au gratin	1 pie	690	19	50	1300	4	46.0	30
pot pie, frozen	1 pkg	999	25	88	2078	na	61.1	28
pot pie, frozen	1 serving	501	12	44	1041	na	30.6	14
pot pie, w/broccoli	1 pie	670	16	54	1000	4	43.0	25
sweet and sour	14 oz	530	25	86	700	1	9.0	35
(Michelina's)								
primavera, w/spirals, 'Lean 'n Tasty'	1 entrée	250	13	32	860	2	7.0	35
teriyaki, w/rice 'Lean 'n Tasty'	1 entrée	290	9	65	1140	2	3.0	15
(Mrs. Paterson's) pie, hand held pie, frozen, 'Aussie Pie'	1 serving	434	15	40	799	na	24.0	48
(Mountain House) stew, freeze-dried, prepared	1 cup	230	9	30	209	0	8.0	0
(Myers)								
à la king, frozen	3.5 oz	137	9	6	357	0	9.0	0
and noodles, frozen	3.5 oz	136	8	9	399	0	8.0	0
creamed, frozen	3.5 oz	151	12	5	372	0	10.0	0
croquettes, frozen	3.5 oz	168	16	10	364	0	7.0	0
frozen, à la gratin, frozen	3.5 oz	129	9	9	276	0	7.0	0
pie, frozen	3.5 oz	129	7	10	253	0	7.0	0
(Pierre)								
barbecue, frozen, 'Chix-B-Q' product 9845	1 piece	137	14	6	418	1	5.8	36
breaded, frozen, 'Two-Fers' product 1870	1 piece	92	5	4	194	0	6.5	12
breast, breaded, frozen, cooked, product 1881	1 piece	95	5	3	193	0	6.6	14
breast patty, fillet-shaped, flame-broiled, 'Caboose' product 9863	1 piece	121	15	3	320	1	5.4	35
breast patty, fillet-shaped, flame-broiled, product 9820	1 piece	157	21	4	473	1	6.0	49
breast patty, fillet-shaped, flame-broiled, product 9916	1 piece	152	19	4	417	1	6.3	47
breast patty, mesquite, fillet-shaped, flame-broiled, product 9816	1 piece	149	18	1	382	1	7.4	45
nuggets, breaded, frozen, product 3800	1 piece	47	2	2	99	0	3.3	6
patty, breaded, frozen, product 1915	1 piece	185	9	7	390	1	13.1	25

Food Name	Serv. Size	Total Cal.	Prot. gms	Carbs gms	Sod. mgs	Fiber gms	Fat gms	Chol. mgs
patty, cutlet-shaped, flame-broiled, frozen, product 9835	1 piece	145	18	4	379	1	6.2	47
patty, cutlet-shaped, honey mustard, flame-broiled, frozen, product 9852	1 piece	167	18	8	611	1	7.1	47
patty, cutlet-shaped, mesquite, flame-broiled, frozen, product 9805	1 piece	138	18	1	337	1	6.3	47
patty, cutlet-shaped, rotisserie style, flame-broiled, frozen, product 9878	1 piece	133	19	2	297	1	5.7	45
patty, cutlet-shaped, teriyaki sauce, flame-broiled, frozen, product 9829	1 piece	165	18	7	576	1	6.7	47
patty, fillet-shaped, flame-broiled, frozen, product 9840	1 piece	123	14	3	325	1	5.8	37
(Pilgrim's Pride)								
Cajun style, frozen	3 oz	241	13	9	480	0	17.0	51
primavera, frozen	3 oz	183	14	8	640	0	10.4	21
(Pillsbury)								
casserole, frozen, 'Microwave Classic'	1 pkg	400	21	30	890	0	22.0	0
w/cheese, casserole, 'Microwave Classic'	1 pkg	480	21	33	940	0	29.0	0
(Redi-Serve) nuggets, white meat, breaded and cooked	6 nibblers	270	14	17	610	2	16.0	35
(Rice A Roni)								
w/mushrooms, rice	2.5 oz	203	5	29	835	1	7.9	0
w/vegetable rice	2.5 oz	164	3	29	830	1	4.0	0
(Right Course)								
primavera, sesame, frozen	10 oz	320	25	34	590	0	9.0	50
tenderloins, barbecue, w/sauce, frozen	8.75 oz	270	20	35	590	0	6.0	40
tenderloins, in peanut sauce, frozen	9.25 oz	330	27	32	570	0	10.0	50
(Shanghai) stir-fry, frozen	10.3 oz	190	22	19	1220	0	3.0	30
(Shelton's)								
pie, white flour	1 serving	230	15	18	370	1	10.0	55
pie, whole wheat	1 serving	230	16	18	370	3	10.0	55
(Smart Ones)								
à l'orange, frozen	8 oz	190	12	34	530	0	1.0	15
chow mein	1 entrée	200	12	34	490	3	2.0	25
chow mein, frozen	9 oz	170	14	27	470	1	1.0	20
fiesta	1 entrée	220	12	38	480	5	2.0	25
Francais, w/garlic vegetables, frozen	8.5 oz	150	15	18	400	0	1.0	5
grilled, glazed, w/sauce, frozen	8 oz	130	12	17	540	0	1.0	20
honey mustard	1 entrée	200	13	33	340	6	2.0	30
honey mustard, w/sauce, frozen	7.5 oz	140	11	20	220	0	1.0	10
Marsala	1 entrée	150	10	22	500	6	2.0	25
Mexican, w/Spanish rice, frozen, 'Fiesta'	8 oz	210	14	37	390	0	1.0	20
Mexican style, w/rice, frozen, 'Monterey'	1 pkg	410	23	35	700	4	20.0	75
Mirabella	1 entrée	170	11	26	470	6	2.0	20
picatta	1 entrée	190	10	34	460	3	2.0	25
Szechwan style, spicy, w/vegetables	1 entrée	220	11	39	730	3	2.0	10
(Stouffer's)								
à la king	1 entrée	320	15	43	750	3	10.0	55
à la king, w/rice, frozen	9.5-oz pkg	270	18	38	800	0	5.0	0
and dumplings, frozen, food service product	1 oz	39	2	3	109	0	2.3	9
and noodles, escalloped	1 entrée	450	17	32	1170	1	28.0	50
and noodles, escalloped, frozen	1 entrée	365	17	4	1211	na	31.4	76
and noodles, escalloped, frozen, food service product	1 oz	42	2	3	122	0	2.5	11
and noodles, 'Homestyle'	1 entrée	300	20	25	950	3	13.0	90
and vegetables, w/cream sauce, frozen	1 oz	31	1	2	113	0	2.0	9
baked, w/mashed potatoes, 'Homestyle'	1 entrée	270	22	19	750	2	12.0	75
chow mein, w/rice, frozen	10 3/4 oz pkg	250	13	39	720	0	5.0	0

Food Name	Serv. Size	Total Cal.	Prot. gms	Carbs gms	Sod. mgs	Fiber gms	Fat gms	Chol. mgs
creamed	1 entrée	280	17	8	720	0	20.0	80
creamed, frozen, food service product	1 oz	46	2	1	108	0	3.7	11
divan, frozen	8-oz pkg	220	24	11	610	0	10.0	0
fried, w/mashed potatoes, 'Homestyle'	1 entrée	330	18	29	780	3	16.0	55
grilled, homestyle, w/BBQ sauce, frozen	7 5/8 oz	210	23	14	550	0	7.0	0
Monterey, w/Mexican rice, homestyle, food service product	1 entrée	410	23	35	700	4	20.0	75
noodle, homestyle, frozen, food service product	1 oz	31	2	2	120	0	1.6	6
parmigiana, w/pasta Alfredo, homestyle, frozen	9 7/8 oz	360	31	24	990	0	15.0	0
parmigiana, w/spaghetti, 'Homestyle'	1 entrée	320	27	30	890	4	10.0	75
pie, frozen	1 entrée	572	23	37	942	3	37.1	76
tenders, breaded, w/potatoes, homestyle	8 3/8 oz	430	20	46	950	0	18.0	0
w/dumplings, in broth, frozen, food service product	1 oz	26	2	2	103	0	1.1	11
(Swanson)								
à la king, canned	1 cup	320	15	17	1080	0	22.0	60
à la king, canned	5.25 oz	190	10	9	690	0	12.0	0
and dumplings, canned	1 cup	260	13	22	1120	0	13.0	65
boneless, 'Hungry Man'	1 entrée	630	26	80	1680	9	22.0	55
cacciatore, frozen, 'Homestyle Recipe'	10.95 oz	260	15	33	1030	0	8.0	0
fried, barbecue flavored, frozen	10 oz	540	25	61	1160	0	22.0	0
fried, dark meat	1 entrée	580	24	54	1430	5	30.0	105
fried, dark meat, 'Hungry Man'	1 entrée	780	33	74	1700	8	39.0	105
fried, mostly white meat, 'Hungry Man'	1 entrée	800	35	79	2380	6	39.0	85
fried, white meat	1 entrée	630	26	62	1700	5	31.0	55
grilled, white meat, w/garlic sauce, almonds	10 oz	310	17	39	630	0	9.0	30
nibbles, frozen, 'Homestyle Recipe'	4.25 oz	340	10	29	730	0	20.0	0
nibbles, 'Plump and Juicy'	3.25 oz	300	12	19	690	0	19.0	0
nuggets, 'Plump and Juicy'	3 oz	230	13	14	360	0	14.0	0
nuggets, fried	1 entrée	590	20	71	990	5	25.0	35
nuggets, frozen	8.75 oz	470	19	47	650	0	23.0	0
Parmigiana, frozen, 'Budget'	10 oz	300	7	35	780	0	15.0	0
pie, frozen, 'Homestyle Recipe'	8 oz	410	15	41	1030	0	21.0	0
pot pie	1 pie	410	10	43	780	2	22.0	25
pot pie, 'Hungry Man'	1 pie	650	19	64	1500	3	35.0	65
stew, canned	1 cup	180	11	17	1110	2	8.0	35
(Sweet Sue)								
and dumplings, canned	1 pkg	620	43	65	2683	7	21.1	102
chicken and dumplings, canned	1 serving	218	15	23	946	3	7.4	36
(Swift)								
cordon bleu, frozen, 'International'	6 oz	360	30	23	1010	0	17.0	0
Kiev, frozen, 'International'	6 oz	420	27	22	1030	0	24.0	0
(Top Shelf)								
à la king, packaged	10 oz	360	18	49	890	0	10.0	37
Acapulco, packaged	1 serving	390	28	41	1320	0	13.0	55
cacciatore, packaged	10 oz	210	21	25	810	0	3.0	50
glazed, packaged	10 oz	170	19	19	780	0	2.0	35
sweet and sour, packaged	1 serving	270	24	41	280	0	1.0	60
w/Spanish rice, packaged	10 oz	400	27	38	810	0	15.0	75
(Tyson)								
à l'orange, 'Gourmet Selection' frozen	9.5 oz	300	21	36	670	0	8.0	0
barbecue, frozen	12.5 oz	400	27	56	600	0	8.0	50
barbecue, glazed, frozen, 'Yosemite Sam'	7.38 oz	230	12	28	510	0	8.0	45
barbecue, w/potato and vegetable medley	1 entrée	560	19	73	1190	9	21.0	30
blackened, w/Spanish rice and corn	1 entrée	260	17	36	480	4	5.0	30
breast patty, breaded	1 piece	80	10	9	430	1	0.0	0
breast patty, breaded, Southern fried	1 entrée	180	11	8	360	0	12.0	30
chunks, frozen, 'Chick'n Chunks'	2.6 oz	220	10	11	500	0	15.0	35

Food Name	Serv. Size	Total Cal.	Prot. gms	Carbs gms	Sod. mgs	Fiber gms	Fat gms	Chol. mgs
chunks, frozen, 'Looney Tunes Bugs Bunny'	7.7 oz	290	17	31	480	0	11.0	28
chunks, Southern fried 'Chick'n Chunks'	2.6 oz	220	10	11	540	0	15.0	35
cordon bleu, wholesale club item, 'Mini Cordon Bleu'	1 piece	90	8	5	210	0	4.0	17
cordon bleu, wholesale club item, frozen	7 oz	480	40	28	1030	0	22.0	0
divan, w/candied carrots and pasta	1 entrée	370	20	38	530	2	15.0	50
drummettes, frozen, ' Tazmanian Devil'	8 oz	310	14	31	480	0	14.0	40
drumsticks, roasted, w/skin	3 med pieces	330	40	1	870	0	18.0	225
Francais, frozen, 'Gourmet Selection'	9.5 oz	280	19	20	1130	0	14.0	0
fried, w/mashed potatoes, gravy, corn	1 entrée	360	16	30	5	4	15.0	4
glazed, w/sauce 'Gourmet Selections'	9.25 oz	240	22	29	930	0	4.0	44
grilled, w/corn O'Brien and ranch beans	1 entrée	230	19	30	590	7	4.0	30
grilled, w/Italian style w/pasta and vegetable medley	1 entrée	190	21	19	440	3	3.5	30
'Herb Chicken Meal' frozen	13.75 oz	340	32	43	550	0	4.0	50
honey Dijon, w/pasta and peas	1 entrée	340	20	49	900	6	7.0	25
'Honey Mustard Chicken Meal' frozen	13.75 oz	390	31	52	520	0	6.0	50
honey roasted, frozen, 'Gourmet Selections'	9 oz	220	26	23	500	0	4.0	48
Italian, grilled, 'Gourmet Selections'	9 oz	210	28	19	420	0	3.0	40
'Italian Style Chicken Meal' frozen	13.75 oz	310	30	38	600	0	4.0	50
Kiev, w/rice pilaf, broccoli, carrots	1 entrée	440	18	36	900	2	25.0	85
'Looney Tunes Road Runner' frozen	6.7 oz	300	8	42	490	0	11.0	24
marinara, frozen	13.75 oz	340	31	37	590	0	7.0	45
Marsala, w/carrots and red potatoes	1 entrée	180	15	19	520	4	5.0	30
mesquite breast tenders, boneless, frozen	2.75 oz	110	17	4	420	0	3.0	45
mesquite, w/barbecue sauce, corn, potato	1 entrée	321	18	45	793	4	7.8	26
mesquite, w/corn, pea, and au gratin	1 entrée	320	18	44	780	4	8.0	25
'Mesquite Chicken Meal' frozen	13.25 oz	330	34	38	600	0	5.0	45
nuggets, frozen, 'Microwave'	3.5 oz	220	10	11	0	0	15.0	0
Oriental, breast strips, boneless, frozen	2.75 oz	110	14	6	250	0	3.0	40
Oriental, frozen, 'Gourmet Selection'	10.25 oz	270	20	32	1140	0	7.0	0
parmigiana, frozen, 'Gourmet Selection'	11.25 oz	380	19	37	1100	0	17.0	0
picatta, w/broccoli and parslied potatoes	1 entrée	190	17	18	500	5	6.0	35
pie, premium, frozen	9 oz	390	16	36	1065	0	20.0	43
pie, white meat, premium, frozen	9 oz	400	22	33	783	0	20.0	56
primavera	1 entrée	350	25	48	610	5	6.0	30
roasted, frozen, 'Gourmet Selections'	9 oz	200	21	21	430	0	2.0	42
roasted, w/garlic sauce, pasta, vegetable	1 entrée	214	17	22	467	4	6.7	28
'Salsa Chicken Meal' frozen	13.75 oz	370	34	52	470	0	6.0	45
sesame, frozen, 'Healthy Portions'	13.5 oz	390	27	58	410	0	5.0	45
stir-fry, w/vegetable, frozen, wholesale club item	3.5 oz	130	11	13	710	0	5.0	45
supreme, frozen, 'Gourmet Selections'	9 oz	230	21	23	480	0	6.0	51
sweet and sour, frozen, 'Gourmet Selection'	11 oz	420	22	50	850	0	15.0	0
tabasco barbecue	1 entrée	260	13	37	610	5	7.0	25
tenders, frozen 'Microwave'	3.5 oz	230	16	19	0	0	11.0	0
w/cheddar, boneless, 'Chick'n Cheddar'	2.6 oz	220	11	11	310	0	15.0	40
wholesale club item, 'Classic Colonial'	3.5 oz	180	13	11	190	0	9.0	40
wings, hot, wholesale club item, frozen 'Wings of Fire'	3.5 oz	220	26	2	390	0	12.0	105
wings, teriyaki style	4 pieces	190	21	2	210	2	12.0	120
(Ultra Slim-Fast)								
and vegetables	12 oz	290	24	45	850	0	3.0	30
chow mein	12 oz	320	25	43	580	0	6.0	60
in mushroom sauce	12 oz	280	25	30	830	0	6.0	55
mesquite	12 oz	350	29	61	300	0	1.0	65
sweet and sour, frozen	12 oz	330	20	57	340	0	2.0	45
(Weaver)								
'Honey Batter Tenders' frozen	3 oz	220	13	14	500	0	12.0	0
'Italian Rondolet' frozen	2.6 oz	190	11	11	560	0	11.0	0
'Original Rondolet' frozen	3 oz	190	13	13	610	0	10.0	0

Food Name	Serv. Size	Total Cal.	Prot. gms	Carbs gms	Sod. mgs	Fiber gms	Fat gms	Chol. mgs
'Premium Tenders' frozen	3 oz	170	12	11	500	0	9.0	0
assorted pieces, frozen, 'Crispy Dutch Frye'	3.6 oz	290	16	16	550	0	18.0	0
breast, frozen 'Crispy Dutch Frye'	4.5 oz	350	22	17	520	0	22.0	0
crispy, light, skinless, frozen	2.9 oz	170	14	9	320	0	9.0	0
croquettes, frozen	2 pieces	280	14	22	780	0	16.0	0
frozen, 'Cheese Rondolet'	2.6 oz	190	11	12	520	0	11.0	0
mini drums, herb and spice, frozen	3 oz	200	13	13	320	0	11.0	0
mini-drums, crispy, frozen	3 oz	210	13	13	480	0	12.0	0
(Weight Watchers)								
barbecue glazed	1 entrée	230	20	33	440	4	2.5	30
barbecue, glazed, w/vegetables, frozen, 'Ultimate 200'	7 oz	200	19	22	450	0	6.0	30
barbecue, w/sauce, mixed vegetables, frozen, 'Ultimate 200'	1 serving	217	19	26	405	na	4.4	48
cordon bleu	1 entrée	230	15	31	650	2	4.5	20
cordon bleu, w/vegetables, frozen, 'Ultimate 200'	7.7 oz	170	19	15	560	0	5.0	40
divan, w/baked potato, frozen	11.25 oz	280	17	38	480	0	7.0	30
glazed	1 entrée	240	18	29	550	4	6.0	20
grilled, glazed, frozen, 'Ultimate 200'	7.5 oz	150	15	17	520	0	2.0	20
grilled, w/Spanish rice, frozen, 'Suiza'	8.6 oz	220	21	18	590	0	7.0	60
Hunan, w/vegetables, frozen, 'Stir Fry'	9 oz	160	15	21	430	0	2.0	15
imperial, frozen, 'Ultimate 200'	8.5 oz	200	18	25	430	0	3.0	25
Kiev, w/vegetables, rice, frozen, 'Ultimate 200'	7 oz	190	14	22	470	0	5.0	15
orange glazed, w/rice, frozen, 'Stir Fry'	9 oz	170	14	25	360	0	2.0	10
parmigiana	1 entrée	310	21	39	500	4	7.0	30
patty, Southern baked, w/vegetables, frozen, 'Ultimate 200'	6.3 oz	170	17	10	520	0	7.0	45
Polynesian, frozen, 'Stir Fry'	9 oz	190	12	34	240	0	1.0	20
sesame, w/lo mein noodles, frozen, 'Stir Fry'	9 oz	200	19	23	420	0	4.0	10
teriyaki, frozen, 'Ultimate 200'	7.6 oz	150	21	7	590	0	4.0	50
teriyaki, w/spring vegetables, frozen, 'Stir Fry'	9 oz	140	13	16	470	0	3.0	20
w/Spanish rice, frozen 'TexMex'	8.3 oz	250	18	33	590	0	5.0	35
(Wonderbites)								
barbecue, flame-broiled, frozen, 'Dippers'	1 piece	41	4	2	127	0	1.7	12
breast, flame-broiled, frozen, 'Dippers'	1 piece	35	4	1	91	0	1.5	11
Buffalo flavored, flame-broiled, frozen, 'Dippers'	1 piece	33	4	1	199	0	1.5	11
chili salsa, breaded, frozen, 'Dippers'	1 piece	69	4	3	121	0	4.8	8
flame-broiled, frozen, 'Dippers'	1 piece	35	4	1	92	0	1.5	11
honey mustard, flame-broiled, frozen, 'Dippers'	1 piece	40	4	2	151	0	1.6	12
Italian, flame-broiled, frozen, 'Dippers'	1 piece	33	4	0	124	0	1.4	11
rotisserie style, flame-broiled, frozen, 'Dippers' product 9896	1 piece	34	5	0	75	0	1.4	11
teriyaki, flame broiled, frozen, 'Dippers' product 3727	1 piece	45	4	2	128	0	2.3	11
teriyaki, flame broiled, frozen, 'Dippers' product 3827	1 piece	45	4	2	127	0	2.4	10
teriyaki, flame broiled, frozen, 'Dippers' product 9879	1 piece	41	4	2	142	0	1.7	12
(Yu Sing)								
lo mein, frozen	1 container	230	13	35	950	3	5.0	15
sweet and sour, w/rice	1 container	300	12	50	480	2	6.0	20
w/almonds, w/rice, frozen	1 container	250	12	33	770	3	8.0	20
CHICKEN DINNER/ENTRÉE MIX								
(Chicken Helper)								
cheesy broccoli, 'Skillet' dry	1/5 pkg	160	4	32	700	0	2.0	5
cheesy broccoli, 'Skillet' prepared	7 oz	310	24	34	790	0	9.0	65
stir-fry, 'Skillet' mix only	1/5 pkg	170	4	36	800	0	1.0	0
stir-fry, 'Skillet' prepared	7 oz	370	25	36	950	0	14.0	145

Food Name	Serv. Size	Total Cal.	Prot. gms	Carbs gms	Sod. mgs	Fiber gms	Fat gms	Chol. mgs
creamy, 'Skillet' mix only	1/5 pkg	170	6	28	720	0	5.0	40
creamy, 'Skillet' prepared	8.25 oz	330	26	29	820	0	13.0	100
fettuccini Alfredo, 'Skillet' mix only	1/5 pkg	160	6	25	690	0	4.0	10
fettuccini Alfredo, 'Skillet' prepared	7.5 oz	320	26	27	780	0	12.0	70
creamy mushroom, 'Skillet' mix only	1/5 pkg	170	5	28	720	0	4.0	30
creamy mushroom, 'Skillet' prepared	8 oz	320	25	31	810	0	11.0	90
(Lipton)								
barbecue, 'Microeasy' mix only	1/4 pkg	110	2	24	980	0	1.0	0
barbecue, 'Microeasy' prepared	1/4 pkg	220	16	24	1020	0	6.0	0
country style, 'Microeasy' mix only	1/4 pkg	80	3	15	840	0	1.0	0
country style, 'Microeasy' prepared	1/4 pkg	190	18	15	880	0	6.0	0
(Skillet Chicken Helper) stir-fried	1/4 cup	140	4	30	690	1	0.5	0
CHICKEN FAT								
	1 cup	1846	0.0	0.0	0	0	204.6	174
	1 oz	178	1.1	0.0	9	0	19.3	16
	1 tbsp	115	0.0	0.0	0	0	12.8	11
kosher, retail rendered *(Empire Kosher)*	1 tbsp	120	0	1	0	0	13.0	0
CHICKEN SALAD SPREAD								
(Libby's) 'Spreadables'	1 pkg	329	11	23	1062	na	21.3	59
(Libby's) 'Spreadables'	1/3 cup	140	7	7	340	2	9.0	25
(Libby's) 'Spreadables'	1 serving	171	6	12	552	na	11.1	31
CHICKEN SEASONING. See under SEASONING MIX.								
CHICKEN SEASONING AND COATING MIX. See under SEASONING AND COATING MIX.								
CHICKEN SPREAD								
(Hormel) canned	0.5 oz	30	2	0	0	0	2.0	0
(Underwood) canned, chunky	2 1/8 oz	150	10	2	440	0	9.0	40
(Underwood) canned, 'Light'	2 1/8 oz	80	11	2	330	0	3.0	30
(Underwood) canned, smoky	2 1/8 oz	150	10	10	290	0	8.0	40
CHICKEN SUBSTITUTE								
(Heartline)								
vegetarian, 'Chicken Fillet Style'	2 oz	176	19	9	260	0	7.0	0
vegetarian, lite, 'Chicken Fillet Style'	0.5 oz	22	5	1	135	3	0.0	0
(Morningstar Farms)'								
nuggets, vegetarian, 'Chik Nuggets'	4 nuggets	160	13	17	670	5	4.0	0
nuggets, vegetarian, homestyle, frozen, 'Country Crisps'	3 oz	250	8	18	480	0	16.0	0
nuggets, vegetarian, zesty, frozen, 'Country Crisps'	3 oz	280	9	17	740	0	19.0	0
patty, vegetarian, 'Chik Patty'	1 patty	177	7	15	536	2	9.8	1
patty, vegetarian, frozen, 'Country Crisps'	2.5 oz	220	8	13	620	0	15.0	0
vegetarian, 'Meatless Chicken'	1 patty	170	8	13	590	0	10.0	0
(Worthington)								
chicken style, vegetarian	1 slice	86	10	1	374	1	4.6	1
diced, vegetarian, 'Diced Chik'	1/4 cup drained	40	7	1	270	1	0.0	0
diced, vegetarian, frozen, 5-lb pkg 'Meatless Chicken'	1/4 cup	50	10	2	400	1	0.0	0
nuggets, vegetarian, 'Chik Stiks'	1 serving	111	9	3	355	2	7.3	1
pie, vegetarian, frozen	8 oz	380	7	43	1200	0	20.0	0
roll, vegetarian, 4-lb pkg, 'Meatless Chicken'	3/8-inch slice	80	9	1	360	<1	4.5	0
roll, vegetarian, frozen, 'Meatless Chicken'	2.5 oz	150	11	4	570	0	10.0	0
sliced, vegetarian, 'Chic-Ketts'	2 3/8-inch slices	120	13	2	390	2	7.0	0
sliced, vegetarian, 'Sliced Chik'	3 slices	70	14	2	430	2	0.5	0
slices, vegetarian, 8-oz pkg, 'Meatless Chicken'	2 slices	80	9	1	370	1	4.5	0
slices, vegetarian, frozen, 'Meatless Chicken' 2 oz	2 slices	130	9	3	460	0	9.0	0
vegetarian, 'Chic-Ketts'	1 slice	121	13	2	390	2	6.5	0
vegetarian, diced, canned drained	1/4 cup	90	4	2	330	0	8.0	0
vegetarian, diced, frozen, 'Meatless Chicken'	1/2 cup	190	13	5	680	0	13.0	0

Food Name	Serv. Size	Total Cal.	Prot. gms	Carbs gms	Sod. mgs	Fiber gms	Fat gms	Chol. mgs
vegetarian, frozen, 'Crispy Chik'	3 oz	280	10	17	500	0	19.0	0
vegetarian, sliced, canned, drained, 2.1 oz	2 slices	90	4	2	330	0	8.0	0
CHICKEN SUBSTITUTE DINNER/ENTRÉE								
(Loma Linda)								
croquette, loaf, or patty, vegetarian, dry mix, 'Chicken Supreme'	1/3 cup	90	15	6	720	4	1.0	0
fried chicken style, vegetarian, 'Fried Chik'n with Gravy'	2 pieces	160	12	4	440	2	10.0	0
nuggets, vegetarian, 'Meatless Chik-Nuggets'	5 pieces	240	12	13	710	5	16.0	0
(Morningstar Farms)								
wings, vegetarian, 'Meat-Free Buffalo Wings'	5 nuggets	200	13	16	730	3	9.0	0
(Worthington)								
croquettes, vegetarian, 'Golden Croquettes'	4 pieces	210	14	14	600	3	10.0	0
drumsticks, vegetarian, 'Chik Stiks'	1 piece	110	9	3	360	2	7.0	0
fried chicken style, vegetarian, 'FriChik'	2 pieces	120	10	1	430	1	8.0	0
fried chicken style, vegetarian, low-fat, 'Low Fat FriChik'	2 pieces	80	18	21	870	11	1.0	0
patties, vegetarian, lightly breaded, seasoned, 'Crispy Chik Patties'	1 pattie	150	8	15	600	2	6.0	0
CHICKPEA/ceci/garbanzo								
Canned								
	1 cup	286	12	54	718	11	2.7	0
(A&P)	1/2 cup	100	6	17	270	0	1.0	0
(Allens)	1/2 cup	110	5	18	320	0	1.0	0
(Bush's Best)	1/2 cup	80	5	21	350	6	0.0	0
(Finast)	8 oz	210	10	35	250	0	3.0	0
(Green Giant)	1/2 cup	90	6	18	320	5	2.0	0
(Old El Paso)	1/2 cup	190	5	16	250	0	1.0	0
(Progresso)	1/2 cup	110	9	22	200	6	1.0	0
'Nutradiet' *(S&W)*	1/2 cup	100	5	19	5	0	1.0	0
dry beans in brine *(Green Giant)*	1/2 cup	110	6	18	380	5	1.5	0
50% less salt *(Green Giant)*	1/2 cup	90	6	18	160	5	2.0	0
50% less salt *(Joan of Arc)*	1/2 cup	90	6	18	160	5	2.0	0
large 'Lite 50% Less Salt' *(S&W)*	1/2 cup	110	6	21	295	0	1.0	0
organic, no salt added *(Eden Foods)*	1/2 cup	90	6	17	10	4	1.0	0
organic, w/liquid *(Eden Foods)*	1/2 cup	110	6	17	15	4	2.0	0
Fresh								
mature seed, boiled	1 cup	269	15	45	11	12	4.2	0
mature seed, raw	1 cup	728	39	121	48	35	12.1	0
mature seed, raw	1 tbsp	46	2	8	3	2	0.8	0
raw *(Arrowhead Mills)*	2 oz	200	12	35	9	7	3.0	0
Jarred, organically grown *(Eden Foods)*	1/2 cup	110	7	20	95	4	1.0	0
CHICKPEA FLOUR. See under FLOUR.								
CHICORY								
trimmed	1 oz	7	0.5	1.3	13	(mq)	0.1	0
trimmed, chopped	1/2 cup	21	1.5	4.2	41	3.6	0.3	0
untrimmed	1 lb	87	6.3	17.5	167	(mq)	1.1	0
CHICORY, WITLOOF								
raw	1/2 cup	8	0.4	1.8	1	1.4	0.0	0
raw, medium, approx 2.1 oz	1 head	9	0.5	2.1	1	1.6	0.1	0
trimmed	1 oz	4	0.3	0.9	2	(mq)	<.1	0
untrimmed	1 lb	61	4.0	12.9	28	(mq)	0.4	0
CHICORY ROOT								
raw, medium, approx 2.6 oz	1 root	44	0.8	10.5	30	>1.2 c	0.1	0
raw, 1-inch pieces	1/2 cup	33	0.6	7.9	23	>.9 c	0.1	0
trimmed	1 oz	21	0.4	5.0	14	>.6 c	0.1	0
untrimmed	1 lb	272	5.2	65.1	186	>7.3 c	0.7	0
CHILE PEPPER. See PEPPER, CHILI.								

Food Name	Serv. Size	Total Cal.	Prot. gms	Carbs gms	Sod. mgs	Fiber gms	Fat gms	Chol. mgs
CHILI								
(Armour)								
hot, w/beans, canned	7.5 oz	390	13	27	1080	0	26.0	0
w/beans, canned	7.5 oz	390	13	27	1080	0	26.0	0
w/beans, canned, 'Premium Lite'	7.5 oz	260	16	27	1110	0	10.0	0
w/beans, microwave	7.5 oz	300	16	26	1120	0	14.0	0
w/o beans, canned	7.5 oz	390	13	14	1150	0	31.0	0
(Bearitos)								
black bean, low-fat, 'Premium'	1 cup	150	9	20	550	5	1.0	0
original, lowfat, 'Premium'	1 cup	190	10	36	550	6	1.0	0
spicy, lowfat, 'Premium'	1 cup	190	10	36	550	5	1.0	0
(Chef Boyardee)								
beef, w/beans, canned	7.5 oz	330	15	30	1005	0	17.0	0
'Chili Mac' canned	7.5 oz	230	8	26	1410	0	11.0	0
(Chili Bowl) homestyle	1 cup	680	24	12	1210	8	59.0	10
(Cimmaron)								
beef, w/beans, canned	7.5 oz	230	17	21	0	0	9.0	35
chicken, w/beans, canned	7.5 oz	180	12	22	970	0	5.0	60
(Dennison's)								
chunky, w/beans, canned	7.5 oz	310	16	28	780	10	14.0	0
hot, w/beans, 15-oz can	7.5 oz	310	16	26	910	7	16.0	0
w/beans, 15-oz can	7.5 oz	310	16	27	875	8	15.0	0
'Cook-Off' w/beans, canned	7.5 oz	340	17	25	915	8	19.0	0
w/o beans, 15-oz can	7.5 oz	300	17	15	1380	0	19.0	0
(El Rio)								
con carne, w/o beans, canned	1 pkg	497	25	26	1322	6	32.7	81
con carne, w/o beans, canned	1 serving	305	15	16	812	4	20.1	50
(Estee) w/beans, canned	7.5 oz	370	16	27	125	0	20.0	60
(Featherweight) w/beans, canned	7.5 oz	280	19	29	440	0	10.0	30
(Gebhardt)								
hot, w/beans, canned	1 cup	470	16	47	1000	6	27.0	65
hot, w/beans, canned	4 oz	189	7	9	497	2	14.2	17
longhorn, w/beans	1 cup	450	18	32	1089	8	31.4	33
plain	1 cup	412	20	15	1324	7	30.4	40
plain, w/o beans	1 cup	530	21	20	990	1	41.0	150
vegetarian, canned	4 oz	219	10	7	555	0	17.1	0
w/beans	1 cup	322	15	32	673	15	14.9	29
(Hain)								
w/chicken, canned	7.5 oz	130	11	19	1030	0	2.0	40
spicy Tempeh, vegetarian, canned	7.5 oz	160	7	24	1350	0	4.0	0
vegetarian, spicy, canned	7.5 oz	160	7	29	1060	0	1.0	0
vegetarian, spicy, canned, 'Reduced Sodium'	7.5 oz	170	7	31	200	0	1.0	0
(Health Valley)								
three-bean, vegetarian, mild, fat-free	5 oz	90	10	12	180	9	0.0	0
w/beans, vegetarian, mild, canned, 'No Salt Added'	4 oz	130	8	16	25	8	3.0	0
w/beans, vegetarian, spicy, canned, 'No Salt Added'	4 oz	130	8	16	25	8	3.0	0
w/black beans, vegetarian, mild, fat-free	5 oz	140	11	23	290	12	0.0	0
w/black beans, vegetarian, spicy, canned	5 oz	70	7	9	180	8	0.0	0
w/lentils, vegetarian, mild, 'No Salt Added'	4 oz	130	8	16	50	8	3.0	0
w/lentils, vegetarian, mild, canned	4 oz	130	8	16	200	8	3.0	0
(Heinz)								
'Chili Con Carne' canned	7.75 oz	350	15	27	1000	0	21.0	0
'Chili Mac' canned	7.5 oz	250	10	26	860	0	12.0	0
hot, w/beans, canned	7.75 oz	330	15	30	1140	0	16.0	0
(Hormel)								
'Chili Mac' microwave	7.5 oz	192	10	18	977	0	9.0	22
chunky, w/beans, canned	7.5 oz	290	15	25	780	0	14.0	50

Food Name	Serv. Size	Total Cal.	Prot. gms	Carbs gms	Sod. mgs	Fiber gms	Fat gms	Chol. mgs
hot, w/beans, 15-oz can	7.5 oz	310	16	24	1121	0	16.0	0
hot, w/beans, microwave	7.38 oz	250	15	24	977	0	11.0	49
hot, w/o beans, 15-oz can	7.5 oz	370	17	12	985	0	28.0	0
microwave	1 cup	220	15	27	1050	6	6.0	30
turkey, w/beans, canned	1 cup	203	19	26	1198	6	2.8	35
vegetarian, w/beans, canned	1 cup	205	12	38	778	10	0.7	0
w/beans, canned	1 cup	240	17	34	1163	8	4.4	25
w/beans, 15-oz can	7.5 oz	310	17	23	1127	0	17.0	0
w/beans, 40-oz can	8 oz	320	17	25	1135	0	17.0	0
w/beans, microwave	7.5 oz	250	15	23	980	0	11.0	65
w/o beans, canned	10.5 oz	540	24	19	1384	0	41.0	0
w/o beans, canned	1 cup	194	17	18	970	3	6.6	35
w/o beans, 15-oz can	7.5 oz	370	17	12	1012	0	28.0	0
w/o beans, microwave	7.38 oz	290	18	15	830	0	17.0	60
(Just Rite)								
hot, w/beans, hot, canned	4 oz	195	11	16	495	1	10.0	33
vegetarian, w/beans, canned	4.55 oz	190	9	15	616	6	13.3	18
w/beans, canned	4 oz	200	10	16	500	1	11.0	33
w/o beans, canned	4 oz	180	13	9	515	1	11.0	41
(Lean Cuisine) 3-bean, frozen, food service product	1/2 cup	80	4	12	340	4	2.0	0
(Legume) chicken style, vegetarian	1 cup	160	10	29	460	7	1.0	0
(Libby's)								
w/beans, 15-oz can	7.5 oz	270	13	25	810	0	13.0	0
w/beans, microwave, 'Diner'	7.75 oz	280	15	29	820	4	12.0	40
w/o beans, canned	7.5 oz	390	18	11	800	0	30.0	0
(Luck's) hot, w/pinto beans	1/2 cup	120	6	20	310	6	1.0	0
(Lunch Bucket) w/beans, microwave	7.5 oz	300	16	26	1120	0	14.0	45
(Marie Callender's) w/cornbread	1 cup	350	14	45	1380	5	13.0	30
(Michelina's) black bean, 'Lean 'n Tasty'	1 entrée	400	13	77	480	10	5.0	0
(Mountain House)								
w/beans, freeze-dried, prepared	1 cup	390	20	38	153	0	16.0	0
w/beef, freeze-dried, prepared	1 cup	250	12	31	115	0	8.0	0
(Nalley's)								
chunky, w/o beans, canned, 'Big Chunk'	7.5 oz	270	17	14	810	0	16.0	0
con carne, w/beans, canned	1 serving	281	40	12	1231	13	8.0	26
hot jalapeño, w/beans, canned	7.5 oz	260	14	29	920	0	10.0	0
hot, w/beans, canned	7.5 oz	280	17	30	810	0	10.0	0
w/beans	7.5 oz	260	17	27	880	0	9.0	0
w/beans, canned, 'Thick'	7.5 oz	260	16	29	840	0	9.0	0
(Natural Touch)								
vegetarian, 'Low Fat Vegetarian Chili'	1 cup	170	18	21	870	11	1.0	0
vegetarian, spicy, canned	2/3 cup	230	12	19	890	0	12.0	0
(Nestlé)								
spicy, w/beans, canned, 'Chef Mate'	1 cup	423	17	33	1485	4	24.7	56
w/beans, canned 'Chef Mate'	1 cup	412	18	29	1171	11	25.0	56
w/o beans, canned, 'Chef Mate'	1 cup	430	19	18	1588	3	31.6	85
(Norpac) w/beans, vegetarian, lowfat. 'Soup Supreme'	1 cup	130	7	27	1150	8	1.0	0
(Old El Paso)	1 serving	249	18	22	588	10	10.3	36
(Open Range)								
vegetarian, plain, canned	4.41 oz	176	9	9	608	3	12.8	24
vegetarian, w/beans, canned	4.5 oz	136	9	13	645	5	8.0	13
w/beans, food service product	1 cup	281	17	25	1291	10	16.0	26
w/o beans, food service product	1 cup	353	18	19	1216	6	25.6	48
(Right Course) vegetarian, frozen	9.75 oz	280	9	45	590	0	7.0	0
(Shelton's)								
chicken, mild or spicy	1 cup	210	21	26	970	7	3.0	45
turkey, mild or spicy	1 cup	210	19	26	990	4	4.0	45

Food Name	Serv. Size	Total Cal.	Prot. gms	Carbs gms	Sod. mgs	Fiber gms	Fat gms	Chol. mgs
(Stagg)								
chicken, w/beans, canned	7.5 oz	200	14	21	0	0	6.0	0
chicken, w/beans, canned, 'Ranch House'	7.5 oz	210	17	26	0	0	5.0	0
country, w/beans, canned	7.5 oz	270	14	25	0	0	12.0	0
w/beans, canned, 'Chunkero'	1 cup	330	19	28	880	16	15.0	40
w/beans, canned, 'Classic'	1 cup	324	17	29	825	7	16.3	42
w/beans, canned, 'Country'	1 cup	319	15	29	1131	6	15.8	40
w/beans, canned, 'Dynamite'	1 cup	333	18	31	862	8	15.4	44
w/beans, canned, 'Laredo'	7.5 oz	260	15	22	0	0	12.0	0
w/beans, canned, 'Ranchhouse'	1 cup	284	19	32	813	9	8.9	47
w/beans, canned, 'Silverado'	1 cup	227	18	33	865	8	2.8	40
w/o beans, canned, 'Steak House'	7.5 oz	300	16	17	0	0	19.0	0
(Stouffer's)								
con carne, w/beans, frozen	8.75 oz	280	20	28	910	0	10.0	0
con carne, w/beans, frozen, food service product	4 oz	128	8	12	376	4	4.8	23
w/beans	1 entrée	270	15	29	1130	8	10.0	35
(Swanson) con carne, frozen, 'Homestyle Recipe'	8.25 oz	270	20	26	740	0	10.0	0
(Top Shelf) con carne suprema, packaged	1 serving	320	24	30	1140	0	12.0	65
(Tyson) chicken, frozen, wholesale club item	3.5 oz	105	8	11	420	0	3.0	0
(Van Camp's)								
w/beans, canned	1 cup	352	15	21	1215	2	23.2	0
w/franks, w/o beans, canned, 'ChileeWeenee'	1 cup	309	14	28	1057	2	15.7	0
w/o beans, canned	1 cup	412	15	12	1499	2	33.5	0
(Wolf Brand)								
extra spicy, w/beans, canned	7.75 oz	324	14	21	926	2	20.6	0
extra spicy, w/o beans, canned	7.5 oz	363	19	15	962	2	24.9	0
w/beans, canned	8 oz	345	15	22	1013	2	22.0	0
w/o beans, canned	8 oz	387	21	16	1042	2	26.6	0
w/o beans, canned, 'Chili-Mac'	7.75 oz	317	12	23	854	1	19.9	0
(Worthington)								
vegetarian, 'Chili'	1 cup	290	19	21	1130	9	15.0	0
vegetarian, 'Low Fat Chili'	1 cup	170	18	21	870	11	1.0	0
CHILI BEANS. See BEANS, CHILI, CANNED.								
CHILI MIX								
(Gebhardt) 'Chili Quik' mix only	1.5 oz pkt	82	3	17	2784	3	1.1	0
(Mountain House)								
w/beans, freeze-dried, prepared	1 cup	390	20	38	153	0	16.0	0
w/beef, freeze-dried, 'Chili Mac' prepared	1 cup	250	12	31	115	0	8.0	0
(Old El Paso)								
'Chili con Carne' prepared	1 cup	162	19	8	510	2	7.0	47
w/beans, prepared	1 cup	217	15	17	480	6	10.0	32
CHILI PEPPER. See PEPPER, CHILI. See also under PEPPER, GROUND.								
CHILI POWDER. See under SEASONING MIX.								
CHILI SEASONING. See under SEASONING MIX.								
CHIMICHANGA								
(Banquet)	1 entrée	500	13	56	1180	9	24.0	20
(Fiesta Cafe) beef and bean, frozen	1 serving	422	24	56	804	6	11.6	36
(Marquez) shredded beef 'Primera'	1 chimichanga	380	13	42	890	2	17.0	30
(Old El Paso)								
bean and cheese, frozen	1 pkg	380	12	40	610	0	19.0	20
beef, frozen	1 piece	370	12	34	470	0	21.0	0
beef and cheese, frozen, 'Festive Dinners'	11 oz	510	22	53	1400	0	23.0	0
beef and pork, frozen	1 pkg	340	13	35	700	0	16.0	0
beef, frozen, 'Festive Dinners'	11 oz	540	23	65	1200	0	21.0	0
chicken, frozen	1 piece	360	13	33	470	0	20.0	0
CHINESE APPLE. See POMEGRANATE.								

Food Name	Serv. Size	Total Cal.	Prot. gms	Carbs gms	Sod. mgs	Fiber gms	Fat gms	Chol. mgs
CHINESE BROCCOLI. See BROCCOLI, CHINESE.								
CHINESE CABBAGE. See BOK CHOY.								
CHINESE DATE								
dried	1 oz	81	1.0	20.1	3	>.9 c	0.3	0
raw, seeded	1 oz	22	0.3	5.7	1	>.4 c	0.1	0
raw, w/seeds	1 lb	331	5.1	85.3	11	>5.9 c	0.8	0
CHINESE FUNGUS/Jew's ear/pepeao								
approx 0.2 oz	1 piece	2	0.0	0.4	0	0	(tr)	0
dried	1 cup	72	1	19	17	na	0.1	0
sliced	1/2 cup	13	0.2	3.3	5	0	(tr)	0
trimmed	1 oz	7	0.1	1.9	3	0	na	0
untrimmed	1 lb	111	2.1	30.0	41	0	0.2	0
CHINESE GOOSEBERRY. See KIWI FRUIT.								
CHINESE JUJUBE. See JUJUBE, CHINESE.								
CHINESE NOODLE. See under NOODLE								
CHINESE PARSLEY LEAF. See CORIANDER LEAF.								
CHINESE PARSLEY SEED. See CORIANDER SEED.								
CHINESE PEA PODS. See PEAS, SNOW.								
CHINESE PEAR. See ASIAN PEAR.								
CHINESE RADISH. See DAIKON.								
CHINESE WATERMELON. See GOURD, WHITE.								
CHINESE YAM. See JICAMA.								
CHIVES								
Fresh								
raw	1 oz	7	0.8	1.1	2	0.9	0.2	0
raw, chopped	1 tbsp	1	0.1	0.1	0	0.1	0.0	0
raw, chopped	1 tsp	0	0.0	0.0	0	na	0.0	0
Dried (McCormick/Schilling)	1 tsp	1	0	0	0	0	0.0	0
Freeze-dried								
	1/4 cup	2	0.2	0.5	1	>.1 c	0.0	0
	1 tbsp	1	0.0	0.1	0	tr	0.0	0
(McCormick/Schilling)	1 tsp	1	0	0	0	0	0.0	0
(Tone's)	1 tsp	1	0	0	0	0	0.0	0
CHOCOLATE. See CHOCOLATE, BAKING. See also under CANDY.								
CHOCOLATE, BAKING								
Bars								
bittersweet (Ghirardelli)	1 bar	551	7	63	8	9	39.3	0
dark, dark (Ghirardelli)	1 bar	570	5	68	6	6	38.0	0
semisweet (Baker's)	1/2 bar	70	1	8	0	1	4.5	0
semisweet (Ghirardelli)	1 bar	555	6	66	7	8	38.1	9
semisweet (Nestlé)	1 oz	160	2	16	0	0	9.0	0
semisweet, 'Premium' (Hershey's)	1 oz	140	1	16	0	0	8.0	0
unsweetened (Baker's)	1/2 bar	70	2	4	0	2	7.0	0
unsweetened (Ghirardelli)	1 serving	571	14	33	16	17	59.9	0
unsweetened (Hershey's)	1 oz	190	4	7	5	0	16.0	0
unsweetened (Nestlé)	1 oz	180	4	9	0	0	14.0	0
unsweetened, 'Premium' (Hershey's)	1 oz	190	4	7	5	0	16.0	0
white (Baker's)	1/2 bar	80	1	8	15	0	4.5	3
white, classic (Ghirardelli)	1 bar	627	6	66	111	0	39.5	13
white, 'Premier' (Nestlé)	1 oz	150	2	18	15	0	9.0	0
Chips								
less fat (Hershey's)	1 tbsp	60	1	10	0	0	3.5	0
milk chocolate (Baker's)	1/2 oz	70	1	9	10	0	4.0	0
milk chocolate (Hershey's)	1/4 cup	220	2	27	55	0	12.0	10
milk chocolate (Hershey's)	1 oz	150	2	27	55	0	12.0	10
milk chocolate (Hershey's)	1 tbsp	79	1	9	16	0	4.2	2

Food Name	Serv. Size	Total Cal.	Prot. gms	Carbs gms	Sod. mgs	Fiber gms	Fat gms	Chol. mgs
chips, milk chocolate, 'Big Chips' *(Baker's)*	1/4 cup	240	3	30	40	0	13.0	10
milk chocolate, 'Mini Baking Bits' *(M&M Mars)*	1 oz	142	2	20	20	0	6.6	4
mint chocolate *(Hershey's)*	1.5 oz	230	2	28	1	0	12.0	0
semisweet *(Baker's)*	1/2 oz	60	1	9	0	1	3.5	0
semisweet *(Hershey's)*	1.5 oz	220	2	27	0	0	12.0	0
semisweet, 'Big Chips' *(Baker's)*	1/4 cup	220	2	31	0	0	13.0	0
semisweet, mini, approx 1/4 cup *(Hershey's)*	1.5 oz	220	2	26	5	0	12.0	0
semisweet, 'Mini Baking Bits' *(M&M Mars)*	1 oz	146	2	18	0	2	7.4	0
white *(Hershey's)*	1.5 oz	240	3	25	65	0	14.0	0
Chunks								
milk chocolate *(Hershey's)*	12 pieces	160	2	16	25	0	9.0	10
semisweet *(Hershey's)*	1 oz	140	1	15	0	0	8.0	0
semisweet *(Saco Foods)*	12-oz bag	466	4	67	26	0	26.5	0
white, 'Premier Treasures' *(Nestlé)*	1 oz	160	2	15	25	0	10.0	0
Liquid, unsweetened, premelted, 'Choco Bake' *(Nestlé)*	1 oz	190	4	7	0	0	16.0	0
Shreds *(Tone's)*	1 tsp	21	0	2	1	0	1.4	0
Squares, Mexican	1 square	85	1	15	1	1	3.1	0
CHOCOLATE FLAVORED DRINK. See also CHOCOLATE MILK.								
(Frostee) canned	8 fl oz	200	2	30	160	0	8.0	0
(Yoo-Hoo)	9 fl oz	140	3	27	130	0	1.0	0
CHOCOLATE FLAVORED DRINK MIX								
(Butterfinger) Butterfinger flavored, w/vitamins A and D,								
prepared w/2% milk	8 fl oz	200	8	30	120	1	5.0	20
(Hershey's)								
'Hershey's Genuine' prepared	8 fl oz	150	5	28	85	0	2.0	0
'Hershey's Chocolate Milk Mix' mix only	3 heaping tsp	90	1	22	40	0	1.0	0
(Nestlé)								
chocolate raspberry truffle, prepared	8 fl oz	180	15	23	280	6	2.0	0
classic chocolate chip, prepared	8 fl oz	180	15	24	300	6	2.0	0
classic chocolate chip, mix only	1.13 oz	90	7	12	170	6	2.0	0
creamy milk chocolate, prepared	8 fl oz	180	15	24	280	6	2.0	0
creamy milk chocolate, mix only	1.13 oz	90	7	12	150	6	2.0	0
dark chocolate fudge, mix only	1.13 oz	90	7	11	150	6	2.0	0
'Quik' prepared w/1 cup skim milk	8 fl oz	170	9	31	150	0	1.0	0
'Quik' prepared w/1 cup whole milk	8 fl oz	230	9	31	150	0	9.0	0
sugar-free, 'Quik' prepared w/1 cup 2% milk	8 fl oz	140	9	15	150	0	5.0	0
sugar-free, 'Quik' dry, mix only	1 heaping tsp	18	1	3	35	0	1.0	0
(Swiss Miss) 'Chocolate Milk Maker'	0.67 oz	73	1	17	55	0	0.3	0
(Weight Watchers) chocolate fudge shake mix	1 serving	80	6	12	140	2	1.0	0
CHOCOLATE MILK								
1% fat	1 quart	630	32	104	607	5	10.0	29
1% fat	1 cup	158	8	26	152	1	2.5	7
2% fat	1 quart	715	32	104	602	5	20.0	68
2% fat	1 cup	179	8	26	151	1	5.0	17
2% fat	1 fl oz	22	1	3	19	0	0.6	2
2% fat, vitamin A and D enriched *(Lucerne)*	1 cup	200	8	29	200	0	5.0	25
2% low-fat *(Darigold)*	1 cup	190	8	28	210	0	5.0	17
2% low-fat *(Hershey's)*	1 cup	190	8	29	130	0	5.0	20
2% low-fat, 'Dutch Brand' *(Borden)*	1 cup	180	8	25	180	0	5.0	0
3.5% fat *(Hershey's)*	1 cup	210	7	28	120	0	8.0	0
whole	1 quart	834	32	103	596	8	33.9	122
whole	1 cup	208	8	26	149	2	8.5	31
whole	1 fl oz	26	1	3	19	0	1.1	4
whole, ready to drink, 'Quik' *(Nestlé)*	1 cup	230	7	31	120	0	9.0	30
whole, vitamin D added *(Meadow Gold)*	1 cup	210	8	25	240	0	8.0	0
CHOCOLATE TOPPING. See also DESSERT TOPPING; FUDGE TOPPING.								
(Kraft)	2 tbsp	110	2	26	30	1	0.0	0

Food Name	Serv. Size	Total Cal.	Prot. gms	Carbs gms	Sod. mgs	Fiber gms	Fat gms	Chol. mgs
(Mrs. Richardson's)								
fudge, dark	2 tbsp	130	1	19	55	0	6.0	0
fudge, dark, microwaveable	2 tbsp	130	1	19	55	0	6.0	0
(Nestlé)								
milk, w/almonds, 'Candytops'	1.25 oz	230	2	14	15	0	18.0	0
milk, w/crisps, 'Crunch Candytops'	2 tbsp	220	2	16	40	0	17.0	0
white, w/almonds, 'Candytops'	1.25 oz	230	3	12	20	0	19.0	0
(Smucker's)								
dark, 'Special Recipe'	2 tbsp	130	1	31	45	0	1.0	0
fudge, 'Magic Shell'	2 tbsp	190	1	16	50	0	15.0	0
fudge, milk, Swiss	2 tbsp	140	3	31	70	0	1.0	0
'Magic Shell'	2 tbsp	190	1	16	25	0	15.0	0
nut, 'Magic Shell'	2 tbsp	200	2	25	40	0	16.0	0
CHOP SUEY SEASONING. See under SEASONING MIX.								
CHORIZO. See under SAUSAGE.								
CHOW MEIN SEASONING. See under SEASONING MIX.								
CHRYSANTHEMUM GARLAND								
boiled, drained, 1-inch pieces	1 cup	20	2	4	53	2	0.1	0
raw, 1-inch pieces	1 cup	5	0	1	13	1	0.0	0
raw, whole, approx 8.75-inch long	1 stem	3	0	1	7	0	0.0	0
CHRYSANTHEMUM LEAVES								
raw, whole	1 leaf	4	1	1	21	1	0.1	0
raw, chopped	1 cup	12	2	2	60	2	0.3	0
CHUB/cisco								
raw	3 oz	83	16	0	47	0	1.6	43
smoked	3 oz	150	14	0	409	0	10.1	27
smoked	1 oz	50	5	0	136	0	3.4	9
CHURRO. See under PASTRY.								
CIDER								
APPLE								
(Alpine) spiced	8 fl oz	80	0	21	20	0	0.0	0
(Indian Summer) canned or bottled	6 fl oz	80	1	20	10	0	1.0	0
(Knudsen) and spice	8 fl oz	110	1	28	0	0	0.0	0
(Krusteaz) spiced	8 fl oz	16	0	4	30	0	0.0	0
(Lucky Leaf)								
canned or bottled	6 fl oz	90	0	21	0	0	0.0	0
sparkling, canned or bottled	6 fl oz	80	0	18	45	0	0.0	0
(Musselman's) canned or bottled	6 fl oz	90	0	21	0	0	0.0	0
(Tree Top) canned or frozen, prepared	6 fl oz	90	0	22	10	0	0.0	0
APPLE CHERRY *(Indian Summer)*	6 fl oz	100	1	25	10	0	1.0	0
APPLE CINNAMON *(Indian Summer)* canned or bottled	6 fl oz	90	1	21	10	0	1.0	0
APPLE CRANBERRY *(Indian Summer)*	6 fl oz	100	1	24	10	0	1.0	0
CHERRY								
(Knudsen)								
	8 fl oz	100	1	24	0	0	0.0	0
blend	8 fl oz	130	0	33	35	na	0.0	0
CIDER MIX								
APPLE								
spiced, instant *(Alpine)*	1 pouch	80	0	19	20	0	0.0	0
spiced, instant, sugar-free *(Alpine)*	1 pouch	15	0	4	25	0	0.0	0
(Swiss Miss)	0.78 oz	84	0	20	58	1	0.3	0
CILANTRO LEAF								
dried *(McCormick/Schilling)*	1 tsp	2	0	0	4	0	0.0	0
dried *(Tone's)*	1 tsp	2	0	0	1	0	0.1	0
raw, chopped	1 cup	11	1	2	25	1	0.2	0
raw, minced	1 tsp	0	0	0	1	0	0.0	0
CILANTRO SEED *(Spice Islands)*	1 tsp	6	0	1	1	0	0.3	0

Food Name	Serv. Size	Total Cal.	Prot. gms	Carbs gms	Sod. mgs	Fiber gms	Fat gms	Chol. mgs
CINNAMON								
ground	1 tbsp	18	0	5	2	4	0.2	0
ground	1 tsp	6	0	2	1	1	0.1	0
ground *(McCormick/Schilling)*	1 tsp	6	0	1	0	1	0.0	0
ground *(Spice Islands)*	1 tsp	6	0	1	1	0	0.1	0
ground *(Tone's)*	1 tsp	6	0	2	1	1	0.1	0
ground, fresh *(Durkee)*	1 tsp	8	0	0	0	0	0.0	0
ground, fresh *(Laurel Leaf)*	1 tsp	8	0	0	0	0	0.0	0
CISCO, RAW. See CHUB.								
CITRONELLA. See LEMONGRASS.								
CLAM								
Canned								
baby *(S&W)*	1/4 cup	50	8	2	260	0	1.5	40
baby, smoked *(S&W)*	2 oz	130	9	2	220	0	10.0	20
baby, smoked, in cottonseed oil *(Crown Prince)*	1/3 cup	90	10	2	330	2	5.0	43
chopped *(Gorton's)*	1/2 can	70	12	4	640	0	1.0	0
chopped *(Progresso)*	1/2 cup	70	12	2	140	0	1.0	31
chopped *(S&W)*	1/4 cup	20	4	1	360	0	0.0	0
chopped, w/liquid *(Doxsee)*	6.5 oz	100	14	8	1160	0	1.0	0
chopped, w/liquid *(Orleans)*	6.5 oz	100	14	8	1160	0	1.0	0
minced *(Gorton's)*	1/2 can	70	12	4	640	0	1.0	0
minced *(Progresso)*	1/2 cup	70	12	2	140	0	1.0	31
minced *(S&W)*	1/4 cup	20	8	1	360	0	0.0	0
minced, in clam juice *(Gorton's)*	1/4 cup	20	4	1	360	0	0.0	10
minced, w/liquid *(Doxsee)*	6.5 oz	100	14	8	1160	0	1.0	0
minced, w/liquid *(Orleans)*	6.5 oz	100	14	8	1160	0	1.0	0
mixed species, drained	1 cup	237	41	8	179	0	3.1	107
mixed species, drained	3 oz	126	22	4	95	0	1.7	57
Fresh								
mixed species, boiled or steamed	3 oz	126	22	4	95	0	1.7	57
mixed species, boiled or steamed, small	20 clams	281	49	10	213	0	3.7	127
mixed species, breaded, fried	3 oz	172	12	9	309	na	9.5	52
mixed species, breaded, fried, small	20 clams	380	27	19	684	na	21.0	115
mixed species, raw	3 oz	63	11	2	48	0	0.8	29
mixed species, raw, large	9 clams	133	23	5	101	0	1.7	61
mixed species, raw, large	1 clam	15	3	1	11	0	0.2	7
mixed species, raw, medium	1 clam	11	2	0	8	0	0.1	5
mixed species, raw, small	1 clam	7	1	0	5	0	0.1	3
CLAM DISH/ENTRÉE								
(Gorton's) 'Crunchy Clam Strips' microwave, 5.8-oz pkg	1/2 pkg	270	8	20	350	0	17.0	20
(Matlaw's) stuffed, New England style	2 clams	180	8	21	730	3	8.0	0
CLAM JUICE								
(Doxsee)	3 fl oz	4	1	0	110	0	0.0	0
(S&W)	9.6 fl oz	0	8	0	740	0	0.0	0
(Snow's)	3 fl oz	4	1	0	110	0	0.0	0
all natural *(Reese)*	1 tbsp	0	1	0	100	0	0.0	0
CLAM-TOMATO JUICE								
canned	5.5-oz can	80	1	18	601	0	0.3	0
canned	1 fl oz	14	0	3	109	0	0.1	0
CLARIFIED BUTTER. See GHEE.								
CLOUD EAR FUNGUS								
dried	1 cup	80	3	20	10	20	0.2	0
dried, whole	1 medium	13	0	3	2	3	0.0	0
CLOVES								
ground	1 tbsp	21	0	4	16	2	1.3	0
ground	1 tsp	7	0	1	5	1	0.4	0

Food Name	Serv. Size	Total Cal.	Prot. gms	Carbs gms	Sod. mgs	Fiber gms	Fat gms	Chol. mgs
ground *(McCormick/Schilling)*	1 tsp	5	0	1	4	0	0.3	0
ground *(Spice Islands)*	1 tsp	7	0	1	4	0	0.2	0
ground *(Tone's)*	1 tsp	7	0	1	5	0	0.4	0
ground, fresh *(Durkee)*	1 tsp	9	0	0	0	0	0.0	0
ground, fresh *(Laurel Leaf)*	1 tsp	9	0	0	0	0	0.0	0

COATING MIX. See SEASONING AND COATING MIX.

COBBLER

Fresh

(Awrey's)

Food Name	Serv. Size	Total Cal.	Prot. gms	Carbs gms	Sod. mgs	Fiber gms	Fat gms	Chol. mgs
apple, deep dish	1/8 cobbler	320	2	48	300	1	14.0	0
blueberry, deep dish	1/8 pie	310	2	45	360	2	14.0	0

Frozen

(Pet-Ritz)

Food Name	Serv. Size	Total Cal.	Prot. gms	Carbs gms	Sod. mgs	Fiber gms	Fat gms	Chol. mgs
apple, 4.33-oz pkg	1/6 pkg	290	1	50	0	0	9.0	0
blackberry, 4.33-oz pkg	1/6 pkg	250	2	39	0	0	10.0	0
blueberry, 4.33-oz pkg	1/6 pkg	370	3	50	0	0	12.0	0
cherry, 4.33-oz pkg	1/6 pkg	280	2	46	0	0	10.0	0
peach, 4.33-oz pkg	1/6 pkg	260	2	46	0	0	10.0	0
strawberry, 4.33-oz pkg	1/6 pkg	290	1	50	0	0	9.0	0

(Stilwell)

Food Name	Serv. Size	Total Cal.	Prot. gms	Carbs gms	Sod. mgs	Fiber gms	Fat gms	Chol. mgs
apple, 'Deli'	1/8 cobbler	240	2	39	370	3	9.0	0
apple, light, 'Deli Lite'	1/8 cobbler	140	3	22	300	2	4.5	0
apple, 'Thrifty House'	1/22 cobbler	290	4	45	190	2	11.0	0
apricot	1/8 cobbler	240	3	39	230	3	9.0	0
berry, 'Festival of Berry'	1/8 cobbler	250	3	42	250	3	9.0	0
berry, light, 'Festival of Berry-Lite'	1/8 cobbler	140	3	22	140	2	4.5	0
blackberry, 'Deli'	1/8 cobbler	250	3	39	230	4	9.0	0
blackberry, light, 'Deli Lite'	1/8 cobbler	150	3	24	150	2	4.5	0
blackberry, 'Thrifty House'	1/22 cobbler	320	3	46	105	2	14.0	0
blueberry	1/18 cobbler	270	3	42	250	4	10.0	0
cherry, 'Deli'	1/8 cobbler	250	3	39	280	3	9.0	0
cherry, light, 'Deli Lite'	1/8 cobbler	150	3	24	170	1	4.5	0
cherry, 'Thrifty House'	1/22 cobbler	330	3	47	125	2	14.0	0
peach, 'Deli'	1/8 cobbler	240	3	38	250	3	9.0	0
peach, light, 'Deli Lite'	1/8 cobbler	140	3	22	150	1	4.5	0
peach, 'Thrifty House'	1/22 cobbler	300	4	43	170	0	12.0	0
pecan	1/6 cobbler	440	5	66	310	3	17.0	50
strawberry	1/8 cobbler	260	3	41	200	3	9.0	0

COBNUT. See HAZELNUT.

COCA-COLA. See under SOFT DRINKS AND MIXERS.

COCKTAIL. See also COCKTAIL MIX; LIQUEUR; SHERRY; VERMOUTH; WINE.

DAIQUIRI

Food Name	Serv. Size	Total Cal.	Prot. gms	Carbs gms	Sod. mgs	Fiber gms	Fat gms	Chol. mgs
canned	6.8 fl oz	259	0	32	83	0	0.0	0
canned	1 fl oz	38	0	5	12	0	0.0	0

PIÑA COLADA

Food Name	Serv. Size	Total Cal.	Prot. gms	Carbs gms	Sod. mgs	Fiber gms	Fat gms	Chol. mgs
canned	6.8 fl oz	526	1	61	158	0	16.9	0
canned	1 fl oz	77	0	9	23	0	2.5	0

TEQUILA SUNRISE

Food Name	Serv. Size	Total Cal.	Prot. gms	Carbs gms	Sod. mgs	Fiber gms	Fat gms	Chol. mgs
canned	6.8 fl oz	232	1	24	120	0	0.2	0
canned	1 fl oz	34	0	4	18	0	0.0	0
TOM COLLINS	1 fl oz	16	0.0	0.4	5	0	0.0	0

WHISKEY SOUR

Food Name	Serv. Size	Total Cal.	Prot. gms	Carbs gms	Sod. mgs	Fiber gms	Fat gms	Chol. mgs
canned	6.8 fl oz	249	0	28	92	0	0.0	0
canned	1 fl oz	37	0	4	14	0	0.0	0

COCKTAIL MIX

BLOODY MARY

Food Name	Serv. Size	Total Cal.	Prot. gms	Carbs gms	Sod. mgs	Fiber gms	Fat gms	Chol. mgs
(Holland House) bottled 'Smooth 'N' Spicy'	1 fl oz	3	0	1	329	0	0.0	0

Food Name	Serv. Size	Total Cal.	Prot. gms	Carbs gms	Sod. mgs	Fiber gms	Fat gms	Chol. mgs
(Mr. & Mrs. T)								
bottled	4.5 fl oz	20	1	4	670	0	0.0	0
bottled, rich and spicy	4.5 fl oz	30	1	6	500	0	0.0	0
(V8)	8 fl oz	49	2	9	1256	1	0.0	0
DAIQUIRI								
(Bacardi)								
banana, frozen, prepared w/rum	7 fl oz	210	0	35	0	0	1.0	0
banana, frozen, prepared w/water	7 fl oz	150	0	35	0	0	1.0	0
lime, shelf-stable, prepared w/rum	7 fl oz	210	0	33	10	0	0.0	0
lime, shelf-stable, prepared w/water	7 fl oz	130	0	33	10	0	0.0	0
peach, frozen, prepared w/rum	7 fl oz	200	0	33	5	0	0.0	0
peach, frozen, prepared w/water	7 fl oz	130	0	33	5	0	0.0	0
strawberry, frozen, prepared w/rum	7 fl oz	200	0	34	0	0	0.0	0
strawberry, frozen, prepared w/water	7 fl oz	140	0	34	0	0	0.0	0
strawberry, shelf-stable, prepared w/rum	7 fl oz	200	0	31	15	0	0.0	0
strawberry, shelf-stable, prepared w/water	7 fl oz	130	0	31	15	0	0.0	0
(Holland House)								
bottled	1 fl oz	36	0	9	111	0	0.0	0
instant, dry	0.56 oz	65	0	16	21	0	0.0	0
prepared w/liquor	3.5 fl oz	177	0	18	50	0	0.0	0
raspberry, bottled	1 fl oz	30	0	7	4	0	0.0	0
strawberry, bottled	1 fl oz	31	0	7	3	0	0.0	0
GRENADINE SYRUP *(Roses)*	1 fl oz	65	0	16	27	0	0.0	0
MAI TAI								
(Holland House)								
bottled	1 fl oz	32	0	8	60	0	0.0	0
instant, dry	0.56 oz	64	0	16	4	0	0.0	0
MANHATTAN *(Holland House)* bottled	1 fl oz	28	0	7	5	0	0.0	0
MARGARITA								
(Bacardi)								
frozen, prepared w/rum	7 fl oz	160	0	24	5	0	0.0	0
frozen, prepared w/water	7 fl oz	90	0	24	0	0	0.0	0
shelf stable, prepared w/rum	7 fl oz	210	0	33	10	0	0.0	0
shelf stable, prepared w/water	7 fl oz	130	0	33	10	0	0.0	0
(Holland House)								
bottled	1 fl oz	27	0	6	92	0	0.0	0
instant, dry	0.5 oz	57	0	14	4	0	0.0	0
strawberry, bottled	1 fl oz	31	0	7	3	0	0.0	0
strawberry, instant, dry	0.56 oz	66	0	16	1	0	0.0	0
(Mr. & Mrs. T)								
bottled	3 fl oz	80	1	20	35	0	1.0	0
strawberry, bottled	3.5 fl oz	100	1	24	10	0	1.0	0
OLD-FASHIONED DRINK *(Holland House)* bottled	1 fl oz	33	0	8	6	0	0.0	0
PIÑA COLADA								
(Bacardi)								
frozen, prepared w/rum	7 fl oz	260	1	37	25	0	6.0	0
frozen, prepared w/water	7 fl oz	200	1	37	25	0	6.0	0
shelf-stable, prepared w/rum	7 fl oz	240	0	36	20	0	2.0	0
shelf-stable, prepared w/water	7 fl oz	170	0	36	20	0	2.0	0
(Holland House)								
bottled	1 fl oz	33	0	8	4	0	0.0	0
instant, dry	0.56 oz	82	0	12	1	0	3.0	0
(Mr. & Mrs. T) bottled	4 fl oz	150	1	39	120	0	1.0	0
RUM RUNNER								
(Bacardi)								
shelf-stable, prepared w/rum	7 fl oz	210	0	33	15	0	0.0	0
shelf-stable, prepared w/water	7 fl oz	140	0	33	15	0	0.0	0

Food Name	Serv. Size	Total Cal.	Prot. gms	Carbs gms	Sod. mgs	Fiber gms	Fat gms	Chol. mgs
STRAWBERRY COLADA								
(Bacardi)								
shelf-stable, prepared w/rum	7 fl oz	230	0	34	15	0	1.0	0
shelf-stable, prepared w/water	7 fl oz	150	0	34	15	0	1.0	0
SWEET AND SOUR DRINK								
(Holland House) liquid	1 fl oz	34	0	8	107	0	0.0	0
(Mr. & Mrs. T) bottled	3 fl oz	70	1	17	45	0	1.0	0
TOM COLLINS								
(Holland House)								
bottled	1 fl oz	47	0	11	96	0	0.0	0
instant, dry	0.56 oz	65	0	16	14	0	0.0	0
WHISKEY SOUR								
bottled	1 fl oz	26	0	7	32	0	0.0	0
bottled, w/added potassium and sodium	1 fl oz	27	0	7	11	0	0.0	0
instant, dry	1 pkt	64	0	16	46	0	0.0	0
(Bar-Tender's) powder, prepared w/whiskey	3.5 fl oz	177	0	18	50	0	0.0	0
(Holland House)								
bottled	1 fl oz	37	0	9	105	0	0.0	0
instant, dry	0.56 oz	64	0	16	16	0	0.0	0
COCKTAIL ONIONS. See under ONION.								
COCOA								
baking, 'Premium' *(Saco Foods)*	1 tbsp	15	2	4	51	0	0.9	0
100% *(Nestlé)*	1 oz	80	7	5	5	10	5.0	0
powder *(Bensdorp)*	1 oz	130	6	8	5	0	7.0	1
powder *(Nestlé)*	1.5 oz	180	11	21	6	0	6.0	0
unsweetened, European style *(Hershey's)*	1 cup	332	20	45	42	25	8.0	0
unsweetened, European style *(Hershey's)*	1 tbsp	19	1	3	2	1	0.5	0
unsweetened, powder	1 cup	197	17	47	18	29	11.8	0
unsweetened, powder	1 tbsp	12	1	3	1	2	0.7	0
unsweetened, processed w/alkali, powder	1 cup	191	16	47	16	26	11.3	0
unsweetened, processed w/alkali, powder	1 tbsp	12	1	3	1	2	0.7	0
COCOA, HOT, MIX								
(Alba '66)								
milk chocolate flavor, mix only	0.68 oz	60	6	10	160	0	0.0	0
milk chocolate flavor, w/marshmallows, mix only	0.68 oz	60	6	10	160	0	0.0	0
w/aspartame, mix only	1 pkt	61	5	11	214	0	0.6	2
(Carnation)								
chocolate fudge flavor, mix only	1 pkt	110	1	24	135	0	1.3	1
mocha flavor, 'Sugar-free' mix only	1 pkt	50	3	9	140	0	0.3	2
rich, mix only	1 pkt	112	1	24	102	1	1.1	2
'70-Calorie' mix only	1 pkt	70	3	16	135	0	0.3	1
sugarless, mix only	1 pkt	55	4	8	142	1	0.4	3
w/marshmallows, mix only	1 pkt	112	1	24	96	1	1.0	2
(Featherweight)								
mix only	0.44 oz	50	2	8	110	0	1.0	0
(Finast)								
regular, prepared	6 fl oz	110	2	24	150	0	1.0	0
w/mini marshmallows, prepared	6 fl oz	110	2	24	150	0	1.0	0
(Hills Bros)								
regular, mix only	2 tbsp	110	3	23	55	0	1.0	0
'Sugar-free' mix only	3 tbsp	60	2	9	145	0	2.0	0
(Land O'Lakes)								
chocolate and mint 'Cocoa Classics' mix only	1 pkt	160	4	24	160	0	5.0	0
chocolate and raspberry, 'Cocoa Classics' mix only	1 pkt	160	4	25	160	0	5.0	0
chocolate cinnamon, mix only	1.25 oz pkt	160	4	25	180	0	5.0	0
chocolate mint, mix only	1.25-oz pkt	160	4	25	180	0	5.0	0
chocolate raspberry, mix only	1.25-oz pkt	160	4	25	180	0	5.0	0

Food Name	Serv. Size	Total Cal.	Prot. gms	Carbs gms	Sod. mgs	Fiber gms	Fat gms	Chol. mgs
chocolate supreme, 'Cocoa Classics' mix only ..... 1.25-oz pkt		160	4	25	160	0	5.0	0
(Pathmark)								
chocolate flavor, mix only .... 1 oz		110	2	24	110	0	1.0	0
w/mini marshmallows, mix only .... 1 oz		110	2	24	140	0	1.0	0
(Saco Foods)								
milk chocolate flavor, mix only .... 1 oz		110	2	24	150	0	1.0	0
sugar-free, sweetened w/NutraSweet, mix only .... 1 pkt		50	3	9	150	0	1.0	0
(Swiss Miss)								
Amaretto creme flavor, mix only .... 1.25 oz		150	2	29	220	0	3.0	0
Bavarian chocolate, mix only .... 1 oz		110	1	20	170	0	3.0	2
chocolate Bavarian mint, mix only .... 1.23 oz		142	2	28	231	2	2.3	1
chocolate flavor, mix only .... 1 oz		110	1	24	125	0	1.0	0
chocolate flavor, 'Sugar-free' mix only .... 0.5 oz		50	2	9	130	0	1.0	1
chocolate praline and crème, mix only .... 1.23 oz		142	3	29	223	2	2.3	1
diet, mix only .... 0.26 oz		20	2	3	180	0	1.0	1
double rich chocolate flavor, mix only .... 1 oz		110	2	24	125	0	1.0	0
fat-free, mix only .... 1 serving		50	3	9	197	1	0.3	2
light, mix only .... 0.75 oz		74	1	17	197	2	0.5	0
'Marshmallow Lovers' 'Hot Cocoa Mix' mix only .... 1.2 oz		132	2	24	167	1	1.5	2
milk chocolate, 'Hot Cocoa Mix' mix only .... 1.2 oz		133	2	29	169	1	1.5	2
milk chocolate, sugar-free, mix only .... 1 serving		49	2	10	179	1	0.2	0
milk chocolate, w/marshmallows, 'Hot Cocoa Mix' mix only .... 1.2 oz		132	2	29	181	1	1.5	1
milk chocolate flavor, mix only .... 1-oz pkt		110	1	20	170	0	3.0	1
sugar free, mix only .... 1 serving		51	1	11	159	1	0.6	1
vending machine product, 'Hot Cocoa Mix' .... 1.34 oz		146	2	32	185	1	1.7	2
w/aspartame, w/added calcium or phosphorus, w/o added salt or vitamin A, mix only .... 1 pkt		48	4	9	98	0	0.5	1
w/aspartame, w/added salt and vitamin A, w/o added calcium or phosphorus, mix only .... 1 pkt		48	4	9	168	0	0.5	1
w/mini marshmallows, 'Sugar-Free' mix only .... 0.5-oz pkt		50	3	9	120	0	1.0	0
(Weight Watchers) rich milk flavor, w/marshmallows, mix only .... 1 pkt		60	6	10	160	0	0.0	0
COCOA BUTTER OIL								
.... 1 cup		1927	0	0	0	0	218.0	0
.... 1 tbsp		120	0	0	0	0	13.6	0
COCONUT								
Dried								
meat, creamed .... 1 oz		194	2	6	10	na	19.6	0
meat, sweetened, flaked, canned .... 1 cup		341	3	32	15	3	24.4	0
meat, sweetened, flaked, canned .... 4 oz		505	4	47	23	5	36.1	0
meat, sweetened, flaked, packaged .... 1 cup		351	2	35	189	3	23.8	0
meat, sweetened, flaked, packaged .... 1 oz		134	1	13	73	1	9.1	0
meat, sweetened, flaked, packaged, 'Snowflake' *(Finast)* ... 1 oz		137	1	12	1	0	9.0	0
meat, sweetened, shredded .... 1 cup		466	3	44	244	4	33.0	0
meat, sweetened, shredded .... 7-oz pkg		997	6	95	521	9	70.6	0
meat, sweetened, shredded, 'Angel Flake' *(Baker's)* ..... 2 tbsp		70	1	6	45	1	5.0	0
meat, sweetened, shredded, canned, 'Angel Flake' *(Baker's)* .... 2 tbsp		70	1	6	0	1	6.0	0
meat, sweetened, shredded, premium *(Baker's)* .... 2 tbsp		70	1	6	45	1	5.0	0
meat, sweetened, toasted .... 1 oz		168	2	13	10	na	13.3	0
meat, sweetened, toasted, flaked, packaged *(Baker's)* .... 1/3 cup		200	2	17	85	0	17.0	0
meat, unsweetened .... 1 oz		187	2	7	10	5	18.3	0
Fresh								
mature kernel, in shell .... 1 lb		834	7.9	35.9	47	21.2	79.0	0
mature kernel, shelled .... 1 oz		100	0.9	4.3	6	2.6	9.5	0

Food Name	Serv. Size	Total Cal.	Prot. gms	Carbs gms	Sod. mgs	Fiber gms	Fat gms	Chol. mgs
mature kernel, shelled, grated, packed	1 cup	460	4.3	19.8	26	11.7	43.5	0
meat, raw, shredded	1 cup	283	2.7	12.2	16	7.2	26.8	0
meat, raw, 2 x 2 x 1/2-inch pieces	1 piece	159	1	7	9	4	15.1	0
meat, raw, whole, medium	1 coconut	1405	13	60	79	36	133.0	0
COCONUT CREAM								
Canned								
liquid expressed from grated meat	1 cup	568	8	25	148	7	52.5	0
liquid expressed from grated meat	1 tbsp	36	1	2	10	0	3.4	0
sweetened *(Coco Lopez)*	2 tbsp	120	0	20	10	0	5.0	0
Fresh								
liquid expressed from grated meat, raw	1 cup	792	9	16	10	5	83.2	0
liquid expressed from grated meat, raw	1 tbsp	50	1	1	1	0	5.2	0
COCONUT MILK								
Canned								
liquid expressed from grated meat and water	1 cup	445	5	6	29	na	48.2	0
liquid expressed from grated meat and water	1 tbsp	30	0	0	2	na	3.2	0
Fresh								
liquid expressed from grated meat and water, raw	1 cup	552	5	13	36	5	57.2	0
liquid expressed from grated meat and water, raw	1 tbsp	35	0	1	2	0	3.6	0
Frozen								
liquid expressed from grated meat and water	1 cup	485	4	13	29	na	49.9	0
liquid expressed from grated meat and water	1 tbsp	30	0	1	2	na	3.1	0
COCONUT OIL								
	1 cup	1879	0	0	0	0	218.0	0
	1 tbsp	117	0	0	0	0	13.6	0
(Hain)	1 tbsp	120	0	0	0	0	14.0	0
COCONUT WATER								
liquid from coconuts	1 cup	46	2	9	252	3	0.5	0
liquid from coconuts	1 tbsp	3	0	1	16	0	0.0	0
COD								
Frozen								
(Booth) fillet, 'Individually Wrapped'	4 oz	90	20	0	80	0	1.0	0
(Finast) fillet, skinless	4 oz	80	18	0	200	0	1.0	0
(SeaPak) fillet	4 oz	90	20	0	135	0	1.0	0
(Van de Kamp's) fillet, light	1 piece	250	17	20	510	0	11.0	35
(Van de Kamp's) fillet, natural	4 oz	90	20	0	90	0	1.0	25
ALASKAN/sablefish/skil								
Fresh								
baked, broiled, grilled, or microwaved	3 oz	213	15	0	61	0	16.7	54
raw	3 oz	166	11	0	48	0	13.0	42
smoked	3 oz	218	15	0	626	0	17.1	54
ATLANTIC								
Canned, w/liquid	3 oz	89	19	0	185	0	0.7	47
Dried/salted								
	1 oz	82	18	0	1992	0	0.7	43
	3 oz	247	53	0	5973	0	2.0	129
Fresh								
baked, broiled, grilled, or microwaved	3 oz	89	19	0	66	0	0.7	47
raw	3 oz	70	15	0	46	0	0.6	37
PACIFIC								
baked, broiled, grilled, or microwaved	3 oz	89	20	0	77	0	0.7	40
raw	3 oz	70	15	0	60	0	0.5	31
COD DISH/ENTRÉE								
(Gorton's) cod cakes, canned	4 oz	100	8	16	640	0	0.5	15
(Booth)								
fillet, au gratin, frozen	9.5 oz	280	27	18	1160	0	11.0	0
fillet, Florentine, frozen	9.5 oz	244	20	29	880	0	6.0	0

Food Name	Serv. Size	Total Cal.	Prot. gms	Carbs gms	Sod. mgs	Fiber gms	Fat gms	Chol. mgs
fillet, w/lemon butter sauce and rice, frozen . . . . 9.5 oz		567	22	27	1330	0	38.0	0
fillet, w/mushroom sauce and rice, frozen . . . . 9.5 oz		280	27	19	1010	0	11.0	0
COD LIVER OIL. See under FISH OIL.								
COFFEE								
Brewed								
decaffeinated, prepared w/tap water . . . . 6 fl oz		4	0	1	4	0	0.0	0
regular, prepared w/distilled water . . . . 6 fl oz		4	0	1	2	0	0.0	0
regular, prepared w/tap water . . . . 6 fl oz		4	0	1	4	0	0.0	0
Instant								
regular, powder, mix only . . . . 1 rounded tsp		4	0	1	1	0	0.0	0
regular, powder, mix only . . . . 1 tsp		2	0	0	0	0	0.0	0
regular, powder, prepared . . . . 6 fl oz		4	0	1	5	0	0.0	0
w/chicory, powder, prepared . . . . 6 fl oz		7	0	1	11	0	0.0	0
(Brim) decaffeinated mix only . . . . 1 tsp		4	1	1	0	0	0.0	0
(Kava) regular, powder, mix only . . . . 1 tsp		2	0	1	5	0	0.0	0
(Nescafé)								
decaffeinated, 'Decaf' prepared . . . . 8 fl oz		4	1	1	0	0	1.0	0
regular, prepared . . . . 8 fl oz		4	1	1	0	0	1.0	0
regular, 'Brava' prepared . . . . 8 fl oz		4	1	1	0	0	1.0	0
regular, 'Classic' prepared . . . . 8 fl oz		4	1	1	0	0	1.0	0
regular, 'Silka' prepared . . . . 8 fl oz		4	1	1	0	0	1.0	0
w/chicory, 'Mountain Blend' prepared . . . . 8 fl oz		6	1	1	0	0	1.0	0
(Sanka)								
decaffeinated, mix only . . . . 1 tsp		4	1	1	0	0	0.0	0
decaffeinated, prepared . . . . 8 fl oz		3	0	1	0	0	0.0	0
(Sunrise) w/chicory, prepared . . . . 8 fl oz		6	1	1	0	0	1.0	0
(Taster's Choice)								
dark roast, decaffeinated, freeze-dried, 'Maragor'								
prepared . . . . 8 fl oz		4	1	1	0	0	1.0	0
dark roast, freeze-dried, 'Maragor' prepared . . . . 8 fl oz		4	1	1	0	0	1.0	0
decaffeinated, freeze-dried, 'Original' prepared . . . . 8 fl oz		4	1	1	0	0	1.0	0
regular, freeze-dried, 'Colombian Select' prepared . . . . . . 8 fl oz		4	1	1	0	0	1.0	0
regular, freeze-dried, 'Original' prepared . . . . 8 fl oz		4	1	1	0	0	1.0	0
(Yuban) regular, mix only . . . . 1 tsp		4	1	1	0	0	0.0	0
FLAVORED								
Instant								
(General Foods)								
Belgian café, 'International Coffees' mix only . . . . 1 1/3 tbsp		70	1	12	65	0	2.0	0
café Amaretto, mix only . . . . 1 1/3 tbsp		60	1	8	105	0	3.5	0
café Francais, 'International Coffees' mix only . . . . 1 1/3 tbsp		60	1	7	25	0	3.5	0
café Francais, 'International Coffees' prepared . . . . 6 fl oz		62	1	7	93	0	3.5	0
cafe Francais, sugar-free, 'International Coffees'								
prepared . . . . 6 fl oz		35	0	3	30	0	2.0	0
café Vienna, 'International Coffees' mix only . . . . 1 1/3 tbsp		70	1	11	110	0	2.5	0
café Vienna, sugar-free, 'International Coffees'								
mix only . . . . 1 1/3 tbsp		30	1	3	75	0	1.5	0
cappuccino, Italian, mix only . . . . 1 1/3 tbsp		50	1	10	50	0	1.5	0
cappuccino, sugar-free, mix only . . . . 1 1/3 tbsp		30	1	3	75	0	1.5	0
double Dutch chocolate, 'International Coffees,								
prepared . . . . 6 fl oz		50	0	8	15	0	2.0	0
Dutch chocolate mint, 'International Coffees'								
prepared . . . . 6 fl oz		50	0	8	80	0	2.0	0
French vanilla, sugarless, 'International Coffees'								
mix only . . . . 1 1/3 tbsp		35	1	4	55	0	2.0	0
French vanilla, sugarless, 'International Coffees'								
prepared . . . . 8 fl oz		25	0	5	65	0	0.0	0
Irish crème café, 'International Coffees' prepared . . . . 6 fl oz		50	0	8	15	0	2.0	0

Food Name	Serv. Size	Total Cal.	Prot. gms	Carbs gms	Sod. mgs	Fiber gms	Fat gms	Chol. mgs
Kahlua café, mix only	1 1/3 tbsp	60	1	10	55	0	2.0	0
Suisse mocha, 'International Coffees' mix only	1 1/3 tbsp	60	1	8	50	0	2.5	0
Suisse mocha, decaffeinated, 'International Coffees' mix only	1 1/3 tbsp	60	1	8	40	0	3.0	0
Suisse mocha, decaffeinated, sugar-free, 'International Coffees' mix only	1 1/3 tbsp	30	1	4	35	0	1.5	0
Suisse mocha, sugar-free, 'International Coffees' mix only	1 1/3 tbsp	30	1	4	30	0	2.0	0
Suisse mocha, sugar-free, 'International Coffees' prepared	8 fl oz	25	0	5	35	1	0.0	0
Viennese chocolate, 'International Coffees' mix only	1 1/3 tbsp	60	1	10	30	0	2.0	0
(Hills Bros)								
café Vienna, 'Cafe Coffees' prepared	6 fl oz	60	1	9	35	0	2.0	0
Capri orange, 'Cafe Coffees' prepared	6 fl oz	60	1	9	30	0	2.0	0
Swiss mocha, 'Cafe Coffees' prepared	6 fl oz	60	1	8	10	0	2.0	0
Swiss mocha, sugarless, 'Cafe Coffees' prepared	6 fl oz	40	1	5	25	0	2.0	0
(Maxwell House)								
'Cinnamon Hot Cappuccino' prepared	6 fl oz	60	2	11	100	0	1.0	0
'Coffee Hot Cappuccino' prepared	6 fl oz	60	1	12	110	0	1.0	0
'Mocha Hot Cappuccino' prepared	6 fl oz	70	2	12	80	0	2.0	0
(MJB)								
mocha, banana nut, sugar-free, prepared	6 fl oz	39	1	5	60	0	1.8	0
mocha, cherry, prepared	6 fl oz	53	1	10	17	0	1.4	0
mocha, fudge, sugar-free, prepared	6 fl oz	39	1	5	88	0	1.8	0
mocha, mint, prepared	6 fl oz	53	0	10	16	0	1.3	0
mocha, mint, sugar-free, prepared	6 fl oz	37	1	6	43	0	1.3	0
mocha, prepared	6 fl oz	52	1	10	54	0	1.3	0
mocha, vanilla, sugar-free, prepared	6 fl oz	39	1	5	50	0	1.7	0
(Superior) cappuccino, mix only	1 serving	90	1	13	75	0	3.0	0
Ready to drink								
(Cappio)								
cappuccino, cinnamon, iced	8 fl oz	130	2	25	70	0	3.0	15
cappuccino, coffee-flavored, iced	8 fl oz	120	2	23	75	0	3.0	15
cappuccino, mocha, iced	8 fl oz	130	2	25	65	0	2.0	15
cappuccino, vanilla, iced	8 fl oz	130	2	25	65	0	2.0	15
COFFEE SUBSTITUTE								
cereal grain beverage, mix only	1 tsp	8	0	2	2	0	0.1	0
cereal grain beverage, prepared w/milk	6 fl oz	120	6	10	91	0	6.1	24
cereal grain beverage, prepared w/water	6 fl oz	9	0	2	7	0	0.0	0
(Cafix)								
all natural, 100% caffeine-free	1.5 grams	6	0	1	3	0	0.0	0
(Inka)								
grain beverage, caffeine-free, instant, 'Naturalis' mix only *(Inka)*	1 tsp	0	1	1	3	0	1.0	0
(Kaffree Roma)								
cereal grain beverage, coffee flavor, prepared	8 fl oz	6	0	1	0	0	0.0	0
(Pero)								
cereal grain beverage, caffeine-free, mix only	1 serving	4	1	1	2	0	0.0	0
cereal grain beverage, caffeine-free, prepared	5 fl oz	4	1	1	2	0	0.0	0
(Pionier)								
cereal grain beverage, coffee flavor, mix only	1 serving	6	0	1	0	0	0.0	0
(Postum)								
cereal grain beverage, coffee flavor, 'Instant' prepared ...	6 fl oz	12	0	3	0	0	0.0	0
COLE. See KALE.								
COLESLAW								
fresh	1/2 cup	41	1	7	14	1	1.6	5
fresh	1 tbsp	6	0	1	2	0	0.2	1

Food Name	Serv. Size	Total Cal.	Prot. gms	Carbs gms	Sod. mgs	Fiber gms	Fat gms	Chol. mgs
COLESLAW DRESSING. See under SALAD DRESSING								
COLEWORT. See KALE.								
COLLARDS								
Canned								
chopped *(Allens)*	1/2 cup	20	2	2	15	0	1.0	0
chopped, greens *(Bush's Best)*	1/2 cup	30	2	5	320	0	0.0	0
seasoned w/pork *(Luck's)*	1 cup	60	2	5	290	2	3.0	3
Fresh								
boiled, drained, chopped	1 cup	49	4	9	17	5	0.7	0
raw, chopped	1 cup	11	1	2	7	1	0.2	0
Frozen								
chopped *(Flav-R-Pac)*	1/2 cup	30	2	2	20	2	0.0	0
chopped *(Seabrook)*	3.3 oz	25	3	4	45	1	0.0	0
chopped *(Southern)*	3.5 oz	30	3	5	60	0	0.4	0
chopped, unprepared	3-lb pkg	449	37	88	653	49	5.0	0
chopped, unprepared	10-oz pkg	94	8	18	136	10	1.1	0
no salt added, chopped, drained	1 cup	61	5	12	85	5	0.7	0
COLLINS MIXER. See under SOFT DRINKS AND MIXERS.								
COLORADO PINYON. See PINE NUT.								
COOKIE								
(Archway)								
'Aunt Bea's Pound Cake' 'Home Style'	1 serving	105	1	16	83	0	4.1	15
hermits, 'Home Style'	1 serving	95	1	17	147	1	2.7	5
'Select Assortment'	1 piece	50	1	7	40	0	2.0	5
windmill, old fashioned, 'Home Style'	1 serving	91	1	14	93	1	3.5	0
(Break Cake)								
'Hermit'	1 cookie	230	3	38	280	0	7.0	10
'Striper Wafer'	1 wafer	190	2	23	80	0	10.0	0
(Carr's) 'Hob-Nobs'	1 piece	72	1	10	78	0	3.2	0
(Featherweight) double	1 piece	45	1	6	0	0	2.0	0
(Frookie) 'Trolls'	11 cookies	60	1	10	65	0	2.0	0
(Glenny's) 'Nookie'	1.5 oz	180	3	18	24	0	12.0	0
(Lu)								
'Crokine'	2 cookies	35	1	7	70	0	0.0	0
'Little Schoolboy'	1 cookie	70	1	8	35	0	4.0	0
'Marie Lu'	1 cookie	50	1	8	45	0	2.0	0
'Marie Lu' mini	5 cookies	50	1	8	45	0	2.0	0
'Pims'	2 cookies	95	1	18	25	0	2.0	0
wafer, creme filled	3 cookies	110	1	11	50	0	7.0	0
(Made 'em Myself) ready-to-decorate	0.25 oz piece	45	0	7	35	0	2.0	0
(Mother's)								
dinosaur, original, mini	7 cookies	60	1	9	40	0	1.0	0
wafer, checkerboard	5 cookies	85	1	13	15	0	4.0	0
(Nabisco) wafer, striped, 'Cookies, 'N Fudge'	1 piece	70	1	8	25	0	4.0	0
(Oven Lovin')								
candy	1 cookie	70	0	10	40	0	3.0	0
w/Reese's Pieces	1 cookie	70	1	9	50	0	3.0	5
(Stella D'oro)								
'Angel Bars'	1 piece	76	1	7	0	0	4.7	0
'Angel Wings'	1 piece	74	1	7	0	0	4.7	0
'Angelica Goodies'	1 piece	106	2	16	0	0	4.0	0
'Como Delight'	1 piece	145	2	18	0	0	7.2	0
'Holiday Trinkets'	1 piece	38	1	5	0	0	1.9	0
'Hostess' assorted	1 piece	42	1	6	0	0	2.0	0
'Lady Stella' assorted	1 piece	42	1	6	0	0	2.0	0
'Love Cookies'	1 piece	106	1	13	0	0	5.2	0
'Royal Nuggets'	1 piece	2	0	0	0	0	0.1	0

Food Name	Serv. Size	Total Cal.	Prot. gms	Carbs gms	Sod. mgs	Fiber gms	Fat gms	Chol. mgs
ALMOND								
(Ener-G Foods)								
amaretti, gluten-free	1 serving	141	4	14	36	2	4.7	0
butter, gluten-free	2 cookies	119	2	13	85	1	6.1	3
French, gluten-free	1 serving	104	2	17	31	1	3.6	0
macaroon, gluten-free	1 serving	109	2	16	13	1	4.1	5
(Mother's) shortbread	2 cookies	120	1	13	50	0	7.0	0
(Natures Warehouse) butter	2 cookies	122	2	19	41	0	4.1	0
(Stella D'oro)								
'Breakfast Treats'	1 cookie	101	2	15	0	0	3.6	0
'Chinese Dessert'	1 cookie	169	2	20	0	0	8.9	0
toast, 'Mandel'	1 piece	58	1	10	0	0	1.4	0
AMARANTH								
(Hansa) whole grain, biscuit, organic	1 cookie	120	3	22	50	3	3.0	5
(Health Valley)	1 cookie	90	2	12	30	2	3.0	0
ANIMAL CRACKERS								
(Barbara's Bakery) vanilla	1 oz	145	2	18	85	0	7.0	0
(Barnum's)	12 cookies	141	2	23	160	1	4.0	0
(Finast)	5 cookies	120	2	22	110	0	3.0	0
(Frookie) cinnamon, 'Animal Frackers'	6 cookies	60	1	9	45	0	2.0	0
(Glenny's) peanut butter, 'Noah 'N Friends Animal Cookies'	0.5 oz	65	1	9	35	0	3.0	0
(Grandma's) candied	5 cookies	140	1	20	80	0	6.0	0
(Keebler)	5 cookies	70	1	11	75	0	2.0	0
(Mother's) circus animals	4 cookies	110	1	14	40	0	6.0	0
(Ralston)	12 cookies	130	2	22	80	1	3.0	1
(Sunshine)	14 cookies	140	2	24	125	1	4.0	0
ANISE								
(Biscotti Thins) fat- and cholesterol-free, low-sodium	5 cookies	80	1	20	25	0	0.0	0
(Stella D'oro)								
'Anisette Sponge'	1 piece	51	1	10	0	0	0.8	0
'Anisette Toast'	1 piece	46	1	9	0	0	0.6	0
'Anisette Toast Jumbo'	1 piece	109	2	23	0	0	1.0	0
APPLE								
(Archway) cinnamon 'Home Style'	1 serving	106	1	17	132	0	3.7	0
(Bakery Wagon)								
oatmeal, filled	1 cookie	90	1	14	115	0	4.0	2
w/cinnamon	1 cookie	100	1	17	100	0	3.0	2
w/walnuts and raisins	1 cookie	100	2	17	110	0	3.0	2
(Estee) w/cinnamon, 'Snack Crisps'	0.66 oz	80	1	15	75	0	2.0	0
(Frookie)								
'Fruitins'	1 cookie	60	1	12	25	0	1.0	0
w/spice, nonfat	1 cookie	50	1	11	80	1	0.0	0
(Great Cakes)	4.5 oz	260	10	40	20	21	6.0	0
(Health Valley)								
raspberry, nonfat	2 cookies	67	1	16	33	2	0.0	0
spice, nonfat	1 serving	33	1	8	17	1	0.0	0
w/cinnamon, nonfat 'Mini Fruit Centers'	3 cookies	75	2	17	60	3	0.0	0
w/raisin, nonfat, 'Fruit Chunks'	3 cookies	85	2	19	80	3	0.0	0
(Healthy Times) organic, 'Hugga Bears'	1 oz	120	2	17	38	0	3.0	0
(Nabisco) nonfat, 'Newton's'	2 cookies	100	1	24	60	1	0.0	0
(Natures Warehouse) cinnamon	1 bar	54	1	10	10	0	1.0	0
(Stella D'oro)								
bar, Dutch	1 piece	112	1	19	0	0	3.3	0
pastry, dietetic	1 piece	86	1	13	10	0	3.3	0
(Sunshine) low-fat, 'Golden Fruit'	1 serving	70	1	15	60	1	1.0	0
(Weight Watchers) fruit-filled	1 cookie	80	1	21	35	0	1.0	0

Food Name	Serv. Size	Total Cal.	Prot. gms	Carbs gms	Sod. mgs	Fiber gms	Fat gms	Chol. mgs
APPLE RAISIN								
(Archway)								
'Apple n' Raisin'	1 piece	120	2	20	169	1	3.0	10
filled, 'Home Style'	1 serving	100	1	16	80	0	3.5	7
gourmet, 'Home Style'	1 serving	111	1	17	121	1	4.2	5
(Health Valley)								
almond, 'Fancy Fruit Chunks'	2 pieces	90	2	14	45	2	4.0	0
apple, nonfat, 'Fruit Chunks'	3 cookies	85	2	19	80	3	0.0	0
delight, nonfat	1 serving	33	1	8	17	1	0.0	0
nonfat, 'Fruit Centers'	1 cookie	80	2	17	80	2	0.0	0
nonfat, jumbo	1 serving	80	2	19	35	3	0.0	0
(Pepperidge Farm) raspberry, 'Zurich'	1 piece	60	1	10	30	0	2.0	0
ARROWROOT *(Nabisco)* 'National Arrowroot'	1 oz	130	2	21	85	0	4.0	10
BANANA								
(Break Cake) creme	1 cookie	240	2	37	200	0	9.0	5
(Frookie) nonfat	1 cookie	45	1	10	90	1	0.0	0
(Health Valley) spice, nonfat	2 cookies	67	1	16	33	2	0.0	0
(Natures Warehouse)								
all natural, nonfat	1 cookie	75	1	17	69	0	0.4	0
wheat-free, nonfat	1 cookie	80	1	19	65	1	0.0	0
BLUEBERRY *(Great Cakes)*	4.5 oz	260	10	40	20	21	6.0	0
BRAN *(Archway)* w/raisin	1 piece	100	2	18	95	1	3.0	5
BROWNIE								
(Break Cake) creme	1 cookie	240	2	38	150	0	8.0	5
(Eagle) chocolate fudge, 'Gourmet'	1 cookie	330	5	42	120	3	16.0	15
(Pepperidge Farm)								
chocolate nut, 'Old Fashioned'	2 pieces	110	1	11	45	0	7.0	5
cream sandwich, 'Capri'	1 piece	80	0	10	45	0	5.0	0
BUTTER								
(Barbara's Bakery) pecan, bites, 'Small Indulgences'	1 oz	140	2	16	95	0	8.0	20
(Delicious) frosted, made w/Land O'Lakes butter	1 cookie	88	1	11	44	0	5.0	10
(Fifty 50)								
fructose-sweetened	4 cookies	160	2	20	65	1	8.0	25
fructose-sweetened, low-sodium	1 cookie	40	1	5	20	0	2.0	5
(Hansa) biscuit, whole-grain, organic	1 cookie	130	3	24	75	3	3.5	10
(Keebler)								
chocolate coated, 'Baby Bear'	3 pieces	70	1	10	55	0	2.0	0
chocolate coated, 'E.L. Fudge'	2 pieces	80	1	10	40	0	4.0	5
(Lu) 'Petit Beurre'	1 cookie	40	1	7	45	0	1.0	0
(Mother's)	5 cookies	140	2	20	130	0	6.0	0
CARAMEL								
(Barbara's Bakery) apple minis, nonfat	6 cookies	110	2	24	125	1	0.0	0
(FFV) patties	2 pieces	150	1	20	125	0	7.0	0
(Little Debbie) bar	1 bar	160	1	22	85	0	8.0	0
(Natures Warehouse)								
crisp, all natural, nonfat	1 cookie	80	1	19	55	2	0.0	0
wheat-free, crisp, nonfat	1 cookie	80	1	19	55	2	0.0	0
(Snackwell's) 'Caramel Delights'	1 serving	69	1	13	33	0	2.0	0
CAROB								
(Great Cakes) w/cherry	4.5 oz	280	10	40	20	21	8.0	0
(Heaven Scent) fudge, wheat-free	1 cookie	70	2	15	55	1	1.0	0
(Jennies) macaroon, gluten- and lactose-free	1 cookie	310	2	41	20	6	15.0	0
(Natures Warehouse) fudge	2 cookies	116	1	21	78	0	3.1	0
(Westbrae) 'Rice Malt Snap'	1 oz	140	2	18	70	0	7.0	0
CARROT								
(Archway) cake, gourmet, 'Home Style'	1 serving	120	1	18	176	1	5.0	4

Food Name	Serv. Size	Total Cal.	Prot. gms	Carbs gms	Sod. mgs	Fiber gms	Fat gms	Chol. mgs
(Pepperidge Farm) w/walnut, lowfat, soft, 'Wholesome Choice'	1 cookie	60	1	11	45	0	1.0	0
CHERRY								
(Archway) filled, 'Home Style'	1 serving	100	1	16	83	0	3.5	7
(Natures Warehouse)								
all natural, nonfat	1 cookie	72	1	17	69	0	0.4	0
wheat-free, nonfat	1 cookie	80	1	18	60	1	0.5	0
CHOCOLATE								
(Archway)								
devil's food, nonfat, 'Home Style'	1 serving	68	1	16	79	1	0.2	0
mud pie, 'Home Style'	1 serving	107	1	15	103	1	4.9	5
(Auburn Farms)								
chewy, nonfat	2 cookies	80	2	19	65	2	0.5	0
w/mint, nonfat	2 cookies	90	1	20	95	2	0.0	0
(Barbara's Bakery)								
double chocolate, minis, nonfat	6 cookies	100	2	23	135	1	0.0	0
w/raspberry, 'Cookies & Creme'	2 cookies	120	2	18	80	0	5.0	15
(Betty Crocker) w/peanut butter creme, 'Dunkaroos'	1 tray	140	3	15	140	0	8.0	0
(Biscotti Thins) fat- and cholesterol-free, low sodium	5 cookies	80	1	20	25	0	0.0	0
(Break Cake) wafer	4 wafers	200	2	30	95	0	9.0	0
(Cookietree) fudge, nonfat	1 cookie	120	2	27	180	1	0.0	0
(Delicious) wafer	1 wafer	34	1	2	5	0	2.0	0
(Drake's)	2 pieces	130	2	19	85	0	5.0	0
(Ener-G Foods)								
nut, gluten-free	1 serving	102	2	12	7	1	4.5	0
walnut, gluten-free	1 serving	109	1	11	107	1	6.8	5
(Estee) 'Snack Crisps'	0.66 oz	80	1	15	65	0	2.0	0
(FFV) devil's food, 'Trolley Cakes' 2 oz serving	2 pieces	120	2	25	80	0	2.0	0
(Frookie)								
'Animal Frackers'	6 cookies	60	1	9	70	0	2.0	0
'Funky Monkeys'	8 cookies	60	1	10	60	0	2.0	0
(Grandma's) cookie bits	1 oz	140	2	19	180	0	6.0	0
(Health Valley) fudge, nonfat	2 cookies	70	2	17	20	3	0.0	0
(Heaven Scent) wheat-free	1 cookie	71	2	15	54	1	1.0	0
(Keebler) devil's food, fat free, 'Elfin Delights'	1 serving	70	1	14	110	0	0.0	0
(Lu)								
'Chocolatiers'	2 cookies	85	1	10	10	0	4.0	0
dipped, 'Chocolatiers'	2 cookies	105	1	12	15	0	6.0	0
(M&M Mars) fudge, and crunchy, 'Twix'	1 bar	100	1	11	35	0	6.0	0
(Nabisco)								
'Pure Chocolate Middles'	0.5 oz piece	80	1	9	35	0	5.0	5
cake, 'Mallomars'	1 piece	60	1	8	20	0	3.0	0
devil's food, cakes	1 piece	70	1	15	40	0	1.0	0
w/peanut butter, 'Ideal Bars'	0.5 oz piece	90	1	10	80	0	5.0	0
(Snackwell's) devil's food	1 serving	49	1	12	28	0	0.2	0
(Stella D'oro)								
'Castelets'	1 piece	64	1	9	0	0	2.8	0
'Margherite'	1 piece	72	1	10	0	0	3.1	0
(Tastykake) 'Soft, 'n Chewy'	1.4 oz	171	2	26	111	1	7.0	3
(Weight Watchers)	3 cookies	80	1	13	70	0	3.0	0
CHOCOLATE CHIP								
(Almost Home)	0.5 oz piece	60	1	8	45	0	3.0	2
(Archway)								
	1 piece	50	1	7	40	0	3.0	5
and toffee, gourmet, 'Home Style'	1 serving	131	1	18	124	1	6.1	6
drop, 'Home Style'	1 serving	101	1	15	78	0	3.7	14
ice box, 'Home Style'	1 serving	117	1	15	59	0	5.7	8

Food Name	Serv. Size	Total Cal.	Prot. gms	Carbs gms	Sod. mgs	Fiber gms	Fat gms	Chol. mgs
no sugar, 'Home Style'	1 serving	108	1	16	64	0	5.3	0
rocky road, gourmet, 'Home Style'	1 serving	127	2	18	71	1	5.9	11
rocky road, sugarless, 'Home Style'	1 serving	101	1	15	66	1	4.9	0
(Barbara's Bakery) crisp, 'Small Indulgences'	1 oz	140	2	18	105	0	7.0	15
(Break Cake)	5 cookies	140	2	20	115	0	6.0	5
(Drake's)	2 pieces	140	1	18	110	0	6.0	0
(Duncan Hines) milk chocolate	2 pieces	110	1	15	85	0	5.0	0
(Eagle)								
	1 cookie	190	2	26	170	1	8.0	15
peanut butter, 'Gourmet'	1 cookie	360	7	39	110	4	20.0	15
(Ener-G Foods) potato, gluten-free	1 serving	91	1	12	34	0	3.9	4
(Entenmann's)	3 cookies	140	1	19	85	0	7.0	0
(Estee)	3 cookies	110	1	13	20	0	5.0	0
(Featherweight)	1 piece	45	1	6	0	0	2.0	0
(Fifty 50) fructose sweetened	1 cookie	35	1	4	10	0	2.0	0
(Finast)	1 oz	90	1	18	60	0	7.0	0
(Frookie)								
Mandarin	1 cookie	45	1	7	35	0	2.0	0
mint	1 cookie	45	1	7	35	0	2.0	0
(Grandma's)								
'Big Cookies'	1 serving	200	2	28	125	1	9.0	15
'Rich'N Chewy'	3 cookies	140	1	20	80	0	6.0	5
(Keebler)								
bakery crisp, 'Chips Deluxe'	1 cookie	60	1	7	45	0	3.0	0
chewy, 'Elfin Delights'	1 cookie	65	1	11	55	0	2.0	0
'Chips Deluxe'	1 piece	80	1	10	75	0	4.0	5
'Coconut Chocolate Drop'	1 cookie	80	1	10	60	0	5.0	0
food service product, 'Old Fashioned'	1 serving	80	1	10	60	0	4.0	0
less fat, 'Chips Deluxe'	1 serving	70	1	11	70	0	3.0	0
rainbow chips 'Chips Deluxe'	1 piece	80	1	11	45	0	3.0	5
regular, enriched, 'Rich, 'n Chips'	1 large	67	1	9	44	0	3.2	0
'Soft Batch'	1 serving	80	1	10	70	1	3.5	0
(Mother's)								
	1 cookie	70	1	10	55	0	3.0	0
angel	2 cookies	120	1	14	45	0	8.0	0
(Nabisco)								
'Chips Ahoy'	1 cookie	68	1	9	45	0	3.2	0
chunky, 'Chips Ahoy!'	0.5 oz piece	90	1	10	65	0	5.0	10
chunky, 'Chips Ahoy!'	1 serving	80	1	11	60	1	4.0	10
mini, 'Chips Ahoy!'	0.5 oz	70	1	9	50	0	3.0	0
mini, 'Chips Ahoy!'	1 cookie	11	0	1	7	0	0.5	0
pecan, 'Selections' 'Chips Ahoy!'	0.5 oz piece	100	1	10	65	0	6.0	10
'Rockers' 'Chips Ahoy!'	1 cookie	60	1	8	40	0	3.0	0
walnut, 'Selections' 'Chips Ahoy!'	0.5 oz piece	100	1	9	70	0	6.0	5
walnut, w/white fudge chunks 'Chips Ahoy!'	1 cookie	90	1	11	75	0	5.0	5
(Oven Lovin')	1 cookie	70	0	9	50	0	3.0	5
(Pepperidge Farm)								
'Family Request'	2 cookies	90	1	15	55	0	5.0	5
'Old Fashioned'	2 pieces	100	1	12	45	0	5.0	5
w/pecan, regular, enriched	1 cookie	58	1	8	38	0	2.7	0
(Pillsbury)	1 serving	130	1	17	85	1	6.0	3
(Snackwell's) less fat	13 cookies	130	2	22	170	1	3.5	0
(Soft Batch)	1 piece	80	1	10	70	0	4.0	0
(Tastykake)								
bar	1 piece	193	3	28	97	1	8.4	4
'Soft 'n Chewy'	1.4 oz	174	2	26	168	1	7.3	10

Food Name	Serv. Size	Total Cal.	Prot. gms	Carbs gms	Sod. mgs	Fiber gms	Fat gms	Chol. mgs
CHOCOLATE CHOCOLATE CHIP								
(Lady J.) 100% natural	1 cookie	120	2	15	85	1	7.0	0
(Natures Warehouse)	2 cookies	130	3	16	69	0	6.1	0
(Pillsbury) 'Pillsbury's Best'	1 cookie	70	1	9	35	0	3.0	0
CINNAMON								
(Archway) honey hearts, nonfat, 'Home Style'	1 serving	106	1	25	123	0	0.2	0
(Biscotti Thins) fat- and cholesterol-free, low sodium	5 cookies	80	1	20	25	0	0.0	0
(Natures Warehouse) w/nuts	2 cookies	113	1	19	71	0	3.6	0
COCOA								
(Archway) Dutch, 'Home Style'	1 serving	98	1	17	87	1	3.3	3
(Barbara's Bakery) mocha, minis, nonfat	6 cookies	100	2	23	125	1	0.0	0
(Westbrae)								
'Rice Malt Snap'	1 oz	140	2	17	70	0	7.0	0
w/cocoa chip, 'Rice Malt Snap'	1 oz	130	2	18	60	0	7.0	0
COCONUT								
(Archway) macaroon, 'Home Style'	1 serving	106	1	12	38	1	6.1	0
(Break Cake) macaroon	2 cookies	270	2	34	160	0	14.0	0
(Drake's)	2 pieces	130	2	20	95	0	5.0	0
(Estee)	3 cookies	110	1	14	15	0	5.0	0
(Fifty 50) fructose-sweetened	4 cookies	160	2	18	0	1	10.0	0
(Glenny's) w/almonds and raisins, 'Nookie Bar'	1.15 oz	138	2	18	0	0	3.0	0
(Jennies) macaroon, gluten- and lactose-free	1 cookie	270	2	34	20	5	14.0	0
(Mother's)								
'Cocadas'	4 cookies	120	2	17	150	0	6.0	0
macaroon	1 cookie	80	1	8	40	0	5.0	0
(Mrs. Denson's) macaroon, quinoa	2 cookies	150	2	14	25	2	12.0	0
(Pepperidge Farm) chocolate-filled, 'Tahiti'	1 piece	90	0	9	25	0	6.0	5
(Stella D'oro)								
dietetic	1 piece	52	1	7	10	0	2.4	0
macaroon	1 piece	60	1	7	0	0	3.4	0
COFFEE-FLAVORED								
(Barbara's Bakery) cake crunch, 'Small Indulgences'	1 oz	130	2	18	140	0	6.0	20
(Pepperidge Farm) chocolate, praline-filled,								
'Cappuccino'	1 piece	50	0	6	20	0	3.0	5
CRANBERRY								
(Frookie) orange, nonfat	1 cookie	45	1	10	75	1	0.0	0
(Nabisco) nonfat, 'Newton's'	2 cookies	100	1	23	95	1	0.0	0
(Pepperidge Farm) honey, soft, 'Wholesome Choice'	1 cookie	60	1	11	50	0	2.0	0
(Sunshine) low-fat, 'Golden Fruit'	1 serving	70	1	15	60	1	1.0	0
CREAM								
(Break Cake)								
'Chips & Creme'	1 cookie	140	1	21	130	0	6.0	2
devil's food creme	1 cookie	130	1	20	120	0	5.0	0
w/raisins	1 cookie	140	1	22	120	0	5.0	2
(Delicious) mini	1 wafer	24	1	3	2	0	1.0	0
(Eagle)								
lemon	6 sandwiches	260	3	37	190	0	11.0	0
vanilla	6 sandwiches	260	3	37	170	0	11.0	0
DATE								
(Ener-G Foods) gluten-free	1 serving	76	1	13	75	1	2.3	3
(Health Valley)								
almond, 'Fruit Jumbos'	1 cookie	70	2	10	30	1	3.0	0
delight	1 serving	33	1	8	17	1	0.0	0
granola, nonfat	2 cookies	67	1	16	33	2	0.0	0
w/pecan, 'Fancy Fruit Chunks'	2 pieces	90	2	15	45	2	4.0	0
(Lady J.)								
w/almond, 100% natural	1 cookie	120	2	14	75	2	6.0	0

Food Name	Serv. Size	Total Cal.	Prot. gms	Carbs gms	Sod. mgs	Fiber gms	Fat gms	Chol. mgs
w/pecan, 100% natural	1 cookie	110	1	16	90	2	5.0	0
(Pepperidge Farm) w/pecan, 'Kitchen Hearth'	2 pieces	110	1	15	40	0	5.0	10
EGG BISCUIT								
(Estee) 'Original Sandwich'	1 cookie	45	1	6	5	0	2.0	0
(FFV)								
'Kreem Pilot Bread'	1 piece	60	1	9	60	0	2.0	0
'Royal Dainty' 7 oz serving	2 pieces	120	1	14	90	0	6.0	0
'T.C. Rounds' 1 oz serving	2 pieces	160	1	20	65	0	8.0	0
'Tango' 1.2 oz serving	2 pieces	160	1	26	50	0	5.0	0
(Stella D'oro)								
'Anginetti'	1 piece	31	1	5	0	0	1.0	0
dietetic	1 piece	43	2	7	10	0	1.1	0
dietetic, 'Kitchen'	1 piece	8	0	1	10	0	0.5	0
'Jumbo'	1 piece	47	1	9	0	0	0.7	0
'Roman'	1 piece	137	3	20	0	0	5.0	0
sugared	1 piece	75	2	14	0	0	1.4	0
FIG								
(Estee) bar	2 cookies	90	1	21	60	0	1.0	0
(FFV)								
w/vanilla, bar	1 piece	70	1	12	55	0	1.0	0
whole wheat, bar	1 piece	70	1	11	50	0	2.0	0
(Figaroo) bar	1 cookie	150	2	30	151	2	3.1	0
(Frookie)								
'Fruitins'	1 cookie	60	1	12	25	0	1.0	0
nonfat, 'Fruitins'	2 cookies	90	1	21	75	1	0.0	0
(Keebler) bar	1 piece	60	1	11	70	0	2.0	0
(Little Debbie) snack squares, 'Figaroos'	1 cookie	150	2	31	110	1	3.5	0
(Mother's)								
bar	2 cookies	110	1	23	85	0	2.0	0
whole wheat	2 cookies	120	2	25	105	0	2.0	0
(Nabisco)								
'Newton's'	2 cookies	110	1	20	120	1	2.5	0
nonfat, 'Newton's'	2 cookies	100	1	22	125	2	0.0	0
(Natures Warehouse)								
fruit juice sweetened	1 bar	70	1	12	20	1	1.5	1
wheat-free, bar	1 oz	98	1	19	18	0	2.0	0
wheat-free, fruit juice sweetened	1 bar	54	1	10	10	0	1.0	0
whole wheat, bar	1 oz	98	1	19	18	0	2.0	0
w/apple and cinnamon, bar, wheat-free	1 oz	98	1	19	18	0	2.0	0
w/raspberry, bar, wheat-free	1 oz	98	1	19	18	0	2.0	0
(Stella D'oro) pastry, dietetic	1 piece	89	1	13	10	0	3.7	0
(Weight Watchers) filled	1 serving	70	1	16	50	0	0.0	0
FORTUNE								
(La Choy) food service product	1 serving	112	2	26	11	1	0.2	0
(Umeya)	30 grams	110	4	24	90	1	0.0	0
FRUIT								
(Archway) and honey, bar, 'Home Style'	1 serving	103	1	18	107	0	3.3	6
(Bakery Wagon) honey, bar	1 cookie	100	1	16	70	0	3.0	2
(Barbara's Bakery) w/nuts	1 oz	140	2	18	55	0	6.0	0
(Hansa) whole grain, organic, biscuit, 'Fruit, 'n Nut'	1 cookie	120	2	20	45	1	3.5	5
(Health Valley)								
'Fruit & Fitness'	5 pieces	200	4	40	249	4	6.0	0
Hawaiian, nonfat	1 serving	33	1	8	17	1	0.0	0
tropical, 'Fancy Fruit Chunks'	2 pieces	80	2	13	45	2	3.0	0
tropical, 'Fruit Jumbos'	1 piece	70	1	10	26	2	2.0	0
tropical, nonfat, 'Fruit Centers'	1 cookie	80	2	17	80	2	0.0	0
(Nabisco) chewy, nonfat, 'Newton's'	2 cookies	100	1	22	115	1	0.0	0

Food Name	Serv. Size	Total Cal.	Prot. gms	Carbs gms	Sod. mgs	Fiber gms	Fat gms	Chol. mgs
(Stella D'oro) slices .... 1 piece		60	1	9	0	0	2.2	0
FUDGE								
(Almost Home) w/chocolate chips .... 0.5 oz piece		70	1	9	50	0	3.0	2
(Eagle) w/chocolate chips .... 1 cookie		260	3	36	120	3	11.0	20
(Estee) .... 1 cookie		30	1	4	0	0	1.0	0
(Grandma's)								
'Big Cookies' .... 2 pieces		350	4	54	380	0	13.0	5
w/chocolate chips, 'Big Cookies' .... 1 serving		190	2	28	80	1	7.0	10
(Mother's) wafer, 'Flaky Flix' .... 2 cookies		130	1	14	30	0	9.0	0
(Nabisco)								
middles .... 0.5 oz piece		80	1	9	35	0	5.0	5
mini bites, 'Little Fudgies' 'Chips Ahoy!' .... 1 oz		230	3	27	105	0	12.0	0
snaps .... 4 pieces		70	1	11	75	0	2.0	2
wafer, 'Famous Wafers' .... 5 pieces		70	1	11	110	0	2.0	2
w/caramel and peanuts, 'Heyday Bars' .... 0.75 oz		110	2	13	40	1	6.0	0
(Stella D'oro) 'Swiss' .... 1 piece		68	1	9	0	0	3.4	0
(Tastykake) bar .... 1.8 oz		205	2	35	155	1	6.8	6
GINGER								
(Archway)								
snap, 54 per package .... 1 piece		35	0	6	30	0	1.0	0
snap, 80 per package .... 1 piece		25	1	4	20	0	1.0	0
snap, iced, 'Home Style' .... 1 serving		172	1	26	132	0	7.0	0
snap, less fat, 'Home Style' .... 1 serving		136	1	25	141	0	3.6	0
(Break Cake) snap .... 5 cookies		130	2	20	110	0	5.0	0
(Delicious) snap .... 0.5 oz		64	1	11	78	0	1.7	1
(Eagle) 'Gourmet' .... 1 cookie		240	4	49	180	0	3.5	20
(Ener-G Foods) gluten-free .... 1 serving		75	1	12	134	1	2.7	3
(FFV) boys .... 1.25 oz pkg		150	2	26	210	0	5.0	0
(Frookie) spice .... 1 cookie		45	1	7	35	0	2.0	0
(Little Debbie) .... 1 cookie		90	1	15	60	0	3.0	5
(Sunshine) snap .... 5 pieces		100	1	16	120	0	3.0	0
(Westbrae) 'Rice Malt Snap' .... 1 oz		130	2	20	140	0	5.0	0
GRAHAM								
(Betty Crocker)								
cinnamon, w/vanilla frosting, 'Dunkaroos' .... 1 serving		130	1	21	60	0	4.5	0
w/chocolate frosting, 'Dunkaroos' .... 1 tray		130	1	19	70	0	5.0	0
w/vanilla frosting, 'Dunkaroos' .... 1 tray		130	1	21	60	0	5.0	0
(Carafection)								
honey, carob coated, 'Original' .... 1 oz		139	2	17	26	0	7.0	0
mint honey, carob coated .... 1 oz		139	2	17	26	0	7.0	0
(Carr's) wheat and honey, 'Home Wheat Graham' .... 1 piece		74	1	11	1	0	3.3	0
(Delicious)								
w/cinnamon .... 0.5 oz		60	1	11	50	0	2.0	0
w/honey .... 0.5 oz		60	1	11	50	0	2.0	0
(Eagle) peanut butter .... 6 sandwiches		250	4	36	200	1	10.0	0
(Health Valley)								
amaranth, nonfat .... 8 pieces		100	4	23	30	3	0.0	0
honey, 'Fancy' .... 7 pieces		130	3	21	89	4	5.0	0
oat bran, nonfat .... 1 serving		13	1	3	4	0	0.0	0
(Honey Grahams) honey .... 4 pieces		70	1	12	85	0	2.0	0
(Keebler)								
.... 4 crackers		70	1	12	85	0	2.0	0
chocolate, 'Selects' .... 4 cookies		60	1	9	55	0	3.0	0
chocolate, 'Selects' .... 4 crackers		60	1	9	55	0	3.0	0
chocolate, 'Thin Bits' .... 12 pieces		70	1	9	75	0	3.0	0
cinnamon, 'Alpha Grahams' .... 6 pieces		70	1	10	55	0	2.0	0
cinnamon, 'Cinnamon Crisp' .... 4 pieces		70	1	11	85	0	2.0	0

Food Name	Serv. Size	Total Cal.	Prot. gms	Carbs gms	Sod. mgs	Fiber gms	Fat gms	Chol. mgs
cinnamon, fudge covered, 'Deluxe'	2 pieces	90	1	11	60	0	4.0	0
cinnamon, 'Thin Bits'	12 pieces	70	1	10	50	0	3.0	0
honey nut, 'Selects'	4 cookies	60	1	9	70	0	3.0	0
(Mi-Del) 100% whole wheat	1 cracker	60	1	12	110	1	1.5	0
(Mother's)								
cinnamon, dinosaurs	1 cookie	80	1	12	50	0	3.0	0
cinnamon, dinosaurs, mini's	7 cookies	70	1	9	40	0	2.0	0
dinosaurs, original	1 cookie	70	1	12	50	0	2.0	0
(Nabisco)								
	1 serving	119	2	21	185	1	2.8	0
	2 pieces	60	1	11	90	1	1.0	0
apple cinnamon,'Honey Maid Graham Bites'	11 crackers	60	1	11	80	0	2.0	0
brown sugar, 'Honey Maid Graham Bites'	11 crackers	60	1	11	80	0	2.0	0
'Bugs Bunny'	0.5 oz	60	1	11	70	0	2.0	0
chocolate	11 pieces	60	1	10	90	0	2.0	0
chocolate, 'Bugs Bunny'	0.5 oz	60	1	10	80	0	2.0	0
chocolate, w/vanilla creme, 'Bearwichs' 'Teddy Grahams'	4 pieces	70	1	10	60	0	3.0	0
'Chocolate Grahams'	0.5 oz piece	150	3	17	80	0	7.0	0
cinnamon, 'Bearwichs' 'Teddy Grahams'	0.5 oz	70	1	10	60	0	3.0	0
cinnamon, 'Bugs Bunny'	0.5 oz	60	1	11	80	0	2.0	0
cinnamon, 'Honey Maid'	2 pieces	60	1	12	85	0	1.0	0
cinnamon, w/fudge, 'Cookies'N Fudge'	1 piece	45	1	6	35	0	2.0	0
honey, 'Honey Maid'	2 pieces	60	1	11	90	0	1.0	0
honey vanilla	11 pieces	60	1	10	75	0	2.0	0
oat bran, w/honey, 'Graham Bites' 'Honey Maid'	0.5 oz	60	1	11	55	0	2.0	0
vanilla and honey, 'Bearwichs' 'Teddy Grahams'	4 pieces	70	1	10	65	0	3.0	0
(Pepperidge Farm)								
cinnamon, 'Goldfish'	1 oz	130	2	19	130	0	7.0	10
'Goldfish'	1 oz	140	2	18	140	0	7.0	10
honey hazelnut, 'Old Fashioned'	2 pieces	110	1	15	75	0	6.0	0
(Regal)	2 crackers	140	1	19	120	0	7.0	0
(Rokeach)	8 crackers	120	2	21	0	0	3.0	0
(Sunshine)								
cinnamon	1 piece	70	1	11	95	0	3.0	0
'Grahamy Bears'	9 crackers	130	2	21	160	0	5.0	0
GRANOLA								
(Health Valley) 'Healthy'	3 cookies	75	2	17	60	3	0.0	0
(Incredibites)								
w/chocolate filling	1 pouch	170	2	24	150	0	7.0	0
w/peanut butter	1 pouch	170	2	23	160	0	8.0	0
w/vanilla creme	1 pouch	170	2	24	180	0	7.0	0
HONEY								
(Health Valley)								
w/cinnamon, crisp, 'Honey Jumbos'	1 piece	70	1	10	35	3	2.0	0
w/oat bran, fancy, 'Honey Jumbos'	1 piece	70	1	10	22	2	2.0	0
w/peanut butter, crisp, 'Honey Jumbos'	1 piece	70	2	10	24	2	2.0	0
JELLY (Delicious) jelly top	0.8 oz	112	2	14	34	0	5.3	1
LEMON								
(Archway)								
drop, 'Home Style'	1 serving	93	1	15	95	0	3.3	9
frosty, 'Home Style'	1 serving	112	1	17	95	0	4.4	0
nuggets, nonfat, 'Home Style'	1 serving	115	1	27	117	0	0.2	0
snap, 'Home Style'	1 serving	152	2	20	117	0	7.3	7
(Cookietree) poppyseed, nonfat	1 cookie	130	2	28	150	1	0.0	0
(Estee)								
	3 cookies	100	1	14	15	0	5.0	0

Food Name	Serv. Size	Total Cal.	Prot. gms	Carbs gms	Sod. mgs	Fiber gms	Fat gms	Chol. mgs
'Snack Crisps'	0.66 oz	80	1	15	75	0	2.0	0
(Featherweight)	1 piece	45	1	6	0	0	2.0	0
(Westbrae) 'Rice Malt Snap'	1 oz	130	2	20	70	0	6.0	0
MACADAMIA								
(Eagle) w/coconut, 'Gourmet Cookie'	1 cookie	330	5	42	230	3	16.0	20
(Pepperidge Farm) 'Special Collection'	1 piece	70	1	8	35	0	4.0	5
MARSHMALLOW								
(Nabisco)								
cake, chocolate-coated, 'Mallomars'	0.5-oz piece	60	1	9	20	0	3.0	0
cake, chocolate-coated, 'Pinwheels'	1 piece	130	1	20	35	0	5.0	0
(Suddenly S'Mores) fudge graham	0.75-oz piece	100	1	15	90	0	4.0	0
MINT								
(Girl Scout) thin	4 cookies	160	1	20	140	2	9.0	0
(Little Debbie) creme, wafers	1 wafer	150	1	18	40	1	9.0	0
(Snackwell's) creme	1 serving	108	1	19	72	1	3.6	0
(Soft Batch)	1 piece	80	1	10	70	0	4.0	0
MOLASSES								
(Archway)								
	1 piece	100	1	18	155	2	2.0	10
dark, 'Home Style'	1 serving	115	1	20	154	0	3.4	0
iced, 'Home Style'	1 serving	114	1	20	130	0	3.6	0
old fashioned, 'Home Style'	1 serving	105	1	18	138	0	3.0	8
3.5–4-inch diam	1 cookie	138	2	24	147	0	4.1	0
(Bakery Wagon) iced	1 cookie	100	1	17	120	0	4.0	5
(Little Debbie)	1 cookie	86	1	15	92	0	2.6	0
(Nabisco) 'Pantry'	0.5 oz piece	80	1	13	75	0	3.0	0
MUESLI (Carr's)	1 piece	84	1	11	30	1	4.1	0
OAT BRAN								
(Awrey's) w/raisins	1 piece	100	1	14	115	1	4.0	0
(Frookie) muffin cookie	1 cookie	45	1	7	35	0	2.0	0
(Health Valley)								
animal cookies	7 pieces	110	3	20	50	3	4.0	0
w/fruit and nuts	2 pieces	110	3	17	70	3	4.0	0
w/fruit, 'Oat Bran Fruit Jumbos'	1 piece	70	1	10	22	2	2.0	0
w/raisins, 'Fancy Fruit Chunks'	2 pieces	90	2	15	95	2	3.0	0
(Natures Warehouse)								
w/chocolate chips	2 cookies	139	4	17	55	0	6.0	0
wheat-free	2 cookies	129	2	16	54	0	6.2	0
OATMEAL								
(Almost Home) w/raisins	0.5 oz piece	70	1	10	40	1	3.0	2
(Archway)								
	1 piece	110	2	19	90	1	3.0	5
apple-filled	1 piece	90	1	18	115	1	1.0	5
apple-filled, 'Home Style'	1 serving	99	1	16	103	1	3.2	2
date-filled	1 piece	100	1	18	105	1	2.0	5
date-filled, 'Home Style'	1 serving	99	1	17	98	1	3.1	3
golden, gourmet, 'Ruth's' 'Home Style'	1 serving	122	2	18	107	1	5.0	4
'Home Style'	1 serving	106	2	17	87	1	3.8	3
iced	1 piece	140	2	22	107	2	5.0	5
pecan, gourmet, 'Home Style'	1 serving	134	2	16	103	1	6.8	5
raisin, 'Home Style'	1 serving	107	1	17	98	1	3.5	3
raisin, nonfat, 'Home Style'	1 serving	106	1	24	165	1	0.5	0
raspberry, nonfat, 'Home Style'	1 serving	109	1	25	166	1	0.5	0
'Ruth's Golden'	1 piece	120	2	20	122	1	4.0	5
sugar-free, 'Home Style'	1 serving	106	1	16	74	0	5.0	0
w/raisins	1 piece	50	1	7	20	0	2.0	0
(Auburn Farms) raisin, nonfat, 'Jammers'	2 cookies	80	2	19	70	2	0.5	0

Food Name	Serv. Size	Total Cal.	Prot. gms	Carbs gms	Sod. mgs	Fiber gms	Fat gms	Chol. mgs
(Bakers Bonus)	0.5 oz piece	80	1	12	65	0	3.0	0
(Bakery Wagon)								
date-filled	1 cookie	90	1	15	100	0	3.0	2
soft	1 cookie	100	2	15	105	0	5.0	2
w/chocolate chunks	1 cookie	100	2	17	80	0	3.0	2
w/walnuts and raisins	1 cookie	100	2	16	80	0	4.0	2
(Barbara's Bakery)								
raisin, minis, nonfat	6 cookies	110	2	24	105	2	0.0	0
w/raisins	1 oz	100	2	19	50	0	2.0	0
(Break Cake)								
	5 cookies	140	1	20	60	0	6.0	0
w/creme	1 cookie	140	1	21	140	0	5.0	2
(Cookietree) raisin, nonfat	1 cookie	120	2	27	110	1	0.0	0
(Drake's)	2 pieces	120	2	19	50	0	4.0	0
(Duncan Hines) w/raisins	2 pieces	110	1	15	85	0	5.0	0
(Eagle)								
creme pie	1 cookie	310	4	46	340	2	12.0	5
fudge stripe, creme pie	1 cookie	310	3	47	180	2	12.0	5
'Gourmet Oatmeal Raisin Cookie'	1 cookie	330	5	40	190	4	17.0	10
iced	1 cookie	170	2	28	110	1	5.0	0
w/raisins	3 cookies	100	2	14	15	0	4.0	0
(Fifty 50) hearty, fructose sweetened	1 cookie	35	1	5	15	0	1.0	0
(Frookie)								
7-grain	1 cookie	45	1	7	35	0	2.0	0
w/raisins	1 cookie	45	1	7	35	0	2.0	0
w/raisins, nonfat	1 cookie	50	1	11	75	1	0.0	0
(Glenny's) wheat-free, 'Noah, 'N Friends Animal'	0.5 oz	65	1	10	20	0	2.0	0
(Grandma's)								
raisin, 'Big Cookies'	1 serving	180	2	30	240	1	6.0	3
w/apple and spice, 'Big Cookies'	2 pieces	330	5	51	570	0	12.0	10
(Health Valley)								
raisin, nonfat	1 serving	33	1	8	17	1	0.0	0
w/raisins and cinnamon, nonfat, 'Fruit Chunks'	3 cookies	85	2	19	80	3	0.0	0
w/raisins, nonfat	3 cookies	80	2	18	80	3	0.0	0
(Keebler)								
caramel, oatmeal, w/apple, 'Elfin Delights'	1 cookie	65	1	12	55	0	2.0	0
food service product, 'Old Fashioned'	1 serving	80	1	10	75	0	3.5	0
raisin, 'Soft Batch'	1 serving	70	1	10	65	1	3.0	0
w/caramel and apple, 50% less fat, 'Elfin Delights'	1 cookie	70	1	13	80	1	1.5	0
(Little Debbie)	2.75 oz	340	5	52	440	0	12.0	2
(Magic Middles) chocolate-filled	1 piece	80	1	8	30	0	5.0	0
(Mother's)								
	1 cookie	60	1	8	80	0	3.0	0
iced	1 cookie	70	1	10	70	0	3.0	0
w/chocolate chips	1 cookie	70	1	10	85	0	3.0	0
w/walnuts and chocolate chips	1 cookie	70	1	9	60	0	3.0	0
(Nabisco) w/chocolate chips, 'Selections'								
'Chips Ahoy!'	0.5 oz piece	90	1	10	60	0	5.0	5
(Natures Warehouse) w/raisins	2 cookies	135	2	17	44	0	6.4	0
(Pepperidge Farm)								
'Family Request'	2 cookies	90	1	13	70	0	4.0	10
w/chocolate chunks, 'Dakota'	1 piece	110	1	15	70	1	6.0	5
(Raisin Ruckus)								
w/chocolate-covered raisins	1 cookie	70	1	11	70	0	3.0	0
w/raisins, chewy	1 cookie	70	1	10	45	0	3.0	0
(Snackwell's) oatmeal w/raisins, less fat	2 cookies	110	2	20	135	1	2.5	0

Food Name	Serv. Size	Total Cal.	Prot. gms	Carbs gms	Sod. mgs	Fiber gms	Fat gms	Chol. mgs
(Weight Watchers) spice . . . . 3 cookies	3 cookies	80	1	13	75	0	2.0	0
(Westbrae) 'Rice Malt Snap' . . . . 1 oz	1 oz	130	2	19	130	0	5.0	0
ORANGE								
(Archway) frosty, 'Home Style' . . . . 1 serving	1 serving	113	1	17	94	0	4.6	0
(Biscotti Thins) fat and cholesterol free, low sodium . . . . 5 cookies	5 cookies	80	1	20	25	0	0.0	0
(Ener-G Foods) almond, gluten-free . . . . 1 cookie	1 cookie	74	2	9	39	1	3.7	0
(Health Valley) pineapple, nonfat, 'Mini Fruit Centers' . . . 3 cookies	3 cookies	75	2	17	60	3	0.0	0
(Lady J.) pineapple, 100% natural . . . . 1 cookie	1 cookie	100	2	16	175	2	4.0	0
PEACH								
(FFV)								
apricot, whole wheat, bar . . . . 1 piece	1 piece	70	1	11	50	0	2.0	0
apricot, w/vanilla, bar . . . . 1 piece	1 piece	70	1	14	50	0	1.0	0
(Great Cakes) . . . . 4.5 oz	4.5 oz	260	10	40	20	21	6.0	0
(Health Valley) apricot, nonfat . . . . 2 cookies	2 cookies	70	2	19	25	2	0.0	0
(Stella D'oro)								
apricot, pastry . . . . 1 piece	1 piece	93	1	14	0	0	3.8	0
apricot, pastry, dietetic . . . . 1 piece	1 piece	87	1	12	10	0	3.7	0
PEANUT								
(Archway) jumble, 'Home Style' . . . . 1 serving	1 serving	116	2	13	77	1	6.2	4
(Cookietree) crunchy, nonfat . . . . 1 cookie	1 cookie	130	3	28	100	1	0.0	0
(Health Valley) chunky, 'Fancy Peanut Chunks' . . . . 2 pieces	2 pieces	100	2	14	585	2	3.0	0
(Nabisco) creme, 'Nutter Butter Patties' . . . . 0.5 oz	0.5 oz	80	2	8	45	0	4.0	0
PEANUT BUTTER								
(Archway)								
gourmet, old fashioned, 'Home Style' . . . . 1 serving	1 serving	117	2	14	118	1	5.9	9
'Home Style' . . . . 1 serving	1 serving	101	2	12	85	1	5.1	8
(Auburn Farms) nonfat, natural, 'P'nutty crisp' . . . . 2 cookies	2 cookies	90	1	19	90	2	0.0	0
(Bakery Wagon) w/oatmeal . . . . 1 cookie	1 cookie	110	3	12	150	0	7.0	2
(Break Cake)								
. . . . 1 cookie	1 cookie	140	2	18	110	0	7.0	0
wafer, w/peanut butter . . . . 1 wafer	1 wafer	180	2	24	75	0	9.0	0
(Delicious) made w/Skippy peanut butter . . . . 1 cookie	1 cookie	80	2	7	65	1	5.0	0
(Eagle) bar . . . . 1 bar	1 bar	170	2	19	75	1	10.0	0
(Ener-G Foods) gluten-free . . . . 1 serving	1 serving	94	2	11	108	1	4.6	0
(Featherweight) . . . . 1 piece	1 piece	40	1	5	10	0	2.0	0
(Fiber Classic) . . . . 1 serving	1 serving	220	3	36	320	7	9.0	0
(Fifty 50) fructose-sweetened . . . . 1 cookie	1 cookie	40	1	5	10	0	2.0	0
(Grandma's)								
'Big Cookies' . . . . 1 serving	1 serving	200	4	24	200	1	10.0	10
cookie bits . . . . 1 oz	1 oz	140	3	19	125	0	6.0	0
(Keebler) food service product, 'Old Fashioned' . . . . 1 serving	1 serving	80	1	9	80	0	4.5	0
(Little Debbie)								
bar . . . . 1 bar	1 bar	270	4	32	190	1	15.0	0
wafer, w/peanut butter, chocolate covered . . . . 1 serving	1 serving	312	5	31	127	na	18.7	na
(Natures Warehouse)								
. . . . 2 cookies	2 cookies	128	4	18	29	0	6.1	0
w/chocolate chips, ... 2 cookies	2 cookies	139	4	14	50	0	8.5	0
(Pepperidge Farm) w/chocolate chunks, 'Cheyenne' . . . . . 1 piece	1 piece	110	2	13	80	1	6.0	5
(Planters) crispy, 'P.B. Crisps' . . . . 1 oz	1 oz	140	3	17	125	0	7.0	0
(Soft Batch)								
w/chocolate chips . . . . 1 piece	1 piece	80	1	9	55	0	5.0	0
w/nuts . . . . 1 piece	1 piece	80	1	9	60	0	4.0	0
PECAN								
(Archway)								
crunch . . . . 1 piece	1 piece	60	1	8	45	0	3.0	5
iced, 'Home Style' . . . . 1 serving	1 serving	120	1	15	75	0	6.3	6
(FFV) praline . . . . 1 piece	1 piece	40	1	10	40	0	2.0	5

Food Name	Serv. Size	Total Cal.	Prot. gms	Carbs gms	Sod. mgs	Fiber gms	Fat gms	Chol. mgs
(Keebler)								
shortbread, less fat, 'Sandies'	1 serving	70	1	10	50	0	3.0	0
shortbread, rich, 'Sandies'	1 serving	80	1	9	75	1	5.0	3
(Pepperidge Farm)								
chunk, 'Chesapeake'	1 piece	120	1	14	60	1	7.0	5
chunk, 'Special Collection'	1 piece	70	0	8	25	0	4.0	10
PRUNE *(Stella D'oro)* pastry, dietetic	1 piece	95	1	15	10	0	3.4	0
RAISIN								
(Almost Home)	0.5 oz piece	70	1	10	40	0	3.0	2
(Archway)	1 piece	100	2	18	107	1	3.0	5
(Entenmann's) nonfat	2 pieces	80	1	17	120	0	0.0	0
(Featherweight)	1 piece	45	1	6	0	0	2.0	0
(Grandma's) soft, 'Big Cookies'	2 pieces	320	3	54	280	0	10.0	10
(Health Valley)								
jumbo, nonfat	1 serving	80	2	19	35	3	0.0	0
w/nuts, 'Fruit Jumbos'	1 piece	70	2	10	35	1	.3.0	0
(Keebler) iced, bar	1 piece	80	1	11	85	0	4.0	0
(Mother's) iced	1 cookie	80	1	11	45	0	4.0	0
(Pepperidge Farm)								
'Old Fashioned'	2 pieces	110	1	15	115	0	5.0	10
'Santa Fe'	1 piece	100	1	16	70	1	4.0	5
w/bran, 'Kitchen Hearth'	2 pieces	110	1	13	55	0	5.0	5
(Soft Batch)	1 piece	70	1	10	65	0	3.0	0
(Stella D'oro) 'Golden Bars'	1 piece	109	2	16	0	0	4.3	0
(Sunshine)								
	2 pieces	110	1	16	125	0	5.0	0
'Golden Fruit'	1 serving	80	1	15	50	1	1.5	0
(Tastykake)								
bar	1.8 oz	212	3	32	255	1	8.3	17
'Soft'n Chewy'	1.4 oz	161	3	27	158	1	5.4	3
(Weight Watchers) w/spice	3 cookies	80	1	13	75	0	2.0	0
RASPBERRY								
(Archway) filled, 'Home Style'	1 serving	101	1	16	84	0	3.5	7
(Bakery Wagon) filled	1 cookie	90	1	16	125	0	3.0	2
(Frookie) nonfat, 'Fruitins'	2 cookies	90	1	21	75	1	0.0	0
(Great Cakes)	4.5 oz	260	10	40	20	21	6.0	0
(Health Valley)								
center, nonfat	1 serving	70	2	18	20	2	0.0	0
jumbo, nonfat	1 serving	80	2	19	35	3	0.0	0
(Nabisco) nonfat, 'Newton's'	2 cookies	100	1	23	115	1	0.0	0
(Natural Nectar) swirl, 'Incredible Edible Novelties'	1 cookie	220	4	33	115	0	8.0	20
(Natures Warehouse)								
all natural, nonfat	1 cookie	80	2	19	60	1	0.0	0
wheat-free, nonfat	1 cookie	80	2	19	60	1	0.0	0
(Pepperidge Farm)								
filled, 'Chantilly'	1 piece	80	1	14	35	0	2.0	5
filled, w/chocolate, 'Chantilly'	1 piece	90	1	14	35	0	3.0	5
tart, lowfat, 'Wholesome Choice'	1 cookie	60	1	11	35	0	1.0	0
(Weight Watchers) filled	1 serving	70	1	16	45	0	0.0	0
SANDWICH								
(Break Cake) apple	1 cookie	90	1	15	70	0	3.0	5
(Delicious) peanut butter, w/jelly, 'Skippy & Welchs'	1 cookie	120	2	15	90	1	6.0	0
(Ener-G Foods) lemon, gluten-free	1 serving	194	0	30	55	2	8.2	0
(Estee)								
chocolate	1 cookie	50	1	7	15	0	2.0	0
original	2 cookies	110	1	17	25	0	4.0	0
vanilla	2 cookies	110	1	17	20	0	4.0	0

Food Name	Serv. Size	Total Cal.	Prot. gms	Carbs gms	Sod. mgs	Fiber gms	Fat gms	Chol. mgs
w/peanut butter	1 cookie	50	1	5	35	0	3.0	0
(FFV)								
mint	2 pieces	160	2	22	50	0	7.0	0
w/peanut butter	2 pieces	170	2	21	110	0	8.0	0
(Frookie)								
chocolate, 'Frookwich'	1 cookie	50	1	7	30	0	2.0	0
chocolate, w/vanilla filling, 'Frookwich'	1 cookie	50	1	7	30	0	2.0	0
lemon, 'Frookwich'	1 cookie	50	1	7	30	0	2.0	0
vanilla, 'Frookwich'	1 cookie	50	1	7	30	0	2.0	0
w/peanut butter, 'Frookwich'	1 cookie	50	1	7	30	0	2.0	0
(Great Cakes) peanut butter, w/jelly	4.5 oz	280	10	40	20	21	8.0	0
(Keebler)								
butter flavor, w/fudge creme, 'E.L. Fudge'	3 cookies	170	2	24	105	1	8.0	5
chocolate, 'E.L. Fudge'	1 cookie	70	1	9	50	0	3.0	0
chocolate, w/chocolate filling, 'E.L. Fudge'	1 cookie	60	1	8	35	0	3.0	5
chocolate, w/fudge creme, 'Elfin Delights'	1 cookie	55	1	10	50	0	2.0	0
chocolate, w/fudge creme, 50% less fat, 'Elfin Delights'	3 cookies	150	2	27	135	1	3.5	0
chocolate, w/peanut butter, 'E.L. Fudge'	1 cookie	50	1	7	50	0	3.0	0
chocolate, w/vanilla creme, 'E.L. Fudge'	3 cookies	170	2	23	125	1	8.0	0
chocolate, w/vanilla creme, 50% less fat, 'Elfin Delights'	3 cookies	150	2	26	170	1	3.5	0
chocolate-filled sandwich creme, 50% less fat, 'Elfin Delights'	3 cookies	150	1	27	125	1	3.5	0
fudge 'E.L. Fudge'	3 cookies	160	2	23	100	1	7.0	0
fudge, food service product	1 serving	80	1	12	70	0	3.5	0
less fat, 'Elfin Delights'	2 cookies	110	1	19	100	1	2.5	0
praline cream, 'Sandies'	1 cookie	80	1	9	35	0	6.0	0
vanilla, French, 'Classic Collection'	1 serving	80	1	12	65	0	3.5	0
vanilla, French, food service product	1 serving	80	1	12	85	0	3.5	0
(Little Debbie) chocolate	1.8 oz	250	3	35	260	0	12.0	1
(Mother's)								
duplex	2 cookies	105	1	15	70	0	5.0	0
English tea	1 cookie	100	1	14	60	0	4.0	0
fudge, double	2 cookies	100	2	15	75	0	4.0	0
taffy	1 cookie	100	1	12	60	0	6.0	0
w/peanut butter, 'Gaucho'	1 cookie	90	1	12	75	0	5.0	0
(Nabisco)								
chocolate, w/creme filling, 'Big Stuf Oreo'	0.25-oz piece	200	2	27	220	1	9.0	5
chocolate, w/creme filling, 'Oreo'	1 oz	140	1	20	170	0	6.0	0
peanut butter, 'Nutter Butter'	0.5-oz piece	70	1	9	50	0	3.0	0
vanilla, w/creme, 'Cameo'	0.5-oz piece	70	1	10	50	0	3.0	0
vanilla, w/vanilla creme, 'Cameo'	0.5-oz piece	70	1	10	50	0	3.0	0
vanilla, w/vanilla creme, 'Cookie Break'	1 piece	50	1	7	35	0	2.0	0
vanilla, w/vanilla creme, 'Giggles'	2 cookies	60	1	8	20	0	3.0	2
(Pepperidge Farm)								
butter, chocolate filled, 'Brussels'	2 cookies	110	1	13	65	0	5.0	0
butter, chocolate filled, 'Double Chocolate Milano'	2 cookies	150	2	18	45	0	8.0	10
butter, chocolate filled, 'Hazelnut Milano'	2 cookies	130	2	15	30	0	8.0	5
butter, chocolate filled, 'Lido'	1 cookie	90	1	10	30	0	5.0	5
butter, chocolate filled, 'Milano'	2 cookies	120	1	15	45	0	6.0	5
butter, chocolate filled, 'Orleans'	2 cookies	120	1	14	40	0	8.0	5
butter, chocolate mint filled, 'Brussels Mint'	2 cookies	130	1	17	40	0	7.0	0
butter, chocolate mint filled, 'Mint Milano'	2 cookies	150	1	17	60	0	7.0	5
butter, chocolate orange filled, 'Orange Milano'	2 cookies	150	1	17	60	0	7.0	5
(Pitter Patter) peanut butter, cream filled	1 cookie	90	2	12	115	0	4.0	0
(Tastykake) shortbread, w/vanilla creme	0.4 oz	55	1	6	31	0	3.0	0

Food Name	Serv. Size	Total Cal.	Prot. gms	Carbs gms	Sod. mgs	Fiber gms	Fat gms	Chol. mgs
SESAME								
(Glenny's) bite size, 'Nookie'	0.5 oz	60	1	6	8	0	4.0	0
(Stella D'oro)								
dietetic, 'Regina'	1 piece	41	1	5	10	0	2.0	0
'Regina'	1 piece	48	1	6	0	0	2.2	0
SHORTBREAD								
(Archway) sugarless, 'Home Style'	1 serving	107	1	16	47	0	5.4	0
(Break Cake)	5 cookies	140	1	19	70	0	6.0	5
(Ener-G Foods) lemon, gluten-free	1 serving	110	0	16	18	4	5.0	0
(FFV) country style	1 piece	70	1	9	45	0	4.0	5
(Keebler)								
fudge-covered, 'Toffee Toppers'	2 cookies	60	1	10	50	0	4.0	0
pecan, bite size, 'Sandies'	4 cookies	90	1	9	50	0	5.0	5
pecan, 'Sandies'	1 piece	80	1	9	75	0	5.0	5
toffee, 'Sandies'	2 cookies	130	1	16	90	1	7.0	1
w/toffee pieces, 'Sandies'	1 cookie	70	1	8	45	0	4.0	0
(Magic Middles) w/chocolate center	1 piece	80	1	9	25	0	5.0	5
(Mother's) striped	2 cookies	100	1	14	55	0	5.0	0
(Nabisco)								
fudge-striped, 'Cookies, 'n Fudge'	0.5 oz piece	60	1	7	50	0	3.0	0
pecan, supreme, low-cholesterol	1 cookie	80	1	9	45	0	5.0	2
(Pepperidge Farm) pecan, 'Old Fashioned'	1 piece	70	1	7	15	0	5.0	0
SPICE								
(Stella D'oro) drops, 'Pfeffernusse'	1 piece	35	1	7	0	0	0.8	0
(Westbrae) 5-spice wafer	4 1/2 wafers	40	1	8	30	0	0.0	0
STRAWBERRY								
(Archway) filled, 'Home Style'	1 serving	100	1	16	84	0	3.5	7
(Health Valley) nonfat, 'Mini Fruit Centers'	3 cookies	75	2	17	60	3	0.0	0
(Healthy Times) organic, 'Hugga Bears'	1 oz	120	2	17	38	0	3.0	0
(Little Debbie) fruits	1 cookie	130	1	33	105	1	0.0	0
(Nabisco) nonfat, 'Newton's'	2 cookies	100	1	23	115	1	0.0	0
(Natural Nectar) swirl, 'Incredible Edible Novelties'	1 cookie	220	4	33	115	0	8.0	20
(Suddenly S'Mores)	0.75-oz piece	100	1	15	90	0	4.0	0
SUGAR								
(Almost Home) 'Old Fashioned'	0.5 oz piece	70	1	10	80	0	3.0	2
(Archway)								
'Home Style'	1 serving	98	1	17	162	0	3.1	5
nonfat, 'Home Style'	1 serving	71	1	17	80	0	0.2	0
(Cookietree) butter, 'Thaw & Serve'	1 cookie	120	2	18	120	0	4.5	10
(Ener-G Foods) crisp, gluten-free	1 serving	93	3	14	218	2	3.1	2
(Keebler) food service product, 'Old Fashioned'	1 serving	80	1	10	45	0	4.0	0
(Mother's)	1 cookie	70	1	8	35	0	4.0	0
(Pepperidge Farm) cinnamon, 'Family Request'	2 cookies	80	1	12	40	0	4.0	15
SUGAR WAFER								
(Break Cake) strawberry	4 wafers	220	1	28	100	0	11.0	0
(Delicious)								
chocolate, w/strawberry creme	1 wafer	35	1	3	4	0	2.0	0
lemon	1 wafer	35	1	4	3	0	2.0	0
strawberry	1 wafer	35	1	4	3	0	2.0	0
vanilla w/strawberry	1 wafer	35	1	4	3	0	2.0	0
(Estee)								
chocolate, w/chocolate creme	4 wafers	90	1	11	0	0	5.0	0
strawberry	3 wafers	100	1	14	0	0	5.0	0
vanilla	3 wafers	100	1	14	0	0	5.0	0
w/vanilla creme	4 wafers	90	1	12	0	0	4.0	0
(Featherweight)								
chocolate, w/chocolate creme	1 piece	20	0	3	0	0	1.0	0

Food Name	Serv. Size	Total Cal.	Prot. gms	Carbs gms	Sod. mgs	Fiber gms	Fat gms	Chol. mgs
peanut butter	1 piece	25	1	3	0	0	1.0	0
w/strawberry cream	1 piece	20	0	3	0	0	1.0	0
w/vanilla creme	1 piece	20	0	3	0	0	1.0	0
(Fifty 50)								
chocolate, cream filled, sugarless	1 wafer	35	1	4	10	0	2.0	0
w/vanilla creme filled, sugarless	1 wafer	35	1	4	5	0	2.0	0
(Tastykake) vanilla	10 pieces	34	0	4	11	0	1.9	0
TEA BISCUIT *(Nabisco)* 'Social Tea'	0.5 oz	60	1	11	60	0	2.0	5
TOFFEE								
(Delicious) w/Heath English toffee	1 cookie	90	1	10	45	1	5.0	8
(Nabisco) Heath chunk, 'Selections' 'Chips Ahoy!'	1 piece	90	1	5	85	0	5.0	5
(Pepperidge Farm) 'Old Fashioned'	2 pieces	100	1	12	75	0	5.0	5
TOFU *(Health Valley)* 'The Great Tofu Cookie'	2 pieces	90	2	16	29	1	3.0	0
VANILLA								
(Archway) wafer	1 piece	30	0	6	30	0	1.0	0
(Biscotti Thins) fat- and cholesterol-free, low sodium	5 cookies	80	1	20	25	0	0.0	0
(Break Cake) wafer	4 wafers	220	1	28	105	0	11.0	0
(Delicious) wafer	1 wafer	35	1	4	3	0	2.0	0
(Estee)	3 cookies	100	1	14	15	0	5.0	0
(Featherweight)	1 piece	45	1	6	0	0	2.0	0
(FFV) wafer	8 cookies	130	1	19	100	0	5.0	5
(Fiber Classic) 'Original'	1 serving	210	3	37	280	0	8.0	0
(Frookie) 'Funky Monkeys'	8 cookies	60	1	10	60	0	2.0	0
(Glenny's) 'Noah, 'N Friends Animal Cookies'	0.5 oz	65	1	10	35	0	2.0	0
(Keebler)								
wafer, 'Keebler Golden'	1 serving	147	2	22	120	na	6.0	na
wafer, golden, 30% less fat	8 wafers	130	2	25	140	1	3.5	0
(Mother's) wafer, 'Flaky Flix'	2 cookies	115	1	18	25	0	5.0	0
(Nabisco)								
wafer, 'Nilla Wafers'	3 1/2 cookies	60	1	11	45	0	2.0	5
wafer, w/cinnamon, 'Nilla Wafers'	3 1/2 cookies	60	1	11	45	0	2.0	5
(Pepperidge Farm)								
chocolate nut coated, 'Geneva'	2 pieces	130	1	14	50	0	6.0	0
chocolate-coated, 'Orleans'	3 pieces	90	0	11	30	0	6.0	0
chocolate-laced, 'Pirouettes'	2 pieces	70	1	8	20	0	4.0	5
'Goldfish'	1 oz	140	2	19	50	0	7.0	15
'Pirouettes'	2 pieces	70	0	9	35	0	4.0	5
(Stella D'oro)								
'Castelets'	1 piece	72	1	10	0	0	3.1	0
'Margherite'	1 piece	72	1	11	0	0	2.8	0
VANILLA CHIP *(Mrs. Denson's)* macaroon	2 cookies	150	2	14	30	2	11.0	0
WALNUT								
(Archway) black, ice box, 'Home Style'	1 serving	119	1	15	77	0	6.2	10
(Mother's) w/fudge	1 cookie	70	1	8	50	0	4.0	0
(Soft Batch)	1 piece	80	1	10	70	0	4.0	0
WHOLE WHEAT *(Lu)* w/cinnamon, 'Marie Lu'	1 cookie	45	1	8	55	0	1.0	0
COOKIE CRUMB TOPPING								
(Nabisco) 'Oreo Crunchies'	1 serving	52	1	8	58	0	2.4	na
COOKIE CRUMBS								
graham cracker *(Sunshine)*	3 tbsp	80	2	13	150	1	2.0	0
graham cracker, food service product *(Keebler)*	1 cup	550	8	81	480	3	23.0	0
'Nilla' *(Nabisco)*	2 tbsp	70	1	13	55	1	2.5	3
'Oreo' *(Nabisco)*	2 tbsp	80	1	13	140	1	3.0	0
COOKIE DOUGH								
(Pillsbury)								
dinosaurs, ready to bake, prepared	2 cookies	120	2	17	95	1	5.0	5
holiday, ready to bake, prepared	2 cookies	130	1	16	105	0	7.0	5

Food Name	Serv. Size	Total Cal.	Prot. gms	Carbs gms	Sod. mgs	Fiber gms	Fat gms	Chol. mgs
teddy bears, ready to bake, prepared .... 2 cookies	2 cookies	120	1	18	105	0	5.0	5
CANDY *(Pillsbury)* ready to bake .... 1 oz	1 oz	130	1	18	80	1	6.0	5
CHOCOLATE CHIP								
(Mrs. Goodcookie) gourmet, ready to bake, prepared ... 2 cookies	2 cookies	120	1	15	80	0	6.0	0
(Nestlé) ready to bake .... 2 tbsp	2 tbsp	150	2	23	120	1	6.0	10
(Pillsbury)								
.... 1 serving	1 serving	127	1	18	88	1	5.7	na
ready to bake, prepared .... 1 cookie	1 cookie	70	1	9	55	0	3.0	5
(Toll House)								
double chips.................................... 1.2 oz	1.2 oz	150	2	19	60	0	7.0	0
ready to bake .... 1.2 oz	1.2 oz	150	1	20	115	0	7.0	0
w/nuts, ready to bake .... 1.2 oz	1.2 oz	160	2	19	90	0	8.0	0
CHOCOLATE CHOCOLATE CHIP *(Nestlé)* .... 2 tbsp	2 tbsp	150	2	21	110	2	6.0	10
OATMEAL								
(Nestlé) w/Raisinets .... 2 tbsp	2 tbsp	150	2	22	120	2	6.0	10
(Pillsbury)								
w/chocolate chips, ready to bake .... 1 oz	1 oz	120	1	16	95	1	6.0	5
w/raisins, prepared .... 1 cookie	1 cookie	60	1	9	55	0	3.0	0
(Toll House) w/raisins, ready to bake .... 1.2 oz	1.2 oz	130	2	21	55	0	5.0	0
PEANUT BUTTER *(Pillsbury)* prepared .... 1 cookie	1 cookie	70	1	9	75	0	3.0	5
COOKIE MIX								
(Krusteaz) 'Deluxe' prepared .... 1 cookie	1 cookie	120	1	16	126	0	5.0	11
CHOCOLATE CHIP								
(Big Batch) prepared .... 2 cookies	2 cookies	120	1	16	100	0	6.0	0
(Duncan Hines) prepared .... 2 cookies	2 cookies	130	1	20	85	0	5.0	0
(Estee) prepared .... 2 cookies	2 cookies	90	1	13	80	0	4.0	0
(Finast) prepared .... 2 cookies	2 cookies	110	1	16	290	0	5.0	0
(Gluten-Free Pantry) gluten-free, prepared .... 1 serving	1 serving	60	1	12	50	0	1.0	0
(Pillsbury)								
bar, 'Chips Ahoy' mix only .... 1/18 pkg	1/18 pkg	140	1	26	100	1	4.0	0
bar, 'Chips Ahoy' prepared .... 1/18 pkg	1/18 pkg	180	2	26	125	1	7.0	10
(Sweet 'n Low) low-fat, w/ Sweet 'n Low, prepared ..... 4 cookies	4 cookies	120	2	22	30	0	2.5	0
DATE *(Betty Crocker)* bar, prepared .... 1 serving	1 serving	150	1	23	90	1	6.0	0
OATMEAL *(Duncan Hines)* w/raisins, prepared .... 2 cookies	2 cookies	130	2	18	70	0	6.0	0
PEANUT BUTTER *(Duncan Hines)* prepared .... 2 cookies	2 cookies	140	3	15	120	0	7.0	0
SUGAR								
(Duncan Hines) golden, prepared .... 2 cookies	2 cookies	130	1	17	70	0	6.0	0
(Gluten-free Pantry) gluten-free, prepared .... 1 serving	1 serving	130	1	31	130	0	0.0	0
COOKING OIL. See individual listings.								
COOKING SPRAY								
(Canola Harvest) Canola, nonstick .... 0.25 grams	0.25 grams	0	0	0	0	0	0.0	0
(I Can't Believe It's Not Butter) .... 1 spray	1 spray	0	0	0	0	0	0.0	0
(Mazola)								
corn oil .... 2.5-sec spray	2.5-sec spray	6	0	0	0	0	1.0	0
corn oil .... 1 tsp	1 tsp	2	0	0	0	0	0.2	0
(Pam)								
.... 1 serving	1 serving	0	0	0	0	0	0.0	0
butter-flavored .... 1 serving	1 serving	0	0	0	0	0	0.0	0
olive oil .... 1 serving	1 serving	0	0	0	0	0	0.0	0
(Town House) Canola oil .... 0.25 grams	0.25 grams	0	0	0	0	0	0.0	0
(Weight Watchers)								
.... 1-sec spray	1-sec spray	2	0	0	0	0	1.0	0
butter flavor, 'Buttery Spray' .... 1 spray	1 spray	2	0	0	0	0	1.0	0
Canola oil .... 0.33 grams	0.33 grams	2	0	0	0	0	1.0	0
(Wesson)								
.... 0.25 grams	0.25 grams	2	0	0	0	0	0.3	0
lite .... 0.27 grams	0.27 grams	1	0	0	0	0	1.0	0

Food Name	Serv. Size	Total Cal.	Prot. gms	Carbs gms	Sod. mgs	Fiber gms	Fat gms	Chol. mgs
COOKING WINE. See WINE, COOKING.								
CORIANDER LEAF/Chinese parsley leaf								
dried.. 1 tbsp	1 tbsp	5	0	1	4	0	0.1	0
dried.. 1 tsp	1 tsp	2	0	0	1	0	0.0	0
dried *(Tone's)*................................. 1 tsp	1 tsp	2	0	0	1	0	0.1	0
fresh, raw, chopped .... 1/4 cup	1/4 cup	1	0	0	1	0	0.0	0
fresh, raw, whole, med plants .... 9 plants	9 plants	4	0	1	6	0	0.1	0
CORIANDER SEED/Chinese parsley seed								
round *(McCormick/Schilling)* .... 1 tsp	1 tsp	7	0	1	0	1	0.4	0
whole.. 1 tbsp	1 tbsp	15	1	3	2	2	0.9	0
whole.. 1 tsp	1 tsp	5	0	1	1	1	0.3	0
whole *(Durkee)* whole seeds .... 1 tsp	1 tsp	8	0	0	0	0	0.0	0
whole *(Laurel Leaf)* whole seeds .... 1 tsp	1 tsp	8	0	0	0	0	0.0	0
whole *(McCormick/Schilling)* .... 1 tsp	1 tsp	12	0	2	1	2	0.4	0
whole *(Spice Islands)* .... 1 tsp	1 tsp	6	0	1	1	0	0.3	0
CORN. See also CORN DISH/ENTRÉE.								
Canned								
(Del Monte) .... 1/2 cup	1/2 cup	90	3	22	355	0	1.0	0
'Crisp 'N Sweet' *(Freshlike)* .... 1/2 cup	1/2 cup	80	2	18	5	0	1.0	0
'Crisp 'N Sweet' *(Stokely)* .... 1/2 cup	1/2 cup	80	2	13	240	2	1.5	0
'Delicorn' *(Green Giant)* .... 1/2 cup	1/2 cup	80	2	19	350	2	1.0	0
50% less sodium, 'Niblets' *(Green Giant)* .... 1/3 cup	1/3 cup	60	2	14	115	1	0.0	0
in brine, w/liquid *(Green Giant)* .... 1/2 cup	1/2 cup	70	2	18	350	2	0.0	0
kernels, extra sweet, 'Niblets' *(Green Giant)* .... 1/3 cup	1/3 cup	50	2	10	200	2	0.5	0
kernels, 'Niblets' *(Green Giant)* .... 1/2 cup	1/2 cup	80	2	20	310	2	0.0	0
kernels, w/liquid *(A&P)*.......................... 1/2 cup	1/2 cup	80	2	20	350	0	1.0	0
kernels, w/liquid *(Featherweight)* .... 1/2 cup	1/2 cup	80	2	16	10	0	1.0	0
kernels, w/liquid *(Finast)* .... 1/2 cup	1/2 cup	90	2	20	390	0	1.0	0
kernels, w/liquid *(Green Giant)* .... 1/2 cup	1/2 cup	80	2	18	280	3	0.0	0
kernels, w/liquid, 50% less salt, no sugar *(Green Giant)* .... 1/2 cup	1/2 cup	50	2	11	140	2	1.0	0
kernels, w/liquid, 'No Frills' *(Pathmark)* .... 1 cup	1 cup	160	5	38	550	0	1.0	0
kernels, w/liquid, 'No Salt Added' *(A&P)* .... 1/2 cup	1/2 cup	80	2	18	10	0	1.0	0
kernels, w/liquid, 'No Salt Added' *(Finast)* .... 1/2 cup	1/2 cup	80	3	19	10	0	1.0	0
kernels, w/liquid, 'No Salt Added' *(Pathmark)* .... 1/2 cup	1/2 cup	70	2	16	10	0	1.0	0
kernels, w/liquid, 'Nutradiet' *(S&W)* .... 1/2 cup	1/2 cup	80	2	15	0	0	1.0	0
no salt or sugar added, 'Niblets' *(Green Giant)* .... 1/2 cup	1/2 cup	80	2	18	0	2	1.0	0
sweet *(TenderSweet)*............................. 1/2 cup	1/2 cup	100	2	20	340	1	1.0	0
sweet, select *(Green Giant)* .... 1/2 cup	1/2 cup	60	2	15	280	3	1.0	0
vacuum pack, w/liquid, 'No Salt Added' *(Del Monte)* .... 1/2 cup	1/2 cup	90	3	22	10	0	1.0	0
Dried, approx 4 oz prepared *(John Cope's)* .... 1 oz	1 oz	101	3	21	0	0	1.2	0
Freeze-Dried, prepared *(Mountain House)* .... 1/2 cup	1/2 cup	90	2	18	1	0	1.0	0
Frozen								
(Health Valley) .... 1/2 cup	1/2 cup	76	2	17	4	2	0.0	0
kernels *(Finast)* .... 3.3 oz	3.3 oz	80	3	20	5	0	1.0	0
kernels, cut *(Frosty Acres)* .... 3.3 oz	3.3 oz	80	3	20	3	1	1.0	0
kernels, cut *(Seabrook)* .... 3.3 oz	3.3 oz	80	3	20	3	1	1.0	0
kernels, cut *(Southern)* .... 3.5 oz	3.5 oz	98	3	21	20	0	0.7	0
kernels, cut, petite, 'Deluxe' *(Birds Eye)* .... 2.6 oz	2.6 oz	70	2	16	0	2	1.0	0
kernels, cut, 'Portion Pack' *(Birds Eye)* .... 3 oz	3 oz	70	3	18	0	2	1.0	0
kernels, cut, 'Portion Pack' *(Birds Eye)* .... 3 oz	3 oz	70	3	18	0	2	1.0	0
kernels, cut, 'Singles' *(Stokely)* .... 3 oz	3 oz	75	3	18	5	0	1.0	0
kernels, cut, whole *(Flav-R-Pac)* .... 2/3 cup	2/3 cup	80	3	19	10	1	1.0	0
on the cob, half ears. 'Sweet Select' *(Green Giant)* ... 2 half-ears	2 half-ears	90	3	19	10	2	2.0	0
kernels, harvest fresh, 'Niblets' *(Green Giant)* .... 1/2 cup	1/2 cup	80	2	17	40	2	1.0	0
kernels, 'Niblets' *(Green Giant)* .... 1/2 cup	1/2 cup	90	2	19	5	2	1.0	0
kernels, plain polybag, 'Nibblers' *(Green Giant)* .... 1 ear	1 ear	70	2	14	5	1	0.5	0

Food Name	Serv. Size	Total Cal.	Prot. gms	Carbs gms	Sod. mgs	Fiber gms	Fat gms	Chol. mgs
kernels, plain polybag, 'Niblets' *(Green Giant)* .... 1/2 cup		90	2	19	5	2	1.0	0
kernels, supersweet, 'Niblets' *(Green Giant)* .... 1/2 cup		60	2	13	5	2	1.0	0
kernels, 'Sweet' *(Birds Eye)* .... 3.3 oz		80	3	20	0	2	1.0	0
kernels, 'Tender Sweet Deluxe' *(Birds Eye)* .... 3.3 oz		80	3	20	0	2	1.0	0
on the cob *(A&P)* .... 1 ear		120	4	28	0	0	1.0	0
on the cob *(Birds Eye)* .... 1 ear		120	4	29	0	0	1.0	0
on the cob *(Frosty Acres)* .... 1 ear		120	4	29	0	0	1.0	0
on the cob *(Ore-Ida)* .... 1 ear		180	5	39	40	0	2.0	0
on the cob, baby, 'Deluxe' *(Birds Eye)* .... 2.6 oz		25	2	4	10	2	0.0	0
on the cob, 'Big Ears' *(Birds Eye)* .... 1 ear		160	5	37	0	0	1.0	0
on the cob, 'Cob Treats' *(A&P)* .... 2 ears		130	5	28	5	0	1.0	0
on the cob, 5-inch ear *(Seabrook)* .... 1 ear		120	4	29	4	1	1.0	0
on the cob, 5-inch ear *(Southern)* .... 1 ear		140	5	30	0	0	1.0	0
on the cob, 'Little Ears' *(Birds Eye)* .... 2 ears		130	4	30	0	0	1.0	0
on the cob, miniature, 'Mini-Gold' *(Ore-Ida)* .... 2 ears		180	5	39	40	0	2.0	0
on the cob, mini-cob *(Superior Pride)* .... 1 ear		80	3	18	10	1	1.0	0
on the cob, mini-cob *(Trader Joe's)* .... 1/2 cup		90	3	20	230	2	0.5	0
on the cob, 'Niblet Ears' *(Green Giant)* .... 1 ear		120	4	27	10	2	1.0	0
on the cob, 'One Serving' *(Green Giant)* .... 2 half-ears		120	4	26	10	2	1.0	0
on the cob, 'Plain Polybag' *(Green Giant)* .... 1 ear		120	4	22	0	3	2.0	0
on the cob, 6-ear pkg, 'Nibblers' *(Green Giant)* .... 2 ears		120	4	27	10	2	1.0	0
on the cob, supersweet, 'Nibblers' *(Green Giant)* .... 2 ears		90	3	19	10	2	2.0	0
on the cob, supersweet, 'Niblet Ears' *(Green Giant)* ...... 1 ear		90	3	19	10	2	2.0	0
on the cob, sweet, no salt added, mini-cob *(TenderSweet)* .... 1/2 cup		80	2	19	5	0	1.0	0
on the cob, sweet, unprepared, med ears .... 1 ear		123	4	29	6	4	1.0	0
on the cob, 'Sweet Select' *(Green Giant)* .... 1 ear		90	3	19	10	2	2.0	0
sweet *(Birds Eye)* .... 3.3 oz		80	3	20	0	2	1.0	0
sweet, petite, 'Early Harvest' *(C&W)* .... 2/3 cup		80	3	19	10	1	1.0	0
sweet, select, 'Plain Polybag' *(Green Giant)* .... 1/2 cup		60	2	13	5	2	1.0	0
sweet, tender, 'Deluxe' *(Birds Eye)* .... 3.3 oz		80	3	20	0	2	1.0	0
GOLD AND WHITE, canned *(Stokely)* .... 1/2 cup		60	2	10	250	2	1.5	0
GOLDEN								
Canned								
(Pathmark) .... 1/2 cup		90	2	19	330	0	1.0	0
(Stokely) .... 1/2 cup		90	2	20	300	0	0.0	0
50% less salt *(Green Giant)* .... 1/2 cup		70	2	16	175	2	1.0	0
kernels *(Veg-All)* .... 1/2 cup		80	2	19	320	0	1.0	0
kernels, sweet *(Green Giant)* .... 1/2 cup		70	2	18	360	2	0.0	0
kernels, sweet, 50% less salt *(Green Giant)* .... 1/2 cup		70	2	16	180	2	1.0	0
kernels, vacuum packed *(Freshlike)* .... 1/2 cup		100	3	22	260	0	1.0	0
kernels, vacuum packed *(Veg-All)* .... 1/2 cup		100	3	22	260	0	1.0	0
kernels, water pack, w/o salt *(Freshlike)* .... 1/2 cup		80	2	19	5	0	1.0	0
kernels, water pack, w/o sugar, salt *(Freshlike)* .... 1/2 cup		80	2	19	5	0	1.0	0
no salt added *(Del Monte)* .... 1/2 cup		80	2	18	10	0	1.0	0
no salt or sugar added *(Green Giant)* .... 1/2 cup		80	3	18	0	2	1.0	0
no salt or sugar added *(Stokely)* .... 1/2 cup		80	2	16	5	0	0.0	0
'Pantry Express' *(Green Giant)* .... 1/2 cup		80	2	18	210	1	1.0	0
vacuum-packed *(Green Giant)* .... 1/2 cup		80	2	20	330	2	0.0	0
vacuum-packed *(Stokely)* .... 1/2 cup		90	3	22	300	0	0.0	0
w/liquid *(Del Monte)* .... 1/2 cup		70	2	17	355	0	1.0	0
WHITE								
Canned								
(Green Giant) .... 1/2 cup		80	2	20	310	2	0.0	0
(Stokely) .... 1/2 cup		90	3	21	290	0	0.0	0
kernels, sweet, drained .... 1 cup		133	4	30	530	3	1.6	0
kernels, sweet, no salt, vacuum pack .... 1/2 cup		83	3	20	3	2	0.5	0

Food Name	Serv. Size	Total Cal.	Prot. gms	Carbs gms	Sod. mgs	Fiber gms	Fat gms	Chol. mgs
kernels, sweet, no salt, w/liquid	1/2 cup	82	2	20	15	1	0.6	0
kernels, sweet, w/liquid	1/2 cup	82	2	20	273	2	0.6	0
sweet, vacuum packed	1/2 cup	83	3	20	286	2	0.5	0
vacuum-packed (A&P)	1/2 cup	100	2	25	300	0	1.0	0
vacuum-packed (Finast)	4 oz	90	5	20	150	0	1.0	0
vacuum-packed (Green Giant)	1/2 cup	80	2	20	290	2	0.0	0
vacuum-packed (Pathmark)	1/2 cup	120	3	25	350	0	1.0	0
vacuum-packed, 'Niblets' (Green Giant)	1/2 cup	80	3	16	280	2	1.0	0
w/liquid (Del Monte)	1/2 cup	70	2	16	355	0	0.0	0
young, tender, 'Premium' (S&W)	1/2 cup	90	2	20	295	0	1.0	0
Fresh								
kernels, sweet, boiled, drained	1/2 cup	76	3	18	3	2	0.6	0
kernels, sweet, raw	1 cup	132	5	29	23	4	1.8	0
on the cob, sweet, large ears, 7.75 to 9 inches	1 ear	123	5	27	21	4	1.7	0
on the cob, sweet, med ears, 6.75 to 7.5 inches	1 ear	83	3	19	13	2	1.0	0
on the cob, sweet, small ears, 5.5 to 6.5 inches	1 ear	63	2	14	11	2	0.9	0
Frozen								
(Green Giant)	1/2 cup	90	2	19	5	2	1.0	0
(Seabrook)	3.3 oz	80	3	19	3	1	1.0	0
kernels, sweet, boiled, drained	1/2 cup	66	2	16	4	2	0.4	0
kernels, sweet, boiled, drained	10-oz pkg	227	8	56	14	7	1.2	0
kernels, sweet, unprepared	1/2 cup	72	2	17	2	2	0.6	0
kernels, sweet, unprepared	10-oz pkg	250	9	59	9	7	2.2	0
on the cob, sweet, unprepared, med ears	1 ear	123	4	29	6	4	1.0	0
petite, 'Early Harvest' (C&W)	2/3 cup	80	3	19	10	1	1.0	0
shoepeg, 'Harvest Fresh' (Green Giant)	1/2 cup	90	3	19	60	2	1.0	0
shoepeg, 'Select' (Green Giant)	1/2 cup	90	2	19	5	2	1.0	0
YELLOW								
Canned								
kernels, sweet, drained	12-oz can	171	6	39	452	4	2.1	0
kernels, sweet, drained	1 cup	133	4	30	351	3	1.6	0
kernels, sweet, regular pack, w/liquid	1/2 cup	82	2	20	273	2	0.6	0
sweet, no salt, vacuum-packed	1/2 cup	83	3	20	3	2	0.5	0
sweet, no salt, w/liquid	1/2 cup	82	2	20	15	2	0.6	0
Fresh								
baby, sweet, whole, boiled, drained	1 ear	9	0	2	1	0	0.1	0
kernels, sweet, boiled, drained	1/2 cup	76	3	18	3	2	0.6	0
kernels, sweet, raw	1 cup	132	5	29	23	4	1.8	0
on the cob, large ears, 7.75 to 9 inches	1 ear	123	5	27	21	4	1.7	0
on the cob, medium ears, 6.75 to 7.5 inches	1 ear	77	3	17	14	2	1.1	0
on the cob, small ears, 5.5 to 6.5 inches	1 ear	63	2	14	11	2	0.9	0
Frozen								
kernels, sweet, boiled, drained	10 oz pkg	227	8	56	14	7	1.2	0
kernels, sweet, unprepared	10-oz pkg	250	9	59	9	7	2.2	0
kernels, sweet, unprepared	1/2 cup	72	2	17	2	2	0.6	0
CORN, CREAMED. See under CORN DISH/ENTRÉE.								
CORN BRAN, crude	1 cup	170	6	65	5	65	0.7	0
CORN CAKE								
apple cinnamon flavor (Roman Meal)	1 cake	49	1	11	5	0	1.0	0
caramel flavor, nonfat (Roman Meal)	1 cake	50	1	11	5	0	0.0	0
caramel flavored (Quaker)	1 serving	50	1	12	30	0	0.0	0
cheddar flavor (Roman Meal)	1 cake	43	1	9	14	0	1.0	0
natural butter flavor, nonfat (Roman Meal)	1 cake	40	1	8	35	0	0.0	0
popcorn, butter flavor (Chico-San)	1 cake	40	1	8	45	0	0.0	0
popcorn, caramel (Chico-San)	1 cake	50	1	10	55	0	0.0	0
popcorn, lightly salted (Chico-San)	1 cake	40	1	8	45	0	0.0	0
popcorn, white cheddar cheese (Chico-San)	1 cake	50	1	9	65	0	1.0	0

Food Name	Serv. Size	Total Cal.	Prot. gms	Carbs gms	Sod. mgs	Fiber gms	Fat gms	Chol. mgs
popped, butter flavor *(Quaker)*	1 cake	35	1	7	55	0	0.0	0
white cheddar, mild *(Quaker)*	1 serving	40	1	8	100	0	0.0	0
white cheddar flavor, nonfat *(Roman Meal)*	1 cake	45	1	9	15	0	0.0	0

CORN CHIPS AND SNACKS. See also TORTILLA CHIPS.

Food Name	Serv. Size	Total Cal.	Prot. gms	Carbs gms	Sod. mgs	Fiber gms	Fat gms	Chol. mgs
(Arrowhead Mills)								
chips, blue corn, 'Corn Curls'	1 oz	120	3	22	54	4	2.0	0
chips, blue corn, unsalted, 'Corn Curls'	1 oz	120	3	22	1	4	2.0	0
chips, yellow, 'Corn Chips'	0.75 oz	90	2	18	31	3	1.0	0
chips, yellow, w/cheese, 'Corn Chips'	0.75 oz	90	2	15	30	3	2.0	0
(Azteca) chips, 'Unsalted'	1 oz	140	2	18	110	0	7.0	0
(Bachman)								
chips	1 oz	160	2	15	160	0	10.0	0
chips, barbecue	1 oz	150	1	17	230	0	9.0	0
(Barbara's Bakery)								
chips, blue corn	15 chips	140	3	16	40	1	7.0	0
chips, blue corn, no salt added	15 chips	140	3	16	0	1	7.0	0
chips, chipotle chili, 'Potilla'	1 oz	140	2	18	180	0	8.0	0
chips, 'Potilla'	1 oz	140	2	18	120	0	8.0	0
chips, salsa, 'Pinta Puffs'	1 oz	70	2	10	130	0	2.0	0
(Corn Snackers)								
chips	0.5-oz pkg	60	1	10	190	0	2.0	0
chips, nacho cheese	0.5-oz pkg	60	1	10	240	0	2.0	0
(Cornuts)								
nuggets, toasted, barbecue	1 oz	124	3	20	277	2	4.1	0
nuggets, toasted, chili picante	1 oz	120	2	22	260	2	4.0	0
nuggets, toasted, nacho	1 oz	124	3	20	180	2	4.0	1
nuggets, toasted, plain	1 oz	124	2	21	156	2	4.0	0
nuggets, toasted, ranch	1 oz	120	2	20	190	2	4.0	0
nuggets, toasted, unsalted	1 oz	120	2	19	30	3	4.0	0
(Dipsy Doodles) chips, rippled, 'Rippled Corn Chips'	1 oz	160	2	15	180	0	10.0	0
(Doritos)								
chips, 'Nacho Cheesier'	1 oz	140	2	17	360	1	7.0	3
chips, '3-D's'	1 oz	140	2	18	350	1	6.0	3
(Featherweight)								
chips, 'Low-Salt'	1 oz	170	2	15	3	0	11.0	0
puffs, cheese, low-salt 'Cheese Curls'	1 oz	150	2	16	81	0	9.0	0
(Fritos)								
chips, 'Bar-B-Q'	34 pieces	150	2	16	320	0	9.0	0
chips, barbecue, 'Rowdy Rustlers'	34 chips	150	2	17	300	1	9.0	0
chips, chili cheese flavor	34 chips	160	2	15	300	1	10.0	0
chips, 'Dip Size'	13 pieces	150	2	17	210	0	9.0	0
chips, nacho cheese, 'Non-Stop'	34 chips	150	2	16	220	1	9.0	1
chips, original	34 pieces	150	1	16	230	0	9.0	0
chips, 'Wild 'N Mild'	32 chips	160	2	16	240	1	9.0	0
nuggets, toasted	1.38 oz	170	3	29	265	2	5.0	0
(Harry's)								
chips, bean 'Garden Vegetable Chips'	1 oz	144	3	17	1	2	7.0	0
chips, bean, mild, 'Garden Vegetable Chips'	1 oz	144	3	17	74	2	7.0	0
chips, bean, wild, 'Garden Vegetable Chips'	1 oz	141	3	18	51	3	6.0	0
chips, beet-garlic, 'Garden Vegetable Chips'	1 oz	134	2	20	43	2	5.0	0
chips, bell pepper, 'Garden Vegetable Chips'	1 oz	140	2	19	40	2	6.0	0
chips, blue corn, garlic 'Garden Vegetable Chips'	1 oz	129	3	21	28	3	4.0	0
chips, carrot caraway 'Garden Vegetable Chips'	1 oz	131	2	20	31	2	4.0	0
chips, vegetable, 'Garden Vegetable Chips'	1 oz	141	2	18	40	3	7.0	0
(Health Valley)								
chips	1 oz	160	1	13	90	1	11.0	0
chips, 'No Salt Added'	1 oz	160	1	13	1	1	11.0	0

Food Name	Serv. Size	Total Cal.	Prot. gms	Carbs gms	Sod. mgs	Fiber gms	Fat gms	Chol. mgs
puffs, caramel, nonfat, orignal	1 cup	110	2	24	60	2	0.0	0
puffs, caramel corn, peanut flavor	1 oz	100	3	21	65	0	0.0	0
puffs, cheddar cheese	1 oz	160	3	15	120	1	10.0	2
(Jax)								
puffs, cheese 'Crunchy'	1 oz	160	2	14	250	0	11.0	0
puffs, cheese, 'Baked'	1 oz	140	2	17	290	0	7.0	0
(Maine Coast)								
chips, corn-dulse-kelp-onion-garlic, organic	1 oz	146	2	17	65	4	6.6	0
(Peddlers)								
chips, bean 'Offbeat Originals'	1 oz	144	3	17	1	2	7.0	0
chips, bean, mild, 'Offbeat Originals'	1 oz	144	3	17	74	2	7.0	0
chips, bean, wild, 'Offbeat Originals'	1 oz	141	3	18	51	3	6.0	0
chips, beet-garlic 'Offbeat Originals'	1 oz	134	2	20	43	2	5.0	0
chips, bell pepper 'Offbeat Originals'	1 oz	140	2	19	40	2	6.0	0
chips, blue corn, garlic 'Offbeat Originals'	1 oz	129	3	21	28	3	4.0	0
chips, carrot caraway 'Offbeat Originals'	1 oz	131	2	20	31	2	4.0	0
chips, vegetable, 'Offbeat Originals'	1 oz	141	2	18	40	3	7.0	0
(Planters) chips	1 oz	160	2	15	160	0	10.0	0
(Skinny Snacks)								
chips, barbecue	1 cup	60	1	12	140	1	1.0	0
chips, nacho flavor	1 cup	60	1	12	105	1	1.0	0
chips, no salt	1 cup	60	1	12	0	1	1.0	0
chips, salted	1 cup	60	1	12	58	1	1.0	0
chips, sour cream and onion	1 cup	65	1	12	70	1	1.0	0
(Snyder's)								
chips	1 oz	160	2	14	150	0	11.0	0
(Tio Sancho) nachos	0.5 oz	70	4	1	282	0	5.7	0
(Ultra Slim-Fast) curls, cheese, 'Great Tasting'	1 oz	110	2	20	360	3	3.0	0
(Wise)								
corn chips	1 oz	160	2	15	180	0	10.0	0
chips, ridged	1 oz	160	2	15	180	0	10.0	0
crunchies	1 oz	160	2	15	180	0	10.0	0
puffs, cheese, fried, 'Cheez Doodles Corn Puffs'	1 oz	160	2	15	220	0	10.0	0
puffs, cheese, baked, 'Cheez Doodles Corn Puffs'	1 oz	150	2	17	360	0	8.0	0
spirals	1 oz	160	2	15	125	0	10.0	0
twists	1 oz	160	2	15	125	0	10.0	0
CORN DISH/ENTRÉE								
(A&P)								
cream style, canned	1/2 cup	100	2	25	330	0	1.0	0
kernels, cream style, frozen	3.3 oz	80	3	18	0	0	1.0	0
(Del Monte)								
cream style, no salt added, canned	1/2 cup	90	2	20	10	2	1.0	0
golden, cream style, canned	1/2 cup	80	2	18	355	0	1.0	0
golden, cream style, no salt added, canned	1/2 cup	80	2	20	10	0	1.0	0
(Diamond A) sweet, cream style, canned	1 cup	245	5	50	650	0	1.0	0
(Finast) cream style, canned	1/2 cup	105	2	25	350	0	1.0	0
(Flav-R-Pac)								
cream style, frozen	1/2 cup	130	3	24	380	2	3.0	0
w/buttery sauce, frozen	1/2 cup	130	3	24	420	2	3.0	0
(Freshlike)								
and peppers, vacuum packed	1/2 cup	90	3	23	300	0	1.0	0
golden, cream style, canned	1/2 cup	110	2	25	290	0	1.0	0
golden, cream style, no salt added, canned	1/2 cup	110	2	25	15	0	1.0	0
(Green Giant)								
cream style, canned	1/2 cup	100	2	24	390	2	1.0	0
w/peppers, canned, 'Mexicorn'	1/2 cup	80	2	19	450	2	1.0	0
(IGA) golden, sweet, cream style, canned	1/2 cup	70	2	16	10	0	1.0	0

Food Name	Serv. Size	Total Cal.	Prot. gms	Carbs gms	Sod. mgs	Fiber gms	Fat gms	Chol. mgs
(Pathmark)								
cream style, canned, 'No Frills'	1 cup	210	5	51	700	0	1.0	0
golden, cream style, canned	1/2 cup	100	2	25	350	0	1.0	0
(S&W)								
cream style, canned	1/2 cup	100	2	24	340	1	1.0	0
cream style, canned, 'Nutradiet'	1/2 cup	100	3	21	0	0	1.0	0
cream style, no starch added, canned, 'Premium Homestyle'	1/2 cup	120	3	24	285	0	1.0	0
cream style, starch added, canned, 'Premium Homestyle'	1/2 cup	105	2	25	435	0	1.0	0
(Stokely)								
gold and white, cream style, canned	1/2 cup	100	2	23	380	0	0.0	0
gold and white, w/red peppers, canned	1/2 cup	60	2	10	250	2	1.5	0
white, cream style, canned	1/2 cup	100	2	21	400	1	1.0	0
(Stouffer's)								
pudding, frozen, food service product	1 oz	38	1	5	126	0	1.7	15
soufflé	1/2 cup	170	5	21	490	1	7.0	65
(Veg-All)								
golden, cream style, canned	1/2 cup	110	2	25	290	0	1.0	0
w/peppers, vacuum packed	1/2 cup	90	3	23	300	0	1.0	0
CORN DOG. See under FRANKFURTER.								
CORN FLOUR. See under FLOUR. See also CORNMEAL.								
CORN OIL								
(Hain)	1 tbsp	120	0	0	0	0	14.0	0
(Kroger)	1 tbsp	122	0	0	0	0	13.6	0
(Mazola)	1 tbsp	120	0	0	0	0	14.0	0
(Wesson)	1 tbsp	122	0	0	0	0	13.6	0
'No Frills' *(Pathmark)*	1 tbsp	130	0	0	0	0	14.0	0
pure pressed, organic *(Spectrum)*	1 tbsp	120	0	0	0	0	14.0	0
CORN SYRUP								
dark	1 cup	925	0	251	508	0	0.0	0
dark	1 tbsp	56	0	15	31	0	0.0	0
dark *(Karo)*	1 tbsp	60	0	15	40	0	0.0	0
high-fructose	1 cup	871	0	236	6	0	0.0	0
high-fructose	1 tbsp	53	0	14	0	0	0.0	0
light	1 cup	925	0	251	397	0	0.0	0
light	1 tbsp	56	0	15	24	0	0.0	0
light *(Karo)*	1 tbsp	60	0	15	30	0	0.0	0
table blend, w/sugar	1 cup	1008	0	265	224	0	0.0	0
table blend, w/sugar	1 tbsp	64	0	17	14	0	0.0	0
CORNBREAD. See under BREAD, QUICK.								
CORNBREAD MIX. See under BREAD, QUICK, MIX.								
CORNED BEEF. See BEEF, CORNED.								
CORNED BEEF HASH. See under HASH.								
CORNISH GAME HEN								
meat and skin, raw	1/2 medium	336	29	0	102	0	23.6	170
meat and skin, roasted	1/2 medium	335	29	0	83	0	23.5	169
meat only, raw	1/2 medium	139	24	0	82	0	4.0	109
meat only, roasted	1/2 medium	147	26	0	69	0	4.3	117
(Tyson)								
meat and skin, frozen	3.5 oz	250	27	1	80	0	15.0	155
meat only, frozen	3.5 oz	240	28	0	70	0	14.0	75
CORNISH GAME HEN DINNER/ENTRÉE								
(Tyson) w/wild rice, wholesale club item	3.5 oz	190	19	6	125	0	11.0	85
CORNMEAL								
organic, stone ground, gluten free *(Hodgson Mill)*	1/4 cup	100	3	22	0	3	1.0	0
whole-grain, high-lysine *(Arrowhead Mills)*	2 oz	210	4	43	1	7	2.0	0
whole-grain, stone-ground *(Hodgson Mill)*	1/4 cup	100	3	22	0	3	1.0	0

Food Name	Serv. Size	Total Cal.	Prot. gms	Carbs gms	Sod. mgs	Fiber gms	Fat gms	Chol. mgs
BLUE								
(Arrowhead Mills)	1/4 cup	120	3	27	0	3	1.0	0
whole-grain (Arrowhead Mills)	2 oz	210	6	41	1	6	3.0	0
WHITE								
Regular								
(Albers)	1 oz	100	2	22	0	2	1.0	0
bolted (Aunt Jemima)	1/6 cup	99	2	21	337	0	0.7	0
enriched (Aunt Jemima)	3 tbsp	102	2	22	1	1	0.5	0
enriched, degermed	1 cup	505	12	107	4	10	2.3	0
unenriched, degermed	1 cup	505	12	107	4	10	2.3	0
whole-grain	1 cup	442	10	94	43	9	4.4	0
whole-grain, stone-ground (Hodgson Mill)	1/4 cup	100	3	22	0	3	1.0	0
Self-rising								
(Aunt Jemima)	1/6 cup	98	2	21	381	0	0.5	0
bolted, plain, enriched	1 cup	407	10	86	1521	8	4.1	0
bolted, w/wheat flour added, enriched	1 cup	592	14	125	2242	11	4.8	0
buttermilk (Aunt Jemima)	3 tbsp	101	3	20	439	0	1.1	0
enriched, degermed	1 cup	490	12	103	1860	10	2.4	0
YELLOW								
Regular								
(Albers)	1 oz	100	2	22	0	2	1.0	0
bolted (Tone's)	1 tsp	9	0	2	0	0	0.1	0
degermed, unenriched	1 cup	505	12	107	4	10	2.3	0
enriched (Aunt Jemima)	3 tbsp	102	2	22	1	1	0.5	0
enriched, degermed	1 cup	505	12	107	4	10	2.3	0
whole-grain	1 cup	442	10	94	43	9	4.4	0
whole-grain (Arrowhead Mills)	2 oz	210	4	43	1	7	2.0	0
Self-rising								
(Aunt Jemima)	3 tbsp	100	2	21	490	0	1.0	0
bolted, plain, enriched	1 cup	407	10	86	1521	8	4.1	0
bolted, w/wheat flour added, enriched	1 cup	592	14	125	2242	11	4.8	0
enriched, degermed	1 cup	490	12	103	1860	10	2.4	0
whole-grain (Hodgson Mill)	1/4 cup	90	3	21	260	3	1.0	0
CORNSTARCH								
	1 cup	488	0	117	12	1	0.1	0
(Argo)	1 tbsp	30	0	7	0	0	0.0	0
(Cream)	1 tbsp	29	0	7	0	0	0.0	0
(Kingsford)	1 tbsp	30	0	7	0	0	0.0	0
(Tone's)	1 tsp	10	0	2	0	0	0.1	0
100% pure (Hodgson Mill)	2 tsp	35	0	9	0	0	0.0	0
COTTAGE CHEESE. See under CHEESE.								
COTTONSEED FLOUR. See under FLOUR.								
COTTONSEED KERNELS								
roasted	1 cup	754	49	33	37	8	54.1	0
roasted	1 tbsp	51	3	2	3	1	3.6	0
COTTONSEED MEAL, partially defatted	1 oz	104	14	11	10	na	1.4	0
COTTONSEED OIL								
	1 cup	1927	0	0	0	0	218.0	0
	1 tbsp	120	0	0	0	0	13.6	0
(Wesson)	1 tbsp	122	0	0	0	0	13.6	0
w/sesame oil, seasoned, 'Mongolian Fire Oil' (House of Tsang)	1 tsp	45	0	0	0	0	5.0	0
COUSCOUS								
cooked	1 cup	176	6	36	8	2	0.3	0
savory, prepared (Fantastic Foods)	2/3 cup	160	6	33	300	3	0.7	0
uncooked	1 cup	591	20	123	26	7	0.8	0

Food Name	Serv. Size	Total Cal.	Prot. gms	Carbs gms	Sod. mgs	Fiber gms	Fat gms	Chol. mgs
uncooked	1 oz	96	3	20	4	1	0.1	0
uncooked *(Near East)*	1.25 oz	120	4	26	5	0	0.0	0
uncooked 'Elegant Grains' *(Fantastic Foods)*	1/4 cup	210	7	43	5	3	0.0	0
whole wheat, prepared w/2 tbsp salted butter *(Fantastic Foods)*	1/2 cup	111	4	20	23	0	2.0	0
whole wheat, uncooked, 'Elegant Grains' *(Fantastic Foods)*	1/4 cup	210	8	45	0	7	1.0	0
COUSCOUS DISH/ENTRÉE								
pilaf, cooked *(Casbah)*	3/4 cup	220	8	40	480	1	0.5	0
pilaf, savory, prepared w/2 tbsp salted butter *(Quick Pilaf)*	1/2 cup	124	4	19	254	0	3.0	0
pilaf, savory, prepared w/o additional ingredients *(Quick Pilaf)*	1/2 cup	94	4	19	215	0	0.0	0
pilaf, uncooked *(Casbah)*	28 grams	100	4	20	280	1	0.0	0
w/lentils, cooked *(Fantastic Foods)*	1 serving	220	12	47	140	9	1.0	0
w/lentils, uncooked *(Fantastic Foods)*	2.3 oz	220	12	47	140	9	1.0	0
CRAB								
ALASKA KING								
boiled, poached, or steamed	1 med leg	130	26	0	1436	0	2.1	71
boiled, poached, or steamed	3 oz	82	16	0	911	0	1.3	45
raw	1 med leg	144	31	0	1438	0	1.0	72
raw	3 oz	71	16	0	711	0	0.5	36
BLUE								
Canned								
	1 cup	134	28	0	450	0	1.7	120
	3 oz	84	17	0	283	0	1.0	76
	1 oz	28	6	0	94	0	0.3	25
drained	6.5-oz can	124	26	0	416	0	1.5	111
Fresh								
boiled, poached, or steamed	3 oz	87	17	0	237	0	1.5	85
boiled, poached, or steamed, flakes and pieces	1 cup	120	24	0	329	0	2.1	118
boiled, poached, or steamed, pieces	1 cup	138	27	0	377	0	2.4	135
boiled, poached, or steamed, w/o shell	1 oz	29	6	0	79	0	0.5	28
raw	1 med crab	18	4	0	62	0	0.2	16
raw	3 oz	74	15	0	249	0	0.9	66
DUNGENESS								
Canned *(S&W)*	1/3 cup	80	18	0	310	0	1.0	60
Fresh								
boiled, poached, or steamed	1 med crab	140	28	1	480	0	1.6	97
boiled, poached, or steamed	3 oz	94	19	1	321	0	1.1	65
raw	1 med crab	140	28	1	481	0	1.6	96
raw	3 oz	73	15	1	251	0	0.8	50
MIXED SPECIES								
15% leg meat, canned *(Crown Prince)*	1/2 can	50	12	1	300	0	0.0	75
white meat, canned *(Crown Prince)*	1/2 can	50	12	0	340	0	0.0	70
QUEEN								
boiled, poached, or steamed	3 oz	98	20	0	587	0	1.3	60
raw	3 oz	77	16	0	458	0	1.0	47
SNOW								
frozen *(Wakefield)*	3 oz	60	13	0	270	0	1.0	0
raw, Opilio, clusters *(Peter Pan Seafoods)*	3.5 oz	91	21	0	539	0	1.2	55
raw, Opilio, scored, 'Snap 'n' Eat' *(Peter Pan Seafoods)*	3.5 oz	91	21	0	539	0	1.2	55
SOFTSHELL								
boiled	4 oz	116	22.9	0.0	316	0	2.0	113
boiled, approx 4.75 oz	1 cup	138	27.3	0.0	376	0	2.4	135
poached	4 oz	116	22.9	0.0	316	0	2.0	113
poached, approx 4.75 oz	1 cup	138	27.3	0.0	376	0	2.4	135

Food Name	Serv. Size	Total Cal.	Prot. gms	Carbs gms	Sod. mgs	Fiber gms	Fat gms	Chol. mgs
raw	1 lb	395	81.9	0.2	1329	0	4.9	355
raw	1 oz	25	5.1	<.1	83	0	0.3	22
raw, approx 0.7 oz	1 crab	18	3.8	<.1	62	0	0.2	16
steamed	4 oz	116	22.9	0.0	316	0	2.0	113
steamed, approx 4.75 oz	1 cup	138	27.3	0.0	376	0	2.4	135
CRAB ENTRÉE/DINNER *(Wakefield)* w/shrimp, frozen	3 oz	60	13	0	210	0	1.0	0
CRAB SUBSTITUTE								
Alaska King style, made from surimi	3 oz	87	10	9	715	0	1.1	17
made from surimi	1 oz	28	4	2	41	0	0.3	9
made from surimi	3 oz	84	13	6	122	0	0.8	26
(Icicle Brand)	3.5 oz	99	12	11	900	0	0.1	10
(Peter Pan Seafoods)								
leg style, made from surimi and 10% crab, 'Classic Seablends'	3.5 oz	85	10	0	890	0	0.4	31
leg style, made from surimi, 'Standard Seablends'	3.5 oz	88	9	0	845	0	0.4	34
salad style made from surimi and 10% crab, 'Classic Seablends Combo'	3.5 oz	85	10	0	890	0	0.4	31
salad style, made from surimi 'Standard Seablends Combo'	3.5 oz	88	9	0	845	0	0.4	34
(Trader Joe's) made from surimi	1/2 cup	80	6	14	670	0	1.0	15
CRABAPPLE, raw, sliced	1 cup	84	0	22	1	na	0.3	0
CRACKER								
(Adrienne's)								
lahvosh, 'Classic Island'	7 crackers	140	4	21	290	1	4.0	25
lahvosh, onion	4 crackers	66	2	10	120	0	1.9	10
lahvosh, 10-grain	4 crackers	59	2	10	120	0	1.6	0
(Ak-Mak) wheat, 100% stone ground, w/sesame	5 crackers	116	5	19	214	4	2.3	0
(American Classic)								
butter flavor	4 crackers	70	1	9	140	0	3.0	2
cracked wheat	4 crackers	70	1	8	140	0	4.0	0
golden, w/sesame	4 crackers	70	1	9	120	0	3.0	0
onion, minced	4 crackers	70	1	10	120	0	3.0	0
toasted poppy	4 crackers	70	1	9	140	0	3.0	0
(Auburn Farms)								
onion, 7-grain, nonfat, bite size	0.5 oz	60	2	12	105	1	0.0	0
7-grain, bite size	1 oz	120	2	24	220	2	0.0	0
vegetable, 7-grain, nonfat, bite size	1 oz	120	4	24	210	2	0.0	0
(Barbara's Bakery)								
'Wheatines' less salt	1 serving	50	1	10	110	1	1.5	0
'Wheatines' unsalted tops	0.5 oz	60	2	9	45	0	2.0	0
'Wheatines' sesame, less salt	1 serving	50	1	10	110	1	1.5	0
'Wheatines,' w/pepper	1 serving	50	1	10	110	1	1.5	0
'Wheatine' bits	0.5 oz	60	2	9	132	0	2.0	0
(Breton)								
low-sodium	3 crackers	70	2	8	30	0	3.0	0
sesame	3 crackers	80	2	9	120	0	3.5	0
(Cabaret)	3 crackers	70	1	9	160	0	3.5	0
(Carr's)								
'Monterey' savory wheat	3 crackers	70	<1	9	95	1	2.5	0
'Monterey' hearty wheat	3 crackers	60	1	9	100	<1	2.0	0
'Monterey' sesame and onion	3 crackers	70	<1	9	110	<1	3.0	0
'Monterey' roasted vegetable	3 crackers	60	<1	10	160	<1	2.0	0
'Table Water'	5 crackers	70	1	13	100	<1	1.5	0
'Table Water' w/toasted sesame seeds	5 crackers	70	1	13	95	<1	1.5	0
'Table Water' w/cracked pepper	5 crackers	70	1	13	100	<1	1.5	0
'Table Water' w/roasted garlic and herbs	5 crackers	70	1	13	140	<1	1.5	0
(Cheddar Wedges) cheese flavor, bite size	31 pieces	70	1	9	150	0	3.0	0

Food Name	Serv. Size	Total Cal.	Prot. gms	Carbs gms	Sod. mgs	Fiber gms	Fat gms	Chol. mgs
(Cheez-It)								
cheese flavor	12 crackers	70	2	7	135	0	4.0	2
hot and spicy	12 crackers	70	1	8	160	0	4.0	2
low-salt	12 crackers	70	2	7	65	0	4.0	2
party mix	1/2 cup	140	4	19	270	1	5.0	0
white cheddar	12 crackers	76	1	9	160	0	4.0	2
(Club Partners) garlic bread flavor	4 crackers	60	1	10	140	0	2.0	0
(Crackups)								
cheddar	0.5 oz	70	1	10	100	0	3.0	0
salsa	0.5 oz	70	1	9	100	0	3.0	0
(Crisp & Light)								
'Crackerbread'	1 slice	17	1	3	25	0	1.0	0
'Crackerbread' salt-free	1 slice	17	1	3	1	0	1.0	0
(Dandy) soup and oyster, 5 oz serving	20 crackers	60	1	10	220	0	2.0	0
(Dar-Vida)								
crispbread, regular	1 cracker	20	1	4	40	0	1.0	0
crispbread, sesame	1 cracker	22	1	4	40	0	1.0	0
sesame, 'Crispbread'	1 cracker	22	1	4	40	0	1.0	0
(Delicious)								
bacon flavor	0.5 oz	70	1	10	190	0	3.0	0
bite size	0.5 oz	70	1	9	135	0	3.0	1
cheese flavor, 'Big'	25 crackers	140	3	19	220	1	6.0	5
'Crackerdiles'	0.5 oz	70	1	9	135	0	3.0	1
garden vegetable	0.5 oz	70	1	10	220	0	3.0	0
garlic 'Discos'	0.5 oz	78	1	6	184	0	5.0	0
low-sodium, bite size	0.5 oz	70	1	9	55	0	3.0	0
nacho cheese	0.5 oz	89	1	8	150	0	5.0	0
onion, 'Discos'	0.5 oz	76	1	7	156	0	5.0	0
pumpernickel	0.5 oz	70	1	9	160	0	3.0	0
'Regency'	0.5 oz	70	1	9	100	0	3.0	0
'Snackers'	0.5 oz	70	1	9	90	0	3.0	0
sour cream, w/onion, 'Discos'	0.5 oz	79	1	6	162	0	5.0	0
sourdough	0.5 oz	70	1	9	160	0	3.0	0
'Wheat On'	0.5 oz	68	1	8	86	0	3.0	0
wheat wafer, w/sesame	0.5 oz	80	1	9	170	0	4.0	0
'Wheatstone'	0.5 oz	70	2	9	180	0	3.0	0
(Devonsheer)								
Melba toast, honey bran	1 cracker	16	1	3	25	0	0.4	0
Melba toast, honey bran, 'Rounds'	0.5 oz	52	2	10	98	1	0.9	0
Melba toast, plain	1 cracker	16	1	3	30	0	0.4	0
Melba toast, plain, 'Rounds'	0.5 oz	53	2	11	111	1	0.6	0
Melba toast, plain, 'Unsalted'	1 cracker	16	1	3	5	0	0.4	0
Melba toast, plain, 'Unsalted Rounds'	0.5 oz	52	2	11	5	1	0.6	0
Melba toast, rye	1 cracker	16	1	3	30	0	0.4	0
Melba toast, rye, 'Rounds'	0.5 oz	53	2	11	130	1	0.6	0
Melba toast, rye, 'Unsalted'	1 cracker	16	1	3	5	0	0.4	0
Melba toast, sesame	1 cracker	16	1	3	25	0	0.5	0
Melba toast, sesame, 'Rounds'	0.5 oz	57	2	9	131	1	1.8	0
Melba toast, w/onion, 'Rounds'	0.5 oz	51	2	11	120	1	0.6	0
Melba toast, w/vegetable	1 cracker	16	1	3	25	0	0.4	0
Melba toast, whole wheat	1 cracker	16	1	3	30	0	0.4	0
Melba toast, whole wheat, unsalted	1 cracker	16	1	3	5	0	0.4	0
(Distinctive)								
cracked wheat	3 crackers	100	2	14	180	1	4.0	0
'English Water Biscuit'	4 crackers	70	2	13	100	0	1.0	0
sesame	4 crackers	80	2	12	140	2	4.0	0
thins	4 crackers	70	1	10	115	0	3.0	5

Food Name	Serv. Size	Total Cal.	Prot. gms	Carbs gms	Sod. mgs	Fiber gms	Fat gms	Chol. mgs
toasted wheat	4 crackers	80	2	12	140	0	3.0	0
wheat	4 crackers	100	2	13	140	1	5.0	0
(Eagle)								
'Cheese on Cheese'	6 crackers	210	3	24	390	1	11.0	5
peanut butter and cheese sandwich	6 crackers	230	6	25	320	1	12.0	0
peanut butter on toast	6 crackers	210	5	23	430	1	10.0	0
wheat, w/cheddar cheese	6 crackers	200	4	24	400	1	10.0	5
(Eden Foods)								
nori maki	15 crackers	110	3	24	160	2	0.0	0
rice, brown	5 crackers	120	3	22	230	2	2.0	0
(Escort) butter flavor	3 crackers	70	1	9	115	0	4.0	0
(Estee)								
Melba toast, wheat, '6-calorie'	1 cracker	6	1	1	5	0	1.0	0
Melba toast, wheat, 'Snax'	1 oz	100	4	22	15	0	1.0	0
saltine, unsalted	4 crackers	60	1	9	0	0	2.0	0
ranch flavor 'Snack Crisps'	0.66 oz	80	2	13	135	0	2.0	0
(Euphrates)								
wheat	1 cracker	19	0	3	32	0	0.8	0
wheat, low-salt	1 cracker	19	0	3	11	0	0.8	0
(Featherweight) low-salt	2 pieces	30	0	5	1	0	1.0	0
(FFV)								
'Schooners'	0.5 oz	60	1	10	130	0	2.0	0
sesame, 'Crisp'	1 cracker	60	1	10	120	0	2.0	0
soda, 'Ocean Crisps'	1 cracker	60	1	10	120	0	2.0	0
stoned wheat	4 crackers	60	1	10	170	0	2.0	0
wafer, w/sesame, 'Crisp'	4 crackers	60	2	9	140	0	2.0	0
wheat, 'Crispy Wafer'	6 crackers	70	1	9	80	0	3.0	0
(FiberRich) bran	1 cracker	18	1	6	10	3	1.0	0
(Finast)								
snack	12 crackers	70	1	9	135	0	3.0	0
wheat, 'Snacks'	7 crackers	70	1	9	85	0	3.0	0
(Finn Crisp)								
crispbread, dark	2 crackers	38	1	9	130	2	1.0	0
crispbread, light, 'Hi-Fiber'	1 cracker	35	1	8	60	0	1.0	0
crispbread, regular	2 crackers	38	1	9	130	2	1.0	0
crispbread, rye, original, 'Hi-Fiber'	1 cracker	40	1	10	95	0	0.0	0
crispbread, w/caraway	2 slices	38	1	9	130	2	1.0	0
(Flavor Tree)								
sesame chips	1/4 cup	163	3	11	380	0	9.2	0
sesame sticks	1/4 cup	133	3	11	358	0	9.1	0
sesame sticks, no salt	1/4 cup	131	3	13	7	0	8.1	0
(Frito-Lay's)								
cheddar	0.5 oz	70	1	8	150	0	4.0	0
cheese-filled	1.5 oz	210	4	24	470	0	10.0	5
Italian, zesty	0.5 oz	70	1	9	115	0	3.0	0
peanut butter, bar	1.75 oz	270	2	30	65	0	16.0	0
peanut butter filled	6 crackers	210	6	24	450	0	10.0	0
(Frookie)								
garlic, w/herbs, nonfat, 'Gourmet'	4 crackers	35	1	7	120	0	0.0	0
pepper, nonfat, 'Gourmet'	4 crackers	35	1	7	40	0	0.0	0
water, nonfat, 'Gourmet'	4 crackers	35	1	7	60	0	0.0	0
whole wheat, nonfat, 'Gourmet'	4 crackers	35	1	7	60	0	0.0	0
(Garden Crisps) vegetables	15 crackers	130	2	22	290	1	3.5	0
(Grand Union) cheese flavor, 'Big'	25 crackers	140	3	19	220	1	6.0	5
(Hain)								
cheese flavor	1 oz	130	3	17	180	0	6.0	0
onion flavor	1 oz	130	3	17	160	0	6.0	0

Food Name	Serv. Size	Total Cal.	Prot. gms	Carbs gms	Sod. mgs	Fiber gms	Fat gms	Chol. mgs
onion flavor, no salt added	1 oz	130	3	17	5	0	6.0	0
'Rich'	1 oz	130	3	18	160	0	5.0	0
'Rich' no salt added	1 oz	130	3	18	15	0	5.0	0
rye	1 oz	120	3	19	200	0	4.0	0
rye, no salt added	1 oz	120	3	19	10	0	4.0	0
sesame	1 oz	140	3	16	210	0	7.0	0
sesame, no salt added	1 oz	140	3	16	5	0	7.0	0
sour cream, w/chive	1 oz	130	3	15	150	0	6.0	0
sour cream, w/chive, no salt added	1 oz	130	3	15	25	0	6.0	0
sourdough	0.5 oz	65	2	9	100	0	3.0	0
sourdough, low-salt	1 oz	130	3	18	10	0	5.0	0
vegetable, no salt added	1 oz	130	3	10	50	0	5.0	0
(Health Valley)								
cheese, organic, nonfat	0.5 oz	40	1	9	80	2	0.0	0
cheese, whole wheat, nonfat	5 crackers	50	2	11	80	2	0.0	0
herb, organic, nonfat	0.5 oz	40	1	9	80	2	0.0	0
onion, organic, nonfat	0.5 oz	40	1	9	80	2	0.0	0
rice bran	7 crackers	130	4	19	64	2	4.0	0
7-grain, stoned wheat	13 crackers	120	3	17	125	3	5.0	0
7-grain, stoned wheat, no salt added	13 crackers	120	3	17	20	3	5.0	0
7-grain, w/vegetable, organic	0.5 oz	40	1	9	80	2	0.0	0
stoned wheat	13 crackers	120	3	17	85	4	6.0	0
stoned wheat, no salt added	13 crackers	120	3	17	10	4	6.0	0
stoned wheat, w/herbs, no salt added	13 crackers	120	3	17	30	4	6.0	0
stoned wheat, w/sesame	13 crackers	130	3	16	150	3	6.0	0
stoned wheat, w/sesame, no salt added	13 crackers	130	3	17	20	3	6.0	0
whole wheat, nonfat	5 crackers	50	2	11	80	2	0.0	0
whole wheat, w/herbs, nonfat	5 crackers	50	2	11	80	2	0.0	0
whole wheat, w/onions, nonfat	5 crackers	50	2	11	80	2	0.0	0
whole wheat, w/vegetables, nonfat	5 crackers	50	2	11	80	2	0.0	0
(Hickory Farms)								
cracked wheat wafers	8 crackers	100	2	17	290	0	3.0	0
'Old Fashioned' *(Hickory Farms)*	10 pieces	90	2	16	170	0	3.0	0
'Rounds O' Rye' barbecue flavor	1 oz	153	3	13	60	0	10.6	0
'Rounds O' Rye' garlic	1 oz	147	3	15	126	0	8.9	0
'Rounds O' Rye' natural	1 oz	156	3	12	93	0	10.9	0
'Rounds O'Rye' sour cream	1 oz	155	3	13	130	0	10.7	0
rye wafers	8 crackers	90	2	17	250	0	2.0	0
rye wafers, salt-free	8 crackers	90	2	18	0	0	1.0	0
stoned wheat wafers, salt-free	8 crackers	100	2	18	0	0	2.0	0
'Wheat Mill Wafers' salt-free	4 crackers	50	1	9	0	0	1.0	0
(Kavli)								
Norwegian crispbread, thick	1 slice	35	1	8	31	2	0.3	0
Norwegian crispbread, thin	2 slices	40	1	8	32	6	0.3	0
(Keebler)								
cheese, sandwich, w/peanut butter	2 crackers	70	2	9	150	0	3.0	0
'Club' low-salt	4 crackers	60	1	9	75	0	3.0	0
'Hi Ho'	5 crackers	70	1	10	140	1	2.5	0
'Krispy' saltine	5 crackers	60	1	11	210	0	1.0	0
'Krispy' saltine, mild cheddar	5 crackers	60	2	10	180	0	2.0	2
'Krispy' saltine, unsalted tops	5 crackers	60	1	11	120	0	1.0	0
peanut butter and toast sandwich	2 crackers	70	2	9	120	0	3.0	0
sesame breadstix, food service product	2 pieces	26	1	4	47	0	0.8	0
'Toasteds' bacon flavor	4 crackers	60	1	8	125	0	3.0	0
'Toasteds' buttercrisp	4 crackers	60	1	8	125	0	3.0	0
'Toasteds' cheddar, juniors	8 pieces	80	1	8	95	0	4.0	5
'Toasteds' onion flavor	4 crackers	60	1	9	140	0	3.0	0

Food Name	Serv. Size	Total Cal.	Prot. gms	Carbs gms	Sod. mgs	Fiber gms	Fat gms	Chol. mgs
'Toasteds' rye	4 crackers	60	1	8	140	0	3.0	0
'Toasteds' sesame	4 crackers	60	1	8	130	0	3.0	0
'Town House'	4 crackers	70	1	8	120	0	4.0	0
'Town House' 50% less fat	5 crackers	70	1	11	180	1	2.0	0
'Town House' food service product	2 crackers	35	0	4	60	0	2.0	0
'Town House' low-salt	4 crackers	70	1	8	60	0	4.0	0
'Town House' sandwich, cheddar	1 cracker	70	1	6	105	0	4.0	5
'Waldorf' no salt, food service product	2 crackers	30	1	5	1	0	1.0	0
wheat, sandwich, w/American cheese	1 cracker	70	1	7	85	0	4.0	5
wheats, whole grain, food service product	2 crackers	35	1	5	50	0	1.5	0
'Wheatables'	12 crackers	70	1	9	140	0	3.0	0
'Wheatables' low-salt	1 cracker	5	0	1	3	0	0.2	0
'Wheatables' reduced-fat	29 crackers	130	3	21	320	1	3.5	0
'Zesta' saltine	5 crackers	60	1	10	190	0	2.0	0
'Zesta' saltine, 50% less salt	5 crackers	60	1	11	95	1	2.0	0
'Zesta' saltine, food service product	2 crackers	25	1	4	80	0	1.0	0
'Zesta' saltine, low-salt	5 crackers	60	1	10	95	0	2.0	0
'Zesta' saltine, nonfat	5 crackers	50	1	11	90	1	0.0	0
'Zesta' saltine, unsalted tops	5 crackers	60	1	10	85	0	2.0	0
'Zesta' saltine, unsalted tops, food service product	2 crackers	25	1	4	35	0	1.0	0
'Zesta' saltine, wheat	5 crackers	60	1	10	190	0	2.0	0
(Kraft)								
'Handi-Snacks' bacon flavor, w/cheese	1 pkg	130	4	8	410	0	9.0	20
'Handi-Snacks' peanut butter and cheese sandwich	1 pkg	190	6	11	180	0	14.0	0
(Lite 'N Krispy)								
rice sticks	6 sticks	40	1	8	150	1	0.5	0
rice sticks, no salt	6 sticks	40	1	8	0	1	0.5	0
(Little Debbie) wheat, w/cheddar cheese	1 serving	140	3	15	230	0	8.0	3
(M&M Mars)								
'Combos' cheese flavor	1.8 oz	240	5	34	580	0	10.0	0
'Combos' peanut butter	1.8 oz	240	6	30	360	0	10.0	0
(Manischewitz)								
'Tam Tams'	10 crackers	147	2	17	171	0	8.0	0
'Tam Tams' no salt	10 crackers	138	2	18	10	0	7.0	0
'Garlic Tams'	10 crackers	153	2	19	165	0	8.0	0
matzo, American	1 matzo	115	3	22	168	0	1.9	0
matzo, board, 'Daily Unsalted'	1 oz	110	3	24	1	0	0.3	0
matzo, board, 'Passover'	1.1 oz	129	3	27	5	0	0.4	0
matzo, board, thin	0.9 oz	100	3	21	0	0	0.3	0
matzo, dietetic, thin	0.8 oz	91	3	19	1	0	0.4	0
matzo, egg and onion, board	1 oz	112	3	23	180	0	1.0	15
matzo, egg, board, 'Passover'	1.2 oz	132	4	27	5	0	2.0	25
matzo, egg, miniature, 'Passover'	10 crackers	108	3	20	10	0	2.0	20
matzo, miniature	10 crackers	90	2	20	10	0	1.0	0
matzo, tea, thin	1 matzo	100	3	22	3	0	0.3	0
matzo, whole wheat, w/bran, board	1 oz	110	4	21	1	1	0.6	0
'Onion Tams'	10 crackers	150	2	18	157	0	8.0	0
'Wheat Tams'	10 crackers	150	2	18	180	0	8.0	0
(McCrakens)								
cheddar, tangy	1 oz	140	2	18	170	0	8.0	0
country butter flavor	1 oz	140	2	18	170	0	8.0	0
sour cream w/chive flavor	1 oz	140	2	18	170	0	8.0	0
wheat, toasted	1 oz	140	2	18	170	0	8.0	0
(Meal Mates)								
bread wafer, w/sesame	3 crackers	70	1	9	160	0	3.0	0
crispbread, w/sesame	3 crackers	70	1	9	160	0	3.0	0
(Musso's) garlic toast, w/cheese	3 pieces	70	2	11	180	1	2.5	0

Food Name	Serv. Size	Total Cal.	Prot. gms	Carbs gms	Sod. mgs	Fiber gms	Fat gms	Chol. mgs
(Nabisco)								
bacon-flavored	15 crackers	160	3	19	460	0	8.0	0
'Bran Thins' *(Nabisco)*	7 crackers	60	1	9	70	0	3.0	0
cheese, sandwich, w/peanut butter	4 pieces	130	3	15	320	0	7.0	0
'Cheese Nips'	13 pieces	70	1	9	130	0	3.0	0
'Chicken in a Biskit'	7 pieces	80	1	8	130	0	5.0	0
'Crown Pilot'	1 cracker	70	1	13	85	1	1.5	0
'Harvest Crisps' oat	6 crackers	60	1	10	135	0	2.0	0
'Harvest Crisps' rice	6 crackers	60	1	11	135	1	2.0	0
'Harvest Wheat'	4 crackers	60	1	8	95	0	3.0	0
'Harvest Wheat' low-salt	1 cracker	14	0	2	8	0	0.6	0
'Oat Thins'	18 crackers	140	3	20	190	2	6.0	0
'Oysterettes' soup and oyster	18 crackers	60	1	10	140	0	1.0	0
'Premium' saltine, low salt	5 crackers	60	1	10	35	1	1.0	0
'Premium' saltine, multigrain	5 crackers	60	1	10	150	1	1.5	0
'Premium' saltine, original	5 crackers	59	2	10	178	0	1.4	0
'Premium' saltine, unsalted tops	5 crackers	60	1	10	135	1	1.5	0
'Premium' saltine, wheat	4 crackers	60	1	10	130	1	2.0	0
'Royal Lunch' milk biscuit	1 cracker	60	1	10	80	1	2.0	0
'Royal Lunch' soda	0.5 oz	60	1	17	125	0	3.0	0
'Ritz'	4 crackers	70	1	9	140	0	4.0	0
'Ritz' low-salt	5 crackers	80	1	10	35	1	4.0	0
'Ritz' wheat	1 cracker	14	0	2	24	0	0.6	0
'Ritz' wheat, low salt	1 cracker	14	0	2	8	0	0.6	0
'Ritz' whole wheat	5 crackers	70	1	9	135	0	3.0	0
'Ritz Bits' cheese flavor	22 pieces	70	1	8	130	0	4.0	0
'Ritz Bits Sandwiches' w/peanut butter	12 crackers	80	2	8	80	0	4.0	0
'Ritz Bits Sandwiches' w/cheese	6 crackers	80	1	7	135	0	5.0	0
Swiss cheese, 'Naturally Flavored'	7 crackers	70	1	9	170	0	3.0	0
'Toast Sandwich' w/peanut butter	4 pieces	130	3	15	300	0	7.0	0
'Triscuit' wheat	10 bits	44	1	7	66	1	1.7	0
'Triscuit' wheat, low-salt	3 crackers	60	1	10	35	0	2.0	0
'Triscuit Bits'	15 pieces	60	1	10	85	0	3.0	0
'Triscuit Bits' wheat	8 crackers	60	1	10	75	0	2.0	0
'Twigs' cheese	1 cracker	10	0	1	20	0	0.5	0
'Uneeda Biscuits' no salt tops	2 crackers	60	1	10	100	0	2.0	0
'Waverly Wafer'	4 crackers	70	1	10	160	0	3.0	0
'Waverly Wafer' low-salt	4 crackers	70	1	10	80	0	3.0	0
'Wheat Thins'	16 crackers	140	2	19	170	2	6.0	0
'Wheat Thins'	7 crackers	70	1	9	170	0	4.0	0
'Wheat Thins' less fat	18 crackers	120	2	21	220	2	4.0	0
'Wheat Thins' low-salt	1 cracker	14	0	2	8	0	0.6	0
'Wheat Thins' multigrain	17 crackers	130	2	21	291	2	4.0	0
'Wheatsworth'	1 cracker	14	0	2	24	0	0.6	0
'Wheatsworth' low-salt	1 cracker	14	0	2	8	0	0.6	0
(Nature's Path)								
unleavened bread, carrot raisin, flourless, sprouted, organic	2 oz	130	5	22	5	0	1.0	0
unleavened bread, millet-rice, flourless, sprouted, organic	2 oz	140	5	23	0	0	1.0	0
unleavened bread, rye, w/carrot and raisin, organic	1 slice	120	3	26	0	6	0.0	0
unleavened bread, salt-free, organic, 'Sun Seed'	1 slice	160	6	29	3	7	2.0	0
unleavened bread, w/apple and spice, organic	1 slice	130	5	9	6	5	0.0	0
unleavened bread, w/fruit and nuts, organic	1 slice	140	6	27	7	6	0.0	0
unleavened bread, whole rye, flourless, sprouted, organic	2 oz	140	5	23	0	0	1.0	0

Food Name	Serv. Size	Total Cal.	Prot. gms	Carbs gms	Sod. mgs	Fiber gms	Fat gms	Chol. mgs
unleavened bread, whole wheat, flourless,								
sprouted, organic .... 2 oz	140	5	23	0	0	1.0	0
(North Castles) soda, 'English' .... 1 cracker	10	0	3	14	0	0.0	0
(Old London)								
Melba toast, bacon, 'Rounds' .... 0.5 oz	53	2	10	126	1	1.0	0
Melba toast, garlic, 'Rounds' .... 0.5 oz	56	2	10	132	1	1.2	0
Melba toast, pumpernickel .... 0.5 oz	54	2	11	156	1	0.6	0
Melba toast, rye .... 0.5 oz	52	2	11	132	1	0.7	0
Melba toast, rye, 'Rounds' .... 0.5 oz	52	2	11	132	1	0.7	0
Melba toast, sesame .... 0.5 oz	55	2	9	148	1	1.8	0
Melba toast, sesame, 'Rounds' .... 0.5 oz	56	2	9	149	1	1.8	0
Melba toast, sesame, unsalted .... 0.5 oz	55	2	9	5	1	1.8	0
Melba toast, wheat .... 0.5 oz	51	2	11	121	1	0.7	0
Melba toast, white .... 0.5 oz	51	2	10	111	1	0.6	0
Melba toast, white, 'Rounds' .... 0.5 oz	48	2	10	111	1	0.6	0
Melba toast, white, unsalted .... 0.5 oz	51	2	11	4	1	0.6	0
Melba toast, whole grain .... 0.5 oz	52	2	10	116	1	0.9	0
Melba toast, whole grain, 'Rounds' .... 0.5 oz	54	2	10	102	1	1.2	0
Melba toast, whole grain, unsalted .... 0.5 oz	53	2	10	4	1	1.0	0
(Orchard Crisps)								
apple cinnamon .... 0.5 oz	60	1	11	40	0	2.0	0
banana walnut *(Orchard Crisps)* .... 0.5 oz	60	1	11	40	0	2.0	0
(OTC) soup and oyster .... 1 cracker	25	1	4	65	0	1.0	0
(Pacific Grain)								
barbecue, baked, 94% fat-free .... 30 grams	120	2	25	140	1	1.5	0
potato, 100% natural, baked, 94% fat-free, ... 30 grams	120	2	26	150	1	0.5	0
potato, au gratin flavored, baked, 94% nonfat .... 1 oz	120	2	24	140	1	2.0	0
sour cream, w/chive, baked, 94% fat-free .... 30 grams	120	2	24	140	1	2.0	0
(Pepperidge Farm)								
'Flutters' .... 0.75 oz	100	2	15	150	0	4.0	5
'Flutters' garden herb .... 0.75 oz	100	2	14	190	0	4.0	0
'Flutters' golden, w/sesame .... 0.75 oz	110	2	13	150	0	5.0	0
'Flutters' toasted wheat .... 0.75 oz	110	2	13	170	0	5.0	0
'Goldfish' cheddar .... 1 oz	120	4	19	230	1	4.0	5
'Goldfish' cheddar, original .... 1 oz	130	3	18	190	1	5.0	0
'Goldfish' Parmesan cheese .... 1 oz	120	4	19	330	1	4.0	5
'Goldfish' pizza .... 1 oz	130	4	19	220	1	5.0	5
'Goldfish Snack' honey nut, w/roasted								
cashews and almonds .... 1/2 cup	180	5	20	330	2	9.0	25
'Goldfish Snack' w/roasted peanuts .... 1/2 cup	170	5	21	360	2	8.0	5
'Goldfish Thins' cheddar .... 4 crackers	50	1	8	160	0	2.0	0
'Guppies' cheddar .... 12 pieces	40	1	5	95	0	2.0	0
'Snack Sticks' .... 8 crackers	130	4	19	400	1	5.0	0
'Snack Sticks' pumpernickel .... 8 crackers	140	3	20	330	1	6.0	0
'Snack Sticks' sesame .... 8 crackers	140	4	19	280	1	5.0	0
(Premier Japan)								
rice, sembei, 'Fire & Spice' .... 4 crackers	50	1	10	150	1	1.0	0
rice sembei, w/sesame, wheat-free, lowfat .... 4 crackers	60	1	10	260	1	1.0	0
(Ralston)								
'Oat Bran Krisps' .... 0.5 oz	60	1	9	140	3	3.0	0
'Oat Krisp' .... 0.5 oz	50	1	7	140	3	2.0	0
vegetable .... 17 crackers	150	2	19	270	1	7.0	na
vegetable, less fat .... 21 crackers	120	2	23	280	1	3.0	0
wheat, w/sesame, 'Jacquet' .... 8 crackers	140	2	18	150	1	6.0	na
(Red Oval Farms)								
stoned wheat, w/toasted sesame, mini .... 19 crackers	140	4	21	440	2	4.0	0

Food Name	Serv. Size	Total Cal.	Prot. gms	Carbs gms	Sod. mgs	Fiber gms	Fat gms	Chol. mgs
(Rokeach)								
cheese flavor	1 oz	140	3	16	0	0	8.0	0
saltine	10 pieces	120	2	20	0	0	3.0	0
snack	9 crackers	130	2	19	0	0	5.0	0
(Roman Meal)								
wheat, w/onion, baked	6 crackers	70	1	9	120	1	3.0	0
wheat, w/sesame, baked	6 crackers	70	1	9	120	0	3.0	0
whole wheat, baked	6 crackers	70	2	9	105	0	3.0	0
whole wheat, rye and bran, baked	6 crackers	70	1	9	140	0	3.0	0
(RyKrisp)								
'Rykrisp Twindividuals' 2 triple pieces	0.5 oz	45	1	11	105	3	1.0	0
crispbread, original	2 crackers	60	2	8	75	4	0.0	0
crispbread, rye, triple cracker	1 wafer	92	2	21	66	4	0.3	0
crispbread, rye, w/sesame, 2 triple pieces	0.5 oz	50	1	10	105	3	2.0	0
crispbread, seasoned	2 crackers	60	1	10	90	3	1.5	0
crispbread, sesame	2 crackers	60	2	11	80	3	1.5	0
(Ryvita)								
crispbread, dark rye	1 cracker	26	1	6	35	1	1.0	0
crispbread, high-fiber, 'Crisp Bread'	1 cracker	23	1	4	10	2	1.0	0
crispbread, high-fiber, 'Snackbread'	1 cracker	14	1	3	25	1	1.0	0
crispbread, light	1 cracker	26	1	6	20	1	1.0	0
crispbread, rye, light	1 cracker	26	1	6	20	1	1.0	0
crispbread, rye, dark	1 cracker	26	1	6	35	1	1.0	0
crispbread, rye, w/sesame	1 cracker	31	1	5	10	1	1.0	0
wheat, 'Original Snackbread'	1 cracker	20	1	4	20	1	1.0	0
(Snackwell's)								
cheese, zesty	1 serving	129	2	23	315	1	3.0	1
cracked pepper	7 crackers	61	1	10	117	0	1.6	0
French onion	1 serving	128	2	23	275	1	3.0	1
golden, reduced fat	6 crackers	60	1	11	140	0	1.0	0
Italian ranch	1 serving	128	2	23	311	1	3.0	1
salsa, snack	1 serving	128	2	23	321	1	3.0	1
wheat	1 serving	62	1	12	150	1	1.5	na
wheat, nonfat	5 crackers	60	2	12	170	1	0.0	0
wheat thins, baked	1 serving	136	2	20	168	1	5.8	0
(Spicer's)								
diet, natural, for weight control	1 oz	100	4	11	65	9	4.0	0
w/onion, for weight control	1 oz	100	4	12	150	6	4.0	0
wheat, barbecue, for weight control	1 oz	100	5	12	75	9	5.0	0
(Stop & Shop) cheese flavor, 'Big'	25 crackers	140	3	19	220	1	6.0	5
(Sunshine)								
heart shaped	1 cracker	9	0	1	6	0	0.4	0
soup and oyster	16 crackers	60	1	11	190	0	1.0	0
wheat	8 crackers	70	1	9	170	1	4.0	0
wheat, heart shaped	1 cracker	9	0	1	16	0	0.4	0
(Valley Bakery)	8 crackers	110	3	21	140	1	1.0	0
'Janet Saghatelian's Hearts'	8 crackers	110	3	21	140	1	1.0	0
lahvosh, 5-inch rounds	1.2 oz	140	5	26	180	1	1.5	0
lahvosh, 5-Inch wheat rounds	1.2 oz	130	5	26	180	2	1.5	0
lahvosh, hearts	1 oz	110	4	21	140	1	1.0	0
lahvosh, 'Sweet-heart Crispies'	1 oz	120	3	22	130	1	2.5	0
lahvosh, 3-inch rounds	1 oz	110	4	21	140	1	1.0	0
lahvosh, 3-inch wheat rounds	1 oz	110	4	20	140	2	1.0	0
lahvosh, 2-inch rounds	1 oz	110	4	21	140	1	1.0	0
rounds, hors d'oeurvre size	1 cracker	28	1	6	41	0	0.3	0
rounds, snack size	2 crackers	130	4	26	170	1	1.0	0
w/sesame seed, original, Armenian	1 slice	190	6	37	250	1	2.0	0

Food Name	Serv. Size	Total Cal.	Prot. gms	Carbs gms	Sod. mgs	Fiber gms	Fat gms	Chol. mgs
(Vivant) vegetable	3 crackers	70	1	9	125	0	3.0	0
(Wasa)								
crispbread, 'Extra Crisp'	1 cracker	25	1	5	40	0	0.0	0
crispbread, cinnamon toast	1 slice	60	2	11	65	1	1.0	0
crispbread, corn, original, gluten- and wheat-free	1 slice	40	1	7	90	0	1.0	0
crispbread, light, 'Crisp 'N Light'	1 cracker	25	1	5	40	1	0.0	0
crispbread, multigrain, original	1 slice	45	2	8	85	2	0.0	0
crispbread, rye	1 crispbread	37	1	8	26	2	0.1	0
crispbread, rye, fiber	1 slice	30	1	4	60	2	1.0	0
crispbread, rye, golden	1 cracker	35	1	7	55	1	0.0	0
crispbread, rye, hearty	1 slice	45	1	9	40	2	0.0	0
crispbread, rye, light	1 slice	25	1	5	40	1	0.0	0
crispbread, rye, organic, salt-free	1 slice	25	1	7	50	1	0.0	0
crispbread, rye, original	1 slice	30	1	7	0	2	0.0	0
crispbread, sesame, savory	1 cracker	30	2	4	40	2	1.0	0
crispbread, sourdough rye, light, 'Crisp 'N Light'	3 pieces	60	2	12	120	1	0.0	0
crispbread, sourdough rye, original	1 slice	35	1	7	55	1	0.0	0
crispbread, sourdough, crisp	3 pieces	50	2	11	100	2	0.0	0
crispbread, wheat, light, 'Crisp 'N Light'	2 crackers	50	2	10	100	1	0.0	0
crispbread, wheat, toasted, original	1 slice	50	2	8	85	1	1.5	0
crispbread, wheat, w/sesame	1 cracker	50	2	8	65	1	2.0	0
crispbread, whole wheat	1 slice	30	2	4	40	2	1.0	0
crispbread, whole wheat, original	1 slice	50	2	11	55	1	0.5	0
(Weight Watchers)								
crispbread, garlic flavor	2 crackers	30	1	7	55	0	0.0	0
crispbread, harvest rice	2 crackers	30	1	7	55	0	0.0	0
(Westbrae)								
no salt, wafer	4 1/2 wafers	40	1	8	0	0	0.0	0
onion garlic, wafer	4 1/2 wafers	40	1	8	50	0	0.0	0
tamari, wafer	4 1/2 wafers	40	1	8	60	0	0.0	0
w/sesame, wafer	4 1/2 wafers	40	1	8	60	0	0.0	0
(Wheat Krisp) wheat	0.5 oz	50	2	11	220	0	1.0	0
(Zings)								
cracker chips, cheddar, baked	0.5 oz	70	1	9	140	0	3.0	2
cracker chips, ranch flavor, baked	0.5 oz	70	1	9	140	0	3.0	2
CRACKER CRUMBS								
'Ritz' *(Nabisco)*	1/3 cup	140	2	17	270	1	7.0	0
'Premium' *(Nabisco)*	1/4 cup	100	3	23	0	1	0.0	0
CRACKER MEAL								
	1 cup	440	11	93	32	3	2.0	0
	1 oz	109	3	23	8	1	0.5	0
(Golden Dipt)	1 oz	100	3	22	0	0	0.0	0
(Nabisco)	1/4 cup	110	3	24	10	1	0.0	0
extra fine, food service product *(Keebler)*	4 tbsp	130	3	23	0	1	0.0	0
matzo *(Manischewitz)*	1/2 cup	243	6	54	7	2	0.3	0
matzo, 'Farfel' *(Manischewitz)*	1 cup	280	7	60	2	0	0.8	0
matzo, 'Daily' *(Manischewitz)*	1 cup	514	13	109	3	1	1.4	0
CRANBERRY								
Fresh								
raw, chopped	1 cup	54	0	14	1	5	0.2	0
raw, whole	1 cup	47	0	12	1	4	0.2	0
CRANBERRY BEAN. See BEAN, CRANBERRY.								
CRANBERRY JUICE								
(J. Hungerford) 100% juice	9.03 fl oz	133	0	33	19	0	0.0	0
(Knudsen)								
	8 fl oz	60	0	14	25	na	0.0	0
'Just Cranberry'	8 fl oz	40	1	10	0	0	0.0	0
'Yankee'	8 fl oz	120	0	30	25	na	0.0	0

Food Name	Serv. Size	Total Cal.	Prot. gms	Carbs gms	Sod. mgs	Fiber gms	Fat gms	Chol. mgs
(Lucky Leaf)	6 fl oz	110	0	26	10	0	0.0	0
(Ocean Spray) 'Crantastic'	6 fl oz	100	0	26	15	0	0.0	0
(Santa Cruz Natural) organic, 'Sparkling'	8 fl oz	90	1	22	0	0	1.0	0
CRANBERRY JUICE COCKTAIL. See under FRUIT JUICE DRINK.								
CRANBERRY SAUCE								
Canned								
(A&P)	2 oz	100	1	25	15	0	1.0	0
(Knudsen)	1 oz	30	1	8	0	0	1.0	0
jellied *(Finast)*	2 oz	90	0	22	10	0	0.0	0
jellied *(Ocean Spray)*	2 oz	80	0	22	10	0	0.0	0
jellied *(Pathmark)*	2 oz	90	0	22	10	0	0.0	0
jellied *(S&W)*	1/4 cup	100	0	26	15	1	0.0	0
jellied, 'Old Fashioned' *(S&W)*	1/2 cup	90	0	22	20	0	0.0	0
sweetened, 1/2-inch slices	1 slice	86	0	22	17	1	0.1	0
sweetened	1 cup	418	1	108	80	3	0.4	0
whole berry *(Finast)*	2 oz	90	0	22	10	0	0.0	0
whole berry *(Ocean Spray)*	2 oz	80	0	21	10	0	0.0	0
whole berry *(S&W)*	1/4 cup	100	0	26	15	1	0.0	0
whole berry, 'Old Fashioned' *(S&W)*	1/2 cup	90	0	22	20	0	0.0	0
CRAPPIE. See SUNFISH.								
CRAYFISH								
mixed species, farmed, cooked	3 oz	74	15	0	82	0	1.1	116
mixed species, farmed, raw	3 oz	61	13	0	53	0	0.8	91
mixed species, wild, cooked	3 oz	70	14	0	80	0	1.0	113
mixed species, wild, raw	3 oz	65	14	0	49	0	0.8	97
CRAYFISH DINNER/ENTRÉE								
(Cajun Cookin') crayfish etouffee, frozen	12 oz	390	23	51	1110	0	10.0	0
CREAM								
half and half	1 cup	315	7	10	98	0	27.8	89
half and half	1 fl oz	39	1	1	12	0	3.5	11
half and half	1 tbsp	20	0	1	6	0	1.7	6
half and half *(Crowley)*	1 fl oz	35	1	1	10	0	3.0	15
half and half *(Darigold)*	8 fl oz	310	8	11	120	0	27.0	89
half and half *(Knudsen)*	4 fl oz	150	4	5	60	0	13.0	0
half and half *(Rockview)*	2 tbsp	35	1	0	15	0	3.0	15
Hawaiian macadamia flavored *(International Delight)*	1 tbsp	30	0	7	5	0	0.0	0
heavy, whipping	8 fl oz	821	5	7	89	0	88.1	326
heavy, whipping	1 fl oz	103	1	1	11	0	11.0	41
heavy, whipping	1 tbsp	52	0	0	6	0	5.5	21
heavy, whipping *(Crowley)*	1 oz	110	1	1	10	0	11.0	40
heavy, whipping *(Darigold)*	1 cup	790	6	8	90	0	81.0	290
heavy, whipping, 'Classic' *(Darigold)*	1 cup	858	5	7	77	0	90.0	334
heavy, whipping, ultra-pasteurized *(Darigold)*	1 cup	790	6	8	90	0	81.0	290
light	1 cup	469	6	9	95	0	46.3	159
light	1 fl oz	59	1	1	12	0	5.8	20
light	1 tbsp	29	0	1	6	0	2.9	10
light, whipping	1 cup	699	5	7	82	0	73.9	265
light, whipping	1 tbsp	44	0	0	5	0	4.6	17
CREAM CHEESE. See under CHEESE.								
CREAM OF TARTAR								
	1 tsp	8	0	2	2	0	0.0	0
	1/2 tsp	4	0	1	1	0	0.0	0
(Tone's)	1 tsp	2	0	1	0	0	0.0	0
CREAM SUBSTITUTE								
Liquid								
(Carnation)								
butter rum flavored, nondairy, nonfat	1 tbsp	25	0	6	20	0	0.0	0
French vanilla flavored, nondairy, nonfat	1 tbsp	25	0	6	20	0	0.0	0

Food Name	Serv. Size	Total Cal.	Prot. gms	Carbs gms	Sod. mgs	Fiber gms	Fat gms	Chol. mgs
Irish cream flavored, nondairy, nonfat	1 tbsp	25	0	6	20	0	0.0	0
(Coffee-Mate)								
	1 tbsp	16	0	2	5	0	1.0	0
French vanilla flavored, nondairy	1 tbsp	40	0	5	5	0	2.0	0
mocha almond flavored, nondairy	2 tsp	60	0	9	20	0	3.0	0
nondairy, 'Amaretto'	1 tbsp	40	0	5	5	0	2.0	0
nondairy, 'Cinnamon Creme'	1 tbsp	40	0	5	5	0	2.0	0
nondairy, 'Hazelnut'	1 tbsp	40	0	5	5	0	2.0	0
nondairy, 'Irish Creme'	1 tbsp	40	0	5	5	0	2.0	0
nondairy, fat-free	1 tbsp	10	0	2	0	0	0.0	0
nondairy, light	1 tbsp	10	0	1	5	0	0.5	0
(Crowley) nondairy	0.5 fl oz	16	1	1	5	0	1.0	5
(Finast) nondairy, frozen	0.5 fl oz	20	0	2	10	0	2.0	0
(International Delight)								
Amaretto flavored, nondairy	1 tbsp	45	0	7	5	0	1.5	0
Hawaiian macadamia flavored, dairy	1 tbsp	30	0	7	5	0	0.0	0
Irish cream flavored, nondairy	1 tbsp	45	0	7	5	0	1.5	0
(Lucerne) nondairy, 100% milk-free	0.5 fl oz	16	1	1	5	0	2.0	0
(Mocha Mix)								
nondairy	1 tbsp	20	0	1	5	0	1.5	0
nondairy, lite	1 tbsp	10	0	1	0	0	1.0	0
(Rich's)								
nondairy, frozen, 'Coffee Rich'	0.5 fl oz	20	0	2	10	0	2.0	0
nondairy, frozen, 'Farm Rich'	0.5 fl oz	20	0	1	5	0	2.0	0
nondairy, frozen, 'Poly Rich'	0.5 fl oz	20	0	2	5	0	1.0	0
(Saco Foods) nondairy, 'Kwik Kream'	1 tbsp	10	0	2	0	0	1.0	0
(Westbrae) nondairy	1 tbsp	10	1	2	10	0	1.0	0
(WestSoy) nondairy, lite, all natural	1 tbsp	10	1	2	10	0	1.0	0
Powder								
(Coffee-Mate)								
nondairy	1 tsp	10	1	1	5	0	1.0	0
nondairy, 'Amaretto'	2 tsp	60	0	9	15	0	3.0	0
nondairy, 'Hazelnut'	2 tsp	60	0	0	15	0	3.0	0
nondairy, 'Irish Creme'	2 tsp	60	0	9	15	0	3.0	0
nondairy, light	1 tsp	10	0	2	0	0	0.0	0
nondairy, nonfat	1 tsp	10	0	2	0	0	0.0	0
(Cremora) nondairy	1 tsp	10	0	1	5	0	1.0	0
(Diehl) nondairy	1 tsp	10	0	1	0	0	1.0	0
(IGA) nondairy	1 tsp	10	0	2	5	0	1.0	0
(Pathmark) nondairy, 'No Frills'	1 tsp	10	0	1	5	0	0.0	0
CREAM TOPPING								
(Birds Eye)								
chocolate, nondairy, frozen, 'Cool Whip'	1 tbsp	12	0	1	0	0	1.0	0
extra creamy, nondairy, frozen, 'Cool Whip Dairy Recipe'	1 tbsp	14	0	1	0	0	1.0	0
nondairy, frozen, 'Cool Whip Lite'	1 tbsp	8	0	1	0	0	1.0	0
nondairy, frozen, 'Cool Whip'	1 tbsp	12	0	1	0	0	1.0	0
(Crowley)								
whipped, pressurized can	1 tbsp	20	1	1	10	0	1.0	5
whipping, heavy	1 oz	110	1	1	10	0	11.0	40
(Darigold)								
whipping, heavy	1 cup	790	6	8	90	0	81.0	290
whipping, heavy, 'Classic'	1 cup	858	5	7	77	0	90.0	334
whipping, heavy, ultra-pasteurized	1 cup	790	6	8	90	0	81.0	290
(Estee) nondairy, prewhipped	1 tbsp	4	1	1	0	0	1.0	0
(Kraft)								
frozen, whipped, 'Real Cream'	1/4 cup	30	0	2	5	0	2.0	10

Food Name	Serv. Size	Total Cal.	Prot. gms	Carbs gms	Sod. mgs	Fiber gms	Fat gms	Chol. mgs
nondairy, frozen, 'Whipped Topping' .... 1/4 cup		35	0	2	10	0	3.0	0
(La Creme) frozen, whipped .... 1 tbsp		16	0	1	5	0	1.0	1
(Pet) nondairy, frozen, 'Whip' .... 1 tbsp		14	0	1	0	0	1.0	0
(Rich's)								
nondairy, pressurized can, 'Richwhip' .... 0.25 oz		20	0	1	5	0	2.0	0
nondairy, prewhipped, 'Richwhip' .... 1 tbsp		12	0	1	0	0	1.0	0
(Saco Foods)								
chocolate, dark, 'Dolci Frutta Con Cioccolatta' .... 1 serving		111	1	14	14	0	6.6	0
white, 'Dolci Frutta Crema Bianca' .... 1 serving		112	1	12	14	0	6.0	0
CREAM TOPPING MIX								
(D-Zerta) prepared .... 1 tbsp		8	0	0	5	0	1.0	0
(Dream Whip)								
mix only .... 1 tbsp		6	0	1	0	0	0.0	0
prepared w/whole milk .... 1 tbsp		10	0	1	0	0	0.0	0
(Featherweight) prepared .... 1 tbsp		4	0	0	5	0	0.0	0
(Rich's) mix only, 'Richwhip' .... 0.25 oz		20	0	1	10	0	2.0	0
CREOLE SEASONING. See under SEASONING MIX.								
CREPE MIX (Krusteaz) prepared, 7-inch diam .... 2 crepes		80	2	14	110	0	1.0	0
CRIMINI MUSHROOM. See MUSHROOM, CRIMINI.								
CROAKER, ATLANTIC								
breaded, fried .... 3 oz		188	15	6	296	0	10.8	71
raw .... 3 oz		88	15	0	48	0	2.7	52
CROISSANT								
(Awrey's)								
butter... 1 oz		100	2	10	90	0	6.0	15
margarine .... 1.25 oz		120	2	13	180	0	7.0	5
wheat .... 2.5 oz		240	4	24	390	1	14.0	5
(Pepperidge Farm)								
butter, petite, frozen .... 1 piece		140	3	13	160	0	7.0	0
'Sandwich Quartet' .... 1 croissant		170	4	22	250	0	7.0	0
(Sara Lee) butter, petite, frozen .... 1 croissant		120	3	13	160	0	6.0	0
CROOKNECK SQUASH. See SQUASH, CROOKNECK. Also see under SQUASH, SUMMER.								
CROUTONS								
(Brownberry)								
Caesar salad flavored .... 0.5 oz		62	2	8	165	1	2.6	1
cheddar cheese flavored .... 0.5 oz		63	2	8	155	0	2.8	3
onion and garlic flavored .... 0.5 oz		60	2	9	190	0	2.2	1
seasoned .... 1/2 oz		59	2	9	155	1	2.2	1
toasted .... 0.5 oz		56	2	10	145	0	1.4	0
(Ener-G Foods)								
Italian, gluten free .... 1 cup		241	4	31	305	4	12.5	4
onion and garlic, gluten free .... 1 cup		147	2	37	267	4	0.4	4
plain, gluten free .... 1 cup		125	1	17	135	3	7.0	0
(Fresh Gourmet)								
Caesar flavor .... 4 croutons		30	1	4	85	0	1.0	0
cheese and garlic flavor, homestyle .... 4 croutons		30	1	4	100	0	1.0	0
herb seasoned .... 4 croutons		30	1	5	90	0	1.0	0
(Hidden Valley Ranch)								
Parmesan, Italian style, 'Salad Crispins' .... 1 serving		30	1	5	80	na	0.9	na
(Just Off Melrose)								
cheese and garlic .... 3 croutons		25	1	3	30	0	1.5	5
garlic .... 3 croutons		30	0	3	25	0	2.0	0
sun-dried tomato and basil .... 3 croutons		30	0	3	25	0	2.0	0
(Other Fine Foods) whole grain, all natural .... 1 oz		110	3	15	115	0	4.0	0
(Pepperidge Farm)								
cheddar and Romano .... 9 croutons		30	1	4	95	0	1.0	0
cheese and garlic .... 9 croutons		35	1	4	80	0	1.5	0

Food Name	Serv. Size	Total Cal.	Prot. gms	Carbs gms	Sod. mgs	Fiber gms	Fat gms	Chol. mgs
onion and garlic	9 pieces	30	1	5	80	0	1.0	0
seasoned	9 croutons	35	1	4	85	0	1.5	0
seasoned, classic style	1 serving	33	1	4	97	na	1.3	na
sour cream and chive	0.5 oz	70	2	9	170	0	3.0	0
(Reese) Caesar salad flavored	0.5 oz	60	2	9	130	0	2.0	0
(Rothbury Farms)								
onion flavor poppy toast, nonfat	9 grams	35	1	7	135	0	0.0	0
seasoned, French style, nonfat	7 grams	25	1	5	105	0	0.0	0
seasoned, nonfat	7 grams	25	1	5	105	0	0.0	0
CROWDER PEA. See under BLACK-EYED PEAS.								
CRUMPET								
(Wolferman's)								
blueberry, low-fat, cholesterol-free	1 crumpet	90	3	21	250	1	1.0	0
brown sugar-cinnamon, lowfat	1 crumpet	110	3	21	220	2	2.0	0
raspberry, low-fat, cholesterol-free	1 crumpet	90	3	20	260	1	1.0	0
CUCUMBER								
Fresh								
peeled, raw, chopped	1 cup	16	1	3	3	1	0.2	0
peeled, raw, sliced	1 cup	14	1	3	2	1	0.2	0
peeled, raw, sticks, 4-inches	1 stick	1	0	0	0	0	0.0	0
peeled, raw, whole, large, 8.25 inches	1 cucumber	34	2	7	6	2	0.4	0
peeled, raw, whole, small 6 3/8 inches	1 cucumber	19	1	4	3	1	0.3	0
w/peel, raw, whole, large, 8.25 inches	1 cucumber	39	2	8	6	2	0.4	0
w/peel, raw, sliced	1/2 cup	7	0	1	1	0	0.1	0
CUMIN SEED								
ground *(McCormick/Schilling)*	1 tsp	11	0	1	5	1	0.4	0
whole	1 tbsp	22	1	3	10	1	1.3	0
whole	1 tsp	8	0	1	4	0	0.5	0
whole *(Durkee)*	1 tsp	10	0	0	0	0	0.0	0
whole *(Laurel Leaf)*	1 tsp	10	0	0	0	0	0.0	0
whole *(McCormick/Schilling)*	1 tsp	16	1	2	7	1	0.8	0
whole *(Spice Islands)*	1 tsp	7	0	1	3	0	0.4	0
whole *(Tone's)*	1 tsp	7	0	1	3	0	0.4	0
CUPU ASSU OIL								
	1 cup	1927	0	0	0	0	218.0	0
	1 tbsp	120	0	0	0	0	13.6	0
CURRANT								
BLACK/European currant, raw	1 cup	71	2	17	2	na	0.5	0
RED OR WHITE, raw	1 cup	63	2	15	1	5	0.2	0
ZANTE								
dried	1 cup	408	6	107	12	10	0.4	0
dried *(Sun-Maid)*	1/4 cup	130	1	31	10	3	0.0	0
dried *(S&W)*	1/4 cup	130	1	31	10	2	0.0	0
CURRY POWDER. See under SEASONING MIX.								
CUSK/torsk/tusk								
baked, broiled, grilled, or microwaved	3 oz	95	21	0	34	0	0.7	45
raw	3 oz	74	16	0	26	0	0.6	35
CUSTARD APPLE/bullock's heart/cherimoya								
Fresh, raw, skin and seeds removed	1 fruit	514	7	131	na	13	2.2	0
CUTTLEFISH								
mixed species, cooked	3 oz	134	28	1	632	0	1.2	190
mixed species, raw	3 oz	67	14	1	316	0	0.6	95

D

Food Name	Serv. Size	Total Cal.	Prot. gms	Carbs gms	Sod. mgs	Fiber gms	Fat gms	Chol. mgs
DAIKON/Chinese radish/Oriental radish								
boiled, drained	4 oz	19	0.8	3.9	15	>.6 c	0.3	0
boiled, drained, sliced	1 cup	25	1	5	19	2	0.4	0
boiled, drained, sliced	1/2 cup	13	0.5	2.5	10	1.2	0.2	0
dried	1 cup	314	9	74	322	na	0.8	0
dried	1/2 cup	157	4.6	36.8	161	>4.9 c	0.4	0
dried	1 oz	77	2.2	18.0	79	>2.4 c	0.2	0
raw, trimmed	1 oz	5	0.2	1.2	6	>.2 c	<.1	0
raw, trimmed *(Frieda's)*	1 lb	86	4.1	19.1	(mq)	(mq)	0.5	0
raw, trimmed *(Frieda's)*	1 oz	5	0.3	1.2	(mq)	(mq)	<.1	0
raw, trimmed, sliced	1/2 cup	8	0.3	1.8	9	0.7	<.1	0
raw, untrimmed	1 lb	65	2.2	14.7	75	>2.3 c	0.4	0
raw, whole, approx 7 inches long, 2 1/4 inch diam	1 daikon	62	2.0	13.9	71	5.4	0.3	0
DAIQUIRI. See under COCKTAIL; COCKTAIL MIX.								
DANDELION GREENS								
boiled, drained, chopped	1 cup	35	2	7	46	3	0.6	0
raw, chopped	1 cup	25	1	5	42	2	0.4	0
DANISH CABBAGE. See CABBAGE, DANISH.								
DANISH PASTRY. See under PASTRY; PASTRY, TOASTER.								
DASHEEN								
cooked	4 oz	161	0.6	39.2	11	>1.0 c	0.1	0
cooked, sliced	1/2 cup	94	0.3	22.8	10	>.6 c	0.1	0
raw, sliced	1/2 cup	56	0.8	13.8	6	>.4 c	0.1	0
raw, trimmed	1 oz	30	0.4	7.5	3	>.2 c	0.1	0
raw, untrimmed	1 lb	419	5.9	103.2	43	>3.1 c	0.8	0
DASHEEN LEAF								
raw	1/2 cup	6	0.7	0.9	1	>.3 c	0.1	0
raw, trimmed	1 oz	12	1.4	1.9	1	>.6 c	0.2	0
raw, untrimmed	1 lb	115	13.5	18.3	8	>5.5 c	2.0	0
steamed	1/2 cup	18	2.0	3.0	2	>.4 c	0.3	0
steamed	4 oz	27	3.1	4.6	2	>.6 c	0.5	0
DASHEEN SHOOTS								
cooked	4 oz	16	0.8	3.6	2	>.6 c	0.1	0
cooked, sliced	1/2 cup	10	0.5	2.2	1	>.4 c	0.1	0
raw, sliced	1/2 cup	5	0.4	1.0	<1	>.3 c	<.1	0
raw, trimmed	1 oz	3	0.3	0.7	<1	>.2 c	<.1	0
raw, untrimmed	1 lb	45	3.7	9.3	4	>2.3 c	0.4	0
DATE								
Domestic, natural and dry								
	1 lb	1123	8.0	300.1	10	20.8	1.8	0
chopped	1/2 cup	245	1.8	65.4	3	4.5	0.4	0
pitted	1 oz	78	0.6	20.8	1	1.4	0.1	0
pitted *(Dole)*	1/2 cup	280	5.0	62.0	0	(mq)	0.0	0
pitted, whole, approx 10 dates	2.9 oz	228	1.6	61.0	2	4.2	0.4	0
Imported, pitted								
(Amport Foods)								
chopped	1.5 oz	135	0.0	36.0	0	5	0.0	0
whole	1.5 oz	135	0.0	36.0	0	5	0.0	0
(Bordo)								
	2 oz	204	1.2	47.2	5	>1.5 c	1.2	0
diced	2 oz	203	1.0	47.5	5	>1.2 c	1.1	0
(Dromedary)								
chopped	1/4 cup	130	1.0	31.0	0	(mq)	0.0	0
whole, approx 5 dates	1 oz	100	1.0	23.0	0	(mq)	0.0	0

Food Name	Serv. Size	Total Cal.	Prot. gms	Carbs gms	Sod. mgs	Fiber gms	Fat gms	Chol. mgs
DATE, INDIAN. See TAMARIND.								
DEER								
raw	1 lb	544	104.1	0.0	231	na	11.0	386
raw	1 oz	34	6.4	0.0	14	na	0.7	24
roasted	3 oz	134	25.7	0.0	46	na	2.7	95
DESSERT TOPPING								
(Nestlé)								
'Butterfinger'	1 cup	835	22	114	345	4	32.5	2
'Butterfinger'	2 tbsp	120	3	16	50	1	4.7	0
'Crunch'	2 tbsp	125	1	16	32	1	6.3	3
crunchy, 'Buncha Crunch'	1 serving	103	1	13	46	0	5.1	3
crunchy, 'Buncha Crunch'	2 lb pkg	4671	52	598	2095	15	230.7	127
crunchy, 'Buncha Crunch'	2 tbsp	103	1	13	46	0	5.1	3
'Rainbow Morsel'	1 pkt	68	1	10	0	1	2.7	0
'Rainbow Morsel'	1 serving	68	1	10	0	1	2.7	0
'Rainbow Morsel'	3 lb pkg	6628	57	1008	41	75	263.8	27
(Snack Pack)								
chocolate fudge	3.88 oz	166	2	25	148	0	6.3	0
chocolate, w/dinosaurs	3.84 oz	163	2	26	167	0	5.8	0
milk chocolate sprinkles	3.88 oz	178	2	28	156	0	6.3	1
vanilla chocolate sprinkles	3.88 oz	166	2	26	132	0	6.1	0
DIET BAR. See under SPORTS AND DIET/NUTRITION BARS.								
DIET DRINK. See under SPORTS AND DIET/NUTRITION DRINKS.								
DILL SEASONING. See under SEASONING MIX.								
DILL SEED								
whole	1 tbsp	20	1	4	1	1	1.0	0
whole	1 tsp	6	0	1	0	0	0.3	0
whole *(Durkee)*	1 tsp	9	0	0	0	0	0.0	0
whole *(Laurel Leaf)*	1 tsp	9	0	0	0	0	0.0	0
whole *(McCormick/Schilling)*	1 tsp	13	0	2	1	2	0.4	0
whole *(Spice Islands)*	1 tsp	9	0	1	1	0	0.4	0
whole *(Tone's)*	1 tsp	6	0	1	2	0	0.3	0
DILL WEED								
dried	1 tbsp	8	1	2	6	0	0.1	0
dried	1 tsp	3	0	1	2	0	0.0	0
dried *(McCormick/Schilling)*	1 tsp	4	0	0	10	0	0.0	0
dried *(Tone's)*	1 tsp	3	0	1	2	0	0.1	0
fresh, sprigs	1 cup sprigs	4	0	1	5	0	0.1	0
fresh, sprigs	5 med sprigs	0	0	0	1	0	0.0	0
DINNER ROLL. See under ROLL.								
DIP								
ACAPULCO *(Ortega)* nonfat	1 oz	8	0	2	0	0	0.0	0
AVOCADO								
(Kraft)	2 tbsp	60	1	4	240	0	4.0	0
(Rod's Dips)	2 tbsp	110	1	2	210	0	11.0	5
BACON AND HORSERADISH								
(Breakstone's)	2 tbsp	70	1	2	270	0	6.0	15
(Kraft)								
	2 tbsp	60	1	3	220	0	5.0	0
'Premium'	2 tbsp	50	1	2	270	0	5.0	15
(Sealtest)	2 tbsp	70	1	2	270	0	6.0	15
BACON AND ONION								
(Breakstone's) 'Gourmet'	2 tbsp	70	1	2	210	0	6.0	15
(Kraft) 'Premium'	2 tbsp	60	1	2	170	0	5.0	15
BEAN								
(Bearitos)								
black bean, vegetarian, organic, fat-free	1 oz	24	2	4	135	0	0.0	0

Food Name	Serv. Size	Total Cal.	Prot. gms	Carbs gms	Sod. mgs	Fiber gms	Fat gms	Chol. mgs
vegetarian, organic, fat-free	1 oz	25	1	5	135	0	0.0	0
(Chi-Chi's) 'Fiesta'	1 oz	30	1	4	126	0	1.0	3
(Eagle)								
black bean	2 tbsp	35	2	5	220	1	1.0	0
mild	2 tbsp	40	2	5	160	2	1.5	0
(Frito-Lay's)								
	2 tbsp	40	2	6	140	0	1.0	0
hot	2 tbsp	40	2	5	170	1	1.0	0
(Garden of Eden)								
Baja black bean, organic	2 tbsp	25	2	5	80	1	0.0	0
chipotle red bean, organic	2 tbsp	25	1	5	90	2	0.0	0
(Guiltless Gourmet)								
barbecue, mild, nonfat	2 tbsp	23	1	4	100	2	0.0	0
barbecue, spicy, nonfat	2 tbsp	35	2	6	125	1	0.0	0
black bean, barbecue, nonfat	2 tbsp	35	2	6	125	1	0.0	0
black bean, spicy, nonfat	2 tbsp	30	2	5	100	1	0.0	0
mild, nonfat	2 tbsp	23	1	4	100	2	0.0	0
pinto bean, barbecue, mild	2 tbsp	27	2	5	100	2	0.0	0
pinto bean, barbecue, spicy	2 tbsp	40	2	7	110	2	0.0	0
pinto bean, mild	2 tbsp	27	2	5	100	2	0.0	0
pinto bean, spicy, nonfat	2 tbsp	35	2	6	100	2	0.0	0
(Hain)								
hot	4 tbsp	70	4	10	250	0	1.0	5
Mexican	4 tbsp	60	4	9	260	0	1.0	5
w/onion	4 tbsp	70	4	10	270	0	1.0	5
(Mi Ranchito)								
low-fat	2 tbsp	30	2	8	100	0	1.0	0
spicy, low-fat	2 tbsp	27	2	7	105	0	1.0	0
(Old El Paso) black bean	2 tbsp	20	1	4	150	1	0.0	0
(Tostitos) black, medium, nonfat	2 tbsp	30	2	6	210	2	0.0	0
BLUE CHEESE								
(Kraft) 'Premium'	2 tbsp	50	1	2	210	0	4.0	10
(Litehouse)								
and dressing, refrigerated, 'Lite'	1 tbsp	33	1	1	86	0	3.0	0
and dressing, refrigerated, Original'	1 tbsp	77	1	0	82	0	8.0	0
country, and dressing, refrigerated	1 tbsp	76	1	0	84	0	8.0	0
CAESAR (Litehouse) and dressing, refrigerated	1 tbsp	57	0	0	84	0	6.0	0
CHEESE								
(Chi-Chi's) 'Fiesta'	1 oz	41	1	3	296	0	3.0	9
(Frito-Lay's) cheddar, mild	2 tbsp	60	1	3	330	0	4.0	5
(Kraft) nacho, 'Premium'	2 tbsp	55	2	2	200	0	4.0	10
(Guiltless Gourmet)								
queso, mild	2 tbsp	20	1	5	150	0	0.0	0
queso, spicy	2 tbsp	20	1	5	150	0	0.0	0
CHEESE AND SALSA								
(Eagle) medium	2 tbsp	40	1	3	300	0	3.0	5
(Old El Paso) mild or medium	2 tbsp	40	1	3	300	0	3.0	3
CHILI (La Victoria)	1 tbsp	6	1	1	90	0	1.0	0
CLAM								
(Breakstone's)								
	2 tbsp	50	1	2	220	0	4.0	15
'Gourmet Chesapeake'	2 tbsp	50	1	2	200	0	4.0	20
(Kraft)	2 tbsp	60	1	3	250	0	4.0	0
(Sealtest)	2 tbsp	50	1	2	220	0	4.0	15
CUCUMBER (Kraft) creamy, 'Premium'	2 tbsp	50	1	2	130	0	4.0	10
CUCUMBER AND ONION								
(Breakstone's)	2 tbsp	50	1	2	160	0	4.0	15

Food Name	Serv. Size	Total Cal.	Prot. gms	Carbs gms	Sod. mgs	Fiber gms	Fat gms	Chol. mgs
(Sealtest)	2 tbsp	50	1	2	160	0	4.0	15
DILL *(Nasoya)* creamy, 'Vegi-Dip'	1 oz	60	2	4	100	0	4.0	0
GARLIC								
(Life) and dressing, w/tofu, 'All Natural'	1 tbsp	70	1	1	75	0	7.1	0
(Nasoya) and herb, 'Vegi-Dip'	1 oz	50	2	6	100	0	2.0	0
GREEN ONION, *(Kraft)*	2 tbsp	60	1	4	190	0	4.0	0
GUACAMOLE								
(Kraft)	2 tbsp	50	1	3	210	0	4.0	0
(Lucerne)	2 tbsp	80	1	1	170	0	8.0	5
(Rod's Dips)	2 tbsp	80	1	1	170	0	8.0	5
HONEY MUSTARD *(Litehouse)* and dressing, refrigerated	1 tbsp	67	0	2	55	0	7.0	0
ITALIAN *(Litehouse)* creamy, and dressing, refrigerated	1 tbsp	60	0	0	76	0	6.0	0
JALAPEÑO								
(Breakstone's) cheddar, 'Gourmet'	2 tbsp	70	2	2	90	0	6.0	15
(Frito-Lay's)								
and cheddar cheese	2 tbsp	50	1	4	300	0	4.0	5
bean	1 oz	30	1	4	115	0	1.0	0
(Hain) bean, medium	4 tbsp	70	4	10	150	0	1.0	5
(Kraft)	2 tbsp	60	1	3	260	0	4.0	0
(Old El Paso) bean, nonfat	1 tbsp	14	1	2	53	1	0.0	0
(Price's) nacho	1 oz	80	3	2	0	0	7.1	0
(Wise) bean, nonfat	2 tbsp	25	1	5	100	0	0.0	0
MUSHROOM *(Breakstone's)* and herb, 'Gourmet'	2 tbsp	50	1	2	150	0	4.0	10
NACHO *(Guiltless Gourmet)* spicy, nonfat	2 tbsp	25	1	5	150	0	0.0	0
ONION								
(Bison) French	1 oz	60	1	2	180	0	5.0	20
(Breakstone's)								
French	2 tbsp	50	1	2	140	0	5.0	15
toasted, 'Gourmet'	2 tbsp	50	1	2	170	0	5.0	10
(Frito-Lay's) French	2 tbsp	60	1	4	230	0	5.0	15
(Heluva Good) French, real sour cream	2 tbsp	50	1	2	160	0	5.0	20
(Kraft)								
creamy, 'Premium'	2 tbsp	45	1	2	160	0	4.0	10
French	2 tbsp	60	1	4	230	0	4.0	0
French, 'Premium'	2 tbsp	45	1	2	150	0	4.0	10
(Lucerne) French	2 tbsp	70	1	2	160	0	6.0	5
(Nasoya) French, 'Vegi-Dip'	1 oz	50	2	4	100	0	3.0	0
(Rod's Dips)								
French	2 tbsp	70	1	2	160	0	6.0	5
French, nonfat	2 tbsp	25	2	3	40	0	0.0	0
French, w/bacon	2 tbsp	70	1	2	180	0	6.0	5
(Sealtest) French	2 tbsp	50	1	2	140	0	5.0	15
PEPPERCORN *(Litehouse)* and dressing, refrigerated	1 tbsp	67	0	0	66	0	7.0	0
PICANTE								
(Frito-Lay's) nonfat	1 oz	10	0	3	160	0	0.0	0
(Tostitos) medium	1 tbsp	8	0	2	125	1	0.0	0
(Wise) nonfat	2 tbsp	12	0	3	130	0	0.0	0
POPPYSEED *(Litehouse)* and dressing, refrigerated	1 tbsp	65	0	3	83	0	6.0	0
RANCH								
(Heluva Good) real sour cream	2 tbsp	60	1	2	180	0	5.0	20
(Litehouse)								
and dressing, refrigerated	1 tbsp	59	0	1	67	0	6.0	0
and dressing, refrigerated, 'Lite'	1 tbsp	35	1	1	80	0	3.0	0
country, and dressing, refrigerated	1 tbsp	61	0	1	75	0	7.0	0
jalapeño, and dressing, refrigerated	1 tbsp	60	0	1	80	0	6.0	0
refrigerated, 'Veggie Dip'	1 tbsp	60	0	1	68	0	7.0	0

Food Name	Serv. Size	Total Cal.	Prot. gms	Carbs gms	Sod. mgs	Fiber gms	Fat gms	Chol. mgs
(Lucerne)	2 tbsp	110	1	2	160	0	11.0	10
(Rod's Dips)								
nonfat	2 tbsp	25	2	3	40	0	0.0	0
w/bacon	2 tbsp	110	1	2	180	0	11.0	5
SALSA								
(Eagle)								
medium	2 tbsp	10	3	2	250	1	0.0	0
mild	2 tbsp	10	3	2	250	1	0.0	0
(Pace)								
medium, 'Chunky'	2 tbsp	4	1	1	102	0	1.0	0
mild, 'Chunky'	2 tbsp	4	1	1	101	0	1.0	0
SOUR CREAM AND CHIVES								
(Litehouse) vinaigrette, and dressing, refrigerated	1 tbsp	63	0	1	72	0	7.0	0
TACO								
(Hain) and sauce	4 tbsp	25	1	5	350	0	1.0	5
(Wise) nonfat	2 tbsp	12	0	3	115	0	0.0	0
THOUSAND ISLAND								
(Litehouse) and dressing, refrigerated	1 tbsp	65	0	1	99	0	7.0	0
VEGETABLE *(Marzetti)* and dressing	1 tbsp	88	0	1	120	0	10.0	2
DIP MIX								
onion and chive *(Knorr)*	1/20 pkg	5	0	1	110	0	0.0	0
sour cream *(Durkee)*	2 tsp	25	1	4	200	0	0.5	0
nacho cheese, 'Microwave Snacks' *(Tio Sancho)*	3.5 oz	247	15	2	995	0	20.0	0
DISHCLOTH GOURD. See GOURD, DISHCLOTH.								
DOCK								
Fresh								
boiled, drained, chopped	3.5 oz	20	1.8	2.9	3	>.7c	0.6	0
boiled, drained, chopped	4 oz	23	2.1	3.3	3	>.8 c	0.7	0
raw, chopped	1 cup	29	3	4	5	4	0.9	0
raw, chopped	1/2 cup	15	1.3	2.1	3	1.94	0.5	0
raw, trimmed	1 oz	6	0.6	0.9	1	>.2 c	0.2	0
raw, untrimmed	1 lb	70	6.4	10.2	13	>2.5 c	2.2	0
DOLPHIN FISH. See MAHI MAHI.								
DOUGHNUT								
(Awrey's)								
crunch	1 doughnut	600	7	65	730	2	34.0	40
plain	1 doughnut	490	6	48	650	1	30.0	35
sugared	1 doughnut	610	7	68	735	2	35.0	40
(Break Cake)								
chocolate, gem	1 doughnut	70	1	7	60	0	4.0	5
chocolate, 1 oz	1 doughnut	130	1	14	115	0	8.0	5
cinnamon, gem	1 doughnut	60	1	8	70	0	3.0	5
cinnamon, 1 oz	1 doughnut	120	1	15	130	0	6.0	5
dunkin stix, 3 oz	2 stix	420	3	43	320	0	27.0	0
powdered sugar, gem	1 doughnut	60	1	8	70	0	3.0	5
powdered sugar, 1 oz	1 doughnut	120	1	16	135	0	5.0	5
(Ener-G Foods) pumpkin, gluten-free	1 serving	128	0	18	7	na	5.9	na
(Entenmann's)								
crumb-topped	1 doughnut	260	3	34	220	0	12.0	0
devil's food crumb	1 doughnut	250	3	34	200	0	12.0	0
frosted, rich	1 doughnut	280	3	27	210	0	18.0	0
(Hostess)								
cinnamon, 'Breakfast Bake Shop Donette Gems'	1 doughnut	60	1	7	70	0	3.0	5
cinnamon, 'Breakfast Bake Shop Family Pack'	1 doughnut	120	2	14	140	1	6.0	5
cinnamon, 'Breakfast Bake Shop Pantry'	1 doughnut	190	3	24	240	1	10.0	10
cinnamon, apple-filled, mini	1 doughnut	70	1	10	70	0	3.0	5
crumb, 'Breakfast Bake Shop'	1 doughnut	160	1	16	140	1	10.0	10

Food Name	Serv. Size	Total Cal.	Prot. gms	Carbs gms	Sod. mgs	Fiber gms	Fat gms	Chol. mgs
frosted, 'Breakfast Bake Shop Donette Gems'	1 doughnut	80	1	8	70	0	5.0	5
frosted, 'Breakfast Bake Shop' 1.5 oz	1 doughnut	190	2	20	180	1	12.0	5
frosted, 'O's'	1 doughnut	260	3	32	240	2	14.0	5
glazed, 'Breakfast Bake Shop Old Fashioned'	1 doughnut	250	3	33	230	1	12.0	15
glazed, whirl, 'Breakfast Bake Shop'	1 doughnut	190	3	27	230	1	7.0	5
honey wheat, 'Breakfast Bake Shop'	1 doughnut	250	3	32	280	1	12.0	25
'Krunch'	1 doughnut	110	1	16	130	0	4.0	4
plain, 'Breakfast Bake Shop Donette Gems'	1 doughnut	60	1	6	80	0	3.0	5
plain, 'Breakfast Bake Shop Family Pack'	1 doughnut	120	2	13	160	1	6.0	5
plain, 'Breakfast Bake Shop Old Fashioned'	1 doughnut	170	3	21	230	1	9.0	10
plain, 'Breakfast Bake Shop Pantry'	1 doughnut	190	3	21	270	1	11.0	10
plain, 'O's'	1 doughnut	230	3	34	230	1	10.0	5
powdered sugar, 'Breakfast Bake Shop Pantry'	1 doughnut	190	2	24	230	1	10.0	10
powdered sugar, mini	1 doughnut	60	1	7	70	0	3.0	5
strawberry-filled, frosted, mini	1 doughnut	80	1	10	70	1	4.0	5
strawberry-filled, powdered sugar, mini	1 doughnut	70	1	10	70	0	3.0	5
(Rich's)								
glazed, frozen, 1.2 oz, 'Ever Fresh'	1 doughnut	141	2	17	0	0	7.0	0
jelly, frozen, 2.17 oz, 'Ever Fresh'	1 doughnut	213	4	26	0	0	9.5	0
(Tastykake)								
cinnamon, mini	1 doughnut	48	1	6	54	0	2.4	4
cinnamon, 1.6 oz	1 doughnut	179	3	25	211	1	8.2	11
frosted, rich, mini	1 doughnut	61	1	8	59	1	3.2	4
frosted, rich, 2 oz	1 doughnut	258	4	28	196	3	16.0	9
honey wheat, mini	1 doughnut	40	1	7	48	0	1.2	3
honey wheat, mini	1 doughnut	40	1	7	48	0	1.2	3
honey wheat, 2 oz	1 doughnut	209	2	33	190	1	7.5	15
orange glazed, 2 oz	1 doughnut	219	3	32	178	1	9.1	10
plain, 1.6 oz	1 doughnut	185	3	22	171	1	10.1	12
powdered sugar, mini	1 doughnut	42	1	7	71	0	1.3	4
powdered sugar, 1.6 oz	1 doughnut	188	3	24	221	1	8.6	10
DOUGHNUT HOLES *(Ener-G Foods)* gluten free	1 serving	17	1	2	69	0	0.6	4

DRAGON'S EYE. See LONGAN.
DREAM WHIP. See under TOPPING.
DRESSING. See SALAD DRESSING; STUFFING.
DRUM, FRESHWATER
Fresh

Food Name	Serv. Size	Total Cal.	Prot. gms	Carbs gms	Sod. mgs	Fiber gms	Fat gms	Chol. mgs
baked, broiled, grilled, or microwaved	3 oz	130	19	0	82	0	5.4	70
raw	3 oz	101	15	0	64	0	4.2	54

DUCK
AVERAGE OF ALL PARTS
Domestic

Food Name	Serv. Size	Total Cal.	Prot. gms	Carbs gms	Sod. mgs	Fiber gms	Fat gms	Chol. mgs
meat and skin, cooked	10 oz	1159	33	0	181	0	112.9	218
meat and skin, roasted, chopped or diced	1 cup	472	27	0	83	0	39.7	118
meat only, raw	4.8 oz	181	25	0	101	0	8.2	105
meat only, roasted, chopped or diced	1 cup	281	33	0	91	0	15.7	125
Wild, meat and skin, raw	8.3 oz	504	42	0	134	0	36.3	191

BREAST
Domestic

Food Name	Serv. Size	Total Cal.	Prot. gms	Carbs gms	Sod. mgs	Fiber gms	Fat gms	Chol. mgs
meat and skin, roasted	3 oz	172	21	0	71	na	9.2	116
meat only, broiled	3 oz	119	23	0	89	na	2.1	122
meat only, broiled, chopped or diced	1 cup	244	48	0	183	na	4.3	249
Wild, meat only, raw	3 oz	102	16	0	47	0	3.5	64

LEG
Domestic

Food Name	Serv. Size	Total Cal.	Prot. gms	Carbs gms	Sod. mgs	Fiber gms	Fat gms	Chol. mgs
meat and skin, braised, chopped or diced	1 cup	310	51	0	188	na	10.4	183
meat and skin, roasted	3 oz	184	23	0	94	na	9.7	97

Food Name	Serv. Size	Total Cal.	Prot. gms	Carbs gms	Sod. mgs	Fiber gms	Fat gms	Chol. mgs
meat only, braised	3 oz	151	25	0	92	na	5.1	89
LIVER, domestic, raw	1 oz	39	5.3	1.0	(mq)	0	1.3	146
DUCK FAT								
	1 cup	1846	0	0	0	0	204.6	205
	1 tbsp	115	0	0	0	0	12.8	13
DULSE. See under SEA VEGETABLE.								
DUMPLING								
(Creamette) egg noodle, w/pasteurized eggs	2 oz	220	8	40	20	0	3.0	70
(Stilwell) apple dumpling, w/3tbsp sauce	1 dumpling	390	4	59	240	3	15.0	0
DUNGENESS CRAB. See under CRAB.								
DURIAN								
raw or frozen, chopped or diced	1 cup	357	4	66	2	9	13.0	0
raw or frozen, whole	1 medium	885	9	163	6	23	32.1	0

E

Food Name	Serv. Size	Total Cal.	Prot. gms	Carbs gms	Sod. mgs	Fiber gms	Fat gms	Chol. mgs
ÉCLAIR. See under PASTRY.								
EEL								
mixed species, baked, broiled, grilled, or microwaved	3 oz	201	20	0	55	0	12.7	137
mixed species, baked, broiled, grilled, or microwaved, 1-inch cubes	1 piece	40	4	0	11	0	2.5	27
mixed species, raw	3 oz	156	16	0	43	0	9.9	107
EGG								
CHICKEN								
Dried								
white, flakes, glucose-reduced	1/2 lb	797	175	9	2624	0	0.1	0
white, powdered, 100% egg whites *(Nutra/Balance)*	1 tbsp	30	6	1	96	0	0.0	0
white, stabilized, glucose-reduced, flakes	1 oz	100	21.8	1.2	328	0	<.1	0
white, stabilized, glucose-reduced, powder	1 cup	402	88.2	4.8	1325	0	<.1	0
white, stabilized, glucose-reduced, powder	1 oz	107	23.4	1.3	351	0	<.1	0
whole	1 tbsp	30	2	0	26	0	2.0	86
whole, powder, glucose-reduced	1 tbsp	53	12	1	173	0	0.0	0
whole, powder, glucose-reduced, sifted	1 cup	402	88	5	1325	0	0.0	0
whole, sifted	1 cup	505	40	4	445	0	34.8	1458
whole, stabilized, glucose-reduced	1 tbsp	31	2	0	27	0	2.2	101
whole, stabilized, glucose-reduced, sifted	1 cup	523	41	2	466	0	37.4	1714
yolk, powdered	1 tbsp	27	1	0	5	0	2.2	93
yolk, powdered, sifted	1 cup	446	23	2	90	0	37.4	1564
Fresh								
white, raw	1 cup	122	25.6	2.5	399	0	0.0	na
white, raw	1 oz	14	3.0	0.3	46	0	0.0	0
white, raw, large	1 white	17	3.5	0.3	55	0	0.0	na
whole, cooked, omelet	1 tbsp	23	2	0	41	0	1.7	53
whole, cooked, omelet-style, large	1 egg	93	6	1	165	0	7.0	214
whole, fried, large	1 egg	92	6	1	162	0	6.9	211
whole, hard-boiled	1 tbsp	13	1	0	11	0	0.9	36
whole, hard-boiled, chopped	1 cup	211	17	2	169	0	14.4	577
whole, hard-boiled, large	1 egg	78	6	1	62	0	5.3	212
whole, poached, large	1 egg	75	6	1	140	0	5.0	212
whole, raw	1 cup	362	30	3	306	0	24.3	1033
whole, raw, brown, grade AA *(Lucerne)*	1 egg	70	6	1	65	0	4.5	215
whole, raw, extra large	1 egg	86	7	1	73	0	5.8	247
whole, raw, extra large, grade AA *(Lucerne)*	1 egg	80	7	1	70	0	5.0	240
whole, raw, jumbo	1 egg	97	8	1	82	0	6.5	276

Food Name	Serv. Size	Total Cal.	Prot. gms	Carbs gms	Sod. mgs	Fiber gms	Fat gms	Chol. mgs
whole, raw, jumbo, grade A *(Lucerne)*	1 egg	90	8	1	80	0	5.0	270
whole, raw, large	1 egg	75	6	1	63	0	5.0	213
whole, raw, medium	1 egg	66	5	1	55	0	4.4	187
whole, raw, medium, grade AA *(Lucerne)*	1 egg	70	6	1	55	0	4.0	190
whole, raw, small	1 egg	55	5	0	47	0	3.7	157
whole, scrambled	1 cup	365	24	5	616	0	26.9	774
whole, scrambled	1 tbsp	23	2	0	38	0	1.7	48
whole, scrambled, large	1 egg	101	7	1	171	0	7.4	215
yolk, raw	1 cup	870	41	4	104	0	75.0	3113
yolk, raw, large	1 yolk	59	3	0	7	0	5.1	213
Frozen								
diced *(Sunny Fresh)*	1 serving	80	6	1	125	0	5.0	215
liquid, 'Country Gold' *(Sunny Fresh)*	1/2 cup	130	12	2	310	0	9.0	315
whole	1/2 lb	688	35	3	152	0	58.1	2440
whole, raw, sugared	1/2 lb	697	31	25	152	0	51.6	2177
Pickled *(Penrose)* approx 2 oz	1 egg	80	8	1	230	0	5.0	0
DUCK								
whole, fresh, raw	1 large	130	9.0	1.0	102	0	9.6	619
whole, fresh, raw	1 oz	52	3.6	0.4	41	0	3.9	251
GOOSE								
whole, fresh, raw	1 large	267	20.0	1.9	199	0	19.1	1227
whole, fresh, raw	1 oz	52	3.9	0.4	na	0	3.8	(mq)
QUAIL								
whole, fresh, raw	1 oz	45	3.7	0.1	na	0	3.1	239
whole, fresh, raw	1 large	14	1.2	0.0	13	0	1.0	76
TURKEY								
whole, fresh, raw	1 large	135	10.8	0.9	120	0	9.4	737
whole, fresh, raw	1 oz	48	3.9	0.3	na	0	3.4	265
EGG DISH/MEAL								
(Aunt Jemima)								
scrambled, w/cheddar cheese and fried potatoes	5.9 oz	250	11	22	910	0	13.0	0
scrambled, w/sausages and hash browns, frozen	5.7 oz	290	12	14	810	0	20.0	0
scrambled, w/sausages and pancakes, frozen	5.2 oz	270	13	21	880	0	14.0	0
(Downyflake)								
scrambled, w/ham and hash browns, frozen	6.25 oz	360	13	17	730	0	26.0	0
scrambled, w/ham and pecan twirl, frozen	6.25 oz	470	15	40	670	0	28.0	0
scrambled, w/hash browns and sausage link	6.25 oz	420	12	17	790	0	34.0	0
scrambled, w/sausages and pecan twirl, frozen	6.25 oz	510	16	39	710	0	33.0	0
(Great Starts) scrambled, w/home fried potatoes	1 pkg	200	7	15	390	2	12.0	190
(Healthy Choice)								
omelet, turkey sausage, on English muffin, frozen	1 serving	210	16	30	470	0	4.0	20
omelet, Western style, on English muffin, frozen	1 serving	200	16	29	480	0	3.0	15
(Mountain House)								
omelet, cheese, freeze-dried, prepared	1/2 pkg	180	13	8	207	0	9.0	0
w/bacon, freeze-dried, prepared	1/2 pkg	170	12	7	165	0	10.0	0
w/bacon, precooked, freeze-dried, prepared	1/2 pkg	180	12	3	0	0	12.0	0
w/butter, freeze-dried, prepared	1/2 pkg	160	11	8	174	0	8.0	0
(Sunny Fresh)								
scrambled, precooked	2 oz	90	7	2	180	0	5.0	215
scrambled, squares	1 serving	60	5	1	50	0	3.5	145
(Swanson)								
omelet w/cheese sauce, w/ham, 'Great Starts'	7 oz	390	19	15	1220	0	29.0	0
scrambled, w/bacon and home fries	5.6 oz	340	11	16	690	0	26.0	0
scrambled, w/cheese and cinnamon pancakes	3.4 oz	290	7	14	380	0	23.0	0
scrambled, w/sausages and hash browns, frozen	6.5 oz	430	13	19	760	0	34.0	0
w/mini oat bran muffins, reduced cholesterol	4.75 oz	250	10	27	400	0	12.0	0
(Weight Watchers)								
ham and cheese omelet, 'Handy'	1 serving	220	13	30	440	2	5.0	30

Food Name	Serv. Size	Total Cal.	Prot. gms	Carbs gms	Sod. mgs	Fiber gms	Fat gms	Chol. mgs
omelet sandwich, 'Classic' .... 1 sandwich		220	15	26	410	2	5.0	20
omelet sandwich, 'Garden' .... 3.60 oz		210	9	28	480	0	6.0	15
EGG DISH/MEAL MIX								
(LaChoy)								
egg foo yung, w/3 oz sauce, 'Dinner Classics'								
prepared .... 2 patties		170	8	20	1390	1	7.0	275
egg foo yung, packaged, 'Dinner Classics' .... 1/4 pkg		85	3	19	1250	1	1.0	0
EGG ROLL								
(Chun King)								
chicken, mini .... 6 egg rolls		210	6	25	650	2	9.0	15
pork and shrimp, mini .... 6 egg rolls		210	6	27	540	2	9.0	15
shrimp, mini .... 6 egg rolls		190	5	28	730	2	6.0	10
(La Choy)								
pork, spicy, frozen, food service product .... 1 roll		196	6	23	537	2	9.4	5
shrimp, frozen, food service product .... 1 roll		187	6	26	400	2	7.1	4
vegetable, food service product .... 1 roll		174	4	28	456	2	5.1	2
(Worthington) vegetarian .... 1 serving		181	6	20	384	2	8.5	1
EGG ROLL WRAPPER								
(Azumaya) square .... 2 wraps		130	4	26	200	1	0.0	5
(Azumaya) wonton .... 5 wraps		100	3	21	160	0	0.0	5
(Nasoya) .... 1 piece		23	1	5	19	0	0.0	0
EGG SUBSTITUTE								
(Best of Egg) 99% egg white product .... 1/4 cup		30	6	1	100	na	0.0	0
(Ener-G Foods) egg-free, gluten-free .... 1 1/2 tsp		15	0	4	7	0	0.0	0
(Fantastic Foods) dry, 'Tofu Scrambler' .... 2 1/2 tbsp		60	3	12	480	3	0.5	0
(Featherweight). .... 2 eggs		120	9	2	250	0	8.0	15
(Fleischmann's)								
cheese omelet mix, 'Egg Beaters' .... 1/2 cup		110	14	2	480	0	5.0	5
'Egg Beaters' .... 1/4 cup		30	6	1	100	0	0.0	0
vegetable omelet mix, 'Egg Beaters' .... 1/2 cup		50	7	5	170	0	0.0	0
(Healthy Choice) 'Cholesterol-Free Egg Product' .... 1/4 cup		30	5	1	90	0	1.0	0
(Morningstar Farms)								
vegetarian, 'Better 'N Eggs' .... 1/4 cup		23	5	0	90	0	0.3	2
vegetarian, 'Scramblers' .... 1/4 cup		37	6	2	97	0	0.4	2
(Nu Laid) nonfat, cholesterol-free .... 1/4 cup		30	6	1	100	0	0.0	0
(Second Nature)								
cholesterol-free, real egg product .... 1/4 cup		60	6	3	110	0	2.0	0
nonfat, real egg product .... 1/4 cup		40	6	3	115	0	0.0	0
(Tofu Scrambler)								
mix, prepared w/tofu .... 1/2 cup		98	11	7	252	0	5.0	0
mix, prepared w/tofu, 3 tbsp salt .... 1/2 cup		158	11	7	335	0	12.0	0
(Tofutti)								
frozen, 'Egg Watchers' .... 2 oz		50	7	2	100	0	2.0	0
nonfat, 'Egg Watchers' .... 1/4 cup		30	6	1	80	0	0.0	0
(Wonder Slim)								
for cooking, baking, and salad dressing .... 1/4 cup		45	0	9	10	1	1.0	0
nonfat, no animal or dairy products .... 1/4 cup		35	1	8	10	1	0.0	0
EGG SUBSTITUTE DISH/MEAL								
(Morningstar Farms)								
frozen, w/hash browns and links 'Scramblers' .... 7 oz		360	16	22	660	0	23.0	0
frozen, w/pancakes and links 'Scramblers' .... 6.8 oz		380	18	33	900	0	19.0	0
EGG WHITE STABILIZER *(Tone's)* .... 1 tsp		12	0	3	1	0	0.0	0
EGGNOG								
Canned								
(Borden) nonalcoholic .... 1/2 cup		160	3	16	80	0	9.0	0
Refrigerated								
(Crowley) nonalcoholic .... 6 fl oz		270	6	34	200	0	13.0	100

Food Name	Serv. Size	Total Cal.	Prot. gms	Carbs gms	Sod. mgs	Fiber gms	Fat gms	Chol. mgs
(Darigold) nonalcoholic	8 fl oz	350	6	43	120	0	17.0	0
(Darigold) nonalcoholic 'Classic'	8 fl oz	390	10	48	170	0	17.0	0
(Lucerne)	1/2 cup	170	5	19	75	0	9.0	75
EGGPLANT/aubergine								
Fresh								
boiled, drained, cubed	1 cup	28	1	7	3	2	0.2	0
raw, cubed	1 cup	21	1	5	2	2	0.1	0
raw, whole, approx 1.25 lb, peeled	1 eggplant	119	5	28	14	11	0.8	0
raw, whole, approx 1.25 lb, unpeeled	1 eggplant	142	6	33	16	14	1.0	0
Frozen								
cutlets *(Celentano)*	3/4 cup	330	7	23	170	7	23.0	45
cutlets, breaded *(Bernardi)*	1/2 cup	180	3	17	220	2	11.0	0
rollettes *(Celentano)*	11 oz	320	14	36	210	0	14.0	0
rollettes, 'Great Choice' *(Celentano)*	10-oz tray	330	11	39	660	7	15.0	55
rollettes, 'Selects' *(Celentano)*	10-oz tray	360	11	27	490	6	23.0	45
EGGPLANT DISH/ENTRÉE								
(Celentano) Parmigiana	10 oz tray	420	14	30	800	23	27.0	45
(Progresso) appetizer, canned, 'Caponata'	2 tbsp	30	0	2	130	2	2.0	0
ELDERBERRY								
Fresh								
raw	1 lb	329	3.0	83.5	na>31.8 c		2.3	0
raw	1 oz	21	0.2	5.2	na >2.0 c		0.1	0
raw	1 cup	106	1.0	26.7	na>10.1 c		0.7	0
ELK								
raw	1 lb	504	104.1	0.0	263	na	6.6	249
raw	1 oz	31	6.4	0.0	16	na	0.4	15
roasted	3 oz	124	25.7	0.0	52	na	1.6	62
roasted	4 oz	166	34.2	0.0	69	0	2.2	83
roasted, diced, approx 4.9 oz	1 cup	204	42.3	0.0	85	0	2.7	102
ENCHILADA/ENCHILADA ENTRÉE								
(Amy's Kitchen)								
black bean and vegetable	1 serving	130	4	20	390	2	4.0	0
cheese	1 serving	210	11	16	390	2	9.0	20
(Banquet)								
	1 entrée	360	10	55	1390	9	11.0	20
chicken	1 entrée	350	12	54	1580	9	10.0	25
beef, frozen	12 oz	500	19	72	1810	0	15.0	0
beef, w/chili and gravy, 'Family Entrées'	7 oz	270	10	28	0	0	13.0	0
cheese	1 entrée	360	12	56	1500	8	10.0	20
cheese, frozen	12 oz	550	22	71	2170	0	19.0	0
(Gebhardt)								
	2 enchiladas	310	5	20	460	2	24.0	58
	5.71 oz	258	4	20	687	3	19.1	25
beef	1 serving	129	2	10	344	2	9.6	13
(Healthy Choice)								
beef, frozen, 13.4 oz	1 serving	370	15	66	450	0	5.0	30
chicken, frozen, 9.5 oz	1 serving	310	14	44	480	0	9.0	35
chicken, frozen, 13.4 oz	1 serving	340	14	61	470	0	5.0	30
chicken, suprema	1 entrée	300	13	46	560	4	7.0	40
chicken, suprema, w/green sauce, rice, corn, apple raspberry	1 serving	298	13	46	563	4	6.7	38
chicken, Suiza	1 entrée	280	14	43	440	5	4.0	40
(Hormel)								
beef, frozen	1 piece	140	6	17	573	0	5.0	0
cheese, frozen	1 piece	151	6	18	676	0	6.0	0
(Le Menu) chicken, frozen, 'Light Style'	8 oz	280	21	32	530	0	8.0	35
(Legume) w/organic tofu, vegetarian	1 serving	270	14	36	390	10	8.0	0

Food Name	Serv. Size	Total Cal.	Prot. gms	Carbs gms	Sod. mgs	Fiber gms	Fat gms	Chol. mgs
(Lean Cuisine)								
beef and bean, frozen	9.25 oz	240	15	32	480	0	6.0	45
chicken enchilada Suiza	1 entrée	280	11	48	520	3	5.0	25
chicken enchilada Suiza, w/sour cream sauce, rice	1 serving	298	11	52	538	4	4.8	20
(Legume) vegetable, w/tofu and sauce, frozen	11 oz	270	14	36	390	10	8.0	0
(Old El Paso)								
beef, frozen	1 pkg	210	8	16	720	0	13.0	10
beef, frozen, 'Festive Dinners'	11 oz	390	24	56	1200	0	8.0	0
cheese, frozen	1 pkg	250	10	24	830	0	12.0	0
cheese, frozen, 'Festive Dinners'	11 oz	590	24	51	1200	0	31.0	0
chicken, frozen	1 pkg	220	8	20	740	0	12.0	0
chicken, frozen, 'Festive Dinners'	11 oz	460	21	54	770	0	18.0	0
chicken, w/sour cream sauce, frozen	1 pkg	280	10	18	520	0	19.0	0
(Patio)								
beef, frozen	13.25 oz	520	16	59	1810	0	24.0	40
cheese, frozen	12.25 oz	380	14	59	2010	0	10.0	20
(Soypreme) tofu, organic, all-natural, frozen	11 oz	370	21	45	490	0	11.0	0
(Stouffer's)								
cheese, frozen, 1 pkg	9.75 oz	490	23	33	550	0	29.0	0
cheese, w/Mexican rice	1 entrée	370	12	48	890	5	14.0	25
chicken, frozen, 1 pkg	10 oz	490	21	31	860	0	31.0	0
chicken enchanadas, frozen, food service product	1 oz	46	2	4	105	0	2.7	10
chicken enchilada, w/Mexican rice, Monterey Jack sauce	1 serving	376	12	48	1002	5	14.7	25
chicken enchiladas, w/Mexican rice	1 entrée	370	16	45	970	3	14.0	30
(Tio Sancho) 'Dinner Kit'	1 shell	80	1	11	2	1	3.5	0
(Ultimate 200) beef, Ranchero, frozen	9.12 oz	190	18	18	500	0	5.0	20
(Van de Kamp's)								
beef, frozen, 'Mexican Dinner'	1/2 pkg	200	8	27	740	0	7.0	0
beef, frozen, 'Mexican Entrées Family Pack'	1/4 pkg	150	7	19	530	0	5.0	0
beef, frozen, 'Mexican Entrées'	1 pkg	270	11	30	1040	0	12.0	0
beef, shredded, frozen, 'Mexican Entrées'	1 pkg	360	20	40	1010	0	14.0	0
cheese, frozen, 'Mexican Dinner'	1/2 pkg	220	8	26	620	0	9.0	0
cheese, frozen, 'Mexican Entrées'	1 pkg	300	11	31	980	0	15.0	0
cheese, frozen, 'Mexican Entrées Family Pack'	1/4 pkg	200	7	19	460	0	10.0	0
chicken, frozen, 'Mexican Entrées'	1 pkg	260	13	27	1010	0	11.0	0
ranchero, frozen, 'Mexican Entrées'	1/2 pkg	260	11	26	630	0	12.0	0
Suiza, frozen, 'Mexican Entrées'	1 pkg	230	12	23	390	0	10.0	0
(Weight Watchers)								
chicken, nacho Grande, frozen 'Mexican Style'	9 oz	280	14	38	590	0	8.0	20
chicken, Suiza, frozen	9 oz	230	16	25	530	0	7.0	40
chicken enchiladas, nacho grande	1 entrée	290	15	42	560	4	8.0	20
chicken enchiladas Suiza	1 entrée	270	14	33	540	4	9.0	40
chicken enchilada Suiza, w/sour cream sauce and cheese	1 serving	283	16	33	518	4	9.7	64

ENCHILADA SEASONING. See under SEASONING MIX.

ENDIVE

Food Name	Serv. Size	Total Cal.	Prot. gms	Carbs gms	Sod. mgs	Fiber gms	Fat gms	Chol. mgs
raw, chopped	1/2 cup	4	0	1	6	1	0.1	0
raw, whole, approx 1.3 lb	1 head	87	6	17	113	16	1.0	0

ENERGY BAR. See under SPORTS AND DIET/NUTRITION BARS.

ENGLISH MUFFIN

Food Name	Serv. Size	Total Cal.	Prot. gms	Carbs gms	Sod. mgs	Fiber gms	Fat gms	Chol. mgs
(Earth Grains)								
oat bran, 12-oz pkg	1 muffin	120	5	24	410	2	1.0	0
plain, 12-oz pkg	1 muffin	120	5	25	390	1	1.0	0
sourdough, 12-oz pkg	1 muffin	120	5	25	390	1	1.0	0
w/raisins, 14-oz pkg	1 muffin	160	5	33	300	1	2.0	0
w/raisins, 15-oz pkg, 'Sun Maid'	1 muffin	160	5	34	180	2	1.0	0

Food Name	Serv. Size	Total Cal.	Prot. gms	Carbs gms	Sod. mgs	Fiber gms	Fat gms	Chol. mgs
wheat berry, 14-oz pkg	1 muffin	140	6	28	470	2	1.0	0
whole wheat, 14-oz pkg	1 muffin	130	6	26	420	4	1.0	0
whole wheat, 15-oz pkg	1 muffin	140	6	28	450	4	2.0	0
(Ener-G Foods) gluten-free	1 serving	203	4	37	1067	14	3.9	0
(Hi Fiber)								
multigrain	1 muffin	120	4	23	240	4	1.0	0
plain	1 muffin	110	5	21	280	5	1.0	0
w/cinnamon and raisins	1 muffin	110	4	21	275	5	1.0	0
(Oatmeal Goodness)								
oatmeal, w/cinnamon and raisins	1 muffin	140	5	26	160	2	2.0	0
oatmeal, w/honey	1 muffin	140	5	26	160	2	2.0	0
(Organic Grains)								
7-grain, sprouted, organic	1 muffin	140	10	29	150	3	2.0	0
w/cinnamon and raisins, organic	1 muffin	170	8	33	165	3	1.0	0
(Oroweat)								
extra crisp	1 muffin	130	4	26	260	0	1.0	0
'Health Nut'	1 muffin	170	6	29	220	1	4.0	0
sourdough	1 muffin	140	4	27	370	0	1.0	0
(Pepperidge Farm)								
plain	1 muffin	140	5	27	220	0	1.0	0
sourdough	1 muffin	135	4	27	260	0	1.0	0
w/cinnamon and apple	1 muffin	140	4	27	210	0	1.0	0
w/cinnamon and raisins	1 muffin	150	4	29	200	0	2.0	0
w/cinnamon chips	1 muffin	160	4	28	180	0	3.0	0
(Roman Meal)								
honey nut, w/oat bran, refrigerated	1/2 muffin	81	3	15	114	1	1.3	0
'Original'	1 muffin	146	6	29	350	3	1.8	0
plain, refrigerated	1/2 muffin	71	2	14	88	1	0.5	0
(Thomas')								
honey wheat	1 serving	110	5	24	190	3	1.0	0
oat bran	1 serving	120	4	26	210	2	1.0	0
plain	1 muffin	130	4	25	206	0	1.3	0
plain, sandwich size	1 serving	190	7	38	280	2	2.0	0
raisin	1 serving	140	4	31	170	1	1.0	0
rye	1 muffin	120	5	27	210	3	1.0	0
sourdough	1 serving	120	4	25	190	1	1.0	0
sourdough, sandwich size	1 muffin	200	7	41	310	2	2.0	0
w/onion, sandwich size	1 muffin	180	6	40	270	2	1.5	0
wheat, sandwich size	1 serving	180	8	39	280	4	1.5	0
(Wonder) plain	1 serving	130	4	25	290	1	1.0	0

ENOKI. See MUSHROOM, ENOKI.
ENSURE. See under MEDICAL NUTRITIONALS.
EPAZOTE

fresh, raw, whole sprigs	1 medium	1	0	0	1	0	0.0	0
fresh, raw, chopped	1 tbsp	0	0	0	0	0	0.0	0

EPPAW, raw .... 1 cup | 150 | 5 | 32 | 12 | na | 1.8 | 0

EUROPEAN CHESTNUT. See CHESTNUT, EUROPEAN.
EUROPEAN CURRANT. See under CURRANT.

F

Food Name	Serv. Size	Total Cal.	Prot. gms	Carbs gms	Sod. mgs	Fiber gms	Fat gms	Chol. mgs
FAJITA/FAJITA ENTRÉE								
(Healthy Choice)								
beef, frozen	7 oz	210	19	26	250	0	4.0	35

FIG 247

Food Name	Serv. Size	Total Cal.	Prot. gms	Carbs gms	Sod. mgs	Fiber gms	Fat gms	Chol. mgs
chicken, fiesta	1 entrée	260	21	36	410	4	4.0	30
chicken, frozen	7 oz	200	17	25	310	0	3.0	35
(Wonderbites)								
beef, flame-broiled, 'Dippers'	1 piece	33	4	1	86	0	1.5	9
beef, flame-broiled, frozen, product 9971	1 piece	51	4	1	106	0	3.6	11
(Chicken By George) refrigerated	5 oz	170	28	2	370	0	6.0	85
FAJITA MIX								
(Hudson) beef, meal kit, prepared	1 fajita	220	11	22	560	1	9.0	35
(Tyson)								
chicken, kit, frozen	1 pkg	915	57	123	2472	na	23.2	91
chicken, kit, frozen	1 serving	129	8	17	350	na	3.3	13
kit	4 oz	80	7	2	240	0	2.0	0
kit, wholesale club item	3.5 oz	160	10	18	420	0	5.0	30
FAJITA SEASONING. See under SEASONING MIX.								
FALAFEL MIX								
(Casbah) mix only	1.5 oz	160	6	20	530	2	3.0	0
(Fantastic Foods) prepared	1/2 cup	250	15	42	610	11	4.0	0
FARINA. See under CEREAL, HOT.								
FAT SUBSTITUTE								
(Wonder Slim) for cooking, baking, and salad dressing	1/4 cup	45	0	9	10	1	1.0	0
(Rokeach) 'Neutral Nyafat'	1 tbsp	99	0	0	0	0	11.0	0
FATHEAD. See SHEEPSHEAD.								
FAVA BEAN. See BEAN, FAVA.								
FEIJOA								
raw, puréed	1 cup	119	3	26	7	na	1.9	0
raw, whole, trimmed	1 medium	25	1	5	2	na	0.4	0
FENNEL/finnochio								
fresh, raw *(Frieda of California)*	1 oz	4	0	1	26	0	0.1	0
fresh, raw, sliced	1 cup	27	1	6	45	3	0.2	0
fresh, raw, whole, bulb	1 medium	73	3	17	122	7	0.5	0
FENNEL SEED								
whole	1 tbsp	20	1	3	5	2	0.9	0
whole	1 tsp	7	0	1	2	1	0.3	0
whole *(Durkee)*	1 tsp	7	0	0	0	0	0.0	0
whole *(Laurel Leaf)*	1 tsp	7	0	0	0	0	0.0	0
whole *(McCormick/Schilling)*	1 tsp	14	1	2	4	1	0.8	0
whole *(Spice Islands)*	1 tsp	8	0	1	2	0	0.2	0
whole *(Tone"s)*	1 tsp	7	0	1	2	0	0.3	0
FENUGREEK SEED								
whole	1 tbsp	36	3	6	7	3	0.7	0
whole	1 tsp	12	1	2	2	1	0.2	0
FETTUCCINE. See under PASTA.								
FETTUCCINE DISH/ENTRÉE. See under PASTA DISH/ENTRÉE.								
FIELD PEAS. See PEAS, FIELD.								
FIG								
Canned								
in extra heavy syrup, w/liquid	1 cup	279	1	73	3	na	0.3	0
in heavy syrup, w/liquid	1 cup	228	1	59	3	6	0.3	0
in heavy syrup, w/liquid	1 medium	25	0	6	0	1	0.0	0
in light syrup, w/liquid	1 cup	174	1	45	3	5	0.3	0
in light syrup, w/liquid	1 medium	19	0	5	0	1	0.0	0
in water, w/liquid	1 cup	131	1	35	2	5	0.2	0
in water, wliquids	1 medium	14	0	4	0	1	0.0	0
Dried								
raw, chopped	1 cup	507	6	130	22	24	2.3	0
raw, whole	1 medium	48	1	12	2	2	0.2	0
stewed	1 cup	280	3	71	13	13	1.3	0

Food Name	Serv. Size	Total Cal.	Prot. gms	Carbs gms	Sod. mgs	Fiber gms	Fat gms	Chol. mgs
Fresh								
raw, large, approx 2.5-inch diam	1 fig	47	0	12	1	2	0.2	0
raw, medium, approx 2.25-inch diam	1 fig	37	0	10	1	2	0.1	0
raw, small, approx 1.5-inch diam	1 fig	30	0	8	0	1	0.1	0
FILBERT. See HAZELNUT.								
FILBERT BUTTER *(Maranatha Natural)* roasted	2 tbsp	180	5	6	5	0	16.0	0
FILO DOUGH. See PHYLLO DOUGH.								
FINNAN HADDIE. See under HADDOCK.								
FINNOCHIO. See FENNEL.								
FIREWEED LEAVES								
raw, chopped	1 cup	24	1	4	8	2	0.6	0
raw, whole	1 med plant	23	1	4	7	2	0.6	0
FISH. See individual listings.								
FISH AND CHIPS. See under FISH DINNER/ENTRÉE.								
FISH BATTER SEASONING MIX. See under SEASONING AND COATING MIX.								
FISH DINNER/ENTRÉE								
(Banquet)								
fillet	1 entrée	290	11	33	820	4	13.0	30
frozen, 'Platters'	8.75 oz	450	31	33	0	0	22.0	95
(Fisher Boy)								
batter-dipped, crispy, frozen	1 fillet	170	7	15	310	0	9.0	20
batter-dipped, crunchy, 'Portions'	1 portion	110	6	10	450	0	6.0	5
sticks, crunchy, frozen	5 sticks	230	12	19	530	2	11.0	15
(Gorton's)								
breaded, garlic and herb, frozen	2 fillets	250	10	20	720	0	14.0	25
breaded, hot and spicy, frozen	2 fillets	270	10	19	630	0	17.0	30
in herb sauce, frozen	1 pkg	190	26	3	450	0	8.0	90
sticks, mini, breaded, frozen	9 sticks	190	8	14	390	0	11.0	20
(Healthy Choice) lemon pepper	1 entrée	320	14	50	480	5	7.0	30
(Kid Cuisine) nuggets, frozen	7 oz	320	13	33	750	0	15.0	45
(Lean Cuisine)								
baked	1 entrée	270	17	36	540	3	6.0	45
fillet, divan, frozen	10 3/8 oz	210	27	13	490	0	5.0	65
fillet, Florentine, frozen	9 5/8 oz	220	26	13	590	0	7.0	65
(Morton) frozen	9.75 oz	370	18	46	910	0	13.0	65
(Mrs. Paul's)								
Dijon, frozen, 'Light'	8.75 oz	200	21	17	650	0	5.0	60
fillet, Florentine, frozen, 'Light'	8 oz	220	25	10	820	0	8.0	95
Mornay, frozen, 'Light'	9 oz	230	24	12	670	0	10.0	80
(Stouffer's) fillet, w/macaroni and cheese, 'Homestyle'	1 entrée	430	24	37	930	2	21.0	70
(Swanson)								
fish 'n chips, battered and fried	1 entrée	490	19	59	1030	5	20.0	45
w/fries, frozen, 'Home Style Recipe'	6.5 oz	340	11	37	670	0	16.0	0
(Tyson) sticks, frozen 'Looney Tunes Sylvester'	7.5 oz	290	13	36	510	0	11.0	17
(Van de Kamp's)								
breaded, baked, 97% fat-free, frozen, 'Crisp and Healthy'	2 fillets	150	12	18	420	0	3.0	25
fillet, baked, breaded, frozen, microwaveable	2 fillets	150	12	18	420	0	3.0	25
fillet, battered, frozen	1 serving	180	8	12	340	0	11.0	20
fillet, breaded	2 pieces	280	11	18	280	0	18.0	35
fillet, breaded, baked, frozen, 'Crisp and Healthy'	2 pieces	150	12	18	350	0	3.0	25
fillet, breaded, frozen, 'Snack Pack'	2 pieces	220	8	13	280	0	10.0	20
fillet, crispy, frozen, microwave	1 piece	140	6	9	210	0	9.0	15
fillet, large, crispy, frozen, microwave	1 piece	290	12	21	640	0	17.0	25
nuggets, battered, frozen	4 pieces	130	5	8	310	0	9.0	10
sticks, battered, frozen	4 pieces	160	8	12	380	0	9.0	20
sticks, breaded, baked, frozen, 'Crisp and Healthy'	4 pieces	120	9	17	330	0	2.0	15

Food Name	Serv. Size	Total Cal.	Prot. gms	Carbs gms	Sod. mgs	Fiber gms	Fat gms	Chol. mgs
sticks, breaded, frozen 'Snack Pack'	4 pieces	170	8	13	270	0	10.0	20
sticks, breaded, frozen 'Value Pack'	4 pieces	170	8	13	270	0	10.0	20
sticks, breaded, frozen	4 pieces	200	9	15	290	0	12.0	20
sticks, crispy, frozen, microwave	3 pieces	130	7	11	280	0	7.0	15
sticks, mini, breaded, frozen, 'Crisp and Healthy'	10 sticks	180	8	14	280	0	10.0	20
(Wakefield)								
gems, fancy style, frozen	4 oz	80	11	11	0	0	1.0	0
gems, salad style, frozen	3 oz	70	10	8	0	0	1.0	0
(Weight Watchers) oven-baked, w/vegetable medley,								
frozen, 'Ultimate 200'	6.64 oz	120	16	10	390	0	2.0	0
FISH OIL								
COD LIVER								
	1 cup	1966	0.0	0.0	0	0	218.0	1243
	1 tbsp	123	0.0	0.0	0	0	13.6	78
(Hain)								
cherry	1 tbsp	120	0	0	0	0	14.0	75
mint	1 tbsp	120	0	0	0	0	14.0	85
regular	1 tbsp	120	0	0	0	0	14.0	85
HERRING								
	1 cup	1966	0	0	0	0	218.0	1670
	1 tbsp	123	0	0	0	0	13.6	104
MENHADEN								
	1 cup	1966	0	0	0	0	218.0	1136
	1 tbsp	123	0	0	0	0	13.6	71
fully hydrogenated	1 cup	1849	0	0	0	0	205.0	1025
fully hydrogenated	1 tbsp	113	0	0	0	0	12.5	63
SALMON								
	1 cup	1966	0	0	0	0	218.0	1057
	1 tbsp	123	0	0	0	0	13.6	66
SARDINE								
	1 cup	1966	0	0	0	0	218.0	1548
sardine	1 tbsp	123	0	0	0	0	13.6	97
FISH PASTE CAKE								
Japanese, block, steamed, 'Kamoboko'	4 oz	111	13.6	11.0	1134	na	1.0	(mq)
Japanese, stick, grilled, 'Chikuwa'	4 oz	143	13.8	15.3	1134	na	2.4	(mq)
FISH SEASONING. See under SEASONING MIX; SEASONING AND COATING MIX.								
FISH STICKS. See under FISH DINNER/ENTRÉE.								
FISH SUBSTITUTE DINNER/ENTRÉE								
(Worthington) vegetarian, 'Fillets'	2 pieces	180	16	8	750	4	10.0	0
(Loma Linda) vegetarian, 'Ocean Platter' dry mix	1/3 cup	90	14	8	450	4	1.0	0
FIVE-SPICE SEASONING. See under SEASONING MIX.								
FLAN MIX. See under PUDDING MIX.								
FLATFISH. See FLOUNDER; HALIBUT; SOLE.								
FLAX OIL								
organic *(Spectrum Naturals)*	1 tbsp	120	0.0	0.0	0	(tr)	14.0	(tr)
organic, cinnamon flavored *(Spectrum Naturals)*	1 tbsp	120	0.0	0.0	0	(tr)	14.0	(tr)
FLAXSEED								
	1 cup	763	30	53	53	43	52.7	0
	1 tbsp	59	2	4	4	3	4.1	0
(Arrowhead Mills)	1 oz	140	5	11	1	6	10.0	0
FLORIDA POMPANO. See POMPANO, FLORIDA.								
FLOUNDER								
Fresh								
baked, broiled, grilled, or microwaved	3 oz	99	20.5	0.0	89	0	1.3	58
raw	3 oz	77	16.0	0.0	69	0	1.0	41
Frozen								
(Finast)	4 oz	90	19	0	150	0	1.0	0

Food Name	Serv. Size	Total Cal.	Prot. gms	Carbs gms	Sod. mgs	Fiber gms	Fat gms	Chol. mgs
(SeaPak)	4 oz	90	20	0	120	0	1.0	0
Atlantic *(Booth)*	4 oz	90	19	0	180	0	1.0	0
fillet *(Van de Kamp"s)*	1 serving	110	22	0	105	0	2.0	45
fillet, 'Light' *(Van de Kamp's)*	1 piece	260	18	21	480	0	12.0	45
'Natural' *(Van de Kamp's)*	4 oz	100	22	0	100	0	2.0	35
FLOUNDER DINNER/ENTRÉE								
(Gorton's) stuffed, 'Microwave Entrées'	1 pkg	350	25	21	850	0	18.0	120
FLOUR. See also individual listings.								
ACORN, full-fat	1 oz	142	2	15	0	na	8.6	0
AMARANTH *(Arrowhead Mills)*	1/4 cup	110	4	19	0	2	1.5	0
ARROWROOT.	1 cup	457	0	113	3	4	0.1	0
BARLEY								
	1 cup	511	16	110	6	15	2.4	0
(Arrowhead Mills)	2 oz	200	7	35	1	7	1.0	0
(Arrowhead Mills)	1.4 cup	75	3	19	0	3	0.5	0
BARLEY MALT.	1 cup	585	17	127	18	12	3.0	0
BUCKWHEAT								
100% stone ground *(Hodgson Mill)*	1/3 cup	160	7	33	10	2	1.0	0
whole-grain *(Arrowhead Mills)*	2 oz	190	7	41	0	7	1.0	0
whole-groat	1 cup	402	15	85	13	12	3.7	0
CAROB								
	1 cup	229	5	92	36	41	0.7	0
	1 tbsp	18	0	7	3	3	0.1	0
CHESTNUT	100 gm	362	6.1	76.2	11	>2.0 c	3.7	0
CHICKPEA								
(Arrowhead Mills)	2 oz	200	12	35	9	7	3.0	0
besan	1 cup	339	21	53	59	10	6.2	0
CORN. See also CORNMEAL.								
masa, enriched	1 cup	416	11	87	6	11	4.3	0
masa harina, enriched *(Quaker)*	1/4 cup	110	3	25	0	2	1.0	0
masa harina de maiz *(Quaker)*	1/3 cup	137	4	27	5	3	1.5	0
masa trigo *(Quaker)*	1/3 cup	149	4	25	794	1	4.0	0
white, masa harina *(Tone's)*	1 tsp	8	0	2	1	0	0.1	0
white, whole grain	1 cup	422	8	90	6	11	4.5	0
yellow, degermed, unenriched	1 cup	473	7	104	1	2	1.8	0
yellow, enriched	1 cup	416	11	87	6	na	4.3	0
yellow, whole grain	1 cup	422	8	90	6	16	4.5	0
COTTONSEED								
low-fat	1 oz	94	14	10	10	na	0.4	0
partially defatted	1 cup	337	39	38	33	3	5.8	0
partially defatted	1 tbsp	18	2	2	2	0	0.3	0
GARBANZO *(Arrowhead Mills)* toasted	1/4 cup	90	5	15	0	3	1.0	0
GRAHAM								
(Hodgson Mill) whole wheat, organic	1/4 cup	100	3	22	0	3	1.0	na
(Hodgson Mill) whole grain, stone ground, organic	1/4 cup	100	3	22	0	3	1.0	0
KAMUT *(Arrowhead Mills)*	1/4 cup	110	4	25	0	4	0.5	0
MILLET *(Arrowhead Mills)*	1/4 cup	110	4	26	0	2	1.0	0
MUSTARD *(McCormick/Schilling)* ground	1 tsp	12	1	0	0	0	0.8	0
OAT								
(Arrowhead Mills)	1/3 cup	120	5	20	0	4	2.0	0
blend *(Gold Medal)*	1 cup	390	14	81	0	4	3.0	0
OAT BRAN								
blend, all natural *(Hodgson Mill)*	1/4 cup	110	3	24	3	3	1.0	0
all-natural *(Hodgson Mill)*	1/4 cup	110	3	23	4	3	2.0	na
organic, wheat-free *(Hodgson Mill)*	1/4 cup	110	3	24	120	3	1.0	0
PEANUT								
defatted	1 cup	196	31	21	108	9	0.3	0

Food Name	Serv. Size	Total Cal.	Prot. gms	Carbs gms	Sod. mgs	Fiber gms	Fat gms	Chol. mgs
defatted	1 oz	93	15	10	51	4	0.2	0
low-fat	1 cup	257	20	19	1	9	13.1	0
low-fat	1 oz	121	10	9	0	4	6.2	0
POTATO								
	1 cup	571	11	133	88	9	0.5	0
gluten-free *(Ener-G Foods)*	1 cup	527	14	136	58	10	1.4	0
QUINOA								
whole-grain, gluten-free *(Ancient Harvest)*	1/4 cup	132	4	24	10	5	2.0	0
whole-grain, gluten-free *(Quinoa)*	1/4 cup	132	4	24	10	5	2.0	0
RICE								
(Featherweight)	1 cup	500	11	113	7	0	1.0	0
brown	1 cup	574	11	121	13	7	4.4	0
brown *(Arrowhead Mills)*	2 oz	200	4	44	3	3	1.0	0
brown, whole-grain, stone ground *(Hodgson Mill)*	1/4 cup	110	3	23	0	1	1.0	0
sweet, gluten-free *(Ener-G Foods)*	1 cup	406	8	91	18	0	1.1	0
white	1 cup	578	9	127	0	4	2.2	0
RICE STARCH								
gluten-free *(Ener-G Foods)*	1 cup	263	0	69	0	0	0.0	0
RYE								
(Krusteaz)	1 cup	351	11	73	1	3	2.0	0
'Bohemian Style' *(Pillsbury)*	1/4 cup	100	3	22	0	2	0.0	0
medium *(Pillsbury)*	1/4 cup	100	3	22	0	2	0.0	0
stone-ground *(Robin Hood)*	1 cup	360	13	86	10	13	2.0	0
dark	1 cup	415	18	88	1	29	3.4	0
light	1 cup	374	9	82	2	15	1.4	0
medium	1 cup	361	10	79	3	15	1.8	0
organic *(Hodgson Mill)*	1/4 cup	90	3	22	0	5	1.0	0
whole-grain *(Arrowhead Mills)*	2 oz	190	9	39	1	8	1.0	0
whole-grain, stone-ground *(Hodgson Mill)*	1/4 cup	90	3	22	0	5	1.0	0
SESAME								
high-fat	1 oz	149	9	8	12	na	10.5	0
low-fat	1 oz	94	14	10	11	na	0.5	0
partially defatted	1 oz	108	11	10	12	na	3.4	0
SOY								
(Arrowhead Mills)	2 oz	250	20	18	1	8	11.0	0
defatted	1 tbsp	20	3	2	1	1	0.1	0
defatted, stirred	1 cup	329	47	38	20	18	1.2	0
full-fat	1 tbsp	23	2	2	1	0	1.1	0
full-fat, roasted, stirred	1 cup	366	29	30	11	8	17.3	0
full-fat, stirred	1 cup	375	30	29	10	8	18.6	0
gluten-free *(Hodgson Mill)*	1/4 cup	80	15	9	10	na	0.0	0
gluten-free, organic *(Hodgson Mill)*	1/4 cup	110	9	9	0	4	5.0	0
low-fat	1 tbsp	20	3	2	1	1	0.4	0
low-fat, stirred	1 cup	327	41	33	16	9	5.9	0
organic *(Hodgson Mill)*	1/4 cup	110	9	9	0	4	5.0	na
SPELT								
(Arrowhead Mills)	1/4 cup	100	4	24	0	5	0.5	0
wheat-free, oragnic, raw *(Hodgson Mill)*	1/4 cup	115	4	22	0	2	1.0	0
SUNFLOWER SEED								
partially defatted	1 cup	209	31	23	2	3	1.0	0
partially defatted	1 tbsp	13	2	1	0	0	0.1	0
TAPIOCA, cassava flour, gluten-free *(Ener-G Foods)*	1 cup	313	0	100	4	0	0.0	0
TEFF, whole-grain *(Arrowhead Mills)*	2 oz	200	7	41	6	8	1.0	0
TRITICALE, whole-grain	1 cup	439	17	95	3	19	2.4	0
WHEAT								
Semolina								
golden, and extra fancy durum *(Hodgson Mill)*	1/4 cup	110	4	22	0	2	1.0	0

Food Name	Serv. Size	Total Cal.	Prot. gms	Carbs gms	Sod. mgs	Fiber gms	Fat gms	Chol. mgs
pasta flour, unbleached *(Bob's Red Mill)*	1/4 cup	150	5	31	0	0	0.5	0
White								
all-purpose *(Ballard)*	1 cup	400	11	87	0	2	1.0	0
all-purpose *(Ceresota)*	4 oz	390	13	83	0	0	1.0	0
all-purpose *(Gold Medal)*	1 cup	400	11	87	0	0	1.0	0
all-purpose *(Heckers)*	4 oz	390	13	83	0	0	1.0	0
all-purpose *(Red Band)*	1 cup	390	10	85	0	0	1.0	0
all-purpose *(Robin Hood)*	1 cup	400	13	85	0	0	1.0	0
all-purpose *(White Deer)*	1 cup	400	11	87	0	0	1.0	0
all-purpose, bleached *(Pillsbury)*	1/4 cup	100	3	23	0	1	0.0	0
all-purpose, bleached, 'Pillsbury's Best' *(Pillsbury)*	1 cup	400	11	87	0	2	1.0	0
all-purpose, unbleached *(Gold Medal)*	1 cup	400	11	87	0	0	1.0	0
all-purpose, unbleached *(Hodgson Mill)*	1/4 cup	100	3	23	0	1	0.0	0
all-purpose, unbleached *(Pillsbury)*	1/4 cup	100	3	21	0	1	0.0	0
all-purpose, unbleached *(Robin Hood)*	1 cup	400	13	85	0	0	1.0	0
all-purpose, unbleached, 'Pillsbury's Best' *(Pillsbury)*	1 cup	400	12	86	0	3	1.0	0
bread *(Hodgson Mill)*	1/4 cup	100	4	22	0	1	0.0	0
bread *(Pillsbury)*	1/4 cup	100	4	22	0	1	0.0	0
bread, 'Better for Bread' *(Gold Medal)*	1 cup	400	14	83	0	0	1.0	0
bread, high-protein, high-gluten *(Hodgson Mill)*	1/4 cup	100	4	22	5	1	0.0	0
bread, 'Pillsbury's Best' *(Pillsbury)*	1 cup	400	14	83	0	0	2.0	0
bread, enriched	1 cup	495	16	99	3	3	2.3	0
cake, enriched	1 cup	496	11	107	3	2	1.2	0
'Drifted Snow *(Red Band)*	1 cup	400	11	87	0	0	1.0	0
enriched bleached	1 cup	455	13	95	3	3	1.2	0
enriched, unbleached	1 cup	455	13	95	3	3	1.2	0
'La Pina' *(Red Band)*	1 cup	400	10	87	0	0	1.0	0
organic, unbleached, *(Hodgson Mill)*	1/4 cup	100	3	23	0	1	0.0	0
self-rising *(Ballard)*	1 cup	380	9	84	1290	0	1.0	0
self-rising *(Gold Medal)*	1 cup	380	10	83	1520	0	1.0	0
self-rising *(Red Band)*	1 cup	380	9	83	1520	0	1.0	0
self-rising, bleached *(Pillsbury)*	1/4 cup	100	3	22	360	1	0.0	0
self-rising, bleached, 'Pillsbury's Best' *(Pillsbury)*	1 cup	380	9	84	1290	2	1.0	0
self-rising, enriched *(Aunt Jemima)*	1/4 cup	109	3	24	368	0	0.3	0
self-rising, unbleached, 'Pillsbury's Best' *(Pillsbury)*	1 cup	380	9	84	1290	2	1.0	0
self-rising, unbleached *(Pillsbury)*	1/4 cup	100	2	22	360	1	0.0	0
shake and blend *(Pillsbury)*	1/4 cup	100	3	23	0	1	0.0	0
'Softasilk' *(Red Band)*	1/4 cup	100	2	23	0	0	0.0	0
tortilla, enriched	1 cup	450	11	75	751	na	11.8	0
unbleached *(Arrowhead Mills)*	2 oz	200	7	53	1	0	1.0	0
unbleached *(Gold Medal)*	1 cup	400	11	87	0	0	1.0	0
unbleached *(Robin Hood)*	1 cup	400	13	85	0	0	1.0	0
unbleached *(Stone-Buhr)*	1 cup	400	11	87	5	0	1.0	0
unenriched	1 cup	455	13	95	3	3	1.2	0
'Wondra' *(Red Band)*	1 cup	400	11	87	0	0	1.0	0
White and whole wheat								
50/50 blend *(Hodgson Mill)*	1/4 cup	100	4	21	0	2	1.0	0
whole grain, blend *(Gold Medal)*	1 cup	380	14	84	0	8	2.0	0
whole wheat blend *(Gold Medal)*	1 cup	380	14	84	0	8	2.0	0
Whole wheat								
	1 cup	407	16	87	6	15	2.2	0
(Gold Medal)	1 cup	350	16	78	0	10	2.0	0
(Krusteaz)	1 cup	450	17	90	5	15	2.0	0
(Pillsbury)	1/4 cup	120	5	22	0	4	1.0	0
100% hard white wheat *(Hodgson Mill)*	1/4 cup	100	4	21	0	3	1.0	0
pastry, organic *(Hodgson Mill)*	1/4 cup	110	3	22	0	3	1.0	0
pastry, stone-ground *(Hodgson Mill)*	1/4 cup	110	3	22	0	3	1.0	na

Food Name	Serv. Size	Total Cal.	Prot. gms	Carbs gms	Sod. mgs	Fiber gms	Fat gms	Chol. mgs
pastry, whole-grain *(Arrowhead Mills)*	2 oz	180	6	41	1	7	1.0	0
whole-grain, stone-ground *(Arrowhead Mills)*	2 oz	200	8	40	1	7	1.0	0
whole-grain *(Ceresota)*	4 oz	400	15	80	0	0	2.0	0
whole-grain *(Gold Medal)*	1 cup	350	16	78	0	10	2.0	0
whole-grain *(Heckers)*	4 oz	400	15	80	0	0	2.0	0
whole-grain, 'Pillsbury's Best' *(Pillsbury)*	1 cup	400	15	80	10	0	2.0	0
WHEAT AND RYE								
'Bohemian Style' *(Pillsbury)*	1 cup	400	11	86	0	0	1.0	0
'Pillsbury's Best' *(Pillsbury)*	1 cup	400	12	83	0	9	2.0	0
FRANKFURTER								
(Armour)								
beef, 25% less sodium	1 frank	180	7	2	470	0	16.0	30
jumbo, 25% less sodium	1 frank	160	7	2	470	0	14.0	50
(Ball Park)								
beef, pork, and chicken, 'Lite'	1 frank	140	7	1	0	0	12.0	0
light	1 serving	110	7	4	730	0	8.0	20
mini-franks on a bun	1 pkg	180	6	15	450	1	10.0	25
nonfat	1 serving	40	6	4	560	0	0.0	0
(Boar's Head)								
beef	1 oz	80	4	1	0	0	7.0	15
pork and beef	1 oz	80	4	1	250	0	7.0	15
(Butcher Boy Meats) turkey	1 serving	134	8	3	651	0	10.2	58
(Butterball)								
nonfat	1 frank	45	6	4	480	0	0.0	0
turkey	1 frank	140	7	2	610	0	11.0	0
(Eckrich)								
beef, 'Bunsize'	1 frank	190	6	2	520	0	17.0	0
beef, 1 lb pkg	1 frank	150	5	2	400	0	14.0	0
'Bun Size'	1 frank	190	6	2	500	0	17.0	0
cheesefurter	1 frank	180	7	2	530	0	16.0	0
'Jumbo Lean Supreme'	1 frank	140	7	2	490	0	12.0	0
1-lb pkg	1 frank	160	5	2	420	0	14.0	0
(Empire Kosher)								
chicken, kosher	1 frank	100	21	46	820	0	23.0	25
turkey, kosher	1 frank	90	0	1	410	0	6.0	35
(Health Valley)								
chicken, 'Weiners'	1 frank	96	5	1	90	0	8.0	49
turkey, 'Weiners'	1 frank	96	5	1	112	0	8.0	35
(Healthy Choice)								
beef, w/natural smoke flavor, low-fat	1 frank	60	7	5	430	0	1.5	15
turkey, pork, and beef, lowfat, bun size	1 frank	60	6	6	430	0	1.5	20
(Healthy Favorites)								
turkey and beef, 97% fat-free	1 frank	60	9	2	570	0	1.5	25
w/turkey	2 oz	57	9	2	572	0	1.6	24
(Hebrew National) beef	1 frank	149	6	1	497	0	14.0	15
(Hillshire Farm)								
beef, bun size	1 serving	180	6	2	530	0	16.0	40
cheesefurter, 'Bun Size Wieners'	2 oz	180	7	2	530	0	16.0	0
hot, 'Hot Franks'	2 oz	190	8	2	530	0	16.0	0
(Hormel)								
batter-wrapped, frozen, 'Corn Dogs'	1 piece	220	7	21	656	0	12.0	0
batter-wrapped, frozen, 'Tater Dogs'	1 piece	210	6	15	170	0	14.0	0
beef, 1-lb pkg	1 frank	140	5	1	463	0	13.0	0
beef, 12-oz pkg	1 frank	100	4	1	362	0	10.0	0
beef, smoked, 'Wranglers'	1 frank	170	7	2	619	0	15.0	0
chili, 'Frank 'n Stuff'	1 frank	165	7	2	517	0	15.0	0
'Light & Lean 97'	1.6 oz	45	6	2	390	0	1.0	15

Food Name	Serv. Size	Total Cal.	Prot. gms	Carbs gms	Sod. mgs	Fiber gms	Fat gms	Chol. mgs
meat, 1-lb pkg	1 frank	140	5	1	486	0	13.0	0
meat, 12-oz pkg	1 frank	110	4	1	378	0	10.0	0
'Mexicali Dogs'	5 oz	400	14	41	952	0	21.0	0
smoked, 'Range Brand Wranglers'	1 frank	170	7	1	600	0	16.0	0
smoked, w/cheese 'Wranglers'	1 frank	180	8	1	546	0	16.0	0
'Wrangler'	1 frank	162	7	1	557	na	14.4	38
(Hygrade) chicken, 'Grillmaster'	1 frank	130	7	3	0	0	11.0	0
(JM)								
10 per lb	1 frank	140	5	1	490	0	13.0	22
beef	1 frank	100	4	1	350	0	9.0	20
beef, 'Jumbo'	1 frank	180	6	2	600	0	16.0	33
beef, 10 per lb	1 frank	140	5	1	480	0	13.0	26
cheesefurter, 'Cheese Franks'	1.6 oz	140	5	2	540	0	13.0	0
'German Brand'	1 frank	160	7	1	620	0	14.0	0
'Jumbo'	1 frank	190	6	2	620	0	17.0	27
1 frank	1.2 oz	110	4	1	370	0	10.0	16
w/cheese, 'German Brand' 1 frank	2 oz	160	8	2	620	0	14.0	37
(Kahn's)								
beef	1 frank	140	5	2	500	0	13.0	0
beef, 'Bun Size Franks'	1 frank	190	6	3	560	0	17.0	0
beef, 'Jumbo'	1 frank	190	6	3	560	0	18.0	0
beef, smoked, 'Bun Size Beef Smokey'	1 frank	190	7	2	530	0	17.0	0
beef, w/cheddar cheddar, 'Beef n' Cheddar'	1 frank	180	7	2	640	0	16.0	0
'Bun Size Frank'	1 frank	190	6	2	560	0	17.0	0
'Cheese Wiener'	1 frank	150	6	1	490	0	13.0	0
'Jumbo'	1 frank	190	6	2	560	0	17.0	0
smoked, 'Big Red Smokey'	1 frank	170	8	2	550	0	14.0	0
smoked, 'Bun Size Smokey'	1 frank	180	8	2	550	0	15.0	0
'Wieners'	1 frank	140	5	1	500	0	13.0	0
(King Kold) beef	2 oz	173	9	1	815	0	16.3	0
(Loma Linda)								
vegetarian, canned, 'Big Franks'	1 pkg	1315	135	17	2489	17	78.7	0
vegetarian, canned, 'Big Franks'	1 link	118	12	2	224	2	7.1	0
(Longacre)								
chicken	1 oz	63	4	1	230	0	5.0	30
turkey	1 oz	66	4	0	260	0	6.0	30
(Louis Rich)								
cheese	1 frank	90	5	2	420	0	7.0	40
turkey	1 frank	101	6	1	505	0	8.2	42
turkey, w/cheese	1 frank	109	6	1	523	0	8.9	44
turkey and chicken	1 frank	85	5	2	511	0	6.1	41
turkey and chicken, bun size	1 frank	110	7	3	630	0	8.0	50
turkey and chicken, w/cheese	1 frank	90	6	2	482	0	6.5	42
(Morningstar Farms)								
corn dog, vegetarian, 'Meat-Free Corn Dogs'	1 corn dog	150	7	22	500	3	4.0	0
corn dog, vegetarian, 'Meat-Free Mini Corn Dogs'	1 corn dog	150	11	21	580	1	4.5	0
hot dog, vegetarian, 'Veggie Dogs'	1 frank	80	11	6	580	1	0.5	0
vegetarian, 'Deli Franks'	1 serving	109	10	3	524	3	6.5	2
(Mr. Turkey)								
turkey, 10 per lb	1 frank	106	6	1	440	0	8.9	31
turkey, w/cheese	1 frank	109	6	1	526	0	9.1	29
(Natural Touch) vegetarian	1 frank	99	10	2	471	2	5.5	1
(OHSE)								
beef	1 oz	85	3	1	280	0	8.0	0
chicken, beef, and pork	1 oz	85	3	1	260	0	8.0	0
'Wieners'	1 oz	90	3	1	300	0	8.0	0
(Oscar Mayer)								
bacon and cheddar cheese, 'Hot Dogs'	1 frank	137	6	1	501	0	12.0	29

Food Name	Serv. Size	Total Cal.	Prot. gms	Carbs gms	Sod. mgs	Fiber gms	Fat gms	Chol. mgs
beef, deli-style, 'Big & Juicy' .... 1 frank		230	9	1	680	0	22.0	50
beef, 'Franks' .... 1 frank		181	6	1	583	0	16.7	35
beef, 'Light Franks' .... 1 frank		131	7	1	594	0	11.1	23
beef, original, 'Big & Juicy' .... 1 frank		240	9	1	700	0	22.0	45
beef, quarter pound, 'Big & Juicy' .... 1 frank		350	13	2	1050	0	33.0	65
beef, w/cheddar, 'Franks' .... 1 frank		163	8	1	655	0	14.3	36
beef, w/garlic, 'Big & Juicy' .... 2.7 oz		239	9	0	652	0	22.5	51
fat free .... 1 frank		35	6	2	490	0	0.0	0
light .... 1 frank		110	6	2	620	0	8.0	30
pork and turkey .... 1 frank		150	5	1	450	0	13.0	30
pork, turkey, and beef, light .... 1 frank		111	7	2	591	0	8.5	35
turkey, w/cheese .... 1 frank		143	5	1	514	0	12.9	33
wiener, hot and spicy, 'Big & Juicy' .... 1 wiener		220	10	1	750	0	20.0	45
wiener, original, 'Big & Juicy' .... 1 wiener		240	9	1	690	0	22.0	45
wiener, smokie link, 'Big & Juicy' .... 1 wiener		220	10	1	770	0	19.0	50
(Pilgrim's Pride)								
1-lb pkg .... 1 frank		118	8	1	456	0	8.8	31
12-oz pkg .... 1 frank		88	6	1	342	0	6.6	24
(Quick Meal) w/chili and cheese .... 4.5 oz		340	14	25	540	0	20.0	80
(Smart Dog) vegetarian, fat-free, 'Lightlife' .... 1.5 oz		40	8	1	290	0	0.0	0
(State Fair) beef, batter-wrapped, on a stick, 'Corn Dogs' .... 2.67 oz		210	6	24	0	0	10.0	0
(Tyson)								
chicken .... 1 frank		115	6	1	700	0	10.0	0
chicken, batter-wrapped, 'Corn Dogs' .... 3.5 oz		280	9	28	70	0	14.0	75
w/cheese .... 1 frank		145	7	1	680	0	11.0	0
(White Wave SoyFood) vegetarian, 'Healthy' .... 1.5 oz		120	7	5	340	0	8.0	0
(Worthington) vegetarian, 'Leanies' .... 1 serving		106	7	2	425	1	7.8	1
FRENCH ARTICHOKE. See under ARTICHOKE.								
FRENCH BEAN. See BEAN, FRENCH.								
FRENCH TOAST								
(Aunt Jemima)								
cinnamon, frozen .... 1 slice		240	10	35	330	2	7.0	90
homestyle, frozen .... 1 slice		240	10	35	310	2	7.0	95
original, frozen .... 3 oz		166	7	27	554	1	4.4	46
sticks, and syrup, frozen, 'Homestyle' .... 5.2 oz		400	7	48	640	0	20.0	0
wedges, and sausages, frozen, 'Homestyle' .... 5.3 oz		360	13	40	780	0	17.0	0
(Downyflake)								
frozen .... 1 slice		130	4	22	270	0	3.0	25
frozen, 'Extra Thick' .... 1 slice		150	5	11	340	0	9.0	0
Texas style, w/sausage, frozen .... 4.25 oz		400	10	37	550	0	24.0	0
(Farm Rich)								
sticks, apple cinnamon .... 3 oz		310	6	39	300	0	15.0	0
sticks, blueberry .... 3 oz		310	6	37	280	0	14.0	0
sticks, original .... 3 oz		300	5	37	280	0	15.0	0
(French Toast Boat) cinnamon .... 1 piece		224	5	28	267	1	11.1	4
(Krusteaz)								
cinnamon swirl, w/sausage, frozen .... 1 pkg		415	13	38	502	2	23.2	98
cinnamon swirl, frozen .... 2 slices		270	10	46	370	0	5.0	120
regular, frozen .... 2 slices		250	11	38	380	0	6.0	120
(Morningstar Farms)								
vegetarian, cinnamon swirl, w/patties, frozen .... 6.5 oz		380	24	37	1220	4	15.0	0
(Pierre) cinnamon, wedge, product 1847 .... 1 piece		118	2	16	163	1	5.1	32
(Stilwell) sticks, frozen, 'Qwik-Krisp' .... 5 pieces		400	6	46	370	1	21.0	40
(Sunny Fresh)								
bagel, w/maple syrup, frozen .... 1 pkg		15196	1120	1678	22623	0	426.4	10263
bagel, w/maple syrup, frozen .... 1 serving		190	14	21	283	0	5.3	128

Food Name	Serv. Size	Total Cal.	Prot. gms	Carbs gms	Sod. mgs	Fiber gms	Fat gms	Chol. mgs
cinnamon swirl, frozen .... 1 serving		190	6	26	220	1	7.0	75
(Swanson)								
cinnamon swirl, w/sausage, frozen, 'Great Starts' .... 5.5 oz		390	12	37	530	0	21.0	0
mini, w/sausage, frozen, 'Great Starts' .... 2.5 oz		190	6	22	320	0	9.0	0
oatmeal, w/lite links, frozen, 'Great Starts' .... 4.65 oz		310	13	35	500	0	13.0	0
sticks, w/syrup, 'Great Starts' .... 1 pkg		320	7	50	260	2	10.0	25
w/sausage, 'Great Starts' .... 1 pkg		410	13	33	580	3	26.0	110
w/sausage, frozen, 'Great Starts' .... 1 entrée		410	13	33	580	3	26.0	110
FRESHWATER BASS. See BASS, FRESHWATER.								
FRIED RICE SEASONING. See under SEASONING MIX, RICE.								
FRITTER								
corn, frozen *(Mrs. Paul's)* .... 2 pieces		240	5	35	560	0	9.0	10
apple, frozen *(Mrs. Paul's)* .... 2 pieces		240	4	35	500	0	9.0	5
FROG								
legs, raw .... 3.5 oz		73	16.4	0.0	58	0	0.3	50
legs, raw .... 1 oz		21	4.6	0.0	(mq)	0	<1.0	(mq)
FROGFISH. See MONKFISH.								
FROSTING								
(Betty Crocker)								
Amaretto almond, 'Creamy Deluxe' .... 1/12 can		160	0	27	50	0	6.0	0
butter pecan 'Creamy Deluxe' .... 1/12 tub		170	0	26	50	0	7.0	0
chocolate, light, 'Creamy Deluxe' .... 1/12 tub		130	1	28	60	0	2.0	0
chocolate, w/dinosaurs, 'Creamy Deluxe Party' .... 1/12 tub		160	1	24	60	0	7.0	0
chocolate, w/red gel 'Creamy Deluxe Party' .... 1/12 tub		160	1	24	50	0	7.0	0
chocolate, w/turbo racers, 'Creamy Deluxe Party' ..... 1/12 tub		160	1	24	50	0	7.0	0
chocolate chip, 'Creamy Deluxe' .... 1/12 tub		170	1	27	30	0	7.0	0
chocolate chip, 'Creamy Deluxe Party' .... 1/12 tub		160	1	24	60	0	7.0	0
chocolate coconut almond, 'Creamy Deluxe' .... 1/12 can		160	1	21	55	0	8.0	0
double chocolate chip, 'Creamy Deluxe' .... 1/12 can		170	1	24	60	0	8.0	0
Dutch fudge, dark, 'Creamy Deluxe' .... 1/12 tub		160	1	22	70	0	7.0	0
milk chocolate 'Creamy Deluxe Light' .... 1/12 tub		140	1	29	60	0	2.0	0
rocky road, 'Creamy Deluxe' .... 1/12 can		150	1	20	50	0	8.0	0
vanilla, 'Creamy Deluxe Light' .... 1/12 tub		140	0	30	30	0	2.0	0
vanilla, w/blue gel, 'Creamy Deluxe Party' .... 1/12 tub		160	0	27	30	0	6.0	0
vanilla, w/teddy bears, 'Creamy Deluxe Party' .... 1/12 tub		160	0	27	25	0	6.0	0
(Duncan Hines)								
chocolate .... 1/12 can		160	0	24	90	0	7.0	0
cream cheese .... 1/12 can		160	0	24	120	0	8.0	0
cream cheese, 'Homestyle' .... 1/12 can		160	0	26	75	0	6.0	0
dark chocolate 'Homestyle' .... 1/12 can		160	0	25	75	0	6.0	0
Dutch fudge .... 1/12 can		160	0	24	95	0	7.0	0
lemon .... 1/24 tub		60	0	9	30	0	3.0	0
milk chocolate .... 1/12 can		160	0	24	85	0	7.0	0
milk chocolate, 'Homestyle' .... 1/12 can		160	0	25	75	0	6.0	0
vanilla .... 1/12 can		160	0	24	80	0	7.0	0
vanilla, 'Homestyle' .... 1/12 can		160	0	26	75	0	6.0	0
wild cherry .... 1 tbsp		140	0	22	60	0	5.0	0
(Finast) milk .... 1/12 can		160	0	25	105	0	6.0	0
(Pathmark)								
chocolate, creamy .... 1/12 can		160	0	25	95	0	6.0	0
fudge, creamy .... 1/12 can		160	0	25	100	0	7.0	0
white, creamy .... 1/12 can		160	0	25	95	0	6.0	0
(Pillsbury)								
butter fudge, 'Frosting Supreme' .... 1/12 pkg		140	1	22	50	0	6.0	0
candy, creamy, 'Creamy Supreme' .... 2 tbsp		150	0	22	95	0	7.0	0
candy, creamy, 'Frosting Supreme' .... 2 tbsp		150	0	22	95	0	7.0	0
caramel pecan, 'Frosting Supreme' .... 1/12 pkg		150	0	20	70	0	8.0	0

Food Name	Serv. Size	Total Cal.	Prot. gms	Carbs gms	Sod. mgs	Fiber gms	Fat gms	Chol. mgs
chocolate, 'Creamy Supreme'	2 tbsp	140	0	21	80	0	6.0	0
chocolate, 'Frost It Hot'	1/8 cake	50	0	12	50	0	0.0	0
chocolate, 'Frosting Supreme'	2 tbsp	140	0	21	75	0	6.0	0
chocolate, 'Funfetti, Creamy Supreme'	2 tbsp	140	0	22	80	0	6.0	0
chocolate, dark, 'Creamy Supreme'	2 tbsp	130	0	20	45	0	6.0	0
chocolate, dark, 'Frosting Supreme'	2 tbsp	130	0	20	45	0	7.0	0
chocolate, double Dutch, 'Frosting Supreme'	1/12 can	140	1	22	45	0	6.0	0
chocolate chip, 'Frosting Supreme'	1/12 can	150	0	27	70	0	5.0	0
chocolate fudge, 'Funfetti' 'Frosting Supreme'	1/12 pkg	140	0	23	80	0	6.0	0
chocolate fudge, 'Frosting Supreme'	1/12 pkg	150	0	22	85	0	6.0	0
chocolate fudge, 'Lovin Lites'	1/12 pkg	130	1	28	95	1	2.0	0
chocolate fudge, lowfat, 'Creamy Supreme'	2 tbsp	140	0	26	85	0	3.5	0
coconut almond, 'Frosting Supreme'	1/12 can	150	1	17	60	0	9.0	0
coconut pecan, 'Frosting Supreme'	1/12 can	160	0	17	60	0	10.0	0
cream cheese, 'Frosting Supreme'	1/12 can	160	0	26	115	0	6.0	0
decorator, all flavors except chocolate	1 tbsp	70	0	12	0	0	2.0	0
decorator, chocolate	1 tbsp	60	0	11	0	0	2.0	0
fudge, 'Frosting Supreme'	1/12 can	150	1	24	80	0	6.0	0
lemon, 'Frosting Supreme'	1/12 can	160	0	26	80	0	6.0	0
milk, 'Frosting Supreme'	1/12 can	150	0	23	60	0	6.0	0
milk chocolate, 'Creamy Supreme'	2 tbsp	140	0	21	60	1	6.0	0
milk chocolate, 'Frosting Supreme'	1/12 pkg	150	0	23	65	0	6.0	0
milk chocolate, 'Lovin' Lites'	2 tbsp	130	0	25	85	1	3.0	0
milk chocolate, w/fudge glaze, 'Creamy Supreme'	2 tbsp	140	0	22	75	1	6.0	0
milk chocolate, w/fudge swirl, 'Frosting Supreme'	1/12 pkg	150	0	23	65	0	6.0	0
mint, 'Frosting Supreme'	1/12 can	150	1	24	80	0	7.0	0
mocha, 'Frosting Supreme'	1/12 can	150	1	24	60	0	6.0	0
Oreo, 'Frosting Supreme'	2 tbsp	150	0	23	75	0	6.0	0
sour cream vanilla, 'Frosting Supreme'	1/12 can	160	0	27	80	0	6.0	0
strawberry, 'Frosting Supreme'	1/12 can	160	0	26	75	0	6.0	0
vanilla	1/8 cake	120	0	19	60	0	5.0	0
vanilla, 'Creamy Supreme'	2 tbsp	150	0	23	70	0	6.0	0
vanilla, 'Frosting Supreme'	1/12 can	160	0	26	75	0	6.0	0
vanilla, 'Funfetti'	2 tbsp	150	0	25	75	0	6.0	0
vanilla, 'Funfetti Pink'	2 tbsp	150	0	24	70	0	6.0	0
vanilla, 'Lovin Lites'	1/12 pkg	130	0	29	70	0	2.0	0
vanilla, French, 'Creamy Supreme'	2 tbsp	150	0	25	80	0	6.0	0
vanilla, French, 'Frosting Supreme'	2 tbsp	160	0	26	75	0	6.0	0
vanilla, pink and white, 'Frosting Supreme'	1/12 can	150	0	24	70	0	6.0	0
vanilla, w/fudge glaze, 'Creamy Supreme'	2 tbsp	150	0	25	75	0	6.0	0
vanilla, w/fudge swirl, 'Frosting Supreme'	1/12 pkg	150	0	25	75	0	6.0	0
white, fluffy	1/12 can	60	0	15	65	0	0.0	0
white, fluffy, 'Frost It Hot'	1/8 cake	50	0	12	50	0	0.0	0
(Weight Watchers)								
chocolate, less fat, 'Sweet Rewards'	2 tbsp	120	1	24	55	0	2.5	0
milk chocolate, less fat, 'Sweet Rewards'	2 tbsp	120	0	24	60	0	2.5	0
vanilla, 'less fat, Sweet Rewards'	2 tbsp	120	0	26	65	0	2.0	0
FROSTING MIX								
(Betty Crocker)								
cherry, creamy, prepared w/margarine	1/12 pkg	180	0	31	100	0	6.0	0
chocolate fudge, creamy, prepared w/1/4 cup butter	1/12 mix	180	1	30	70	0	6.0	10
chocolate fudge, creamy, prepared w/1/4 cup margarine	1/12 mix	180	1	30	70	0	6.0	0
chocolate fudge, sour cream, creamy, prepared w/margarine	1/12 pkg	180	1	30	75	0	6.0	0
coconut pecan, creamy, mix only	1/12 mix	110	1	19	5	0	4.0	0

Food Name	Serv. Size	Total Cal.	Prot. gms	Carbs gms	Sod. mgs	Fiber gms	Fat gms	Chol. mgs
coconut pecan, creamy, prepared w/butter, 2% milk ...	1/12 mix	150	1	19	50	0	8.0	10
coconut pecan, creamy, prepared w/margarine, skim milk	1/12 mix	150	1	19	50	0	8.0	0
milk chocolate, creamy, prepared w/margarine	1/12 pkg	170	1	29	40	0	5.0	0
rainbow chip, creamy, prepared w/margarine	1/12 pkg	190	1	32	50	0	7.0	0
vanilla, creamy, mix only	1/12 mix	150	0	32	5	0	2.0	0
vanilla, creamy, prepared w/1/4 cup butter	1/12 mix	170	0	32	50	0	5.0	10
vanilla, creamy, prepared w/1/4 cup margarine	1/12 mix	170	0	32	50	0	5.0	0
white, sour cream, creamy, prepared w/margarine	1/12 pkg	170	0	31	100	0	5.0	0
(Sweet 'n Low)								
chocolate fudge, low sodium w/'Sweet 'N Low'	3 tbsp	140	2	16	30	0	8.0	0
white, low-sodium w/Sweet 'N Low	3 tbsp	120	2	16	30	0	8.0	0
FRUCTOSE								
(Estee)	1 tsp	16	0	4	0	0	0.0	0
(Featherweight)	1 tsp	12	0	3	0	0	0.0	0
crystalline, pure *(Esculent)*	1 tsp	15	0	4	0	0	0.0	0
crystalline, pure *(Fifty 50)*	1 tsp	15	0	4	0	0	0.0	0
crystalline, pure *(Healthy Edge)*	1 tsp	15	0	4	0	0	0.0	0
liquid *(Sweet Lite)*	1 tsp	20	0	6	0	0	0.0	0
packet *(Estee)*	1 pkt	12	0	3	0	0	0.0	0
FRUIT, MIXED								
(Flav-R-Pac)								
frozen	2/3 cup	60	1	14	0	2	0.0	0
melons, mixed, frozen	3/4 cup	40	1	10	16	1	0.0	0
w/pineapple, frozen	2/3 cup	60	1	15	0	2	0.0	0
FRUIT AND NUT MIX								
(Eden Foods)	1 oz	160	7	10	0	3	10.0	0
(Estee)	14 pieces	70	2	6	15	0	5.0	0
(Fisher)								
'California Style'	1/4 cup	140	2	16	20	2	8.0	0
classic	1/4 cup	150	5	11	70	2	11.0	0
(Planters)								
'Caribbean Crunch'	1 oz	150	3	14	130	0	10.0	0
'Fruit 'n Nut'	1 oz	150	5	13	90	0	9.0	0
FRUIT BAR. See also FRUIT BAR, FROZEN.								
APPLE								
(Health Valley)								
nonfat	1 bar	140	3	35	0	3	0.0	0
nonfat, 'Bakes'	1 bar	70	2	18	30	2	0.0	0
APPLE RAISIN *(Weight Watchers)*	1 bar	70	1	14	60	2	2.0	0
APRICOT, nonfat *(Health Valley)*	1 bar	140	3	35	5	4	0.0	0
BLUEBERRY, nonfat *(Parnasa)*	1 bar	120	1	28	20	0	0.0	0
CRANBERRY, natural *(Hearty Balance)*	1 bar	150	4	30	60	3	0.5	0
DATE								
(Health Valley)								
	1 bar	140	3	34	5	3	0.0	0
nonfat, 'Bakes'	1 bar	70	2	18	30	2	0.0	0
RAISIN								
(Health Valley)								
nonfat	1 bar	140	2	35	5	3	0.0	0
nonfat, 'Bakes'	1 bar	70	2	18	30	2	0.0	0
RASPBERRY *(Parnasa)* nonfat	1 bar	120	1	29	15	1	0.0	0
FRUIT BAR, FROZEN								
(Dole)								
blueberry and cream, 'Fruit & Cream'	1 bar	90	1	19	20	0	1.4	5
cherry, 'Fresh Lites'	1 bar	25	1	6	6	0	1.0	0
chocolate, banana, and cream, 'Fruit & Cream'	1 bar	175	2	22	20	0	9.0	0

Food Name	Serv. Size	Total Cal.	Prot. gms	Carbs gms	Sod. mgs	Fiber gms	Fat gms	Chol. mgs
chocolate, strawberry, and cream, 'Fruit & Cream'	1 bar	140	2	23	20	0	8.0	0
grape, nonfat, no sugar added	1 bar	25	0	6	5	0	0.0	0
grape, 'SunTops'	1 bar	40	1	9	5	0	1.0	0
lemon, 'Fresh Lites'	1 bar	25	1	6	16	0	1.0	0
lemonade, 'SunTops'	1 bar	40	1	9	5	0	1.0	0
orange, tropical, 'SunTops'	1 bar	40	1	9	5	0	1.0	0
peach and cream, 'Fruit & Cream'	1 bar	90	1	19	19	0	1.4	5
piña colada, 'Fruit 'n Juice'	1 bar	90	1	16	2	0	3.0	0
pineapple, 'Fruit & Juice'	1 bar	70	0	17	4	0	0.1	0
pineapple-orange, 'Fresh Lites'	1 bar	25	1	6	7	0	1.0	0
punch, 'SunTops'	1 bar	40	1	9	5	0	1.0	0
raspberry, 'Fresh Lites'	1 bar	25	1	6	6	0	1.0	0
raspberry, 'Fruit & Juice'	1 bar	70	0	16	14	0	0.1	0
raspberry, nonfat, no sugar added	1 bar	25	0	6	5	0	0.0	0
raspberry and cream, 'Fruit & Cream'	1 bar	90	1	20	23	0	1.4	5
strawberry, 'Fruit n' Juice'	1 bar	70	0	16	6	0	0.1	0
strawberry, nonfat, no sugar added	1 bar	25	0	6	5	0	0.0	0
strawberry and cream, 'Fruit & Cream'	1 bar	90	1	19	22	0	1.4	5
(Fruit a Freeze)								
banana, all natural	1 bar	99	2	16	28	1	4.0	10
strawberry, all-natural	1 bar	100	1	18	35	0	3.0	10
(Minute Maid) all flavors, nonfat, 'Fruit Juicee'	1 bar	60	0	14	0	0	0.0	0
(Natural Nectar)								
lemony lime, juice snack, all natural, nonfat	1 bar	70	1	17	10	0	0.0	0
strawberry nectar, juice snack	1 bar	70	1	16	55	0	1.0	0
'Tropical Delight' juice snack, all-natural, nonfat,	1 bar	70	1	16	10	0	0.0	0
(Sunkist)								
coconut	1 bar	170	3	15	70	0	10.0	0
lemonade, nonfat	1 bar	90	0	24	5	0	0.0	0
orange, nonfat, 'Juice Bar'	1 bar	100	0	25	0	0	0.0	0
strawberry and cream	1 bar	90	0	19	30	0	1.0	0
wildberry, nonfat	1 bar	140	0	33	15	0	0.0	0
FRUIT COCKTAIL *(Hunt's)*	1/2 cup	90	0	23	15	1	0.0	0
FRUIT DESSERT MIX								
apple-cinnamon, w/Nutrasweet *(Sans Sucre de Paris)*	1/4 cup	60	0	14	10	1	0.0	0
piña colada, w/Nutrasweet *(Sans Sucre de Paris)*	1/4 cup	70	0	12	10	1	1.5	0

FRUIT DRINK. See also CIDER; FRUIT DRINK MIX; FRUIT JUICE BLEND; FRUIT JUICE DRINK.

Food Name	Serv. Size	Total Cal.	Prot. gms	Carbs gms	Sod. mgs	Fiber gms	Fat gms	Chol. mgs
(A&P)								
cranberry apple	6 fl oz	130	1	32	1	0	0.0	0
grape	6 fl oz	100	1	25	0	0	1.0	0
lemonade, frozen, prepared	8 fl oz	110	1	28	0	0	1.0	0
lemonade, pink, frozen, prepared	8 fl oz	110	1	28	0	0	1.0	0
raspberry, w/cranberry	6 fl oz	110	1	27	0	0	1.0	0
(Awake) orange, frozen concentrate, prepared	6 fl oz	80	0	20	10	0	0.0	0
(Bama)								
fruit punch	8.45 fl oz	130	0	32	15	0	0.0	0
grape	8.45 fl oz	120	0	29	25	0	0.0	0
orange	8.45 fl oz	120	0	29	60	0	0.0	0
(Bel-Air) lemonade, pink, concentrate, prepared	6 fl oz	110	0	27	0	0	0.0	0
(Bright & Early)								
'Bright & Early Fruit Punch' prepared	6 fl oz	90	0	22	5	0	0.0	0
grape, 'Bright & Early Grape'	6 fl oz	100	0	24	0	0	0.0	0
orange, 'Bright & Early Orange'	6 fl oz	90	0	21	20	0	0.0	0
pineapple, 'Bright & Early Pineapple'	6 fl oz	90	0	23	0	0	0.0	0
(Castle Crest)								
fruit punch, artificially flavored	8 fl oz	120	0	31	15	0	0.0	0
grape flavored	8 fl oz	120	0	31	15	0	0.0	0

Food Name	Serv. Size	Total Cal.	Prot. gms	Carbs gms	Sod. mgs	Fiber gms	Fat gms	Chol. mgs
lemonade drink, artificially flavored	8 fl oz	120	0	31	15	0	0.0	0
(Crowley)								
fruit punch	8 fl oz	130	0	32	15	0	0.0	0
grape	8 fl oz	130	0	32	15	0	0.0	0
lemon	8 fl oz	130	0	32	15	0	0.0	0
orange	8 fl oz	130	0	32	15	0	0.0	0
(Del Monte)								
pineapple, w/grapefruit	6 fl oz	90	0	24	50	0	0.0	0
pineapple, w/pink grapefruit	6 fl oz	90	0	24	50	0	0.0	0
pineapple-orange	6 fl oz	90	0	24	20	0	0.0	0
(Finast)								
cranberry grape	6 fl oz	103	0	26	5	0	0.0	0
raspberry, w/cranberry	6 fl oz	110	0	27	10	0	0.0	0
(Five Alive)								
berry citrus drink	6 fl oz	90	0	22	5	0	0.0	0
tropical citrus	6 fl oz	90	0	21	0	0	0.0	0
(Flav-R-Pac) lemonade	8 fl oz	110	0	27	0	0	0.0	0
(Frostee) strawberry-flavored	8 fl oz	180	2	27	150	0	7.0	0
(Fruit Corners) soda pop snacks "soda Licious"	1 pouch	100	1	22	20	0	1.0	0
(Hawaiian Punch)								
fruit punch, red, 'Fruit Juicy Lite'	6 fl oz	60	0	15	30	0	0.0	0
fruit punch, red, 'Fruit Juicy'	6 fl oz	90	0	22	20	0	0.0	0
fruit punch, tropical	6 fl oz	90	0	22	30	0	0.0	0
fruit punch, tropical, wild fruit	6 fl oz	90	0	23	35	0	0.0	0
fruit punch cocktail, island fruit	6 fl oz	90	0	22	30	0	0.0	0
orange	6 fl oz	100	0	24	20	0	0.0	0
'Very Berry'	6 fl oz	90	0	22	30	0	0.0	0
(Hi-C)								
'Boppin' Berry'	6 fl oz	90	0	23	25	0	0.0	0
'Candy Apple Cooler'	6 fl oz	94	0	23	17	0	0.1	0
cherry, aseptic box	6 fl oz	100	0	24	25	0	0.0	0
'Double Fruit Cooler'	6 fl oz	93	0	23	18	0	0.1	0
'Ecto Cooler'	6 fl oz	95	0	23	17	0	0.1	0
'Fruity Bubble Gum'	6 fl oz	90	0	22	20	0	0.0	0
grape	6 fl oz	90	0	23	25	0	0.0	0
'Hula Cooler'	6 fl oz	97	0	24	17	0	0.1	0
'Hula Punch'	6 fl oz	87	0	21	17	0	0.1	0
'Jammin' Apple Drink' aseptic box	6 fl oz	90	0	23	20	0	0.0	0
lemonade	8.45 fl oz	109	0	27	73	0	0.1	0
orange	6 fl oz	95	0	23	17	0	0.1	0
peach	6 fl oz	100	0	24	20	0	0.0	0
'Stompin' Banana Berry'	6 fl oz	90	0	22	25	0	0.0	0
wild berry	6 fl oz	92	0	23	17	0	0.1	0
(J. Hungerford)								
fruit punch, 20% plus juice	9.03 fl oz	43	0	11	32	0	0.0	0
grape, 20% plus juice	9.03 fl oz	41	0	11	31	0	0.0	0
lemon, 20% plus juice	9.03 fl oz	41	0	11	38	0	0.0	0
lemonade, pink, 20% plus juice	9.03 fl oz	41	0	11	39	0	0.0	0
orange, 20% plus juice	9.03 fl oz	41	0	11	23	0	0.0	0
punch juice	9.03 fl oz	133	0	33	2	0	0.0	0
(Juicy Juice)								
fruit punch	6 fl oz	100	1	23	10	0	0.0	0
tropical	6 fl oz	100	1	24	5	0	0.0	0
(Kern's)								
apple-strawberry nectar, canned or bottled	6 fl oz	110	0	26	0	0	0.0	0
apricot-mango nectar	11.5 fl oz	220	1	53	10	0	0.0	0
apricot nectar, canned or bottled	6 fl oz	110	1	27	0	0	0.0	0

Food Name	Serv. Size	Total Cal.	Prot. gms	Carbs gms	Sod. mgs	Fiber gms	Fat gms	Chol. mgs
apricot-pineapple nectar	11.5 fl oz	220	1	53	5	2	0.0	0
banana-pineapple nectar	11.5 fl oz	220	1	52	5	0	0.0	0
coconut-pineapple nectar, can or bottle	6 fl oz	140	1	26	25	0	4.0	0
(Knudsen)								
apricot nectar	8 fl oz	105	1	24	0	0	0.0	0
blueberry nectar	8 fl oz	135	1	34	0	0	0.0	0
boysenberry nectar	8 fl oz	110	1	33	0	0	0.0	0
calamansi punch, 'Rain Forest'	8 fl oz	115	1	27	0	0	0.0	0
cherry lemonade	8 fl oz	120	0	29	35	na	0.0	0
coconut nectar	8 fl oz	140	1	26	55	na	5.0	na
guanabana punch, 'Rain Forest'	8 fl oz	125	1	29	0	0	0.0	0
hibiscus cooler	8 fl oz	95	1	24	0	0	0.0	0
lime cactus cooler blend *(Knudsen)*	8 fl oz	120	0	29	35	na	0.0	0
lemonade, 'Natural'	8 fl oz	100	1	26	0	0	0.0	0
lime, tropical	8 fl oz	130	1	32	0	0	0.0	0
papaya, concentrate	1.5 fl oz	90	1	22	37	0	0.0	0
passionfruit, tropical	8 fl oz	80	1	20	0	0	0.0	0
rainforest punch, cupu assu	8 fl oz	110	1	25	0	0	0.0	0
rainforest punch, fruit juice sweetened	8 fl oz	120	1	29	20	0	0.0	0
raspberry float	8 fl oz	130	2	31	0	0	0.0	0
raspberry lemonade	8 fl oz	110	1	28	0	0	0.0	0
strawberry lemonade	8 fl oz	90	1	21	0	0	0.0	0
tropical punch	8 fl oz	120	0	29	20	na	0.0	0
(Kool-Aid)								
cherry, 'Koolers'	8.45 fl oz	140	0	38	10	0	0.0	0
grape, 'Koolers'	8.45 fl oz	140	0	35	10	0	0.0	0
grape-berry, 'Kool-Aid Splash'	1 serving	116	0	31	35	0	0.0	0
'Great Bluedini' 'Koolers'	8.45 fl oz	110	0	29	10	0	0.0	0
mountain berry punch, 'Koolers'	8.45 fl oz	140	0	37	10	0	0.0	0
rainbow punch, 'Koolers'	8.45 fl oz	130	0	36	10	0	0.0	0
'Rock-A-Dile Red' 'Koolers'	8.45 fl oz	130	0	34	10	0	0.0	0
tropical punch, 'Koolers'	8.45 fl oz	130	0	35	10	0	0.0	0
tropical, 'Kool-Aid Burst'	1 serving	90	0	24	29	0	0.0	0
(Lemonade Chillers) 'Key Lime'	8 fl oz	110	0	26	0	0	0.0	0
(Libby's)								
apricot nectar	5.5 fl oz	105	0	25	5	0	0.0	0
banana nectar	8 fl oz	132	0	33	24	0	0.0	0
banana nectar	6 fl oz	110	0	26	15	0	0.0	0
(Minute Maid)								
apple punch, prepared	6 fl oz	90	0	23	20	0	0.0	0
berry punch	6 fl oz	90	0	23	20	0	0.0	0
berry punch, frozen concentrate, prepared	6 fl oz	90	0	23	0	0	0.0	0
cranberry lemonade	6 fl oz	90	0	23	20	0	0.0	0
cranberry lemonade, frozen, concentrate, prepared	6 fl oz	90	0	22	0	0	0.0	0
lemonade, country style	6 fl oz	80	0	21	20	0	0.0	0
lemonade, country style, frozen concentrate, prepared	6 fl oz	90	0	22	0	0	0.0	0
lemonade, pink	6 fl oz	80	0	21	20	0	0.0	0
lemonade, pink, frozen concentrate, prepared	6 fl oz	90	0	22	0	0	0.0	0
limeade, frozen concentrate, prepared	6 fl oz	70	0	19	0	0	0.0	0
orange punch	6 fl oz	80	0	20	20	0	0.0	0
raspberry lemonade	6 fl oz	90	0	23	20	0	0.0	0
raspberry lemonade, frozen concentrate, prepared	6 fl oz	90	0	22	0	0	0.0	0
tropical punch	6 fl oz	90	0	22	20	0	0.0	0
(Mott's)								
apple cranberry	10 fl oz	176	0	44	3	0	0.0	0
apple raspberry drink	10 fl oz	158	0	40	17	0	0.0	0
punch	9.5 fl oz	161	0	40	4	0	0.0	0

Food Name	Serv. Size	Total Cal.	Prot. gms	Carbs gms	Sod. mgs	Fiber gms	Fat gms	Chol. mgs
grape-apple	10 fl oz	167	0	42	1	0	0.0	0
(Mountain Sun)								
cherry lemonade, organic	8 fl oz	101	0	25	0	0	0.0	0
lemonade, organic	8 fl oz	110	0	27	0	0	0.0	0
(Natural Choice)								
apple cranberry, 5% juice, vitamin C added	1 cup	120	0	30	20	0	0.0	0
(Nestlé) strawberry-flavored, ready to drink, 'Quik'	1 cup	230	7	31	100	0	9.0	30
(Ocean Spray)								
'Cran-Apple'	6 fl oz	120	0	31	15	0	0.0	0
'Cran-Apple Low-calorie'	6 fl oz	35	0	9	15	0	0.0	0
cranberry, citrus 'Refreshers'	6 fl oz	100	0	26	15	0	0.0	0
'Cran-Grape'	6 fl oz	120	0	31	15	0	0.0	0
'Cranicot'	6 fl oz	120	0	29	15	0	0.0	0
'Cran-Blueberry'	6 fl oz	120	0	31	10	0	0.0	0
'Cran-Raspberry' low-calorie	6 fl oz	40	0	9	15	0	0.0	0
'Cran-Raspberry'	6 fl oz	110	0	27	15	0	0.0	0
'Cran-Strawberry'	6 fl oz	110	0	27	15	0	0.0	0
guava-passionfruit, Hawaiian, 'Mauna La'i'	6 fl oz	100	0	25	10	0	0.0	0
lemonade drink, w/cranberry juice	8 fl oz	110	0	26	35	0	0.0	0
orange-cranberry, 'Refreshers'	6 fl oz	100	0	26	15	0	0.0	0
peach, citrus, 'Refreshers'	6 fl oz	90	0	23	15	0	0.0	0
(Orange Julius)								
piña colada flavored	16 fl oz	300	2	71	15	0	1.0	0
raspberry cream supreme	16 fl oz	510	4	76	40	0	23.0	0
strawberry, regular	16 fl oz	340	1	82	15	0	1.0	0
tropical cream supreme	16 fl oz	510	5	67	40	0	25.0	95
(Orlando Sun)								
pineapple-orange-banana	8 fl oz	110	1	29	0	0	0.0	0
strawberry-guava	8 fl oz	110	1	29	0	0	0.0	0
(P&Q) cranberry apple	6 fl oz	130	1	32	1	0	0.0	0
(Pathmark)								
cranberry-apple	6 fl oz	130	0	32	10	0	0.0	0
cranberry-grape	6 fl oz	103	0	26	5	0	0.0	0
fruit punch	6 fl oz	90	0	22	0	0	0.0	0
grape	6 fl oz	90	0	22	0	0	0.0	0
guava-passionfruit, Hawaiian, 'Hawaii'	6 fl oz	100	0	25	10	0	0.0	0
orange, 'No Frills Sodium-free'	6 fl oz	80	0	22	0	0	0.0	0
pineapple, w/grapefruit	6 fl oz	80	0	21	0	0	0.0	0
raspberry, w/cranberry	6 fl oz	110	0	27	10	0	0.0	0
raspberry, w/cranberry, 'Sodium-free'	6 fl oz	110	0	27	0	0	0.0	0
(Red Cheek) apple punch drink	6 fl oz	113	0	28	7	0	0.0	0
(S&W)								
apricot nectar, canned or bottled	8 fl oz	140	1	35	15	1	0.0	0
apricot nectar, canned or bottled	5.5 fl oz	100	1	24	10	1	0.0	0
apricot-pineapple nectar	4 fl oz	35	0	12	20	0	0.0	0
(Santa Cruz Natural)								
apricot nectar, certified organic	8 fl oz	150	1	38	25	0	0.0	0
berry nectar, organic	8 fl oz	90	1	22	0	0	1.0	0
cherry lemonade, dark, sweet, organic	8 fl oz	60	1	20	0	0	1.0	0
cranberry guava nectar, certified organic	8 fl oz	110	1	24	25	0	0.0	0
lemonade, certified organic	8 fl oz	120	1	29	35	0	0.0	0
lemonade, organic	8 fl oz	60	1	21	0	0	1.0	0
lemonade, organic, 'Sparkling'	8 fl oz	85	1	20	0	0	1.0	0
limeade, organic, 'Sparkling'	8 fl oz	60	1	23	0	0	1.0	0
orangeade, organic	8 fl oz	90	1	22	0	0	1.0	0
orangeade, organic, 'Sparkling'	8 fl oz	90	1	24	0	0	1.0	0
organic, 'Kauai Punch'	8 fl oz	120	1	28	0	0	1.0	0

Food Name	Serv. Size	Total Cal.	Prot. gms	Carbs gms	Sod. mgs	Fiber gms	Fat gms	Chol. mgs
raspberry lemonade, organic	8 fl oz	60	1	20	0	0	1.0	0
raspberry lemonade, organic, 'Sparkling'	8 fl oz	85	1	20	0	0	1.0	0
red raspberry, organic, 'Cruz'	8 fl oz	120	1	28	0	0	1.0	0
strawberry lemonade, organic	8 fl oz	60	1	20	0	0	1.0	0
tropical punch, organic	8 fl oz	110	1	26	0	0	1.0	0
(Shasta) lemonade	12 fl oz	146	0	39	106	0	0.0	0
(Squeezit)								
'Berry B. Wild'	6.75 fl oz	120	0	29	5	0	0.0	0
'Chucklin' Cherry'	1 serving	110	0	28	0	0	0.0	0
'Grumpy Grape'	1 serving	110	0	28	0	0	0.0	0
'Mean Green Puncher'	6.75 fl oz	100	0	25	5	0	0.0	0
orange fruit, 'Smarty Arty'	1 serving	110	0	27	45	0	0.0	0
'Rockin Red Puncher'	6.75 fl oz	110	0	28	5	0	0.0	0
'Silly Billy Strawberry'	6.75 fl oz	90	0	23	5	0	0.0	0
strawberry	1 serving	110	0	29	0	0	0.0	0
(Sunkist)								
lemonade	8 fl oz	141	0	36	0	0	0.0	0
lemonade, frozen, prepared	8 fl oz	92	0	24	1	0	0.0	0
(Sunny Delight) orange, 'California Style'	8 fl oz	130	0	31	130	0	0.0	0
(Tang)								
berry blend drink, 'Fruit Box'	8.45 fl oz	140	0	36	10	0	0.0	0
orange, tropical, 'Fruit Box'	8.45 fl oz	150	0	37	10	0	0.0	0
strawberry-flavored	8.45 fl oz	120	0	32	10	0	0.0	0
(10-K)								
apple	8 fl oz	60	0	15	55	0	0.0	0
fruit punch	8 fl oz	60	0	15	55	0	0.0	0
grape, 'Clear'	8 fl oz	60	0	15	55	0	0.0	0
lemonade, pink	8 fl oz	60	0	15	55	0	0.0	0
lemon-lime	8 fl oz	60	0	15	55	0	0.0	0
orange	8 fl oz	60	0	15	55	0	0.0	0
strawberry	8 fl oz	60	0	15	55	0	0.0	0
(Thick & Easy)								
apple, honey consistency	1/2 cup	70	0	17	30	0	0.0	0
cranberry, honey consistency	1/2 cup	70	0	17	20	0	0.0	0
cranberry, nectar consistency	1/2 cup	60	0	15	20	0	0.0	0
orange, honey consistency	1/2 cup	60	0	16	25	0	0.0	0
orange, nectar consistency	1/2 cup	60	0	15	25	0	0.0	0
(Tree Top) fruit punch, 100%	8 fl oz	119	0	30	24	0	0.0	0
(Tropicana)								
apple, 'Single Serve'	10 fl oz	175	0	43	3	0	0.0	0
berry, 'Berries & Berries'	6 fl oz	90	1	23	20	0	1.0	0
cranberry raspberry, w/strawberry	8 fl oz	120	0	31	5	na	0.0	0
cranberry raspberry, w/strawberry, light	8 fl oz	45	0	11	10	na	0.0	0
fruit punch, 'Single Serve'	10 fl oz	148	0	37	3	0	0.0	0
grape	6 fl oz	90	1	22	10	0	1.0	0
lemonade, 'Single Serve'	8 fl oz	120	0	30	3	0	0.0	0
orange, 'Single Serve'	10 fl oz	132	0	33	3	0	0.0	0
pineapple, w/grapefruit	6 fl oz	100	1	24	10	0	1.0	0
(Veryfine)								
fruit punch, '100% Juice Punch'	8 fl oz	122	1	30	10	0	0.0	0
grape	8 fl oz	130	0	34	10	0	0.0	0
guava-strawberry, 'Refresher'	8 fl oz	120	0	30	25	0	0.0	0
lemonade	8 fl oz	120	0	30	25	0	0.0	0
lemon-lime	8 fl oz	120	0	30	10	0	0.0	0
orange	8 fl oz	130	1	33	70	0	0.0	0
papaya punch	8 fl oz	120	1	30	10	0	0.0	0
pineapple-orange	8 fl oz	130	0	32	10	0	0.0	0

Food Name	Serv. Size	Total Cal.	Prot. gms	Carbs gms	Sod. mgs	Fiber gms	Fat gms	Chol. mgs
(Welch's)								
cranberry-apple cocktail, frozen, prepared .... 6 fl oz		120	0	30	0	0	0.0	0
cranberry-grape cocktail, frozen, prepared .... 6 fl oz		110	0	27	0	0	0.0	0
fruit punch cocktail, 'Orchard Fruit Harvest Punch' ..... 10 fl oz		180	0	45	0	0	0.0	0
raspberry cocktail, 'Orchard' *(Welch's)* .... 10 fl oz		160	0	40	10	0	0.0	0
(Wyler's)								
fruit punch, tropical, 'Fruit Slush' .... 4 fl oz		157	0	39	10	0	0.0	0
'Fruit Tea Punch' .... 12 fl oz		118	0	30	1	0	0.0	0
grape, 'Fruit Slush' .... 4 fl oz		157	0	39	10	0	0.0	0
lemonade .... 6 fl oz		64	0	17	33	0	0.0	0
lemonade, pink, 'Fruit Slush' .... 4 fl oz		157	0	39	10	0	0.0	0
orange, 'Fruit Slush' .... 4 fl oz		157	0	39	10	0	0.0	0
FRUIT DRINK MIX								
(Continental Mills) apple flavored, instant, powdered .... 1 pouch		83	0	21	0	na	0.0	na
(Country Time)								
lemonade, pink, sugar-free, w/vitamin C, mix only ... 1/8 cap/tub		5	0	2	0	na	0.0	na
lemonade, w/vitamin C, mix only .... 1/8 cap/tub		64	0	18	13	na	0.2	na
lemonade drink, pink, prepared .... 8 fl oz		80	0	20	20	0	0.0	0
lemonade drink, pink, sugar-free, prepared .... 8 fl oz		4	0	0	0	0	0.0	0
lemonade drink, pink, sugar-sweetened, prepared ...... 8 fl oz		80	0	20	20	0	0.0	0
lemonade drink, pink, w/NutraSweet, prepared .... 8 fl oz		4	0	0	0	0	0.0	0
lemonade drink, prepared .... 8 fl oz		80	0	20	20	0	0.0	0
lemonade punch, prepared .... 8 fl oz		80	0	20	15	0	0.0	0
lemonade punch, sugar-sweetened, prepared .... 8 fl oz		80	0	20	15	0	0.0	0
(Crystal Light)								
berry blend, sugar-free, prepared .... 8 fl oz		4	0	0	0	0	0.0	0
cherry, cranberry, low-calorie, sugarless .... 1/8 pkt		5	0	0	0	0	0.0	0
fruit punch, sugar-free, prepared .... 8 fl oz		4	0	0	0	0	0.0	0
lemonade drink, low-calorie, prepared .... 8 fl oz		5	0	0	20	0	0.0	0
lemonade drink, mix only .... 1 serving		5	0	0	0	0	0.0	0
lemonade drink, sugar-free, prepared .... 8 fl oz		4	0	0	0	0	0.0	0
lemonade drink, w/NutraSweet, prepared .... 8 fl oz		4	0	0	0	0	0.0	0
lemon-lime, mix only .... 1 serving		5	0	0	0	0	0.0	0
lemon-lime, sugar-free, prepared .... 8 fl oz		4	0	0	0	0	0.0	0
(Finast)								
cherry, prepared .... 8 fl oz		80	0	21	15	0	0.0	0
grape, prepared .... 8 fl oz		80	0	21	15	0	0.0	0
lemonade drink, prepared .... 8 fl oz		80	0	20	15	0	0.0	0
orange, breakfast, prepared .... 8 fl oz		80	0	20	15	0	0.0	0
(Kool-Aid)								
berry blend, sugar-free, w/NutraSweet, mix, prepared ... 8 fl oz		4	0	0	5	0	0.0	0
berry blue, mix, prepared w/sugar .... 8 fl oz		100	0	25	0	0	0.0	0
berry blue, mix, sugar-sweetened, prepared .... 8 fl oz		80	0	21	5	0	0.0	0
berry blue, mix, unsweetened, preparedd .... 8 fl oz		2	0	0	0	0	0.0	0
black cherry, prepared w/sugar .... 8 fl oz		100	0	25	0	0	0.0	0
black cherry, unsweetened, prepared .... 8 fl oz		2	0	0	0	0	0.0	0
cherry, sugar-free, prepared .... 8 fl oz		4	0	0	0	0	0.0	0
cherry, sugar-sweetened, prepared .... 8 fl oz		80	0	20	0	0	0.0	0
cherry, unsweetened, prepared .... 8 fl oz		2	0	0	0	0	0.0	0
cherry, w/aspartame and vitamin C, sugarless .... 1/8 envelope		3	0	1	5	na	0.0	na
grape, sugar-free, prepared .... 8 fl oz		4	0	0	0	0	0.0	0
grape, sugar-sweetened .... 8 fl oz		80	0	20	25	0.0	0	
grape, unsweetened .... 8 fl oz		2	0	0	0	0	0.0	0
'Great Bluedini' prepared w/sugar .... 8 fl oz		100	0	25	0	0	0.0	0
'Great Bluedini' sugar-free, prepared .... 8 fl oz		4	0	0	0	0	0.0	0
'Great Bluedini' unsweetened, prepared .... 8 fl oz		2	0	0	0	0	0.0	0
'Incrediberry' sugar-free, mix only .... 1/8 envelope		5	0	0	0	0	0.0	0

Food Name	Serv. Size	Total Cal.	Prot. gms	Carbs gms	Sod. mgs	Fiber gms	Fat gms	Chol. mgs
lemonade drink, pink, prepared w/sugar	8 fl oz	100	0	25	0	0	0.0	0
lemonade drink, pink, unsweetened, prepared	8 fl oz	2	0	0	0	0	0.0	0
lemonade drink, w/NutraSweet, prepared	8 fl oz	4	0	0	0	0	0.0	0
lemonade drink, sugar-sweetened, prepared	8 fl oz	80	0	20	0	0	0.0	0
lemon-lime, prepared w/sugar	8 fl oz	100	0	25	0	0	0.0	0
lemon-lime, unsweetened, prepared	8 fl oz	2	0	0	0	0	0.0	0
mountain berry punch, prepared w/sugar	8 fl oz	100	0	25	15	0	0.0	0
mountain berry punch, sugar-free, prepared	8 fl oz	4	0	0	35	0	0.0	0
mountain berry punch, sugar-sweetened, prepared	8 fl oz	80	0	20	15	0	0.0	0
mountain berry punch, unsweetened, prepared	8 fl oz	2	0	0	15	0	0.0	0
orange, prepared w/sugar	8 fl oz	100	0	25	0	0	0.0	0
orange, sugar-free, prepared	8 fl oz	4	0	0	0	0	0.0	0
orange, sugar-sweetened, prepared	8 fl oz	80	0	20	0	0	0.0	0
orange, unsweetened, prepared	8 fl oz	2	0	0	0	0	0.0	0
'Purplesaurus Rex' prepared w/sugar	8 fl oz	100	0	25	5	0	0.0	0
'Purplesaurus Rex' sugar-free, prepared	8 fl oz	4	0	0	5	0	0.0	0
'Purplesaurus Rex' unsweetened, prepared	8 fl oz	2	0	0	5	0	0.0	0
rainbow punch, prepared w/sugar	8 fl oz	100	0	25	0	0	0.0	0
rainbow punch, sugar-sweetened, prepared	8 fl oz	80	0	21	20	0	0.0	0
rainbow punch, unsweetened, prepared	8 fl oz	2	0	0	0	0	0.0	0
raspberry punch, prepared w/sugar	8 fl oz	100	0	25	25	0	0.0	0
raspberry punch, sugar-sweetened, prepared	8 fl oz	80	0	20	25	0	0.0	0
raspberry punch, unsweetened, prepared	8 fl oz	2	0	0	25	0	0.0	0
'Rock-A-Dile Red' prepared w/sugar	8 fl oz	100	0	25	0	0	0.0	0
'Rock-A-Dile Red' sugar-free, prepared	8 fl oz	4	0	0	0	0	0.0	0
'Rock-A-Dile Red' unsweetened, prepared	8 fl oz	2	0	0	0	0	0.0	0
'Sharkleberry Fin' prepared w/sugar	8 fl oz	100	0	25	0	0	0.0	0
'Sharkleberry Fin' sugar-free, prepared	8 fl oz	4	0	0	0	0	0.0	0
'Sharkleberry Fin' sugar-sweetened, prepared	8 fl oz	80	0	21	0	0	0.0	0
'Sharkleberry Fin' unsweetened, prepared	8 fl oz	2	0	0	0	0	0.0	0
strawberry punch, prepared w/sugar	8 fl oz	100	0	25	25	0	0.0	0
strawberry punch, sugar-sweetened, prepared	8 fl oz	80	0	20	0	0	0.0	0
strawberry punch, unsweetened, prepared	8 fl oz	2	0	0	25	0	0.0	0
strawberry-flavored, prepared	8 fl oz	100	0	25	25	0	0.0	0
strawberry-flavored, presweetened, prepared	8 fl oz	80	0	20	0	0	0.0	0
'Surfin' Berry' prepared w/sugar	8 fl oz	100	0	25	25	0	0.0	0
'Surfin' Berry' sugar-free, prepared	8 fl oz	4	0	0	10	0	0.0	0
'Surfin' Berry' unsweetened, prepared	8 fl oz	2	0	0	25	0	0.0	0
tropical punch, sugar-sweetened, mix only	1 serving	64	0	16	2	0	0.0	0
tropical punch, sugar-sweetened, prepared	8 fl oz	80	0	21	0	0	0.0	0
tropical punch, unsweetened, mix only	1 serving	1	0	0	15	0	0.0	0
tropical punch, unsweetened, prepared	8 fl oz	2	0	0	0	0	0.0	0
(Kroger)								
lemonade drink, light, diet, 15% vitamin C, mix only	1/8 pkt	5	0	1	0	0	0.0	0
lemonade drink, sugar, 10% vitamin C, no preservatives, mix only	1 1/2 tbsp	65	0	16	40	0	0.0	0
lemon-lime, light, diet, 15% vitamin C	1/8 pkt	6	0	2	0	0	0.0	0
(Minute Maid)								
grape punch, chilled	6 fl oz	90	0	23	20	0	0.0	0
grape punch, frozen concentrate, prepared	6 fl oz	90	0	23	0	0	0.0	0
(Nestlé)								
strawberry-flavored, 'Quik' mix only	0.75 oz	80	0	21	0	0	0.0	0
strawberry-flavored, 'Quik' prepared w/skim milk	8 fl oz	160	8	32	125	0	0.0	0
strawberry-flavored, 'Quik' prepared wwhole milk	8 fl oz	220	8	32	120	0	8.0	0
(Pathmark)								
cherry, 'No Frills' prepared	8 fl oz	90	0	22	65	0	0.0	0
fruit punch, 'No Frills' prepared	8 fl oz	90	0	22	85	0	0.0	0

Food Name	Serv. Size	Total Cal.	Prot. gms	Carbs gms	Sod. mgs	Fiber gms	Fat gms	Chol. mgs
grape, 'No Frills Sodium-free' prepared	6 fl oz	80	0	22	0	0	0.0	0
grape, 'No Frills' prepared	8 fl oz	90	0	22	20	0	0.0	0
lemon, 'No Frills' prepared	8 fl oz	90	0	20	55	0	0.0	0
orange, breakfast, 'No Frills' prepared	4 fl oz	60	0	15	0	0	0.0	0
mango flavor, prepared	6 fl oz	80	0	20	0	0	0.0	0
(Tang)								
orange, mix only	2 tbsp	100	0	24	0	0	0.0	0
orange, prepared	8 fl oz	90	0	23	0	0	0.0	0
orange, sugar-free, 'Breakfast Beverage Crystals'								
prepared	6 fl oz	6	0	1	0	0	0.0	0
orange, sugar-free, prepared	6 fl oz	6	0	1	0	0	0.0	0
orange-flavored, mix only	2 tbsp	92	0	25	2	0	0.0	0
orange-flavored, prepared	8 fl oz	92	0	25	2	0	0.0	0
orange-flavored, sugarless, prepared	8 fl oz	5	0	2	2	0	0.0	0
orange, 'Breakfast Beverage Crystals' prepared	6 fl oz	90	0	22	0	0	0.0	0
(Welch's) grape, frozen concentrate, 'Welchade'	2 fl oz	130	0	31	10	0	0.0	0
(Wyler's)								
cherry, 'Fruit Slush' prepared	4 fl oz	157	0	39	10	0	0.0	0
fruit punch, tropical, 'Crystals' prepared	8 fl oz	85	0	21	18	0	0.1	0
lemonade drink, 'Crystals' prepared	8 fl oz	92	0	20	44	0	1.5	0
strawberry-flavored, 'Crystals' prepared	8 fl oz	85	0	21	43	0	0.3	0
FRUIT JUICE BLEND. See also CIDER; FRUIT DRINK; FRUIT JUICE DRINK.								
AMBROSIA *(Knudsen)*	8 fl oz	110	1	27	0	0	0.0	0
APPLE APRICOT *(Knudsen)*	8 fl oz	120	0	30	35	na	0.0	0
APPLE BANANA *(Knudsen)*	8 fl oz	120	0	30	25	na	0.0	0
APPLE BLACKBERRY								
(Knudsen)	8 fl oz	100	1	24	0	0	0.0	0
organic *(Santa Cruz Natural)*	8 fl oz	120	1	29	0	0	1.0	0
APPLE BOYSENBERRY								
organic *(Santa Cruz Natural)*	8 fl oz	120	1	29	0	0	1.0	0
(Knudsen)	8 fl oz	120	0	30	25	na	0.0	0
APPLE CARROT 100% pure juice *(Vruit)*	8.45 fl oz	120	1	28	60	na	0.0	na
APPLE CHERRY								
'Breakfast Cocktail' *(Musselman's)*	6 fl oz	100	1	26	5	0	0.0	0
'Naturally 100%' *(Red Cheek)*	6 fl oz	113	0	28	11	0	0.0	0
100% juice 'Junior' *(McCain)*	4.2 fl oz	50	0	13	5	0	0.0	0
APPLE CITRUS, canned or frozen *(Tree Top)*	6 fl oz	90	1	22	10	0	0.0	0
APPLE CRANBERRY								
(Apple & Eve)	6 fl oz	80	0	19	5	0	0.0	0
(Knudsen)	8 fl oz	120	0	30	25	na	0.0	0
(Lucky Leaf)	6 fl oz	130	0	32	10	0	0.0	0
(Mott's)	6 fl oz	83	0	24	17	0	0.0	0
(Santa Cruz Natural) organic	8 fl oz	115	1	28	0	0	1.0	0
(Smucker's) 'Naturally 100%'	8 fl oz	120	0	32	10	0	0.0	0
(Tree Top) canned or frozen	6 fl oz	100	0	25	10	0	0.0	0
(Veryfine) cocktail	8 fl oz	130	0	33	10	0	0.0	0
APPLE CRANBERRY RASPBERRY *(Ultra Slim Fast)*	8 fl oz	153	5	32	167	3	1.0	7
APPLE GRAPE CHERRY								
(Welch's) frozen, 'Orchard Cocktail'	6 fl oz	90	0	22	10	0	0.0	0
(Welch's) 'Orchard Cocktails-In-A-Box'	8.45 fl oz	150	0	38	20	0	0.0	0
APPLE GRAPE								
(Juicy Juice)	6 fl oz	90	0	22	10	0	0.0	0
(Mott's)	6 fl oz	86	0	23	17	0	0.0	0
(Musselman's) 'Breakfast Cocktail'	6 fl oz	110	0	28	5	0	0.0	0
(Red Cheek)	6 fl oz	109	0	27	9	0	0.0	0
(Tree Top) 100%	8 fl oz	130	0	32	30	0	0.0	0
(Welch's) 'Orchard Cocktail'	6 fl oz	110	0	27	20	0	0.0	0

Food Name	Serv. Size	Total Cal.	Prot. gms	Carbs gms	Sod. mgs	Fiber gms	Fat gms	Chol. mgs
APPLE GRAPE RASPBERRY								
(Welch's) 'Orchard Cocktail' frozen, prepared	6 fl oz	90	0	22	10	0	0.0	0
(Welch's) 'Orchard Cocktails-In-A-Box'	8.45 fl oz	140	0	35	20	0	0.0	0
APPLE ORANGE PINEAPPLE								
(Welch's) 'Orchard Tropical Cocktails'	6 fl oz	100	0	25	20	0	0.0	0
APPLE PEACH *(Knudsen)*	8 fl oz	120	0	30	25	na	0.0	0
APPLE PEAR *(Tree Top)* 100%	8 fl oz	120	0	29	25	0	0.0	0
APPLE RASPBERRY								
(Knudsen)	8 fl oz	120	0	30	25	na	0.0	0
(Mott's)	6 fl oz	83	0	22	48	0	0.0	0
(Red Cheek)	6 fl oz	113	0	28	8	0	0.0	0
(Santa Cruz Natural) organic	8 fl oz	120	1	29	0	0	1.0	0
(Tree Top) 100%	8 fl oz	116	0	28	22	0	0.0	0
(Veryfine) cocktail	8 fl oz	110	0	27	15	0	0.0	0
APPLE STRAWBERRY								
(Knudsen)	8 fl oz	120	0	30	25	na	0.0	0
(Santa Cruz Natural) organic	8 fl oz	120	1	29	0	0	1.0	0
APPLE WHITE GRAPE								
(Welch's) cocktail, frozen 'No Sugar Added'	6 fl oz	40	0	10	5	0	0.0	0
BERRY								
(Juicy Juice) bottled	6 fl oz	90	1	22	10	0	0.0	0
CRANBERRY BLUEBERRY								
(Knudsen)	8 fl oz	115	1	36	0	0	0.0	0
CRANBERRY RASPBERRY								
(Knudsen)	8 fl oz	140	0	36	35	na	0.0	0
(Welch's) light, frozen, prepared	6 fl oz	40	0	10	0	0	0.0	0
GRAPE *(Juicy Juice)* juice blend	6 fl oz	100	0	25	5	0	0.0	0
GUAVA CRANBERRY								
(Santa Cruz Natural) organic 'Cruz'	8 fl oz	130	1	30	0	0	1.0	0
HIBISCUS CRANBERRY *(Knudsen)*	8 fl oz	120	0	30	35	na	0.0	0
LEMON GINGER *(Santa Cruz Natural)* organic 'Cruz'	8 fl oz	125	1	29	0	0	1.0	0
MANGO PEACH *(Knudsen)*	8 fl oz	120	0	30	50	na	0.0	0
ORANGE *(Minute Maid)* blend, 'Juices To Go'	6 fl oz	90	1	22	20	0	0.0	0
ORANGE APRICOT *(Musselman's)* 'Breakfast Cocktail'	6 fl oz	90	0	21	20	0	0.0	0
ORANGE BANANA *(Smucker's)* 'Naturally 100%'	8 fl oz	120	0	30	10	0	0.0	0
ORANGE CRANBERRY *(Santa Cruz Natural)*								
organic 'Cruz'	8 fl oz	125	1	29	0	0	1.0	0
ORANGE GRAPEFRUIT								
(Kraft) chilled, 'Pure 100%'	6 fl oz	80	1	19	0	0	0.0	0
(Tropicana) ruby red, 'Pure Premium'	8 fl oz	120	1	28	0	1	0.0	na
ORANGE KIWI PASSIONFRUIT								
(Tropicana) 100% pure	6 fl oz	80	1	17	35	0	1.0	0
(Tropicana) 'Pure Premium'	8 fl oz	100	1	26	15	1	0.0	na
ORANGE MANGO								
(Knudsen)	8 fl oz	120	0	30	50	na	0.0	0
(Tropicana) 'Twister'	6 fl oz	90	1	21	45	0	1.0	0
ORANGE PASSIONFRUIT *(Tropicana)* 'Twister'	6 fl oz	80	1	19	35	0	1.0	0
ORANGE PEACH *(Tropicana Twister)*	8 fl oz	120	0	31	20	na	0.0	0
ORANGE PEACH MANGO								
(Tropicana) 100% pure	6 fl oz	80	1	19	20	0	1.0	0
(Tropicana) 'Pure Premium'	8 fl oz	110	1	28	15	1	0.0	na
ORANGE PINEAPPLE								
(Kraft) 'Pure 100%'	6 fl oz	80	1	19	0	0	0.0	0
(Musselman's) 'Breakfast Cocktail'	6 fl oz	90	1	23	15	0	0.0	0
(Tropicana) 100% pure	6 fl oz	80	1	19	15	0	1.0	0
(Tropicana) 'Pure Premium'	8 fl oz	110	1	27	15	1	0.0	na
(Ultra Slim-Fast)	8 fl oz	153	5	33	181	3	1.0	7

Food Name	Serv. Size	Total Cal.	Prot. gms	Carbs gms	Sod. mgs	Fiber gms	Fat gms	Chol. mgs
ORANGE STRAWBERRY BANANA								
(Tropicana) 100% pure	6 fl oz	80	1	18	25	0	1.0	0
(Ultra Slim-Fast)	8 fl oz	153	5	33	167	3	1.0	7
PAPAYA LIME (Knudsen)	8 fl oz	115	1	29	0	0	0.0	0
PASSIONFRUIT RASPBERRY (Knudsen)	8 fl oz	130	1	32	0	0	0.0	0
PINEAPPLE COCONUT (Knudsen)	8 fl oz	130	0	32	50	na	0.0	0
PINEAPPLE GRAPEFRUIT								
(Dole) frozen, prepared	6 fl oz	90	1	22	10	0	0.0	0
(Dole) w/pink grapefruit	6 fl oz	101	0	25	0	0	0.1	0
PINEAPPLE ORANGE								
(Dole)	6 fl oz	90	0	22	10	0	0.0	0
(Dole) w/banana	6 fl oz	100	0	23	10	0	0.0	0
(Dole) w/guava	6 fl oz	100	1	21	10	0	0.0	0
(Minute Maid)	6 fl oz	90	1	23	0	0	0.0	0
PINEAPPLE PASSIONFRUIT (Dole) w/banana	6 fl oz	100	1	21	10	0	0.0	0
RASPBERRY								
(Apple & Eve) w/cranberry	6 fl oz	90	0	21	10	0	0.0	0
(Dole) blend, 'Pure & Light Country Raspberry'	6 fl oz	87	0	24	15	0	0.2	0
(Knudsen) blend, 'Razzleberry'	8 fl oz	90	1	21	0	0	0.0	0
RASPBERRY PEACH (Knudsen)	8 fl oz	120	0	31	25	na	0.0	0
STRAWBERRY BANANA (Knudsen)	8 fl oz	120	0	30	25	na	0.0	0
STRAWBERRY GUAVA (Knudsen)	8 fl oz	105	1	26	0	0	0.0	0
TOMATO-BEEF COCKTAIL (Beefamato)	6 fl oz	80	1	19	240	0	0.0	0
TOMATO-CHILE COCKTAIL (Snap-E-Tom)	6 fl oz	40	2	8	500	1	0.0	0
TOMATO-CLAM COCKTAIL (Clamato)	6 fl oz	96	1	23	815	0	0.0	0
FRUIT JUICE DRINK								
(A&P)								
cranberry juice cocktail, bottled	6 fl oz	100	1	26	0	0	1.0	0
(Capri Sun)								
fruit punch	1 serving	100	0	26	20	0	0.0	0
'Pacific Cooler'	1 serving	100	0	26	20	0	0.0	0
Maui punch	1 serving	100	0	27	20	0	0.0	0
wild cherry	1 serving	110	0	30	20	0	0.0	0
(Citrus Hill)								
grapefruit, 'Plus Calcium'	6 fl oz	70	1	19	10	0	1.0	0
orange, 'Lite Premium'	6 fl oz	60	1	14	10	0	1.0	0
(Clinical Resource)								
orange	8 fl oz	180	9	36	70	na	0.0	0
peach	8 fl oz	180	9	36	70	na	0.0	0
wild berry	8 fl oz	180	9	36	70	na	0.0	0
(Del Monte) apricot nectar	6 fl oz	100	1	26	10	0	0.0	0
(Hi-C)								
cherry	8.45 fl oz	141	0	35	24	0	0.1	0
grape	6 fl oz	96	0	24	17	0	0.1	0
(IGA) pink grapefruit	6 fl oz	80	0	20	15	0	0.0	0
(J. Hungerford)								
cranberry juice cocktail	9.03 fl oz	141	1	36	0	0	0.0	0
cranberry juice cocktail, 50% juice	9.03 fl oz	134	0	35	7	0	0.1	0
fruit punch, 50% juice	9.03 fl oz	107	0	27	7	0	0.0	0
fruit punch, 100% juice	9.03 fl oz	116	1	30	11	0	0.0	0
grape, 50% juice	9.03 fl oz	135	0	34	0	0	0.0	0
grapefruit, 50% juice	9.03 fl oz	109	1	27	0	0	0.0	0
pineapple, 50% juice	9.03 fl oz	123	0	31	0	0	0.0	0
(Kern's)								
guava nectar	11.5 fl oz	216	0	55	7	0	0.0	0
mango nectar	11.5 fl oz	216	0	52	7	52	0.0	0
mango-orange nectar	8 fl oz	140	0	35	10	0	0.0	0

Food Name	Serv. Size	Total Cal.	Prot. gms	Carbs gms	Sod. mgs	Fiber gms	Fat gms	Chol. mgs
orange-banana nectar	6 fl oz	110	1	25	0	0	0.0	0
orange-guava nectar	8 fl oz	150	0	36	10	0	0.0	0
papaya nectar	11.5 fl oz	210	1	51	10	0	0.0	0
peach nectar	11.5 fl oz	210	1	52	5	0	0.0	0
peach-passionfruit nectar	11.5 fl oz	220	1	53	5	2	0.0	0
pear nectar	11.5 fl oz	220	0	54	5	3	0.0	0
pineapple-orange-passionfruit nectar	8 fl oz	146	2	33	7	0	0.0	0
strawberry nectar	6 fl oz	110	0	28	0	0	0.0	0
strawberry-banana nectar	8 fl oz	150	0	36	5	0	0.0	0
tropical nectar	11.5 fl oz	210	3	48	10	0	0.0	0
(Knudsen)								
breakfast juice, natural	8 fl oz	110	1	27	35	na	0.0	0
breakfast juice, natural, concentrate, prepared	8 fl oz	110	1	27	35	na	0.0	0
kiwi nectar	8 fl oz	60	1	14	0	0	0.0	0
orange juice float	8 fl oz	140	1	33	60	na	0.0	0
papaya nectar	8 fl oz	130	0	34	35	na	0.0	0
peach nectar	8 fl oz	120	0	30	25	na	0.0	0
pineapple juice float	8 fl oz	130	2	31	0	0	0.0	0
raspberry nectar, concentrate, prepared	8 fl oz	120	0	30	25	na	0.0	0
red raspberry nectar	8 fl oz	120	1	30	0	0	0.0	0
strawberry juice float	8 fl oz	130	2	32	0	0	0.0	0
strawberry nectar	8 fl oz	120	0	30	25	na	0.0	0
(Kool-Aid) orange, 'Koolers'	8.45 fl oz	110	0	30	10	0	0.0	0
(Libby's)								
guanabana nectar	8 fl oz	147	0	35	17	0	0.0	0
guava nectar	8 fl oz	153	0	38	7	0	0.0	0
mango nectar	6 fl oz	110	0	26	0	0	0.0	0
papaya nectar	6 fl oz	110	0	28	10	0	0.0	0
peach nectar	6 fl oz	100	0	24	5	0	0.0	0
pineapple nectar	6 fl oz	110	0	27	30	0	0.0	0
strawberry nectar	6 fl oz	110	0	27	0	0	0.0	0
(Minute Maid) pink grapefruit, 'Juices To Go'	6 fl oz	80	0	20	20	0	0.0	0
(Mott's) orange	10 fl oz	144	1	35	6	0	0.0	0
(Musselman's) w/grapefruit juice, 'Breakfast Cocktail'	6 fl oz	90	1	22	20	0	0.0	0
(Ocean Spray)								
cranberry juice cocktail, bottled	6 fl oz	110	0	26	10	0	0.0	0
cranberry juice cocktail, bottled, 'Low-calorie'	6 fl oz	40	0	9	15	0	0.0	0
cranberry juice drink, citrus, 'Refreshers'	6 fl oz	100	0	26	15	0	0.0	0
pink grapefruit	6 fl oz	80	0	20	15	0	0.0	0
orange juice cocktail	6 fl oz	100	0	25	15	0	0.0	0
pineapple cocktail, w/grapefruit juice	6 fl oz	110	0	26	5	0	0.0	0
(Orange Julius) orange	16 fl oz	265	1	66	15	0	1.0	0
(P&Q) cranberry juice cocktail, bottled	6 fl oz	100	1	24	0	0	1.0	0
(Pathmark)								
cranberry juice cocktail, bottled, 'No Frills'	6 fl oz	100	0	26	10	0	0.0	0
pink grapefruit	6 fl oz	80	0	20	15	0	0.0	0
(Santa Cruz Natural)								
papaya nectar, certified organic	8 fl oz	110	1	28	35	0	0.0	0
red raspberry nectar, certified organic	8 fl oz	100	1	26	35	0	0.0	0
strawberry-guava nectar, certified organic	8 fl oz	100	1	24	25	0	0.0	0
(Snapple)								
'Apple Crisp' *(Snapple)*	10 fl oz	140	0	36	30	0	0.0	0
'Cranberry Royale'	10 fl oz	150	0	37	25	0	0.0	0
'Passion Supreme'	10 fl oz	160	0	39	20	0	0.0	0
(Sunkist)								
cranberry juice cocktail, bottled	6 fl oz	110	0	28	8	0	0.1	0
cranberry juice cocktail, frozen, prepared	6 fl oz	110	0	28	0	0	0.1	0

Food Name	Serv. Size	Total Cal.	Prot. gms	Carbs gms	Sod. mgs	Fiber gms	Fat gms	Chol. mgs
grape, frozen, prepared	6 fl oz	69	0	17	3	0	0.1	0
(Tang)								
cherry, 'Fruit Box'	8.45 fl oz	130	0	34	10	0	0.0	0
grape, 'Fruit Box'	8.45 fl oz	130	0	34	10	0	0.0	0
mixed fruit, 'Fruit Box'	8.45 fl oz	140	0	36	10	0	0.0	0
orange, 'Fruit Box'	8.45 fl oz	130	0	32	10	0	0.0	0
strawberry, 'Fruit Box'	8.45 fl oz	120	0	32	10	0	0.0	0
(TreeSweet) pink grapefruit 'Lite'	6 fl oz	40	1	10	15	0	0.0	0
(Tropic Isle) fruit punch, vitamin-enriched	6 fl oz	90	0	22	5	0	0.0	0
(Tropicana)								
apple raspberry blackberry drink, 'Twister'	8 fl oz	130	0	31	20	na	0.0	0
cranberry juice drink, 'Season's Best' 'Medley'	10 fl oz	140	1	35	30	1	0.0	na
cranberry juice drink, 'Season's Best' 'Medley'	8 fl oz	120	1	29	20	1	0.0	na
'Cranberry Orchard Juice Sparkler'	8 fl oz	120	0	30	20	0	0.0	0
grapefruit, 'Juice Sparkler'	8 fl oz	110	0	26	50	0	0.0	0
pink grapefruit, 'Twister'	8 fl oz	110	0	28	1	0	0.0	0
grapefruit, ruby red w/cranberry, 'Twister'	8 fl oz	120	0	30	20	na	0.0	na
Mandarin orange-papaya, 'Twister'	6 fl oz	90	1	21	30	0	1.0	0
orange-cranberry, 'Twister'	8 fl oz	130	0	32	45	na	0.0	0
orange-cranberry, light, 'Twister'	8 fl oz	30	0	7	20	na	0.0	0
orange-raspberry, 'Twister'	6 fl oz	80	1	20	30	0	1.0	0
orange-raspberry, light, 'Twister'	8 fl oz	35	0	9	20	na	0.0	0
orange-strawberry-banana, 'Twister'	8 fl oz	130	0	32	45	na	0.0	0
orange-strawberry-banana, light, 'Twister'	8 fl oz	35	1	9	20	na	0.0	0
orange-strawberry-guava, 'Twister'	8 fl oz	120	0	29	20	na	0.0	0
pineapple, w/grapefruit juice, 'Twister'	8 fl oz	125	0	32	2	0	0.0	0
pineapple-grapefruit, 'Twister'	8 fl oz	120	0	29	20	na	0.0	0
pineapple-grapefruit, light, 'Twister'	8 fl oz	35	0	9	20	na	0.0	0
'Season's Best' 'Medley'	8 fl oz	130	1	32	25	1	0.0	na
wild berry, 'Juice Sparkler'	8 fl oz	110	0	27	15	0	0.0	0
(Veryfine)								
apple cherry berry	8 fl oz	130	0	33	25	0	0.0	0
cranberry juice cocktail, bottled	8 fl oz	160	1	40	10	0	0.0	0
'Passionfruit Refresher' w/orange, tropical	8 fl oz	110	1	26	25	0	0.0	0
pink grapefruit	8 fl oz	120	1	29	15	0	0.0	0
(Welch's)								
cranberry juice cocktail, frozen, diluted as directed	6 fl oz	100	0	26	0	0	0.0	0
cranberry juice cocktail, no sugar added, frozen, prepared	6 fl oz	40	0	10	5	0	0.0	0
cranberry juice cocktail, w/raspberry, frozen, prepared	6 fl oz	110	0	28	0	0	0.0	0
cranberry juice cocktail, w/blueberry, frozen, prepared	6 fl oz	110	0	27	0	0	0.0	0
cranberry juice cocktail, lite, frozen, prepared	6 fl oz	40	0	10	20	0	0.0	0
grape juice cocktail, no sugar added, frozen concentrate, prepared	6 fl oz	40	0	10	5	0	0.0	0
grape juice cocktail, 'Orchard Cocktails-In-A-Box'	8.45 fl oz	150	0	38	20	0	0.0	0
grape juice cocktail, 'Orchard'	6 fl oz	110	0	27	20	0	0.0	0
orange juice cocktail, 'Orchard'	10 fl oz	150	0	37	0	0	0.0	0
'Orchard Harvest Blend Cocktails-In-A-Box'	8.45 fl oz	150	0	38	20	0	0.0	0
'Orchard Harvest Blend' frozen, prepared	6 fl oz	110	0	27	10	0	0.0	0
passionfruit cocktail, 'Orchard Tropical Cocktails-In-A-Box'	8.45 fl oz	140	0	34	20	0	0.0	0
passionfruit cocktail, 'Orchard Tropicals' frozen, prepared	6 fl oz	100	0	25	20	0	0.0	0
pineapple cocktail, w/banana, 'Orchard Tropicals'	6 fl oz	100	0	24	20	0	0.0	0
pineapple cocktail, w/banana, 'Orchard Tropicals'	8.45 fl oz	140	0	34	20	0	0.0	0
(Wyler's)								
grapefruit, 'Fruit Slush'	4 fl oz	157	0	39	10	0	0.0	0

Food Name	Serv. Size	Total Cal.	Prot. gms	Carbs gms	Sod. mgs	Fiber gms	Fat gms	Chol. mgs
strawberry, 'Fruit Slush' .... 4 fl oz		157	0	39	10	0	0.0	0

FRUIT ROLL. See FRUIT SNACK.
FRUIT SNACK
(Betty Crocker)

Food Name	Serv. Size	Total Cal.	Prot. gms	Carbs gms	Sod. mgs	Fiber gms	Fat gms	Chol. mgs
all flavors, 'Berry Bears' .... 1 pouch		100	1	22	20	0	1.0	0
all flavors, 'Fruit Roll-Ups Peel-Outs' .... 1 roll		50	1	12	40	0	1.0	0
assorted flavors, 'Bugs Bunny & Friends' 1 pouch 90		1	21	30	0	1.0	0.0	9%
assorted flavors, 'Tasmanian Devil' .... 1 pouch		90	1	21	30	0	1.0	0
berry fruit roll-up, w/vitamin C .... 2 rolls		104	0	24	89	na	1.0	na
blueberry, 'Wild Blue' 'Garfield & Friends' .... 1 roll		50	1	12	20	0	1.0	0
cherry, 'Fruit by the Foot' .... 1 roll		80	1	17	45	0	2.0	0
cherry, 'Fruit Roll-Ups' .... 0.5 oz roll		50	1	12	40	0	1.0	0
crazy colors, 'Fruit Roll-Ups' .... 0.5 oz roll		50	1	12	40	0	1.0	0
grape, 'Fruit by the Foot' .... 1 roll		80	1	17	45	0	2.0	0
grape, 'Fruit Roll-Ups' .... 0.5 oz roll		50	1	12	40	0	1.0	0
grape, 'Gushin Grape Gushers' .... 1 pouch		90	1	21	45	0	1.0	0
raspberry, 'Fruit Roll-Ups' .... 0.5 oz roll		50	1	12	40	0	1.0	0
strawberry, 'Fruit by the Foot' .... 1 roll		80	1	17	45	0	2.0	0
strawberry, 'Fruit Roll-Ups' .... 0.5-oz roll		50	1	12	40	0	1.0	0
strawberry, 'Gushers' .... 1 pouch		90	1	21	45	0	1.0	0
wild cherry, 'Gushers' .... 1 pouch		90	1	21	40	0	1.0	0

(Farley)

Food Name	Serv. Size	Total Cal.	Prot. gms	Carbs gms	Sod. mgs	Fiber gms	Fat gms	Chol. mgs
assorted flavors, 'Dinosaurs' .... 1 oz		90	1	22	0	0	1.0	0
assorted flavors, 'Teenage Mutant Ninja Turtles' .... 1 oz		90	1	22	0	0	1.0	0
assorted flavors, 'Trolls' .... 1 oz		90	1	22	0	0	1.0	0
w/vitamins A, C, and E .... 1 pouch		89	1	21	9	na	0.0	na

(Flavor Tree)

Food Name	Serv. Size	Total Cal.	Prot. gms	Carbs gms	Sod. mgs	Fiber gms	Fat gms	Chol. mgs
apple roll .... 1 piece		75	0	19	17	0	0.0	0
apricot roll .... 1 piece		76	0	18	17	0	0.5	0
assorted flavors, 'Fruit Circus Fruit Bears' .... 1.05 oz		117	0	25	12	0	1.6	0
cherry roll .... 1 piece		75	0	18	18	0	0.1	0
grape roll .... 1 piece		76	0	19	13	0	0.1	0
raspberry roll .... 1 piece		75	0	18	20	0	0.1	0
strawberry roll .... 1 piece		74	0	18	11	0	0.1	0

(Fruit Parade)

Food Name	Serv. Size	Total Cal.	Prot. gms	Carbs gms	Sod. mgs	Fiber gms	Fat gms	Chol. mgs
assorted flavors, 'Chip 'N Dale Rescue Rangers' ...... 1 pouch		100	0	22	10	0	1.0	0
assorted flavors, 'Darkwing Duck' .... 1 pouch		100	0	22	10	0	1.0	0
assorted flavors, 'Tale Spin' .... 1 pouch		100	0	22	10	0	1.0	0
(Rokeach) compote .... 4 oz		120	1	31	4	0	1.0	0

(Stretch Island)

Food Name	Serv. Size	Total Cal.	Prot. gms	Carbs gms	Sod. mgs	Fiber gms	Fat gms	Chol. mgs
'Berry Blackberry' 100% fruit .... 1 oz		90	0	24	0	2	0.0	0
'Chunky Cherry' 100% fruit .... 1 oz		90	0	24	0	2	0.0	0
'Great Grape' 100% fruit .... 1 oz		90	0	24	0	2	0.0	0
'Rave Raspberry' 100% fruit .... 1 oz		90	0	24	0	2	0.0	0
apple, 100% fruit, 'Snappy Apple' .... 1 oz		90	0	25	0	2	0.0	0
apricot, 'Tangy Apricot' 100% fruit .... 1 oz		90	1	23	0	2	0.0	0

(Sunkist)

Food Name	Serv. Size	Total Cal.	Prot. gms	Carbs gms	Sod. mgs	Fiber gms	Fat gms	Chol. mgs
assorted flavors, 'Fun Fruits Fantastic Fruit' .... 1 pouch		100	0	22	10	0	1.4	0
assorted flavors, all shapes, 'Fun Fruits' .... 1 pouch		100	0	22	10	0	1.4	0
berry, 'Fun Fruits Berry Bunch' .... 1 pouch		100	0	22	10	0	1.4	0
cherry, 'Fun Fruits' .... 1 pouch		100	0	22	10	0	1.4	0
grape, 'Fun Fruits' .... 1 pouch		100	0	22	10	0	1.4	0
orange, 'Fun Fruits' .... 1 pouch		100	0	22	10	0	1.4	0
strawberry roll, w/vitamins A, C, and E .... 1 roll		72	0	17	23	2	0.2	na
strawberry, 'Fun Fruits' .... 1 pouch		100	0	22	10	0	1.4	0
strawberry, yogurt-coated, 'Creme Supremes' .... 1 pouch		114	0	20	19	0	3.6	0
(Sun-Maid) raisin, muscat, seeded .... 1/2 cup		270	2	67	25	0	1.0	0

Food Name	Serv. Size	Total Cal.	Prot. gms	Carbs gms	Sod. mgs	Fiber gms	Fat gms	Chol. mgs
(Weight Watchers)								
apple	1 pouch	50	1	13	75	0	1.0	0
apple chips	0.75 oz	70	0	19	110	0	0.0	0
cinnamon flavor	1 pouch	50	1	13	75	0	1.0	0
peach	0.5 oz	50	1	13	75	0	1.0	0
strawberry	1 pouch	50	1	13	75	0	1.0	0
FRUIT SPREAD. See also JAM AND PRESERVES.								
(Fifty 50)								
apple, no sugar added	1 tsp	2	0	1	5	0	0.0	0
grape, no sugar added	1 tsp	2	0	1	5	0	0.0	0
grape spread, no sugar added, contains phenylalanine	1 tbsp	10	0	3	10	0	0.0	0
orange marmalade, no sugar added	1 tsp	2	0	1	5	0	0.0	0
raspberry, no sugar added	1 tsp	2	0	1	5	0	0.0	0
strawberry, no sugar added	1 tsp	2	0	1	5	0	0.0	0
(Knott's Berry Farm)								
apricot-pineapple	1 tsp	16	0	4	0	0	0.0	0
apricot-pineapple, 'Light'	1 tsp	8	0	2	0	0	0.0	0
apricot-pineapple, portion pack	0.5 oz	35	0	9	0	0	0.0	0
blackberry	1 tsp	16	0	4	0	0	0.0	0
blackberry, 'Light'	1 tsp	8	0	2	0	0	0.0	0
blackberry, portion pack	0.5 oz	35	0	9	0	0	0.0	0
boysenberry	1 tsp	16	0	4	0	0	0.0	0
boysenberry, 'Light'	1 tsp	8	0	2	0	0	0.0	0
boysenberry, portion pack	0.5 oz	35	0	9	0	0	0.0	0
orange marmalade	1 tsp	16	0	4	0	0	0.0	0
orange marmalade, 'Light'	1 tsp	8	0	2	0	0	0.0	0
orange marmalade, portion pack	0.5 oz	35	0	9	0	0	0.0	0
red raspberry	1 tsp	16	0	4	0	0	0.0	0
red raspberry, 'Light'	1 tsp	8	0	2	0	0	0.0	0
red raspberry, portion pack	0.5 oz	35	0	9	0	0	0.0	0
strawberry, 'Light'	1 tsp	8	0	2	0	0	0.0	0
(Knudsen)								
calamansi, 'Tropical Rainforest'	2 tsp	35	0	8	0	0	0.0	0
guanabana, 'Tropical Rainforest'	2 tsp	35	0	8	0	0	0.0	0
(Polaner)								
apricot, 'All Fruit Spreadable Fruit'	1 tsp	14	0	4	0	0	0.0	0
black cherry, 'All Fruit Spreadable Fruit'	1 tsp	14	0	4	0	0	0.0	0
blueberry, 'All Fruit Spreadable Fruit'	1 tsp	14	0	4	0	0	0.0	0
grape, 'All Fruit Spreadable Fruit'	1 tsp	14	0	4	0	0	0.0	0
orange, 'All Fruit Spreadable Fruit'	1 tsp	14	0	4	0	0	0.0	0
raspberry, seedless, 'All Fruit Spreadable Fruit'	1 tsp	14	0	4	0	0	0.0	0
strawberry, 'All Fruit Spreadable Fruit'	1 tsp	14	0	4	0	0	0.0	0
(Smucker's)								
all flavors, 'Homestyle'	1 tsp	15	0	3	0	0	0.0	0
all flavors, 'Slenderella'	1 tsp	7	0	2	0	0	0.0	0
apricot, low-sugar	1 tsp	8	0	2	10	0	0.0	0
apricot, 'Simply Fruit'	1 tsp	16	0	4	0	0	0.0	0
black raspberry, 'Simply Fruit'	1 tsp	16	0	4	0	0	0.0	0
blackberry, low-sugar	1 tsp	8	0	2	10	0	0.0	0
blackberry, 'Simply Fruit'	1 tsp	16	0	4	0	0	0.0	0
blueberry, 'Simply Fruit'	1 tsp	16	0	4	0	0	0.0	0
boysenberry, low-sugar	1 tsp	8	0	2	10	0	0.0	0
concord grape, low-sugar	1 tsp	8	0	2	0	0	0.0	0
grape, 'Imitation'	1 tsp	2	0	1	2	0	0.0	0
grape, 'Simply Fruit'	1 tsp	16	0	4	0	0	0.0	0
orange marmalade, low-sugar	1 tsp	8	0	2	10	0	0.0	0
orange marmalade, 'Simply Fruit'	1 tsp	16	0	4	0	0	0.0	0

Food Name	Serv. Size	Total Cal.	Prot. gms	Carbs gms	Sod. mgs	Fiber gms	Fat gms	Chol. mgs
peach, 'Simply Fruit'	1 tsp	16	0	4	0	0	0.0	0
red raspberry, low-sugar	1 tsp	8	0	2	0	0	0.0	0
red raspberry, 'Simply Fruit'	1 tsp	16	0	4	0	0	0.0	0
strawberry, 'Imitation'	1 tsp	2	0	1	2	0	0.0	0
strawberry, low-sugar	1 tsp	8	0	2	0	0	0.0	0
strawberry, 'Simply Fruit'	1 tsp	16	0	4	0	0	0.0	0
(Weight Watchers)								
grape	1 tsp	8	0	2	0	0	0.0	0
raspberry	1 tsp	8	0	2	0	0	0.0	0
strawberry	1 tsp	8	0	2	0	0	0.0	0
FRUIT TOPPING, pourable, 'Fruit 'n Maple' *(Knudsen)*	1 oz	105	0	26	0	0	0.0	0
FUDGE. See under CANDY.								
FUDGE TOPPING. See also CHOCOLATE TOPPING.								
(Kraft) hot	2 tbsp	140	1	24	100	1	4.5	0
(Mrs. Richardson's)								
caramel, microwavable	2 tbsp	130	1	28	90	0	2.0	5
hot	2 tbsp	140	1	20	75	0	7.0	0
hot, microwaveable	2 tbsp	140	1	20	75	0	7.0	0
(Smucker's)								
	2 tbsp	130	1	31	50	0	1.0	0
hot	2 tbsp	110	1	18	55	0	4.0	0
hot, 'Light'	2 tbsp	70	2	19	35	0	0.0	0
hot, 'Special Recipe'	2 tbsp	150	2	23	60	0	5.0	0
'Magic Shell'	2 tbsp	190	1	16	50	0	15.0	0
FUKI. See BUTTERBUR.								

G

Food Name	Serv. Size	Total Cal.	Prot. gms	Carbs gms	Sod. mgs	Fiber gms	Fat gms	Chol. mgs
GARBANZO BEAN. See CHICKPEA.								
GARDEN CRESS								
boiled, drained	1 cup	31	3	5	11	1	0.8	0
boiled, drained	1/2 cup	16	1	3	5	0	0.4	0
raw	1 cup	16	1	3	7	1	0.3	0
GARLIC AND HERB SEASONING. See under SEASONING MIX.								
GARLIC								
Fresh								
raw, chopped	1 cup	203	9	45	23	3	0.7	0
raw, chopped	1 tsp	4	0	1	0	0	0.0	0
raw, whole	1 med clove	4	0	1	1	0	0.0	0
raw, whole	3 med cloves	13	1	3	2	0	0.0	0
Jarred								
crushed *Gilroy)*	1 tsp	8	0	2	4	0	0.0	0
dehydrated *(Basic American)*	1 oz	86	5	22	8	1	0.1	0
minced *(Gilroy)*	1 tsp	23	0	2	4	0	1.0	0
GARLIC BREAD. See under BREAD.								
GARLIC OIL *(Hain)*	1 tbsp	120	0	0	0	0	14.0	0
GARLIC POWDER								
	1 tbsp	28	1	6	2	1	0.1	0
	1 tsp	9	0	2	1	0	0.0	0
(Lawry's)	1/4 tsp	0	0	1	0	na	0.0	0
(McCormick/Schilling)	1 tsp	10	0	2	2	1	0.0	0
(Spice Islands)	1 tsp	5	0	1	1	0	0.0	0
(Tone's)	1 tsp	9	1	2	1	0	0.1	0
fresh ground *(Durkee)*	1 tsp	10	0	0	0	0	0.0	0

Food Name	Serv. Size	Total Cal.	Prot. gms	Carbs gms	Sod. mgs	Fiber gms	Fat gms	Chol. mgs
fresh ground *(Laurel Leaf)*	1 tsp	10	0	0	0	0	0.0	0
w/parsley *(Lawry's)*	1 tsp	12	1	2	5	0	0.9	0
GARLIC SALT. See under SEASONING MIX.								
GARLIC TABLETS *(Shaklee)*	2 tablets	5	0	1	0	0	0.0	0
GATORADE. See under SPORTS AND DIET/NUTRITION DRINKS.								
GEFILTE FISH								
(Mother's)								
in jelled broth, 'Old Fashioned' 24-oz jar	1 ball	70	9	5	0	0	1.0	0
in jelled broth, 'Old Fashioned' 12-oz jar	1 ball	54	7	4	0	0	0.8	0
in jelled broth, 'Old World'	1 ball	70	8	7	0	0	1.0	0
in jelled broth, 'Unsalted'	1 ball	45	5	2	0	0	1.0	0
in liquid, 'Old Fashioned' 24- or 31-oz jar	1 ball	70	9	7	0	0	1.0	0
in liquid, 'Old Fashioned' 12-oz'	1 ball	54	7	5	0	0	0.8	0
sweet, 'Old World'	1 ball	54	6	5	0	0	0.8	0
(Rokeach)								
hors d'oeuvres	8 balls	60	8	4	0	0	1.0	0
in jelled broth, 'Old Vienna' 31-oz jar	3 oz	81	9	9	0	0	1.0	0
in jelled broth, 'Old Vienna' 24-oz jar	2.6 oz	70	8	8	0	0	1.0	0
in jelled broth, 'Old Vienna' 12-oz jar	2 oz	54	6	6	0	0	1.0	0
in jelled broth, 'Redi-Jelled'	2 oz	46	6	3	222	0	1.0	0
in natural broth, 24-oz pkg	4 oz	60	8	4	835	0	1.0	0
WHITEFISH								
(Mother's)								
in jelled broth, 12-oz jar	1 ball	46	7	3	0	0	0.8	0
in liquid, 12-oz pkg	1 ball	54	7	5	0	0	0.8	0
WHITEFISH AND PIKE								
(Mother's)								
in jelled broth	1 ball	60	9	4	0	0	1.0	0
in jelled broth, 'Old World'	1 ball	54	6	5	0	0	0.8	0
in liquid	1 ball	70	9	7	0	0	1.0	0
(Rokeach) in jelled broth	2 oz	46	7	3	0	0	1.0	0
GELATIN, unflavored *(Knox)*	1 pkt	25	6	0	10	0	0.0	0
GELATIN DESSERT								
(Estee) all flavors	1/2 cup	8	1	1	0	0	0.0	0
(Jell-O)								
'Berry Blue'	3.5 oz	80	1	18	40	0	0.0	0
cherry	3.5 oz	80	1	18	40	0	0.0	0
cherry, sugar-free	1 snack	10	1	0	50	0	0.0	0
orange, sugar-free	1 snack	10	1	0	50	0	0.0	0
raspberry, sugar-free	1 snack	10	1	0	50	0	0.0	0
strawberry	3.5 oz	80	1	18	40	0	0.0	0
strawberry, sugar-free	1 snack	10	1	0	50	0	0.0	0
GELATIN DESSERT MIX								
(D-Zerta) all flavors, except strawberry, low-calorie, prepared	1/2 cup	8	2	0	0	0	0.0	0
(Featherweight) all flavors, except lemon, prepared	1/2 cup	10	2	1	5	0	0.0	0
APPLE *(Royal)* prepared	1/2 cup	80	2	19	95	0	0.0	0
BANANA *(Ener-G Foods)* low-fat, gluten free, prepared	1/2 cup	249	0	62	28	1	0.0	0
BLACK RASPBERRY *(Jell-O)* prepared	1/2 cup	80	2	19	35	0	0.0	0
BLACKBERRY *(Royal)* prepared	1/2 cup	80	2	19	95	0	0.0	0
CHERRY								
(Jell-O) sugar-free, prepared	1/2 cup	8	1	0	80	0	0.0	0
(Royal)								
prepared	1/2 cup	80	2	19	95	0	0.0	0
sugar-free, mix only	1 serving	8	1	1	90	0	0.0	0
CHOCOLATE *(Ener-G Foods)* prepared	1/2 cup	231	0	56	47	4	0.6	0

Food Name	Serv. Size	Total Cal.	Prot. gms	Carbs gms	Sod. mgs	Fiber gms	Fat gms	Chol. mgs
GRAPE								
(Jell-O) Concord, prepared	1/2 cup	80	2	19	35	0	0.0	0
(Royal) Concord, prepared	1/2 cup	80	2	19	130	0	0.0	0
LEMON								
(Ener-G Foods) prepared	1/2 cup	246	0	63	30	1	0.0	0
(Featherweight) prepared	1/2 cup	10	2	1	4	0	0.0	0
(Jell-O) sugar-free, prepared	1/2 cup	10	1	0	55	0	0.0	0
(Royal) prepared	1/2 cup	80	2	19	125	0	0.0	0
LEMON-LIME (Royal) prepared	1/2 cup	80	2	19	95	0	0.0	0
LIME								
(Jell-O) sugar-free, prepared	1/2 cup	8	1	0	65	0	0.0	0
(Royal)								
prepared	1/2 cup	80	2	19	125	0	0.0	0
sugar-free, mix only	1 serving	8	1	1	100	0	0.0	0
MIXED BERRY (Royal) prepared	1/2 cup	80	2	19	90	0	0.0	0
MIXED FRUIT								
(Jell-O) sugar-free, prepared	1/2 cup	10	1	0	50	0	0.0	0
(Royal) 'Fruit Punch' prepared	1/2 cup	80	2	19	90	0	0.0	0
ORANGE								
(Ener-G Foods) prepared	1/2 cup	242	0	60	46	1	0.0	0
(Jell-O) sugar-free, prepared	1/2 cup	8	1	0	55	0	0.0	0
(Royal)								
prepared	1/2 cup	80	2	19	95	0	0.0	0
sugar-free, mix only	1 serving	10	1	1	90	0	0.0	0
ORANGE-PINEAPPLE (Jell-O) prepared	1/2 cup	80	2	19	65	0	0.0	0
PEACH (Royal) prepared	1/2 cup	80	2	19	95	0	0.0	0
PINEAPPLE (Royal) mix only	1 serving	80	2	19	95	0	0.0	0
RASPBERRY								
(Ener-G Foods) low-fat, prepared	1/2 cup	248	0	62	29	1	0.0	0
(Jell-O) sugar-free, prepared	1/2 cup	8	1	0	55	0	0.0	0
(Royal)								
prepared	1/2 cup	80	2	19	125	0	0.0	0
sugar-free, mix only	1 serving	8	1	1	90	0	0.0	0
STRAWBERRY								
(D-Zerta) low-calorie, prepared	1/2 cup	10	1	0	55	0	0.0	0
(Jell-O) sugar-free, prepared	1/2 cup	10	1	0	55	0	0.0	0
(Royal)								
prepared	1/2 cup	80	2	19	105	0	0.0	0
sugar-free, mix only	1 serving	8	1	1	90	0	0.0	0
STRAWBERRY-BANANA								
(Jell-O) sugar-free, prepared	1/2 cup	10	1	0	50	0	0.0	0
(Royal)								
prepared	1/2 cup	80	2	19	105	0	0.0	0
sugar-free, mix only	1 serving	8	1	1	85	0	0.0	0
STRAWBERRY-ORANGE (Royal) mix only	1 serving	80	2	19	110	0	0.0	0
TROPICAL FRUIT (Royal) mix only	1 serving	80	2	19	110	0	0.0	0
WATERMELON (Jell-O) sugar-free, prepared	1/2 cup	10	1	0	55	0	0.0	0
GHEE/clarified butter	1 oz	249	0.0	0.0	na	0	28.4	(mq)
GIN								
80 proof	1 fl oz	64	0	0	0	0	0.0	0
86 proof	1 fl oz	70	0	0	0	0	0.0	0
90 proof	1 fl oz	73	0	0	0	0	0.0	0
94 proof	1 fl oz	76	0	0	0	0	0.0	0
100 proof	1 fl oz	82	0	0	0	0	0.0	0
GINGER								
Dried								
ground	1 tbsp	19	0	4	2	1	0.3	0
ground	1 tsp	6	0	1	1	0	0.1	0

Food Name	Serv. Size	Total Cal.	Prot. gms	Carbs gms	Sod. mgs	Fiber gms	Fat gms	Chol. mgs
ground *(Durkee)*	1 tsp	7	0	0	0	0	0.0	0
ground *(Laurel Leaf)*	1 tsp	7	0	0	0	0	0.0	0
ground *(McCormick/Schilling)*	1 tsp	7	0	2	0	0	0.0	0
ground *(Spice Islands)*	1 tsp	6	0	1	1	0	0.1	0
ground *(Tone's)*	1 tsp	6	0	1	1	0	0.1	0
Fresh								
raw, minced	1 tsp	1	0	0	0	0	0.0	0
raw, sliced, 1-inch diam	1/4 cup	17	0	4	3	0	0.2	0
Pickled *(Eden Foods)*	1 tbsp	15	0	3	340	1	0.0	0
GINGERBREAD MIX. See under CAKE, SNACK, MIX.								
GINKGO NUT								
Canned								
approx 78 kernels	1 cup	172	4	34	476	14	2.5	0
approx 14 kernels	1 oz	31	1	6	87	3	0.5	0
Dried	1 oz	99	3	21	4	na	0.6	0
Fresh, raw	1 oz	52	1	11	2	na	0.5	0
GLOBE ARTICHOKE. See under ARTICHOKE.								
GLUTEN. See WHEAT GLUTEN.								
GLUTINOUS RICE. See under RICE.								
GNOCCHI, RAW. See under POTATO DISH/ENTRÉE.								
GOA BEAN. See BEAN, WINGED.								
GOAT								
raw	1 oz	31	6	0	23	0	0.7	16
roasted	3 oz	122	23	0	73	0	2.6	64
GOATFISH								
raw	1 lb	435	92.5	0.0	(mq)	0	4.5	(mq)
raw	1 oz	27	5.8	0.0	(mq)	0	0.3	(mq)
GOAT'S MILK. See under MILK.								
GOBO. See BURDOCK ROOT.								
GOOSE.								
AVERAGE OF ALL PARTS								
meat and skin, raw	1 oz	105	4.5	0.0	21	0	9.5	23
meat and skin, roasted	4 oz	346	28.5	0.0	79	0	24.9	103
meat only, raw	1 oz	46	6.4	0.0	25	0	2.0	24
meat only, roasted	4 oz	270	32.9	0.0	86	0	14.4	109
GIBLETS, raw	3.5 oz	156	21.1	0.6	70	0	7.0	350
GIZZARD, raw	3.5 oz	139	21.4	0.0	65	0	5.3	145
LIVER. See also PÂTÉ.								
raw	1 med liver	125	15	6	132	0	4.0	484
GOOSE FAT								
	1 cup	1846	0	0	0	0	204.6	205
	1 tbsp	115	0	0	0	0	12.8	13
GOOSEBERRY								
Canned, in light syrup, w/liquid	1 cup	184	2	47	5	6	0.5	0
Fresh, raw	1 cup	66	1	15	2	6	0.9	0
GOOSEFISH. See MONKFISH.								
GORDITA, low-fat *(La Tortilla)*	1 serving	150	4	29	175	2	2.5	0
GOURD, BOTTLE/calabash gourd/white-flowered gourd								
boiled, drained, cubed	1 cup	22	1	5	3	na	0.0	0
raw, cubed	1/2 cup	8	0	2	1	na	0.0	0
raw, whole	1 gourd	108	5	26	15	na	0.2	0
GOURD, CALABASH. See GOURD, BOTTLE.								
GOURD, DISHCLOTH/loofah gourd/rag gourd/sponge gourd/towelgourd/vegetable sponge								
boiled, drained, chopped, 1-inch pieces	1 cup	100	1	26	37	na	0.6	0
boiled, drained, sliced, 1-inch slices	1/2 cup	50	1	13	19	na	0.3	0
raw, chopped, 1-inch pieces	1 cup	19	1	4	3	na	0.2	0
raw, whole	1 medium	36	2	8	5	na	0.4	0

Food Name	Serv. Size	Total Cal.	Prot. gms	Carbs gms	Sod. mgs	Fiber gms	Fat gms	Chol. mgs
GOURD, LOOFAH. See GOURD, DISHCLOTH.								
GOURD, RAG. See GOURD, DISHCLOTH.								
GOURD, SPONGE. See GOURD, DISHCLOTH.								
GOURD, WAX								
boiled, drained, cubed	1 cup	23	1	5	187	2	0.3	0
raw, cubed	1 cup	17	1	4	147	4	0.3	0
raw, whole	1 medium	741	23	171	6327	165	11.4	0
GOURD, WHITE/Chinese watermelon/tunka								
boiled, drained	4 oz	15	0.5	3.4	121	>.6 c	0.2	0
boiled, drained, cubed	1/2 cup	11	0.4	2.6	93	>.4 c	0.2	0
raw, cubed	1 cup	17	0.5	4.0	147	>.7 c	0.3	0
raw, trimmed	1 oz	4	0.1	0.9	31	.2	0.1	0
raw, untrimmed	1 lb	42	1.3	9.7	358	1.9	0.6	0
GOURD, WHITE-FLOWERED. See GOURD, BOTTLE.								
GOVERNOR PLUM, trimmed	1 oz	31	0.1	8.4	na	>.1 c	0.0	0
GRAHAM CRACKER. See under COOKIE.								
GRAHAM CRACKER CRUMBS, FS. See under COOKIE CRUMBS.								
GRAHAM FLOUR, ORGANIC. See under FLOUR.								
GRAIN CAKE								
(Great Cakes)								
w/summer fruits, 'Nature Cake'	4 oz	250	9	45	10	21	3.5	0
w/tropical fruits, 'Nature Cake'	4 oz	245	9	47	5	21	2.5	0
carob, 'Nature Cake'	4 oz	255	8	45	10	21	5.0	0
w/raspberry, 'Nature Cake'	4 oz	235	9	47	5	21	2.5	0
GRANADILLA. See PASSIONFRUIT.								
GRANOLA. See under CEREAL, HOT; CEREAL, READY-TO-EAT.								
GRANOLA/CEREAL BAR								
(Barbara's Bakery)								
apple-filled, nonfat	1 bar	110	2	27	90	2	0.0	0
blueberry-filled, nonfat	1 bar	110	2	27	90	2	0.0	0
carob chip, no cholesterol	1 bar	80	2	16	5	2	2.0	0
cinnamon and oats	1 bar	260	6	31	105	2	15.0	0
cinnamon-raisin, no cholesterol	1 bar	80	2	16	5	3	2.0	0
coconut-almond	1 bar	290	6	23	20	3	20.0	0
oats and honey, no cholesterol	1 bar	80	2	15	5	2	2.0	0
peanut butter	1 bar	260	9	28	75	3	15.0	0
peanut butter, no cholesterol	1 bar	80	2	14	5	2	3.0	0
raspberry-filled, nonfat	1 bar	110	2	27	110	2	0.0	0
strawberry-filled, nonfat	1 bar	110	2	27	110	2	0.0	0
(Bear Valley)								
carob-cocoa, food bar, 'Pemmican'	3.75 oz	440	16	68	80	7	12.0	0
coconut almond, 'Meal Pack'	3.75 oz	400	16	56	80	6	12.0	0
fruit and nut, 'Pemmican'	3.75 oz	420	17	59	90	9	13.0	0
sesame lemon, 'Meal Pack'	3.75 oz	410	17	57	85	4	13.0	0
(Ener-G Foods) gluten-free	1 serving	335	7	29	115	4	21.3	0
(Glenny's)								
'Bee Pollen Sunrise'	1.5 oz	190	5	22	0	0	8.0	0
'Ginseng Sunrise'	1.5 oz	160	1	24	0	0	7.0	0
'Spirulina Sunrise'	1.5 oz	140	3	21	0	0	5.0	0
almond, toasted, w/oat bran, 'Brown Rice Treats'	1 bar	200	4	34	20	2	5.0	0
carob mint, w/oat bran, 'Brown Rice Treats'	1 bar	180	3	37	20	2	2.0	0
cinnamon and raisin, 'Brown Rice Treats'	1.75 oz	170	2	38	30	0	1.0	0
coconut almandine ,'Moist & Chewy'	1.5 oz	190	3	22	20	0	10.0	0
oatmeal raisin, 'Moist & Chewy'	1.5 oz	160	3	30	25	0	3.0	0
peanut and raisin, 'Brown Rice Treats'	2 oz	210	4	39	29	0	5.0	0
peanut snack, 'Moist & Chewy'	1.5 oz	180	5	24	20	0	7.0	0
raisin bran, 'Brown Rice Treats'	1.75 oz	170	2	38	17	0	1.0	0

Food Name	Serv. Size	Total Cal.	Prot. gms	Carbs gms	Sod. mgs	Fiber gms	Fat gms	Chol. mgs
rice, plain and fancy, 'Brown Rice Treats'	1.25 oz	120	1	28	29	0	1.0	0
sunflower, 'Moist & Chewy'	1.5 oz	180	5	24	15	0	7.0	0
(Golden Temple)								
cashew almond, 'Wha Guru Chew Bar'	1 bar	164	3	15	63	1	11.0	0
peanut cashew, 'Wha Guru Chew Bar'	1 bar	167	4	14	62	1	11.0	0
sesame almond, 'Wha Guru Chew Bar'	1 bar	160	3	15	61	1	10.0	0
(Health Valley)								
blueberry apple, nonfat	1 bar	140	3	33	10	4	0.0	0
blueberry, nonfat	1 bar	140	2	35	5	3	0.0	0
chocolate chip, nonfat	1 bar	140	2	35	5	3	0.0	0
date-almond, nonfat	1 bar	140	2	35	5	3	0.0	0
raisin, nonfat	1 bar	140	2	35	5	3	0.0	0
strawberry, nonfat	1 bar	140	2	35	5	3	0.0	0
(Hershey's)								
chocolate chip, chocolate coated	1.2-oz bar	170	2	22	50	0	8.0	0
cocoa creme, chocolate-coated	1.2-oz bar	180	2	22	50	0	9.0	5
cookies and creme, chocolate-coated	1.2-oz bar	170	2	22	50	0	8.0	0
peanut butter, chocolate-coated	1.2-oz bar	180	4	19	65	0	10.0	5
(Kellogg's)								
almond and brown sugar, low-fat, crunchy	1 bar	80	2	16	60	1	1.5	0
apple spice, crunchy, low-fat	1 bar	80	2	16	60	1	1.5	0
raspberry-filled 'Common Sense Smart Start'	1 bar	170	2	28	160	1	6.0	0
(M&M Mars)								
chocolate chip, 'Kudos'	1 bar	180	3	21	60	0	9.0	0
chocolate chunk, 'Simply Kudos'	1 bar	100	1	13	50	0	4.0	0
fudge, nutty, 'Kudos'	1 bar	190	4	19	60	0	11.0	0
honey nut, 'Simply Kudos'	1 bar	100	2	13	55	0	4.0	0
oatmeal raisin, 'Simply Kudos'	1 bar	90	1	13	55	0	4.0	0
peanut butter, chocolate coated, 'Kudos'	1.3-oz bar	190	4	18	70	0	12.0	0
(Nature Valley)								
chocolate chip, crunchy	2 bars	210	4	32	120	2	9.0	0
cinnamon	2 bars	180	4	29	180	2	6.0	0
oat bran-honey graham	0.8-oz bar	110	2	16	90	1	4.0	0
oats and honey	2 bars	180	4	29	180	2	6.0	0
peanut butter	2 bars	190	5	28	180	2	6.0	0
(Nature's Choice)								
carob chip	0.75-oz bar	90	2	15	15	0	3.0	0
cinnamon-raisin	0.75-oz bar	90	2	15	10	0	3.0	0
oats 'n honey	0.75-oz bar	90	2	15	15	0	3.0	0
peanut butter	0.75-oz bar	90	2	14	25	0	3.0	0
(Nutri-Grain)								
blueberry, 'Smart Start'	1.5-oz bar	180	2	26	170	1	8.0	0
corn, mixed berry-filled, 'Smart Start'	1 bar	170	2	27	160	1	7.0	0
raisin bran, 'Smart Start'	1.5-oz bar	160	2	28	170	2	5.0	0
Rice Krispies, w/almonds, 'Smart Start'	1-oz bar	130	2	18	65	1	6.0	0
strawberry, 'Smart Start'	1.5-oz bar	180	2	26	170	1	8.0	0
(Quaker)								
apple berry, chewy	1-oz bar	120	2	20	95	0	4.0	0
Butterfinger, chewy	1 bar	160	2	29	100	1	4.0	0
caramel apple, chewy low-fat	1 bar	120	2	21	80	1	3.5	0
caramel nut, 'Granola Dipps'	1-oz bar	148	2	21	81	1	6.4	2
chocolate chip, 'Chewy'	1 bar	128	2	19	90	1	4.7	0
chocolate chip, 'Granola Dipps'	1-oz bar	139	2	19	78	1	6.3	1
chocolate chunk, low-fat, chewy	1 bar	110	1	22	110	1	2.0	0
chocolate fudge 'Granola Dipps'	1-oz bar	160	2	20	74	0	7.9	0
crunch, chewy	1 bar	160	2	28	95	1	5.0	0
honey and oats, 'Chewy'	1-oz bar	125	2	19	95	1	4.4	1

Food Name	Serv. Size	Total Cal.	Prot. gms	Carbs gms	Sod. mgs	Fiber gms	Fat gms	Chol. mgs
nut and raisin, chunky, 'Chewy'	1-oz bar	131	3	17	86	2	5.8	1
peanut butter chocolate chip, 'Chewy'	1-oz bar	131	3	17	112	1	5.7	0
peanut butter chocolate chip, 'Granola Dipps'	1 bar	174	4	17	102	0	10.0	0
peanut butter, 'Chewy'	1-oz bar	128	3	18	116	1	4.9	1
peanut butter, 'Granola Dipps'	1-oz bar	170	4	19	74	1	9.1	2
raisin cinnamon, 'Chewy'	1-oz bar	128	2	19	92	1	5.0	0
S'mores, 'Chewy'	1-oz bar	126	2	20	108	1	4.4	0
trail mix, 'Chewy'	1 oz	130	2	18	105	0	5.0	0
(Sunbelt)								
apple bar, baked	1.31 oz	130	1	28	130	1	2.0	0
chocolate chip, chewy	1.25 oz	150	3	23	75	2	7.0	2
chocolate chip, fudge-dipped, chewy	1.5 oz	210	2	26	55	4	10.0	2
oats and honey, chewy	1-oz bar	130	2	18	35	0	5.0	1
oats and honey, fudge-dipped, chewy	1.38-oz bar	190	2	24	55	0	10.0	1
w/almonds, chewy	1-oz bar	120	3	18	65	0	6.0	1
w/chocolate chips, chewy	1.75-oz bar	220	4	32	105	0	9.0	1
w/peanuts, fudge-dipped, chewy	1.38-oz bar	190	2	24	55	0	10.0	1
w/peanuts, fudge-dipped, chewy	1.5-oz bar	200	4	24	60	4	12.0	2
w/peanuts, fudge-dipped, chewy	2.25-oz bar	300	6	36	90	0	18.0	1
w/raisins, chewy	1.25-oz bar	150	2	24	65	2	6.0	0
w/raisins, fudge-dipped, chewy	1.5-oz bar	200	4	24	60	0	12.0	1

GRANOLA SNACK. See under CEREAL SNACK. Also see GRANOLA/CEREAL BAR.

GRAPE
AMERICAN (Concord, Delaware, Niagara)
Fresh

Food Name	Serv. Size	Total Cal.	Prot. gms	Carbs gms	Sod. mgs	Fiber gms	Fat gms	Chol. mgs
(Dole)	1.5 cup	85	1.0	24.0	3	2.0	0.0	na
slipskin, peeled and seeded	1 oz	18	0.2	4.9	<1	>.2 c	0.1	0
slipskin, trimmed	10 medium	15	0.2	4.1	0	>.2 c	0.1	0
slipskin, untrimmed	1 lb	165	1.7	45.1	4	>2.0 c	0.9	0
slipskin, untrimmed	1 cup	58	0.6	15.8	2	>.9 c	0.3	0

EUROPEAN (Muskat, Tokay, Thompson)
Canned

Food Name	Serv. Size	Total Cal.	Prot. gms	Carbs gms	Sod. mgs	Fiber gms	Fat gms	Chol. mgs
Thompson, seedless, in heavy syrup, w/liquid	1 cup	187	1	50	13	1	0.3	0
Thompson, seedless, in water, w/liquid	1 cup	98	1	25	15	2	0.3	0

Fresh

Food Name	Serv. Size	Total Cal.	Prot. gms	Carbs gms	Sod. mgs	Fiber gms	Fat gms	Chol. mgs
adherent skin, w/seeds	1/2 cup	57	0.5	14.2	2	0.6	0.5	0
adherent skin, w/seeds	1 oz	20	0.2	5.0	1	0.2	0.2	0
adherent skin, w/o seeds	1/2 cup	57	0.5	14.2	2	0.6	0.5	0
adherent skin, w/o seeds	1 oz	20	0.2	5.0	1	0.2	0.2	0
adherent skin, w/o seeds, approx 1.75 oz	10 medium	36	0.3	8.9	1	0.4	0.3	0

GRAPE DRINK. See under FRUIT DRINK; FRUIT JUICE BLEND; FRUIT JUICE DRINK.
GRAPE JUICE
Canned, bottled, or boxed

Food Name	Serv. Size	Total Cal.	Prot. gms	Carbs gms	Sod. mgs	Fiber gms	Fat gms	Chol. mgs
(Flav-R-Pac)	1 cup	130	0	33	10	0	0.0	0
(IGA) unsweetened	6 fl oz	120	0	30	5	0	0.0	0
(J. Hungerford)								
100% juice	9.03 fl oz	155	1	39	11	0	0.0	0
regular	9.03 fl oz	160	0	40	0	0	0.0	0
(Juicy Juice)	6 fl oz	90	1	22	5	0	0.0	0
(Knudsen)								
	8 fl oz	150	1	37	30	na	0.0	0
Concord	8 fl oz	130	1	32	0	0	0.0	0
(Kraft) 'Pure 100% Unsweetened'	6 fl oz	104	1	25	0	0	0.0	0
(Lucky Leaf)	6 fl oz	130	0	32	0	0	0.0	0
(Minute Maid)	6 fl oz	100	1	24	20	0	1.0	0
(Pathmark)								
'No Frills'	6 fl oz	113	0	27	10	0	0.0	0

Food Name	Serv. Size	Total Cal.	Prot. gms	Carbs gms	Sod. mgs	Fiber gms	Fat gms	Chol. mgs
unsweetened	6 fl oz	120	0	30	10	0	0.0	0
(S&W) Concord, unsweetened	6 fl oz	100	1	25	9	0	0.0	0
(Sippin' Pak)	8.45 fl oz	130	1	32	25	0	0.0	0
(Squeezit 100) 100% natural, 'Caped Grape'	6.75 fl oz	100	0	24	20	0	0.0	0
(Tree Top) 100%	8 fl oz	160	0	38	22	0	0.0	0
(Tropicana) 'Season's Best'	8 fl oz	160	1	39	25	1	0.0	na
(Veryfine) '100%'	8 fl oz	153	1	37	20	0	0.0	0
(Welch's)								
purple	6 fl oz	120	0	30	10	0	0.0	0
red	6 fl oz	120	0	30	15	0	0.0	0
red, sparkling	6 fl oz	128	0	30	30	0	0.0	0
white	6 fl oz	120	0	30	15	0	0.0	0
white, sparkling	6 fl oz	120	0	30	30	0	0.0	0
Refrigerated or frozen								
(Minute Maid)	6 fl oz	90	0	24	0	0	0.0	0
(Sunkist) concentrate, prepared	6 fl oz	69	0	17	3	0	0.1	0
(Welch's)								
purple, concentrate, prepared	6 fl oz	100	0	25	0	0	0.0	0
white, concentrate, prepared	6 fl oz	100	0	25	0	0	0.0	0
GRAPE LEAVES								
raw	1 cup	13	1	2	1	2	0.3	0
raw, whole	1 medium	3	0	1	0	0	0.1	0
whole (Reese)	1 leaf	5	0	0	110	0	0.0	0
GRAPEFRUIT								
PINK								
Fresh								
Arizona, sections, w/juice	1 cup	85	1	22	2	na	0.2	0
Arizona, whole, approx 3.75-inch diam	1/2 fruit	46	1	12	1	na	0.1	0
California, sections, w/juice	1 cup	85	1	22	2	na	0.2	0
California, whole, approx 3.75-inch diam	1/2 fruit	46	1	12	1	na	0.1	0
Florida, sections, w/juice	1 cup	69	1	17	0	3	0.2	0
Florida, whole, approx 3.75-inch diam	1/2 fruit	37	1	9	0	1	0.1	0
whole, approx 4.5-inch diam	1/2 fruit	53	1	13	0	2	0.2	0
whole, approx 4-inch diam	1/2 fruit	41	1	10	0	1	0.1	0
whole, approx 3.5-inch diam	1/2 fruit	32	1	8	0	1	0.1	0
RED								
Fresh								
Arizona, sections, w/juice	1 cup	85	1	22	2	na	0.2	0
Arizona, whole, approx 3.75-inch diam	1/2 fruit	46	1	12	1	na	0.1	0
California, sections, w/juice	1 cup	85	1	22	2	na	0.2	0
California, whole, approx 3.75-inch diam	1/2 fruit	46	1	12	1	na	0.1	0
Florida, sections, w/juice	1 cup	69	1	17	0	3	0.2	0
Florida, whole, approx 3.75-inch diam	1/2 fruit	37	1	9	0	1	0.1	0
whole, approx 4.5-inch diam	1/2 fruit	53	1	13	0	2	0.2	0
whole, approx 4-inch diam	1/2 fruit	41	1	10	0	1	0.1	0
whole, approx 3.5-inch diam	1/2 fruit	32	1	8	0	1	0.1	0
WHITE								
Canned								
sections, in juice, w/liquid	1 cup	92	2	23	17	1	0.2	0
sections, in light syrup, w/liquid	1 cup	152	1	39	5	1	0.3	0
sections, in water, w/liquid	1 cup	88	1	22	5	1	0.2	0
Fresh								
California, sections, w/juice	1 cup	85	2	21	0	na	0.2	0
California, whole, approx 3.75-inch diam	1/2 fruit	44	1	11	0	na	0.1	0
Florida, sections, w/juice	1 cup	74	1	19	0	na	0.2	0
Florida, whole, approx 3.75-inch diam	1/2 fruit	38	1	10	0	na	0.1	0

Food Name	Serv. Size	Total Cal.	Prot. gms	Carbs gms	Sod. mgs	Fiber gms	Fat gms	Chol. mgs
whole, approx 4.5-inch diam	1/2 fruit	53	1	13	0	2	0.2	0
whole, approx 4-inch diam	1/2 fruit	41	1	10	0	1	0.1	0
whole, approx 3.5-inch diam	1/2 fruit	32	1	8	0	1	0.1	0
GRAPEFRUIT JUICE								
Canned, bottled, or boxed								
(Del Monte)	6 fl oz	70	1	17	10	0	0.0	0
(Florida's Natural) ruby red, not from concentrate	8 fl oz	100	1	24	0	0	0.0	0
(J. Hungerford)								
100% juice	9.03 fl oz	98	1	24	6	0	0.0	0
regular	9.03 fl oz	120	0	30	0	0	0.0	0
(Knudsen) pink	8 fl oz	100	2	23	35	na	0.0	0
(Kraft)	6 fl oz	70	1	16	0	0	0.0	0
(Libby's)	6 fl oz	70	1	17	0	0	0.0	0
(Minute Maid) 'Juices To Go'	6 fl oz	70	1	17	20	0	0.0	0
(Mott's)	10 fl oz	124	1	30	5	0	0.0	0
(Ocean Spray)								
	6 fl oz	70	1	16	10	0	0.0	0
'Pink Premium'	6 fl oz	60	1	15	10	0	0.0	0
'Ruby Red'	6 fl oz	100	0	24	15	0	0.0	0
(S&W)	6 fl oz	80	1	18	0	0	0.0	0
(Stokely)	6 fl oz	76	1	18	5	0	1.0	0
(Sunkist) 'Fresh Squeezed'	8 fl oz	96	1	23	3	0	0.2	0
(Tree Top) 100%	8 fl oz	104	0	24	32	0	0.0	0
(TreeSweet)								
pink	6 fl oz	72	0	17	15	0	0.0	0
regular	6 fl oz	72	0	17	15	0	0.0	0
(Tropicana)								
100% pure	6 fl oz	70	1	14	20	0	1.0	0
golden, 'Pure Premium'	8 fl oz	90	1	23	0	0	0.0	na
'Ruby Red' 100% pure	6 fl oz	70	1	14	20	0	1.0	0
ruby red, 'Pure Premium'	8 fl oz	100	1	23	0	1	0.0	na
'Season's Best'	8 fl oz	90	1	22	5	1	0.0	na
'100%'	8 fl oz	101	1	23	10	0	0.0	0
Refrigerated or frozen								
(A&P) concentrate, prepared	6 fl oz	80	1	18	0	0	1.0	0
(Del Monte)	6 fl oz	70	1	17	10	0	0.0	0
(Kraft)	6 fl oz	70	1	16	0	0	0.0	0
(Minute Maid) concentrate, prepared	6 fl oz	80	1	18	0	0	0.0	0
(Ocean Spray)	6 fl oz	70	1	16	10	0	0.0	0
(S&W)	6 fl oz	80	1	18	0	0	0.0	0
(Stokely)	6 fl oz	76	1	18	5	0	1.0	0
(Sunkist) concentrate, prepared	6 fl oz	56	1	13	1	0	0.2	0
(TreeSweet)								
	6 fl oz	72	0	17	15	0	0.0	0
concentrate, prepared	6 fl oz	78	1	18	15	0	0.0	0
(Veryfine) '100%'	8 fl oz	101	1	23	10	0	0.0	0
GRAPESEED OIL								
	1 cup	1927	0	0	0	0	218.0	0
	1 tbsp	120	0	0	0	0	13.6	0
GRAVY								
AU JUS								
(Franco-American)	1/4 cup	10	1	2	310	0	0.5	3
(Heinz) 'HomeStyle'	1/4 cup	18	0	2	350	0	1.0	0
BEEF								
(Franco-American)	1/4 cup	30	1	3	310	0	1.5	3
(Heinz) nonfat	1/4 cup	15	1	3	330	0	0.0	0

Food Name	Serv. Size	Total Cal.	Prot. gms	Carbs gms	Sod. mgs	Fiber gms	Fat gms	Chol. mgs
(Hormel) w/chunky beef. 'Great Beginnings' .... 5 oz		136	12	7	904	0	7.0	0
(Pepperidge Farm)								
hearty .... 1 jar		146	10	21	2145	na	2.4	17
hearty .... 1 serving		26	2	4	379	na	0.4	3
98% fat-free .... 1/4 cup		25	1	4	360	0	1.0	5
BROWN								
(Heinz)								
'HomeStyle' .... 1/4 cup		25	1	3	320	0	1.0	0
savory, 'HomeStyle' .... 1/4 cup		24	1	3	352	na	0.8	2
w/onions, 'HomeStyle' .... 1/4 cup		25	1	3	330	0	1.0	0
(La Choy) .... 1/4 cup		275	3	66	320	0	0.0	0
(McCormick/Schilling) .... 1/3 cup		30	1	5	417	0	1.0	0
(Pillsbury) .... 1/4 cup		10	0	3	270	0	0.0	0
CHICKEN								
(Franco-American)								
.... 1/4 cup		40	0	3	240	0	3.0	3
giblet .... 1/4 cup		30	1	3	310	0	2.0	10
(Heinz)								
classic, homestyle .... 1/4 cup		30	1	3	340	0	1.5	0
'HomeStyle' .... 1/4 cup		35	1	3	350	0	2.0	0
w/mushrooms and onions, 'HomeStyle' .... 1/4 cup		35	1	3	330	0	2.0	1
(Hormel) w/chunky chicken, 'Great Beginnings' .... 5 oz		147	14	5	567	0	8.0	0
(Pepperidge Farm) golden, 98% fat-free .... 2 oz		25	1	3	240	0	1.0	0
(Pillsbury) chicken style .... 1/4 cup		20	1	4	260	0	0.0	0
COUNTRY *(Heinz)* homestyle, 'Blue Ribbon' .... 1/4 cup		25	0	4	210	1	1.0	0
CREAM *(Franco-American)* .... 2 oz		35	0	4	220	0	2.0	0
HOMESTYLE *(Pillsbury)* .... 1/4 cup		10	0	3	270	0	0.0	0
MUSHROOM								
(Franco-American) creamy .... 1/4 cup		20	1	4	310	0	1.0	3
(Heinz) 'HomeStyle' .... 1/4 cup		25	1	3	340	0	1.0	0
PORK								
(Franco-American) golden .... 1/4 cup		45	1	3	340	1	4.0	4
(Heinz) 'HomeStyle' .... 1/4 cup		25	1	3	310	0	1.0	0
(Hormel) w/chunky pork, 'Great Beginnings' .... 5 oz		140	14	5	567	0	8.0	0
SAUSAGE								
(Nestlé)								
country, 'Chef-Mate' .... 1 pkg		4614	137	187	11313	21	369.1	625
country, 'Chef-Mate' .... 1/4 cup		96	3	4	236	0	7.7	13
TURKEY								
(Franco-American) .... 1/4 cup		25	1	3	290	0	1.0	3
(Heinz)								
'HomeStyle' .... 1/4 cup		25	1	3	370	0	1.0	0
nonfat .... 1/4 cup		15	1	3	330	0	0.0	0
roasted, homestyle .... 1/4 cup		25	1	3	360	0	1.0	0
(Hormel) w/chunky turkey, 'Great Beginnings' .... 5 oz		138	11	7	585	0	8.0	0
(Pepperidge Farm) seasoned, 98% fat-free .... 2 oz		25	1	4	320	0	1.0	0
GRAVY MIX								
AU JUS								
(Custom Foods)								
base, 'Red Label' mix only .... 16-oz pkg		867	71	104	84548	14	18.2	27
base, 'Red Label' mix only .... 1 serving		19	2	2	1862	0	0.4	1
instant, 'Superb' mix only .... 4-oz pkg		334	24	45	12501	3	6.8	7
instant, 'Superb' mix only .... 1 serving		20	1	3	741	0	0.4	0
(French's) mix, prepared .... 1/4 cup		10	0	2	260	0	0.0	0
(Lawry's) mix, prepared .... 1 cup		84	6	11	3454	0	1.6	0
(McCormick/Schilling) mix, prepared .... 1/4 cup		20	1	4	786	0	0.3	0
(Nestlé)								
'Trio' mix only .... 7-oz pkg		554	2	115	26334	2	9.9	8

Food Name	Serv. Size	Total Cal.	Prot. gms	Carbs gms	Sod. mgs	Fiber gms	Fat gms	Chol. mgs
'Trio' mix only	1 tsp	8	0	2	399	0	0.1	0
(Tone's) mix only	1 tsp	10	0	1	680	0	0.5	1
BEEF								
(Custom Foods)								
instant, 'Superb' mix only	1 serving	25	1	4	349	0	0.6	1
instant, 'Superb' mix only	16-oz pkg	1675	44	277	23622	20	43.0	50
(McCormick/Schilling) and herb, mix only	2 tsp	30	1	3	290	0	1.0	3
BISCUIT								
(Custom Foods)								
old-fashioned, 'Superb' mix only	1 pkg	3366	45	369	13416	33	190.6	20
old-fashioned, 'Superb' mix only	1 serving	48	1	5	191	0	2.7	0
BROWN								
(Crown Colony) mix only	2 tbsp	15	1	3	310	0	0.0	0
(Custom Foods)								
instant, 'Superb' mix only	1 pkg	1725	39	271	22941	15	53.8	54
instant, 'Superb' mix only	1 serving	25	1	4	339	0	0.8	1
(French's) prepared	1/4 cup	20	1	4	250	0	1.0	0
(Hain) mix only	1/4 cup	16	1	3	600	0	0.0	0
(Lawry's) prepared	1 cup	94	4	17	1500	0	1.4	0
(Loma Linda) vegetarian, 'Gravy Quik' mix only	1 tbsp	20	1	4	367	0	0.2	0
(McCormick/Schilling)								
'Lite' prepared	1/4 cup	10	1	2	450	0	1.0	0
mix only	1 pkg	91	2	14	1251	0	3.0	0
prepared	1/4 cup	23	1	4	313	0	0.8	0
(Nestlé)								
'Trio' mix only	16-oz pkg	1839	47	262	19764	16	67.0	0
'Trio' mix only	1 tbsp	24	1	3	262	0	0.9	0
'Trio Supreme' mix only	16-oz pkg	1843	45	262	22700	0	68.0	14
'Trio Supreme' mix only	1 tbsp	24	1	3	300	0	0.9	0
(Pillsbury)								
mix only	2 tsp	10	0	3	270	0	0.0	0
prepared w/water	1/4 cup	16	0	3	180	0	0.0	0
(Tone's) mix only	1 tsp	10	0	2	239	0	0.2	1
(Weight Watchers)								
prepared	1/4 cup	10	1	2	360	0	0.0	0
w/mushrooms, prepared	1/4 cup	10	1	2	270	0	0.0	0
w/onions, prepared	1/4 cup	10	1	2	310	0	0.0	0
CHICKEN								
(Custom Foods)								
instant, 'Superb' mix only	16-oz pkg	1793	46	257	20907	15	64.6	159
instant, 'Superb' mix only	1 serving	26	1	4	309	0	1.0	2
(French's) prepared w/water	1/4 cup	25	1	4	270	0	1.0	0
(Lawry's) prepared w/water	1 cup	99	3	16	980	0	2.8	0
(Loma Linda) 'Gravy Quik'	1 tbsp	19	1	3	408	0	0.1	0
(McCormick/Schilling) prepared w/water	1/4 cup	22	1	4	300	0	0.4	0
(Nestlé)								
'Trio' mix only	1 pkg	2596	73	405	20833	9	75.6	179
'Trio' mix only	1 tbsp	32	1	5	260	0	0.9	2
'Trio Supreme' mix only	1 pkg	2291	63	357	20219	0	67.2	23
'Trio Supreme' mix only	1 tbsp	32	1	5	285	0	0.9	0
(Pillsbury)								
mix only	2 tsp	20	1	4	260	0	0.0	0
prepared w/water	1/4 cup	25	1	4	230	0	1.0	0
(Tone's) mix only	1 tsp	11	0	2	157	0	0.2	1
(Weight Watchers) prepared	1/4 cup	10	1	2	410	0	0.0	0
COUNTRY								
(Custom Foods)								
'Superb' mix only	1 pkg	3271	55	364	15239	33	177.3	14

Food Name	Serv. Size	Total Cal.	Prot. gms	Carbs gms	Sod. mgs	Fiber gms	Fat gms	Chol. mgs
'Superb' mix only	1 serving	47	1	5	217	0	2.5	0
(Loma Linda) 'Gravy Quik'	1 tbsp	22	1	4	249	0	0.6	0
(Nestlé)								
'Trio' mix only	1 pkg	2702	57	405	15968	56	95.3	37
'Trio' mix only	1 tbsp	35	1	5	205	1	1.2	0
(Tone's) mix only	1 tsp	12	0	2	114	0	0.5	1
(Williams) low-fat, low-cholesterol	0.33 oz	40	1	5	320	0	2.0	0
HOMESTYLE								
(French's) prepared	1/4 cup	20	1	4	250	0	1.0	0
(McCormick/Schilling) prepared	1/4 cup	24	1	4	295	0	0.8	0
(Pillsbury)								
mix only	2 tsp	10	0	3	270	0	0.0	0
prepared w/water, 1/4 cup 2% milk	1/4 cup	25	1	4	170	0	1.0	0
HERB (McCormick/Schilling) prepared	1/4 cup	20	1	3	312	0	0.5	0
MUSHROOM								
(French's) prepared w/water	1/4 cup	20	1	3	250	0	1.0	0
(Loma Linda) 'Gravy Quik' mix only	1 tbsp	16	1	3	304	1	0.3	0
(McCormick/Schilling) mix only	1/4 cup	19	1	3	270	0	0.5	0
ONION								
(French's) prepared w/water	1/4 cup	25	1	4	270	0	1.0	0
(Loma Linda) 'Gravy Quik' mix only	1 tbsp	18	1	3	229	1	0.0	0
(McCormick/Schilling) mix only	2 tsp	20	1	3	340	0	0.5	0
PORK								
(Custom Foods)								
instant, 'Superb' mix only	16-oz pkg	1648	38	294	20289	11	35.8	45
instant, 'Superb' mix only	1 serving	24	1	4	299	0	0.5	1
(French's) prepared w/water	1/4 cup	20	1	4	250	0	1.0	0
(McCormick/Schilling) prepared w/water	1/4 cup	20	1	4	297	0	0.6	0
SOUTHERN								
(Nestlé)								
'Trio' mix only	1 pkg	1770	9	223	10672	0	93.7	7
'Trio' mix only	1 serving	48	0	6	290	0	2.5	0
TURKEY								
(Custom Foods)								
instant, 'Superb' mix only	16-oz pkg	1857	53	261	18569	17	66.6	109
instant, 'Superb' mix only	1 serving	27	1	4	274	0	1.0	2
(Lawry's) prepared w/water	1 cup	102	3	13	1400	0	4.1	0
(McCormick/Schilling) prepared w/water	1/4 cup	22	1	4	353	0	0.5	0
(Nestlé)								
'Trio' mix only	1 pkg	2053	49	409	19204	9	24.6	62
'Trio' mix only	1 serving	29	1	6	271	0	0.3	1

GREAT NORTHERN BEAN. See BEAN, GREAT NORTHERN.
GREEK SEASONING MIX. See under SEASONING MIX.
GREEN BEAN. See BEAN, GREEN; BEAN, FRENCH; BEEN DISH/ENTRÉE.
GREEN ONION. See SCALLION.
GREEN PEAS. See PEAS, GREEN.
GREEN PEPPER. See PEPPER, BELL.
GREEN PEPPER DISH/ENTRÉE. See PEPPER, BELL, DISH/ENTRÉE.
GREEN TURTLE. See TURTLE, GREEN.
GREENLAND HALIBUT. See under HALIBUT.
GRENADINE SYRUP. See under COCKTAIL MIX.
GRITS
CORN
Instant
(Quaker)

butter flavor	1 pkt	101	2	21	323	1	1.4	0

Food Name	Serv. Size	Total Cal.	Prot. gms	Carbs gms	Sod. mgs	Fiber gms	Fat gms	Chol. mgs
cheddar cheese flavor	1 pkt	102	2	21	522	1	1.6	1
plain	1 cup	159	4	37	517	2	0.5	0
plain	1 pkt	96	2	22	305	1	0.3	0
w/imitation bacon bits	1 pkt	94	3	21	331	1	0.5	0
w/imitation ham bits	1 pkt	92	3	20	510	1	0.5	0
w/sausage bits	1 serving	100	3	21	480	2	1.0	0
Quick-cooking								
white, enriched, cooked w/water, w/o salt	1 cup	145	3	31	0	0	0.5	0
white, enriched, cooked w/water, w/o salt	3/4 cup	109	3	24	0	0	0.4	0
white, unenriched, cooked w/water, w/o salt	1 cup	145	3	31	0	0	0.5	0
white, unenriched, cooked w/water, w/o salt	3/4 cup	109	3	24	0	0	0.4	0
white, unenriched, dry	1 cup	579	14	124	2	2	1.9	0
white, unenriched, dry	1 tbsp	36	1	8	0	0	0.1	0
yellow, enriched, cooked w/water, w/o salt	1 cup	145	3	31	0	0	0.5	0
yellow, enriched, cooked w/water, w/o salt	3/4 cup	109	3	24	0	0	0.4	0
yellow, enriched, dry	1 cup	579	14	124	2	2	1.9	0
yellow, enriched, dry	1 tbsp	36	1	8	0	0	0.1	0
yellow, unenriched, cooked w/water, w/o salt	1 cup	145	3	31	0	0	0.5	0
yellow, unenriched, cooked w/water, w/o salt	3/4 cup	109	3	24	0	0	0.4	0
yellow, unenriched, dry	1 cup	579	14	124	2	2	1.9	0
yellow, unenriched, dry	1 tbsp	36	1	8	0	0	0.1	0
(Arrowhead Mills)								
white, dry	2 oz	200	5	43	1	2	1.0	0
yellow, dry	2 oz	200	5	44	1	2	1.0	0
(Aunt Jemima) white, enriched, dry	3 tbsp	101	2	22	1	1	0.2	0
(Quick) yellow, enriched, dry	3 tbsp	101	2	22	1	1	0.2	0
(Tone's) yellow, enriched, dry	1 tsp	12	0	3	0	0	0.1	0
HOMINY								
Canned								
(Allens)								
golden	1/2 cup	80	2	16	370	0	1.0	0
Mexican	1/2 cup	80	2	16	330	0	1.0	0
white	1/2 cup	70	2	16	430	0	1.0	0
(Bush's Best)								
golden	1/2 cup	45	1	11	390	0	0.0	0
white	1/2 cup	45	1	11	450	0	0.0	0
(Juanita's)								
Mexican style	1/2 cup	60	2	10	190	5	0.5	0
(S&W)								
golden, 'Sun-Vista'	1/2 cup	70	2	19	540	3	0.0	0
white	1/2 cup	65	2	18	530	3	0.5	0
white, 'Sun-Vista'	1/2 cup	65	2	18	530	3	0.5	0
(Van Camp's)								
golden	1 cup	128	3	28	701	1	0.6	0
golden, w/red and green peppers	1 cup	129	3	29	685	1	0.5	0
white	1 cup	138	3	30	708	1	0.7	0
Instant								
(Albers) 'Hominy Quick Grits'	1/2 cup	150	4	33	0	0	0.0	0
(Aunt Jemima) white, enriched, 'Quick'	3 tbsp	101	2	22	1	1	0.2	0
(Quaker) w/real cheddar cheese flavor	1 pkt	104	2	22	497	1	1.0	0
Quick-cooking								
(Aunt Jemima) white, enriched, 'Regular'	3 tbsp	101	2	22	1	1	0.2	0
(Quaker)								
white	1/4 cup	130	3	29	0	2	0.5	0
yellow	1/3 cup	133	3	30	0	2	0.5	0

GROUND HUSK TOMATO. See TOMATILLO.

Food Name	Serv. Size	Total Cal.	Prot. gms	Carbs gms	Sod. mgs	Fiber gms	Fat gms	Chol. mgs
GROUPER								
mixed species, baked, broiled, grilled, or microwaved	3 oz	100	21	0	45	0	1.1	40
mixed species, raw	3 oz	78	16	0	45	0	0.9	31
GUACAMOLE. See under DIP.								
GUACAMOLE SEASONING.								
See under SEASONING MIX.								
GUANABANA/soursop								
raw, trimmed	1/2 cup	75	1.1	18.9	16	>1.2 c	0.3	0
raw, untrimmed	1 lb	202	3.0	51.2	42	>3.3 c	0.9	0
raw, whole, approx 2.1 lb	1 medium	416	6.3	105.3	87	>6.9 c	1.9	0
GUAVA								
raw, chopped	1 cup	84	1	20	5	9	1.0	0
raw, whole, trimmed	1 medium	46	1	11	3	5	0.5	0
GUAVA, STRAWBERRY								
raw, chopped	1 cup	168	1	42	90	13	1.5	0
raw, whole, trimmed	1 medium	4	0	1	2	0	0.0	0
GUAVA JUICE								
Frozen *(Welch's)* 'Orchard Tropicals' prepared	6 fl oz	100	0	25	20	0	0.0	0
GUINEA HEN								
giblets, raw	3.5 oz	157	20.8	1.2	70	0	7.0	350
meat and skin, raw	1 lb	567	84.0	0.0	241	0	23.2	266
meat only, raw	1 oz	31	5.9	0.0	(mq)	0	0.7	18
GUM. See under CANDY.								
GUMBO FILE POWDER.								
See under SEASONING MIX.								

H

Food Name	Serv. Size	Total Cal.	Prot. gms	Carbs gms	Sod. mgs	Fiber gms	Fat gms	Chol. mgs
HADDOCK								
Fresh								
baked, broiled, grilled, or microwaved	3 oz	95	21	0	74	0	0.8	63
raw	3 oz	74	16	0	58	0	0.6	48
Frozen								
fillet, 'Fishmarket Fresh' *(Gorton's)*	5 oz	110	25	0	120	0	1.0	0
fillet *(SeaPak)*	4 oz	90	18	0	120	0	1.0	0
fillet *(Van de Kamp's)*	4 oz	90	21	0	125	0	1.0	20
Smoked								
fillet	3 oz	99	21	0	649	0	0.8	65
fillet, boneless	1 oz	33	7	0	216	0	0.3	22
finnian haddie	4 oz	132	28.6	0.0	865	0	1.1	87
HADDOCK, NORWAY. See OCEAN PERCH, ATLANTIC.								
HADDOCK DINNER/ENTRÉE								
(Van de Kamp's)								
fillet, battered, frozen	2 pieces	250	12	19	580	0	15.0	30
fillet, breaded, frozen	2 pieces	270	12	19	290	0	16.0	25
fillet, light, frozen	1 piece	240	15	21	590	0	11.0	35
HAKE, SILVER. See WHITING.								
HALIBUT								
ATLANTIC								
Fresh								
baked, broiled, grilled, or microwaved	4 oz	159	30.3	0.0	78	0	3.3	46
baked, broiled, grilled, or microwaved	3 oz	119	22.7	0.0	59	0	2.5	35
raw	1 lb	497	94.4	0.0	245	0	10.4	146

Food Name	Serv. Size	Total Cal.	Prot. gms	Carbs gms	Sod. mgs	Fiber gms	Fat gms	Chol. mgs
raw	3 oz	94	17.7	0.0	46	0	2.0	27
raw	1 oz	31	5.9	0.0	15	0	0.6	9
Frozen, steaks *(SeaPak)*	6-oz pkg	160	36	0	120	0	1.0	0
GREENLAND								
baked, broiled, grilled, or microwaved	3 oz	203	15.7	0.0	88	0	15.1	50
raw	1 lb	845	65.2	0.0	363	0	62.8	209
raw	3 oz	158	12.2	0.0	68	0	11.8	39
raw	1 oz	53	4.1	0.0	23	0	3.9	13
PACIFIC								
Fresh								
baked, broiled, grilled, or microwaved	4 oz	159	30.3	0.0	78	0	3.3	46
baked, broiled, grilled, or microwaved	3 oz	119	22.7	0.0	59	0	2.5	35
raw	1 lb	497	94.4	0.0	245	0	10.4	146
raw	3 oz	94	17.7	0.0	46	0	2.0	27
raw	1 oz	31	5.9	0.0	15	0	0.6	9
Frozen								
fillet, boneless, skinless, raw *(Peter Pan Seafoods)*	3.5 oz	110	21	0	54	0	2.3	32
loin steaks, raw *(Peter Pan Seafoods)*	3.5 oz	110	21	0	54	0	2.3	32
steaks, standard cut, raw *(Peter Pan Seafoods)*	3.5 oz	110	21	0	54	0	2.3	32
steaks *(SeaPak)*	6 oz pkg	160	36	0	120	0	1.0	0
HALIBUT DINNER/ENTRÉE								
(Van de Kamp's) fillet, battered, frozen	2 pieces	150	8	16	400	0	6.0	10
HAM. See also HAM SUBSTITUTE; PORK.								
Also see under LUNCHEON MEAT.								
CANNED								
chopped	1 oz	68	4.6	0.1	387	0	5.3	14
chopped	0.75-oz slice	50	3.4	0.1	287	0	4.0	10
cured, extra lean, approx 4% fat, baked	3 oz	116	18.0	0.4	965	0	4.2	25
cured, extra lean, approx 4% fat, unheated	1 oz	34	5.2	0.0	356	0	1.3	11
cured, extra lean and regular, baked	3 oz	142	17.8	0.4	908	0	7.2	35
cured, extra lean and regular, unheated	1 oz	41	5.1	0.0	362	0	2.1	11
cured, regular, approx 13% fat, baked	3 oz	192	17.5	0.4	800	0	12.9	53
cured, regular, approx 13% fat, unheated	1 oz	54	4.8	0.0	352	0	3.7	11
(Armour) chopped	3 oz	190	13	1	1260	0	14.0	0
(Black Label) 3-lb can	4 oz	140	20	0	1315	0	7.0	0
(Chi-Chi's) 'Black Label'	1 oz	37	5	2	303	0	1.0	15
(EXL)								
	4 oz	120	22	0	1382	0	4.0	0
'Deli Ham' 10-lb can	4 oz	130	20	0	1368	0	6.0	0
(Holiday Glaze) '3-lb can'	4 oz	130	21	2	0	0	4.0	0
(Hormel)								
'Bone-In'	4 oz	210	17	1	0	0	15.0	0
chopped, 12-oz can	2 oz	120	10	0	703	0	9.0	0
chunk	2.5 oz	110	11	1	780	0	7.0	35
'Cure/81'	4 oz	160	22	0	1322	0	8.0	0
'Curemaster'	4 oz	140	22	1	1361	0	5.0	0
'Light & Lean 97'	2 oz	60	10	1	450	0	2.0	26
patty	1 patty	180	7	0	456	0	16.0	0
patty, w/cheese	1 patty	190	7	0	468	0	18.0	0
roll	4 oz	170	21	0	1338	0	10.0	0
spiced	3 oz	240	13	1	1093	0	21.0	0
(JM) '95% Fat-Free'	2 oz	60	10	1	680	0	2.0	0
(Light & Lean) 'No bone'	2 oz	60	10	0	574	0	2.0	0
(Oscar Mayer) 'Jubilee'	1 oz	29	5	0	287	0	0.9	14
(Rath) hickory smoked, 'Black Hawk'	2 oz	60	10	1	720	0	2.0	0
(Swift) patty, 'Premium Brown 'N Serve'	1 patty	130	3	1	260	0	13.0	0

Food Name	Serv. Size	Total Cal.	Prot. gms	Carbs gms	Sod. mgs	Fiber gms	Fat gms	Chol. mgs
CURED								
(NOTE: TRIMMED = Lean; separable fat removed. UNTRIMMED = Separable fat not removed.)								
Bone in, Boston butt, trimmed								
medium fat, chopped, roasted .... 1 cup		340	38.9	0.0	1393	0	19.3	123
medium fat, roasted .... 9.8 oz		678	77.6	0.0	2777	0	38.5	246
Bone in, whole								
honey glazed, 'Traditional' *(Carving Board)* .... 1 slice		50	8	1	560	0	1.5	25
trimmed, fully cooked, baked .... 3 oz		133	21.3	0.0	1128	0	4.7	47
trimmed, fully cooked, unheated .... 1 oz		42	6.3	0.0	430	0	1.6	15
smoked *(Carving Board)* .... 1 slice		45	8	0	570	0	1.5	20
untrimmed, fully cooked, baked .... 3 oz		207	18.3	0.0	1009	0	14.2	53
untrimmed, fully cooked, unheated .... 1 oz		70	5.2	0.0	364	0	5.3	16
water added, baked *(Carving Board)* .... 1 slice		50	8	1	550	0	1.5	25
Boneless								
breakfast, 'Light AM' *(Healthy Deli)* .... 1 oz		27	4	1	200	0	0.6	11
'Breakfast Ham' *(Oscar Mayer)* .... 1.5 oz slice		47	7	1	582	0	1.5	21
center slice, country-style, trimmed, unheated .... 4 oz		220	31	0	3045	0	9.4	79
center slice, country-style, untrimmed, heated .... 4 oz		229	23	0	1566	0	14.6	61
extra lean, approx 5% fat, baked .... 3 oz		123	17.8	1.3	1023	0	4.7	45
extra lean, approx 5% fat, baked, chopped .... 1 cup		203	29	2	1684	0	7.7	74
extra lean, approx 5% fat, unheated .... 1 oz		37	5.5	0.3	405	0	1.4	13
extra lean and regular, baked .... 3 oz		140	18.7	0.4	1177	0	6.5	48
extra lean and regular, baked, chopped .... 1 cup		231	31	1	1939	0	10.7	80
extra lean and regular, unheated .... 1 oz		46	5.2	0.7	362	0	2.4	15
extra lean and regular, unheated, chopped .... 1 cup		227	26	3	1789	0	11.7	74
extra lean and regular, unheated, 4 x 6 1/4 inch slice .... 1 slice		46	5.2	0.7	362	0	2.4	15
mini *(JM)* .... 3 oz		90	17	0	40	0	3.0	0
regular, approx 11% fat, baked .... 3 oz		151	19.2	0.0	1275	0	7.7	50
regular, approx 11% fat, baked, chopped .... 1 cup		249	32	0	2100	0	12.6	83
regular, approx 11% fat, unheated .... 1 oz		52	5.0	0.9	373	0	3.0	16
steak, dinner sliced *(Oscar Mayer)* .... 1 piece		60	10	0	750	0	2.0	30
steak, unheated .... 2 oz		69	11.1	0.0	720	0	2.4	26
whole *(JM)* .... 3 oz		140	17	0	40	0	8.0	0
w/natural juices, 'EZ Cut' *(JM)* .... 2 oz		70	11	1	660	0	3.0	0
Patty, raw .... 1 oz		89	4	0	308	0	8.0	20
Puréed *(Bryan Foods)* .... 1/3 cup		160	11	0	75	0	12.0	40
HAM DINNER/ENTRÉE								
(Armour) steak, frozen, 'Classics' .... 10.75 oz		270	15	36	1320	0	7.0	50
(Banquet) frozen, 'Platters' .... 10 oz		400	20	43	1180	0	17.0	50
(Cook's)								
hickory-smoked, honey, spiral-sliced .... 3 oz		150	14	2	850	0	10.0	30
hickory-smoked, honey, w/glaze, spiral-sliced, ... 3 oz		160	14	4	850	0	10.0	30
(Hormel) 96% nonfat, water added, cooked, 'Curemaster' ... 3 oz		80	14	0	940	0	3.0	40
(Le Menu) steak, frozen .... 10 oz		300	19	31	1500	0	11.0	0
(Louis Rich) dinner slices, baked, 98% fat-free .... 1 slice		80	16	1	1150	0	1.5	40
(Marie Callender's) steak, honey-smoked, w/macaroni and cheese .... 14 oz		490	29	63	2310	5	13.0	80
(Morton) frozen .... 10 oz		290	15	49	1400	0	4.0	45
(Pillsbury) casserole, w/cheese, 'Microwave Classic' ...... 1 pkg		470	18	34	1300	0	29.0	0
(Stouffer's) w/asparagus .... 1 entrée		520	16	32	1040	2	36.0	75
(Swanson) w/scalloped potatoes, 'Homestyle Recipe' .... 9 oz		300	19	26	1080	0	13.0	0
(West Virginia) boneless, no water added, cooked .... 3 oz		110	15	1	900	0	4.0	40
HAM SPREAD								
(Libby's) salad, 'Spreadables' .... 1/3 cup		110	8	8	621	4	4.5	20
(Hormel)								
deviled .... 1 oz		76	4	1	214	0	6.0	19

Food Name	Serv. Size	Total Cal.	Prot. gms	Carbs gms	Sod. mgs	Fiber gms	Fat gms	Chol. mgs
deviled	1 tbsp	35	2	0	108	0	3.0	0
(Underwood)								
deviled	2 1/8 oz	220	8	1	430	0	19.0	50
deviled, 'Light'	2 1/8 oz	120	11	1	250	0	8.0	35
deviled, smoked	2 1/8 oz	190	9	1	260	0	18.0	65
HAM SUBSTITUTE								
(Worthington) meatless, vegetarian, 'Wham'	1 slice	82	7	1	426	0	5.2	1
HAMBURG PARSLEY. See PARSLEY ROOT.								
HAMBURGER. See under BEEF, GROUND; BEEF DINNER/ENTRÉE. See also HAMBURGER ENTRÉE MIX.								
HAMBURGER BUN. See BUN, HAMBURGER.								
HAMBURGER ENTRÉE MIX								
(Hamburger Helper)								
beef noodle, mix only	1/5 pkg	140	5	26	1000	0	2.0	0
beef noodle, prepared	1 cup	320	20	26	1050	0	15.0	0
beef pasta, prepared	1 cup	270	20	26	910	1	10.0	50
beef Romanoff, prepared	1 cup	280	20	27	920	0	10.0	50
beef taco, prepared	1 cup	310	20	31	930	1	11.0	50
beef teriyaki, mix only	1/5 pkg	180	4	38	1110	0	1.0	0
beef teriyaki, prepared	1 cup	360	20	38	1160	0	14.0	0
cheddar 'n bacon meal, mix only	2/3 cup	170	7	25	810	1	5.0	10
cheddar 'n bacon meal, prepared	1 cup	350	24	28	890	1	16.0	65
cheeseburger macaroni meal, mix only	1/3 cup	180	5	30	860	1	4.0	5
cheeseburger macaroni meal, prepared	1 cup	360	23	33	940	1	15.0	65
cheesy Italian meal, mix only	1/2 cup	150	5	26	850	1	3.0	3
cheesy Italian meal, prepared	1 cup	330	22	29	920	1	14.0	60
chili macaroni meal, mix only	1/3 cup	140	3	30	820	1	1.0	0
chili macaroni meal, prepared	1 cup	290	19	30	870	1	10.0	55
chili tomato meal, mix only	1/5 pkg	150	5	31	1360	0	1.0	0
chili tomato meal, prepared	1 cup	330	20	31	1410	0	14.0	0
chili w/beans meal, mix only	1/4 pkg	130	5	25	1680	0	1.0	0
chili w/beans meal, prepared	1 1/4 cup	350	24	25	1740	0	17.0	0
creamy Stroganoff, prepared w/whole milk	1 cup	390	22	30	870	0	20.0	0
creamy Stroganoff, prepared	1 cup	320	21	30	830	0	13.0	55
hamburger hash meal, mix only	1/5 pkg	140	3	27	970	0	2.0	0
hamburger hash meal, prepared	1 cup	320	18	27	1020	0	15.0	0
hamburger stew meal, mix only	1/5 pkg	120	3	25	960	0	1.0	0
hamburger stew meal, prepared	1 cup	300	18	25	1010	0	14.0	0
lasagna meal, mix only	2/3 cup	140	4	30	950	0	1.0	0
lasagna meal, prepared	1 cup	280	19	30	990	0	10.0	50
meat loaf meal, mix only	1 1/2 tbsp	50	2	10	500	0	0.5	0
mushroom and wild rice meal, mix only	1/5 pkg	180	4	34	880	0	3.0	0
mushroom and wild rice meal, prepared	1 cup	380	21	37	950	0	16.0	0
nacho cheese meal, mix only	1/2 cup	160	5	28	860	1	2.5	0
nacho cheese meal, prepared	1 cup	320	22	30	930	1	13.0	55
pizza dish meal, mix only	1/5 pkg	180	6	37	960	0	1.0	0
pizza dish meal, prepared	1 cup	360	21	37	1010	0	14.0	0
pizza pasta w/cheese topping, mix only	1/2 cup	150	4	30	700	0	1.5	0
pizza pasta w/cheese topping, prepared	1 cup	290	19	31	750	0	10.0	50
pizzabake, mix only	1 serving	140	3	28	670	1	1.5	0
pizzabake, prepared	1 serving	270	17	28	720	1	10.0	45
potato Stroganoff meal, mix only	2/3 cup	120	2	24	810	2	2.0	0
potato Stroganoff meal, prepared	1 cup	270	18	25	870	2	12.0	55
potatoes au gratin meal, mix only	2/3 cup	120	3	23	740	2	2.5	3
potatoes au gratin meal, prepared	1 cup	290	18	24	820	2	14.0	55
rice Oriental meal, mix only	1/4 cup	160	3	35	1000	0	0.5	0
rice Oriental meal, prepared	1 cup	310	19	35	1050	0	10.0	55
sloppy Joe meal, mix only	1/6 pkg	180	5	33	1060	0	3.0	

Food Name	Serv. Size	Total Cal.	Prot. gms	Carbs gms	Sod. mgs	Fiber gms	Fat gms	Chol. mgs
sloppy Joe meal, prepared	5 oz	340	18	33	1100	0	15.0	0
spaghetti meal, mix only	1/2 cup	150	5	29	890	1	1.0	0
spaghetti meal, prepared	1 cup	300	21	29	940	1	11.0	55
Stroganoff meal, mix only	1/5 pkg	190	5	30	800	0	5.0	0
Stroganoff meal, prepared	2/3 cup	160	5	27	760	0	3.0	0
taco meal, 'Tacobake' mix only	1/6 pkg	170	4	31	920	0	4.0	0
taco meal, 'Tacobake' prepared	5.75 oz	320	17	31	940	0	15.0	0
tamale pie meal, mix only	1/5 pkg	200	4	39	890	0	3.0	0
tamale pie meal, prepared	1 cup	380	19	39	940	0	16.0	0
three cheese meal mix, prepared	1/5 pkg	400	24	32	980	0	20.0	0
three cheese meal, mix only	1/5 pkg	210	7	30	910	0	7.0	0
zesty Italian meal, mix only	1/3 cup	160	5	34	840	1	1.0	0
zesty Italian meal, prepared	1 cup	320	21	34	890	1	11.0	55

HAMBURGER RELISH. See under RELISH.
HAMBURGER SUBSTITUTE. See under BEEF SUBSTITUTE DINNER/ENTRÉE.
HARD ROLL. See under ROLL.
HARICOTS. See BEAN, FRENCH.
HASH
CORNED BEEF
(Armour)

Food Name	Serv. Size	Total Cal.	Prot. gms	Carbs gms	Sod. mgs	Fiber gms	Fat gms	Chol. mgs
canned	1 pkg	897	43	22	1539	3	71.0	174
canned	1 serving	498	24	12	854	2	39.4	97
(Hormel) canned	1 cup	387	21	22	1003	3	24.2	76

(Libby's)

Food Name	Serv. Size	Total Cal.	Prot. gms	Carbs gms	Sod. mgs	Fiber gms	Fat gms	Chol. mgs
	1 cup	470	21	25	1200	8	35.0	90
	1/4 cup	120	15	0	490	0	7.0	50

(Nestlé)

Food Name	Serv. Size	Total Cal.	Prot. gms	Carbs gms	Sod. mgs	Fiber gms	Fat gms	Chol. mgs
'Chef Mate'	1 pkg	5823	291	348	19108	73	363.7	1062
'Chef Mate'	1 cup	486	24	29	1594	6	30.3	89

ROAST BEEF

Food Name	Serv. Size	Total Cal.	Prot. gms	Carbs gms	Sod. mgs	Fiber gms	Fat gms	Chol. mgs
(Libby's)	1 cup	460	19	23	1390	3	33.0	80
(Hormel) canned	1 cup	385	21	23	793	4	23.6	73

HAWAIIAN YAM. See under YAM.

Food Name	Serv. Size	Total Cal.	Prot. gms	Carbs gms	Sod. mgs	Fiber gms	Fat gms	Chol. mgs
HAWS/hawthorn tree fruit, scarlet, w/skin, raw	3.5 oz	87	2.0	20.8	0	>2.1	0.7	0

HAZELNUT/cobnut/filbert

Food Name	Serv. Size	Total Cal.	Prot. gms	Carbs gms	Sod. mgs	Fiber gms	Fat gms	Chol. mgs
dried	1 oz	178	4	5	0	3	17.2	0
dried	10 medium	88	2	2	0	1	8.5	0
dried, blanched	1 oz	178	4	5	0	3	17.3	0
dried, chopped	1 cup	722	17	19	0	11	69.9	0
dried, ground	1 cup	471	11	13	0	7	45.6	0
dried, whole	1 cup	848	20	23	0	13	82.0	0
dry-roasted, no salt added	1 oz	183	4	5	0	3	17.7	0
natural, unsalted *(Flanigan Farms)*	1/4 cup	180	4	4	0	2	18.0	0
natural, whole *(Oregon Hazelnuts)*	1/2 cup	396	11	12	1	9	36.8	0

HAZELNUT BUTTER

Food Name	Serv. Size	Total Cal.	Prot. gms	Carbs gms	Sod. mgs	Fiber gms	Fat gms	Chol. mgs
creamy, roasted fresh, no salt added *(Roaster Fresh)*	1 oz	188	4	5	1	0	19.0	0

HAZELNUT OIL

Food Name	Serv. Size	Total Cal.	Prot. gms	Carbs gms	Sod. mgs	Fiber gms	Fat gms	Chol. mgs
	1 cup	1927	0	0	0	0	218.0	0
	1 tbsp	120	0	0	0	0	13.6	0
(International Collection)	1 tbsp	120	0	0	0	0	14.0	0

HAZELNUT SPREAD

Food Name	Serv. Size	Total Cal.	Prot. gms	Carbs gms	Sod. mgs	Fiber gms	Fat gms	Chol. mgs
w/milk and cocoa, 'Nutella' *(Ferrero)*	1 tbsp	80	1	9	10	0	5.0	0

HEAD CHEESE. See under SAUSAGE.
HEART NUT. See CASHEW.
HEARTS OF PALM. See under PALM.
HERB SEASONING MIX. See under SEASONING MIX.

Food Name	Serv. Size	Total Cal.	Prot. gms	Carbs gms	Sod. mgs	Fiber gms	Fat gms	Chol. mgs
HERBAL TEA. See under TEA.								
HERRING								
ATLANTIC								
fillet, baked, broiled, grilled, or microwaved	3 oz	173	20	0	98	0	9.9	65
fillet, kippered, large, approx 7 x 2.25 x 1/4 inch	1 fillet	141	16	0	597	0	8.0	53
fillet, kippered, medium, approx 5 x 1.75 x 1/4 inch	1 fillet	87	10	0	367	0	4.9	33
fillet, kippered, small, approx 2-3/8 x 1-3/8 x 1/4 inch	1 fillet	43	5	0	184	0	2.5	16
fillet, kippered, boneless	1 oz	62	7	0	260	0	3.5	23
fillet, kippered, smoked, salt added (Crown Prince)	1/4 cup	110	11	0	230	0	8.0	35
fillet, kippered, w/naturally smoked wood flavoring (Beach Cliff)	3.3 oz	220	17	1	475	0	17.0	0
pickled	1 cup	367	20	13	1218	0	25.2	18
pickled, approx 1.75 x 7/8 x 1/2 inch	1 piece	39	2	1	131	0	2.7	2
pickled, boneless	1 oz	74	4	3	247	0	5.1	4
raw	3 oz	134	15	0	77	0	7.7	51
raw, boneless	1 oz	45	5	0	26	0	2.6	17
snacks, kippered, w/smoke flavoring, drained (Beach Cliff)	3.3 oz	220	17	1	350	0	17.0	0
steaks, in soybean oil, drained (Beach Cliff)	3 oz	240	16	0	350	0	20.0	0
steaks, in water, drained (Beach Cliff)	3 oz	230	17	1	350	0	18.0	0
steaks, w/mustard, drained (Beach Cliff)	3 oz	227	13	4	350	0	18.0	0
steaks, w/tomato, drained (Beach Cliff)	3 oz	210	15	0	350	0	17.0	0
PACIFIC								
baked, broiled, grilled, or miocrowaved	3 oz	213	18	0	81	0	15.1	84
raw	3 oz	166	14	0	63	0	11.8	65
HERRING OIL. See under FISH OIL.								
HICKORY NUT								
dried	1 cup	788	15	22	1	8	77.2	0
dried	1 oz	186	4	5	0	2	18.2	0
dried	1 medium	20	0	1	0	0	1.9	0
HIRITAKE. See MUSHROOM, OYSTER.								
HIZIKI. See under SEA VEGETABLE.								
HOG PLUM. See JOBO.								
HOMINY. See under GRITS.								
HON SHIMEJI. See MUSHROOM, JAPANESE HONEY.								
HONEY								
(Golden Blossom)	1 tbsp	60	0	16	0	0	0.0	0
(Knott's Berry Farm)	1 tbsp	60	0	17	0	0	0.0	0
(Sioux)	1 tbsp	60	0	16	0	0	0.0	0
mesquite, desert, 100%, raw, wild, unblended (Trader Joe's)	1 tbsp	60	0	17	0	0	0.0	0
strained or extracted	1 cup	1031	1	279	14	1	0.0	0
strained or extracted	1 tbsp	64	0	17	1	0	0.0	0
HONEY BUTTER (Honey Butter)	1 tbsp	50	1	11	5	0	1.0	0
HONEY MUSHROOM. See MUSHROOM, JAPANESE HONEY.								
HONEYDEW MELON. See MELON, HONEYDEW.								
HORSE								
raw	1 oz	38	6	0	15	0	1.3	15
roasted	3 oz	149	24	0	47	0	5.1	58
roasted, boneless, yield from 1 lb raw	11.9 oz	595	96	0	187	0	20.6	231
HORSE BEAN. See BEAN, FAVA.								
HORSERADISH								
Prepared								
	1 tbsp	7	0	2	47	0	0.1	0
	1 tsp	2	0	1	16	0	0.0	0
(Crowley)	1 oz	10	1	2	25	0	1.0	0
(Gold's) hot	1 tsp	4	1	1	60	0	1.0	0

Food Name	Serv. Size	Total Cal.	Prot. gms	Carbs gms	Sod. mgs	Fiber gms	Fat gms	Chol. mgs
(Gold's) red	1 tsp	4	1	1	75	0	0.0	0
(Gold's) white	1 tsp	4	1	1	55	0	1.0	0
(Kraft)	1 tbsp	10	0	1	140	0	0.0	0
(Kraft) cream style	1 tbsp	12	0	1	85	0	0.0	0
(Silver Spring) cream style	1 tsp	0	0	0	10	0	0.0	0
Raw	1 lb	288	10.6	65.3	27	>7.9 c	1.0	0
HORSERADISH, JAPANESE. See WASABI ROOT.								
HORSERADISH SPREAD *(Alouette)* cheese and chive	1 oz	85	2	1	130	0	8.0	28
HORSERADISH TREE								
leafy tips, boiled, drained, chopped	1 cup	25	2	5	4	1	0.4	0
leafy tips, raw, chopped	1 cup	13	2	2	2	0	0.3	0
pods, boiled, drained, sliced	1 cup	42	2	10	51	5	0.2	0
pods, raw, sliced	1 cup	37	2	9	42	3	0.2	0
pods, raw, whole, approx 15 1/3 inch long	1 pod	4	0	1	5	0	0.0	0
HOT COCOA. See COCOA, HOT, MIX.								
HOT DOG. See FRANKFURTER.								
HOT DOG BUN. See BUN, FRANKFURTER.								
HUBBARD SQUASH. See SQUASH, HUBBARD.								
HUMMUS MIX								
(Fantastic Foods) mix only	2 tbsp	60	3	9	220	2	2.0	0
(Casbah) prepared	1 oz	160	5	14	180	1	8.0	0
HUMPBACK SALMON. See under SALMON.								
HUNGARIAN PEPPER. See PEPPER, HUNGARIAN.								
HUSHPUPPY								
(SeaPak) regular, frozen	4 oz	330	6	56	690	0	9.0	0
(Stilwell) jalapeño, frozen	3 pieces	70	2	4	360	2	5.0	0
(Stilwell) regular, frozen	3 pieces	140	2	19	310	2	6.0	0
HUSHPUPPY MIX								
(Golden Dipt)								
deluxe	1.25 oz	120	3	26	520	0	0.0	0
jalapeño	1.25 oz	120	3	27	570	0	0.0	0
w/onion	1.25 oz	120	3	27	520	0	0.0	0
HYACINTH BEAN. See BEAN, HYACINTH.								

I

Food Name	Serv. Size	Total Cal.	Prot. gms	Carbs gms	Sod. mgs	Fiber gms	Fat gms	Chol. mgs
ICE BAR/DESSERT. See also FRUIT BAR, FROZEN; SHERBET; SORBET.								
BAR								
(Cool Creations)								
fruit flavors, nonfat, 'Mickey & Minnie Surprise Pop'	1 pop	60	0	14	5	0	0.0	0
(Crystal Light) all flavors, nonfat	1 bar	14	0	2	10	0	0.0	0
(Eskimo Pie) vanilla, w/dark chocolate coating	1 bar	166	2	12	34	na	12.1	14
(Freezer Pleezer) assorted flavors, nonfat	1 bar	40	0	10	0	0	0.0	0
(Gold Bond) all flavors, nonfat, 'Twin Pop'	1 bar	60	0	14	0	0	0.0	0
(Good Humor)								
all flavors, nonfat, 'Ice Stripes'	1 bar	35	0	9	0	0	0.0	0
cherry, 'Calippo'	1 bar	138	0	35	5	0	0.1	0
cherry, Italian	6 oz	138	0	34	0	0	0.1	0
lemon, 'Calippo'	1 bar	112	0	28	0	0	0.1	0
orange, 'Calippo'	1 bar	111	0	27	0	0	0.2	0
(Jell-O)								
all flavors nonfat, 'Gelatin Pops'	1 bar	35	1	8	25	0	0.0	0
lemon, nonfat, 'Snowburst Bars'	1 bar	45	0	12	10	0	0.0	0
orange, nonfat, 'Snowburst Bars'	1 bar	45	0	12	10	0	0.0	0

Food Name	Serv. Size	Total Cal.	Prot. gms	Carbs gms	Sod. mgs	Fiber gms	Fat gms	Chol. mgs
(Klondike Bar) vanilla, w/chocolate coating . . . . 1 bar		489	6	36	108	na	35.7	40
(Kool-Aid)								
all flavors, 'Cream Pops' . . . . 1 bar		50	1	9	20	0	2.0	5
all flavors, 'Kool Pumps' . . . . 1 snack		80	1	16	25	0	1.0	5
all flavors, nonfat, 'Kool Pops' . . . . 1 bar		40	0	10	10	0	0.0	0
(Mama Tish's)								
Italian ice, cherry, made w/real fruit . . . . 4 oz		120	0	29	0	0	0.0	0
Italian ice, lemon, made w/real fruit . . . . 4 oz		90	0	24	0	0	0.0	0
Italian ice, strawberry, made w/real fruit . . . . 4 oz		80	1	21	5	0	0.0	0
Italian ice, tropical, made w/real fruit . . . . 4 oz		110	0	27	0	0	0.0	0
(Popsicle)								
all flavors, 'All Natural' . . . . 1 bar		60	0	14	0	0	0.0	0
all flavors, except cherry and wildberry, 'Water Ice' . . . . 1 bar		50	0	12	10	0	0.0	0
cherry, cola/cherry, 'Twister' . . . . 1 piece		45	0	10	0	0	0.0	0
cherry, 'Water Ice' . . . . 1 bar		70	0	17	15	0	0.0	0
wildberry, 'Water Ice' . . . . 1 bar		40	0	10	10	0	0.0	0
(Push-ups) assorted, orange, cherry, grape, 'Flintstones' . . 1 tube		100	1	20	25	0	2.0	5
(Tootsie Pop) assorted, cherry, grape, orange . . . . 1 bar		70	2	13	32	0	1.0	4
ITALIAN ICE								
(Luigi's)								
cherry . . . . 1 cup		120	1	28	10	0	0.0	0
chocolate fudge . . . . 1 cup		150	1	38	10	0	0.0	0
grape . . . . 1 cup		110	0	26	10	0	0.0	0
lemon . . . . 1 cup		110	1	25	10	0	0.0	0
strawberry . . . . 1 cup		110	1	26	10	0	0.0	0
ICE CREAM. See also ICE CREAM BAR/DESSERT; ICE CREAM CONE; ICE CREAM MIX; ICE CREAM SUBSTITUTE; ICE CREAM SUBSTITUTE BAR/DESSERT; ICE CREAM SUBSTITUTE MIX; ICE MILK.								
(Borden)								
butter pecan, 'Lady Borden' . . . . 1/2 cup		180	3	16	65	0	12.0	0
chocolate swirl . . . . 1/2 cup		130	2	18	65	0	6.0	0
chocolate, Dutch, 'Olde Fashioned Recipe' . . . . 1/2 cup		130	2	16	65	0	6.0	0
strawberry . . . . 1/2 cup		130	2	18	55	0	6.0	0
strawberry cream, 'Olde Fashioned Recipe' . . . . 1/2 cup		130	2	19	55	0	5.0	0
vanilla, 'Olde Fashioned Recipe' . . . . 1/2 cup		130	2	15	55	0	7.0	0
(Breyers)								
butter almond . . . . 1/2 cup		170	4	15	125	0	10.0	25
butter pecan . . . . 1/2 cup		180	3	15	125	0	12.0	25
cherry vanilla . . . . 1/2 cup		150	3	17	45	0	7.0	20
chocolate . . . . 1/2 cup		160	3	20	30	0	8.0	20
chocolate chip . . . . 1/2 cup		170	3	18	45	0	10.0	35
coffee . . . . 1/2 cup		150	3	16	50	0	8.0	30
cookies and cream . . . . 1/2 cup		170	3	19	60	0	9.0	20
mint chocolate chip . . . . 1/2 cup		170	3	18	45	0	10.0	25
mocha almond fudge . . . . 1/2 cup		190	4	20	60	0	10.0	0
peach, natural . . . . 1/2 cup		130	2	18	35	0	6.0	15
strawberry . . . . 1/2 cup		130	2	16	40	0	6.0	20
vanilla . . . . 1/2 cup		150	3	15	50	0	8.0	25
vanilla fudge twirl . . . . 1/2 cup		160	3	19	55	0	8.0	20
vanilla-chocolate . . . . 1/2 cup		160	3	17	40	0	8.0	25
vanilla-chocolate-strawberry . . . . 1/2 cup		150	3	17	40	0	8.0	20
(Darigold)								
chocolate . . . . 1/2 cup		140	2	17	70	0	7.0	0
chocolate, 'Alpine' . . . . 1/2 cup		140	2	17	70	0	7.0	0
chocolate, 'Classic' . . . . 1/2 cup		180	3	16	30	0	13.0	0
vanilla . . . . 1/2 cup		130	2	15	50	0	7.0	0
vanilla, 'Alpine' . . . . 1/2 cup		130	2	15	50	0	7.0	0
vanilla, 'Classic' . . . . 1/2 cup		180	2	16	40	0	12.0	0

Food Name	Serv. Size	Total Cal.	Prot. gms	Carbs gms	Sod. mgs	Fiber gms	Fat gms	Chol. mgs
(Dreyer's/Edys)								
black cherry vanilla, fat-free	1/2 cup	100	3	22	45	na	0.0	0
black cherry vanilla, sugar-free	1/2 cup	90	3	12	50	na	3.0	10
butter pecan, light	1/2 cup	120	3	16	100	na	5.0	20
caramel cream, dreamy, light	1/2 cup	110	2	18	60	na	3.0	20
chocolate almond fudge, light	1/2 cup	120	3	16	45	na	5.0	20
chocolate chip	1/2 cup	150	3	16	40	0	9.0	30
chocolate fudge, fat-free	1/2 cup	110	3	25	55	na	0.0	0
chocolate fudge mousse, light	1/2 cup	110	3	17	50	na	3.0	20
cookie dough, light	1/2 cup	130	3	19	75	na	5.0	20
cookies and cream	1/2 cup	160	3	18	80	0	9.0	28
cookies and cream, light	1/2 cup	120	3	17	65	na	4.0	20
espresso fudge chip, light	1/2 cup	120	3	18	60	na	4.0	15
'French Silk' light	1/2 cup	120	3	19	55	na	4.0	15
fudge, marble	1/2 cup	150	3	18	50	0	8.0	28
marble fudge, fat-free	1/2 cup	110	3	24	55	na	0.0	0
marble fudge, sugar-free	1/2 cup	90	3	13	60	na	3.0	10
mint fudge, fat free	1/2 cup	110	3	24	55	na	0.0	0
mocha fudge, sugar-free	1/2 cup	90	3	13	60	na	3.0	10
peanut butter cup, light	1/2 cup	130	3	17	55	na	5.0	20
raspberry vanilla, fat free, sugar-free	1/2 cup	90	3	19	45	na	0.0	0
rocky road	1/2 cup	170	3	18	30	0	10.0	30
rocky road, light	1/2 cup	120	3	17	45	na	4.0	20
strawberry, sugar-free	1/2 cup	80	3	11	50	na	3.0	10
triple chocolate, sugar-free	1/2 cup	100	3	13	60	na	3.5	10
vanilla	1/2 cup	160	2	14	30	0	10.0	40
vanilla, fat-free	1/2 cup	100	3	22	45	na	0.0	0
vanilla, light	1/2 cup	100	3	15	50	na	3.0	20
vanilla, sugar-free	1/2 cup	80	3	11	55	na	3.0	10
vanilla and caramel, sugar-free	1/2 cup	90	3	13	60	na	3.0	10
vanilla-chocolate, fat free, sugar-free	1/2 cup	100	4	20	50	na	0.0	0
(Eagle Brand) vanilla, 'Homestyle'	1/2 cup	150	3	16	55	0	9.0	0
(Eskimo Pie) chocolate chip cone, 'Cookie Dough'	1 cone	280	4	33	103	0	14.0	14
(Frusen Gladje)								
butter pecan	1/2 cup	280	5	16	160	0	21.0	85
chocolate chocolate chip	1/2 cup	270	5	21	60	0	18.0	55
chocolate	1/2 cup	240	5	17	65	0	17.0	75
chocolate, Swiss candy almond	1/2 cup	270	6	18	60	0	19.0	55
strawberry	1/2 cup	230	4	20	60	0	15.0	65
vanilla	1/2 cup	230	5	16	70	0	17.0	65
vanilla Swiss almond	1/2 cup	270	6	18	65	0	19.0	65
vanilla toffee chunk	1/2 cup	270	5	22	160	0	17.0	85
(Good Humor)								
vanilla, 'Cup'	3 oz	98	2	12	35	0	5.1	0
vanilla-chocolate cup, 'Combo'	6 oz	201	4	26	80	0	9.2	0
(Haagen-Dazs)								
caramel nut sundae	1/2 cup	310	5	26	100	0	21.0	0
chocolate fudge, deep	1/2 cup	290	5	26	70	0	14.0	0
chocolate mint	1/2 cup	300	5	26	50	0	20.0	0
chocolate, deep	1/2 cup	290	5	26	70	0	14.0	0
chocolate, low-fat	1/2 cup	170	7	29	50	1	2.5	30
chocolate-peanut butter, deep	1/2 cup	330	7	25	90	0	19.0	0
coffee fudge, low-fat	1/2 cup	170	5	32	95	0	2.5	25
'Cookie Dough Dynamo'	4 oz	300	4	31	110	0	18.0	0
strawberry, low-fat	1/2 cup	150	5	28	40	0	2.0	15
vanilla, low-fat	1/2 cup	170	7	29	50	0	2.5	20
vanilla honey	1/2 cup	250	5	22	55	0	16.0	135

Food Name	Serv. Size	Total Cal.	Prot. gms	Carbs gms	Sod. mgs	Fiber gms	Fat gms	Chol. mgs
vanilla-peanut butter swirl	1/2 cup	280	5	19	120	0	21.0	110
(Healthy Choice)								
Black Forest, low-fat	1/2 cup	120	3	23	50	1	2.0	5
Bordeaux cherry, 'Dairy Dessert'	4 oz	120	3	23	50	0	2.0	5
Bordeaux cherry chocolate chip 'Dairy Dessert'	4 oz	120	3	23	50	0	2.0	5
butter pecan crunch, low-fat	1/2 cup	120	3	22	60	1	2.0	3
cappuccino chocolate chunk, low-fat	1/2 cup	120	3	22	60	1	2.0	10
cappuccino mocha fudge, low-fat	1/2 cup	120	3	23	50	1	2.0	3
chocolate, 'Dairy Dessert'	4 oz	130	3	24	70	0	2.0	5
chocolate chip, 'Dairy Dessert'	4 oz	130	3	24	70	0	2.0	5
coffee toffee, 'Dairy Dessert'	4 oz	130	3	25	80	0	2.0	5
cookies and cream, low-fat	1/2 cup	120	3	21	90	1	2.0	3
double fudge swirl, 'Dairy Dessert'	4 oz	130	3	24	70	0	2.0	5
fudge brownie, low-fat	1/2 cup	120	3	22	55	1	2.0	5
fudge brownie à la mode, low-fat	1/2 cup	120	3	22	55	1	2.0	5
mint chocolate chip, low-fat	1/2 cup	120	3	21	50	1	2.0	3
Neapolitan, 'Dairy Dessert'	4 oz	120	3	22	60	0	2.0	5
praline and caramel, low-fat	1/2 cup	130	3	25	70	1	2.0	3
praline caramel cluster, low-fat	1/2 cup	130	3	25	70	1	2.0	3
raspberry swirl, 'Dairy Dessert'	4 oz	120	3	23	60	0	2.0	5
rocky road, 'Dairy Dessert'	4 oz	160	3	32	70	0	2.0	5
strawberry, 'Dairy Dessert'	4 oz	120	2	23	50	0	2.0	5
turtle fudge cake, low-fat	1/2 cup	130	3	25	60	2	2.0	3
vanilla, 'Dairy Dessert'	4 oz	120	4	21	60	0	2.0	5
vanilla, old fashioned, 'Dairy Dessert'	4 oz	120	4	21	60	0	2.0	5
(Nutra/Balance) high-calorie and -protein	1 serving	232	7	25	79	0	12.0	46
(Sealtest)								
butter crunch	1/2 cup	150	2	18	90	0	7.0	25
butter pecan	1/2 cup	160	3	16	125	0	9.0	15
chocolate	1/2 cup	140	2	18	50	0	6.0	20
chocolate chip	1/2 cup	150	2	17	50	0	8.0	15
chocolate triple stripes	1/2 cup	140	2	17	50	0	7.0	0
chocolate-marshmallow sundae	1/2 cup	150	2	21	40	0	6.0	20
coffee	1/2 cup	140	2	16	50	0	7.0	15
fudge Royale	1/2 cup	140	3	19	55	0	7.0	15
heavenly hash	1/2 cup	150	2	19	50	0	7.0	15
maple walnut	1/2 cup	160	3	17	40	0	9.0	20
peanut fudge sundae	1/2 cup	140	3	17	50	0	7.0	20
strawberry	1/2 cup	130	2	18	40	0	5.0	15
vanilla	1/2 cup	140	2	16	50	0	7.0	20
vanilla, French	1/2 cup	140	2	16	50	0	7.0	35
vanilla-chocolate-strawberry 'Cubic Scoops'	1/2 cup	130	2	17	50	0	6.0	20
vanilla-chocolate-strawberry	1/2 cup	140	2	18	50	0	6.0	20
vanilla-orange sherbet, 'Cubic Scoops'	1/2 cup	130	2	22	40	0	4.0	15
vanilla-red raspberry sherbet, 'Cubic Scoops'	1/2 cup	130	2	22	40	0	4.0	15
(TCBY Treats)								
all flavors, hand-dipped	1/2 cup	140	2	17	60	0	7.0	25
all flavors, hand-dipped, low-fat, no added sugar	1/2 cup	100	3	19	60	0	2.5	10
all flavors, hand-dipped, nonfat	1/2 cup	100	2	23	50	1	0.0	0
(Weight Watchers)								
chocolate chip, 'ONE-ders'	4 oz	120	3	19	80	0	4.0	10
'Cookie Dough Craze'	1/2 cup	140	3	24	85	1	3.5	5
heavenly hash 'ONE-ders'	4 oz	130	4	22	90	0	3.0	10
'Oh! So Very Vanilla' light	1/2 cup	120	4	20	65	1	2.5	5
'Positively Praline Crunch' light	1/2 cup	140	3	25	105	0	3.0	5
pralines and creme, 'ONE-ders'	4 oz	120	3	19	110	0	4.0	10
'Reckless Rocky Road'	1/2 cup	140	4	23	75	1	3.0	5

Food Name	Serv. Size	Total Cal.	Prot. gms	Carbs gms	Sod. mgs	Fiber gms	Fat gms	Chol. mgs
'Triple Chocolate Tornado' light	1/2 cup	150	4	26	80	1	3.5	5

ICE CREAM BAR/DESSERT
BAR
(Baker's)

Food Name	Serv. Size	Total Cal.	Prot. gms	Carbs gms	Sod. mgs	Fiber gms	Fat gms	Chol. mgs
chocolate fudge sundae 'Fudgetastic'	1 bar	220	3	23	45	0	15.0	20
chocolate fudge sundae, crunchy, 'Fudgetastic'	1 bar	230	3	24	40	0	14.0	20
(Eskimo Pie)								
vanilla, w/dark chocolate coating	1 bar	180	2	16	35	0	12.0	0
vanilla, w/milk chocolate coating	1 bar	190	5	18	16	0	12.0	0
vanilla, w/milk chocolate coating, almonds	1 bar	140	3	12	35	0	13.0	0
vanilla, w/milk chocolate coating, crisp rice	1 bar	150	4	12	40	0	11.0	0
(Freezer Pleezer) vanilla, w/chocolate flavored coating	1 bar	140	2	13	25	1	9.0	15
(Good Humor)								
'Fat Frog'	1 bar	154	2	16	36	0	9.2	0
'Halo Bar'	1 bar	230	4	23	64	0	13.7	0
'Whammy' assorted flavors	1 bar	95	1	7	17	0	7.2	0
chip candy crunch	1 bar	255	2	21	40	0	17.9	0
chocolate éclair	1 bar	188	2	23	54	0	9.9	0
chocolate fudge cake	1 bar	214	2	18	50	0	15.0	0
strawberry shortcake	1 bar	176	2	24	88	0	8.2	0
toasted almond	1 bar	212	2	24	34	0	11.8	0
vanilla, w/chocolate flavor coating	1 bar	198	2	17	44	0	13.7	0
(Haagen-Dazs)								
caramel almond, 'Crunch Bar'	1 bar	240	3	17	65	0	18.0	40
peanut butter, 'Crunch Bar'	1 bar	270	6	16	55	0	21.0	35
vanilla, 'Crunch Bar'	1 bar	220	3	16	55	0	16.0	40
vanilla, w/milk chocolate-brittle coating	1 bar	370	5	32	160	0	25.0	0
(Heath) 1 bar	1 bar	170	3	16	155	0	13.0	0
(Klondike)								
chocolate	1 bar	270	4	23	60	0	19.0	0
'Krispy'	1 bar	290	4	26	70	0	19.0	0
'Lite'	1 bar	140	3	10	45	0	10.0	10
w/chocolate flavored coating, 'Lite'	1 bar	110	3	14	50	0	6.0	5
(Natural Nectar)								
banana cream, 'Stick Novelties'	1 bar	170	3	22	70	0	8.0	20
cocoa fudge and cream, 'Stick Novelties'	1 bar	170	3	22	70	0	8.0	20
strawberries and cream, 'Stick Novelties'	1 bar	120	2	18	40	0	5.0	15
wildberry cream, 'Stick Novelties'	1 bar	120	2	22	50	0	3.0	15
(Nestlé)								
chocolate, w/milk chocolate coating, 'Quik'	1 bar	210	3	19	40	0	14.0	0
milk chocolate, w/almonds, milk chocolate coated	1 bar	350	6	28	45	0	23.0	5
vanilla, w/chocolate coating, crisp rice, 'Crunch'	1 bar	180	2	15	0	0	13.0	0
vanilla, w/chocolate coating, crisp rice, 'Crunch Lite'	1 bar	120	2	16	50	0	5.0	0
vanilla, w/white chocolate coating, 'Alpine Premium'	1 bar	350	6	25	50	0	25.0	5
(Oh Henry!)								
vanilla, w/caramel peanut, milk chocolate coating	1 bar	320	1	34	75	0	20.0	0
(Weight Watchers)								
chocolate, 'Treat Bars'	1 bar	100	4	18	75	0	1.0	0
chocolate fudge, double	1 bar	60	3	12	50	0	1.0	5
chocolate mousse, sugar-free	1 bar	35	2	9	30	0	1.0	5
CONE								
(Good Humor)								
'King Cone'	5.5 oz	290	5	41	119	0	12.0	0
boysenberry, 'King Cone'	5 oz	340	4	52	151	0	13.1	0
NOVELTY								
(Carnation)								
vanilla nuggets, w/dark chocolate coating, 'Bon Bons'	5 pieces	170	2	15	50	0	11.0	14

Food Name	Serv. Size	Total Cal.	Prot. gms	Carbs gms	Sod. mgs	Fiber gms	Fat gms	Chol. mgs
vanilla nuggets, w/milk chocolate coating, 'Bon Bons' ...	5 pieces	165	2	14	50	0	11.0	16
(Natural Nectar)								
mocha 'Round Novelties'	4 oz	300	4	40	135	0	14.0	10
nectar 'Round Novelties'	4 oz	300	4	38	120	0	15.0	15
SANDWICH								
(Eskimo Pie) vanilla, w/chocolate wafer	1 sandwich	170	4	26	142	0	6.0	0
(Good Humor)								
vanilla	1 sandwich	191	4	31	155	0	5.7	0
vanilla, w/chocolate chip cookie	1 sandwich	246	3	35	181	0	10.5	0
(Klondike)								
vanilla, 'Lite'	1 sandwich	100	2	18	110	0	2.0	5
vanilla	1 sandwich	230	5	33	220	0	9.0	0
(Weight Watchers)								
sandwich snack	1 sandwich	90	2	17	120	0	2.0	0
vanilla	1 sandwich	150	3	28	170	0	3.0	5
ICE CREAM CONE								
(Bozo)								
cake cup	1 cone	16	1	3	13	0	0.0	0
sugar	1 cone	53	1	11	29	0	1.0	0
(Comet)								
sugar	1 cone	50	1	11	40	0	0.0	0
waffle	1 cone	70	1	14	30	1	0.5	0
(Ener-G Foods) gluten free	1 cone	154	0	36	1	1	1.1	0
(Joy)	1 cone	16	1	3	5	0	1.0	0
(Keebler)								
cup, assorted colors	1 cone	15	1	4	20	0	1.0	0
cup, large, food service product	1 serving	15	0	4	20	0	0.0	0
plain	1 cone	15	1	4	20	0	1.0	0
sugar	1 cone	45	1	11	35	0	1.0	0
sugar, food service product	1 serving	47	1	10	28	0	0.2	0
waffle bowl, large, food service product	1 serving	60	1	12	20	0	1.5	1
waffle cone, large, food service product	1 serving	100	2	20	35	0	2.0	0
(Little Debbie) plain, 'Ice Cream Cup'	1 cone	15	0	3	15	0	0.1	1
(Nabisco)								
cup	1 cone	18	1	4	5	0	1.0	0
cup, 'Comet'	1 cone	18	1	4	5	0	1.0	0
sugar	1 cone	50	1	11	40	0	1.0	0
ICE CREAM MIX								
(Salada)								
Dutch chocolate, mix only	1 oz	110	1	26	20	0	0.0	0
Dutch chocolate, prepared	1 cup	310	4	31	75	0	19.0	0
peach, vanilla, mix only	1 oz	110	0	27	10	0	0.0	0
peach, vanilla, prepared	1 cup	310	4	32	60	0	18.0	0
peach, wild strawberry, mix only	1 oz	110	0	27	10	0	0.0	0
peach, wild strawberry, prepared	1 cup	310	4	32	60	0	18.0	0
ICE CREAM SANDWICH. See under ICE CREAM BAR/DESSERT.								
ICE CREAM SUBSTITUTE. See also YOGURT, FROZEN.								
(Freezees Nutcreem)								
butter pecan, nondairy, 100% natural	3 oz	131	4	17	78	0	7.0	0
cashew vanilla, nondairy, 100% natural	3 oz	131	4	17	78	0	7.0	0
lemon, nondairy, 100% natural	3 oz	131	4	17	78	0	7.0	0
orange, nondairy, 100% natural	3 oz	131	4	17	78	0	7.0	0
peanut, nondairy, 100% natural, 'Delight'	3 oz	131	4	17	78	0	7.0	0
strawberry, nondairy, 100% natural	3 oz	131	4	17	78	0	7.0	0
(Ice Bean)								
almond espresso, nondairy	4 oz	150	3	13	60	0	10.0	0
chocolate, nondairy, nonfat, 'Thunder'	1/2 cup	110	1	27	30	1	0.0	0

Food Name	Serv. Size	Total Cal.	Prot. gms	Carbs gms	Sod. mgs	Fiber gms	Fat gms	Chol. mgs
peanut butter carob chip, nondairy	4 oz	200	3	18	100	0	13.0	0
'Raspberry Patch' nondairy, nonfat	1/2 cup	110	1	27	30	1	0.0	0
'Vanilla Wavy' nondairy, nonfat	1/2 cup	110	1	27	30	1	0.0	0
(Living Rightly)								
almond pecan, nondairy	1/2 cup	140	3	21	75	0	5.0	0
carob peppermint, nondairy	1/2 cup	100	2	21	30	0	1.5	0
chocolate almond, nondairy	1/2 cup	140	3	21	75	0	5.0	0
vanilla, nondairy	1/2 cup	110	2	22	15	0	1.0	0
vanilla Swiss almond, nondairy	1/2 cup	140	3	21	75	0	5.0	0
(Low, Lite 'n Luscious)								
chocolate chip	1/2 cup	100	3	19	80	0	2.0	4
Jamoca Swiss almond	1/2 cup	90	3	19	100	0	2.0	4
pineapple coconut	1/2 cup	90	3	19	70	0	1.0	3
strawberry	1/2 cup	80	3	17	70	0	1.0	3
(Mocha Mix)								
strawberry swirl, nondairy, 100% milk-free	1/2 cup	140	1	20	55	0	6.0	0
vanilla, nondairy, 100% milk-free	1/2 cup	140	1	18	70	0	7.0	0
(Rice Dream)								
cappuccino flavor, nondairy	1/2 cup	130	1	17	80	0	5.0	0
carob almond, nondairy	1/2 cup	140	1	20	85	2	6.0	0
carob chip, nondairy	1/2 cup	130	1	20	70	1	6.0	0
carob, nondairy	1/2 cup	130	1	20	80	0	5.0	0
cocoa marble fudge, nondairy	1/2 cup	140	1	19	80	0	6.0	0
cookies and cream, nondairy	1/2 cup	130	1	21	80	0	5.0	0
lemon, nondairy	1/2 cup	130	1	17	80	0	5.0	0
mint carob chip, nondairy	1/2 cup	130	1	20	70	1	6.0	0
Neapolitan, nondairy	1/2 cup	130	1	21	80	0	5.0	0
peanut butter cup, nondairy	1/2 cup	130	2	21	75	1	6.0	0
peanut butter fudge, nondairy	1/2 cup	160	3	19	100	0	7.0	0
vanilla fudge, nondairy	1/2 cup	130	1	20	70	1	5.0	0
vanilla Swiss almond, nondairy	1/2 cup	130	1	20	70	1	6.0	0
vanilla, nondairy	1/2 cup	130	1	19	70	1	5.0	0
wildberry, nondairy	1/2 cup	130	1	17	80	0	5.0	0
(Sealtest)								
black cherry, nonfat, 'Free'	1/2 cup	100	2	25	45	0	0.0	0
chocolate, nonfat, 'Free'	1/2 cup	100	3	23	50	0	0.0	0
peach, nonfat, 'Free'	1/2 cup	100	2	23	45	0	0.0	0
strawberry, nonfat, 'Free'	1/2 cup	100	2	23	40	0	0.0	0
vanilla, nonfat, 'Free'	1/2 cup	100	3	24	45	0	0.0	0
vanilla-chocolate strawberry, nonfat, 'Free'	1/2 cup	100	3	23	40	0	0.0	0
vanilla-fudge royale, nonfat, 'Free'	1/2 cup	100	3	24	50	0	0.0	0
vanilla-strawberry royale, nonfat, 'Free'	1/2 cup	100	3	25	35	0	0.0	0
(Simple Pleasures)								
chocolate	1/2 cup	140	9	25	15	0	1.0	0
coffee	4 oz	120	8	22	15	0	1.0	0
peach	4 oz	135	9	24	5	0	1.0	0
rum raisin	4 oz	130	7	25	10	0	1.0	0
strawberry	4 oz	120	8	22	55	0	1.0	11
(Sweet Nothings)								
berry blackberry, nondairy, nonfat	1/2 cup	110	0	26	10	0	0.0	0
'Black Leopard' nondairy, nonfat	1/2 cup	100	1	23	5	0	0.0	0
chocolate Mandarin, nondairy, nonfat	1/2 cup	100	1	23	5	0	0.0	0
chocolate, nondairy, nonfat	1/2 cup	100	1	23	5	0	0.0	0
espresso fudge, nondairy, nonfat	1/2 cup	110	1	25	5	0	0.0	0
mango raspberry, nondairy, nonfat	1/2 cup	110	0	26	10	0	0.0	0
raspberry swirl, nondairy, nonfat	1/2 cup	110	0	26	10	0	0.0	0
'Tiger Stripes' nondairy, nonfat	1/2 cup	110	1	25	5	0	0.0	0

Food Name	Serv. Size	Total Cal.	Prot. gms	Carbs gms	Sod. mgs	Fiber gms	Fat gms	Chol. mgs
vanilla, nondairy, nonfat	1/2 cup	110	1	25	5	0	0.0	0
(Tofutti)								
all flavors, 'Lite Lite'	1/2 cup	90	2	20	80	0	1.0	0
all flavors, nondairy, 'Fruitti'	1/2 cup	100	2	20	90	na	0.0	0
butter pecan, nondairy	1 fl oz	55	0	6	50	0	3.3	0
chocolate cookie, nondairy, 'Supreme'	1 fl oz	53	1	7	25	0	2.8	0
chocolate fudge, nondairy, 'Better Than Yogurt'	1/2 cup	120	2	25	98	0	2.0	0
chocolate supreme, nondairy	1/2 cup	210	3	20	130	0	13.0	0
coffee marshmallow, nondairy, 'Better Than Yogurt'	1/2 cup	100	1	24	77	0	1.0	0
passion island fruit, nondairy, 'Better Than Yogurt'	1/2 cup	100	1	21	100	0	1.0	0
peach mango, nondairy, 'Better Than Yogurt'	1/2 cup	100	1	23	102	0	1.0	0
strawberry banana, nondairy, 'Better Than Yogurt'	1/2 cup	100	1	23	92	0	1.0	0
vanilla almond bark, nondairy	1 fl oz	53	1	5	33	0	3.3	0
vanilla fudge, nondairy, 'Better Than Yogurt'	1/2 cup	120	2	24	90	0	2.0	0
vanilla, nondairy	1 fl oz	48	1	5	53	0	2.8	0
'Wildberry Supreme' nondairy	1 fl oz	48	1	6	48	0	2.3	0
(Weight Watchers)								
'Arctic D'Lights'	1 serving	130	3	14	20	0	7.0	5
berries 'n creme mousse	1 serving	35	2	4	38	1	0.8	0
chocolate, nonfat	1/2 cup	80	3	19	75	0	0.0	5
chocolate swirl, nonfat	1/2 cup	90	3	22	75	0	0.0	5
chocolate treat	1 serving	100	3	21	150	1	1.0	10
Neapolitan, nonfat	1/2 cup	80	3	19	75	0	0.0	5
vanilla, nonfat	1/2 cup	80	3	20	75	0	0.0	5

ICE CREAM SUBSTITUTE BAR/DESSERT. See also YOGURT BAR, FROZEN BAR

Food Name	Serv. Size	Total Cal.	Prot. gms	Carbs gms	Sod. mgs	Fiber gms	Fat gms	Chol. mgs
(Crystal Light)								
Amaretto chocolate swirl, 'Cool N'Creamy'	1 bar	60	2	10	60	0	2.0	0
chocolate vanilla, 'Cool N'Creamy'	1 bar	50	2	7	55	0	2.0	0
double chocolate fudge, 'Cool N'Creamy'	1 bar	50	2	7	60	0	2.0	0
orange vanilla, 'Cool N'Creamy'	1 bar	30	1	5	25	0	1.0	0
(Freezer Pleezer)								
fudge flavored	1 bar	100	2	20	75	1	1.0	5
orange cream treats	1 bar	80	1	16	20	1	1.5	10
(Good Humor)								
chocolate fudge	1 bar	127	4	27	91	0	0.6	0
'Cool Shark'	1 bar	68	0	17	7	0	0.1	0
'Jumbo Jet Star'	1 bar	85	0	20	0	0	0.7	0
'Milky Pop'	1 bar	45	1	8	25	0	0.0	0
strawberry finger	1 bar	49	0	12	0	0	0.1	0
(Light n' Lively)								
chocolate mousse, nonfat	1 bar	50	2	12	45	0	0.0	0
double chocolate fudge, nonfat	1 bar	50	2	11	45	0	0.0	0
orange vanilla, nonfat	1 bar	40	1	10	15	0	0.0	0
strawberry, nonfat	1 bar	80	2	12	25	0	0.0	0
vanilla, chocolate dipped	1 bar	110	2	14	35	0	6.0	0
(Rice Dream)								
chocolate, nondairy	1 bar	270	1	33	115	0	16.0	0
chocolate, nutty, nondairy	1 bar	330	5	29	110	0	23.0	0
strawberry, nondairy	1 bar	260	1	31	110	0	14.8	0
vanilla, nondairy	1 bar	275	1	33	120	0	15.8	0
vanilla, nutty, nondairy	1 bar	330	5	29	100	0	23.0	0
(Sealtest)								
chocolate, w/fudge swirl, nonfat, 'Free'	1 bar	80	3	19	55	0	0.0	0
vanilla, w/fudge swirl, nonfat, 'Free'	1 bar	80	2	18	55	0	0.0	0
vanilla, w/strawberry swirl, nonfat, 'Free'	1 bar	70	2	17	60	0	0.0	0

Food Name	Serv. Size	Total Cal.	Prot. gms	Carbs gms	Sod. mgs	Fiber gms	Fat gms	Chol. mgs
(Trix)								
assorted flavors, nonfat	1 bar	40	0	10	0	0	0.0	0
'Fudge N' Fruity'	1 bar	80	2	17	60	0	1.0	5
(Weight Watchers)								
chocolate dip	1 bar	100	3	21	150	1	1.0	10
'Crispy Pralines & Creme'	1 bar	120	2	13	45	0	6.0	5
NOVELTY								
(Rice Dream)								
'Dream Pie' mint, nondairy	1 pie	380	3	47	225	0	19.0	0
'Dream Pie' vanilla, nondairy	1 pie	380	3	47	225	0	19.0	0
(Tofutti)								
'Love Drops' cappuccino flavored	1/2 cup	230	3	26	120	0	12.0	0
'Love Drops' chocolate	1/2 cup	230	3	26	100	0	13.0	0
'Love Drops' vanilla	1/2 cup	220	3	26	100	0	12.0	0
'O's' vanilla, chocolate dipped	1 piece	40	1	4	20	0	2.0	0
(Weight Watchers)								
'ONE-ders' brownies and creme	4 oz	130	4	20	115	0	4.0	10
parfait, double fudge brownie	1 serving	190	6	39	170	2	2.5	5
parfait, praline toffee crunch	1 serving	190	5	40	140	2	3.0	5
parfait, strawberry royale	1 serving	180	5	35	100	0	2.0	10
SUNDAE								
(Weight Watchers)								
chocolate chip cookie dough	1 serving	180	3	33	115	2	4.0	5
hot caramel fudge	4.5 oz	160	5	27	140	0	4.0	15
hot chocolate fudge	4.5 oz	160	6	26	115	0	4.0	15
hot mocha fudge	4.5 oz	160	5	24	120	0	5.0	15
ICE CREAM SUBSTITUTE MIX								
(Tofutti)								
soft serve	1 oz	48	1	5	24	0	1.0	0
soft serve, light	1 oz	23	1	5	20	0	0.3	0
ICE MILK								
(Borden)								
chocolate	1/2 cup	100	3	18	80	0	2.0	0
strawberry	1/2 cup	90	2	17	65	0	2.0	0
vanilla	1/2 cup	90	2	17	60	0	2.0	0
(Breyers)								
chocolate, 'Light'	1/2 cup	120	3	18	55	0	4.0	15
chocolate chocolate chip, 'Light'	1/2 cup	140	4	20	55	0	5.0	25
chocolate fudge twirl, 'Light'	1/2 cup	130	4	21	60	0	4.0	10
heavenly hash, 'Light'	1/2 cup	150	3	21	55	0	5.0	10
praline almond, 'Light'	1/2 cup	130	3	19	70	0	5.0	10
strawberry, 'Light'	1/2 cup	110	3	18	50	0	3.0	15
Swiss almond fudge twirl	1/2 cup	150	4	21	65	0	6.0	0
toffee fudge parfait, 'Light'	1/2 cup	140	3	22	90	0	5.0	10
vanilla, 'Light'	1/2 cup	120	3	18	60	0	4.0	10
vanilla-chocolate-strawberry, 'Light'	1/2 cup	120	3	18	55	0	4.0	15
vanilla-raspberry parfait, 'Light'	1/2 cup	130	3	23	50	0	3.0	15
(Darigold)								
chocolate, 'Lite'	1/2 cup	110	3	19	65	0	3.0	0
vanilla	1/2 cup	110	2	18	66	0	3.0	0
(Light n' Lively)								
caramel nut	1/2 cup	120	3	18	85	0	4.0	10
chocolate chip	1/2 cup	120	3	18	35	0	4.0	10
coffee	1/2 cup	100	3	16	40	0	3.0	10
cookies and cream	1/2 cup	110	3	18	65	0	3.0	10
heavenly hash	1/2 cup	120	3	20	35	0	4.0	10
vanilla	1/2 cup	100	3	16	40	0	3.0	10
vanilla, w/chocolate covered almonds	1/2 cup	120	3	17	45	0	4.0	10

Food Name	Serv. Size	Total Cal.	Prot. gms	Carbs gms	Sod. mgs	Fiber gms	Fat gms	Chol. mgs
vanilla-chocolate-strawberry	1/2 cup	100	2	17	35	0	3.0	10
vanilla-fudge twirl	1/2 cup	110	3	18	45	0	3.0	10
vanilla-raspberry swirl	1/2 cup	110	3	19	35	0	3.0	10
(Ponderosa)								
chocolate	3.5 oz	152	4	30	70	0	2.9	22
vanilla	3.5 oz	150	4	30	58	0	2.6	20
(Weight Watchers)								
chocolate, 'Grand Collection'	1/2 cup	110	4	18	75	0	3.0	10
chocolate chip, 'Grand Collection'	1/2 cup	120	3	19	75	0	4.0	10
chocolate swirl, 'Grand Collection'	1/2 cup	120	3	19	75	0	3.0	5
Neapolitan, 'Grand Collection'	1/2 cup	110	3	18	75	0	3.0	10
pecan pralines and creme, 'Grand Collection'	1/2 cup	120	3	20	80	0	4.0	10
vanilla, 'Grand Collection'	1/2 cup	100	3	16	75	0	3.0	10
ICE MILK BAR/DESSERT								
bar, 'Chocolate Almond Crunch' *(Weight Watchers)*	1 bar	120	2	12	45	0	7.0	5
cone, w/nuts 'Olde Nut Sundae' *(Gold Bond)*	3 oz	230	5	36	0	0	8.0	0

ICEBERG LETTUCE. See LETTUCE, ICEBERG.
ICED TEA. See TEA, ICED.
IMBU. See JOBO.
INDIAN DATE. See TAMARIND.
INDIAN FRY BREAD. See under BREAD.
INFANT FORMULA. See under BABY FOOD, FORMULA.
IRISH MOSS. See under SEA VEGETABLE.
ITALIAN BEAN. See BEAN, ITALIAN.
ITALIAN CHESTNUT. See CHESTNUT, EUROPEAN.
ITALIAN MUSHROOM. See MUSHROOM, CRIMINI.
ITALIAN SEASONING. See under SEASONING MIX.
ITALIAN STONE PINE NUT. See PINE NUT.

J

Food Name	Serv. Size	Total Cal.	Prot. gms	Carbs gms	Sod. mgs	Fiber gms	Fat gms	Chol. mgs
JACK BEAN. See BEAN, FAVA.								
JACK MACKEREL. See under MACKEREL.								
JACKFRUIT								
Fresh, raw, sliced	1 cup	155	2	40	5	3	0.5	0
Canned, in syrup, drained	1 cup	164	1	43	20	2	0.2	0
JALAPEÑO. See PEPPER, JALAPEÑO.								
JAM AND PRESERVES. See also FRUIT SPREAD.								
(Estee) all flavors	1 tsp	2	0	0	10	0	0.0	0
(Featherweight) all flavors	1 tsp	4	0	1	0	0	0.0	0
(Kraft) all flavors	1 tsp	17	0	4	0	0	0.0	0
(S&W) all flavors, 'Nutradiet'	1 tsp	4	0	1	0	0	0.0	0
APRICOT								
(Finast)	2 tsp	35	0	9	1	0	0.0	0
(Knott's Berry Farm) pure preserves	1 tsp	18	0	4	0	0	0.0	0
(Polaner)	2 tsp	35	0	9	5	0	0.0	0
(Smucker's) natural ingredients	1 tsp	18	0	4	0	0	0.0	0
APRICOT-PINEAPPLE								
(Knott's Berry Farm) pure preserves	1 tsp	18	0	4	0	0	0.0	0
(Knudsen)	2 tsp	35	1	8	0	0	1.0	0
(Smucker's) natural ingredients	1 tsp	18	0	4	0	0	0.0	0
BLACK CHERRY *(Knudsen)*	2 tsp	35	1	8	0	0	1.0	0
BLACKBERRY								
(Finast)	2 tsp	16	0	4	5	0	0.0	0

Food Name	Serv. Size	Total Cal.	Prot. gms	Carbs gms	Sod. mgs	Fiber gms	Fat gms	Chol. mgs
(Knott's Berry Farm) seedless, pure preserves	1 tsp	18	0	4	0	0	0.0	0
(Knudsen)								
....	2 tsp	35	1	8	0	0	1.0	0
organic	2 tsp	25	1	7	0	0	1.0	0
(Polaner) seedless	2 tsp	35	0	9	5	0	0.0	0
(Smucker's) natural ingredients	1 tsp	18	0	4	0	0	0.0	0
(Stilwell) freezer jam	1 tbsp	36	0	8	0	0	0.0	na
BLUEBERRY								
(Finast)	2 tsp	16	0	4	5	0	0.0	0
(Knott's Berry Farm) pure preserves	1 tsp	18	0	4	0	0	0.0	0
(Knudsen)								
....	2 tsp	35	1	8	0	0	1.0	0
organic	2 tsp	25	1	7	0	0	1.0	0
(Polaner)	2 tsp	35	0	9	5	0	0.0	0
(Smucker's) natural ingredients	1 tsp	18	0	4	0	0	0.0	0
BOYSENBERRY								
(Knott's Berry Farm) pure preserves	1 tsp	18	0	4	0	0	0.0	0
(Knudsen)	2 tsp	35	1	8	0	0	1.0	0
(Smucker's) natural ingredients	1 tsp	18	0	4	0	0	0.0	0
CHERRY								
(Finast)	2 tsp	25	0	9	5	0	0.0	0
(Knott's Berry Farm)								
Bing, pure preserves	1 tsp	18	0	4	0	0	0.0	0
red, pure preserves	1 tsp	18	0	4	0	0	0.0	0
(Smucker's) natural ingredients	1 tsp	18	0	4	0	0	0.0	0
FIG *(Knott's Berry Farm)* Kadota, pure preserves	1 tsp	18	0	4	0	0	0.0	0
GRAPE								
(Finast)								
....	2 tsp	35	0	9	5	0	0.0	0
Concord	2 tsp	35	0	9	5	0	0.0	0
(Knudsen) Concord	2 tsp	35	1	8	0	0	1.0	0
(Polaner)	2 tsp	35	0	9	5	0	0.0	0
(Smucker's) Concord, natural ingredients	1 tsp	18	0	4	0	0	0.0	0
(Welch's)	2 tsp	35	0	9	5	0	0.0	0
ORANGE								
(Fifty 50) no sugar added	1 tsp	2	0	1	5	0	0.0	0
(Finast) marmalade	2 tsp	35	0	9	0	0	0.0	2
(Knott's Berry Farm) marmalade, w/NutraSweet, 'Light'	1 tsp	8	0	2	0	0	0.0	0
(Knudsen) marmalade	2 tsp	35	1	8	0	0	1.0	0
(Smucker's)								
marmalade	1 tsp	18	0	4	0	0	0.0	0
marmalade, low-sugar	1 tsp	8	0	2	0	0	0.0	0
marmalade, 'Simply Fruit'	1 tsp	16	0	4	0	0	0.0	0
marmalade, sweet, natural ingredients	1 tsp	18	0	4	0	0	0.0	0
(Polaner) marmalade	2 tsp	35	0	9	5	0	0.0	0
PEACH								
(Bama)	2 tsp	30	0	8	5	0	0.0	0
(Finast)	2 tsp	35	0	9	1	0	0.0	0
(Knudsen)	2 tsp	35	1	8	0	0	1.0	0
(Polaner)	2 tsp	35	0	9	5	0	0.0	0
(Smucker's) natural ingredients	1 tsp	18	0	4	0	0	0.0	0
PINEAPPLE								
(Finast)	2 tsp	35	0	9	1	0	0.0	0
(Polaner)	2 tsp	35	0	9	5	0	0.0	0
(Smucker's) natural ingredients	1 tsp	18	0	4	0	0	0.0	0
PLUM								
(Bama) red	2 tsp	30	0	8	5	0	0.0	0

Food Name	Serv. Size	Total Cal.	Prot. gms	Carbs gms	Sod. mgs	Fiber gms	Fat gms	Chol. mgs
(Smucker's) natural ingredients	1 tsp	18	0	4	0	0	0.0	0
RASPBERRY								
(Finast) red	2 tsp	35	0	9	3	0	0.0	0
(Knott's Berry Farm) seedless, pure preserves	1 tsp	18	0	4	0	0	0.0	0
(Knudsen)								
red	2 tsp	35	1	8	0	0	1.0	0
red, organic	2 tsp	25	1	7	0	0	1.0	0
(Polaner)								
red	2 tsp	35	0	9	5	0	0.0	0
red, seedless	2 tsp	35	0	9	5	0	0.0	0
(Smucker's)								
black, natural ingredients	1 tsp	18	0	4	0	0	0.0	0
red, seedless, natural ingredients	1 tsp	18	0	4	0	0	0.0	0
(Stilwell) freezer jam	1 tbsp	33	0	8	0	0	0.0	na
RASPBERRY-APPLE *(Welch's)*	2 tsp	35	0	9	5	0	0.0	0
STRAWBERRY								
(Bama)	2 tsp	30	0	8	5	0	0.0	0
(Finast)	2 tsp	35	0	9	3	0	0.0	0
(Knott's Berry Farm) seedless, pure preserves	1 tsp	18	0	4	0	0	0.0	0
(Knudsen)								
	2 tsp	35	1	8	0	0	1.0	0
organic	2 tsp	25	1	7	0	0	1.0	0
(Kraft) reduced calorie	1 tsp	6	0	2	5	0	0.0	0
(Piedmont)	2 tsp	35	0	9	10	0	0.0	0
(Polaner) strawberry	2 tsp	35	0	9	5	0	0.0	0
(Smucker's) seedless, natural ingredients	1 tsp	18	0	4	0	0	0.0	0
(Stilwell) freezer jam	1 tbsp	37	0	9	0	0	0.0	na
(Welch's)	2 tsp	35	0	9	5	0	0.0	0
TOMATO *(Smucker's)* natural ingredients	1 tsp	18	0	4	0	0	0.0	0

JAMAICAN BREADNUT. See BREADNUT TREE SEEDS.

JAMBALAYA. See under SHRIMP DISH/ENTRÉE.

JAMBERRY, fresh *(Frieda's)*	3.5 oz	25	1.4	4.2	na	(mq)	0.5	0

JAMBOLAN. See JAVA PLUM.

JAPANESE HONEY MUSHROOM. See MUSHROOM, JAPANESE HONEY.

JAPANESE MEDLAR. See LOQUAT.

JASMINE RICE. See under RICE.

JAVA PLUM/jambolan

cut up	1 cup	81	1	21	19	na	0.3	0
whole	3 med fruits	5	0	1	1	na	0.0	0

JELL-O. See under GELATIN DESSERT; GELATIN DESSERT MIX.

JELLY. See also FRUIT SPREAD; JAM AND PRESERVES.

(Estee) all flavors	1 tsp	2	0	0	10	0	0.0	0
(Featherweight) all flavors, except grape	1 tsp	4	0	1	0	0	0.0	0
(Kraft) all flavors	1 tsp	17	0	4	0	0	0.0	0
APPLE								
(Bama)	2 tsp	30	0	8	5	0	0.0	0
(Finast)	2 tsp	35	0	9	2	0	0.0	0
(Lucky Leaf)	1 oz	80	0	20	5	0	0.0	0
(Musselman's)	1 oz	80	0	20	5	0	0.0	0
(Polaner)	2 tsp	35	0	9	5	0	0.0	0
(Smucker's)								
cinnamon-flavored, natural ingredients	1 tsp	18	0	4	0	0	0.0	0
mint-flavored, natural ingredients	1 tsp	18	0	4	0	0	0.0	0
natural ingredients	1 tsp	18	0	4	0	0	0.0	0
APPLE BLACKBERRY *(Musselman's)*	1 oz	80	0	19	0	0	0.0	0
APPLE CHERRY *(Musselman's)*	1 oz	80	0	19	5	0	0.0	0

Food Name	Serv. Size	Total Cal.	Prot. gms	Carbs gms	Sod. mgs	Fiber gms	Fat gms	Chol. mgs
APPLE GRAPE								
(Musselman's)	1 oz	80	0	20	5	0	0.0	0
(Welch's)	2 tsp	35	0	9	5	0	0.0	0
APPLE RASPBERRY (Musselman's)	1 oz	80	0	19	0	0	0.0	0
APPLE STRAWBERRY (Musselman's)	1 oz	80	0	20	5	0	0.0	0
APRICOT-PINEAPPLE								
(Knott's Berry Farm) w/NutraSweet, 'Light'	1 tsp	8	0	2	0	0	0.0	0
BLACKBERRY								
(Bama)	2 tsp	30	0	8	5	0	0.0	0
(Knott's Berry Farm) w/NutraSweet, 'Light'	1 tsp	8	0	2	0	0	0.0	0
(Smucker's) natural ingredients	1 tsp	18	0	4	0	0	0.0	0
BOYSENBERRY								
(Knott's Berry Farm) w/NutraSweet, 'Light'	1 tsp	8	0	2	0	0	0.0	0
CHERRY (Smucker's) natural ingredients	1 tsp	18	0	4	0	0	0.0	0
CRABAPPLE (Smucker's) natural ingredients	1 tsp	18	0	4	0	0	0.0	0
CURRANT								
(Finast)	2 tsp	35	0	9	2	0	0.0	0
(Polaner)	2 tsp	35	0	9	5	0	0.0	0
(Smucker's) natural ingredients	1 tsp	18	0	4	0	0	0.0	0
ELDERBERRY (Smucker's) natural ingredients	1 tsp	18	0	4	0	0	0.0	0
GRAPE								
(Bama)	2 tsp	30	0	8	5	0	0.0	0
(Featherweight)	1 tsp	4	0	1	5	0	0.0	0
(Finast)	2 tsp	35	0	9	5	0	0.0	0
(Kraft) reduced calorie	1 tsp	6	0	2	5	0	0.0	0
(Musselman's)	1 oz	80	0	20	0	0	0.0	0
(Polaner)	2 tsp	35	0	9	5	0	0.0	0
(Smucker's) Concord, natural ingredients	1 tsp	18	0	4	0	0	0.0	0
(Welch's)	2 tsp	35	0	9	5	0	0.0	0
GREEN PEPPER (Great Impressions)	1 tbsp	50	0	13	1	0	0.0	0
GUAVA (Smucker's) natural ingredients	1 tsp	18	0	4	0	0	0.0	0
JALAPEÑO								
(Great Impressions)	1 tbsp	58	0	15	51	0	0.0	0
(Knott's Berry Farm) pure	1 tsp	18	0	4	0	0	0.0	0
MINT								
(Finast)	2 tsp	35	0	9	2	0	0.0	0
(Polaner)	2 tsp	35	0	9	5	0	0.0	0
MIXED FRUIT (Smucker's) natural ingredients	1 tsp	18	0	4	0	0	0.0	0
PLUM (Smucker's) natural ingredients	1 tsp	18	0	4	0	0	0.0	0
QUINCE (Smucker's) natural ingredients	1 tsp	18	0	4	0	0	0.0	0
RASPBERRY								
(Knott's Berry Farm) red, w/NutraSweet, 'Light'	1 tsp	8	0	2	0	0	0.0	0
(Polaner) raspberry	2 tsp	35	0	9	5	0	0.0	0
(Smucker's)								
black, natural ingredients	1 tsp	18	0	4	0	0	0.0	0
red, natural ingredients	1 tsp	18	0	4	0	0	0.0	0
RED PEPPER (Great Impressions)	1 tbsp	50	0	13	9	0	0.0	0
STRAWBERRY								
(Finast)	2 tsp	35	0	9	2	0	0.0	0
(Knott's Berry Farm) w/NutraSweet, 'Light'	1 tsp	8	0	2	0	0	0.0	0
(Polaner)	2 tsp	35	0	9	5	0	0.0	0
(Smucker's) natural ingredients	1 tsp	18	0	4	0	0	0.0	0
STRAWBERRY APPLE (Polaner)	2 tsp	35	0	9	5	0	0.0	0

JELLYBEAN. See under CANDY.

JERKY. See BEEF JERKY; BEEF SUBSTITUTE JERKY; TURKEY JERKY.

JERUSALEM ARTICHOKE. See ARTICHOKE, JERUSALEM.

JEW'S EAR. See CHINESE FUNGUS.

Food Name	Serv. Size	Total Cal.	Prot. gms	Carbs gms	Sod. mgs	Fiber gms	Fat gms	Chol. mgs
JICAMA/Chinese yam/Mexican potato/sicama/yambean tuber								
raw, sliced	1 cup	46	1	11	5	6	0.1	0
raw, trimmed *(Frieda of California)*	1 oz	13	0	3	0	0	0.1	0
raw, whole	1 medium	250	5	58	26	32	0.6	0
JOBO/hog plum/imbu/yellow mombin								
seeded	1 oz	20	0.2	3.9	na	0.3	0.6	0
JUICE. See FRUIT JUICE BLEND; individual listings.								
JUJUBE, CHINESE								
dried	3.5 oz	287	3.7	73.6	9	3.0	1.1	0
dried	1 oz	81	1.0	20.1	3	0.9	0.3	0
raw	3.5 oz	79	1.2	20.2	3	1.4	0.1	0
raw	1 oz	22	0.3	5.7	1	0.4	0.1	0
JUNKET MIX								
CHOCOLATE								
mix only *(Junket)*	3/8 oz	40	1	10	5	0	0.0	0
prepared w/nonfat milk *(Junket)*	1/2 cup	90	5	15	70	0	0.0	0
prepared w/whole milk *(Junket)*	1/2 cup	120	5	15	65	0	4.0	0
RASPBERRY								
mix only *(Junket)*	3/8 oz	40	0	10	0	0	0.0	0
prepared w/nonfat milk *(Junket)*	1/2 cup	90	4	16	65	0	0.0	0
prepared w/whole milk *(Junket)*	1/2 cup	120	4	16	60	0	4.0	0
STRAWBERRY								
mix only *(Junket)*	3/8 oz	40	0	10	0	0	0.0	0
prepared w/nonfat milk *(Junket)*	1/2 cup	90	4	16	65	0	0.0	0
prepared w/whole milk *(Junket)*	1/2 cup	120	4	16	60	0	4.0	0
VANILLA								
mix only *(Junket)*	3/8 oz	40	0	10	5	0	0.0	0
prepared w/nonfat milk *(Junket)*	1/2 cup	90	4	16	70	0	0.0	0
prepared w/whole milk *(Junket)*	1/2 cup	120	4	16	65	0	4.0	0
JUTE POTHERB								
boiled, drained	1 cup	32	3	6	10	2	0.2	0
raw	1 cup	10	1	2	2	na	0.1	0

K

Food Name	Serv. Size	Total Cal.	Prot. gms	Carbs gms	Sod. mgs	Fiber gms	Fat gms	Chol. mgs
KAISER ROLL. See under ROLL.								
KALE/borecole/cole/colewort								
Canned, chopped *(Allens)*	1/2 cup	25	2	3	15	0	1.0	0
Fresh								
boiled, drained	4 oz	36	2.2	6.4	26	>.9 c	0.5	0
boiled, drained, chopped	1 cup	42	2.5	7.3	30	2.6	0.5	0
raw, chopped	1 cup	34	2	7	29	1	0.5	0
raw, chopped *(Dole)*	1/2 cup	17	1	3	15	0	0.5	0
boiled, drained, chopped	1 cup	36	2	7	30	3	0.5	0
Frozen								
boiled, drained, chopped	1 cup	39	4	7	20	3	0.6	0
boiled, drained, chopped or diced	1/2 cup	20	2	3	10	1	0.3	0
chopped *(Frosty Acres)*	3.3 oz	25	3	5	15	1	0.0	0
chopped *(Seabrook)*	3.3 oz	25	3	5	14	1	0.0	0
chopped *(Southern)*	3.5 oz	30	3	5	30	0	0.5	0
unprepared	10-oz pkg	80	8	14	43	6	1.3	0
KALE, SCOTCH								
boiled, drained, chopped	1 cup	36	2	7	59	2	0.5	0
raw, chopped	1 cup	28	2	6	47	1	0.4	0

Food Name	Serv. Size	Total Cal.	Prot. gms	Carbs gms	Sod. mgs	Fiber gms	Fat gms	Chol. mgs
KANPYO/dried gourd strips . . . . .1/2 cup	70	2	18	4	na	0.2	0
KANTEN								
raw . . . . 1 lb	116	2.5	30.6	40 >2.0 c		0.1	0
raw . . . . 1 oz	7	0.2	1.9	3 >.1 c		tr	0
KASHA. See BUCKWHEAT GROATS, ROASTED.								
KATSUO. See under TUNA, SKIPJACK.								
KATURAY/sesbania flower								
flowers, raw, whole . . . . 1 cup	5	0	1	3	na	0.0	0
flowers, raw, whole . . . . 1 medium	1	0	0	0	na	0.0	0
flowers, steamed . . . . 1 cup	23	1	5	11	na	0.1	0
KEFIR								
black cherry flavored, cultured (*Alta Dena*) . . . . 1 cup	200	9	24	120	0	9.0	0
boysenberry flavored, cultured (*Alta Dena*) . . . . 1 cup	200	9	24	120	0	9.0	0
peach flavored, cultured (*Alta Dena*) . . . . 1 cup	200	9	24	120	0	9.0	0
plain, cultured, including acidophilus (*Alta Dena*) . . . . 1 oz	70	1	1	40	0	6.0	0
red raspberry flavored, cultured (*Alta Dena*) . . . . 1 cup	200	9	24	120	0	9.0	0
KELP. See under SEA VEGETABLE.								
KETA SALMON. See under SALMON.								
KETCHUP. See CATSUP.								
KIDNEY BEAN. See BEAN, KIDNEY.								
KIELBASA. See under SAUSAGE.								
KING CRAB. See under CRAB.								
KING MACKEREL. See under MACKEREL.								
KING SALMON. See under SALMON.								
KIWI FRUIT/Chinese gooseberry								
Fresh								
raw, cut up . . . . 1 cup	108	2	26	9	6	0.8	0
raw, peeled . . . . 1 large	56	1	14	5	3	0.4	0
raw, peeled . . . . 1 medium	46	1	11	4	3	0.3	0
KOHLRABI/cabbage turnip								
boiled, drained, sliced . . . . 1 cup	48	3	11	35	2	0.2	0
raw, sliced . . . . 1 cup	36	2	8	27	5	0.1	0
KOMBU. See under SEA VEGETABLE.								
KOLBASSY. See under SAUSAGE.								
KOOL-AID. See under FRUIT DRINK; FRUIT DRINK MIX.								
KOTTERIN MIRIN. See under SEASONING MIX.								
KUMQUAT								
raw, trimmed . . . . 1 med fruit	12	0	3	1	1	0.0	0
raw, w/seeds . . . . 1 lb	266	3.8	69.3	25	15.6	0.4	0

L

Food Name	Serv. Size	Total Cal.	Prot. gms	Carbs gms	Sod. mgs	Fiber gms	Fat gms	Chol. mgs
LAMB, AUSTRALIAN								
(NOTE: All USDA choice grade. TRIMMED = Lean; separable fat removed. UNTRIMMED = Separable fat not removed.)								
COMPOSITE CUTS								
Trimmed								
cooked . . . . 3 oz	171	23	0	68	na	8.2	74
raw . . . . 3 oz	121	17	0	71	na	5.3	54
raw . . . . 1 oz	40	6	0	24	na	1.8	18
Untrimmed								
cooked . . . . 3 oz	218	21	0	65	na	14.3	74
raw . . . . 3 oz	195	15	0	63	na	14.4	56
raw . . . . 1 oz	65	5	0	21	na	4.8	19

Food Name	Serv. Size	Total Cal.	Prot. gms	Carbs gms	Sod. mgs	Fiber gms	Fat gms	Chol. mgs
LEG/CENTER SLICE								
Trimmed								
center slice, raw	9.8 oz	403	58	0	180	na	17.1	180
center slice, w/bone, broiled	3 oz	156	23	0	56	na	6.5	72
center slice, w/bone, raw	1 oz	41	6	0	18	na	1.7	18
Untrimmed								
center slice, broiled	3 oz	183	22	0	55	na	10.0	72
center slice, raw	11 oz	616	61	0	193	na	39.7	205
center slice, w/bone, raw	1 oz	55	5	0	17	na	3.6	18
LEG/FORESHANK								
Trimmed								
braised	3 oz	140	23	0	85	na	4.4	78
raw	3 oz	105	18	0	90	na	3.2	56
raw	1 oz	35	6	0	30	na	1.1	19
Untrimmed								
braised	3 oz	201	21	0	79	na	12.3	77
raw	3 oz	166	16	0	82	na	10.8	57
raw	1 oz	55	5	0	27	na	3.6	19
LEG/SHANK								
Trimmed								
raw	3 oz	113	17	0	69	na	4.3	54
raw	1 oz	38	6	0	23	na	1.4	18
roasted	3 oz	155	23	0	59	na	6.2	71
Untrimmed								
raw	3 oz	171	16	0	64	na	11.5	56
raw	1 oz	57	5	0	21	na	3.8	19
roasted	3 oz	196	21	0	57	na	11.6	71
LEG/SIRLOIN								
Trimmed								
raw	3 oz	117	17	0	68	na	4.8	54
raw	1 oz	39	6	0	23	na	1.6	18
roasted	3 oz	183	24	0	71	na	9.1	89
Untrimmed								
raw	3 oz	216	15	0	60	na	17.0	56
raw	1 oz	72	5	0	20	na	5.7	19
roasted	3 oz	239	21	0	66	na	16.5	87
LEG/WHOLE								
Trimmed								
raw	3 oz	115	17	0	69	na	4.4	54
raw	1 oz	38	6	0	23	na	1.5	18
roasted	3 oz	162	23	0	61	na	6.9	76
Untrimmed								
raw	3 oz	183	16	0	62	na	12.9	56
raw	1 oz	61	5	0	21	na	4.3	19
roasted	3 oz	207	21	0	60	na	12.9	75
LOIN								
Trimmed								
broiled	3 oz	163	23	0	68	na	7.4	69
broiled, yield from 1 med chop	3.7 oz	111	15	0	46	na	5.1	47
raw	3 oz	124	18	0	64	na	5.3	54
raw	1 oz	41	6	0	21	na	1.8	18
Untrimmed								
broiled	3 oz	186	22	0	66	na	10.4	70
broiled, yield from 1 med chop	2.2 oz	136	16	0	48	na	7.6	51
raw	3 oz	173	16	0	60	na	11.4	56
raw	1 oz	58	5	0	20	na	3.8	19

Food Name	Serv. Size	Total Cal.	Prot. gms	Carbs gms	Sod. mgs	Fiber gms	Fat gms	Chol. mgs
RIB								
Trimmed								
raw	3 oz	136	17	0	69	na	7.0	56
raw	1 oz	45	6	0	23	na	2.3	19
roasted	3 oz	179	21	0	70	na	9.9	68
Untrimmed								
raw	3 oz	246	14	0	58	na	20.6	58
raw	1 oz	82	5	0	19	na	6.9	19
roasted	3 oz	235	19	0	65	na	17.2	68
SHOULDER/ARM								
Trimmed								
braised	3 oz	264	25	0	62	na	17.3	90
braised, yield from 1 med chop	6.5 oz	289	28	0	68	na	19.0	99
raw	3 oz	116	17	0	71	na	4.9	53
raw	1 oz	39	6	0	24	na	1.6	18
Untrimmed								
raw	1 oz	69	5	0	20	na	5.4	18
raw	3 oz	207	15	0	61	na	16.1	55
SHOULDER/BLADE								
Trimmed								
broiled	3 oz	196	20	0	80	na	12.2	72
raw	3 oz	139	16	0	77	na	7.7	54
raw	1 oz	46	5	0	26	na	2.6	18
Untrimmed								
broiled	3 oz	247	18	0	75	na	18.7	71
raw	3 oz	223	14	0	66	na	18.1	57
raw	1 oz	74	5	0	22	na	6.0	19
SHOULDER/WHOLE								
Trimmed								
cooked	3 oz	198	22	0	77	na	11.4	77
raw	3 oz	132	16	0	75	na	6.8	54
raw	1 oz	44	5	0	25	na	2.3	18
Untrimmed								
cooked	3 oz	252	20	0	72	na	18.4	76
raw	3 oz	218	14	0	65	na	17.4	56
raw	1 oz	73	5	0	22	na	5.8	19
SIRLOIN CHOP								
Trimmed								
broiled	3 oz	200	22	0	54	na	11.8	72
broiled, yield from 1 med chop	5.3 oz	247	27	0	67	na	14.5	89
raw	1 oz	59	5	0	17	na	4.1	19
Untrimmed								
broiled	3 oz	160	23	0	56	na	6.6	72
broiled, yield from 1 med chop	5.3 oz	179	26	0	63	na	7.4	81
raw	1 oz	37	6	0	18	na	1.4	18
LAMB, NEW ZEALAND								
COMPOSITE CUTS								
Trimmed								
cooked	4 oz	234	33.6	0.0	57	0	10.0	124
raw	1 oz	36	5.9	0.0	13	0	1.3	21
Untrimmed								
raw	1 oz	182	2.0	0.0	6	0	19.2	25
LEG/FORESHANK								
Trimmed								
braised	3 oz	158	26.1	0.0	42	0	5.1	86
braised, diced	1 cup	260	43.1	0.0	69	0	8.5	141
raw	1 lb	535	94.4	0.0	227	0	14.9	304

Food Name	Serv. Size	Total Cal.	Prot. gms	Carbs gms	Sod. mgs	Fiber gms	Fat gms	Chol. mgs
raw	1 oz	33	5.8	0.0	14	0	0.9	19
stewed	4 oz	211	34.9	0.0	56	0	6.8	115
stewed, diced	1 cup	260	43.1	0.0	69	0	8.5	141
Untrimmed								
braised	3 oz	219	22.9	0.0	40	0	13.5	87
braised, diced	1 cup	361	37.8	0.0	66	0	22.2	143
raw	1 lb	1012	81.8	0.0	204	0	73.3	322
raw	1 oz	62	5.1	0.0	13	0	4.5	20
stewed	4 oz	293	30.6	0.0	53	0	18.0	116
stewed, diced	1 cup	361	37.8	0.0	66	0	22.2	143
LEG/WHOLE								
Trimmed								
raw	1 lb	558	94.6	0.0	200	0	17.2	331
raw	1 oz	34	5.8	0.0	12	0	1.1	20
roasted	3 oz	154	23.5	0.0	38	0	6.0	85
roasted, diced	1 cup	253	38.8	0.0	63	0	9.8	140
Untrimmed								
raw	1 lb	980	83.2	0.0	181	0	69.4	345
raw	1 oz	60	5.1	0.0	11	0	4.3	21
roasted	3 oz	209	21.1	0.0	37	0	13.2	86
roasted, diced	1 cup	344	34.7	0.0	60	0	21.8	141
LOIN								
Trimmed								
broiled	4 oz	226	33.2	0.0	62	0	9.3	129
raw	1 oz	36	5.9	0.0	13	0	1.2	22
roasted	3 oz	169	24.9	0.0	47	0	7.0	97
Untrimmed								
broiled	3 oz	268	19.9	0.0	42	0	20.3	95
raw	1 oz	85	4.6	0.0	10	0	7.3	23
RIB								
Trimmed								
raw	1 lb	644	92.9	0.0	236	0	27.5	345
raw	1 oz	40	5.7	0.0	15	0	1.7	21
roasted	3 oz	167	20.8	0.0	41	0	8.6	80
Untrimmed								
raw	1 lb	1569	67.7	0.0	181	0	142.0	367
raw	1 oz	97	4.2	0.0	11	0	8.8	23
roasted	3 oz	289	16.1	0.0	37	0	24.4	85
SHOULDER/WHOLE								
Trimmed								
braised	3 oz	242	29.0	0.0	48	0	13.2	108
braised, diced	1 cup	399	47.7	0.0	78	0	21.7	178
raw	1 lb	612	91.8	0.0	213	0	24.6	322
raw	1 oz	38	5.8	0.0	13	0	1.5	20
stewed	6.5 oz	522	62.3	0.0	103	0	28.3	232
stewed, diced	1 cup	399	47.7	0.0	78	0	21.7	178
Untrimmed								
braised	3 oz	303	24.0	0.0	43	0	22.3	106
braised, diced	1 cup	491	40.2	0.0	73	0	35.5	172
raw	1 lb	1234	75.5	0.0	186	0	100.8	340
stewed	4 oz	398	32.5	0.0	59	0	28.8	139
stewed, diced	1 cup	491	40.2	0.0	73	0	35.5	172
LAMB, U.S.								

(NOTE: All USDA choice grade. TRIMMED = Lean; separable fat removed. UNTRIMMED = Separable fat not removed.)

Food Name	Serv. Size	Total Cal.	Prot. gms	Carbs gms	Sod. mgs	Fiber gms	Fat gms	Chol. mgs
BRAIN								
braised	3 oz	123	10.7	0.0	114	0	8.6	1737
braised, yield from 1 lb raw	12.25 oz	503	43.5	0.0	465	0	35.3	7089

Food Name	Serv. Size	Total Cal.	Prot. gms	Carbs gms	Sod. mgs	Fiber gms	Fat gms	Chol. mgs
pan-fried	3 oz	232	14.4	0.0	133	0	18.9	2128
raw	4 oz	138	11.8	0.0	127	0	9.7	1533
COMPOSITE CUTS/LEG AND SHOULDER								
Trimmed								
braised, cubed	3 oz	190	28.6	0.0	59	0	7.5	92
broiled, cubed	3 oz	158	23.9	0.0	65	0	6.2	77
broiled, ground	3 oz	241	21.0	0.0	69	na	16.7	82
raw, cubed	1 lb	608	91.7	0.0	295	0	24.0	295
raw, cubed	1 oz	38	5.7	0.0	18	0	1.5	18
raw, ground	1 lb	1279	75.1	0.0	268	na	106.2	331
raw, ground	1 oz	79	4.6	0.0	17	na	6.6	20
stewed, cubed	4 oz	253	38.2	0.0	79	0	10.0	122
GROUND								
broiled	3 oz	241	21	0	69	0	16.7	82
raw	4 oz	319	19	0	67	0	26.5	82
raw	1 oz	80	5	0	17	0	6.6	21
HEART								
braised	3 oz	157	21.2	1.6	54	0	6.7	212
raw	4 oz	138	18.7	0.2	101	0	6.4	153
simmered	4 oz	210	28.3	2.2	71	0	9.0	282
KIDNEYS								
braised	3 oz	116	20.1	0.8	128	0	3.1	480
raw	4 oz	110	17.8	0.9	177	0	3.3	382
LEG/FORESHANK								
Trimmed								
braised	3 oz	159	26.4	0.0	63	0	5.1	88
braised	1 oz	53	8.8	0.0	21	0	1.7	29
braised, diced	1 cup	262	43.4	0.0	104	0	8.4	146
broiled, ground	1 cup	328	28.7	0.0	94	0	23.1	113
broiled, ground	4 oz	321	28.1	0.0	92	0	22.3	110
raw	1 lb	544	95.6	0.0	358	0	14.9	313
raw	1 oz	34	5.9	0.0	22	0	0.9	19
raw, ground	1 cup	637	37.4	0.0	133	0	52.9	165
stewed	4 oz	212	35.2	0.0	84	0	6.8	118
stewed	1 oz	53	8.8	0.0	21	0	1.7	29
stewed, diced	1 cup	262	43.4	0.0	104	0	8.4	146
Untrimmed								
braised	3 oz	207	24.1	0.0	61	0	11.4	90
braised	1 oz	69	8.0	0.0	20	0	3.8	30
braised, diced	1 cup	340	39.7	0.0	101	0	18.8	148
raw	1 lb	912	85.8	0.0	327	0	60.7	327
raw	1 oz	56	5.3	0.0	20	0	3.8	20
stewed	1 oz	69	8.0	0.0	20	0	3.8	30
stewed, diced	1 cup	340	39.7	0.0	101	0	18.8	148
LEG/SHANK								
Trimmed								
raw	1 lb	567	93.1	0.0	277	0	19.0	290
raw	1 oz	35	5.8	0.0	17	0	1.2	18
roasted	3 oz	153	23.9	0.0	56	0	5.7	74
roasted	1 oz	51	8.0	0.0	19	0	1.9	25
roasted, diced	1 cup	252	39.4	0.0	92	0	9.3	122
Untrimmed								
raw	1 lb	912	84.3	0.0	259	0	61.2	304
raw	1 oz	56	5.2	0.0	16	0	3.8	19
roasted	3 oz	191	22.5	0.0	55	0	10.6	77
roasted	1 oz	64	7.5	0.0	18	0	3.5	26
roasted, diced	1 cup	315	37.0	0.0	91	0	17.4	126

Food Name	Serv. Size	Total Cal.	Prot. gms	Carbs gms	Sod. mgs	Fiber gms	Fat gms	Chol. mgs
LEG/SIRLOIN								
Trimmed								
raw	1 lb	608	93.2	0.0	290	0	23.0	299
raw	1 oz	38	5.8	0.0	18	0	1.4	18
roasted	3 oz	173	24.1	0.0	60	0	7.8	78
roasted	1 oz	58	8.0	0.0	20	0	2.6	26
roasted, diced	1 cup	286	39.7	0.0	99	0	12.8	129
Untrimmed								
raw	1 lb	1234	76.8	0.0	254	0	100.3	327
raw	1 oz	76	4.7	0.0	16	0	6.2	20
roasted	3 oz	248	20.9	0.0	58	0	17.6	82
roasted	1 oz	83	7.0	0.0	19	0	5.9	27
roasted, diced	1 cup	409	34.5	0.0	95	0	28.9	136
LEG/WHOLE								
Trimmed								
raw	1 lb	581	93.3	0.0	281	0	20.5	290
raw	1 oz	36	5.8	0.0	17	0	1.3	18
roasted	3 oz	162	24.1	0.0	58	0	6.6	76
roasted	1 oz	54	8.0	0.0	19	0	2.2	25
roasted, diced	1 cup	267	39.6	0.0	95	0	10.8	125
Untrimmed								
raw	1 lb	1043	81.2	0.0	254	0	77.4	313
raw	1 oz	64	5.0	0.0	16	0	4.8	19
roasted	3 oz	219	21.7	0.0	56	0	14.0	79
roasted	1 oz	73	7.2	0.0	19	0	4.7	26
roasted, diced	1 cup	361	35.8	0.0	92	0	23.0	130
LIVER								
braised	3 oz	187	26.0	2.2	48	na	7.5	426
pan-fried	3 oz	202	21.7	3.2	105	na	10.8	419
raw	4 oz	158	23.1	2.0	79	na	5.7	421
LOIN								
Trimmed								
broiled	3 oz	184	25.5	0.0	71	0	8.3	81
raw	1 oz	40	5.8	0.0	19	0	1.7	18
roasted	3 oz	172	22.6	0.0	56	0	8.3	74
Untrimmed								
broiled	3 oz	269	21.4	0.0	65	0	19.6	85
roasted	3 oz	263	19.2	0.0	54	0	20.0	81
LUNGS								
braised	3 oz	96	16.9	0.0	71	0	2.6	241
raw	4 oz	108	18.9	0.0	178	0	3.0	na
PANCREAS								
braised	3 oz	199	19.4	0.0	44	0	12.8	340
raw	4 oz	172	16.8	0.0	85	0	11.1	295
RIB								
Trimmed								
broiled	3 oz	200	23.6	0.0	72	0	11.0	77
raw	1 lb	767	90.6	0.0	327	0	41.9	299
raw	1 oz	47	5.6	0.0	20	0	2.6	18
roasted	3 oz	197	22.2	0.0	69	0	11.3	75
Untrimmed								
broiled	3 oz	307	18.8	0.0	65	0	25.1	84
raw	1 lb	1687	65.9	0.0	254	0	156.0	345
raw	1 oz	104	4.1	0.0	16	0	9.6	21
roasted	3 oz	305	18.0	0.0	62	0	25.3	82
SHOULDER/ARM								
Trimmed								
braised	3 oz	237	30.2	0.0	65	0	12.0	103

Food Name	Serv. Size	Total Cal.	Prot. gms	Carbs gms	Sod. mgs	Fiber gms	Fat gms	Chol. mgs
broiled	3 oz	170	23.5	0.0	70	0	7.7	78
raw	1 oz	37	5.6	0.0	19	0	1.5	18
roasted	3 oz	163	21.6	0.0	57	0	7.9	73
Untrimmed								
braised	3 oz	294	25.8	0.0	61	0	20.4	102
broiled	3 oz	239	20.8	0.0	65	0	16.6	82
raw	1 oz	73	4.7	0.0	17	0	5.8	20
roasted	3 oz	237	19.1	0.0	55	0	17.2	78
SHOULDER/BLADE								
Trimmed								
braised	1 oz	81	9.1	0.0	22	0	4.7	33
broiled	3 oz	179	21.7	0.0	75	0	9.6	77
raw	3 oz	128	16.4	0.0	59	0	6.5	57
roasted	3 oz	178	20.9	0.0	58	0	9.8	74
Untrimmed								
braised	3 oz	293	24.2	0.0	64	0	21.0	99
broiled	3 oz	236	19.6	0.0	70	0	17.0	81
raw	1 lb	1175	75.4	0.0	281	0	94.6	327
raw	1 oz	73	4.7	0.0	17	0	5.8	20
roasted	3 oz	239	18.9	0.0	56	0	17.5	78
SHOULDER/WHOLE								
Trimmed								
braised	4 oz	321	37.2	0.0	90	0	10.0	133
braised, diced	1 cup	396	45.9	0.0	111	0	22.2	164
broiled	4 oz	238	30.8	0.0	94	0	11.9	105
roasted	4 oz	231	28.3	0.0	77	0	12.2	99
roasted, diced	1 cup	286	34.9	0.0	95	0	15.1	122
stewed	4 oz	321	37.2	0.0	90	0	10.0	133
stewed, diced	1 cup	396	45.9	0.0	111	0	22.2	164
Untrimmed								
braised, diced	1 cup	482	40.2	0.0	105	0	34.4	162
broiled	4 oz	315	27.7	0.0	88	0	21.8	110
broiled, diced	1 cup	389	34.2	0.0	109	0	27.0	136
roasted	4 oz	313	25.5	0.0	75	0	22.6	104
roasted, diced	1 cup	386	31.5	0.0	92	0	28.0	129
stewed	4 oz	390	32.5	0.0	85	0	27.8	132
stewed, diced	1 cup	482	40.2	0.0	105	0	34.4	162
SPLEEN								
braised	3 oz	133	22.5	0.0	49	0	4.1	327
raw	4 oz	115	19.5	0.0	95	0	3.5	283
TONGUE								
braised	3 oz	234	18.3	0.0	57	0	17.2	161
raw	4 oz	252	17.8	0.0	88	0	19.5	177
LAMB DINNER/ENTRÉE								
(Stouffer's) shepherd's pie, frozen, food service product	1 oz	36	2	3	122	na	1.8	3
LAMB'S QUARTERS								
Fresh								
boiled, drained	4 oz	36	3.6	5.7	(mq)	>2.0 c	0.8	0
boiled, drained, chopped	1 cup	58	5.8	9.0	52	>3.2 c	1.3	0
raw	3.5 oz	43	4.2	7.3	43	>4.0	0.8	0
raw, trimmed	1 lb	195	19.1	33.1	(mq)	>9.5 c	3.6	0
raw, trimmed	1 oz	12	1.2	2.1	(mq)	>.6 c	0.2	0
LARD								
	1 cup	1849	0	0	0	0	205.0	195
	1 tbsp	115	0	0	0	0	12.8	12
LASAGNA/LASAGNA ENTRÉE								
(Amy's Kitchen)								
tofu and vegetable	1 serving	300	18	41	630	6	10.0	0

Food Name	Serv. Size	Total Cal.	Prot. gms	Carbs gms	Sod. mgs	Fiber gms	Fat gms	Chol. mgs
vegetable, w/cheese	1 serving	300	15	39	680	5	10.0	15
(Banquet)								
frozen, 'Extra Helping'	16.5 oz	645	24	88	1582	0	23.0	38
w/meat sauce	1 entrée	260	10	38	820	5	8.0	10
(Bernardi)								
'Solito'	1 cup	380	22	33	760	5	18.0	60
'Supreme'	1 cup	310	18	32	930	3	13.0	40
supreme, portioned	1 1/4 cup	369	21	38	1108	4	15.0	45
vegetable, 'Supreme'	1 cup	360	20	35	870	2	17.0	65
(Budget Gourmet)								
sausage, Italian	1 entrée	430	20	40	730	4	21.0	60
three cheese	1 entrée	370	20	38	870	5	16.0	60
vegetable, 'Light'	1 entrée	290	15	36	780	5	9.0	15
w/cheese and meat sauce	1 entrée	326	20	35	687	4	12.0	46
w/Italian sausage	1 entrée	456	21	40	903	3	23.8	48
w/meat sauce, 'Light'	1 entrée	250	15	31	690	3	7.0	30
(Buitoni)								
in sauce, frozen, 'Family Style'	7.3 oz	370	13	30	940	0	13.0	55
meat, frozen, 'Single Serving'	9 oz	580	23	57	820	0	19.0	110
(Celentano)								
....	10-oz tray	400	18	51	650	7	14.0	80
....	1 cup	320	14	41	520	6	11.0	65
frozen, 14-oz tray	7 oz	280	15	33	660	8	10.0	75
low-fat, frozen, 'Great Choice'	10-oz tray	260	18	42	650	2	2.5	20
primavera, 'Great Choice'	10-oz tray	240	17	33	600	0	7.0	0
primavera, 'Selects'	10-oz tray	220	12	32	510	5	5.0	5
(Chef Boyardee)								
....	1 cup	270	10	41	680	3	8.0	20
hearty, microwave cup, 'Main Meals'	10.5 oz	290	13	41	0	0	8.0	0
in garden vegetable sauce, canned, microwave	7.5 oz	170	5	14	940	0	1.0	3
microwave	7.5 oz	230	7	31	1080	0	9.0	18
(Contadina)								
chicken, food service product, frozen	1 oz	44	2	3	116	na	2.6	6
classic, frozen, food service product	1 oz	39	2	4	119	1	1.6	8
precut, classic, frozen, food service product	1 oz	39	2	3	88	0	2.2	5
(Dining Lite)								
cheese, frozen	9 oz	260	14	36	800	0	6.0	30
w/meat sauce, frozen	9 oz	240	13	36	800	0	5.0	25
(Dinty Moore)								
w/meat sauce, packaged, 'American Classics'	10 oz	320	16	33	870	0	14.0	35
(Freezer Queen) w/meat sauce, 'Deluxe Family Suppers' ...	7 oz	200	8	28	730	0	6.0	0
(Green Giant) frozen, 'Entrées'	12 oz	490	33	44	1660	0	20.0	0
(Healthy Choice)								
Roma, w/meat sauce	1 entrée	400	26	59	580	9	7.0	15
w/meat sauce, frozen	10 oz	260	18	37	420	0	5.0	20
zucchini, frozen	11.5 oz	250	14	41	400	0	3.0	15
(Hormel) microwave cup	7.5 oz	250	8	25	949	0	13.0	23
(Le Menu)								
garden vegetable, 'Light Style'	10.5 oz	260	11	35	500	0	8.0	25
w/meat sauce, frozen, 'LightStyle'	10 oz	290	19	36	510	0	8.0	30
(Lean Cuisine)								
chicken, scaloppini, frozen, 'Café Classics'	1 pkg	290	20	34	560	4	8.0	40
classic	1 entrée	290	20	38	560	5	6.0	30
5-cheese, frozen, food service product	1 oz	27	2	3	68	0	0.7	3
'Hearty Portions'	1 entrée	440	26	64	830	6	9.0	30
tuna, w/spinach noodles, frozen	9.75 oz	240	16	29	520	0	7.0	20
vegetable	1 entrée	260	15	35	590	5	7.0	20

Food Name	Serv. Size	Total Cal.	Prot. gms	Carbs gms	Sod. mgs	Fiber gms	Fat gms	Chol. mgs
w/meat sauce	1 entrée	290	20	35	560	6	8.0	35
w/meat sauce, frozen	10.25 oz	280	20	36	560	0	6.0	25
(Legume)								
vegetable, w/tofu and sauce	12 oz	240	14	26	520	6	8.0	0
vegetarian, nondairy, classic, w/organic pasta and tofu	1 serving	340	20	37	560	11	13.0	0
vegetable, vegetarian, nondairy, w/organic pasta and tofu	1 serving	210	13	24	480	5	7.0	0
(Libby's) w/meat sauce, microwave cup, 'Diner'	7.75 oz	200	9	29	790	2	5.0	15
(Lunch Bucket) w/meat sauce, microwave lunch cup	7.5 oz	220	8	38	870	0	4.0	30
(Lunch Express)								
casserole, cheese	1 entrée	270	14	38	590	5	7.0	15
w/meat sauce	1 entrée	330	18	42	910	5	10.0	40
(Marie Callender's)								
extra cheese	1 cup	350	16	36	720	4	16.0	20
w/meat sauce	15 oz	370	17	34	740	4	18.0	35
w/meat sauce, frozen, family size	1 cup	350	17	32	770	3	16.0	50
(Mrs. Paul's) seafood, frozen, 'Light'	9.5 oz	290	14	39	750	0	8.0	57
(Nalley's) canned	7.5 oz	180	10	24	720	0	5.0	0
(Smart Ones)								
Alfredo	1 entrée	300	14	46	680	3	7.0	20
Florentine	1 entrée	200	10	34	590	5	2.0	10
w/meat sauce	1 entrée	240	13	43	520	4	2.0	10
(Stouffer's)								
fiesta, w/meat, frozen, food service product	1 oz	43	2	4	105	na	2.0	4
frozen, 96-oz pkg	9 3/5 oz	400	30	37	940	0	14.0	0
frozen, 10-oz pkg	10 oz	340	18	40	840	0	12.0	0
frozen, 21-oz pkg	10.5 oz	360	28	33	1020	0	13.0	0
vegetable	1 entrée	450	20	41	980	5	23.0	40
vegetable, frozen, 96-oz pkg	9.6 oz	400	23	33	760	0	20.0	0
w/meat and sauce, frozen	1 pkg	768	52	73	2035	9	29.8	113
w/meat and sauce	1 serving	277	19	26	735	3	10.8	41
w/meat and sauce, frozen, food service product	1 entrée	40	3	4	94	0	1.7	5
w/meat sauce	1 entrée	360	27	34	780	5	13.0	50
w/meat sauce, frozen, food service product	1 oz	39	3	3	95	0	1.6	5
(Swanson)								
w/meat sauce	1 entrée	340	22	37	940	5	12.0	30
w/meat sauce, frozen, 'Homestyle Recipe'	10.5 oz	400	26	39	1070	0	15.0	0
(Top Shelf)								
Italian, packaged	10 oz	350	23	30	840	0	16.0	60
vegetable, packaged	10.6 oz	275	18	34	1024	0	8.0	35
(Tyson) frozen 'Gourmet Selection'	11.5 oz	380	20	47	840	0	14.0	0
(Ultra Slim-Fast)								
vegetable	12 oz	240	17	39	730	0	4.0	15
w/meat sauce	12 oz	330	28	38	980	0	9.0	55
(Weight Watchers)								
Bolognese	1 entrée	300	16	45	590	4	7.0	20
cheese, Italian	1 entrée	300	20	38	550	5	8.0	30
garden	1 entrée	270	14	36	4	5	7.0	30
w/cheese, meat, and tomato sauce	11-oz entrée	358	22	38	755	4	13.2	50
w/meat sauce	1 entrée	270	14	38	570	6	7.0	35

LASAGNA NOODLE. See under PASTA.
LAVER. See under SEA VEGETABLE.
LEEK
Fresh

boiled, drained, chopped	1/4 cup	8	0	2	3	0	0.1	0
boiled, drained, whole	1 medium	38	1	9	12	1	0.2	0

Food Name	Serv. Size	Total Cal.	Prot. gms	Carbs gms	Sod. mgs	Fiber gms	Fat gms	Chol. mgs
raw, chopped	1 cup	54	1	13	18	2	0.3	0
raw, whole	1 medium	54	1	13	18	2	0.3	0
Freeze-dried								
bulb/lower leaf portion	1/4 cup	3	0	1	0	0	0.0	0
bulb/lower leaf portion	1 tbsp	1	0	0	0	0	0.0	0
LEMON								
Fresh								
raw, sectioned, w/o peel	1 cup	61	2	20	4	6	0.6	0
raw, sliced, w/o peel, 1/8 of 2 1/8 inch diam lemon	1 wedge	2	0	1	0	0	0.0	0
raw, whole, w/o peel, 2 1/8 inch diam	1 lemon	17	1	5	1	2	0.2	0
raw, w/peel, w/o seeds, 2 3/8 inch diam	1 lemon	22	1	12	3	5	0.3	0
LEMON HERB SEASONING. See under SEASONING MIX.								
LEMON JUICE								
Canned or bottled								
....	1 cup	51	1	16	51	1	0.7	0
....	1 fl oz	6	0	2	6	0	0.1	0
....	1 tbsp	3	0	1	3	0	0.0	0
unsweetened, single strength	1 cup	54	1	16	2	1	0.8	0
unsweetened, single strength	1 fl oz	7	0	2	0	0	0.1	0
(A&P) reconstituted, natural strength	1 fl oz	6	1	2	0	0	1.0	0
(Lucky Leaf)	6 fl oz	30	1	6	35	0	0.0	0
(ReaLemon)								
reconstituted, natural strength	1 fl oz	6	0	2	10	0	0.0	0
reconstituted, '100%'	1 fl oz	6	0	2	5	0	0.0	0
Fresh								
....	1 cup	61	1	21	2	1	0.0	0
....	1 fl oz	8	0	3	0	0	0.0	0
juice of 1/8 of 2 1/8 inch-diam lemon	0.2 oz	1	0	1	0	0	0.0	0
juice of 2 1/8 inch-diam lemon	1.6 oz	12	0	4	0	0	0.0	0
Frozen								
(Minute Maid) concentrate, prepared	6 fl oz	8	0	2	0	0	0.0	0
(Sunkist)	1 fl oz	7	0	2	1	0	0.1	0
LEMON PEEL								
raw, grated	1 tbsp	3	0	1	0	1	0.0	0
raw, grated	1 tsp	1	0	0	0	0	0.0	0
raw, grated *(Tone's)*	1 tsp	0	0	0	0	0	0.0	0
LEMON PEPPER. See under SEASONING MIX.								
LEMONADE. See under FRUIT DRINK; FRUIT DRINK MIX.								
LEMONGRASS/citronella								
raw	1 cup	66	1	17	4	na	0.3	0
raw	1 tbsp	5	0	1	0	na	0.0	0
LEMON-LIME DRINK. See under FRUIT DRINK.								
LENTIL								
Canned, organic *(Eden Foods)*	1/2 cup	90	8	13	210	4	0.0	0
Dried								
boiled *(A&P)*	1 cup	210	16	39	0	0	1.0	0
green, raw *(Arrowhead Mills)*	2 oz	190	13	35	9	9	1.0	0
mature seeds, boiled	1 cup	230	18	40	4	16	0.8	0
mature seeds, boiled	1 tbsp	14	1	2	0	1	0.0	0
mature seeds, raw	1 cup	649	54	110	19	59	1.8	0
mature seeds, raw	1 tbsp	41	3	7	1	4	0.1	0
pink, raw	1 cup	664	48	114	13	21	4.2	0
red, raw *(Arrowhead Mills)*	2 oz	195	14	34	10	9	1.0	0
Sprouted, raw	1 cup	82	7	17	8	na	0.4	0
LENTIL DISH/ENTRÉE								
(Casbah) pilaf, prepared	3/4 cup	240	9	38	400	2	0.5	0

Food Name	Serv. Size	Total Cal.	Prot. gms	Carbs gms	Sod. mgs	Fiber gms	Fat gms	Chol. mgs
(Health Valley) canned, w/garden vegetables, nonfat,								
canned, 'Fast Menu'	7.5 oz	160	13	18	204	16	4.0	0
(Natural Touch) lentil rice loaf	1 slice	166	8	15	366	4	8.6	2

LETTUCE
BIBB, BOSTON, OR BUTTERHEAD

Food Name	Serv. Size	Total Cal.	Prot. gms	Carbs gms	Sod. mgs	Fiber gms	Fat gms	Chol. mgs
leaf, large	1 leaf	2	0	0	1	0	0.0	0
leaf, medium	1 leaf	1	0	0	0	0	0.0	0
leaf, small	1 leaf	1	0	0	0	0	0.0	0
shredded	1 cup	7	1	1	3	1	0.1	0
whole *(Dole)*	1 med head	21	2	4	8	2	0.1	0
whole, approx 5-inch diam	1 head	21	2	4	8	2	0.4	0

COS

Food Name	Serv. Size	Total Cal.	Prot. gms	Carbs gms	Sod. mgs	Fiber gms	Fat gms	Chol. mgs
inner leaf, whole	1 med leaf	1	0	0	1	0	0.0	0
shredded	1/2 cup	4	0	1	2	0	0.1	0

ICEBERG

Food Name	Serv. Size	Total Cal.	Prot. gms	Carbs gms	Sod. mgs	Fiber gms	Fat gms	Chol. mgs
leaf, large	1 leaf	2	0	0	1	0	0.0	0
leaf, medium	1 leaf	1	0	0	1	0	0.0	0
leaf, small	1 leaf	1	0	0	0	0	0.0	0
shredded or chopped	1 cup	7	1	1	5	1	0.1	0
wedge, 1/6 of med head *(Dole)*	1 wedge	20	1	4	10	1	0.0	0
whole, approx 6-inch diam	1 head	65	5	11	49	8	1.0	0
LEAF, shredded *(Dole)*	1.5 cup	12	1	1	40	1	0.0	0

LOOSELEAF

Food Name	Serv. Size	Total Cal.	Prot. gms	Carbs gms	Sod. mgs	Fiber gms	Fat gms	Chol. mgs
leaf, medium	1 leaf	2	0	0	1	0	0.0	0
shredded	1/2 cup	5	0	1	3	1	0.1	0

ROMAINE

Food Name	Serv. Size	Total Cal.	Prot. gms	Carbs gms	Sod. mgs	Fiber gms	Fat gms	Chol. mgs
inner leaf, whole	1 leaf	1	0	0	1	0	0.0	0
shredded	1/2 cup	4	0	1	2	0	0.1	0
shredded *(Dole)*	1.5 cup	18	1	2	40	1	1.0	0

LICHI. See LITCHI.
LIMA BEAN. See BEAN, LIMA; BEAN DISH/ENTRÉE.
LIME

Food Name	Serv. Size	Total Cal.	Prot. gms	Carbs gms	Sod. mgs	Fiber gms	Fat gms	Chol. mgs
fresh, raw, peeled and seeded	1 oz	9	02	3.0	1	>.1 c	0.1	0
fresh, raw, whole, approx 2-inch dia	1 lime	20	0	7	1	2	0.1	0

LIME DRINK. See under FRUIT DRINK.
LIME JUICE
Canned or bottled

Food Name	Serv. Size	Total Cal.	Prot. gms	Carbs gms	Sod. mgs	Fiber gms	Fat gms	Chol. mgs
unsweetened	1 cup	52	1	16	39	1	0.6	0
unsweetened	1 fl oz	6	0	2	5	0	0.1	0
(ReaLime)								
original, unsweetened	1 tbsp	0	0	0	0	0	0.0	0
reconstituted, natural strength	1 fl oz	6	0	2	10	0	0.0	0
(Roses)	1 fl oz	48	0	12	6	0	0.0	0
(Santa Cruz Natural) organic, 'Cruz'	8 fl oz	120	1	27	0	0	1.0	0
Fresh								
	1 cup	66	1	22	2	1	0.2	0
	1 fl oz	8	0	3	0	0	0.0	0
juice of 2 1/8 inch-diam lime	1.3 oz	10	0	3	0	0	0.0	0
juice of 1/8 of 2 1/8 inch-diam lime	0.2 oz	1	0	0	0	0	0.0	0

LIMEADE. See under FRUIT DRINK.
LING

Food Name	Serv. Size	Total Cal.	Prot. gms	Carbs gms	Sod. mgs	Fiber gms	Fat gms	Chol. mgs
baked, broiled, grilled, or microwaved	3 oz	94	21	0	147	0	0.7	43
raw	3 oz	74	16	0	115	0	0.5	34

LINGCOD

Food Name	Serv. Size	Total Cal.	Prot. gms	Carbs gms	Sod. mgs	Fiber gms	Fat gms	Chol. mgs
baked, broiled, grilled, or microwaved	3 oz	93	19	0	65	0	1.2	57
raw	3 oz	72	15	0	50	0	0.9	44

LINGUINE. See under PASTA.

Food Name	Serv. Size	Total Cal.	Prot. gms	Carbs gms	Sod. mgs	Fiber gms	Fat gms	Chol. mgs
LINGUINE DISH/ENTRÉE. See under PASTA DISH/ENTRÉE.								
LIQUEUR								
COFFEE								
w/cream, 34 proof	1 fl oz	102	1	7	29	0	4.9	5
53 proof	1 fl oz	117	0	16	3	0	0.1	0
63 proof	1 fl oz	107	0	11	3	0	0.1	0
CRÈME DE MENTHE								
72 proof	1 fl oz	125	0	14	2	0	0.1	0
LIQUOR. See individual listings.								
LITCHI/lychee								
dried	3.5 oz	277	3.8	70.7	3	>1.4 c	1.2	0
dried	1 oz	79	1.1	20.0	1	4.6	0.3	0
dried	1 medium	7	0	2	0	0	0.0	0
raw	1 cup	125	2	31	2	2	0.8	0
raw, shelled and seeded	1/2 cup	63	0.8	15.7	1	>.2 c	0.4	0
raw, shelled and seeded	1 oz	19	0.2	4.7	<1	>.1 c	0.1	0
raw, trimmed, approx 0.6 oz	1 medium	6	0	2	0	0	0.0	0
raw, untrimmed	1 lb	179	2.3	45.0	2	>.6 c	1.2	0
LIVER. See under individual meat listings. Also see PÂTÉ, CANNED.								
LIVERWURST. See under LUNCHEON MEAT.								
LOBSTER								
NORTHERN								
boiled, poached, or steamed	1 cup	142	29.7	1.9	551	0	0.9	104
boiled, poached or steamed	4 oz	111	23.2	1.5	431	0	0.7	82
raw	1 lb	410	85.3	2.3	(mq)	0	4.1	432
raw	3 oz	77	16.0	0.4	252	0	0.8	81
raw	1 oz	26	5.3	0.1	(mq)	0	0.3	27
SPINY, MIXED SPECIES								
boiled, poached or steamed	3 oz	122	22.5	2.7	193	0	1.6	77
raw	1 lb	506	93.4	11.0	803	0	6.9	318
raw	3 oz	95	17.5	2.1	150	0	1.3	59
raw	1 oz	32	5.8	0.7	50	0	0.4	20
LOGANBERRY								
Fresh								
raw, trimmed	1 lb	281	4.5	67.6	5	(mq)	2.7	0
raw, trimmed	1 cup	89	1.4	21.5	1	>4.3 c	0.9	0
raw, untrimmed	1 lb	267	4.3	64.2	4	(mq)	2.6	0
Frozen								
	1 cup	81	2.2	19.1	1	7.2	0.5	0
	4 oz	62	1.7	14.8	1	(mq)	0.4	0
LONGAN/dragon's eye								
Dried	1 oz	81	1.4	21.0	14	13.4	0.1	0
Fresh								
raw, approx 0.2 oz	1 medium	2	<.1	0.5	tr	<.1	tr	0
raw, shelled and seeded	1 oz	17	0.4	4.3	tr	>.1 c	<.1	0
raw, untrimmed	1 lb	144	3.2	36.4	1	>1.0 c	0.2	0
LONGBEAN								
Fresh								
boiled, drained	4 oz	53	2.9	10.4	5	>1.7 c	0.1	0
boiled, drained, sliced	1/2 cup	25	1.3	4.8	2	>.8 c	0.1	0
boiled, drained, 13 1/4 inches long x 1/4 inch diam	1 pod	7	0.4	1.3	1	>.2 c	<.1	0
raw, sliced	1/2 cup	22	1.3	3.8	2	(mq)	0.2	0
raw, 13 1/4 inches long x 1/4 inch diam	1 pod	6	0.3	1.0	tr	(mq)	0.1	0
raw, trimmed	1 oz	13	0.8	2.4	1	(mq)	0.1	0
raw, untrimmed	1 lb	203	12.1	36.0	17	(mq)	1.7	0
Dried								
boiled	1/2 cup	102	7.1	18.1	4	>1.4 c	0.4	0

Food Name	Serv. Size	Total Cal.	Prot. gms	Carbs gms	Sod. mgs	Fiber gms	Fat gms	Chol. mgs
boiled .... 4 oz		134	9.4	23.9	6	>1.8 c	0.5	0
raw .... 1/2 cup		292	20.4	52.0	14	>4.0 c	1.1	0
raw .... 1 oz		98	6.9	17.6	5	>1.4 c	0.4	0

LOOFAH GOURD. See GOURD, DISHCLOTH.

LOQUAT/Japanese medlar

raw, cubed .... 1 cup		70	1	18	1	3	0.3	0
raw, whole, large .... 1 fruit		9	0	2	0	0	0.0	0
raw, whole, medium .... 1 fruit		8	0	2	0	0	0.0	0
raw, whole, small .... 1 fruit		6	0	2	0	0	0.0	0

LOTTE. See MONKFISH.

LOTUS ROOT

boiled, drained, sliced .... 1/2 cup		40	1	10	27	2	0.0	0
raw, whole, 9.5-inch long .... 1 root		85	3	20	46	6	0.1	0

LOTUS SEED

dried .... 1 cup		106	5	21	2	na	0.6	0
dried, whole, approx 42 kernels .... 1 oz		94	4	18	1	na	0.6	0
raw .... 1 oz		25	1	5	0	na	0.1	0

LOX. See under SALMON.

LUNCH COMBINATION, PACKAGED

(Eckrich)

ham and Swiss, crackers, 'Lunch Makers' .... 1 piece		40	2	2	170	0	2.0	5
turkey and cheddar, crackers, 'Lunch Makers' .... 1 piece		40	2	2	160	0	2.0	5

(Hillshire Farm)

bologna and American, cracker, Snickers, 6-oz drink ... 1 lunch		590	15	55	1130	0	34.0	0
bologna and American, cracker, Snickers, w/o drink .... 1 lunch		490	15	31	1110	0	34.0	0
chicken and Monterey Jack, cracker, Snickers .... 1 lunch		400	19	31	1080	0	23.0	0
ham and cheddar, cracker, Snickers, w/o drink .... 1 lunch		400	17	32	1010	0	23.0	0
ham and cheddar, cracker, Snickers, 6 oz drink .... 1 lunch		500	17	56	1030	0	23.0	0
ham and Swiss, cracker, Oreo, 'Lunch'n Munch' .... 1 lunch		370	16	30	1160	0	21.0	0
turkey and cheddar, cracker, brownie .... 1 lunch		400	17	34	1240	0	22.0	0

(Louis Rich)

turkey breast and cheddar cheese, 'Lunch Breaks' ...... 1 pkg		410	22	23	1715	0	26.0	70
turkey ham and Swiss cheese, 'Lunch Breaks' .... 1 pkg		380	24	25	1875	0	22.0	75
turkey salami and cheddar cheese, 'Lunch Breaks' ...... 1 pkg		430	22	25	1595	0	29.0	85
turkey, w/Monterey Jack cheese, 'Lunch Breaks' .... 1 pkg		400	21	27	1665	0	25.0	75

(Oscar Mayer)

bologna and American lunch, 'Lunchables' .... 1 lunch		470	17	22	1670	1	35.0	90
bologna and wild cherry lunch, 'Lunchables' .... 1 lunch		530	12	60	1140	1	28.0	70
chicken and turkey lunch, 'Deluxe' 'Lunchables' .... 1 lunch		390	21	25	1830	1	23.0	70
chicken w/Monterey Jack, cracker, pudding, 'Lunchables' .... 1 lunch		380	19	32	1200	0	21.0	45
ham and cheddar lunch, 'Lunchables' .... 1 lunch		360	20	21	1750	1	22.0	75
ham and Swiss lunch, 'Lunchables' .... 1 lunch		340	21	20	1780	1	20.0	70
ham w/American cheese, cracker, pudding, 'Lunchables' .... 1 lunch		410	19	33	1380	0	23.0	45
ham w/fruit punch, 'Lunchables' .... 1 lunch		440	15	54	1270	1	20.0	50
ham w/Surfer Cooler, low-fat, 'Lunchables' .... 1 lunch		390	17	58	1350	1	11.0	35
ham w/Swiss, cracker, cookie, 'Lunchables' .... 1 lunch		380	18	29	1370	0	23.0	50
ham w/fruit punch, low-fat, 'Lunchables' .... 1 lunch		330	17	48	1120	1	9.0	35
pepperoni pizza, 'Lunchables' .... 1 lunch		310	15	30	790	2	15.0	35
pepperoni pizza and orange, 'Lunchables' .... 1 lunch		460	16	62	830	2	16.0	35
pizza lunch, extra cheesy, 'Lunchables' .... 1 lunch		300	17	30	690	2	13.0	30
pizza lunch, extra cheesy, w/fruit punch, 'Lunchables' ... 1 lunch		450	17	63	720	2	15.0	30
smokie links sausage, 'Lunchables' .... 1 lunch		130	5	1	430	0	12.0	25
turkey, lowfat, w/Pacific Cooler, 'Lunchables' .... 1 lunch		360	15	56	1190	1	9.0	30
turkey, w/Pacific Cooler, 'Lunchables' .... 1 lunch		450	15	54	1340	1	20.0	50
turkey, w/Surfer Cooler, 'Lunchables' .... 1 lunch		430	13	61	1250	0	15.0	45

Food Name	Serv. Size	Total Cal.	Prot. gms	Carbs gms	Sod. mgs	Fiber gms	Fat gms	Chol. mgs
turkey and cheddar, 'Lunchables'	1 lunch	350	20	22	1760	1	20.0	70
turkey and ham, deluxe, 'Lunchables'	1 lunch	370	21	25	1940	1	21.0	65
turkey w/cheddar, cracker, trail mix	1 lunch	460	20	41	1230	0	26.0	40
turkey w/Monterey Jack, wheat cracker, 'Lunchables'	1 lunch	360	21	18	1600	0	22.0	75
(Star-Kist) 'Charlie's Lunch Kit' w/1 mayo packet	4.6 oz	290	24	16	780	0	15.0	0
LUNCHEON MEAT								
BARBECUE LOAF (Oscar Mayer)	1 oz	46	5	2	333	0	2.3	14
BEEF								
(Boar's Head)								
roast, top round, oven-roasted	1 oz	40	7	1	30	0	1.0	20
roast, top round, oven-roasted, 'Deluxe'	1 oz	45	7	1	40	0	2.0	20
(Carl Budding)								
peppered, smoked, sliced, chopped, 'Lean'	1 oz	40	5	1	0	0	2.0	0
smoked, sliced	1 pkg	99	14	0	1016	0	4.6	48
smoked, sliced	2 oz	79	11	0	811	0	3.7	38
smoked, sliced, chopped, 'Lean'	1 oz	40	5	1	0	0	2.0	0
(Eckrich) 'Slender Sliced'	1 oz	35	6	1	270	0	1.0	0
(Healthy Deli)								
roast	1 oz	30	6	0	130	0	0.4	13
roast, Italian	1 oz	31	6	0	140	0	0.6	16
(Hillshire Farm) roast, cured 'Deli Select'	1 oz	31	6	1	270	0	0.5	0
(Hormel)								
jellied, 'Perma-Fresh'	2 slices	90	14	0	900	0	4.0	0
smoked, cured	1 oz	50	5	0	315	0	2.0	0
smoked, cured, dried	1 oz	45	8	0	822	0	1.0	0
(Oscar Mayer)								
'Deli Thin'	4 slices	60	11	1	530	0	1.5	25
roast, 'Thin Sliced'	0.4 oz	14	2	0	55	0	0.4	5
smoked	0.5 oz	14	3	0	173	0	0.3	7
BOLOGNA								
(Bar-S) chicken, 'Tasty Bolony'	1 slice	70	3	3	330	0	5.0	30
(Boar's Head)								
beef	1 oz	74	4	1	270	0	7.0	17
ham	1 oz	40	5	1	0	0	2.0	15
pork and beef	1 oz	80	4	1	250	0	7.0	15
(Butterball)								
'Turkey Variety Pak'	3/4 oz	50	3	1	280	0	4.0	0
turkey 'Deli/Slice 'n Serve'	1 oz	70	4	2	370	0	6.0	0
turkey, 'Cold Cuts'	1 oz	70	4	2	370	0	6.0	0
(Eckrich)								
	1 oz	100	3	1	240	0	9.0	0
beef	1 oz	90	3	1	230	0	8.0	0
beef, 'Thick Sliced'	1.5 oz	130	4	2	340	0	12.0	0
garlic	1 oz	90	3	1	230	0	9.0	0
'German Brand'	1 oz	80	4	1	300	0	7.0	0
'Lean Supreme'	1 oz	70	4	1	240	0	6.0	0
'Sandwich'	1 oz	100	3	1	240	0	9.0	0
'Smorgas Pac'	1 oz	100	3	1	240	0	9.0	0
thick sliced, 1-lb pkg	1.8 oz	170	5	2	430	0	15.0	0
w/cheese	1 oz	90	3	1	250	0	9.0	0
(Empire Kosher)								
chicken, kosher	3 slices	200	7	2	360	0	7.0	40
turkey, kosher, sliced	3 slices	90	8	3	430	0	5.5	30
(Grillmaster) chicken	1 slice	70	3	1	350	0	6.0	30
(Health Valley) chicken	1 slice	85	4	1	329	0	8.0	13
(Healthy Choice)								
beef, low-fat, 'Cold Cuts'	1 slice	35	4	3	240	0	1.0	10

Food Name	Serv. Size	Total Cal.	Prot. gms	Carbs gms	Sod. mgs	Fiber gms	Fat gms	Chol. mgs
low-fat, 'Deli-Thin'	4 slices	60	8	5	480	0	1.5	30
turkey, pork and beef, low-fat, 'Cold Cuts'	1 slice	30	4	3	240	0	1.0	15
(Healthy Deli) beef and pork	1 oz	41	4	1	200	0	2.0	9
(Healthy Favorites) sliced	21 grams	20	3	1	239	0	0.3	5
(Hebrew National) beef, 'Original Deli Style'	1 oz	90	3	1	330	0	3.0	15
(Hillshire Farm)								
'Large'	1 oz	90	3	1	0	0	8.0	0
'Ring'	1 oz	89	3	1	0	0	8.0	0
(Hormel)								
beef, 'Coarse Ground, 1 lb.'	2 oz	160	8	1	576	0	14.0	0
beef, 'Perma-Fresh'	2 slices	170	6	1	592	0	16.0	0
'Fine Ground, 1-lb.'	2 oz	170	7	1	596	0	16.0	0
'Perma-Fresh'	2 slices	180	7	0	599	0	16.0	0
(JM)								
'German Brand'	1 oz	70	4	1	270	0	6.0	0
beef	1 oz	90	3	1	350	0	8.0	0
garlic	1 oz	90	3	1	350	0	8.0	0
(Kahn's)								
beef	1 slice	90	3	1	300	0	8.0	0
beef, 'Family Pack'	1 slice	70	2	1	230	0	6.0	0
beef, 'Giant'	1 slice	90	3	1	300	0	8.0	0
beef, 'Pounder'	1 slice	90	3	1	300	0	8.0	0
beef and cheddar	1 slice	90	4	1	320	0	8.0	0
'Deluxe Club Family Pack'	1 slice	70	2	1	220	0	6.0	0
'Deluxe Club'	1 slice	90	3	1	290	0	8.0	0
garlic	1 slice	90	3	1	290	0	8.0	0
'Giant Deluxe'	1 slice	90	3	1	290	0	8.0	0
'Giant Thick Deluxe'	1 slice	110	4	1	330	0	10.0	0
'Thick Deluxe'	1 slice	140	5	1	450	0	13.0	0
'Thin Sliced Deluxe'	1 slice	60	2	1	190	0	5.0	0
(Light and Lean)								
	2 slices	140	6	2	0	0	12.0	0
'Thin Sliced'	2 slices	70	3	1	0	0	6.0	0
(Longacre) turkey, sliced	1 oz	61	4	0	270	0	5.0	25
(Louis Rich)								
turkey, mild	1 oz	59	4	1	298	0	4.5	18
turkey	1 slice	52	3	1	270	0	3.7	19
(Mr. Turkey) turkey	1 slice	67	3	1	377	0	5.6	25
(Norbest) turkey, 'Blue Label' 2–2.5 lb	1 oz	68	4	1	331	0	5.6	0
(OHSE)								
	1 slice	130	4	1	430	0	11.0	30
	1 oz	75	3	3	280	0	6.0	0
beef	1 oz	85	3	1	310	0	8.0	0
'15% Chicken'	1 oz	90	3	1	320	0	8.0	0
turkey	1 oz	70	3	2	300	0	6.0	0
(Oscar Mayer)								
	1 slice	90	3	1	290	0	8.0	30
beef	1 slice	89	3	1	310	0	8.2	20
beef, Lebanon	0.8 oz	46	5	0	302	0	2.9	16
beef, light	1 slice	55	3	2	314	0	4.0	13
chicken, pork, and beef	1 slice	89	3	1	289	0	8.2	29
fat-free	1 slice	22	4	2	274	0	0.2	7
garlic	1 slice	130	5	1	420	0	12.0	40
light	1 slice	60	3	2	310	0	4.0	15
pork, chicken, and beef, light	1 slice	56	3	2	312	0	4.1	15
Wisconsin made ring	1 slice	175	7	1	463	0	15.9	35
w/cheese	0.8 oz	74	3	1	232	0	6.8	15

Food Name	Serv. Size	Total Cal.	Prot. gms	Carbs gms	Sod. mgs	Fiber gms	Fat gms	Chol. mgs
(Pilgrim's Pride)	1 oz	59	4	1	228	0	4.4	16
(Smok-a-Roma) chicken, pork, and beef	1 slice	80	4	1	340	0	6.0	20
(Tyson) chicken	1 slice	44	2	4	185	0	0.5	0
CHICKEN BREAST								
(Carl Budding)								
smoked, sliced, chopped, 'Lean'	1 oz	50	5	1	0	0	3.0	0
smoked, w/dark meat, sliced	1 pkg	117	13	0	677	0	7.2	38
smoked, w/dark meat, sliced	2 oz	94	10	0	541	0	5.7	30
(Healthy Choice)								
roasted, 'Cold Cuts'	1 slice	25	5	2	240	0	0.0	0
roasted, 'Fresh Trak'	1 slice	35	5	2	240	0	1.0	10
smoked, 'Cold Cuts'	1 slice	30	5	2	240	0	1.0	15
(Healthy Favorites)								
oven-roasted, fat-free, thin sliced	4 slices	40	9	1	620	0	0.0	25
oven-roasted, thin sliced	1 slice	12	2	1	110	0	1.0	5
(Hillshire Farm) smoked, boneless, 'Deli Select'	1 slice	31	6	1	290	0	0.2	0
(Land O'Frost) smoked, thin sliced	2.5 oz	120	12	0	930	0	7.0	65
(Longacre) 'Premium'	1 slice	45	4	1	280	0	3.0	20
(Louis Rich)								
baked, 'Classic Baked Grill'	1 slice	44	9	2	514	0	0.2	23
baked, thin sliced, 'Classic Baked Grill'	1 slice	22	4	1	251	0	0.1	11
hickory smoked, boneless	1 slice	30	5	1	356	0	0.8	14
hickory smoked, boneless, 97% fat-free	1 slice	30	5	1	370	0	1.0	15
honey glazed, 'Carving Board'	1 slice	23	5	1	265	0	0.3	13
roasted, 'Cold Cuts'	1 slice	36	5	1	335	0	1.6	17
roasted, deluxe, 'Cold Cuts'	1 slice	28	5	1	333	0	0.6	14
roasted, thin sliced, 'Deli Thin'	1 slice	15	2	1	155	0	0.4	6
(Mr. Turkey)								
boneless	1 slice	32	5	1	242	0	1.1	9
smoked, 'Deli Cut'	3 slices	28	5	2	357	0	0.1	13
(Oscar Mayer)								
honey glazed, roasted	1 slice	57	10	2	721	0	0.7	28
honey glazed, roasted, thin sliced	1 slice	14	3	1	180	0	0.2	7
oven-roasted	1 slice	29	5	1	414	0	0.7	15
roasted, fat-free	1 slice	44	10	1	646	0	0.3	23
roasted, fat-free, thin sliced	1 slice	11	2	0	161	0	0.1	6
smoked	1 slice	25	5	0	397	0	0.4	15
'Thin Sliced'	1 slice	13	2	0	151	0	0.4	5
(Tyson)								
breast, hickory smoked	1 slice	25	4	1	195	0	1.0	0
honey flavored	1 slice	25	4	1	0	0	1.0	0
mesquite, oven-roasted	1 slice	25	4	1	0	0	1.0	0
oven-roasted	1 slice	25	4	1	185	0	0.5	0
CHICKEN ROLL								
(Longacre) sliced	1 slice	60	4	1	210	0	5.0	25
(Pilgrim's Pride)	1 slice	35	5	0	260	0	1.2	15
(Tyson)	1 slice	26	3	1	153	0	0.5	0
CORNED BEEF LOAF								
jellied	1 slice	43	6	0	270	0	1.7	13
(Carl Budding)								
chopped, pressed	1 pkg	101	14	1	953	0	4.8	46
chopped, pressed	2 oz	81	11	1	761	0	3.9	37
DUTCH LOAF								
(Eckrich)								
'Lean Supreme'	1 slice	60	4	2	250	0	4.0	0
'Smorgas Pac'	1 slice	70	3	2	300	0	6.0	0
(Kahn's)	1 slice	80	3	1	280	0	7.0	0

Food Name	Serv. Size	Total Cal.	Prot. gms	Carbs gms	Sod. mgs	Fiber gms	Fat gms	Chol. mgs
HAM								
(Boar's Head)								
boiled, 'Deluxe'	1 oz	28	5	1	275	0	1.0	15
'Lower Salt'	1 slice	28	5	1	250	0	1.0	15
(Butterball)								
turkey, 'Cold Cuts'	1 oz	35	5	1	390	0	1.0	0
turkey, honey cured, chopped 'Cold Cuts'	1 oz	35	5	2	290	0	1.0	0
turkey, honey cured, 'Cold Cuts'	1 oz	35	5	1	380	0	1.0	0
turkey, honey cured, 'Slice 'n Serve'	1 oz	40	5	1	370	0	2.0	0
turkey, 'Slice 'n Serve'	1 oz	35	5	1	340	0	2.0	0
turkey, sliced, 'Deli Thin'	1 oz	35	5	1	390	0	1.0	0
(Carl Budding)								
honey, smoked, sliced, chopped, 'Lean'	1 slice	50	5	1	0	0	3.0	0
smoked, sliced	1 pkg	116	13	1	981	0	6.6	39
smoked, sliced	2 oz	92	10	1	783	0	5.3	31
smoked, sliced, chopped, 'Lean'	1 slice	50	5	1	0	0	3.0	0
(Danola)								
Danish, premium, 97% fat-free	1 slice	30	5	1	0	0	1.0	15
Danish, premium, 97% fat-free, thin sliced	2 slices	45	8	0	650	0	1.0	25
(Decker) chopped	1 slice	100	6	2	500	0	8.0	20
(Eckrich)								
chopped	1 slice	45	5	1	350	0	2.0	0
chopped, 'Lean Supreme'	1 slice	35	10	1	350	0	2.0	0
smoked, 'Slender Sliced'	1 slice	40	5	1	360	0	2.0	0
(Healthy Choice)								
baked, water added, 'Cold Cuts'	1 slice	30	5	1	240	0	1.0	10
cooked, water added, 'Fresh Trak'	1 slice	30	5	1	240	0	1.0	15
honey, water added, 'Cold Cuts'	1 slice	30	5	1	240	0	1.0	10
honey, water added, 'Fresh Trak'	1 slice	30	5	1	240	0	1.0	10
smoked, water added, 'Cold Cuts'	1 slice	30	5	1	240	0	1.0	10
(Healthy Deli)								
baked, Virginia	1 slice	34	5	2	245	0	0.9	12
baked, Virginia, less salt	1 slice	32	5	1	19	0	0.9	13
Black Forest	1 slice	32	6	0	220	0	0.6	16
cooked, fresh	1 slice	33	6	0	120	0	0.8	13
'Deluxe'	1 slice	31	5	1	245	0	0.9	12
honey, 'Honey Valley'	1 slice	31	5	1	26	0	0.8	10
jalapeño	1 slice	25	4	1	260	0	0.6	11
'Lessalt'	1 slice	32	5	1	190	0	0.9	13
'Taverne'	1 slice	31	5	0	210	0	0.8	15
(Healthy Favorites)								
baked, 98% fat-free	4 slices	50	9	1	600	0	1.0	25
boiled, thin sliced	1 slice	12	2	1	115	0	1.0	5
chicken, smoked, w/natural juices, thin sliced	1 slice	13	2	0	116	0	0.4	7
honey, thin sliced	1 slice	14	2	1	115	0	1.0	5
honey, water added, 'Breakfast'	1 slice	30	5	1	346	0	0.9	14
honey baked, 98% fat-free, thin sliced	4 slices	50	9	2	630	0	1.5	25
smoked, cooked, thin sliced	1 slice	14	2	1	115	0	1.0	5
(Hormel)								
'Cure 81'	1 slice	89	15	0	872	na	3.0	43
deli, cooked	1 slice	29	4	1	344	0	1.0	11
chopped, 'Black Label'	1 slice	70	4	1	326	0	6.0	16
chopped, 'Perma-Fresh'	2 slices	88	11	0	685	0	5.0	0
(Jennie-O)								
turkey, cooked, natural smoked flavoring, cured	2 oz	80	8	1	610	0	4.5	35
turkey, cooked, smoke flavoring, lean, 20% water added	2 oz	70	9	0	670	0	3.5	40

Food Name	Serv. Size	Total Cal.	Prot. gms	Carbs gms	Sod. mgs	Fiber gms	Fat gms	Chol. mgs
(JM)								
chopped	1 slice	80	4	1	370	0	7.0	0
cooked	1 slice	30	4	1	360	0	1.0	0
'Slice 'n Eat 93% Fat-Free'	2 oz	70	10	1	630	0	3.0	24
'Slice 'n Eat 95% Fat-Free Presliced'	2 slices	60	9	1	620	0	2.0	30
smoked, golden	2 slices	80	8	1	630	0	5.0	0
smoked, golden, water added	2 slices	70	8	4	810	0	2.0	23
(Jones Dairy Farm)								
'Farm'	1 slice	50	9	0	381	0	1.1	21
'Farm Family Ham'	1 slice	35	6	0	298	0	1.2	14
hickory smoked, 97% fat-free, 'Lean Choice'	2 slices	50	9	0	420	0	1.5	30
(Kahn's)								
low-salt	1 slice	30	5	1	290	0	1.0	0
chopped	1 slice	50	5	1	360	0	3.0	0
cooked, sliced	1 slice	30	5	1	360	0	1.0	0
(Light and Lean)								
barbecue	2 slices	50	8	0	0	0	2.0	0
black peppered	2 slices	50	9	0	0	0	2.0	0
chopped	2 slices	70	8	0	0	0	4.0	0
cooked, sliced	2 slices	50	9	0	0	0	2.0	0
glazed	2 slices	50	9	0	0	0	2.0	0
red peppered	2 slices	50	9	0	0	0	2.0	0
smoked, cooked	2 slices	50	9	0	0	0	2.0	0
(Longacre)								
turkey, chunk	1 oz	37	5	0	360	0	2.0	25
turkey, lean, lite, 'Deli'	1 oz	37	6	0	150	0	2.0	25
turkey, sliced	1 oz	33	6	0	310	0	1.0	20
(Louis Rich)								
baked, dinner slices	1 slice	80	16	1	1150	0	1.5	40
turkey, chopped	1 oz	46	5	0	289	0	2.8	19
turkey, cured	1 oz	25	4	1	217	0	0.7	14
turkey, 'Deli Thin'	1 slice	15	3	0	145	0	0.4	9
turkey, 15% water added, 'Cold Cuts'	1 slice	45	5	1	300	0	2.5	20
turkey, honey cured, 'Cold Cuts' 15% water added	1 slice	30	5	1	290	0	1.0	20
turkey, 96% fat-free, 'Deli-Thin'	1 slice	15	2	1	110	0	1.0	5
turkey, 96% fat-free, square	1 slice	25	4	1	215	0	1.0	15
turkey, 'Round'	1 oz	34	5	0	300	0	1.2	19
turkey, 'Square'	1 slice	24	4	0	213	0	0.7	14
turkey, 10% water added, 'Cold Cuts'	1 slice	35	5	0	310	0	1.0	20
turkey, 10% water added, 'Square'	1 serving	32	5	0	316	0	1.1	19
turkey, thin sliced	1 slice	12	2	0	111	0	0.4	7
turkey, water added	1 oz	33	5	0	294	0	1.4	19
turkey, water added, 94% fat-free	1 oz	35	5	1	300	0	2.0	20
turkey, water added, 95% fat-free, round	1 slice	30	5	1	325	0	1.0	20
(Mr. Turkey)								
turkey	1 slice	33	5	0	322	0	1.4	20
turkey, chopped	1 oz	37	5	0	301	0	1.6	17
turkey, smoked	1 slice	33	5	0	322	0	1.4	20
turkey, smoked, breakfast	1 oz	33	5	0	306	0	1.3	16
turkey, smoked, buffet style	1 oz	32	5	0	340	0	1.3	17
turkey, smoked, 'Chub'	1 oz	32	5	0	340	0	1.3	17
(Norbest)								
turkey, dark meat, hickory smoked	1 oz	39	5	0	335	0	2.2	0
turkey, thigh meat, cured, Canadian style	1 oz	35	5	0	331	0	1.4	0
turkey, thigh meat, cured, 'Gold Label'	1 oz	27	6	0	297	0	0.7	0
turkey, thigh meat, cured, half, 'Tavern'	1 oz	29	5	1	312	0	0.8	0
turkey, thigh meat cured, whole, 'Tavern'	1 oz	27	5	0	311	0	0.8	0

Food Name	Serv. Size	Total Cal.	Prot. gms	Carbs gms	Sod. mgs	Fiber gms	Fat gms	Chol. mgs
(OHSE)								
chopped	1 slice	65	4	1	260	0	5.0	0
cooked	1 slice	30	5	1	260	0	1.0	0
pit	1 slice	40	4	1	300	0	2.0	0
smoked, 95% fat-free	1 slice	30	5	1	310	0	1.0	0
turkey	1 oz	30	4	2	370	0	1.0	0
(Oscar Mayer)								
baked	1 slice	21	4	0	238	0	0.5	11
baked, water added, 96% fat free	1 slice	65	10	1	765	0	2.3	30
baked, water added, 96% fat free, thin sliced	1 slice	22	3	0	255	0	0.8	10
black peppered, cracked	1 slice	22	4	0	284	0	0.8	11
boiled	1 slice	23	4	0	275	0	0.7	12
boiled, thin sliced	1 slice	13	2	0	157	0	0.4	7
boiled, water added, thin sliced	4 slices	50	9	0	680	0	2.0	25
chopped	1 slice	50	4	1	340	0	3.0	15
chopped, w/natural juice	1 slice	52	5	1	327	0	3.4	na
honey, thin sliced	1 slice	13	2	0	153	0	0.4	7
'Jubilee'	1 slice	43	5	0	365	0	2.4	15
peppered, chopped	1 slice	55	4	1	312	0	3.7	16
smoked, 40% ham/water product	1 slice	34	7	1	509	0	0.3	18
smoked, 40% ham/water product, thin sliced	1 slice	12	2	0	173	0	0.1	6
water added, boiled	1 slice	22	3	0	283	0	0.8	10
water added, smoked, cooked	1 slice	21	3	0	255	0	0.8	10
(Pilgrim's Pride) chicken	1 slice	35	4	1	430	0	1.8	18
(Smok-a-Roma) cooked, 95% fat-free	1 slice	35	5	0	410	0	1.5	15
(Swift)								
'Premium Hostess'	1 slice	30	5	0	330	0	1.0	0
'Premium Sugar Plum'	1 slice	30	5	1	280	0	1.0	0
(Tyson) turkey	1 slice	23	3	1	182	0	0.2	0
HAM LOAF *(Eckrich)*	1 slice	50	5	1	290	0	4.0	0
HAM AND CHEESE LOAF								
(Eckrich)	1 oz slice	50	4	1	300	0	4.0	0
(Hormel)								
canned, 8-lb	3 oz	260	13	1	1135	0	22.0	0
'Perma-Fresh'	2 slices	110	11	0	668	0	7.0	0
(Kahn's)	1 slice	70	4	1	310	0	6.0	0
(Light and Lean)	2 slices	90	8	0	0	0	6.0	0
(OHSE)	1 oz	65	4	2	190	0	5.0	0
(Oscar Mayer)	1 slice	66	4	1	358	0	5.0	19
HEAD CHEESE *(Oscar Mayer)*	1 slice	52	4	0	300	0	3.8	25
HONEY LOAF								
(Eckrich) 'Smorgas Pac'	1 oz slice	35	4	2	280	0	1.0	0
(Hormel) 'Perma-Fresh'	2 slices	90	1	0	584	0	5.0	0
(Kahn's)	1 slice	40	4	1	320	0	2.0	0
(Oscar Mayer)	1 slice	34	5	1	378	0	1.0	16
IOWA BRAND LOAF *(Hormel)* 'Perma-Fresh'	2 slices	90	10	0	607	0	6.0	0
JALAPEÑO LOAF *(Kahn's)*	1 slice	70	3	2	340	0	6.0	0
LIVER CHEESE								
(JM)	1 oz slice	70	4	1	0	0	6.0	0
(Oscar Mayer) pork fat wrapped	1 slice	114	6	1	419	0	9.9	80
LIVER LOAF								
(Hormel) 'Perma-Fresh'	2 slices	160	9	1	704	0	13.0	0
(Kahn's)	1 slice	170	6	3	370	0	15.0	0
LIVERWURST								
(Hickory Farms)	1 oz	97	4	1	249	0	9.0	74
(Hormel) canned	0.5 oz	35	2	0	0	0	3.0	0
(Jones Dairy Farm)								
'Farm Club'	1 oz	80	5	0	254	0	6.3	43

Food Name	Serv. Size	Total Cal.	Prot. gms	Carbs gms	Sod. mgs	Fiber gms	Fat gms	Chol. mgs
'Farm Slices'	1 slice	75	4	0	186	0	6.6	43
(Oscar Mayer)								
Braunschweiger, sliced	1 slice	94	4	1	324	0	8.5	49
Braunschweiger, tube	1 serving	191	8	1	626	0	17.1	90
(Underwood) canned	2 1/8 oz	180	8	4	470	0	15.0	90
LOAF								
(Armour)								
canned, 'Treet'	2 oz	200	6	3	840	0	17.0	0
low-salt, canned, 'Treet'	2 oz	190	6	3	610	0	16.0	0
(Hormel)								
pork w/chicken, light, 'Spam'	2 oz	108	9	1	578	na	7.8	42
pork w/ham, 'Spam'	2 oz	172	7	1	789	na	15.6	39
pork w/ham, less salt, 'Spam'	2 oz	176	8	1	550	0	15.0	38
pork w/ham, light, 'Spam'	2 oz	140	8	1	560	0	12.0	43
pork w/ham, smoke-flavored, 'Spam'	2 oz	170	8	0	774	0	15.0	0
pork w/ham, w/cheese chunks, 'Spam'	2 oz	170	8	0	811	0	16.0	0
(JM) 'P&B'	1 slice	70	3	2	330	0	5.0	0
(Kahn's) 'P&B'	1 slice	40	5	1	270	0	2.0	0
(OHSE)								
	1 slice	100	5	2	440	0	8.0	30
	1 oz	75	3	1	320	0	6.0	0
(Oscar Mayer) spiced	1 slice	70	4	2	340	0	5.0	20
(Smok-a-Roma)								
	2 slices	90	4	0	200	0	8.0	10
spiced	1 slice	90	4	2	370	0	7.0	20
MACARONI AND CHEESE LOAF								
(Eckrich)	1 slice	75	3	3	320	0	6.0	0
(OHSE)	1 slice	60	4	4	310	0	3.0	0
OLD FASHIONED LOAF *(Oscar Mayer)*	1 slice	65	4	2	332	0	4.6	17
OLIVE LOAF								
(Eckrich)	1 slice	80	3	2	320	0	6.0	0
(Hormel) 'Perma-Fresh'	2 slices	110	7	5	810	0	7.0	0
(Oscar Mayer) chicken, pork, turkey	1 slice	74	3	2	369	0	6.1	20
PASTRAMI								
(Boar's Head) 'Round'	1 slice	40	6	1	270	0	1.5	16
(Butterball)								
turkey, 'Cold Cuts'	1 oz	30	5	0	290	0	1.0	0
turkey, 'Slice 'n Serve'	1 oz	35	5	1	320	0	1.0	0
(Carl Budding)								
beef, smoked, chopped, pressed	1 pkg	100	14	1	750	0	4.6	46
beef, smoked, chopped, pressed	2 oz	80	11	1	599	0	3.7	37
smoked, sliced, chopped, 'Lean'	1 slice	40	5	1	0	0	2.0	0
(Empire Kosher) turkey, kosher, sliced	3 slices	60	9	0	270	1	2.0	30
(Healthy Deli) 'Deli Round'	1 slice	34	5	1	195	0	1.1	14
(Longacre) turkey, sliced	1 oz	32	5	0	260	0	1.0	25
(Louis Rich)								
turkey	1 slice	30	5	0	320	0	1.0	20
turkey, 96% fat-free, 'Deli-Thin'	1 slice	10	2	1	125	0	1.0	5
turkey, 96% fat-free, square	1 oz slice	25	4	1	260	0	1.0	15
turkey, 'Round'	1 oz	32	5	0	288	0	1.1	18
turkey, 'Square'	1 oz	24	4	0	262	0	0.7	14
turkey, thin sliced	1 oz	11	2	0	125	0	0.4	7
(Mr. Turkey)								
turkey	1 slice	31	4	1	298	0	1.0	17
turkey, sliced, 'Deli Cut'	3 slices	36	5	1	260	0	1.4	21
(Norbest) turkey, 3 lb	1 oz	29	5	0	302	0	0.8	0
(Oscar Mayer) thin sliced	1 slice	16	3	0	217	0	0.3	7

Food Name	Serv. Size	Total Cal.	Prot. gms	Carbs gms	Sod. mgs	Fiber gms	Fat gms	Chol. mgs
PEPPERED LOAF								
(Eckrich)	1 slice	35	5	2	340	0	1.0	0
(Kahn's)	1 slice	40	5	1	340	0	2.0	0
(Oscar Mayer)	1 slice	39	5	1	367	0	1.5	14
PICKLE AND PIMIENTO LOAF								
(Oscar Mayer)								
	1 slice	80	3	3	360	0	6.0	20
w/chicken	1 serving	75	3	3	357	0	6.0	22
PICKLE LOAF								
(Eckrich) 'Smorgas Pac'	1 slice	80	3	2	270	0	6.0	0
(Hormel) 'Perma-Fresh'	2 slices	102	8	3	752	0	7.0	0
(Kahn's)								
	1 slice	80	3	2	280	0	7.0	0
beef 'Family Pack'	1 slice	60	2	1	210	0	5.0	0
'Family Pack'	1 slice	70	3	2	220	0	6.0	0
(Light and Lean)	2 slices	100	8	3	0	0	6.0	0
(OHSE)	1 oz	60	3	2	330	0	4.0	0
(Smok-a-Roma) w/turkey and pork	1 slice	90	5	4	300	0	6.0	15
PORK (Eckrich) 'Slender Sliced'	1 oz	45	5	1	320	0	2.0	0
SALAMI								
(Boar's Head) beef	1 oz	60	5	1	288	0	4.0	20
(Eckrich)								
beer	1 slice	70	4	1	330	0	6.0	0
cotto	1 slice	70	4	1	380	0	6.0	0
cotto, beef	1.3 oz	100	5	2	460	0	8.0	0
(Gallo Salame)								
dry, Italian, light, w/turkey, pork, and beef	7 slices	70	8	1	360	0	5.0	30
(Hebrew National) beef, 'Original Deli Style'	1 oz	80	7	1	230	0	7.0	15
(Hickory Farms)								
dry or hard	1 oz	120	6	0	535	0	10.0	30
Genoa	1 oz	110	6	0	540	0	10.0	20
(Hormel)								
beef, 'Perma-Fresh'	2 slices	50	3	0	219	0	5.0	0
cotto, 'Club'	1 oz	100	5	0	385	0	5.0	0
cotto, 'Perma-Fresh'	2 slices	105	9	1	750	0	7.0	0
dry or hard	1 oz	110	7	0	468	0	10.0	0
dry or hard, 'Homeland'	1 oz	117	6	2	448	0	10.0	29
dry or hard, 'National Brand'	1 oz	120	6	0	463	0	11.0	0
dry or hard, 'Perma-Fresh'	2 slices	80	4	0	339	0	7.0	0
dry or hard, 'Sliced'	1 oz	110	6	0	483	0	10.0	0
Genoa	1 oz	110	6	0	456	0	10.0	0
Genoa, 'DiLusso'	1 oz	100	6	0	443	0	8.0	0
Genoa, 'Gran Valore'	1 oz	110	6	0	453	0	10.0	0
Genoa, 'San Remo Brand'	1 oz	118	7	0	541	0	10.0	0
'Party'	1 oz	90	5	0	399	0	8.0	0
piccolo, 'Stick'	1 oz	120	6	0	512	0	11.0	0
(JM)								
cotto	1 oz slice	80	4	2	270	0	6.0	0
dry or hard	1 oz slice	110	6	1	580	0	9.0	0
Genoa	1 oz slice	100	6	1	540	0	8.0	0
(Kahn's)								
beef	1 slice	70	3	1	250	0	6.0	0
beef, 'Family Pack'	1 slice	60	2	1	190	0	5.0	0
cooked	1 slice	60	4	1	300	0	4.0	0
cotto, 'Family Pack'	1 slice	45	3	1	230	0	3.0	0
(Light and Lean) cotto	2 slices	80	6	0	0	0	6.0	0
(Mr. Turkey) cotto, turkey	1 slice	49	4	1	239	0	3.3	21

Food Name	Serv. Size	Total Cal.	Prot. gms	Carbs gms	Sod. mgs	Fiber gms	Fat gms	Chol. mgs
(OHSE) cooked	1 oz	65	4	1	330	0	5.0	0
(Oscar Mayer)								
beef, 'Machiaeh Brand'	1 slice	60	3	0	265	0	5.0	15
beer	1 slice	52	3	0	283	0	4.2	16
cotto	1 slice	70	3	1	280	0	5.0	25
cotto, beef	1 slice	47	3	0	301	0	3.6	19
cotto, beef, pork, and chicken	1 slice	56	3	1	252	0	4.7	18
Genoa	1 slice	35	2	0	164	0	3.0	9
hard	1 slice	36	2	0	169	0	2.8	9
SPICE LOAF								
(Hormel)								
canned	3 oz	280	11	2	1110	0	26.0	0
'Perma-Fresh'	2 slices	118	9	1	702	0	9.0	0
(JM)	1 slice	70	4	1	370	0	6.0	0
(Kahn's)								
beef, 'Family Pack'	1 slice	60	2	1	200	0	5.0	0
'Family Pack'	1 slice	70	3	1	180	0	6.0	0
'Luncheon Loaf'	1 slice	80	3	1	240	0	7.0	0
(Oscar Mayer)	1 serving	66	4	2	343	0	4.7	19
TURKEY BREAST								
(Boar's Head)								
golden	1 oz	35	6	1	200	0	1.0	20
golden, skinless	1 oz	30	6	1	0	0	1.0	10
(Butterball)								
barbecue seasoned, 'Slice 'n Serve'	1 oz	40	5	1	210	0	2.0	0
'Cold Cuts'	1 oz	30	5	1	230	0	1.0	0
hickory smoked, 'Slice 'n Serve'	1 oz	35	5	1	250	0	1.0	0
no salt added, 'Deli'	1 oz	45	7	0	15	0	2.0	0
'Slice 'n Serve'	1 oz	35	5	1	230	0	1.0	0
smoked, 'Cold Cuts'	1 oz	35	5	0	190	0	1.0	0
smoked, 'Turkey Variety Pak'	3/4 oz	25	4	1	160	0	1.0	0
(Carl Budding)								
and dark meat, smoked, sliced	1 pkg	114	12	1	778	0	6.5	40
and dark meat, smoked, sliced	2 oz	91	10	1	621	0	5.2	32
smoked, sliced, chopped, 'Lean'	1 oz	50	5	1	0	0	3.0	0
(Carving Board)								
hickory-smoked	1 slice	40	9	0	540	0	0.5	20
traditional	1 slice	40	9	0	540	0	0.5	20
(Empire Kosher)								
oven prepared, kosher, sliced	3 slices	50	10	1	200	0	0.5	15
smoked, kosher, sliced	3 slices	40	8	0	350	0	0.0	15
(Healthy Choice)								
and white meat, honey roasted and smoked, 'Cold Cuts'	1 slice	35	5	2	240	0	1.0	15
honey roasted and smoked	1 slice	35	6	1	230	0	1.0	15
honey roasted and smoked, 'Fresh Trak'	1 slice	35	5	2	240	0	1.0	15
roasted, 'Cold Cuts'	1 slice	30	5	1	240	0	1.0	15
roasted, 'Fresh Trak'	1 slice	30	5	1	240	0	1.0	15
roasted, 97% fat-free	1 slice	30	6	1	290	0	1.0	10
smoked, 'Cold Cuts'	1 slice	30	5	2	240	0	1.0	15
(Healthy Deli)								
'Gourmet'	1 oz	28	5	1	170	0	0.6	9
honey	1 oz	28	5	1	170	0	0.5	9
'Lessalt'	1 oz	25	5	0	140	0	0.5	9
oven cooked	1 oz	26	5	0	180	0	0.2	8
smoked 'Gourmet'	1 oz	31	6	0	170	0	0.5	11
smoked, 3-lb	1 oz	29	5	0	180	0	0.5	8

Food Name	Serv. Size	Total Cal.	Prot. gms	Carbs gms	Sod. mgs	Fiber gms	Fat gms	Chol. mgs
(Healthy Favorites)								
oven-roasted	1 slice	12	2	1	100	0	1.0	5
oven-roasted, fat-free	4 slices	40	8	2	610	0	0.0	15
smoked	1 slice	12	2	1	80	0	1.0	5
(Hormel)								
'Perma-Fresh'	2 slices	60	9	0	484	0	2.0	0
smoked, 'Perma-Fresh'	2 slices	60	10	0	540	0	2.0	0
(Land O'Frost) smoked, thin sliced	2.5 oz	110	12	0	990	0	7.0	55
(Light and Lean) breast	2 slices	60	8	0	0	0	2.0	0
(Longacre)								
and white meat, browned and roasted	1 oz	40	5	1	240	0	2.0	15
and white meat, 'Deli Chef'	1 oz	35	5	1	240	0	1.0	15
and white meat, skinless 'Deli Chef'	1 oz	40	4	1	240	0	2.0	15
browned, glazed, 'Gourmet'	1 oz	35	5	1	240	0	1.0	15
browned, glazed, 'Premium'	1 oz	30	4	1	300	0	1.0	10
browned, roasted, 'Gourmet'	1 oz	35	5	1	260	0	1.0	15
browned, roasted, 'Premium'	1 oz	30	4	1	300	0	1.0	10
'Catering'	1 oz	35	6	1	280	0	1.0	15
'Gourmet'	1 oz	35	5	1	300	0	1.0	15
lean, lite, 'Deli'	1 oz	35	6	0	160	0	1.0	15
lean, lite, skinless, 'Deli'	1 oz	35	6	0	160	0	1.0	15
lean, lite, smoked, 'Deli'	1 oz	35	6	0	160	0	1.0	15
low-salt, 'Gourmet'	1 oz	30	6	1	150	0	1.0	10
'Premium'	1 oz	30	4	1	250	0	1.0	10
'Salt Watchers'	1 oz	32	7	0	10	0	1.0	15
skinless, 'Catering'	1 oz	35	6	1	280	0	1.0	15
skinless, 'Gourmet'	1 oz	30	5	1	260	0	1.0	15
skinless, 'Premium'	1 oz	30	4	1	250	0	1.0	10
sliced	1 oz	30	5	1	280	0	1.0	10
smoked	1 oz	35	6	0	240	0	1.0	15
smoked, sliced	1 oz	26	5	1	260	0	1.0	10
(Louis Rich)								
and white meat, roasted	1 serving	27	5	1	309	0	0.5	11
and white meat, smoked	1 serving	28	5	1	257	0	0.6	12
'Carving Board'	22 grams	21	5	0	272	0	0.3	9
cooked, barbecued, no skin	1 oz	30	6	1	280	0	1.0	10
hickory smoked	1 slice	60	11	2	640	0	0.0	0
hickory smoked, nonfat, 'Cold Cuts'	1 slice	25	4	1	300	0	0.0	0
honey roasted, 95% fat-free	1 slice	35	5	1	315	0	1.0	10
nonfat, 'Deli-Thin'	4 slices	40	8	2	608	0	0.0	0
oven-roasted	1 oz	31	5	1	323	0	0.8	11
oven-roasted, 97% fat-free, 'Deli-Thin'	1 slice	10	2	1	125	0	1.0	5
roasted	1 slice	50	11	1	620	0	0.0	0
roasted, fat-free	1 slice	24	4	1	334	0	0.2	9
roasted, nonfat, 'Cold Cuts'	1 slice	25	4	1	330	0	0.0	0
roasted, thin sliced	1 slice	12	2	0	127	0	0.3	4
smoked	1 slice	21	5	0	211	0	0.3	9
smoked, 'Carving Board'	1 slice	21	4	0	264	0	0.2	9
smoked, 98% fat-free	1 slice	20	4	1	210	0	1.0	10
smoked, 97% fat-free, 'Deli-Thin'	1 slice	10	2	1	110	0	1.0	5
smoked, 96% fat-free'	1 oz	35	6	1	270	0	1.0	10
smoked, thin sliced	0.4 oz slice	11	2	0	111	0	0.1	5
white, smoked, 'Cold Cuts'	1 slice	30	5	0	280	0	1.0	15
(Mr. Turkey)								
	1 oz	31	6	0	233	0	0.7	10
smoked	1 oz	31	6	0	332	0	0.7	10
honey roasted, 'Deli Cut'	3 slices	30	5	2	309	0	0.5	15

Food Name	Serv. Size	Total Cal.	Prot. gms	Carbs gms	Sod. mgs	Fiber gms	Fat gms	Chol. mgs
roasted	1 slice	33	5	2	274	0	0.8	13
roasted, quartered	3.5 oz	94	15	3	1035	0	2.2	40
smoked, 'Deli Cut'	3 slices	24	4	2	354	0	0.2	11
smoked, quartered	3.5 oz	89	17	4	1275	0	0.5	31
(Norbest)								
and thigh,'Blue Label'	1 oz	31	6	0	238	0	0.9	0
skinless, 'Blue Label'	1 oz	24	4	1	253	0	0.3	0
skinless, 'Orange Label'	1 oz	26	5	1	239	0	0.2	0
skinless, 'Tan Label'	1 oz	24	4	1	354	0	0.5	0
skinless, 'Yellow Label'	1 oz	24	4	0	284	0	0.5	0
skinless, salt-free, 'Blue Label'	1 oz	33	8	0	13	0	0.3	0
smoked, 'Gold Label'	1 oz	29	6	0	270	0	0.6	0
w/skin, 'Blue Label'	1 oz	28	5	0	239	0	0.7	0
w/skin, 'Orange Label'	1 oz	26	5	0	256	0	0.3	0
w/skin, 'Yellow Label'	1 oz	25	5	0	244	0	0.5	0
w/skin, prebrowned, 'Orange Label'	1 oz	29	5	0	259	0	0.8	0
w/skin, salt-free, 'Blue Label'	1 oz	35	8	0	13	0	0.5	0
w/skin, smoked, 'Orange Label'	1 oz	30	5	1	284	0	0.5	0
(OHSE)								
oven cooked	1 oz	30	5	1	190	0	1.0	0
smoked	1 oz	30	5	1	340	0	1.0	0
(Oscar Mayer)								
cooked, oven-roasted, thin sliced	1 slice	12	2	0	151	0	0.2	5
smoked	1 slice	20	4	0	300	0	0.2	9
roasted	4 slices	50	9	2	580	0	1.0	20
roasted, nonfat	4 slices	40	8	2	670	0	0.0	0
smoked, fat-free	1 slice	10	2	0	142	0	0.1	4
smoked, honey roasted	4 slices	60	10	2	520	0	1.0	20
smoked, nonfat	4 slices	40	8	2	570	0	0.0	0
white, roasted	1 slice	30	4	1	300	0	1.0	10
(Tyson) breast	1 slice	20	4	0	136	0	0.4	0
TURKEY HAM. See under LUNCHEON MEAT, HAM.								
TURKEY LOAF								
(Louis Rich) 89% fat-free	1 oz	45	5	0	270	0	2.8	16
(Mr. Turkey) spiced	1 oz	51	4	1	292	0	3.6	11
TURKEY ROLL								
(Norbest)								
	1 oz	31	5	1	346	0	1.1	0
white and dark meat, 'Orange Label'	1 oz	36	4	0	314	0	2.0	0
white meat, diced	1 oz	31	4	1	318	0	0.9	0
white meat, 'Orange Label'	1 oz	29	4	1	299	0	0.9	0
LUNCHEON MEAT SPREAD								
(Hormel)								
deviled, 'Spam'	1 oz	78	4	2	260	0	7.0	20
deviled, 'Spam'	1 tbsp	35	2	0	125	0	3.0	0
LUNCHEON MEAT SUBSTITUTE								
(White Wave)								
chicken style, sandwich sliced *(White Wave)*	1 slice	80	12	8	260	0	0.0	0
pastrami style, vegetarian, sandwich sliced	1 slice	90	14	8	270	1	0.0	0
(Worthington)								
bologna style, vegetarian, 'Bolono'	3 slices	79	10	2	717	2	3.3	2
salami style, vegetarian, 'Meatless Salami'	3 slices	130	12	2	930	2	8.0	0
smoked turkey style slices, vegetarian *(Worthington)*	3 slices	142	10	3	618	3	9.9	1
vegetarian, 'Numete'	3/8-inch slice	130	6	5	270	3	10.0	0
vegetarian, 'Protose'	3/8-inch slice	131	13	5	283	3	6.7	0
LUPIN								
mature seeds, boiled	1 cup	198	26	16	7	5	4.8	0
mature seeds, raw	1 cup	668	65	73	27	na	17.5	0

M

Food Name	Serv. Size	Total Cal.	Prot. gms	Carbs gms	Sod. mgs	Fiber gms	Fat gms	Chol. mgs
MACADAMIA NUT								
dried, whole, 10–12 kernels	1 oz	204	2	4	1	2	21.5	0
dried, whole or halves	1 cup	962	11	19	7	12	101.5	0
dry-roasted, salted, whole, 10-12 kernels	1 oz	203	2	4	75	2	21.6	0
dry-roasted, salted, whole or halves	1 cup	959	10	17	355	11	101.9	0
dry-roasted, unsalted, whole, 10-12 kernels	1 oz	204	2	4	1	2	21.6	0
dry-roasted, unsalted, whole or halves	1 cup	962	10	18	5	11	101.9	0
salted *(Mauna Loa)*	1 oz	210	2	4	75	0	21.0	0
shelled, salted *(Mauna Loa)*	1 oz	210	2	4	75	0	21.0	0
unsalted, natural *(Flanigan Farms)*	1/4 cup	200	2	4	0	1	21.0	0
MACADAMIA NUT BUTTER								
roasted *(Maranatha Natural)*	2 tbsp	200	2	6	5	0	19.0	0
roasted, organic *(Maranatha Natural)*	2 tbsp	230	3	5	0	3	24.0	0
MACARONI. See under PASTA.								
MACARONI DISH/ENTRÉE. See under PASTA DISH ENTRÉE.								
MACE								
ground	1 tbsp	25	0	3	4	1	1.7	0
ground	1 tsp	8	0	1	1	0	0.6	0
ground *(Durkee)*	1 tsp	10	0	0	0	0	0.0	0
ground *(Laurel Leaf)*	1 tsp	10	0	0	0	0	0.0	0
ground *(McCormick/Schilling)*	1 tsp	8	0	1	2	0	0.4	0
ground *(Spice Islands)*	1 tsp	10	0	1	1	0	0.7	0
ground *(Tone's)*	1 tsp	8	0	1	1	0	0.6	0
MACKEREL								
ATLANTIC								
baked, broiled, grilled, or microwaved	4 oz	297	27.0	0.0	94	0	20.2	85
baked, broiled, grilled, or microwaved	3 oz	223	20.3	0.0	71	0	15.1	64
raw	1 lb	929	84.4	0.0	408	0	63.0	318
raw	3 oz	174	15.8	0.0	77	0	11.8	59
JACK, mixed species								
Canned								
drained	1 cup	296	44.1	0.0	720	0	12.0	150
drained	4 oz	177	26.3	0.0	430	0	7.1	90
Fresh								
baked, broiled, grilled, or microwaved	3 oz	171	21.9	0.0	94	0	8.6	51
raw	1 lb	712	91.0	0.0	391	0	35.8	213
raw	3 oz	134	17.1	0.0	73	0	6.7	40
KING								
baked, broiled, grilled, or microwaved	3 oz	114	22.1	0.0	173	0	2.2	58
raw	1 lb	475	92.0	0.0	717	0	9.1	242
raw	3 oz	89	17.2	0.0	134	0	1.7	45
PACIFIC, mixed species								
baked, broiled, grilled, or microwaved	3 oz	171	21.9	0.0	94	0	8.6	51
raw	1 lb	712	91.0	0.0	391	0	35.8	213
raw	3 oz	134	17.1	0.0	73	0	6.7	40
SPANISH								
baked, broiled, grilled, or microwaved	5.1-oz fillet	231	34.4	0.0	96	0	9.2	107
baked, broiled, grilled, or microwaved	4 oz	179	26.8	0.0	75	0	7.2	83
baked, broiled, grilled, or microwaved	3 oz	134	20.0	0.0	56	0	5.4	62
raw	1 lb	631	87.5	0.0	266	0	28.6	345
raw	3 oz	118	16.4	0.0	50	0	5.3	65
MAHI MAHI/dolphin fish								
Fresh								
baked, broiled, grilled, or microwaved	3 oz	93	20	0	96	0	0.8	80

Food Name	Serv. Size	Total Cal.	Prot. gms	Carbs gms	Sod. mgs	Fiber gms	Fat gms	Chol. mgs
raw	3 oz	72	16	0	75	0	0.6	62
Frozen *(Peter Pan Seafoods)* fillets, boneless, skinless	3.5 oz	85	19	0	88	0	0.7	73
MAI TAI. See under COCKTAIL MIX.								
MALABAR SPINACH. See SPINACH, MALABAR.								
MALACCA APPLE, w/o seeds	1 oz	9	0.2	2.3	na	>.2 c	<.1	0
MALT, dry	1 oz	103	3.7	21.7	22	>1.6 c	0.5	0
MALT EXTRACT, dried	1 oz	103	1.7	25.0	22	0	0.0	0
MALT SYRUP. See under SYRUP.								
MALTED MILK FLAVOR DRINK MIX								
CHOCOLATE FLAVOR								
w/added nutrients, powder, mix only	1 cup	279	4	66	463	1	2.7	4
w/added nutrients, powder, prepared w/milk	8 fl oz	225	9	29	244	0	8.7	34
w/o added nutrients, powder, mix only	1 envelope	79	1	18	53	0	0.8	1
w/o added nutrients, powder, prepared w/milk	8 fl oz *(1 cup)*	228	9	30	172	0	9.0	34
(Kraft) powder, 'Instant' mix only	3 tsp	90	1	18	45	0	1.0	0
NATURAL FLAVOR								
w/added nutrients, powder, prepared	8 fl oz *(1 cup)*	231	10	28	204	0	8.7	34
w/o added nutrients, powder, prepared	8 fl oz *(1 cup)*	236	10	27	223	0	9.8	37
(Kraft) powder, 'Instant'	3 tsp	90	3	16	100	0	2.0	0
MAMMY APPLE								
peeled, w/o seeds	1 oz	14	0.1	3.5	4	.9	0.1	0
raw	3 1/2 oz	51	0.5	12.5	15	3.0	0.5	0
raw, trimmed, whole, approx 3.1 lb	1 medium	431	4.2	105.8	127	25.4	4.2	0
raw, untrimmed	1 lb	139	1.4	34.0	41	>2.7 c	1.4	0
MANDARIN ORANGE. See also TANGERINE.								
Canned								
in juice	1 cup	92	2	24	12	2	0.1	0
in light syrup	1 cup	154	1	41	15	2	0.3	0
MANGO								
Canned or jarred, sliced, chilled *(Sun Fresh)*	3.5 oz	89	0.5	21.0	11	1.9	0.3	1
Fresh								
raw, peeled, w/o seed	1 oz	18	0.1	4.8	1	.3	0.1	0
raw, sliced	1 cup	107	0.8	28.1	3	3.0	0.5	0
raw, trimmed, whole, medium, approx 10.6 oz	1 mango	135	1.1	35.2	4	3.7	0.6	0
raw, untrimmed	1 lb	204	1.6	53.2	6	3.4	0.9	0
MANGOSTEEN								
Canned								
in syrup	1 cup	158	1	39	15	4	1.3	0
in syrup, drained	1 cup	143	1	35	14	4	1.1	0
MANHATTAN. See under COCKTAIL MIX.								
MANICOTTI/MANICOTTI ENTRÉE								
(Bernardi)								
cheese	2 pieces	300	15	27	340	1	14.0	45
cheese, large	1 piece	170	8	16	230	1	8.0	45
(Budget Gourmet)								
cheese, w/meat sauce	1 entrée	420	18	38	810	4	22.0	85
frozen, w/meat sauce, frozen	1 entrée	440	20	34	780	5	26.0	90
(Buitoni) frozen 'Single Serving' one package	9 oz	470	18	45	830	0	14.0	130
(Celentano)								
	10-oz tray	450	24	41	910	9	21.0	85
Florentine, 'Great Choice'	10-oz tray	210	15	29	600	5	6.0	35
Florentine, 'Selects'	10-oz tray	230	14	29	670	4	7.0	5
mini	4.8 oz	280	17	32	500	13	12.0	66
w/sauce	8 oz	320	17	28	690	6	15.0	75
w/o sauce	7 oz	410	20	40	630	7	19.0	100
(Contadina) cheese, frozen	1 oz	31	2	3	95	0	1.4	3

Food Name	Serv. Size	Total Cal.	Prot. gms	Carbs gms	Sod. mgs	Fiber gms	Fat gms	Chol. mgs
(Healthy Choice)								
cheese, frozen	9.25 oz	220	15	34	310	0	3.0	30
w/three cheeses	1 entrée	300	15	40	550	5	9.0	35
(Le Menu) three cheese, frozen	11.75 oz	390	19	44	870	0	15.0	0
(Lean Cuisine) cheese and spinach, 'Hearty Portions'	1 entrée	340	18	52	790	10	7.0	40
(Legume)								
cheese, w/spinach, tofu, and sauce, frozen	11 oz	260	18	30	650	9	7.0	0
classic, vegetarian, nondairy, w/organic pasta and tofu	1 serving	360	23	40	510	10	13.0	0
Florentine, nondairy, w/organic pasta and tofu	1 serving	300	19	39	540	11	8.0	0
(Stouffer's) cheese	1 entrée	340	18	32	810	7	16.0	50
(Weight Watchers)								
cheese	1 entrée	260	17	31	570	5	7.0	30
cheese, frozen	9.25 oz	260	17	31	510	0	8.0	25

MANICOTTI NOODLE. See under PASTA.

MANIOC. See CASSAVA.

MAPLE SYRUP. See under SYRUP.

MARGARINE

Food Name	Serv. Size	Total Cal.	Prot. gms	Carbs gms	Sod. mgs	Fiber gms	Fat gms	Chol. mgs
coconut, hydrogenated and regular, w/safflower and hydrogenated palm	1 stick	815	1	1	1070	0	91.3	0
coconut, hydrogenated and regular, w/safflower and hydrogenated palm	1 tsp	34	0	0	44	0	3.8	0
corn, hydrogenated	1 stick	815	1	1	1070	0	91.3	0
corn, hydrogenated	1 tsp	34	0	0	44	0	3.8	0
corn, hydrogenated and regular	1 stick	815	1	1	1070	0	91.3	0
corn, hydrogenated and regular	1 tsp	34	0	0	44	0	3.8	0
corn, hydrogenated and regular, soft	1 cup	1626	2	1	2449	0	182.5	0
corn, hydrogenated and regular, soft	1 tsp	34	0	0	51	0	3.8	0
corn, w/hydrogenated soybean and cottonseed	1 stick	815	1	1	1070	0	91.3	0
corn, w/hydrogenated soybean and cottonseed	1 tsp	34	0	0	44	0	3.8	0
corn, w/hydrogenated soybean and cottonseed, unsalted	1 stick	810	1	1	2	0	91.1	0
corn, w/hydrogenated soybean and cottonseed, unsalted	1 tsp	34	0	0	0	0	3.8	0
lard, hydrogenated	1 stick	831	1	1	1070	0	91.3	58
lard, hydrogenated	1 tsp	34	0	0	44	0	3.8	2
safflower, hydrogenated and regular	1 cup	1626	2	1	2449	0	182.5	0
safflower, hydrogenated and regular	1 tsp	34	0	0	51	0	3.8	0
safflower, w/hydrogenated cottonseed and peanut, soft	1 cup	1626	2	1	2449	0	182.5	0
safflower, w/hydrogenated cottonseed and peanut, soft	1 tsp	34	0	0	51	0	3.8	0
safflower, w/hydrogenated soybean	1 stick	815	1	1	1070	0	91.3	0
safflower, w/hydrogenated soybean	1 tsp	34	0	0	44	0	3.8	0
safflower, w/hydrogenated soybean and cottonseed	1 stick	815	1	1	1070	0	91.3	0
safflower, w/hydrogenated soybean and cottonseed	1 tsp	34	0	0	44	0	3.8	0
soybean, hydrogenated	1 stick	812	1	1	1066	0	91.0	0
soybean, hydrogenated	1 tsp	34	0	0	44	0	3.8	0
soybean, hydrogenated and regular	1 stick	815	1	1	1070	0	91.3	0
soybean, hydrogenated and regular	1 tsp	34	0	0	44	0	3.8	0
soybean, hydrogenated and regular, soft, salted	1 cup	1626	2	1	2449	0	182.5	0
soybean, hydrogenated and regular, soft, salted	1 tsp	34	0	0	51	0	3.8	0
soybean, hydrogenated and regular, soft, unsalted	1 cup	1626	2	2	63	0	182.3	0
soybean, hydrogenated and regular, soft, unsalted	1 tsp	34	0	0	1	0	3.8	0
soybean, hydrogenated, w/corn and hydrogenated cottonseed	1 stick	815	1	1	1070	0	91.3	0
soybean, hydrogenated, w/corn and hydrogenated cottonseed	1 tsp	34	0	0	44	0	3.8	0
soybean, hydrogenated, w/cottonseed	1 stick	815	1	1	1070	0	91.3	0

Food Name	Serv. Size	Total Cal.	Prot. gms	Carbs gms	Sod. mgs	Fiber gms	Fat gms	Chol. mgs
soybean, hydrogenated, w/cottonseed .... 1 tsp		34	0	0	44	0	3.8	0
soybean, hydrogenated, w/cottonseed, soft .... 1 cup		1626	2	1	2449	0	182.5	0
soybean, hydrogenated, w/cottonseed, soft .... 1 tsp		34	0	0	51	0	3.8	0
soybean, hydrogenated, w/hydrogenated and regular palm .... 1 stick		815	1	1	1070	0	91.3	0
soybean, hydrogenated, w/hydrogenated and regular palm.. 1 tsp		34	0	0	44	0	3.8	0
soybean, hydrogenated, w/hydrogenated and regular palm, soft .... 1 cup		1626	2	1	2449	0	182.5	0
soybean, hydrogenated, w/hydrogenated and regular palm, soft....................................... 1 tsp		34	0	0	51	0	3.8	0
soybean, hydrogenated, w/safflower, soft .... 1 cup		1626	2	1	2449	0	182.5	0
soybean, hydrogenated, w/safflower, soft .... 1 tsp		34	0	0	51	0	3.8	0
soybean and cottonseed, hydrogenated .... 1 stick		815	1	1	1070	0	91.3	0
soybean and cottonseed, hydrogenated .... 1 tsp		34	0	0	44	0	3.8	0
soybean and cottonseed, hydrogenated, soft .... 1 cup		1626	2	1	2449	0	182.5	0
soybean and cottonseed, hydrogenated, soft .... 1 tsp		34	0	0	51	0	3.8	0
soybean and cottonseed, hydrogenated, soft, salted ..... 1 cup		1626	2	1	2449	0	182.5	0
soybean and cottonseed, hydrogenated, soft, salted ..... 1 tsp		34	0	0	51	0	3.8	0
soybean and cottonseed, hydrogenated, soft, unsalted ... 1 cup		1626	2	2	63	0	182.3	0
soybean and cottonseed, hydrogenated, soft, unsalted ... 1 tsp		34	0	0	1	0	3.8	0
soybean and cottonseed, hydrogenated and regular, liquid .... 1 cup		1637	4	0	1773	0	183.0	0
soybean and cottonseed, hydrogenated and regular, liquid .... 1 tsp		34	0	0	37	0	3.8	0
soybean and palm, hydrogenated .... 1 stick		815	1	1	1070	0	91.3	0
soybean and palm, hydrogenated .... 1 tsp		34	0	0	44	0	3.8	0
sunflower, w/hydrogenated cottonseed and peanut, soft .. 1 cup		1626	2	1	2449	0	182.5	0
sunflower, w/hydrogenated cottonseed and peanut, soft ... 1 tsp		34	0	0	51	0	3.8	0
sunflower, w/hydrogenated soybean and cottonseed .... 1 stick		815	1	1	1070	0	91.3	0
sunflower, w/hydrogenated soybean and cottonseed ..... 1 tsp		34	0	0	44	0	3.8	0
(A&P)								
premium .... 1 tbsp		100	1	1	110	0	11.0	0
quarters, corn oil .... 1 tbsp		100	1	1	105	0	11.0	0
soft, bowl .... 1 tbsp		100	1	1	105	0	11.0	0
(Blue Bonnet)								
soft... 1 tbsp		100	0	0	95	0	11.0	0
stick .... 1 tbsp		100	0	0	95	0	11.0	0
whipped, stick .... 1 tbsp		70	0	0	70	0	7.0	0
(Cannola) soft .... 1 tbsp		100	0	0	95	0	11.0	0
(Canoleo) 100% Canola oil, all natural, dairy-free .... 1 tbsp		100	0	0	120	0	11.0	0
(Chiffon)								
soft, cup .... 1 tbsp		90	0	0	95	0	10.0	0
soft, stick .... 1 tbsp		100	0	0	105	0	11.0	0
soft, unsalted .... 1 tbsp		90	0	0	0	0	10.0	0
whipped .... 1 tbsp		70	0	0	80	0	8.0	0
(Country Morning)								
light, stick...................................... 1 tsp		20	0	0	30	0	2.0	3
light, tub .... 1 tsp		20	0	0	25	0	2.0	3
regular, stick.................................... 1 tsp		35	0	0	35	0	4.0	5
regular, tub..................................... 1 tsp		30	0	0	25	0	3.0	5
unsalted, stick .... 1 tsp		35	0	0	0	0	4.0	4
unsalted, tub .... 1 tsp		30	0	0	0	0	3.0	5
(Fleischmann's)								
diet, lower calorie .... 1 tbsp		50	0	0	50	0	6.0	0
40% corn oil, less fat, stick .... 1 tbsp		52	0	1	77	0	5.6	0
regular, soft .... 1 tbsp		100	0	0	95	0	11.0	0

Food Name	Serv. Size	Total Cal.	Prot. gms	Carbs gms	Sod. mgs	Fiber gms	Fat gms	Chol. mgs
regular, stick	1 tbsp	100	0	0	95	0	11.0	0
sweet, unsalted, soft	1 tbsp	100	0	0	0	0	11.0	0
sweet, unsalted, stick	1 tbsp	100	0	0	0	0	11.0	0
whipped, lightly salted	1 tbsp	70	0	0	60	0	7.0	0
whipped, unsalted	1 tbsp	70	0	0	0	0	7.0	0
(Hain)								
safflower	1 tbsp	100	0	0	170	0	11.0	0
safflower, soft	1 tbsp	100	0	0	170	0	11.0	0
safflower, unsalted	1 tbsp	100	0	0	5	0	11.0	0
(Hollywood)								
safflower	1 tbsp	100	0	0	130	0	11.0	0
safflower, unsalted	1 tbsp	100	0	0	2	0	11.0	0
(I Can't Believe It's Not Butter)	1 tbsp	90	0	0	0	0	10.0	0
(Imperial)								
lower calorie, 'Diet'	1 tbsp	50	0	0	140	0	6.0	0
soft	1 tbsp	100	0	0	95	0	11.0	0
(Land O'Lakes)								
corn oil, premium, stick	1 tbsp	35	0	0	35	0	4.0	0
regular, stick	1 tsp	35	0	0	35	0	4.0	0
soy oil, regular, stick	1 tbsp	35	0	0	35	0	4.0	0
soy oil, soft	1 tbsp	35	0	0	35	0	4.0	0
tub	1 tsp	35	0	0	35	0	4.0	0
(Mazola)								
	1 tbsp	100	0	0	100	0	11.0	0
lower calorie	1 tbsp	50	0	0	135	0	5.5	0
unsalted	1 tbsp	100	0	0	0	0	11.0	0
(Miracle Brand)								
whipped, cup	1 tbsp	60	0	0	70	0	7.0	0
whipped, stick	1 tbsp	70	0	0	65	0	7.0	0
(Fleischmann's) 'Move Over Butter'	1 tbsp	60	0	0	75	0	6.0	0
(Nucoa)								
	1 tbsp	100	0	0	160	0	11.0	0
'Heart Beat'	1 tbsp	25	0	0	110	0	3.0	0
soft	1 tbsp	90	0	0	150	0	10.0	0
unsalted, 'Heart Beat'	1 tbsp	24	0	0	0	0	3.0	0
(P&Q) quarters, 60% vegetable oil	1 tbsp	80	1	1	105	0	8.0	0
(Parkay)								
	1 tbsp	100	0	0	105	0	11.0	0
diet, soft	1 tbsp	50	0	0	110	0	6.0	0
regular, soft	1 tbsp	100	0	0	105	0	11.0	0
squeezable	1 tbsp	90	0	0	110	0	10.0	0
whipped, cup	1 tbsp	70	0	0	70	0	7.0	0
whipped, stick	1 tbsp	70	0	0	65	0	7.0	0
(Saffola) soft	1 tbsp	100	0	0	95	0	11.0	0
(Smart Beat)								
super light	1 tbsp	20	0	0	105	0	2.0	0
trans fat-free, lactose-free	1 tbsp	20	0	0	105	0	2.0	0
(Weight Watchers)								
light	1 tbsp	45	0	2	70	0	4.0	0
stick	1 tbsp	60	0	0	130	0	7.0	0
tub	1 tbsp	50	0	0	130	0	6.0	0
unsalted	1 tbsp	50	0	0	0	0	6.0	0
MARGARINE SPREAD								
margarine-butter blend, 60% corn oil margarine, 40% butter	1 stick	811	1	1	1014	0	91.2	99

Food Name	Serv. Size	Total Cal.	Prot. gms	Carbs gms	Sod. mgs	Fiber gms	Fat gms	Chol. mgs
margarine-butter blend, 60% corn oil margarine, 40% butter	1 tsp	36	0	0	45	0	4.0	4
(Blue Bonnet)								
48% vegetable oil	1 tbsp	60	1	1	115	0	6.0	5
75% vegetable oil	1 tbsp	90	0	0	95	0	11.0	0
soft, 'Better Blend'	1 tbsp	90	0	0	95	0	11.0	0
stick, 'Better Blend'	1 tbsp	90	0	0	95	0	11.0	0
unsalted, 'Better Blend'	1 tbsp	90	0	0	0	0	11.0	5
whipped, 60% vegetable oil	1 tbsp	80	0	0	100	0	8.0	0
(Brummel & Brown)								
58% vegetable oil, 10% yogurt	1 tbsp	70	0	0	95	0	8.0	0
35% vegetable oil, 25% yogurt	1 tbsp	50	0	0	95	0	5.0	0
(Country Crock)								
48% vegetable oil	1 tbsp	60	0	0	110	0	7.0	0
48% vegetable oil, churn style	1 tbsp	60	0	0	60	0	7.0	0
52% vegetable oil	1 tbsp	60	0	0	110	0	7.0	0
52% vegetable oil, churn style, stick	1 tbsp	80	0	0	55	0	9.0	0
64% vegetable oil, stick	1 tbsp	80	0	0	110	0	9.0	0
squeezable	1 tbsp	80	0	0	115	0	9.0	0
(Fleischmann's)								
'Move Over Butter'	1 tbsp	90	0	0	100	0	10.0	0
72% vegetable oil w/cream buttermilk, tub, whipped, 'Move Over Butter'	1 tbsp	60	0	0	75	0	7.0	0
72% vegetable. oil w/sweet cream buttermilk, stick, 'Move Over Butter'	1 tbsp	90	0	0	100	0	10.0	0
(Hollywood) soft	1 tbsp	90	0	1	135	0	10.0	0
(I Can't Believe It's Not Butter)								
	1 tbsp	90	0	0	0	0	10.0	0
40% vegetable oil w/cream buttermilk, tub	1 tbsp	50	0	0	90	0	6.0	0
52% vegetable oil w/cream buttermilk, quarters	1 tbsp	60	0	0	110	0	7.0	0
single portion	1 tbsp	90	0	0	95	0	10.0	0
68% vegetable oil w/buttermilk, squeezable	1 tbsp	90	0	0	90	0	10.0	0
70% vegetable oil w/cream buttermilk, stick	1 tbsp	90	0	0	90	0	10.0	0
70% vegetable oil w/cream buttermilk, tub	1 tbsp	90	0	0	95	0	10.0	0
light	1 tbsp	60	0	0	110	0	7.0	0
(Imperial) 45% vegetable oil, 'Light'	1 tbsp	60	0	0	110	0	6.0	0
(Kraft)								
bowl, 'Touch of Butter'	1 tbsp	50	0	0	110	0	6.0	0
stick, 'Touch of Butter'	1 tbsp	90	0	0	110	0	10.0	0
(Land O'Lakes)								
w/sweet cream, stick	1 tsp	30	0	0	35	0	4.0	0
w/sweet cream, tub	1 tsp	25	0	0	25	0	3.0	0
w/sweet cream, unsalted	1 tsp	30	0	0	0	0	4.0	0
lightly salted, soft, 'Country Morning Blend'	1 tbsp	30	0	0	25	0	3.0	5
lightly salted, soft, 'Country Morning Light'	1 tbsp	20	0	0	30	0	3.0	3
lightly salted, soft, 64% soy oil	1 tbsp	25	0	0	25	0	3.0	0
lightly salted, soft, w/sweet cream	1 tbsp	25	0	0	25	0	3.0	0
lightly salted, stick, 'Country Morning Blend'	1 tbsp	35	0	0	35	0	4.0	5
lightly salted, stick, 'Country Morning Light'	1 tbsp	20	0	0	30	0	3.0	3
lightly salted, stick, w/sweet cream	1 tbsp	30	0	0	35	0	4.0	0
unsalted, soft, 'Country Morning Blend'	1 tbsp	30	0	0	0	0	3.0	5
unsalted, stick, 'Country Morning Blend'	1 tbsp	35	0	0	35	0	4.0	5
unsalted, stick, w/sweet cream	1 tbsp	30	0	0	0	0	4.0	0
(Parkay) 50% vegetable oil	1 tbsp	60	0	0	110	0	7.0	0
(Promise)								
24% vegetable oil, 'Ultra'	1 tbsp	30	0	0	55	0	3.5	0
40% vegetable oil, soft	1 tbsp	50	0	0	55	0	6.0	0

Food Name	Serv. Size	Total Cal.	Prot. gms	Carbs gms	Sod. mgs	Fiber gms	Fat gms	Chol. mgs
40% vegetable oil, stick	1 tbsp	50	0	0	55	0	6.0	0
68% vegetable oil	1 tbsp	90	0	0	90	0	10.0	0
extra light	1 tbsp	50	0	0	50	0	6.0	0
lower calorie	1 tbsp	70	0	0	70	0	7.0	0
w/Canola oil, 'Ultra'	1 tbsp	35	0	0	50	0	4.0	0
whipped	1 tbsp	60	0	0	45	0	7.0	0
(Shedd's Spread) 52% vegetable oil	1 tbsp	60	0	0	110	0	7.0	0
(Touch of Butter) 47% vegetable oil and dairy spread	1 tbsp	60	0	0	110	0	7.0	0
(Weight Watchers)								
extra light, sweet, no salt, 'Country Cottage'	1 tbsp	50	0	0	0	0	6.0	0
extra light, tub 'Country Cottage Farms'	1 tbsp	45	0	2	75	0	4.0	0
light, 'Country Cottage Farms'	1 tbsp	50	0	0	130	0	6.0	0
light, stick	1 tbsp	60	0	0	130	0	7.0	0
MARGARINE SUBSTITUTE								
corn, hydrogenated and regular, 40% fat	1 cup	801	1	1	2226	0	90.0	0
corn, hydrogenated and regular, 40% fat	1 tsp	17	0	0	46	0	1.9	0
soybean, hydrogenated, 40% fat	1 cup	801	1	1	2226	0	90.0	0
soybean, hydrogenated, 40% fat	1 tsp	17	0	0	46	0	1.9	0
soybean, hydrogenated, w/cottonseed, 40% fat	1 cup	801	1	1	2226	0	90.0	0
soybean, hydrogenated, w/cottonseed, 40% fat	1 tsp	17	0	0	46	0	1.9	0
soybean, hydrogenated, w/hydrogenated and regular palm, 40% fat	1 cup	801	1	1	2226	0	90.0	0
soybean, hydrogenated/w.hydrogenated and regular palm, 40% fat	1 tsp	17	0	0	46	0	1.9	0
soybean, hydrogenated, w/hydrogenated and regular palm, 60% fat, tub	1 cup	1236	1	0	2276	0	139.2	0
soybean, hydrogenated, w/hydrogenated and regular palm, 60% fat, tub	1 tsp	26	0	0	48	0	2.9	0
soybean and cottonseed, hydrogenated, 40% fat	1 cup	801	1	1	2226	0	90.0	0
soybean and cottonseed, hydrogenated, 40% fat	1 tsp	17	0	0	46	0	1.9	0
soybean and cottonseed, hydrogenated, 60% fat, tub	1 cup	1236	1	0	2276	0	139.2	0
soybean and cottonseed, hydrogenated, 60% fat, tub	1 tsp	26	0	0	48	0	2.9	0
soybean and palm, hydrogenated, 60% fat, stick	1 cup	1236	1	0	2276	0	139.2	0
soybean and palm, hydrogenated, 60% fat, stick	1 tsp	26	0	0	48	0	2.9	0
(Promise Ultra) nonfat	1 tbsp	5	0	1	90	0	0.0	0
MARGARITA. See under COCKTAIL MIX.								
MARINADE								
(DiGiorno) refrigerated	5 oz	110	3	12	680	0	6.0	5
CALCUTTA MASALA (TAJ Cuisine of India)	4 oz	100	2	13	510	2	5.0	5
FAJITA								
(Old El Paso)	1/8 jar	14	0	3	450	0	0.0	0
(Tone's)	1 tsp	9	0	2	963	0	0.1	0
FOR MEAT (Crown Colony)	1/2 tsp	5	0	1	420	0	0.0	0
FRENCH (Litehouse) country herb, refrigerated	1 tbsp	54	0	2	196	0	5.0	0
KASHMIR TANDOOKI (TAJ Cuisine of India)	2 oz	50	2	5	260	1	3.0	0
Lemon Herb (Golden Dipt)	1 oz	130	0	2	210	0	14.0	0
LEMON PEPPER (Lawry's)	1 oz	20	0	2	800	0	1.1	0
MESQUITE (S&W)	1 tbsp	10	0	3	400	0	0.0	0
OYSTER AND SHRIMP (Caribbean Clipper)	1 tsp	10	0	2	140	na	0.0	na
SEAFOOD (Golden Dipt) honey soy, nonfat	1 tbsp	30	0	5	360	0	0.0	0
STIR-FRY (La Choy) food service product	1 tbsp	25	1	5	672	0	0.1	0
TERIYAKI								
(Golden Dipt) ginger	1 oz	120	1	12	920	0	7.0	0
(Kikkoman)								
....	1 tbsp	15	1	2	610	0	0.0	0
light	1 tbsp	15	1	3	320	0	0.0	0
(LaChoy)	1 oz	30	1	5	1640	0	0.0	0

Food Name	Serv. Size	Total Cal.	Prot. gms	Carbs gms	Sod. mgs	Fiber gms	Fat gms	Chol. mgs
(Lawry's)								
....	2 tbsp	72	6	11	7100	0	0.4	0
barbecue	1/4 cup	164	8	27	12330	0	2.3	0
barbecue	1/8 cup	82	4	14	6115	0	1.1	0
(S&W)								
....	1 tbsp	25	1	5	480	0	0.0	0
light	1 tbsp	25	1	5	220	0	0.0	0
WHITE WINE DIJON *(Golden Dipt)*	1 tbsp	10	0	1	100	0	0.0	0
WINE AND GARLIC *(Charcoal Companion)* glaze, spray ...	2 tbsp	40	1	4	230	0	0.0	0
MARINADE MIX								
BARBECUE *(Adolph's)* 'Marinade in Minutes'	1/2 tsp	5	0	1	310	0	0.0	0
BEEF								
(Durkee)	1/2 tsp	0	0	1	220	0	0.0	0
(Lawry's)	1 pkg	49	1	11	7284	0	0.2	0
(Marinade Magic)	1/2 tsp	10	1	2	400	1	0.0	0
CAJUN								
(Adolph's) 'Marinade in Minutes'	1/2 tsp	5	0	1	170	0	0.0	0
(Luzianne)	1/4 tsp	0	0	0	260	0	0.0	0
(Tone's)	1 tsp	9	0	2	215	1	0.2	0
CHICKEN								
(Adolph's)								
....	3/4 tsp	5	0	1	291	0	0.0	0
salt-free	3/4 tsp	5	0	2	0	0	0.0	0
(McCormick/Schilling) mesquite, 'Sauce Blends'	1 pkg	132	2	24	2068	0	3.0	0
(Schilling) mesquite	1/6 pkg	20	0	4	460	0	0.0	0
CITRUS *(Lawry's)* grill	2 tbsp	34	4	3	3350	0	0.4	0
FAJITA								
(Marinade Magic)	1/2 tsp	5	1	1	100	0	0.0	0
(McCormick/Schilling)	2 tsp	15	1	3	280	1	0.0	0
FOR MEAT								
(Adolph's)								
....	1/2 tsp	5	0	1	390	0	0.0	0
no salt	1/2 tsp	5	0	2	0	0	0.0	0
(French's)	1/8 pkg	10	0	2	540	0	0.0	0
(Kikkoman)	1 tsp	10	0	2	590	0	0.0	0
(McCormick/Schilling)	1 tsp	15	0	2	240	0	0.0	0
GARLIC								
(Adolph's)								
Dijon, 'Marinade in Minutes'	3/4 tsp	10	0	1	210	0	0.0	0
'Marinade in Minutes'	1/2 tsp	0	0	1	460	0	0.0	0
HERB								
(Adolph's)								
Italian, 'Marinade in Minutes'	1/4 tsp	0	0	1	270	0	0.0	0
lemon, 'Marinade in Minutes'	1/2 tsp	10	0	2	170	0	0.0	0
Parmesan, 'Marinade in Minutes'	3/4 tsp	10	0	1	230	0	0.0	0
(Lawry's) herb and garlic, w/lemon	2 tbsp	36	4	4	3688	0	1.0	0
(Marinade Magic) lemon	1/2 tsp	5	1	1	200	0	0.0	0
HICKORY *(Adolph's)* grill, 'Marinade in Minutes'	1 tbsp	20	0	4	200	0	0.5	0
HOT AND SPICY *(Adolph's)* 'Marinade in Minutes'	3/4 tsp	5	0	1	130	0	0.0	0
LEMON GARLIC *(Adolph's)* 'Marinade in Minutes'	1 tbsp	30	0	2	80	0	2.5	0
LEMON PEPPER *(Adolph's)* 'Marinade in Minutes'	1/2 tsp	10	0	2	180	0	0.0	0
MESQUITE								
(Adolph's)								
'Marinade in Minutes' dry	3/4 tsp	10	0	2	230	0	0.0	0
'Marinade in Minutes' liquid	1 tsp	45	0	5	270	0	2.5	0
(Lawry's)	2 tbsp	24	3	3	4142	0	0.4	0
SCAMPI *(Adolph's)* 'Marinade in Minutes'	1/2 tsp	10	0	2	240	0	0.0	0

Food Name	Serv. Size	Total Cal.	Prot. gms	Carbs gms	Sod. mgs	Fiber gms	Fat gms	Chol. mgs
STEAK *(Adolph's)* 'Marinade in Minutes'	1/4 tsp	0	0	1	350	0	0.0	0
TERIYAKI								
(Adolph's)								
'Marinade in Minutes' dry	1 1/2 tsp	15	0	3	380	0	0.0	0
'Marinade in Minutes' liquid	1 tbsp	20	0	5	740	0	0.0	0
MARIONBERRY TOPPING *(Flav-R-Pac)*	2 tbsp	40	0	10	0	2	0.0	0
MARJORAM								
dried	1 tbsp	5	0	1	1	1	0.1	0
dried	1 tsp	2	0	0	0	0	0.0	0
dried *(Durkee)*	1 tbsp	7	0	0	0	0	0.0	0
dried *(Durkee)*	1 tsp	2	0	0	0	0	0.0	0
dried *(Laurel Leaf)*	1 tbsp	7	0	0	0	0	0.0	0
dried *(McCormick/Schilling)*	1 tsp	4	0	1	1	0	0.0	0
dried *(Laurel Leaf)*	1 tsp	2	0	0	0	0	0.0	0
dried *(Spice Islands)*	1 tsp	4	0	1	1	0	0.1	0
dried *(Tone's)*	1 tsp	2	0	0	1	0	0.1	0
MARMALADE. See under JAM AND PRESERVES.								
MARMALADE PLUM. See SAPOTE.								
MARROW BEAN. See BEAN, MARROW.								
MARROW SQUASH. See SQUASH, MARROW.								
MARSHMALLOW. See under CANDY.								
MARSHMALLOW TOPPING								
(Finast) creme	1 oz	95	0	23	45	0	0.0	0
(Kraft) creme	1 oz	90	0	23	20	0	0.0	0
(Marshmallow Fluff)	1 tsp	59	0	15	12	0	0.0	0
(Smucker's)	2 tbsp	120	0	29	0	0	0.0	0
MASA HARINA. See under FLOUR.								
MATAI. See under WATER CHESTNUT.								
MATZO. See under CRACKER.								
MATZO MEAL. See under CRACKER MEAL.								
MAYONNAISE								
(Bama)	1 tbsp	100	0	0	65	0	11.0	0
(Bennett's) 'Real'	1 tbsp	110	0	1	65	0	12.0	0
(Best Foods)								
cholesterol-free	1 tbsp	50	0	1	80	0	5.0	0
light	1 tbsp	50	0	1	115	0	5.0	5
low-fat	1 tbsp	25	0	4	140	0	1.0	0
'Real'	1 tbsp	100	0	0	80	0	11.0	5
(Blue Plate)								
less fat, cholesterol-free	1 tbsp	50	0	1	90	0	5.0	0
100% natural, no additives	1 tbsp	100	0	0	80	0	11.0	10
(Cains)	1 tbsp	100	0	0	80	0	11.0	10
(Estee)								
lower calorie	1 tbsp	50	0	1	80	0	5.0	0
lower calorie	1 packet	15	0	2	35	0	1.0	0
(Featherweight)								
lower calorie	1 tbsp	30	0	3	40	0	2.0	10
soy, 'Soyamaise'	1 tbsp	100	0	0	3	0	11.0	5
(Finast)								
. . . .	1 tbsp	100	0	0	80	0	11.0	10
lower calorie, 'Lite'	1 tbsp	40	0	1	100	0	4.0	5
(Hain)								
Canola	1 tbsp	100	0	1	100	0	11.0	5
cold processed	1 tbsp	110	0	0	70	0	12.0	5
less fat, no salt added, 'Real'	1 tbsp	110	0	0	0	0	12.0	5
lower calorie, low sodium, 'Light'	1 tbsp	60	0	2	95	0	6.0	10

Food Name	Serv. Size	Total Cal.	Prot. gms	Carbs gms	Sod. mgs	Fiber gms	Fat gms	Chol. mgs
low-sodium, all natural	1 tbsp	110	0	0	70	0	12.0	5
no salt added, 'Real'	1 tbsp	110	0	0	0	0	12.0	5
safflower	1 tbsp	110	0	0	70	0	12.0	5
(Hellmann's)								
cholesterol-free	1 tbsp	50	0	1	80	0	5.0	0
lower calorie, 'Light'	1 tbsp	50	0	1	115	0	5.0	5
low-fat	1 tbsp	25	0	4	140	0	1.0	0
'Real'	1 tbsp	100	0	0	80	0	11.0	5
(Hollywood)								
	1 tbsp	110	0	0	80	0	12.0	5
Canola	1 tbsp	100	0	1	100	0	11.0	5
safflower	1 tbsp	100	0	0	75	0	12.0	5
(Janet Lee) lower calorie, 'Light'	1 tbsp	50	0	1	115	0	5.0	5
(JFG)								
'Creamy Velvet'	1 tbsp	100	0	0	70	0	11.0	10
less fat, cholesterol free	1 tbsp	50	0	0	85	0	5.0	0
(Kraft)								
light	1 tbsp	50	0	2	90	0	5.0	5
lower calorie, 'Light'	1 tbsp	50	0	1	110	0	5.0	0
nonfat	1 tbsp	10	0	2	120	0	0.0	0
'Real'	1 tbsp	100	0	0	75	0	11.0	5
w/lime juice, 'Mayonesa'	1 tbsp	64	0	0	60	0	12.0	10
(Pathmark)								
	1 tbsp	100	0	0	70	0	11.0	5
lower calorie	1 tbsp	40	0	1	100	0	4.0	5
low-sodium	1 tbsp	100	0	0	70	0	11.0	5
'No Frills'	1 tbsp	100	0	0	75	0	11.0	10
(Rokeach)	1 tbsp	100	0	0	70	0	11.0	10
(Smart Beat) lower calorie, 'Golden Corn Light'	1 tbsp	40	0	1	110	0	4.0	0
(Spectrum) Canola, eggless, lite	1 tbsp	35	0	1	60	0	3.0	0
(Weight Watchers)								
light	1 tbsp	25	0	1	40	0	2.0	5
lower calorie	1 tbsp	50	0	1	100	0	5.0	5
lower calorie, low-sodium	1 tbsp	50	0	1	45	0	5.0	5
(Westbrae)								
	1 tbsp	100	0	0	75	0	11.0	5
Canola	1 tbsp	100	0	0	75	0	11.0	5
MAYONNAISE SUBSTITUTE								
(Best Foods) vegetarian	1 tbsp	50	0	2	170	0	5.0	5
(Hain)								
Canola, lower calorie	1 tbsp	60	0	2	160	0	5.0	0
eggless, no salt added	1 tbsp	110	0	0	5	0	12.0	0
(Hellmann's)								
cholesterol-free	1 tbsp	50	0	1	80	0	5.0	0
vegetarian	1 tbsp	50	0	2	170	0	5.0	5
(Kraft) vegetarian	1 tbsp	50	0	3	95	0	5.0	5
(Life) sunflower, all natural	1 tbsp	71	1	1	3	0	8.0	0
(Nasoya) 'Nayonaise'	1 tbsp	35	1	1	104	0	3.3	0
(Nayonnaise) vegetable dressing and dip	1 tbsp	35	0	1	100	0	3.0	0
(Nucoa) 'Heart Beat'	1 tbsp	40	0	1	110	0	4.0	0
(Weight Watchers) cholesterol-free	1 tbsp	50	0	1	90	0	5.0	0
MEAT LOAF DINNER/ENTRÉE								
(Banquet) w/tomato sauce, potatoes, carrots in sauce, frozen, 'Extra Helping'	1 pkg	612	29	34	1943	6	40.0	113
(Healthy Choice) traditional, w/potato, vegetable, apple praline	1 pkg	316	15	52	459	6	5.0	37

Food Name	Serv. Size	Total Cal.	Prot. gms	Carbs gms	Sod. mgs	Fiber gms	Fat gms	Chol. mgs
(Lean Magic) flame broiled	1 piece	148	17	4	400	1	7.2	41
(Lean Magic 30) flame broiled	1 piece	110	15	4	449	1	3.6	35
(Stouffer's) w/gravy, frozen, food service product	1 oz	40	3	2	96	0	2.4	11
MEAT LOAF SEASONING. See under SEASONING MIX.								
MEAT STICKS, SMOKED								
	1 oz	156	6	2	420	na	14.1	38
	1 stick	109	4	1	293	na	9.8	26
MEAT SUBSTITUTE. See also individual meat substitute listings.								
(Heartline) vegetarian, unflavored, lite	0.5 oz	22	5	1	135	3	0.0	0
(Worthington)								
multigrain cutlets, vegetarian	1 slice	99	15	5	384	4	1.8	0
vegetarian, 'Choplets'	1 slice	94	17	3	500	2	1.6	0
vegetarian, cutlets	1 slice	66	11	3	340	2	1.1	0
vegetarian, 'Diced Chik'	1/4 cup	57	5	1	236	1	3.5	1
vegetarian, 'Numete'	1 slice	132	6	5	272	3	9.6	0
vegetarian, patties, 'Crispychik'	1 serving	175	8	15	596	4	9.4	1
MEAT TENDERIZER								
(Adolph's)								
seasoned, '100% Natural'	1/4 tsp	0	0	0	450	0	0.0	0
sodium-free, '100% Natural'	1/4 tsp	0	0	1	0	0	0.0	0
spiced, sodium-free, '100% Natural'	1/4 tsp	0	0	1	0	0	0.0	0
unseasoned, '100% Natural'	1/4 tsp	0	0	0	420	0	0.0	0
(Tone's)								
seasoned	1 tsp	7	0	1	1650	0	0.2	0
unseasoned	1 tsp	7	0	1	1760	0	0.2	0
MEATBALL DINNER/ENTRÉE								
(Armour)								
Swedish, 'Classics'	11.25 oz	330	19	23	1140	0	18.0	80
Swedish, beef, 'Classics'	11.25 oz	360	20	32	1170	0	17.0	65
(Banquet) Swedish, beef, frozen	11 oz	440	26	27	770	0	27.0	85
(Bernardi) meatballs	6 meatballs	270	12	5	630	2	22.0	65
(Budget Gourmet)								
Swedish, beef, frozen	11.2 oz	450	23	40	1110	0	22.0	70
Swedish, w/cream sauce and noodles, frozen	1 entrée	550	22	40	1050	3	34.0	150
(Chef Boyardee) stew, canned	8 oz	350	9	24	1315	0	24.0	0
(Dinty Moore)								
stew	8 oz	240	11	14	980	0	16.0	30
stew, microwave cup	7.5 oz	240	11	14	980	0	16.0	30
(Freezer Queen) Swedish, beef, frozen	10 oz	350	19	26	910	0	19.0	0
(Healthy Choice)								
Italian style, 'Hearty Handfuls'	1 entrée	320	18	51	590	6	5.0	15
Swedish, frozen	1 entrée	280	22	35	590	3	6.0	50
(Lean Cuisine)								
Swedish	1 entrée	280	20	33	590	3	7.0	50
Swedish, w/pasta, frozen	1 entrée	290	22	32	590	3	8.0	55
Swedish, w/pasta, frozen	1 pkg	276	22	31	562	3	7.2	46
(Lunch Express) Swedish, w/pasta, frozen	1 entrée	530	19	41	1010	3	32.0	65
(Marie Callender's) Swedish, frozen	12.5 oz	520	28	44	1020	3	26.0	65
(Morton) Swedish, beef, frozen	10 oz	310	11	26	1520	0	17.0	50
(Smart Ones) Swedish	1 entrée	300	19	33	510	2	10.0	50
(Stouffer's)								
Swedish, frozen	1 entrée	440	23	36	840	3	23.0	85
Swedish, w/gravy, food service product	1 oz	48	3	2	150	0	3.3	9
(Swanson) Swedish, beef, frozen	10 oz	350	26	37	700	0	11.0	0
(Weight Watchers) Swedish, frozen	1 entrée	280	18	34	510	3	8.0	30
MEATBALL SEASONING. See under SEASONING MIX.								

Food Name	Serv. Size	Total Cal.	Prot. gms	Carbs gms	Sod. mgs	Fiber gms	Fat gms	Chol. mgs
MEDICAL NUTRITIONALS								
CARBOHYDRATE SUPPLEMENT								
(Mead Johnson Nutritionals)								
'Moducal, 100% maltodextrin, powder .... 1/2 cup	1/2 cup	240	0	64	na	na	0.0	na
(Ross)								
'Polycose' for oral or tube feeding (not parenteral use), kosher, gluten- and lactose-free, low-residue, liquid ... 100 ml	100 ml	200	0	50	70	na	0.0	na
'Polycose' for oral or tube feeding (not parenteral use), kosher, gluten- and lactose-free, low-residue, powder ... 100 gm	100 gm	380	0	94	110	na	0.0	na
CRITICAL CARE SUPPORT								
(Nestlé Clinical Nutrition)								
'Crucial' for tube feeding, lactose- and gluten-free, low-residue, ready to use .... 1000 ml	1000 ml	1500	94	135	1168	na	68.0	na
'Crucial' for tube feeding, lactose- and gluten-free, low-residue, ready to use .... 250 ml	250 ml	375	24	34	292	na	16.9	na
(Novartis [Sandoz])								
'Impact' ready to use .... 1000 ml	1000 ml	1000	56	130	1100	na	28.0	na
'Impact' ready to use, 1 can, ... 250 ml	250 ml	250	14	33	267	na	6.9	na
'Impact 1.5' for fluid restriction or high caloric needs, ready to use, ... 1000 ml	1000 ml	1500	80	140	1280	na	69.0	na
'Impact 1.5' for fluid restriction or high caloric needs, ready to use, 1 can .... 250 ml	250 ml	375	21	35	320	na	17.2	na
'Impact with Fiber' ready to use .... 1000 ml	1000 ml	1000	56	140	1100	na	28.0	na
'Impact with Fiber' ready to use, 1 can, ... 250 ml	250 ml	250	14	34	267	na	6.9	na
(Ross)								
'Perative' for tube feeding (not parenteral use), kosher, gluten- and lactose-free, low-residue, ready to use, ... 1 liter	1 liter	1300	67	177	1040	na	37.4	na
'Perative' for tube feeding (not parenteral use), kosher, gluten- and lactose-free, low-residue, ready to use ..... 8 fl oz	8 fl oz	308	16	42	250	na	8.8	na
DIABETES/GLUCOSE INTOLERANCE SUPPORT								
(Mead Johnson Nutritionals)								
'Choice DM' for oral or tube feeding, ready to use ..... 1000 ml	1000 ml	1060	45	106	850	14	51.0	na
'Choice DM' for oral or tube feeding, ready to use .... 8 fl oz	8 fl oz	250	11	25	200	3	12.0	na
(Nestlé Clinical Nutrition)								
'Glytrol with Fiber' for oral or tube feeding, kosher, sucrose-, lactose-, and gluten-free, ready to use ..... 1000 ml	1000 ml	1000	45	100	740	15	47.5	na
'Glytrol with Fiber' for oral or tube feeding, kosher, sucrose-, lactose-, and gluten-free, ready to use ...... 250 ml	250 ml	250	11	25	185	4	11.9	na
(Novartis [Sandoz])								
'Diabetisource with Fiber' ready to use .... 1000 ml	1000 ml	1000	50	90	1000	4	49.0	na
'Diabetisource with Fiber' ready to use, 1 can .... 250 ml	250 ml	250	13	23	250	1	12.2	na
'Resource Diabetic with Fiber' for oral or tube feeding, ready to use .... 1000 ml	1000 ml	1060	63	99	970	13	47.0	na
'Resource Diabetic with Fiber' for oral or tube feeding, ready to use .... 237 ml	237 ml	250	15	23	230	3	11.1	na
(Ross)								
'Glucerna with Fiber' for oral or tube feeding (not parenteral use), kosher, gluten- and lactose-free, low-residue, ready to use .... 1 liter	1 liter	1000	42	96	930	14	54.4	na
'Glucerna with Fiber' for oral or tube feeding (not parenteral use), kosher, gluten- and lactose-free, low-residue, ready to use .... 8 fl oz	8 fl oz	237	10	23	220	3	12.9	na
ELEMENTAL DIET								
(B. Braun/McGaw)								
'Immun-Aid' for oral or tube feeding, high-nitrogen, powder, prepared, daily dose .... 2000 ml	2000 ml	2000	160	240	1150	na	44.0	na

Food Name	Serv. Size	Total Cal.	Prot. gms	Carbs gms	Sod. mgs	Fiber gms	Fat gms	Chol. mgs
'Immun-Aid' for oral or tube feeding, high-nitrogen, powder, prepared, 1 serving	500 ml	500	40	60	290	na	11.0	na
(Mead Johnson Nutritionals)								
'Criticare HN' high-nitrogen, ready to use	1000 ml	1060	38	220	630	na	5.3	na
'Criticare HN' high-nitrogen, ready to use	8 fl oz	250	9	51	150	na	1.3	na
(Nestlé Clinical Nutrition)								
'Peptamen' for tube feeding, isotonic, lactose- and gluten-free, low-residue, ready to use	1000 ml	1000	40	127	560	na	39.0	na
'Peptamen' for tube feeding, isotonic, lactose- and gluten-free, low-residue, ready to use	250 ml	250	10	32	140	na	9.8	na
'Peptamen Oral' oral, lactose- and gluten-free, low-residue, ready to use	1000 ml	1000	40	127	560	na	39.0	na
'Peptamen Oral' oral, lactose- and gluten-free, low-residue, ready to use	250 ml	250	10	32	140	na	9.8	na
'Peptamen VHP' for tube feeding, very high protein, isotonic, lactose- and gluten-free, low-residue, ready to use	1000 ml	1000	63	105	560	na	39.0	na
'Peptamen VHP' for tube feeding, very high protein, isotonic, lactose- and gluten-free, low-residue, ready to use	250 ml	250	16	26	140	na	9.8	na
'Peptamen VHP' oral, very high protein, lactose- and gluten-free, low-residue, ready to use	1000 ml	1000	63	105	560	na	39.0	na
'Peptamen VHP' oral, very high protein, lactose- and gluten-free, low-residue, ready to use	250 ml	250	16	26	140	na	9.8	na
'Reabilan' for tube feeding, lactose and gluten-free, low-residue, ready to use	1000 ml	1000	32	132	700	na	40.5	na
'Reabilan' for tube feeding, lactose and gluten-free, low-residue, ready to use	375 ml	375	12	49	262	na	15.2	na
'Reabilan HN' for tube feeding, high-nitrogen, lactose- and gluten-free, low-residue, ready to use	1000 ml	1333	58	158	1000	na	54.0	na
'Reabilan HN' for tube feeding, high-nitrogen, lactose- and gluten-free, low-residue, ready to use	375 ml	500	22	59	380	na	20.2	na
(Novartis [Sandoz])								
'Tolerex' powder, prepared	1000 ml	1000	21	230	470	na	1.5	na
'Tolerex' powder, prepared, 1 packet	300 ml	300	6	68	141	na	0.4	na
'Vivonex Plus' high-nitrogen, powder, prepared	1000 ml	1000	45	190	610	na	6.7	na
'Vivonex Plus' high-nitrogen, powder, prepared	300 ml	300	14	57	183	na	2.0	na
'Vivonex T.E.N' for gastrointestinal impairment, powder, prepared	1000 ml	1000	38	210	460	na	2.8	na
'Vivonex T.E.N' for gastrointestinal impairment, powder, prepared, 1 packet	300 ml	300	12	62	138	na	0.8	na
FAT MALABSORPTION SUPPORT								
(Mead Johnson Nutritionals)								
'Lipisorb' lactose-free, low-residue, powder, prepared	8 fl oz	480	17	56	352	na	23.0	na
'Lipisorb' lactose-free, low-residue, ready to use	1000 ml	1350	57	161	1350	na	57.0	na
'Lipisorb' lactose-free, low-residue, ready to use	8 fl oz	320	14	38	320	na	13.4	na
GASTROINTESTINAL SUPPORT								
(Nestlé Clinical Nutrition)								
'Elementra' for oral or tube feeding, elemental protein, powder, 2 scoops	6.6 gm	25	5	0	10	na	0.3	na
(Novartis [Sandoz])								
'Sandosource Peptide' semi-elemental, low-fat, ready to use	1000 ml	1000	50	160	1200	na	17.0	na
'Sandosource Peptide' semi-elemental, low-fat, ready to use	250 ml	250	13	41	300	na	4.4	na
(Ross)								
'Alitraq' for oral or tube feeding (not parenteral use), kosher, gluten-free, low-residue, powder, prepared	1 liter	1000	53	165	1000	na	15.5	na

Food Name	Serv. Size	Total Cal.	Prot. gms	Carbs gms	Sod. mgs	Fiber gms	Fat gms	Chol. mgs
'Alitraq' for oral or tube feeding (not parenteral use), kosher, gluten-free, low-residue, powder, prepared .... 300 ml	300 ml	300	16	50	300	na	4.7	na
'Vital High Nitrogen' for oral or tube feeding (not parenteral use), kosher, gluten- and lactose-free, low-residue, powder, prepared .... 1 liter	1 liter	1000	42	185	566	na	10.8	na
'Vital High Nitrogen' for oral or tube feeding (not parenteral use), kosher, gluten- and lactose-free, low-residue, powder, prepared .... 300 ml	300 ml	300	13	55	170	na	3.3	na
GENERAL PURPOSE								
(Mead Johnson Nutritionals)								
'Boost' oral, milk-based, cholesterol- and lactose-free .... 8 fl oz	8 fl oz	240	10	41	130	0	4.2	na
'Sustacal' oral, milk-based, lactose-free cholesterol-free, powder, prepared .... 8 fl oz	8 fl oz	200	13	36	190	0	0.7	na
'Sustacal' oral, milk-based, moderate protein, fiber-free, lactose-free, low-residue, ready to use .... 8 fl oz	8 fl oz	240	15	33	220	0	5.5	na
'Sustacal Pudding' lactose-free, fiber-free .... 8 fl oz	8 fl oz	240	7	32	120	na	9.5	na
'Sustacal with Fiber' oral, milk-based, w/fiber, lactose-free, ready to use .... 8 fl oz	8 fl oz	250	11	33	170	3	8.3	na
(Novartis [Sandoz])								
'Resource' fruit beverage, low-electrolyte, fat-free ..... 1000 ml	1000 ml	760	37	150	230	na	0.0	na
'Resource' fruit beverage, low-electrolyte, fat-free, 1 Brik Pak .... 237 ml	237 ml	180	9	36	55	na	0.0	na
(Ross)								
'Ensure' for oral or tube feeding (not parenteral use), kosher, gluten- and lactose-free, low-residue, powder, prepared .... 1 liter	1 liter	1060	37	145	846	na	37.2	na
'Ensure' for oral or tube feeding (not parenteral use), kosher, gluten- and lactose-free, low-residue, powder, prepared .... 8 fl oz	8 fl oz	250	9	34	200	na	8.8	na
'Ensure' for oral or tube feeding (not parenteral use), kosher, gluten- and lactose-free, low-residue, ready to use .... 1 liter	1 liter	1060	37	169	845	na	25.8	na
'Ensure' for oral or tube feeding (not parenteral use), kosher, gluten- and lactose-free, low-residue, ready to use .... 8 fl oz	8 fl oz	250	9	40	200	na	6.1	na
'Ensure Pudding' oral, patients w/swallowing impairments, kosher, gluten-free, 9.2 g lactose/serving .... 5 oz can	5 oz can	250	7	34	240	na	9.7	na
'Ensure with Fiber' for oral or tube feeding (not parenteral use), fiber-fortified, kosher, gluten- and lactose-free, low-residue, ready to use .... 1 liter	1 liter	1100	40	162	846	14	37.2	na
'Ensure with Fiber' for oral or tube feeding (not parenteral use), fiber-fortified, kosher, gluten- and lactose-free, low-residue, ready to use .... 8 fl oz	8 fl oz	260	9	38	200	3	8.8	na
GERIATRIC								
(Nestlé Clinical Nutrition)								
'Probalance with Fiber' for oral or tube feeding, high-fiber, kosher, lactose- and gluten-free, ready to use .... 1000 ml	1000 ml	1200	54	156	763	10	40.6	na
'Probalance with Fiber' for oral or tube feeding, high-fiber, kosher, lactose- and gluten-free, ready to use .... 250 ml	250 ml	300	14	39	191	3	10.2	na
HEALING SUPPORT								
(Mead Johnson Nutritionals)								
'Protain XL' for tube feeding, high-protein, w/fiber, ready to use .... 1000 ml	1000 ml	1000	57	129	920	na	30.0	na
'Protain XL' for tube feeding, high-protein, w/fiber, ready to use .... 8 fl oz	8 fl oz	237	14	31	220	na	7.1	na

Food Name	Serv. Size	Total Cal.	Prot. gms	Carbs gms	Sod. mgs	Fiber gms	Fat gms	Chol. mgs
'Traumacal' for oral or tube feeding, high-calorie, high-nitrogen	1000 ml	1500	82	142	1180	na	68.0	na
'Traumacal' for oral or tube feeding, high-calorie, high-nitrogen	8 fl oz	355	20	34	280	na	16.2	na
(Nestlé Clinical Nutrition)								
'Replete' isotonic, kosher, lactose- and gluten-free, low-residue, ready to use	1000 ml	1000	63	113	876	na	34.0	na
'Replete' isotonic, kosher, lactose- and gluten-free, low-residue, ready to use	250 ml	250	16	28	219	na	8.5	na
'Replete with Fiber' for oral or tube feeding, isotonic, high-fiber, kosher, lactose- and gluten-free, ready to use	1000 ml	1000	63	113	876	14	34.0	na
'Replete with Fiber' for oral or tube feeding, isotonic, high-fiber, kosher, lactose- and gluten-free, ready to use	250 ml	250	16	28	219	4	8.5	na
(Ross)								
'Ensure' oral, coffee flavored, canned	8 fl oz	250	9	34	0	0	8.8	0
'Promote' for oral or tube feeding, high-protein, kosher, gluten- and lactose-free, low-residue, ready to use	1 liter	1000	63	130	1000	na	26.0	na
'Promote' for oral or tube feeding, high-protein, kosher, gluten- and lactose-free, low-residue, ready to use	8 fl oz	237	15	31	240	na	6.2	na
'Promote with Fiber' for oral or tube feeding, high-protein, kosher, gluten- and lactose-free, low-residue, ready to use	1 liter	1000	63	139	1300	na	28.2	na
'Promote with Fiber' for oral or tube feeding, high-protein, kosher, gluten- and lactose-free, low-residue, ready to use	8 fl oz	237	15	33	310	na	6.7	na
HEPATIC SUPPORT								
(B. Braun/McGaw)								
'Hepatic-Aid II' for oral or tube feeding, amino acid and calories, powder, prepared	340 ml	400	15	57	na	na	12.3	na
(Nestlé Clinical Nutrition)								
'Nutrihep' for oral or tube feeding, kosher, lactose- and gluten-free, ready to use	1000 ml	1500	40	290	320	na	21.2	na
'Nutrihep' for oral or tube feeding, kosher, lactose- and gluten-free, ready to use	250 ml	375	10	73	80	na	5.3	na
HIV/AIDS SUPPORT								
(Ross)								
'Advera with Fiber' for oral or tube feeding (not parenteral use), kosher, gluten- and lactose-free, ready to use	1 liter	1280	60	216	1013	9	22.8	na
'Advera with Fiber' for oral or tube feeding (not parenteral use), kosher, gluten- and lactose-free, ready to use	8 fl oz	303	14	51	240	2	5.4	na
HYDRATION SUPPORT								
(Ross)								
'Equalyte' enteral rehydration solution	8 fl oz	24	0	7	432	0	0.0	0
'Equalyte' rehydration solution, for oral or tube feeding (not parenteral use), kosher, gluten- and lactose-free, ready to use	1 liter	100	na	25	1800	na	na	na
'Introlite' rehydration solution, for tube feeding (not parenteral use), low calorie, kosher, gluten- and lactose-free, low-residue, ready to use	1 liter	530	22	71	930	na	18.4	na
'Pedialyte' for children	8 fl oz	24	0	6	244	0	0.0	0
HYPEROSMOLAR SENSITIVITY SUPPORT								
(Ross)								
for oral or tube feeding (not parenteral use), kosher, gluten- and lactose-free, low-residue, ready to use	1 liter	1060	37	152	640	na	34.7	na

Food Name	Serv. Size	Total Cal.	Prot. gms	Carbs gms	Sod. mgs	Fiber gms	Fat gms	Chol. mgs
for oral or tube feeding (not parenteral use), kosher, gluten- and lactose-free, low-residue, ready to use	8 fl oz	250	9	36	150	na	8.2	na

INTACT PROTEIN DIET
(Mead Johnson Nutritionals)

Food Name	Serv. Size	Total Cal.	Prot. gms	Carbs gms	Sod. mgs	Fiber gms	Fat gms	Chol. mgs
'Comply' for tube feeding, high-calorie, lactose-free, ready to use	1000 ml	1500	60	180	1200	na	61.0	na
'Comply' for tube feeding, high-calorie, lactose-free, ready to use	8 fl oz	355	14	43	280	na	14.5	na
'Deliver 2.0' for oral or tube feeding, high-calorie, high-nitrogen, lactose-free	1000 ml	2000	75	200	800	na	102.0	na
'Deliver 2.0' for oral or tube feeding, high-calorie, high-nitrogen, lactose-free	8 fl oz	470	18	47	190	na	24.0	na
'Isocal' for tube feeding, lactose-free, low-residue, ready to use	1000 ml	1060	34	135	530	na	44.0	na
'Isocal' for tube feeding, lactose-free, low-residue, ready to use	8 fl oz	250	8	32	125	na	10.5	na
'Isocal HN' for tube feeding, high-nitrogen, isotonic, low-residue, ready to use	1000 ml	1060	44	123	930	na	145.0	na
'Isocal HN' for tube feeding, high-nitrogen, isotonic, low-residue, ready to use	8 fl oz	250	10	29	220	na	10.7	na
'Ultracal with Fiber' for tube feeding, high-nitrogen, w/fiber, ready to use	1000 ml	1060	44	123	930	14	45.0	na
'Ultracal with Fiber' for tube feeding, high-nitrogen, w/fiber, ready to use	8 fl oz	250	10	29	220	3	10.7	na

(Nestlé Clinical Nutrition)

Food Name	Serv. Size	Total Cal.	Prot. gms	Carbs gms	Sod. mgs	Fiber gms	Fat gms	Chol. mgs
'Nubasics' oral, low-sodium, kosher, lactose-, gluten-, and cholesterol-free, low-residue, ready to use	250 ml	250	9	33	219	na	9.2	na
'Nubasics Complete Nutrition Bar' oral, low-sodium, kosher, lactose- and gluten-free	1 bar	125	4	17	135	na	4.6	na
'Nubasics Complete Nutrition Soup' oral, low-cholesterol, lactose- and gluten-free, low-residue, 1 envelope	56 g	250	9	33	390	na	9.2	na
Nubasics Decaffeinated Coffee Beverage' oral, kosher, lactose-, gluten-, and cholesterol-free, powder	2 scoops level	125	6	19	120	na	2.8	na
'Nubasics Juice Drink' oral, kosher, lactose-, gluten-, and cholesterol-free; low-residue	163 ml	163	6	34	50	na	0.1	na
'Nubasics Plus' oral, high-calorie, low-sodium, kosher, lactose-, gluten-, and cholesterol-free, low-residue, ready to use	250 ml	375	13	44	292	na	16.2	na
'Nubasics 2.0' oral, very high calorie; kosher, lactose- and gluten-free, low-residue, ready to use	250 ml	500	20	49	325	na	26.5	na
'Nubasics VHP' oral, high-protein, low-sodium, kosher, lactose-, gluten-, and cholesterol-free, ready to use	250 ml	250	16	28	219	na	8.3	na
'Nubasics with Fiber' oral, high-protein with fiber, low-sodium, kosher, lactose-, gluten-, and cholesterol-free, low-residue, ready to use	250 ml	250	9	33	219	4	9.2	na
'Nutren 1.0' for oral or tube feeding, kosher, lactose- and gluten-free, low-residue, ready to use	250 ml	250	10	32	219	na	9.5	na
'Nutren 1.0' for oral or tube feeding, kosher, lactose- and gluten-free, low-residue, ready to use	1000 ml	1000	40	127	876	na	38.0	na
'Nutren 1.0 with Fiber' for oral or tube feeding, high-fiber, kosher, lactose- and gluten-free, ready to use	1000 ml	1000	40	127	876	14	38.0	na
'Nutren 1.0 with Fiber' for oral or tube feeding, high-fiber, kosher, lactose- and gluten-free, ready to use	250 ml	250	10	32	219	4	9.5	na
'Nutren 1.5' for oral or tube feeding, high-calorie, kosher, lactose- and gluten-free, low-residue, ready to use	1000 ml	1500	60	169	1170	na	67.6	na
'Nutren 1.5' for oral or tube feeding, high-calorie, kosher, lactose- and gluten-free, low-residue, ready to use	250 ml	375	15	42	292	na	16.9	na

Food Name	Serv. Size	Total Cal.	Prot. gms	Carbs gms	Sod. mgs	Fiber gms	Fat gms	Chol. mgs
'Nutren 2.0' for oral or tube feeding, very high calorie, kosher, lactose- and gluten-free, low-residue, ready to use	1000 ml	2000	80	196	1300	na	106.0	na
'Nutren 2.0' for oral or tube feeding, very high calorie, kosher, lactose- and gluten-free, low-residue, ready to use	250 ml	500	20	49	325	na	26.5	na
(Novartis [Sandoz])								
'Citrotein' fruit-flavored, lactose-free, low-residue, powder, prepared, 1 serving	254 ml	170	11	31	170	na	0.4	na
'Citrotein' fruit-flavored, lactose-free, low-residue, powder, prepared	100 ml	670	41	120	670	na	1.6	na
'Compleat' for tube feeding, blenderized, ready to use	1000 ml	1070	43	130	1300	4	43.0	na
'Compleat' for tube feeding, blenderized, ready to use, 1 can	250 ml	265	11	32	317	1	10.7	na
'Compleat Modified with Fiber' for tube feeding, blenderized, lactose-free, isotonic, ready to use	1000 ml	1070	43	140	1000	4	37.0	na
'Compleat Modified with Fiber' for tube feeding, blenderized, lactose-free, isotonic, ready to use, 1 can	250 ml	265	11	35	250	1	9.2	na
'Fibersource HN' for oral or tube feeding, high-fiber, high-nitrogen, lactose- and gluten-free, ready to use	1000 ml	1200	53	160	1100	7	41.0	na
'Fibersource HN' for oral or tube feeding, high-fiber, high-nitrogen, lactose- and gluten-free, ready to use, 1 can	250 ml	300	13	40	283	2	10.4	na
'Fibersource' for oral or tube feeding, high-fiber, lactose- and gluten-free, ready to use	1000 ml	1200	43	170	1100	10	41.0	na
'Fibersource' for oral or tube feeding, high-fiber, lactose- and gluten-free, ready to use, 1 can	250 ml	300	11	42	283	3	10.4	na
'Isosource HN' for oral or tube feeding, protein maintenance, lactose-, gluten-, and fiber-free, ready to use	1000 ml	1200	53	160	1100	na	41.0	na
'Isosource HN' for oral or tube feeding, protein maintenance, lactose-, gluten-, and fiber-free, ready to use	250 ml	300	13	39	267	na	10.4	na
'Isosource 1.5 with Fiber' high-calorie, high-nitrogen, ready to use	1000 ml	1500	170	68	1300	8	65.0	na
'Isosource 1.5 with Fiber' high-calorie, high-nitrogen, ready to use, 1 can	250 ml	375	42	17	322	2	16.2	na
'Isosource Standard' for oral or tube feeding, protein maintenance, lactose-, gluten-, and fiber-free, ready to use	1000 ml	1200	43	170	1200	na	41.0	na
'Isosource Standard' for oral or tube feeding, protein maintenance, lactose-, gluten-, and fiber-free, ready to use	250	300	11	42	300	na	10.4	na
'Isosource VHN with Fiber' for oral or tube feeding, w/fiber, ready to use	1000 ml	1000	62	130	1300	10	29.0	na
'Isosource VHN with Fiber' for oral or tube feeding, w/fiber, ready to use	250 ml	250	16	32	320	3	7.2	na
'Resource Plus' for oral or tube feeding, high-calorie, lactose- and gluten-free, ready to use	1000 ml	1500	55	200	1300	na	53.0	na
'Resource Plus' for oral or tube feeding, high-calorie, lactose- and gluten-free, ready to use, 1 Brik Pak	237 ml	355	13	47	300	na	12.6	na
'Resource Standard' maintenance protein and calorie, lactose- and gluten-free, ready to use	1000 ml	1100	37	140	890	na	37.0	na

Food Name	Serv. Size	Total Cal.	Prot. gms	Carbs gms	Sod. mgs	Fiber gms	Fat gms	Chol. mgs
'Resource Standard' maintenance protein and calorie, lactose- and gluten-free, ready to use, 1 Brik Pak	237 ml	250	9	34	210	na	8.8	na
(Ross)								
'Ensure High Protein' oral (not parenteral use), kosher, gluten- and lactose-free, low-residue, ready to use	8 fl oz	225	12	31	290	na	6.0	na
'Ensure Plus' for oral or tube feeding (not parenteral use), high-calorie, kosher, gluten- and lactose-free, low-residue, ready to use	1 liter	1500	55	200	1050	na	53.3	na
'Ensure Plus' for oral or tube feeding (not parenteral use), high-calorie, kosher, gluten- and lactose-free, low-residue, ready to use	8 fl oz	355	13	47	250	na	12.6	na
'Ensure Plus HN' for oral or tube feeding (not parenteral use), high calorie, kosher, gluten- and lactose-free, low-residue, ready to use	1 liter	1500	63	200	1180	na	50.0	na
'Ensure Plus HN' for oral or tube feeding (not parenteral use), high calorie, kosher, gluten- and lactose-free, low-residue, ready to use	8 fl oz	355	15	47	280	na	11.8	na
'Jevity with Fiber' for tube feeding (not parenteral use), fiber-fortified, isotonic, kosher, gluten-and lactose-free, low-residue, ready to use	1 liter	1060	44	154	930	14	34.7	na
'Jevity with Fiber' for tube feeding (not parenteral use), fiber-fortified, isotonic, kosher, gluten-and lactose-free, low-residue, ready to use	8 fl oz	250	11	36	220	3	8.2	na
'Jevity Plus with Fiber' for tube feeding (not parenteral use), high-nitrogen, kosher, gluten- and lactose-free, ready to use	1 liter	1200	56	175	1350	12	39.3	na
'Jevity Plus with Fiber' for tube feeding (not parenteral use), high-nitrogen, kosher, gluten- and lactose-free, ready to use	8 fl oz	285	13	42	275	3	9.3	na
'Osmolite' for oral or tube feeding (not parenteral use), high-nitrogen, isotonic, kosher, gluten- and lactose-free, low-residue, ready to use	1 liter	1060	44	144	930	na	34.7	na
'Osmolite' for oral or tube feeding (not parenteral use), high-nitrogen, isotonic, kosher, gluten- and lactose-free, low-residue, ready to use	8 fl oz	250	11	34	220	na	8.2	na
'Osmolite HN Plus' for tube feeding (not parenteral use), high-calorie, high-nitrogen, kosher, gluten- and lactose-free, low-residue, ready to use	1 liter	1200	56	158	1420	na	39.3	na
'Osmolite HN Plus' for tube feeding (not parenteral use), high-calorie, high-nitrogen, kosher, gluten- and lactose-free, low-residue, ready to use	8 fl oz	285	13	38	340	na	9.3	na
'Twocal HN' for oral or tube feeding (not parenteral use), high-calorie, high-protein, kosher, gluten- and lactose-free, ready to use	1 liter	2000	84	217	1456	na	90.9	na
'Twocal HN' for oral or tube feeding (not parenteral use), high-calorie, high-protein, kosher, gluten- and lactose-free, low-residue, ready to use	8 fl oz	475	20	51	345	na	21.5	na
PARENTERAL SUPPORT (NUTRIENT INJECTIONS)								
(B. Braun/McGaw)								
'Freamine HBC' 6.9% amino acids, sterile, nonpyrogenic, hypertonic solution	100 ml	na	na	na	na	na	na	na
'Freamine III' 8.5% amino acids, nonpyrogenic, hypertonic solution	100 ml	na	na	na	na	na	na	na

Food Name	Serv. Size	Total Cal.	Prot. gms	Carbs gms	Sod. mgs	Fiber gms	Fat gms	Chol. mgs
'Freamine III' 10% amino acids, sterile, nonpyrogenic, hypertonic solution, w/electrolytes	100 ml	na	na	na	na	na	na	na
'Freamine III with Electrolytes' 8.5% amino acids, sterile, nonpyrogenic, hypertonic solution, w/electrolytes	100 ml	na	na	na	na	na	na	na
'Freamine II' 3% amino acids, sterile, nonpyrogenic, slightly hypertonic solution, w/electrolytes	100 ml	na	na	na	0	na	na	na
'Hepatamine' 8% amino acids, for patients w/cirrhosis or hepatitis, sterile, nonpyrogenic, hypertonic solution ..	500 ml	na	na	na	na	na	na	na
'Hepatamine' 8% amino acids, for patients w/hepatic encephalopathy-injection	100 ml	na	na	na	na	na	na	na
'Procalamine' 3% amino acids, 3% glycerine, sterile, nonpyrogenic, moderately hypertonic injection, w/electrolytes	100 ml	na	na	na	0	na	na	na
'Trophanine' 10% amino acids, sterile, nonpyrogenic, hypertonic solution, w/electrolytes	100 ml	na	na	na	na	na	na	na
'Trophanine' 6% amino acids, sterile, nonpyrogenic, hypertonic solution, w/electrolytes	100 ml	na	na	na	na	na	na	na
PEDIATRIC								
(Mead Johnson Nutritionals)								
'Kindercal with Fiber' for oral or tube feeding, lactose-free, isotonic, ready to use	1000 ml	1060	34	135	370	6	44.0	na
'Kindercal with Fiber' for oral or tube feeding, lactose-free, isotonic, ready to use	8 fl oz	250	8	32	88	2	10.5	na
'Portagen' for GI disorders, children under 2 years, powder, prepared	5 fl oz	100	4	12	55	na	4.8	na
(Nestlé Clinical Nutrition)								
'Nutren Junior' for oral or tube feeding, children 1–10 years, kosher, lactose- and gluten-free, low-residue, ready to use	1000 ml	1000	30	128	460	na	42.0	na
'Nutren Junior' for oral or tube feeding, children 1–10 years, kosher, lactose- and gluten-free, low-residue, ready to use	250 ml	250	8	32	115	na	10.5	na
'Nutren Junior with Fiber' for oral or tube feeding, children 1–10 years, kosher, lactose- and gluten-free, low-residue, ready to use	1000 ml	1000	30	128	460	6	42.0	na
'Nutren Junior with Fiber' for oral or tube feeding, children 1–10 years, kosher, lactose- and gluten-free, low-residue, ready to use	250 ml	250	8	32	115	2	10.5	na
'Peptamen Junior' for tube feeding, GI patients, children 1-10 years, lactose- and gluten-free, low-residue, ready to use	1000 ml	1000	30	138	460	na	38.5	na
'Peptamen Junior' for tube feeding, GI patients, children 1-10 years, lactose- and gluten-free, low-residue, ready to use	250 ml	250	8	34	115	na	9.6	na
'Peptamen Junior Oral' oral, for children 1-10 years, lactose- and gluten-free, low-residue, ready to use ...	1000 ml	1000	30	138	460	na	38.5	na
'Peptamen Junior Oral' oral, for children 1-10 years, lactose- and gluten-free, low-residue, ready to use	250 ml	250	8	34	115	na	9.6	na
(Novartis [Sandoz])								
'Vivonex Pediatric' for oral or tube feeding, children 1–10 years, powder, prepared	1000 ml	800	24	130	400	na	24.0	na
'Vivonex Pediatric' for oral or tube feeding, children 1–10 years, powder, prepared	250 ml	200	6	32	100	na	5.9	na
(Ross)								
'Pediasure with Fiber' for oral or tube feeding (not parenteral use), kosher, gluten- and lactose-free, ready to use, not for children with galactosemia	1 liter	1000	30	114	380	na	49.7	na

Food Name	Serv. Size	Total Cal.	Prot. gms	Carbs gms	Sod. mgs	Fiber gms	Fat gms	Chol. mgs
'Pediasure with Fiber' for oral or tube feeding (not parenteral use), kosher, gluten- and lactose-free, ready to use, not for children with galactosemia	8 fl oz	237	7	27	90	na	11.8	na
'Pediasure' for oral or tube feeding (not parenteral use) kosher, gluten- and lactose-free, low-residue, not for children with galactosemia	1 liter	1000	30	110	380	na	49.7	na
'Pediasure' for oral or tube feeding (not parenteral use) kosher, gluten- and lactose-free, low-residue, not for children with galactosemia	8 fl oz	237	7	26	90	na	11.8	na
PROTEIN SUPPLEMENT								
(Mead Johnson Nutritionals)								
'Casec'	100 gm	380	90	0	100	na	2.0	na
(Novartis [Sandoz])								
'Meritene' oral, powder, prepared	1000 ml	1100	69	120	1100	na	34.0	na
'Meritene' oral, powder, prepared, 1 serving	275 ml	275	18	31	280	na	8.8	na
(Ross)								
for oral or tube feeding (not parenteral use), powder, gluten-free, low-residue, kosher, 2 scoops	6.6 gm	28	5	1	15	na	0.6	na
PULMONARY SUPPORT								
(Mead Johnson Nutritionals)								
'Respalor' for oral or tube feeding, high-nitrogen, high-calorie, ready to use	1000 ml	1520	76	148	1270	na	71.0	na
'Respalor' for oral or tube feeding, high-nitrogen, high-calorie, ready to use	8 fl oz	360	18	35	300	na	16.8	na
(Nestlé Clinical Nutrition)								
'Nutrivent' for tube feeding, kosher, lactose- and gluten-free, low-residue, ready to use	1000 ml	1500	68	100	1170	na	94.0	na
'Nutrivent' for tube feeding, kosher, lactose- and gluten-free, low-residue, ready to use	250 ml	375	17	25	292	na	23.7	na
(Ross)								
'Pulmocare' for oral or tube feeding (not parenteral use), kosher, gluten- and lactose-free, low-residue, ready to use	1 liter	1500	63	106	1310	na	93.3	na
'Pulmocare' for oral or tube feeding (not parenteral use), kosher, gluten- and lactose-free, low-residue, ready to use	8 fl oz	355	15	25	310	na	22.1	na
RENAL SUPPORT								
(Mead Johnson Nutritionals)								
'Magnacal' for oral or tube feeding, high-calorie, ready to use	1000 ml	2000	75	200	800	na	101.0	na
'Magnacal' for oral or tube feeding, high-calorie, ready to use	8 fl oz	470	18	47	190	na	24.0	na
(Nestlé Clinical Nutrition)								
'Renalcal Diet' for oral or tube feeding, patients w/renal failure, high-calorie, kosher, lactose- and gluten-free, low-residue, ready to use	1000 ml	2000	34	290	na	na	82.4	na
'Renalcal Diet' for oral or tube feeding, patients w/renal failure, high-calorie, kosher, lactose- and gluten-free, low-residue, ready to use	250 ml	500	9	73	na	na	20.6	na
(Ross)								
'Nepro' for oral or tube feeding (not parenteral use), dialzed patients, kosher, gluten- and lactose-free, low-residue, ready to use	1 liter	2000	70	222	842	na	95.6	na
'Nepro' for oral or tube feeding (not parenteral use), dialzed patients, kosher, gluten- and lactose-free, low-residue, ready to use	8 fl oz	475	17	52	200	na	22.7	na

Food Name	Serv. Size	Total Cal.	Prot. gms	Carbs gms	Sod. mgs	Fiber gms	Fat gms	Chol. mgs
'Suplena' for oral or tube feeding (not parenteral use), predialyzed patients, kosher, gluten- and lactose-free, low-residue, ready to use	1 liter	2000	30	255	783	na	95.6	na
'Suplena' for oral or tube feeding (not parenteral use), predialyzed patients, kosher, gluten- and lactose-free, low-residue, ready to use	8 fl oz	475	7	61	186	na	22.7	na
MEDLAR, JAPANESE. See LOQUAT.								
MELBA TOAST. See under CRACKER.								
MELON, CANTALOUPE/muskmelon								
Fresh								
balls	1 cup	62	2	15	16	1	0.5	0
balls	10 balls	48	1	12	12	1	0.4	0
cubed	1 cup	56	1	13	14	1	0.4	0
diced	1 cup	55	1	13	14	1	0.4	0
wedges, 1/8 of large melon	1 wedge	36	1	9	9	1	0.3	0
wedges, 1/8 of medium melon	1 wedge	24	1	6	6	1	0.2	0
wedges, 1/8 of small melon	1 wedge	19	0	5	5	0	0.2	0
whole, large, approx 6 1/2 inch diam	1 melon	285	7	68	73	7	2.3	0
whole, medium, approx 5-inch diam	1 melon	193	5	46	50	4	1.5	0
whole, small, approx 4 1/4 inch diam	1 melon	154	4	37	40	4	1.2	0
Frozen, balls *(Flav-R-Pac)*	3/4 cup	40	1	10	16	0	0.0	0
MELON, CASABA								
cubed	1 cup	44	2	11	20	1	0.2	0
sliced, medium	1/10 melon	43	1	10	20	1	0.2	0
whole, medium	1 melon	426	15	102	197	13	1.6	0
MELON, HONEYDEW								
Fresh								
balls	1 cup	62	1	16	18	1	0.2	0
diced	1 cup	60	1	16	17	1	0.2	0
wedges, 1/8 of 5.25-inch diam melon	1 wedge	44	1	11	13	1	0.1	0
wedges, 1/8 of 6- to 7-inch diam melon	1 wedge	56	1	15	16	1	0.2	0
whole, approx 5.25-inch diam	1 melon	350	5	92	100	6	1.0	0
whole, 6- to 7-inch diam	1 melon	448	6	118	128	8	1.3	0
Frozen								
balls, *(Flav-R-Pac)*	3/4 cup	45	1	11	16	1	0.0	0
balls, unthawed	1 cup	57	1	14	54	1	0.4	0
MENHADEN OIL. See under FISH OIL.								
MENUDO MIX. See under SEASONING MIX.								
MESQUITE SEASONING. See under MARINADE MIX; SEASONING MIX.								
MEXICAN OREGANO. See OREGANO, MEXICAN.								
MEXICAN POTATO. See JICAMA.								
MEXICAN SEASONING. See under SEASONING MIX.								
MEXICAN STYLE DINNER/ENTRÉE. See also individual listings.								
(Amy's Kitchen) tamale pie	1 serving	220	10	41	480	11	3.0	0
(Banquet)								
combination, frozen	12 oz	520	20	72	1980	0	17.0	0
frozen	12 oz	490	18	62	2000	0	18.0	0
(Morton) Mexican style, frozen	10 oz	300	9	44	1390	0	10.0	20
(Patio)								
'Fiesta' frozen	12.25 oz	470	16	55	2040	0	20.0	30
frozen	13.25 oz	540	15	64	1940	0	25.0	45
w/tamale, beef enchilada, beans, rice	1 pkg	508	14	68	1812	8	19.9	26
(Stouffer's) 'Mexi-Mac' frozen, food service product	1 oz	26	1	4	142	1	0.9	3
(Swanson) 'Hungry Man'	1 entrée	690	26	87	2170	13	27.0	35
(Van de Kamp's) frozen	1/2 pkg	220	7	25	640	0	10.0	0

Food Name	Serv. Size	Total Cal.	Prot. gms	Carbs gms	Sod. mgs	Fiber gms	Fat gms	Chol. mgs
MILK								
COW								
Canned								
Low-fat								
(Carnation)	1/2 cup	110	9	12	130	0	3.0	0
Nonfat/skim								
(Carnation)	1/2 cup	100	9	14	147	0	0.3	0
(Diehl)	1/2 cup	100	9	14	150	0	1.0	0
(Finast)	1/2 cup	100	9	14	150	0	1.0	0
(Pathmark)	1/2 cup	100	9	14	15	0	0.0	0
(Pet)	1/2 cup	100	9	14	150	0	1.0	10
Whole								
(Carnation)	1/2 cup	110	9	12	130	0	3.0	0
Condensed								
sweetened, canned	1 cup	982	24	166	389	0	26.6	104
sweetened, canned	1 fl oz	123	3	21	49	0	3.3	13
sweetened, canned (Borden)	1/3 cup	320	7	54	115	0	8.0	0
sweetened, canned (Carnation)	1/3 cup	320	7	56	110	0	8.0	0
sweetened, canned (Eagle)	1/2 cup	320	7	52	120	0	9.0	0
sweetened, canned, 'Jerzee' (Diehl)	1/3 cup	320	7	52	120	0	9.0	0
sweetened, freeze-dried (Crystalac)	1 oz	139	3	22	na	na	3.4	51
Evaporated								
Low-fat								
(Carnation)	1/2 cup	110	8	12	140	0	3.0	10
canned (Pathmark)	1/2 cup	100	9	14	15	0	0.0	0
Nonfat/skim								
	1 cup	199	19	29	294	0	0.5	9
	1/2 cup	100	10	15	147	0	0.3	5
	1 fl oz	25	2	4	37	0	0.1	1
(Carnation)	1/2 cup	100	9	14	150	0	1.0	5
(Pet)	1/2 cup	100	9	14	150	0	1.0	10
Whole								
	1 cup	339	17	25	267	0	19.1	74
	1/2 cup	169	9	13	133	0	9.5	37
	1 fl oz	42	2	3	33	0	2.4	9
(Finast)	1/2 cup	170	8	12	135	0	10.0	0
(IGA)	1/2 cup	170	8	12	140	0	10.0	0
(Pathmark)	1/2 cup	170	8	12	140	0	10.9	0
(Pet)	1/2 cup	170	8	12	140	0	10.0	36
canned (Carnation)	1/2 cup	170	8	12	135	0	10.0	0
canned (Diehl)	1/2 cup	170	8	12	135	0	10.0	0
filled (Pet)	1/2 cup	150	8	12	140	0	8.0	5
imitation, filled (Diehl)	1/2 cup	150	8	12	135	0	8.0	5
vitamin A, canned	1/2 cup	169	9	13	133	0	9.5	37
vitamin A, canned	1 fl oz	42	2	3	33	0	2.4	9
Dry								
Nonfat/skim								
calcium reduced	1 oz	100	10	15	646	0	0.1	1
calcium reduced	1/4 lb	400	40	59	2576	0	0.2	2
extra grade, instant (Saco Foods)	5 tbsp	80	8	12	125	0	1.0	5
instant	1 cup	244	24	35	373	0	0.5	12
instant	1/3 cup	82	8	12	126	0	0.2	4
instant (Carnation)	5 tbsp	80	8	12	125	0	0.2	5
instant, 'Dairy Creamer' (Weight Watchers)	1 pkt	10	1	1	15	0	0.0	0
instant, 'Dairy Fresh' (Sanalac)	0.8 oz	80	8	12	85	0	0.1	5
instant, prepared (Alba)	8 fl oz	80	8	12	190	0	0.0	0
low lactose (Nutra/Balance)	1/4 cup	20	2	3	31	0	0.1	na

Food Name	Serv. Size	Total Cal.	Prot. gms	Carbs gms	Sod. mgs	Fiber gms	Fat gms	Chol. mgs
regular	1 cup	435	43	62	642	0	0.9	24
regular	1/4 cup	109	11	16	161	0	0.2	6
vitamin A	1 cup	435	43	62	642	0	0.9	24
vitamin A	1/4 cup	109	11	16	161	0	0.2	6
Whole								
	1 cup	635	34	49	475	0	34.2	124
	1/4 cup	159	8	12	119	0	8.5	31
Fresh								
Low-fat, 1% fat								
(Crowley)	1 cup	100	8	11	130	0	2.0	10
protein fortified (A&P)	1 cup	100	8	12	120	0	3.0	0
protein fortified (Borden)	1 cup	100	8	11	130	0	2.0	0
protein fortified (Crowley)	1 cup	100	8	11	130	0	2.0	10
protein fortified (Darigold)	1 cup	100	8	13	130	0	2.0	10
protein fortified 'Nice n' Light' (Knudsen)	1 cup	130	10	15	153	0	3.0	0
protein fortified, calcium added (Darigold)	1 cup	100	8	11	130	0	2.0	10
protein fortified, lactose added, 'Lactaid' (Crowley)	1 cup	100	8	11	125	0	2.0	10
vitamin A	1 quart	409	32	47	493	0	10.3	39
vitamin A	1 cup	102	8	12	123	0	2.6	10
vitamin A, protein fortified	1 quart	477	39	54	574	0	11.5	39
vitamin A, protein fortified	1 cup	119	10	14	143	0	2.9	10
vitamin A, school milk carton	1/2 pint	102	8	12	123	0	2.6	10
vitamin A, w/added nonfat milk solids	1 quart	418	34	49	514	0	9.5	39
vitamin A, w/added nonfat milk solids	1 cup	104	9	12	128	0	2.4	10
vitamin A and D enriched (Lucerne)	1 cup	110	9	13	130	0	2.5	15
Low-fat, 2% fat								
(Lucerne) vitamin A and D enriched	1 cup	130	8	13	125	0	5.0	20
protein fortified (A&P)	1 cup	120	8	12	120	0	5.0	0
protein fortified (Crowley)	1 cup	120	8	11	125	0	5.0	15
protein fortified (Darigold)	1 cup	120	8	11	130	0	5.0	18
protein fortified (Finast)	1 cup	130	9	12	130	0	5.0	0
protein fortified (Knudsen)	1 cup	140	10	13	150	0	5.0	0
protein fortified (Viva)	1 cup	120	8	11	125	0	5.0	0
protein fortified, 'Hi-Protein' (Borden)	1 cup	140	10	13	150	0	5.0	0
protein fortified, 'Nutrish Acidophilus' (Darigold)	1 cup	120	8	11	130	0	5.0	18
protein fortified, 'Sweet Acidophilus' (Knudsen)	1 cup	140	10	13	150	0	5.0	0
protein fortified, 'Tone Acidophilus' (Crowley)	1 cup	120	8	11	125	0	5.0	15
vitamin A	1 quart	485	33	47	487	0	18.7	73
vitamin A	1 cup	121	8	12	122	0	4.7	18
vitamin A, protein fortified	1 quart	546	39	54	579	0	19.5	76
vitamin A, protein fortified	1 cup	137	10	14	145	0	4.9	19
vitamin A, school milk carton	1/2 pint	121	8	12	122	0	4.7	18
vitamin A, w/added nonfat milk solids	1 quart	500	34	49	514	0	18.8	74
vitamin A, w/added nonfat milk solids	1 cup	125	9	12	128	0	4.7	18
w/added nonfat milk solids	1 quart	544	39	54	576	0	19.4	75
w/added nonfat milk solids	1 cup	136	10	13	144	0	4.9	19
Nonfat/skim								
	1 quart	343	33	48	510	0	1.8	20
	1 cup	86	8	12	127	0	0.4	5
protein fortified (A&P)	1 cup	90	8	12	125	0	1.0	0
protein fortified (Crowley)	1 cup	90	9	12	130	0	1.0	1
protein fortified (Knudsen)	1 cup	80	9	12	130	0	0.0	0
protein fortified (Weight Watchers)	1 cup	90	9	13	140	0	1.0	0
protein fortified, 'Skim-Line' (Borden)	1 cup	100	10	13	150	0	1.0	0
protein fortified, 'Trim' (Darigold)	1 cup	80	8	11	130	0	1.0	4
vitamin A, nonfat	1 quart	342	33	48	505	0	1.8	18
vitamin A, nonfat	1 cup	86	8	12	126	0	0.4	4

Food Name	Serv. Size	Total Cal.	Prot. gms	Carbs gms	Sod. mgs	Fiber gms	Fat gms	Chol. mgs
vitamin A, protein fortified, nonfat	1 quart	400	39	55	578	0	2.5	20
vitamin A, protein fortified, nonfat	1 cup	100	10	14	144	0	0.6	5
vitamin A, w/added nonfat milk solids	1 quart	361	35	49	519	0	2.5	20
vitamin A, w/added nonfat milk solids	1 cup	90	9	12	130	0	0.6	5
vitamin A and D enriched (Lucerne)	1 cup	90	9	13	130	0	0.0	15
Whole								
(Carnation)	1 cup	150	8	12	120	0	8.0	33
low-salt	1 quart	594	30	44	24	0	33.8	133
low-salt	1 cup	149	8	11	6	0	8.4	33
low-sodium (A&P)	1 cup	150	8	11	120	0	8.0	0
low-sodium (Borden)	1 cup	150	8	11	130	0	8.0	0
low-sodium (Crowley)	1 cup	150	8	11	125	0	8.0	30
low-sodium (Darigold)	1 cup	150	8	11	125	0	8.0	33
low-sodium (Knudsen)	1 cup	160	9	12	180	0	8.0	0
low-sodium, 'Hi-Calcium' (Borden)	1 cup	150	8	11	130	0	8.0	0
3.7% fat	1 quart	626	32	45	476	0	35.7	140
3.7% fat	1 cup	157	8	11	119	0	8.9	35
3.25% fat	1 quart	600	32	45	478	0	32.6	133
3.25% fat	1 cup	150	8	11	120	0	8.2	33
3.25% fat	1 tbsp	9	1	1	7	0	0.5	2
3.25% fat, school milk carton	1/2 pint	150	8	11	120	0	8.2	33
vitamin A and D enriched (Lucerne)	1 cup	150	8	12	125	0	8.0	34
vitamin D, homogenized (Borden)	1 cup	150	8	11	130	0	8.0	0
vitamin D, homogenized (Trader Joe's)	1 cup	150	8	11	115	0	8.0	35
GOAT								
Evaporated, canned, undiluted (Meyenberg)	4 fl oz	143	8	10	86	0	7.9	0
Fresh								
	1 quart	672	35	43	486	0	40.4	111
	1 cup	168	9	11	122	0	10.1	28
	1 fl oz	21	1	1	15	0	1.3	3
HUMAN								
	1 cup	171	3	17	42	0	10.8	34
	1 fl oz	21	0	2	5	0	1.3	4
INDIAN BUFFALO								
	1 quart	943	37	51	509	0	67.2	185
	1 cup	236	9	13	127	0	16.8	46
SHEEP								
	1 quart	1057	59	53	432	0	68.6	265
	1 cup	264	15	13	108	0	17.1	66
MILK SUBSTITUTE. See also RICE BEVERAGE; SOYMILK.								
w/lauric acid oil, fluid	1 quart	600	17	60	764	0	33.3	2
w/lauric acid oil, fluid	1 cup	150	4	15	191	0	8.3	0
w/hydrogenated vegetable oils, fluid	1 quart	600	17	60	764	0	33.3	2
w/hydrogenated vegetable oils, fluid	1 cup	150	4	15	191	0	8.3	0
w/hydrogenated vegetable oils, fluid	1 fl oz	19	1	2	24	0	1.0	0
(First Alternative) 1%, lactose-free	1 cup	80	8	6	180	0	2.0	0
(Ener-G Foods) lactose-free	3 tbsp	85	10	7	4	5	1.6	0
MILKFISH. See AWA.								
MILKSHAKE								
(Killer Shake)								
banana, 'Bodacious Bananaberry'	1 carton	420	12	62	250	5	14.0	55
chocolate, 'Totally Chocolate'	1 carton	470	14	65	320	6	17.0	60
(MicroMagic)								
chocolate, frozen	11.5 fl oz	340	5	55	120	0	8.0	40
strawberry, frozen	11.5 fl oz	340	5	54	120	0	9.0	40
vanilla, frozen	11.5 fl oz	380	8	60	150	0	13.0	45

Food Name	Serv. Size	Total Cal.	Prot. gms	Carbs gms	Sod. mgs	Fiber gms	Fat gms	Chol. mgs
MILKSHAKE MIX, CHOCOLATE								
chocolate fudge *(Weight Watchers)*	1 pkt	70	6	11	170	0	1.0	0
orange sherbet *(Weight Watchers)*	1 pkt	70	6	11	210	0	0.0	0
MILLET								
pearl, cooked	1/2 cup	143	4.2	28.4	2	1.6	1.2	0
pearl, cooked	4 oz	135	4.0	26.8	2	1.5	1.1	0
pearl, raw	1/2 cup	378	11.0	72.9	5	8.5	4.2	0
pearl, raw	1 oz	107	3.1	20.7	1	2.4	1.2	0
pearl, raw, hulled *(Arrowhead Mills)*	1 oz	90	3.0	21.0	1	1.8	1.0	0
Proso/hog millet, whole grain	3 1/2 oz	327	9.9	72.9	1	>3.2 c	2.9	0
MINCEMEAT. See under PIE FILLING.								
MISO								
	1 cup	567	32	77	10029	15	16.7	0
barley, mugi, organic *(Eden Foods)*	1 tbsp	25	2	3	760	1	1.0	0
barley, pasteurized *(Westbrae)*	1 tsp	12	1	2	310	0	0.0	0
brown rice, genmai, organic *(Eden Foods)*	1 tbsp	25	2	3	810	1	1.0	0
brown rice, pasteurized *(Westbrae)*	1 tsp	10	1	2	360	0	0.0	0
hacho *(Westbrae)*	1 tsp	14	1	1	240	0	0.0	0
hacho, organic *(Eden Foods)*	1 tbsp	35	3	2	600	1	1.5	0
red, instant *(Westbrae)*	.35 oz	35	3	3	750	0	1.0	0
red, pasteurized *(Westbrae)*	1 tsp	10	1	1	375	0	0.0	0
rice, kome, organic *(Eden Foods)*	1 tbsp	25	2	3	850	1	1.0	0
rice, sweet white shiro, organic *(Eden Foods)*	1 tbsp	35	2	5	410	1	1.0	0
soy and rice, red, kome, organic *(Eden Foods)*	1 tbsp	25	2	3	850	0	1.0	0
soy, hacho, organic *(Eden Foods)*	1 tbsp	35	3	2	600	0	2.0	0
soy, pasteurized *(Westbrae)*	1 tsp	12	1	1	265	0	0.0	0
white, instant *(Westbrae)*	.35 oz	35	2	4	740	0	1.0	0
MOLASSES								
	1 cup	872	0	226	121	0	0.3	0
	1 tbsp	53	0	14	7	0	0.0	0
bead *(LaChoy)*	1/2 tsp	7	1	2	1	0	1.0	0
blackstrap	1 cup	771	0	199	180	0	0.0	0
blackstrap	1 tbsp	47	0	12	11	0	0.0	0
dark *(Br'er Rabbit)*	1 oz	110	0	28	20	0	0.0	0
gold *(Grandma's)*	1 tbsp	70	0	17	28	0	0.0	0
gold, mild flavor *(Grandma's)*	1 tbsp	70	0	17	28	0	0.0	0
green, robust flavor *(Grandma's)*	1 tbsp	70	0	16	57	0	0.0	0
light *(Br'er Rabbit)*	1 oz	110	0	29	15	0	0.0	0
MOMBIN, YELLOW. See JOBO.								
MONKFISH/angler fish/bellyfish/frogfish/goosefish/lotte/sea devil								
baked, broiled, grilled, or microwaved	3 oz	82	16	0	20	0	1.7	27
raw	3 oz	65	12	0	15	0	1.3	21
MONOSODIUM GLUTAMATE								
flavor enhancer, 'MSG' *(Accent)*	0.13 tsp	0	0	0	80	0	0.0	0
flavor enhancer, 'MSG' *(Tone's)*	1 tsp	0	0	0	638	0	0.0	0
MOOSE								
raw	1 oz	29	6	0	18	0	0.2	17
roasted	3 oz	114	25	0	59	0	0.8	66
roasted, boneless, yield from 1 lb raw	11.9 oz	456	100	0	235	0	3.3	265
MOSTACCIOLI. See under PASTA.								
MOSTACCIOLI DISH/ENTRÉE. See under PASTA DISH/ENTRÉE.								
MOTH BEAN. See BEAN, MOTH.								
MOUNTAIN YAM. See under YAM.								
MOUSSE								
(Estee) orange chocolate	1/2 cup	70	3	9	50	0	3.0	0
(Weight Watchers)								
chocolate	1 serving	190	6	31	150	3	5.0	5
pecan praline	1 serving	170	4	31	140	0	3.5	0

Food Name	Serv. Size	Total Cal.	Prot. gms	Carbs gms	Sod. mgs	Fiber gms	Fat gms	Chol. mgs
triple chocolate caramel .... 1 serving	1 serving	200	5	34	120	2	4.0	5
MOUSSE BAR chocolate *(Weight Watchers)* .... 1 bar	1 bar	35	2	9	40	2	0.5	3
MOUSSE MIX								
(Alsa) dark chocolate .... 2.5 tbsp	2.5 tbsp	105	2	13	83	na	5.1	na
(Jell-O)								
chocolate, 'Rich & Luscious' mix only .... 1 pkg	1 pkg	110	3	18	45	0	3.0	0
chocolate, 'Rich & Luscious' prepared w/whole milk .... 1/2 cup	1/2 cup	150	5	21	75	0	6.0	10
chocolate fudge, 'Rich & Luscious' prepared w/whole milk .... 1/2 cup	1/2 cup	140	5	20	75	0	6.0	10
chocolate fudge 'Rich & Luscious' mix only .... 1 pkg	1 pkg	110	3	18	45	0	4.0	0
(Sans Sucre de Paris)								
cheesecake, w/NutraSweet, mix only .... 1/2 cup	1/2 cup	60	4	7	80	0	1.5	5
cheesecake, w/NutraSweet, prepared w/skim milk ..... 1/2 cup	1/2 cup	73	5	10	105	0	1.5	5
chocolate, w/NutraSweet, mix only .... 1/2 cup	1/2 cup	55	1	6	25	0	3.0	0
chocolate, w/NutraSweet, prepared w/skim milk .... 1/2 cup	1/2 cup	75	2	8	45	0	3.0	0
chocolate cheesecake, w/NutraSweet, prepared w/skim milk .... 1/2 cup	1/2 cup	75	5	10	105	0	1.5	5
chocolate cheesecake, w/NutraSweet, mix only .... 1/2 cup	1/2 cup	60	4	7	80	0	1.5	5
key lime, w/NutraSweet, mix only .... 4 oz	4 oz	60	1	6	40	0	4.0	0
key lime w/NutraSweet, prepared w/skim milk .... 4 oz	4 oz	75	1	6	40	0	4.0	0
lemon, w/NutraSweet, mix only .... 1/2 cup	1/2 cup	50	1	7	25	0	2.0	0
lemon, w/NutraSweet, prepared w/skim milk .... 1/2 cup	1/2 cup	70	2	9	45	0	2.0	0
strawberry, w/NutraSweet, mix .... 1/2 cup	1/2 cup	50	1	7	25	0	2.0	0
strawberry, w/NutraSweet, prepared w/skim milk ...... 1/2 cup	1/2 cup	70	2	9	45	0	2.0	0
(Weight Watchers)								
chocolate, prepared w/nonfat milk .... 1/2 cup	1/2 cup	60	3	9	45	0	3.0	0
chocolate cheesecake, prepared w/nonfat milk .... 1/2 cup	1/2 cup	60	4	12	75	0	2.0	0
chocolate raspberry, prepared w/nonfat milk .... 1/2 cup	1/2 cup	60	3	12	75	0	3.0	0
white chocolate, almond, prepared w/nonfat milk ...... 1/2 cup	1/2 cup	60	3	6	50	0	3.0	0
MUFFIN. See also ENGLISH MUFFIN; MUFFIN MIX.								
APPLE								
(Awrey's)								
1.5 oz .... 1 muffin	1 muffin	130	2	17	210	0	6.0	20
streusel, 4.2 oz, 'Grande' .... 1 muffin	1 muffin	340	6	50	540	1	13.0	35
2.5 oz .... 1 muffin	1 muffin	220	3	30	350	1	10.0	35
(Muffin-A-Day) bran, 'Total Health Muffin' .... 1 muffin	1 muffin	120	7	31	140	9	0.0	0
APPLE BANANA NUT								
(Awrey's) 4.2 oz, 'Grande' .... 1 muffin	1 muffin	260	3	27	160	1	16.0	40
(Hostess) w/walnuts, mini .... 5 muffins	5 muffins	160	2	17	90	0	9.0	0
APPLE SPICE								
(Health Valley) nonfat .... 1 muffin	1 muffin	130	4	30	110	5	0.0	0
(Healthy Choice) frozen, 2.5 oz .... 1 muffin	1 muffin	190	3	40	90	0	4.0	0
(Sara Lee) frozen, 2.5 oz .... 1 muffin	1 muffin	220	4	36	280	0	8.0	0
(Weight Watchers) 'Microwave' 2.5 oz .... 1 muffin	1 muffin	160	3	29	260	0	5.0	0
BANANA								
(Health Valley) nonfat .... 1 muffin	1 muffin	130	4	29	110	5	0.0	0
(Hostess) bran, low-fat .... 1 serving	1 serving	240	4	47	270	2	3.0	0
BANANA NUT								
(Break Cake) 5 oz .... 1 muffin	1 muffin	60	1	7	45	0	3.0	10
(Healthy Choice) frozen, 2.5 oz .... 1 muffin	1 muffin	180	3	32	80	0	6.0	0
(Weight Watchers) .... 1 muffin	1 muffin	180	3	34	260	5	4.0	15
BLUEBERRY								
(Awrey's)								
4.2 oz, 'Grande' .... 1 muffin	1 muffin	360	5	52	480	2	14.0	35
1.5 oz .... 1 muffin	1 muffin	130	2	18	180	1	5.0	10
(Break Cake) 5 oz .... 1 muffin	1 muffin	60	1	8	50	0	3.0	10
(Ener-G Foods) gluten-free .... 1 muffin	1 muffin	51	1	8	54	0	1.9	15

Food Name	Serv. Size	Total Cal.	Prot. gms	Carbs gms	Sod. mgs	Fiber gms	Fat gms	Chol. mgs
(Entenmann's)								
....	1 muffin	200	3	29	250	0	8.0	0
nonfat, no cholesterol	1 muffin	120	2	26	220	1	0.0	0
(Healthy Choice) frozen, 2.5 oz	1 muffin	190	3	39	110	0	4.0	0
(Hostess)								
low-fat	1 serving	230	4	47	350	1	2.5	0
mini, 'Breakfast Bake Shop'	5 muffins	240	3	29	180	1	13.0	40
(Muffin-A-Day) bran, 'Total Health Muffin'	1 muffin	120	7	31	140	9	0.0	0
(Natural Ovens) low-fat	1 muffin	160	4	32	190	2	1.0	0
(Pepperidge Farm) frozen, 'Old Fashioned'	1 muffin	170	2	27	250	1	7.0	25
(Sara Lee)								
frozen, 'Free & Light'	1 muffin	120	3	28	140	0	0.0	0
frozen, 2.5 oz	1 muffin	200	3	34	290	0	8.0	0
(Weight Watchers)	1 muffin	180	3	33	270	2	4.0	15
BLUEBERRY APPLE *(Health Valley)* twin pack	1 muffin	140	4	32	100	5	0.0	0
BRAN								
(Awrey's)								
w/raisins, 1.5 oz	1 muffin	110	2	18	170	1	4.0	15
w/raisins, 2.5 oz	1 muffin	190	3	30	280	2	7.0	20
w/raisins, 4.2 oz, 'Grande'	1 muffin	320	5	50	470	3	12.0	35
(Pepperidge Farm) w/raisins, cholesterol-free,								
frozen, 'Old Fashioned'	1 muffin	170	4	30	280	3	6.0	0
(Sara Lee) w/raisins, 2.5 oz, frozen	1 muffin	220	4	37	400	0	7.0	0
(Weight Watchers) 'Harvest Honey'	1 muffin	220	3	42	180	5	4.5	5
BUTTERMILK *(Ener-G Foods)* gluten-free	1 muffin	195	4	30	425	4	6.9	14
CARROT								
(Health Valley) nonfat, twin pack	1 muffin	130	4	30	110	5	0.0	0
(Muffin-A-Day) 'Total Health Muffin'	1 muffin	120	7	31	140	9	0.0	0
(Natural Ovens) low-fat	1 muffin	150	4	30	200	2	2.0	0
CHEESE *(Sara Lee)* streusel, 2.1 oz	1 muffin	220	4	27	170	0	11.0	0
CHOCOLATE CHIP								
(Sara Lee) chocolate chunk, frozen, 2.1 oz	1 muffin	220	3	33	210	0	8.0	0
(Weight Watchers)	1 muffin	200	4	39	250	1	4.0	5
CINNAMON *(Pepperidge Farm)* swirl, frozen,								
'Old Fashioned'	1 muffin	190	2	30	170	1	6.0	35
CORN								
(Awrey's) 1.5 oz	1 muffin	130	2	20	270	0	5.0	15
(Pepperidge Farm) frozen, 'Old Fashioned'	1 muffin	180	3	27	260	2	7.0	30
(Sara Lee) golden, frozen, 2.5 oz	1 muffin	250	4	31	310	0	13.0	0
CRANBERRY								
(Awrey's) 1.5 oz	1 muffin	120	2	20	210	0	4.0	10
(Natural Ovens) low-fat	1 muffin	140	4	26	200	2	2.0	0
OAT BRAN								
(Awrey's)								
2.75 oz	1 muffin	180	5	27	330	2	7.0	0
w/pineapple and raisins, 2.75 oz	1 muffin	180	5	26	320	2	6.0	0
(Health Valley)								
w/almonds and dates	1 muffin	180	4	31	81	8	4.0	0
w/blueberries	1 muffin	180	4	32	99	8	4.0	0
w/raisins	1 muffin	180	4	31	90	8	5.0	0
(Hostess)								
'Breakfast Bake Shop'	1 muffin	160	2	21	150	2	7.0	0
'Snack Cake'	1 serving	160	2	21	150	1	8.0	0
w/banana and nuts, 'Breakfast Bake Shop'	1 muffin	140	2	20	160	1	5.0	0
(Pepperidge Farm) w/apple, cholesterol-free, frozen,								
'Old Fashioned'	1 muffin	190	3	29	200	2	7.0	0

Food Name	Serv. Size	Total Cal.	Prot. gms	Carbs gms	Sod. mgs	Fiber gms	Fat gms	Chol. mgs
(Sara Lee)								
2.5 oz	1 muffin	210	4	35	320	0	8.0	0
w/apple, 2.5 oz	1 muffin	210	4	35	320	0	8.0	0
RAISIN								
(Awrey's)								
bran, 1.5 oz	1 muffin	110	2	18	170	1	4.0	15
bran, 4.2 oz, 'Grande'	1 muffin	320	5	50	470	3	12.0	35
(Health Valley) spice	1 muffin	140	4	32	100	5	0.0	0
(Pepperidge Farm) bran, cholesterol-free, frozen,								
'Old Fashioned	1 muffin	170	4	30	280	3	6.0	0
(Sara Lee) bran, 2.5 oz	1 muffin	220	4	37	400	0	7.0	0
(Wonder) 'Raisin Rounds'	1 muffin	140	4	27	280	1	2.0	0
RASPBERRY *(Health Valley)* nonfat, twin pack	1 muffin	130	4	30	110	5	0.0	0
RICE BRAN								
(Ener-G Foods) gluten-free	1 serving	257	6	32	605	9	11.8	22
(Health Valley) w/raisins	1 muffin	215	5	35	124	6	7.0	0
SOURDOUGH *(Wonder)*	1 muffin	130	4	27	250	1	1.0	0
MUFFIN MIX								
(Gluten-Free Pantry) gluten-free	1 serving	100	1	24	120	0	0.0	0
ALMOND								
(Krusteaz) w/poppyseeds, prepared	1 muffin	167	2	30	242	na	4.0	0
APPLE								
(Betty Crocker)								
cinnamon, prepared w/egg, 2% milk	1/12 pkg	120	2	18	140	0	4.0	25
cinnamon, prepared w/egg white, nonfat milk	1/12 pkg	110	2	18	140	0	3.0	0
streusel, Dutch, prepared w/egg, whole milk	1/12 pkg	200	3	32	240	0	7.0	0
(General Mills)								
and cinnamon, prepared	1 muffin	100	1	17	130	0	3.0	0
and cinnamon, prepared w/egg white, nonfat milk	1 muffin	110	2	18	140	0	3.0	0
and cinnamon, prepared w/2% milk, 1 egg	1 muffin	120	2	18	140	0	4.0	25
(Krusteaz) and cinnamon, prepared	1 muffin	180	3	36	340	0	3.0	4
(Martha White) and cinnamon, prepared w/2% milk	1 muffin	140	2	25	250	0	3.0	2
APPLESAUCE								
(Gold Medal) prepared w/egg, whole milk	1/6 pkg	160	3	26	240	0	5.0	0
(Robin Hood) prepared w/egg, whole milk	1/6 pkg	160	3	26	240	0	5.0	0
BANANA								
(Gold Medal) prepared w/egg, whole milk	1/12 pkg	150	3	24	240	0	5.0	0
(Robin Hood) prepared w/egg, whole milk	1/12 pkg	150	3	24	240	0	5.0	0
BANANA NUT								
(Betty Crocker)								
prepared w/egg, 2% milk	1/12 pkg	120	2	17	140	0	5.0	25
prepared w/egg white, nonfat milk	1/12 pkg	110	2	17	140	0	4.0	0
(General Mills)								
prepared	1 muffin	110	1	17	140	0	4.0	0
prepared w/egg white, nonfat milk	1 muffin	120	2	18	150	0	4.0	0
prepared w/2% milk, 1 egg	1 muffin	120	2	18	150	0	4.0	20
(Martha White) prepared w/2% milk	1 muffin	180	3	23	240	0	8.0	35
BERRY								
(General Mills)								
wild, prepared	1 muffin	100	1	18	140	0	3.0	0
wild, 'Light' prepared	1 muffin	90	1	20	140	0	1.0	0
wild, 'Light' prepared w/1 egg	1 muffin	90	2	20	140	0	1.0	20
wild, prepared w/2% milk, 1 egg	1 muffin	120	2	19	150	0	4.0	20
wild, prepared w/egg white, skim milk	1 muffin	110	2	19	150	0	3.0	0
BLACKBERRY *(Martha White)* prepared	1 muffin	140	2	25	250	0	3.0	2
BLUEBERRY								
(Betty Crocker)								
streusel 'Bake Shop' prepared	1/12 pkg	210	3	31	230	0	8.0	0

Food Name	Serv. Size	Total Cal.	Prot. gms	Carbs gms	Sod. mgs	Fiber gms	Fat gms	Chol. mgs
wild, mix only	1 serving	128	2	26	186	na	1.8	na
wild, prepared w/egg, 2% milk	1/12 pkg	120	2	18	150	0	4.0	25
wild, prepared w/egg white, skim milk	1/12 pkg	110	2	18	150	0	3.0	0
(Duncan Hines)								
bakery style, mix only	1 muffin	180	2	32	245	0	5.0	0
bakery style, prepared	1 muffin	190	2	32	250	0	6.0	0
regular style, mix only	1 muffin	110	2	21	180	0	2.0	0
regular style, prepared	1 muffin	120	2	21	185	0	3.0	0
(General Mills)								
prepared w/egg white, nonfat milk	1 muffin	110	2	18	140	0	3.0	0
prepared w/2% milk, 1 egg	1 muffin	120	2	18	140	0	4.0	20
'Twice the Blueberries' prepared	1 muffin	100	1	17	130	0	3.0	0
'Twice the Blueberries' prepared, cholesterol-free								
recipe	1 muffin	110	2	18	140	0	3.0	0
'Twice the Blueberries' prepared w/2% milk, 1 egg	1 muffin	120	2	18	140	0	4.0	20
(Gold Medal) imitation, mix only	1 serving	127	1	24	205	na	2.7	na
(Krusteaz) prepared	1 muffin	150	3	27	260	1	4.0	27
(Lovin' Lites)								
prepared w/water, 1 egg	1/12 pkg	100	2	21	160	0	1.0	20
prepared w/water, 2 egg whites	1/12 pkg	100	3	21	160	0	1.0	0
(Martha White)								
artificial flavor	1 serving	162	2	30	343	na	3.5	na
prepared	1/6 pkg	140	2	25	260	0	3.0	3
prepared w/2% milk	1 muffin	140	2	25	260	0	3.0	2
(Robin Hood) 'Pouch Mix' prepared w/egg, whole milk	1/6 pkg	170	3	26	240	0	6.0	0
BRAN								
(Duncan Hines) and honey, bakery style, prepared	1 muffin	200	2	32	220	0	7.0	0
(Gold Medal) w/honey, prepared w/egg, whole milk	1/6 pkg	170	5	25	240	0	6.0	0
(Hodgson Mill) stone ground, whole grain	1/4 cup	130	4	27	150	3	1.0	0
(Krusteaz) w/honey, prepared	1 muffin	140	3	23	290	3	4.0	0
(Martha White) prepared w/2% milk	1 muffin	150	3	24	330	0	5.0	35
(Robin Hood) w/honey, prepared w/egg, whole milk	1/6 pkg	170	5	25	240	0	6.0	0
CARAMEL								
(Gold Medal) 'Pouch Mix' prepared w/egg, whole milk	1/6 pkg	150	3	23	250	0	5.0	0
(Robin Hood) 'Pouch Mix', prepared w/egg, whole milk	1/6 pkg	150	3	23	250	0	5.0	0
CARROT NUT								
(Betty Crocker)								
prepared w/egg, 2% milk	1/12 pkg	150	3	22	160	0	5.0	25
prepared w/egg white, nonfat milk	1/12 pkg	150	3	22	160	0	5.0	0
CHOCOLATE CHIP								
(Betty Crocker)								
prepared	1/12 pkg	140	2	22	180	0	5.0	0
prepared w/egg, 2% milk	1/12 pkg	150	2	22	180	0	6.0	20
(Krusteaz)								
chocolate, prepared	1 muffin	200	3	36	340	0	5.0	11
CINNAMON								
(Betty Crocker) streusel, prepared w/egg, 2% milk	1/12 pkg	200	3	27	240	0	9.0	30
(Duncan Hines)								
swirl, bakery style, mix only	1 muffin	190	2	32	240	0	6.0	0
swirl, bakery style, prepared	1 muffin	200	2	32	245	0	7.0	0
(General Mills)								
'Streusel' prepared	1 muffin	190	2	27	220	0	8.0	0
'Streusel' prepared w/2% milk, 1 egg	1 muffin	200	3	27	240	0	9.0	25
CORN								
(Arrowhead Mills) blue, prepared	1 muffin	110	4	15	0	3	4.0	0

Food Name	Serv. Size	Total Cal.	Prot. gms	Carbs gms	Sod. mgs	Fiber gms	Fat gms	Chol. mgs
(Dromedary)								
mix only	3 1/2 tbsp	110	1	20	250	0	3.0	0
prepared	1 muffin	120	3	20	270	0	4.0	0
(Flako)								
mix only	1/3 cup	160	3	29	380	1	4.0	0
prepared	1 muffin	116	2	20	351	1	3.3	0
(Gold Medal) prepared w/egg, whole milk	1/6 pkg	130	3	24	250	0	2.0	0
(Krusteaz) prepared, 1.48 oz	1 muffin	220	4	36	450	0	7.0	5
(Martha White) yellow, prepared w/water	1 muffin	160	2	30	230	0	3.0	1
(Robin Hood) prepared w/egg, whole milk	1/6 pkg	130	3	24	250	0	2.0	0
CRANBERRY ORANGE NUT								
(Duncan Hines) bakery style, prepared	1 muffin	200	2	30	215	0	8.0	0
LEMON								
(Martha White) and poppy seed, prepared w/2% milk	1 muffin	200	2	30	260	0	9.0	35
OAT								
(Gold Medal) prepared w/egg & 2% milk	1/6 pkg	150	4	23	220	0	5.0	45
(Robin Hood) prepared w/egg & 2% milk	1/6 pkg	150	4	23	220	0	5.0	45
OAT BRAN								
(Arrowhead Mills)								
w/apple and spice, prepared	1 muffin	120	6	15	0	5	4.0	0
wheat-free, prepared	1 muffin	100	5	11	0	5	5.0	0
(Betty Crocker)								
prepared w/egg, 2% milk	1/8 pkg	190	4	25	240	0	8.0	35
prepared w/egg white, nonfat milk	1/8 pkg	180	4	25	240	0	7.0	0
w/oatmeal and raisins, prepared w/egg, 2% milk	1/12 pkg	140	3	22	125	0	4.0	25
(General Mills) prepared	1 muffin	170	3	26	230	0	6.0	0
prepared w/nonfat milk, egg white	1 muffin	170	4	26	260	0	6.0	0
prepared w/2% milk, 1 egg	1 muffin	180	4	26	250	0	7.0	35
(Hain)								
w/apple and cinnamon, prepared	1 muffin	140	4	28	200	5	3.0	0
w/banana and nuts, prepared	1 muffin	140	4	26	190	4	4.0	0
w/raspberry and spice, prepared	1 muffin	140	5	27	190	4	3.0	0
(Krusteaz) prepared	1 muffin	190	3	33	310	4	5.0	0
OATMEAL								
(Betty Crocker)								
and raisin, prepared w/egg white, nonfat milk	1/12 pkg	130	3	22	125	0	3.0	0
ORANGE								
(Martha White) and berry, prepared w/2% milk	1 muffin	140	2	25	220	0	3.0	2
PECAN								
(Duncan Hines) crunch, bakery style, prepared	1 muffin	220	3	27	250	0	11.0	0
RASPBERRY								
(Martha White) raspberry, prepared w/2% milk	1 muffin	140	2	25	180	0	3.0	2
STRAWBERRY								
(Arrowhead Mills) wheat bran, prepared	2 muffins	270	10	43	0	11	7.0	0
(Betty Crocker)								
crown, prepared w/egg, 2% milk	1/10 pkg	150	2	24	170	0	5.0	25
crown, prepared w/egg white, nonfat milk	1/10 pkg	140	2	24	170	0	4.0	0
(Martha White)								
prepared	1/6 pkg	140	2	25	270	0	3.0	3
prepared w/2% milk	1 muffin	140	2	25	270	0	3.0	2
WHOLE WHEAT								
(Hodgson Mill) stone ground, whole grain	1/4 cup	130	4	27	560	3	1.0	0
MULBERRY								
fresh, raw	1 cup	60	2	14	14	2	0.5	0
fresh, raw	10 medium	6	0	1	2	0	0.1	0
MULLET, STRIPED								
baked, broiled, grilled, or microwaved	4 oz	170	28.1	0.0	81	0	5.5	71

Food Name	Serv. Size	Total Cal.	Prot. gms	Carbs gms	Sod. mgs	Fiber gms	Fat gms	Chol. mgs
raw	1 lb	530	87.8	0.0	294	0	17.2	224
raw	3 oz	99	16.5	0.0	55	0	3.2	42

MUNG BEAN. See BEAN, MUNG.
MUNGO BEAN. See BEAN, MUNGO.
MUSHROOM, BUTTON. See MUSHROOM, WHITE.

Food Name	Serv. Size	Total Cal.	Prot. gms	Carbs gms	Sod. mgs	Fiber gms	Fat gms	Chol. mgs
MUSHROOM, CRIMINI, brown, Italian, fresh, raw	1 piece	3	0	1	1	0	0.0	0
MUSHROOM, ENOKI								
Fresh								
raw, whole	1 large	2	0	0	0	0	0.0	0
raw, whole	1 medium	1	0	0	0	0	0.0	0
MUSHROOM, JAPANESE HONEY/hon shimeji								
Fresh								
(Frieda of California) trimmed	1 oz	9	1	1	0	0	0.1	0
MUSHROOM, OYSTER/abalone/hiritake/shimeji/tree mushroom								
Fresh								
raw (Frieda of California)	1 oz	7	1	1	1	0	0.1	0
raw, whole	1 large	55	6	9	46	4	0.8	0
raw, whole	1 small	6	1	1	5	0	0.1	0
MUSHROOM, SHIITAKE								
Dried								
whole	4 medium	44	1	11	2	2	0.1	0
whole	1 medium	11	0	3	0	0	0.0	0
Fresh								
cooked, pieces	1 cup	80	2	21	6	3	0.3	0
cooked, whole	4 medium	40	1	10	3	2	0.2	0
MUSHROOM, STRAW								
Canned								
in salt water, imported (Orchids)	11 med pieces	16	2	2	231	2	0.0	0
Oriental (Green Giant)	2 oz	12	1	2	290	1	0.0	0
pieces, drained	1 cup	58	7	8	699	5	1.2	0
pieces, drained	1 med piece	2	0	0	21	0	0.0	0
whole (Green Giant)	1/4 cup	12	1	2	290	1	0.0	0
MUSHROOM, TREE. See MUSHROOM, OYSTER.								
MUSHROOM, WHITE								
Canned								
(B in B)	1/4 cup	12	1	2	240	1	0.0	0
caps, drained	8 caps	11	1	2	200	1	0.1	0
pieces, drained	1 cup	37	3	8	663	4	0.5	0
pieces, drained	1/2 cup	19	1	4	332	2	0.2	0
pieces and stems (Allens)	1/2 cup	20	2	3	450	0	1.0	0
pieces and stems, broiled in butter, 'BinB'								
(Green Giant)	1/2 cup	30	3	4	460	2	0.0	0
sliced (Green Giant)	1/2 cup	30	3	4	440	2	0.0	0
sliced, broiled in butter, 'BinB' (Green Giant)	1/2 cup	30	3	4	460	2	0.0	0
slices, drained	10 slices	10	1	2	170	1	0.1	0
stems and pieces (Brandywine)	1/2 cup	20	2	3	400	1	0.0	0
w/garlic (B in B)	1/4 cup	12	1	2	200	1	0.0	0
whole, broiled in butter, 'BinB' (Green Giant)	1 can	30	3	4	460	2	0.0	0
whole, drained, medium	1 mushroom	3	0	1	51	0	0.0	0
whole, pieces, and stems (Green Giant)	1/4 cup	12	1	2	220	1	0.0	0
Fresh								
boiled, drained, chopped	1 tbsp	3	0	1	0	0	0.0	0
boiled drained, sliced	1 cup	42	3	8	3	3	0.7	0
boiled, drained, sliced	1/2 cup	21	2	4	2	2	0.4	0
boiled, drained, whole, medium	1 mushroom	3	0	1	0	0	0.1	0
raw, pieces or slices	1 cup	18	2	3	3	1	0.2	0
raw, sliced	1/2 cup	9	1	1	1	0	0.1	0

Food Name	Serv. Size	Total Cal.	Prot. gms	Carbs gms	Sod. mgs	Fiber gms	Fat gms	Chol. mgs
raw, whole	1 cup	24	3	4	4	1	0.3	0
raw, whole, medium	1 mushroom	5	1	1	1	0	0.1	0
Frozen								
(Freshlike)	3.5 oz	30	3	4	15	0	0.0	0
(Veg-All)	3.5 oz	30	3	4	15	0	0.0	0
whole, 'Deluxe' (Birds Eye)	2.6 oz	20	2	4	0	2	0.0	0
MUSHROOM DISH/ENTRÉE								
(Empire Kosher) breaded, frozen	7 mushrooms	90	4	16	390	1	1.0	0
(Gardenburger) patty, savory, vegetarian, 'Gourmet'	2.5 oz	120	6	18	270	4	3.0	9
(Green Giant) creamy, 'Right for Lunch'	9.5 oz	220	6	29	860	4	11.0	25
(Stilwell)								
battered, 'Quick Krisp'	5 pieces	90	3	13	190	2	2.5	0
breaded	6 pieces	90	4	17	250	1	0.0	0
MUSKMELON. See MELON, CANTALOUPE.								
MUSKRAT								
raw	1 oz	46	6	0	23	0	2.3	na
roasted	3 oz	199	26	0	81	0	10.0	103
roasted, boneless, yield from 1 lb raw	11 oz	732	94	0	297	0	36.7	379
MUSSEL, BLUE								
boiled, poached, or steamed	3 oz	146	20	6	314	0	3.8	48
raw	1 cup	129	18	6	429	0	3.4	42
raw	3 oz	73	10	3	243	0	1.9	24
raw, large	1 mussel	17	2	1	57	0	0.4	6
raw, medium	1 mussel	14	2	1	46	0	0.4	4
raw, small	1 mussel	9	1	0	29	0	0.2	3
raw, w/o shell	1 oz	24	3	1	81	0	0.6	8
MUSTARD, DRY								
(Spice Islands)	1 tsp	9	1	0	1	0	0.6	0
ground (Durkee)	1 tsp	19	0	0	0	0	0.1	0
ground (Eden Foods)	1 tsp	0	0	1	65	0	0.0	0
ground (Laurel Leaf)	1 tsp	19	0	0	0	0	0.1	0
MUSTARD, PREPARED								
yellow	1 cup	165	10	19	2800	8	7.8	0
yellow	1 tsp	3	0	0	56	0	0.2	0
(Dietsource) lower calorie, low sodium	1 serving	15	0	1	na	na	1.0	na
(Featherweight)	1 tsp	5	0	0	0	0	0.0	0
(French's)								
'Bold'n Spicy'	1 tsp	5	0	0	80	0	0.0	0
Dijon	1 tsp	10	0	0	115	0	0.5	0
horseradish	1 tsp	0	0	0	85	0	0.0	0
Medford	1 tbsp	16	1	1	240	0	1.0	0
w/onion	1 tsp	8	0	2	70	0	0.0	0
yellow	1 tsp	0	0	0	55	0	0.0	0
(Great Impressions) jalapeño	2 tsp	7	0	1	173	0	0.3	0
(Grey Poupon)								
Dijon	1 tsp	6	0	1	28	0	0.4	0
Dijon, country	1 tsp	6	0	0	120	0	0.0	0
Parisian	1 tsp	6	0	0	55	0	0.0	0
(Gulden's)								
hot, 'Diablo'	.25 oz	8	0	0	55	0	0.0	0
mild, yellow, creamy	.25 oz	6	0	0	60	0	0.0	0
spicy, brown	.25 oz	8	0	0	45	0	0.0	0
(Hain)								
stone ground	1 tbsp	14	1	1	185	0	1.0	0
stone ground, no salt added	1 tbsp	14	1	1	10	0	1.0	0
(Heinz)								
mild, yellow	1 tbsp	8	1	1	175	0	1.0	0

Food Name	Serv. Size	Total Cal.	Prot. gms	Carbs gms	Sod. mgs	Fiber gms	Fat gms	Chol. mgs
spicy, brown	1 tbsp	14	1	1	115	0	1.0	0
yellow	1 tsp	3	0	0	55	0	0.2	0
(Kraft)								
horseradish	1 tbsp	14	1	1	135	0	1.0	0
'Pure'	1 tbsp	11	0	1	160	0	1.0	0
(Westbrae)								
Dijon	1 tbsp	16	1	1	195	0	1.0	0
'Mt. Fuji'	1 tbsp	16	1	1	195	0	1.0	0
stone ground, no salt	1 tbsp	16	1	1	195	0	1.0	0
yellow	1 tbsp	16	1	1	195	0	1.0	0
MUSTARD BLEND								
(Best Foods/Hellmann's) blend, 'Creamy Dijonniase'	1 tsp	10	0	1	60	0	1.0	0
(Luzianne) 'Creole' yellow and brown	1 tbsp	10	1	2	320	na	0.0	na
MUSTARD FLOUR. See under FLOUR.								
MUSTARD GREENS								
Fresh								
boiled, drained, chopped	1 cup	21	3	3	22	3	0.3	0
raw, chopped	1 cup	15	2	3	14	2	0.1	0
Canned, chopped *(Allens)*	1/2 cup	20	1	2	35	0	1.0	0
Frozen								
(Frosty Acres)	3.3 oz	20	2	3	20	1	0.0	0
chopped *(Flav-R-Pac)*	1/3 cup	25	2	2	15	2	0.0	0
chopped *(Seabrook)*	3.3 oz	20	2	3	20	1	0.0	0
chopped *(Southern)*	3.5 oz	25	3	4	40	0	0.3	0
chopped, unprepared	1 cup	29	4	5	42	5	0.4	0
unprepared	10-oz pkg	57	7	10	82	9	0.8	0
w/o salt, chopped, drained	1 cup	29	3	5	38	4	0.4	0
w/o salt, drained	10-oz pkg	40	5	7	53	6	0.5	0
w/salt, chopped or diced, drained	1/2 cup	14	2	2	196	2	0.2	0
w/salt, drained	10-oz pkg	40	5	7	553	6	0.5	0
MUSTARD OIL								
	1 cup	1927	0	0	0	0	218.0	na
	1 tbsp	124	0	0	0	0	14.0	na
MUSTARD SEED								
(McCormick/Schilling)	1 tsp	17	1	1	0	0	0.8	0
yellow	1 tbsp	53	3	4	1	2	3.2	0
yellow	1 tsp	15	1	1	0	0	0.9	0
MUSTARD SPINACH/tendergreen								
boiled, drained, chopped	1 cup	29	3	5	25	4	0.4	0
raw, chopped	1 cup	33	3	6	32	4	0.5	0
MUTTON TALLOW								
	1 cup	1849	0	0	0	0	205.0	209
	1 tbsp	115	0	0	0	0	12.8	13
MUTTONFISH. See OCEAN POUT.								

N

Food Name	Serv. Size	Total Cal.	Prot. gms	Carbs gms	Sod. mgs	Fiber gms	Fat gms	Chol. mgs
NACHO CHIPS. See under CORN CHIPS AND SNACKS.								
NACHO SEASONING. See under SEASONING MIX.								
NAPA CABBAGE. See BOK CHOY.								
NAPOLES								
cooked	1 med pad	4	0	1	6	1	0.0	0
cooked, sliced	1 cup	22	2	5	30	3	0.1	0
raw, sliced	1 cup	14	1	3	19	2	0.1	0

Food Name	Serv. Size	Total Cal.	Prot. gms	Carbs gms	Sod. mgs	Fiber gms	Fat gms	Chol. mgs
NATAL PLUM. See CARISSA.								
NATTO. See SOYBEAN, FERMENTED.								
NAVY BEAN. See BEAN, NAVY.								
NECTAR. See under FRUIT DRINK.								
NECTARINE								
Fresh								
raw, pitted .... 1 oz	14	0.3	3.3	tr	.5	0.1	0
raw, sliced .... 1 cup	68	1.3	16.3	0	2.2	0.6	0
raw, trimmed, whole, approx 2.5 inch diam .... 1 nectarine	67	1.3	16.0	0	2.2	0.6	0
raw, untrimmed *(Dole)* .... 1 medium	70	1.0	16.0	0	3.0	1.0	na
raw, whole .... 1 lb	204	3.9	48.6	1	6.6	1.9	0
NEW ZEALAND SPINACH. See SPINACH, NEW ZEALAND.								
NONDAIRY DESSERT, FROZEN. See ICE CREAM SUBSTITUTE; ICE CREAM SUBSTITUTE BAR/DESSERT.								
NONDAIRY DESSERT MIX. See ICE CREAM SUBSTITUTE MIX.								
NOODLE. See also PASTA.								
CELLOPHANE. See under NOODLE, CHINESE.								
CHINESE								
cellophane/long rice, mung bean, dry .... 1 cup	491	0	121	14	1	0.1	0
chow mein .... 1 cup	237	4	26	198	2	13.8	0
chow mein .... 1.5 oz	227	4	25	189	2	13.2	0
rice, cooked .... 1 cup	192	2	44	33	2	0.4	0
(China Boy) chow mein .... 1/2 cup	130	3	16	110	1	5.0	0
(Chun King)								
chow mein, w/almonds .... 1/3 cup	140	4	15	380	1	7.0	0
chow mein, w/sesame bits .... 1/3 cup	140	3	16	460	1	7.0	0
(La Choy)								
chow mein, food service product .... 1/2 cup	140	4	17	209	2	6.1	0
chow mein, wide, crispy .... 1 cup	296	5	32	578	2	16.5	0
rice, canned .... 1 cup	242	5	43	756	1	6.1	0
rice, food service product .... 1/2 cup	122	2	22	362	0	3.1	0
CHOW MEIN. See under NOODLE, CHINESE.								
EGG								
enriched, cooked .... 1 cup	213	8	40	11	2	2.4	53
enriched, dry .... 1 cup	145	5	27	8	1	1.6	36
enriched, dry .... 2 oz	217	8	41	12	2	2.4	54
spinach, enriched, cooked .... 1 cup	211	8	39	19	4	2.5	53
spinach, enriched, dry .... 1 cup	145	6	27	27	3	1.7	36
spinach, enriched, dry .... 2 oz	218	8	40	41	4	2.6	54
unenriched, dry .... 1 cup	145	5	27	8	1	1.6	36
(American Beauty)								
extra wide, enriched, dry .... 2 oz	220	8	42	15	0	3.0	55
fine, enriched, dry .... 2 oz	220	8	42	15	0	3.0	55
medium, enriched, dry .... 2 oz	220	8	42	15	0	3.0	55
wide, enriched, dry .... 2 oz	220	8	42	15	0	3.0	55
(Borden) kluski, enriched, dry .... 1 cup	220	8	40	210	1	3.0	55
(Creamette)								
plain, enriched, dry .... 2 oz	221	8	40	3	1	2.5	70
w/pasteurized eggs, wide, 'Fancy' dry .... 2 oz	220	8	40	20	0	3.0	70
(De Boles)								
Jerusalem artichoke, dry .... 2 oz	210	7	41	0	1	1.0	0
Jerusalem artichoke, garlic and parsley, dry .... 2 oz	210	7	41	5	2	1.0	0
(De Cecco) spinach, dry .... 2 oz	210	7	41	35	0	1.0	0
(Eden Foods)								
bifun, rice .... 2 oz	200	5	44	5	0	0.5	0
fine, dry, 'Herb's' .... 2 oz	220	10	42	5	2	2.0	60
kluski, medium, dry, 'Herb's' .... 2 oz	220	10	42	5	2	2.0	60
kluski, wide, dry, 'Herb's' .... 2 oz	220	10	42	5	2	2.0	60

Food Name	Serv. Size	Total Cal.	Prot. gms	Carbs gms	Sod. mgs	Fiber gms	Fat gms	Chol. mgs
medium, dry, 'Herb's'	2 oz	220	10	42	5	2	2.0	60
(Gioia) plain, dry	2 oz	220	8	40	0	0	3.0	0
(Golden Grain) plain, dry	2 oz	210	8	39	10	2	2.2	65
(Goodman's) plain, 'Country Style' dry	2 oz	220	8	40	15	0	3.0	0
(Hodgson Mill)								
spinach, whole wheat, dry	2 oz	190	10	32	45	5	2.0	30
vegetable, dry	2 oz	200	9	37	25	2	2.0	35
whole wheat, wide, dry	2 oz	190	10	34	20	4	2.0	30
(Hospitality) wide, enriched, 'Valu Pack' dry	1 1/4 cup	235	9	43	5	2	2.5	80
(Mrs. Grass) plain, dry	2 oz	220	8	40	200	0	3.0	0
(Mueller's)								
kluski, dry	2 oz	220	8	38	10	1	3.0	65
plain, dry	2 oz	220	8	40	10	0	3.0	55
(No Yolks) no egg yolks, broad, dry	2 oz	200	8	40	25	0	1.0	0
(P&R) plain, dry	2 oz	220	8	42	15	0	3.0	0
(Prince) plain, dry	2 oz	210	8	40	35	0	2.0	65
(Reames) homestyle, frozen	1/2 cup	170	4	32	10	1	2.0	85
(Ronzoni)								
very low-sodium, dry, 'Egg Pastina'	2 oz	220	8	42	15	0	3.0	65
wide, enriched, 'Country Kitchen Style' dry	2 oz	220	8	42	15	0	3.0	65
(San Giorgio) plain, dry	2 oz	220	8	42	15	0	3.0	0
JAPANESE								
soba, cooked	1 cup	113	6	24	68	na	0.1	0
soba, dry	2 oz	192	8	43	451	na	0.4	0
somen, cooked	1 cup	231	7	48	283	na	0.3	0
somen, dry	2 oz	203	6	42	1049	2	0.5	0
(Eden Foods)								
harusame, mung bean, dry	2 oz	190	0	47	5	0	0.0	0
jinenjo soba, wild yam, dry	2 oz	190	9	37	510	2	0.5	0
kuzu and sweet potato, dry	2 oz	190	0	47	0	0	0.0	0
soba, 40% buckwheat	2 oz	190	8	37	490	3	1.0	0
soba, buckwheat, 100% buckwheat, dry	2 oz	200	5	41	30	3	1.5	0
soba, lotus root	2 oz	190	9	37	470	4	1.0	0
soba, mugwort	2 oz	190	8	37	550	2	0.5	0
soba, traditional	2 oz	190	8	37	490	3	1.0	0
soba, wild yam	2 oz	190	9	37	510	2	0.5	0
udon, brown rice	2 oz	190	8	38	510	2	1.0	0
(Westbrae)								
buckwheat, dry	2 oz	190	7	40	5	0	2.0	0
genmai, dry	2 oz	200	5	41	411	0	1.0	0
somen, whole wheat, dry	2 oz	200	7	41	375	0	1.0	0
traditional, dry	2 oz	190	7	41	198	0	2.0	0
udon, whole wheat, organic, dry	2 oz	200	7	41	375	0	1.0	0
SOBA. See under NOODLE, JAPANESE.								
UDON. See under NOODLE, JAPANESE.								
NOODLE DISH/ENTRÉE See also PASTA DISH/ENTRÉE.								
(Banquet)								
and julienne beef, w/sauce, frozen, 'Family Entrées'	7 oz	170	12	22	0	0	3.0	0
w/beef gravy, frozen, 'Family Entrées'	8 oz	200	13	22	0	0	7.0	0
w/chicken, frozen	10 oz	350	10	42	460	0	15.0	45
w/chicken, frozen, 'Family Favorites'	10 oz	340	11	42	455	0	15.0	45
(Dinty Moore)								
and chicken, packaged, 'American Classics'	10 oz	230	17	24	1020	0	7.0	65
tuna noodle casserole, packaged, 'American Classics'	10 oz	240	16	28	1280	0	7.0	65
(Heinz)								
and chicken, canned	7.5 oz	160	6	19	930	0	7.0	0
w/beef, in sauce, canned	7.5 oz	170	8	17	825	0	8.0	0

Food Name	Serv. Size	Total Cal.	Prot. gms	Carbs gms	Sod. mgs	Fiber gms	Fat gms	Chol. mgs
w/tuna, canned	7.5 oz	170	11	20	950	0	5.0	0
(Hormel) w/chicken, 'Micro-Cup'	7.5 oz	180	7	18	1000	0	8.0	20
(Kid's Kitchen) rings and chicken, microwave cup	7.5 oz	150	11	17	840	0	4.0	25
(La Choy)								
and vegetables	1 cup	131	5	27	1311	3	1.3	0
chow mein, canned	1 cup	300	6	32	440	2	16.0	0
w/beef, bi-pack	1 cup	148	12	24	1101	3	1.2	13
w/beef, vegetables	1 cup	156	7	27	1332	3	3.5	6
w/chicken, bi-pack	1 cup	161	11	23	1163	4	3.8	13
w/chicken, vegetables	1 cup	163	10	24	858	1	3.3	19
(Marie Callender's) w/chicken, escalloped	1 cup	420	13	44	1010	3	21.0	45
(Nalley's)								
and chicken, canned	7 3/8 oz	150	9	17	1000	0	5.0	0
and chicken, w/vegetables, canned	7 3/8 oz	160	10	18	1450	0	5.0	0
(Stouffer's)								
Romanoff	1 entrée	490	18	48	1400	4	25.0	60
Romanoff, frozen, food service product	1 oz	41	2	4	173	0	2.2	5
(Swanson) w/chicken, frozen	10.5 oz	280	7	45	740	0	8.0	40
(Van Camp's) w/franks, canned, 'Noodle Weenee'	1 cup	245	9	33	1245	5	8.5	0
(Weight Watchers) kung pao	1 entrée	260	8	35	690	5	10.0	5
NOODLE DISH/ENTRÉE MIX. See also PASTA DISH/ENTRÉE MIX.								
(Kraft)								
cheese, 'Dinner'	3/4 cup	340	10	37	670	0	17.0	50
chicken flavor, 'Dinner'	3/4 cup	240	8	32	1050	0	9.0	45
(Lipton)								
egg noodles Alfredo, mix only	1 cup	389	14	58	1646	na	11.0	104
egg noodles Alfredo, mix only	1 pkg	518	19	77	2195	na	14.6	139
egg noodles Alfredo, prepared	1 serving	259	10	39	1097	na	7.3	69
(Mountain House) w/chicken, freeze-dried, prepared	1 cup	270	10	34	201	0	10.0	0
(Ultra Slim Fast) w/Alfredo sauce, prepared	8 oz	240	9	47	1110	4	4.0	0
NORI. See under SEA VEGETABLE.								
NORTHERN PIKE. See under PIKE.								
NORWAY HADDOCK. See OCEAN PERCH, ATLANTIC.								
NUT SNACK								
(Fisher)								
crisp, golden, 'Nut 'N Crunchies'	1/4 cup	140	4	15	320	1	7.0	0
fiesta, 'Nut 'N Crunchies'	1/4 cup	140	4	16	330	1	7.0	0
honey crunch, 'Nut 'N Crunchies'	1/4 cup	140	4	17	210	1	6.0	0
NUT TOPPING								
(Fisher)								
fancy	1 oz	170	5	7	60	0	15.0	0
oil roasted, w/peanuts	1 oz	160	6	7	115	0	14.0	0
(Planters)	1 oz	180	5	6	0	0	16.0	0
(Smucker's)								
pecan, in syrup	2 tbsp	130	2	28	0	0	1.0	0
walnut, in syrup	2 tbsp	130	2	27	0	0	1.0	0
NUTMEG								
ground	1 tbsp	37	0	3	1	1	2.5	0
ground	1 tsp	12	0	1	0	0	0.8	0
ground (Durkee)	1 tsp	12	0	0	0	0	0.0	0
ground (Laurel Leaf)	1 tsp	12	0	0	0	0	0.0	0
ground (McCormick/Schilling)	1 tsp	11	0	1	0	0	0.8	0
ground (Spice Islands)	1 tsp	11	0	1	1	0	0.7	0
NUTMEG BUTTER OIL								
	1 cup	1927	0	0	0	0	218.0	0
	1 tbsp	120	0	0	0	0	13.6	0

Food Name	Serv. Size	Total Cal.	Prot. gms	Carbs gms	Sod. mgs	Fiber gms	Fat gms	Chol. mgs
NUTS, MIXED								
(Eagle)								
....	1/4 cup	200	6	6	140	2	17.0	0
lightly salted	1/4 cup	200	6	6	65	2	17.0	0
w/o peanuts, deluxe	1/4 cup	200	5	8	130	2	14.0	0
(Fisher)								
cashews, honey-glazed 'Favorites'	1/4 cup	170	6	9	110	2	13.0	0
cashews, praline-glazed, 'Favorites'	1/4 cup	170	5	11	90	1	12.0	0
cashews, toffee-glazed, 'Favorites'	1/4 cup	170	5	11	90	2	11.0	0
cashews, tropical fruit, 'Favorites'	1/4 cup	140	4	14	90	2	8.0	0
lightly salted	1/4 cup	180	6	5	50	2	16.0	0
salted	1/4 cup	180	6	5	110	2	16.0	0
(Flanigan Farms) natural, unsalted	1 oz	180	4	5	2	na	17.0	0
(Guy's) w/peanuts	1 oz	170	8	3	140	0	14.0	0
(Planters)								
cashews, almonds, and peanuts, 'Select Mix'	1 oz	170	5	7	100	0	14.0	0
cashews, almonds, and pecans, 'Select Mix'	1 oz	180	4	6	85	0	16.0	0
cashews, pecans, and peanuts, 'Select Mix'	1 oz	180	4	6	80	0	16.0	0
Dry-roasted								
(Eden Foods) sunflower, peanuts, cashews, almonds	1 oz	170	8	9	55	3	11.0	0
(Finast)								
lightly salted	1 oz	170	6	7	0	0	15.0	0
salted	1 oz	170	6	7	125	0	15.0	0
salted, w/peanuts, 'No Frills'	1 oz	180	5	7	150	0	14.0	0
w/peanuts, salted, 'No Frills'	1 oz	180	5	7	150	0	14.0	0
(Pathmark) w/peanuts, salted, 'No Frills'	1 oz	180	6	7	220	0	14.0	0
(Planters)								
....	1 oz	160	5	7	250	0	14.0	0
sesame nut mix	1 oz	160	5	8	330	0	12.0	0
unsalted	1 oz	170	6	7	0	0	15.0	0
Honey-roasted								
(Eagle) cashews and peanuts	1/4 cup	180	5	8	130	2	14.0	0
(Fisher) cashews and peanuts	1/4 cup	170	6	8	110	1	13.0	0
(Planters)								
....	1 oz	170	5	9	140	0	13.0	0
cashews and peanuts	1 oz	170	5	9	170	0	12.0	0
Oil-roasted								
(Flavor House)	1 oz	180	5	6	125	0	18.0	0
(Planters)								
....	1 oz	180	5	6	110	0	16.0	0
'Deluxe'	1 oz	180	4	6	110	0	17.0	0
lightly salted	1 oz	180	5	6	80	0	16.0	0
sesame nut mix	1 oz	160	5	8	200	0	13.0	0
unsalted	1 oz	180	5	6	0	0	16.0	0
(Pathmark)								
w/peanuts, salted, 'No Frills'	1 oz	180	6	5	150	0	15.0	0
w/o peanuts, salted, fancy, 'No Frills'	1 oz	180	4	7	150	0	15.0	0

O

Food Name	Serv. Size	Total Cal.	Prot. gms	Carbs gms	Sod. mgs	Fiber gms	Fat gms	Chol. mgs
OAT. See also under CEREAL, HOT.								
....	1 cup	607	26	103	3	17	10.8	0
steel cut *(Arrowhead Mills)*	2 oz	220	10	37	1	3	4.0	0
OAT BRAN								
cooked	1 cup	88	7	25	2	6	1.9	0

Food Name	Serv. Size	Total Cal.	Prot. gms	Carbs gms	Sod. mgs	Fiber gms	Fat gms	Chol. mgs
raw	1 cup	231	16	62	4	14	6.6	0
OAT FLOUR. See under FLOUR.								
OAT MIX, gluten free *(Ener-G Foods)*	1 cup	376	10	7	276	12	7.7	0
OAT VEGETABLE OIL								
	1 cup	1927	0	0	0	0	218.0	0
	1 tbsp	120	0	0	0	0	13.6	0
OCEAN CATFISH. See WOLF FISH.								
OCEAN PERCH, ATLANTIC/Norway haddock/red perch/rose perch								
Fresh								
baked, broiled, or grilled	3 oz	103	20	0	82	0	1.8	46
raw	3 oz	80	16	0	64	0	1.4	36
raw, boneless	1 oz	27	5	0	21	0	0.5	12
Frozen								
(Booth)	4 oz	100	20	0	250	0	1.0	0
fillet, light *(Van de Kamp's)*	1 piece	280	17	21	450	0	14.0	35
'Fishmarket Fresh' *(Gorton's)*	5 oz	140	25	2	100	0	3.0	0
natural *(Van de Kamp's)*	4 oz	130	20	0	65	0	5.0	40
OCEAN POUT/muttonfish								
baked, broiled, or grilled	3 oz	87	18	0	66	0	1.0	57
raw	3 oz	67	14	0	52	0	0.8	44
OCEANIC BONITO. See under TUNA.								
OCTOPUS								
common, boiled, poached, or steamed	3 oz	139	25	4	391	0	1.8	82
common, raw	3 oz	70	13	2	196	0	0.9	41
OHELOBERRY, RAW								
fresh, raw	1 cup	39	1	10	1	na	0.3	0
fresh, raw	10 medium	3	0	1	0	na	0.0	0
OKRA								
Fresh								
boiled, drained, sliced	1/2 cup	26	1	6	4	2	0.1	0
boiled, drained, whole, approx 3-inch long	8 med pods	27	2	6	4	2	0.1	0
raw, sliced	1 cup	33	2	8	8	3	0.1	0
raw, whole, approx 3-inch long	8 med pods	31	2	7	8	3	0.1	0
Frozen								
cut *(Flav-R-Pac)*	3/4 cup	25	2	4	15	3	0.0	0
cut *(Freshlike)*	3.3 oz	25	1	6	5	0	0.0	0
cut *(Pictsweet)*	3/4 cup	25	1	5	35	3	0.0	0
cut *(Seabrook)*	3.3 oz	25	1	6	3	1	0.0	0
cut *(Southern)*	3.5 oz	31	2	7	20	0	0.2	0
cut *(Veg-All)*	3.3 oz	25	1	6	5	0	0.0	0
drained	10-oz pkg	71	5	15	8	7	0.8	0
sliced, drained	1/2 cup	26	2	5	3	3	0.3	0
unprepared	10-oz pkg	85	5	19	9	6	0.7	0
unprepared	3 lb pkg	408	23	90	41	30	3.4	0
whole *(Flav-R-Pac)*	9 pieces	35	1	6	15	4	0.5	0
whole *(Freshlike)*	3.3 oz	30	2	7	5	0	0.0	0
whole *(Seabrook)*	3.3 oz	30	2	7	2	1	0.0	0
whole *(Southern)*	3.5 oz	35	2	7	20	0	0.2	0
whole *(Veg-All)*	3.3 oz	30	2	7	5	0	0.0	0
whole, baby *(Frosty Acres)*	3.3 oz	30	2	7	2	1	0.0	0
OLD-FASHIONED. See under COCKTAIL MIX.								
OLIVE								
all varieties, all sizes, pickled *(S&W)*	1 oz	46	0	0	215	0	5.1	0
mixed sizes, chopped	1 tbsp	10	0	1	73	0	0.9	0
mixed varieties, pickled, chopped *(Lindsay)*	1 oz	29	0	2	249	1	2.7	0
mixed varieties, pickled, pitted *(Vlasic)*	1 oz	37	0	1	230	0	3.9	0
mixed varieties, pickled, sliced *(Lindsay)*	1 oz	29	0	2	249	1	2.7	0

Food Name	Serv. Size	Total Cal.	Prot. gms	Carbs gms	Sod. mgs	Fiber gms	Fat gms	Chol. mgs
salad, pickled *(Progresso)*	1/2 cup	120	1	1	2400	4	15.0	0
whole, large	1 olive	5	0	0	38	0	0.5	0
whole, small	1 olive	4	0	0	28	0	0.3	0
ASCOLANO								
all sizes, pickled, pitted *(Lindsay)*	1 oz	23	0	2	255	1	1.9	0
colossal, pickled, pitted *(Lindsay)*	10 olives	90	1	6	1010	3	7.7	0
jumbo, pickled, pitted *(Lindsay)*	10 olives	66	1	5	745	2	5.7	0
super colossal, pickled, pitted *(Lindsay)*	10 olives	122	2	9	1365	4	10.4	0
BLACK								
colossal, w/pits *(S&W)*	1 piece	15	0	1	80	0	1.5	0
extra large, pitted *(S&W)*	3 pieces	25	0	1	110	0	2.5	0
extra large, pitted, 'Black Pearls' *(Musco)*	3 olives	25	0	1	95	0	2.0	0
jumbo, pitted *(S&W)*	3 pieces	25	0	1	135	0	2.0	0
medium, pitted, 'Black Pearls' *(Musco)*	5 olives	25	0	1	95	0	2.0	0
GREEK								
all sizes, salt-cured, oil-coated, pickled, pitted	1 oz	96	0.6	2.5	932	(mq)	10.2	0
extra large, salt-cured, oil-coated, pickled, w/pits	10 olives	89	0.6	2.3	868	(mq)	9.5	0
extra large, salt-cured, pickled, w/pits	10 olives	89	0.6	2.3	868	(mq)	9.5	0
medium, salt-cured, oil-coated, pickled, w/pits	10 olives	65	0.4	1.7	631	(mq)	6.9	0
medium, salt-cured, pickled, w/pits	10 olives	65	0.4	1.7	631	(mq)	6.9	0
GREEN								
chopped *(Early California)*	14 grams	18	0	1	110	0	2.0	0
extra large, pitted *(Vlasic)*	14 grams	18	0	1	110	0	2.0	0
jumbo	1 olive	7	0	0	75	0	0.6	0
large, pitted *(Vlasic)*	15 grams	25	0	1	115	0	2.5	0
martini, pimento stuffed *(Santa Barbara Olive Co.)*	0.5 oz	25	0	0	95	0	2.0	0
medium, pitted *(Vlasic)*	14 grams	18	0	1	110	0	2.0	0
pimento stuffed *(Golden Gate)*	15 grams	15	0	1	260	0	1.0	0
pitted, pitted *(Vlasic)*	14 grams	18	0	1	110	0	2.0	0
queen *(S&W)*	2 olives	20	0	1	220	0	2.0	0
small, pitted *(Vlasic)*	14 grams	18	0	1	110	0	2.0	0
Spanish, pimento stuffed *(Star)*	15 grams	15	0	1	260	0	1.0	0
super colossal	1 olive	12	0	1	136	0	1.0	0
w/jalapeño *(Santa Barbara Olive Co.)*	0.5 oz	25	0	0	95	0	2.0	0
MANZANILLA								
all sizes, pickled, pitted *(Lindsay)*	1 oz	32	0	2	247	1	3.0	0
extra large, pickled, pitted *(Lindsay)*	10 olives	63	1	4	484	2	5.9	0
large, pickled, pitted *(Lindsay)*	10 olives	50	0	3	388	1	4.8	0
medium, pickled, pitted *(Lindsay)*	10 olives	44	0	2	336	1	4.1	0
small, pickled, pitted *(Lindsay)*	10 olives	37	0	2	283	1	3.5	0
stuffed *(S&W)*	3 olives	25	0	1	240	0	2.0	0
w/pimento *(S&W)*	3 olives	25	0	1	240	0	2.0	0
MISSION								
all sizes, pickled, pitted *(Lindsay)*	1 oz	32	0	2	247	1	3.0	0
extra large, pickled, pitted *(Lindsay)*	10 olives	63	1	4	484	2	5.9	0
large, pickled, pitted *(Lindsay)*	10 olives	50	0	3	388	1	4.8	0
medium, pickled, pitted *(Lindsay)*	10 olives	44	0	2	336	1	4.1	0
small, pickled, pitted *(Lindsay)*	10 olives	37	0	2	283	1	3.5	0
SEVILLANO								
all sizes, pickled, pitted *(Lindsay)*	1 oz	23	0	2	255	1	1.9	0
colossal, pickled, pitted *(Lindsay)*	10 olives	90	1	6	1010	3	7.7	0
jumbo, pickled, pitted *(Lindsay)*	10 olives	66	1	5	745	2	5.7	0
super colossal, pickled, pitted *(Lindsay)*	10 olives	122	2	9	1365	4	10.4	0
OLIVE APPETIZER								
(Progresso)								
	1/2 cup	180	1	6	1600	3	21.0	0
'Condite'	1/2 cup	130	1	5	870	2	14.0	0

Food Name	Serv. Size	Total Cal.	Prot. gms	Carbs gms	Sod. mgs	Fiber gms	Fat gms	Chol. mgs
OLIVE OIL								
salad or cooking	1 cup	1909	0	0	0	0	216.0	0
salad or cooking	1 tbsp	119	0	0	0	0	13.5	0
(Amore)								
'Pure'	1 tbsp	130	0	0	0	0	14.0	0
extra virgin	1 tbsp	130	0	0	0	0	14.0	0
(Bertolli)	1 tbsp	120	0	0	0	0	14.0	0
(Filippo Berio)	1 tbsp	120	0	0	0	0	14.0	0
(Hain)	1 tbsp	120	0	0	0	0	14.0	0
(Pope) Italian, cold press, no salt	1 tbsp	120	0	0	0	0	14.0	0
(Progresso)								
'Riviera Blend'	1 tbsp	120	0	0	0	0	14.0	0
extra mild	1 tbsp	120	0	0	0	0	14.0	0
extra virgin	1 tbsp	120	0	0	0	0	14.0	0
oil cured	6 olives	80	0	3	330	1	6.0	0
(Spectrum) extra virgin, pure pressed, organic	1 tbsp	120	0	0	0	0	14.0	0
(Wesson)	1 tbsp	122	0	0	0	0	13.6	0
OLIVE SALAD *(Progresso)* drained	2 tbsp	25	0	1	360	1	2.5	0
ONION								
COCKTAIL								
large *(S&W)*	8 onions	5	0	1	300	0	0.0	0
lightly spiced *(Vlasic)*	1 oz	4	0	1	365	0	0.0	0
small *(S&W)*	12 onions	5	0	1	300	0	0.0	0
GREEN. See SCALLION.								
RED, WHITE, OR YELLOW								
Canned								
chopped or diced, w/liquid	1/2 cup	21	1	4	416	1	0.1	0
sweet *(Heinz)*	1 oz	40	0	9	165	0	0.0	0
whole, small *(Green Giant)*	1/2 cup	35	1	8	410	1	0.0	0
whole, small *(Pathmark)*	1/2 cup	35	2	7	280	0	0.0	0
whole, w/liquid	1 medium	12	1	3	234	1	0.1	0
Dried								
(Basic American)	1 oz	99	3	22	49	1	0.3	0
minced, w/green onion *(Lawry's)*	1 tsp	7	0	2	1	1	0.2	0
Fresh								
boiled, drained, chopped	1 cup	92	3	21	6	3	0.4	0
boiled, drained, chopped	1 tbsp	7	0	2	0	0	0.0	0
boiled, drained, chopped or diced	1/2 cup	29	1	7	13	2	0.1	0
boiled, drained, chopped or diced	1 tbsp	4	0	1	2	0	0.0	0
boiled, drained, whole, medium, approx 2.5-inch diam	1 onion	41	1	10	3	1	0.2	0
boiled, drained, sliced, medium, 1/8 inch thick	1 slice	5	0	1	0	0	0.0	0
raw, chopped	1 cup	61	2	14	5	3	0.3	0
raw, chopped	1 tbsp	4	0	1	0	0	0.0	0
raw, sliced	1 cup	44	1	10	3	2	0.2	0
raw, sliced, medium, 1/8-inch thick	1 slice	5	0	1	0	0	0.0	0
raw, whole, medium, approx 2.5-inch diam	1 onion	42	1	9	3	2	0.2	0
Frozen								
chopped *(Ore-Ida)*	2 oz	20	0	4	10	0	1.0	0
chopped *(Seabrook)*	1 oz	8	0	2	2	0	0.0	0
diced *(Flav-R-Pac)*	2/3 cup	30	1	6	30	1	0.0	0
diced *(Freshlike)*	3.3 oz	8	0	2	0	0	0.0	0
diced *(Veg-All)*	3.3 oz	8	0	2	0	0	0.0	0
unprepared	10-oz pkg	82	2	19	34	5	0.3	0
whole *(Freshlike)*	3.3 oz	35	1	8	10	0	0.0	0
whole *(Veg-All)*	3.3 oz	35	1	8	10	0	0.0	0
whole, small *(Birds Eye)*	4 oz	40	1	10	10	2	0.0	0
whole, small *(Flav-R-Pac)*	1/2 cup	25	1	7	15	2	0.0	0

Food Name	Serv. Size	Total Cal.	Prot. gms	Carbs gms	Sod. mgs	Fiber gms	Fat gms	Chol. mgs
whole, small *(Seabrook)*	3.3 oz	35	1	8	9	1	0.0	0
WELSH								
trimmed	1 lb	160	8.0	28.8	na	4.8	1.6	0
trimmed	1 oz	10	0.5	1.8	na	0.3	0.1	0
ONION DISH MIX *(Vidalia Sweet)* rings, all purpose	1/4 cup	100	3	21	690	1	na	na
ONION FLAKES								
dehydrated	1 tbsp	17	0	4	1	0	0.0	0
dehydrated	1/4 cup	49	1	12	3	1	0.1	0
minced *(Lawry's)*	1 tsp	7	0	2	1	1	0.2	0
ONION POWDER								
	1 tbsp	23	1	5	3	0	0.1	0
	1 tsp	7	0	2	1	0	0.0	0
ground *(Durkee)*	1 tsp	8	0	0	0	0	0.0	0
ground *(Laurel Leaf)*	1 tsp	8	0	0	0	0	0.0	0
ground *(McCormick/Schilling)*	1 tsp	10	0	2	2	0	0.0	0
ground *(Spice Islands)*	1 tsp	8	0	2	1	0	0.1	0
ground *(Tone's)*	1 tsp	5	0	2	1000	0	0.1	0
ONION SALT								
(Schilling) 'California blend'	1/4 tsp	0	0	0	170	0	0.0	0
(Tone's)	1 tsp	1	0	0	1599	0	0.0	0
ONION SNACK *(Wise)* rings	1 oz	130	1	21	360	0	5.0	0
OPOSSUM								
roasted	3 oz	188	26	0	49	0	8.7	110
roasted, boneless, yield from 1 lb raw	14 oz	882	120	0	231	0	40.7	515
roasted, diced	1 cup	309	42.3	0.0	(mq)	0	14.3	(mq)
ORANGE								
ALL VARIETIES								
raw, peeled, sections	1 cup	85	2	21	0	4	0.2	0
raw, peeled, whole, large, approx 3 1/16 inch diam	1 orange	86	2	22	0	4	0.2	0
raw, peeled, whole, medium, approx 2 5/8 inch diam	1 orange	62	1	15	0	3	0.2	0
raw, peeled, whole, small, approx 2 3/8 inch diam	1 orange	45	1	11	0	2	0.1	0
raw, w/peel	1 cup	68	2	26	3	8	0.5	0
raw, medium, w/peel, w/o seeds	1 orange	64	2	25	3	7	0.5	0
CALIFORNIA								
Navel								
peeled, raw, sections, w/o membranes	1 cup	76	2	19	2	4	0.1	0
peeled, raw, whole, medium, approx 2 7/8 inch diam	1 orange	64	1	16	1	3	0.1	0
Valencia								
peeled, raw, sections, w/o membranes	1 cup	88	2	21	0	5	0.5	0
peeled, raw, whole, medium, approx 2 5/8 inch diam	1 orange	59	1	14	0	3	0.4	0
FLORIDA								
raw, whole, peeled, medium, approx 2 11/16 inch diam	1 orange	69	1	17	0	4	0.3	0
raw, whole, peeled, medium, approx 2 5/8 inch diam	1 orange	65	1	16	0	3	0.3	0
raw, sections, peeled, w/o membranes	1 cup	85	1	21	0	4	0.4	0
ORANGE DRINK. See under FRUIT DRINK; FRUIT JUICE DRINK.								
ORANGE JUICE								
canned or boxed	1 cup	105	1	25	5	0	0.3	0
fresh squeezed	1 cup	112	2	26	2	0	0.5	0
fresh squeezed	1 fl oz	14	0	3	0	0	0.1	0
fresh squeezed, juice from 1 med fruit	3 oz	39	1	9	1	0	0.2	0
(A&P) frozen concentrate, prepared	6 fl oz	80	1	19	0	0	1.0	0
(Citrus Hill)								
'Plus Calcium'	6 fl oz	90	1	20	10	0	1.0	0
'Select'	6 fl oz	90	1	20	10	0	1.0	0
(Crowley)	8 fl oz	110	2	26	5	0	0.0	0
(Del Monte) canned or boxed, 'Unsweetened'	6 fl oz	80	1	19	10	0	0.0	0

Food Name	Serv. Size	Total Cal.	Prot. gms	Carbs gms	Sod. mgs	Fiber gms	Fat gms	Chol. mgs
(Donald Duck)								
100% orange juice, from concentrate	8 fl oz	120	1	29	0	0	0.0	0
100% pure, from concentrate	6 fl oz	90	1	22	0	0	0.0	0
(Flav-R-Pac)	1 cup	120	1	29	0	0	0.0	0
(Florida's Natural)								
homestyle, Florida fruit, not from concentrate	8 fl oz	120	1	29	0	0	0.0	0
(Knudsen)								
	8 fl oz	100	2	23	35	na	0.0	0
float	8 fl oz	120	2	27	0	0	0.0	0
(Kraft) chilled, 'Pure 100% Unsweetened'	6 fl oz	80	1	19	0	0	0.0	0
(Minute Maid)								
calcium-fortified	6 fl oz	80	1	20	20	0	0.0	0
calcium-fortified, frozen concentrate, prepared	6 fl oz	80	1	20	0	0	0.0	0
country style	6 fl oz	80	1	20	20	0	0.0	0
country style, frozen concentrate, prepared	6 fl oz	80	1	20	0	0	0.0	0
premium choice	6 fl oz	90	1	21	0	0	0.0	0
pulp-free	6 fl oz	80	1	20	20	0	0.0	0
pulp-free, frozen concentrate, prepared	6 fl oz	80	1	20	0	0	0.0	0
reduced acid, frozen concentrate, prepared	6 fl oz	80	1	20	0	0	0.0	0
regular	6 fl oz	80	1	20	20	0	0.0	0
regular, frozen concentrate, prepared	6 fl oz	80	1	20	0	0	0.0	0
(Ocean Spray)	6 fl oz	80	0	19	15	0	0.0	0
(S&W)	6 fl oz	90	1	22	0	0	0.0	0
(Sippin' Pak)	8.45 fl oz	110	1	26	25	0	0.0	0
(Stokely) canned or boxed, 'Unsweetened'	6 fl oz	89	1	21	5	0	1.0	0
(Sunkist)								
	6 fl oz	84	1	20	2	0	0.1	0
8–16 servings per pkg, frozen concentrate, prepared	6 fl oz	112	2	27	3	0	0.1	0
'Fresh Squeezed'	6 fl oz	77	1	18	2	0	0.3	0
(Tree Top) 100%	8 fl oz	120	0	28	24	0	0.0	0
(TreeSweet)								
	6 fl oz	78	1	18	15	0	0.0	0
frozen concentrate, prepared	6 fl oz	84	1	20	15	0	0.0	0
(Tropicana)								
from concentrate	60 ml	110	1	27	5	1	0.0	na
homestyle, 'Season's Best'	8 fl oz	110	1	27	5	0	0.0	na
plus calcium, 'Pure Premium'	8 fl oz	110	2	26	0	na	0.0	0
plus calcium, 'Season's Best'	8 fl oz	110	1	27	5	0	0.0	na
plus fiber, 'Pure Premium'	8 fl oz	120	1	30	0	3	0.0	na
plus vitamins, 'Pure Premium'	8 fl oz	110	2	26	0	na	0.0	0
plus vitamins, 'Season's Best'	8 fl oz	110	1	27	5	0	0.0	na
'Pure Premium'	8 fl oz	110	1	26	0	0	0.0	0
reconstituted, 100% pure	6 fl oz	80	1	16	20	0	1.0	0
(Veryfine)								
blend, '100%'	8 fl oz	120	1	30	35	0	0.0	0
'100%'	8 fl oz	121	2	24	10	0	0.0	0
ORANGE JUICE BLEND. See under FRUIT JUICE BLEND.								
ORANGE PEEL								
grated, raw	1 tbsp	6	0	2	0	1	0.0	0
grated, raw	1 tsp	2	0	1	0	0	0.0	0
ORANGE ROUGHY/slimehead								
baked, broiled, or grilled	3 oz	76	16	0	69	0	0.8	22
raw	3 oz	59	12	0	54	0	0.6	17
ORANGEADE. See under FRUIT DRINK.								
OREGANO								
(McCormick/Schilling)	1 tsp	6	0	1	1	1	0.0	0
dried *(Golden Dipt)*	2 grams	6	0	1	88	0	0.0	0

Food Name	Serv. Size	Total Cal.	Prot. gms	Carbs gms	Sod. mgs	Fiber gms	Fat gms	Chol. mgs
dried *(Spice Islands)*	1 tsp	6	0	1	1	0	0.1	0
dried *(Tone's)*	1 tsp	5	0	1	1	0	0.2	0
ground	1 tbsp	14	0	3	1	2	0.5	0
ground	1 tsp	5	0	1	0	1	0.2	0
ground *(Durkee)*	1 tsp	5	0	0	0	0	0.0	0
ground *(Laurel Leaf)*	1 tsp	5	0	0	0	0	0.0	0
OREGANO, MEXICAN *(McCormick/Schilling)*	1 tsp	4	0	1	0	0	0.0	0
ORIENTAL RADISH. See DAIKON.								
ORIENTAL SEASONING MIX. See under SEASONING MIX.								
ORIENTAL STYLE DINNER/ENTRÉE. See also individual listings.								
(Le Menu) Empress, w/seasoned rice, frozen,	8.25 oz	210	16	26	690	0	5.0	30
(Pasta Roni) stir-fry	1 serving	131	3	17	452	1	5.4	0
(Rice A Roni) stir-fry, 'Fast Cook'	2.5 oz	164	3	24	525	1	5.6	0
OYSTER								
ALL SPECIES								
Canned								
(Bumble Bee)	1 cup	218	25	15	185	0	5.3	0
(S&W)	2 oz	70	8	2	160	2	3.0	20
'Fancy' *(S&W)*	2 oz	95	12	4	0	0	3.0	0
cherrywood smoked, petite, in cottonseed oil,								
w/salt *(Reese)*	2 oz	110	8	6	220	0	6.0	50
salt and water added, whole								
(Crown Prince)	3 pieces	70	7	4	150	0	3.0	35
smoked *(S&W)*	2 oz	100	10	6	210	4	6.0	40
smoked, whole, in cottonseed oil								
(Crown Prince)	1 can	170	14	8	280	1	9.0	20
EASTERN								
Canned								
	3 oz	59	6	3	95	0	2.1	47
	1 medium	6	1	0	9	0	0.2	4
drained	1 oz	16	2	1	26	0	0.6	13
drained	1 cup	112	11	6	181	0	4.0	89
w/liquid	12 oz	188	19	11	305	0	6.7	150
w/liquid	1 cup	171	18	10	278	0	6.1	136
Fresh								
breaded and fried	3 oz	167	7	10	354	na	10.7	69
breaded and fried	6 medium	173	8	10	367	na	11.1	71
farmed, cooked	3 oz	67	6	6	139	0	1.8	32
farmed, cooked	6 medium	47	4	4	96	0	1.3	22
farmed, raw	3 oz	50	4	5	151	0	1.3	21
farmed, raw	6 medium	50	4	5	150	0	1.3	21
wild, cooked, dry heat	3 oz	61	7	4	207	0	1.6	42
wild, cooked, dry heat	6 medium	42	5	3	144	0	1.1	29
wild, cooked, moist heat	3 oz	116	12	7	359	0	4.2	89
wild, cooked, moist heat	6 medium	58	6	3	177	0	2.1	44
wild, raw	1 cup	169	17	10	523	0	6.1	131
wild, raw	6 medium	57	6	3	177	0	2.1	45
PACIFIC								
cooked	3 oz	139	16	8	180	0	3.9	85
cooked	1 medium	41	5	2	53	0	1.1	25
raw	3 oz	69	8	4	90	0	2.0	43
raw	1 medium	41	5	2	53	0	1.1	25
OYSTER DISH/ENTRÉE								
(Campbell's) stew, canned, condensed, prepared	8 oz	70	2	5	840	0	5.0	25
OYSTER MUSHROOM. See MUSHROOM, OYSTER.								
OYSTER PLANT. See SALSIFY.								

P

Food Name	Serv. Size	Total Cal.	Prot. gms	Carbs gms	Sod. mgs	Fiber gms	Fat gms	Chol. mgs
PACIFIC COD. See COD, PACIFIC.								
PACIFIC MACKEREL. See MACKEREL, PACIFIC.								
PACIFIC ROCKFISH. See ROCKFISH, PACIFIC.								
PAD THAI SEASONING. See under SEASONING MIX.								
PAK-CHOI. See BOK CHOY.								
PALM, HEARTS OF								
Canned								
	1 cup	41	4	7	622	4	0.9	0
	1 med piece	9	1	2	141	1	0.2	0
Brazilian *(Reese)*	1/3 cup	15	2	1	420	2	1.0	0
PALM KERNEL OIL/babassu oil								
	1 cup	1879	0	0	0	0	218.0	0
	1 tbsp	117	0	0	0	0	13.6	0
	2 tbsp	234	0	0	0	0	27.2	0
PALM OIL								
	1 cup	1909	0	0	0	0	216.0	0
	1 tbsp	120	0	0	0	0	13.6	0
PANCAKE								
(Aunt Jemima)								
homestyle, frozen	3 pancakes	210	6	40	560	2	3.5	20
low-fat, frozen	3 pancakes	150	5	30	530	8	1.5	3
original, frozen, microwave	3 pancakes	211	6	40	801	2	3.6	0
(Downyflake) frozen	3 pancakes	280	5	45	920	0	9.0	0
(Krusteaz) mini, frozen, microwave	6 pancakes	120	3	21	280	0	2.0	4
(Pillsbury) original, frozen, microwave	3 pancakes	240	6	47	550	0	4.0	0
BLUEBERRY								
(Aunt Jemima) frozen	3 pancakes	210	6	40	590	2	3.5	20
(Downyflake) frozen	3 pancakes	290	5	48	920	0	9.0	0
(Krusteaz) frozen, 4.5-oz serving	3 pancakes	280	8	49	710	0	5.0	14
(Pillsbury) frozen, microwave	3 pancakes	250	5	49	540	0	4.0	0
BUTTERMILK								
(Aunt Jemima)								
frozen, microwave	3 pancakes	210	6	40	600	2	3.5	20
frozen, microwave, 'Lite'	3 pancakes	140	7	28	660	0	3.0	0
(Downyflake) frozen	3 pancakes	280	5	45	920	0	9.0	0
(Krusteaz)								
frozen, 4.75-oz serving	3 pancakes	290	8	53	900	0	5.0	14
mini, frozen, microwave	1 serving	116	4	22	290	na	1.6	na
(Pillsbury)								
frozen, microwave	3 pancakes	260	6	51	590	0	4.0	0
mini, frozen, microwave	11 pancakes	230	5	44	550	1	4.0	10
(Weight Watchers) frozen, microwave, 2.5-oz serving	1/2 pkg	140	5	22	270	0	3.0	10
WHOLE WHEAT								
(Krusteaz) whole, and honey, frozen, 4.75-oz serving	3 pancakes	250	8	45	990	1	4.0	12
(Pillsbury) harvest, frozen, microwave	3 pancakes	240	6	48	420	0	4.0	0
PANCAKE BATTER								
(Aunt Jemima)								
blueberry, frozen	3.6 oz	204	5	39	688	2	4.0	27
buttermilk, frozen	3.6 oz	180	6	36	778	2	2.3	27
plain, frozen	3.6 oz	183	6	37	763	2	2.4	19
PANCAKE DISH/MEAL								
(Aunt Jemima)								
and sausages, frozen, 'Homestyle'	6 oz	420	12	57	1140	0	16.0	0

Food Name	Serv. Size	Total Cal.	Prot. gms	Carbs gms	Sod. mgs	Fiber gms	Fat gms	Chol. mgs
breakfast, lite, w/lite syrup, frozen, 'Homestyle'	6 oz	260	10	53	860	0	3.0	0
w/lite links, lite, frozen, 'Homestyle'	6 oz	310	14	43	970	0	10.0	0
(Downyflake) and sausages, frozen	5.5 oz	430	11	47	1170	0	23.0	0
(Great Starts)								
silver dollar sized, w/sausage	1 meal	340	9	36	670	1	18.0	70
w/bacon	1 meal	400	12	42	1030	1	20.0	100
w/sausage	1 meal	490	14	52	950	3	25.0	90
(Swanson) whole wheat, w/lite links, 'Great Starts'	5.5 oz	350	15	39	600	0	16.0	0
PANCAKE MIX. See also PANCAKE/WAFFLE MIX.								
(Betty Crocker) complete, mix only	1/3 cup	200	6	39	540	1	3.0	10
(Gluten Free Pantry) gluten-free, mix only	1 serving	130	3	28	270	1	1.0	5
(Sweet 'n Low) low-salt and -cholesterol,								
w/Sweet 'n Low prepared, 3-inch diam	5 pancakes	160	4	32	20	1	2.0	0
BUCKWHEAT								
(Hodgson Mill) whole grain, stone ground, mix only	1/3 cup	190	5	40	560	3	1.0	0
BUTTERMILK								
(Aunt Jemima) lower calorie, complete, mix only	1/3 cup	131	7	28	477	5	1.4	14
(Betty Crocker) complete, mix only	1/3 cup	200	5	39	540	1	2.5	10
(Hungry Jack)								
complete, mix only	1/3 cup	160	4	32	561	1	1.5	3
mix only	1/3 cup	160	4	33	651	1	1.5	0
(MET-RX Caffe) mix only	1/2 cup	200	12	33	590	2	3.0	0
(Robin Hood) mix only	1/3 cup	180	5	31	510	1	3.0	0
WHOLE WHEAT *(Hodgson Mill)* w/buttermilk, mix only	1/3 cup	120	4	28	550	4	1.0	0
PANCAKE SYRUP. See under SYRUP.								
PANCAKE/WAFFLE MIX								
(Arrowhead Mills)								
'Griddle Lite' mix only	1/2 cup	260	8	50	0	0	3.0	0
original style, mix only	1/4 cup	130	4	24	180	0	2.0	0
(Aunt Jemima)								
'Original' prepared, 4-inch diam	3 pancakes	116	3	25	609	1	0.8	0
complete, mix only	1/3 cup	165	5	34	408	1	1.7	13
(Bisquick) 'Shake 'n Pour' prepared, 4-inch diam	3 pancakes	260	6	48	850	1	5.0	0
(Downyflake) plain, prepared, 'Crisp & Healthy'	1 waffle	80	2	16	180	1	1.0	0
(Estee) prepared, 3-inch diam	3 pancakes	100	3	21	130	0	0.0	0
(Featherweight) prepared, 4-inch diam	3 pancakes	140	6	24	90	1	2.0	5
(Gold Medal) 'Pouch Mix' prepared w/egg	1/8 pouch	100	3	17	280	0	2.0	0
(Hungry Jack)								
'Panshakes' prepared, 4-inch diam	3 pancakes	250	7	43	880	1	6.0	0
light, complete, 'Extra Lights' mix only	1/17 pkg	180	4	38	730	1	3.0	0
light, complete, 'Extra Lights' prepared w/water, 4-inch diam	3 pancakes	180	4	38	730	1	3.0	0
light, complete, 'Extra Lights' prepared, 4-inch diam	3 pancakes	190	4	37	700	0	2.0	0
light, prepared w/3/4 cup skim milk, 2 tbsp oil, 2 egg whites, 4-inch diam	3 pancakes	170	6	28	500	1	4.0	0
light, regular, 'Extra Lights' mix only	1/17 pkg	180	4	38	730	1	3.0	0
light, regular, 'Extra Lights' prepared w/3/4 cup 2% milk, 2 tbsp oil, 1 egg, 4-inch diam	3 pancakes	190	5	28	490	1	6.0	55
light, regular, 'Extra Lights' prepared w/nonfat milk, 2 egg whites, 4-inch diam	3 pancakes	170	6	28	500	1	4.0	0
light, regular, 'Extra Lights' prepared w/water, 4-inch diam	3 pancakes	180	4	38	730	1	3.0	0
light, regular, 'Extra Lights' prepared, 4-inch diam	3 pancakes	210	6	30	490	0	7.0	0
pre-measured, mix only	1/2 pkt	200	5	38	780	1	3.5	0
pre-measured, prepared w/water, 4-inch diam	3 pancakes	180	4	33	650	0	3.0	0
regular, mix only	1/3 cup	150	3	32	640	1	1.5	0

Food Name	Serv. Size	Total Cal.	Prot. gms	Carbs gms	Sod. mgs	Fiber gms	Fat gms	Chol. mgs
(Martha White)								
'FlapStax' prepared w/water .... 1 pancake		80	3	17	320	0	1.0	0
'Light Crust' mix only .... 2 oz		120	4	20	290	0	3.0	25
(Robin Hood) 'Pouch Mix' prepared w/egg .... 1/8 pouch		100	3	17	280	0	2.0	0
APPLE CINNAMON								
(Bisquick) 'Shake 'n Pour' 4", prepared .... 3 pancakes		270	6	49	870	0	5.0	0
(Downyflake) 'Crisp & Healthy' .... 1 waffle		80	2	16	180	1	1.0	0
BLUEBERRY								
(Hungry Jack)								
microwave, mix only .... 3/4 pkg		230	5	47	550	1	4.0	10
prepared, 4-inch diam .... 3 pancakes		320	6	41	820	0	15.0	0
wild, mix only .... 1/5 pkg		170	3	38	780	0	1.0	0
wild, prepared w/ 1 1/4 cup milk, 1/4 cup oil,								
1 egg, 4-inch diam .... 3 pancakes		320	6	41	820	0	14.0	45
(Krusteaz) imitation, prepared, 4 inch diam .... 3 pancakes		205	5	39	660	0	4.0	14
BUCKWHEAT								
(Arrowhead Mills) mix only .... 1/2 cup		270	11	53	0	0	2.0	0
(Aunt Jemima) mix only .... 1/4 cup		105	4	24	488	3	0.9	0
(Don's Chuck Wagon) buckwheat, compete, mix only .... 1/3 cup		160	5	33	550	1	1.0	0
(Krusteaz) buckwheat, prepared, 4-inch diam .... 3 pancakes		215	8	40	770	6	3.0	9
BUTTERMILK								
(Aunt Jemima)								
complete, 'Lite' prepared, 4-inch diam .... 3 pancakes		130	7	25	570	0	2.0	0
complete, mix only .... 1/3 cup		162	5	32	408	2	1.7	93
original, prepared, 4-inch diam .... 3 pancakes		122	4	26	698	1	0.7	1
(Betty Crocker)								
complete, prepared, 4-inch diam .... 3 pancakes		210	5	41	500	0	3.0	0
original, mix only .... 1/2 cup		170	4	36	760	0	1.0	0
original, prepared, 4-inch diam .... 3 pancakes		210	5	41	500	0	3.0	0
original, prepared w/2/3 cup milk, 1 tbsp oil, egg,								
4-inch diam .... 3 pancakes		280	8	39	810	0	10.0	0
(Bob's Red Mill) mix only .... 1/2 cup		190	4	11	26	1	1.0	2
(Downyflake) 'Jumbo' .... 2 waffles		170	4	30	630	0	4.0	0
(Health Valley) 'Biscuit & Pancake' mix only .... 1 oz		100	4	20	170	3	1.0	0
(Hungry Jack) complete, mix only .... 1/17 pkg		180	5	38	720	1	1.0	5
(Hungry Jack)								
complete, packets, prepared, 4-inch diam .... 3 pancakes		180	4	35	680	0	3.0	0
complete, prepared, 4-inch diam .... 3 pancakes		180	4	39	710	0	1.0	0
complete, prepared w/water, 4-inch diam .... 3 pancakes		180	5	38	720	1	1.0	5
microwave, mix ony .... 3/4 pkg		260	5	51	590	1	4.0	10
original, mix only .... 1/25 pkg		120	3	26	530	1	0.0	0
original, prepared, 4-inch diam .... 3 pancakes		240	7	29	570	0	11.0	0
original, prepared w/2/3 cup 2% milk, 2 tbsp oil,								
1 egg, 4-inch diam .... 3 pancakes		210	6	28	560	1	9.0	55
original, prepared w/2/3 cup nonfat milk, 2 tbsp oil,								
2 egg whites, 4-inch diam .... 3 pancakes		200	6	28	570	1	7.0	0
(Krusteaz) prepared, 4-inch diam .... 3 pancakes		200	5	39	770	0	3.0	10
CORN *(Arrowhead Mills)* blue corn, mix only .... 1/3 cup		150	4	28	130	0	2.0	0
MULTIGRAIN *(Arrowhead Mills)* mix only .... 1/2 cup		350	12	70	0	1	2.0	0
OAT BRAN								
(Arrowhead Mills) oat bran, mix only .... 1/2 cup		200	9	64	0	2	2.0	0
(Bisquick) 'Shake 'n Pour' prepared, 4-inch diam .... 3 pancakes		240	7	45	580	1	4.0	0
(Hungry Jack) microwave, mix onlry .... 3/4 pkg		230	6	45	580	3	4.0	10
(Krusteaz) 'Lite' prepared, 4-inch diam .... 3 pancakes		130	5	36	370	10	1.0	0
WHOLE WHEAT								
(Aunt Jemima)								
mix only .... 1/4 cup		120	6	26	519	3	0.5	0

Food Name	Serv. Size	Total Cal.	Prot. gms	Carbs gms	Sod. mgs	Fiber gms	Fat gms	Chol. mgs
prepared, 4-inch diam	3 pancakes	161	7	35	892	4	1.0	0
(Hungry Jack) harvest, microwave, mix only	3/4 pkg	230	6	46	560	3	4.0	10
(Krusteaz) w/honey, prepared, 4' diam	3 pancakes	215	8	42	630	5	1.0	9
(Stone-Buhr) mix only	1/4 cup	120	5	28	330	3	1.0	0
PAPAYA								
raw, cubed	1 cup	55	1	14	4	3	0.2	0
raw, mashed	1 cup	90	1	23	7	4	0.3	0
raw, whole, large, 5.75 inch long, 3.25 inch diam	1 papaya	148	2	37	11	7	0.5	0
raw, whole, medium, 5 1/8 inch long, 3 inch diam	1 papaya	119	2	30	9	5	0.4	0
raw, whole, small, 4.5 inch long, 2.75 inch diam	1 papaya	59	1	15	5	3	0.2	0
PAPAYA DRINK. See under FRUIT DRINK; FRUIT JUICE DRINK.								
PAPAYA JUICE (Knudsen) creamed	8 fl oz	160	0	40	40	na	0.0	0
PAPRIKA								
ground	1 tbsp	20	1	4	2	1	0.9	0
ground	1 tsp	6	0	1	1	0	0.3	0
ground (Durkee)	1 tsp	8	0	0	0	0	0.0	0
ground (Laurel Leaf)	1 tsp	8	0	0	0	0	0.0	0
ground (McCormick/Schilling)	1 tsp	9	0	1	2	1	0.4	0
ground (Spice Islands)	1 tsp	7	0	1	1	0	0.2	0
PARANUT. See BRAZIL NUT.								
PARROTFISH/pollyfish								
raw	1 lb	390	87.5	0.0	(mq)	0	1.8	(mq)
raw	1 oz	24	5.5	0.0	(mq)	0	0.1	(mq)
PARSLEY								
dried	1 tbsp	4	0	1	6	0	0.1	0
dried	1 tsp	1	0	0	1	0	0.0	0
dried (McCormick/Schilling)	1 tsp	2	0	0	2	0	0.0	0
freeze-dried	1/4 cup	4	0	1	5	0	0.1	0
freeze-dried	1 tbsp	1	0	0	2	0	0.0	0
fresh, raw	1 cup	22	2	4	34	2	0.5	0
fresh, raw	10 sprigs	4	0	1	6	0	0.1	0
fresh, raw	1 tbsp	1	0	0	2	0	0.0	0
PARSLEY FLAKES								
(Spice Islands)	1 tsp	4	0	1	6	0	0.1	0
ground (Durkee)	1 tsp	1	0	0	0	0	0.0	0
ground (Laurel Leaf)	1 tsp	1	0	0	0	0	0.0	0
PARSLEY ROOT/Hamburg parsley/turnip-rooted parsley								
fresh	1 lb	50	12.7	10.4	454	5.9	2.7	0
fresh	1 oz	3	0.8	0.7	28	0.4	0.2	0
PARSLEY SEASONING. See under SEASONING MIX.								
PARSNIP								
boiled, drained, sliced	1/2 cup	63	1	15	8	3	0.2	0
boiled, drained, whole, approx 9 inch long	1 parsnip	130	2	31	16	6	0.5	0
raw, sliced	1 cup	100	2	24	13	7	0.4	0
PARTY MIX								
(Michael Season's)								
spicy, low-fat, original	1 oz	110	2	23	280	1	1.5	0
traditional, low-fat	1 oz	120	3	23	320	1	1.5	0
PASSIONFRUIT/granadilla								
purple, raw, sliced	1 cup	229	5	55	66	25	1.7	0
purple, raw, whole, trimmed	1 fruit	17	0	4	5	2	0.1	0
PASSIONFRUIT JUICE								
purple	1 cup	126	1	34	15	0	0.1	0
purple	1 fl oz	16	0	4	2	0	0.0	0
yellow	1 cup	148	2	36	15	0	0.4	0
yellow	1 fl oz	19	0	4	2	0	0.1	0

Food Name	Serv. Size	Total Cal.	Prot. gms	Carbs gms	Sod. mgs	Fiber gms	Fat gms	Chol. mgs
PASTA. See also NOODLE.								
(NOTE: 2 ounces uncooked pasta = approximately 1 cup cooked.)								
(Al Dente) wild mushroom, dry	2 oz	220	8	40	20	0	2.0	0
(Creamette)								
dry	2 oz	210	7	42	0	0	1.0	0
rainbow, dry	2 oz	210	8	42	5	1	1.0	0
vegetable, dry	2 oz	210	8	42	5	1	1.0	0
w/egg, dry	2 oz	221	8	40	3	1	2.5	7
(De Boles)								
rainbow, dry, 'Primavera'	2 oz	200	8	41	8	0	1.0	0
vegetable, dry, 'Primavera' dry	2 oz	200	8	41	8	0	1.0	0
(Golden Grain) dry	2 oz	203	8	41	26	0	0.7	0
(Misura) whole wheat, w/bran, dry	2 oz	197	6	40	16	0	1.0	0
(Mueller's) 'Super Shapes' dry	2 oz	210	7	42	0	1	1.0	0
(Pastamania!)								
beet, spinach, and tomato	2 oz	200	8	40	10	1	1.0	0
oat bran, natural, gourmet, dry	2 oz	209	8	41	7	2	1.0	0
(Ronzoni) dry	2 oz	210	7	41	5	0	1.0	0
ACINI PEPE (Ronzoni) enriched, dry	2 oz	210	7	42	0	0	1.0	0
AGNOLOTTI (Contadina) refrigerated, 'Fresh'	3 oz	270	13	38	230	0	7.0	40
ANGEL HAIR								
(American Beauty) 100% durum wheat semolina, dry	2 oz	210	7	42	0	0	1.0	0
(Contadina)	1 1/4 cup	240	10	43	30	2	3.0	90
(Creamette) enriched, dry	2 oz	210	7	42	0	2	1.0	0
(De Boles)								
Jerusalem artichoke, dry	2 oz	210	7	41	0	1	1.0	0
Jerusalem artichoke, garlic and parsley, dry	2 oz	210	7	41	5	2	1.0	0
Jerusalem artichoke, tomato and basil, dry	2 oz	210	7	41	0	2	1.0	0
Jerusalem artichoke, tomato and lemon pepper, dry	2 oz	200	8	40	10	1	1.0	0
Jerusalem artichoke, whole wheat, dry	2 oz	210	7	40	0	5	2.0	0
(DiGiorno) refrigerated, uncooked	3 oz	250	11	47	140	0	3.0	0
(Hodgson Mill) 100% durum whole wheat flour, dry	2 oz	190	9	34	10	6	1.0	0
(Westbrae) corn, dry	2 oz	210	4	46	10	0	2.0	0
BOW TIE								
(De Cecco) farfelle, enriched, dry	2 oz	210	7	41	0	0	1.0	0
(Garden Time) four-color, dry	2 oz	203	8	41	1	1	1.0	0
(Hodgson Mill) whole wheat, dry	2 oz	190	9	34	10	6	1.0	0
(Mueller's) dry	2 oz	220	8	38	10	1	3.0	65
(Pasta Perfect) dry	1 cup	140	5	26	20	3	2.0	25
(Ronzoni) enriched, dry	2 oz	210	7	42	0	0	1.0	0
(Westbrae) vegetable, dry	2 oz	190	9	39	10	5	2.0	0
CAPELLINI								
(American Beauty) 100% durum wheat semolina, dry	2 oz	210	7	42	0	0	1.0	0
CORN (Westbrae) corn, dry	2 oz	210	4	46	10	0	2.0	0
CURLS (Ancient Harvest) quinoa, wheat-free, dry	2 oz	180	5	35	5	3	2.0	0
FARFALLE. See BOW TIE.								
FETTUCCINE								
(Al Dente)								
basil, dry	2 oz	220	8	40	20	0	2.0	0
curry, dry	2 oz	220	8	40	20	0	2.0	0
dill, dry	2 oz	220	8	40	20	0	2.0	0
spinach, dry	2 oz	220	8	40	20	0	2.0	0
tarragon, dry	2 oz	220	8	40	20	0	2.0	0
whole wheat, dry	2 oz	210	8	42	10	0	1.0	0
(American Beauty)								
spinach and egg, enriched, dry, 'Florentine'	2 oz	220	8	42	35	0	3.0	65
(Antoine's) egg, enriched, dry	2 oz	210	7	41	0	0	1.0	0

Food Name	Serv. Size	Total Cal.	Prot. gms	Carbs gms	Sod. mgs	Fiber gms	Fat gms	Chol. mgs
(Contadina)								
.... 1 1/4 cup		250	10	45	30	2	3.5	85
cholesterol-free .... 1 cup		240	9	46	16	2	3.0	0
(De Boles)								
cholesterol-free, low-sodium, low-fat .... 2 oz		210	7	41	0	2	1.0	0
Jerusalem artichoke, dry .... 2 oz		210	7	41	0	1	1.0	0
Jerusalem artichoke, spinach, dry .... 2 oz		210	9	41	5	0	1.0	0
Jerusalem artichoke, tomato and lemon pepper, dry ...... 2 oz		200	6	40	10	1	1.0	0
Jerusalem artichoke, tomato and pesto, dry .... 2 oz		210	7	41	5	2	1.0	0
(De Cecco) egg, dry, 'Home-Style' .... 2 oz		210	8	40	35	0	3.0	0
(DiGiorno)								
dry, approx 1 1/3 cups cooked .... 3 oz		250	11	47	140	0	3.0	0
spinach, dry, approx 1 1/3 cups cooked .... 3 oz		250	12	46	140	0	3.0	0
(Eden Foods)								
bell pepper basil, dry, 'Herb's' .... 2 oz		220	10	42	5	2	2.0	60
parsley garlic, dry, 'Herb's' .... 2 oz		220	10	42	5	2	2.0	60
spinach, dry, 'Herb's' .... 2 oz		220	10	42	5	2	2.0	60
(Hodgson Mill) whole wheat, dry .... 2 oz		190	9	34	10	6	1.0	0
(Pastamania!)								
durum wheat, dry .... 2 oz		200	8	38	20	1	2.0	30
garlic and parsley, dry .... 2 oz		200	8	38	20	1	2.0	30
garlic, parsley, and basil, dry .... 2 oz		200	8	38	20	1	2.0	30
spinach and durum wheat, dry .... 2 oz		200	8	38	30	1	2.0	35
w/Jerusalem artichoke .... 2 oz		210	8	41	10	2	2.0	na
w/lemon and pepper, dry .... 2 oz		220	8	40	15	2	3.0	35
w/mushrooms, dry .... 2 oz		210	8	41	15	2	2.0	35
(Ronzoni) egg, extra long, enriched, dry .... 2 oz		220	8	42	15	0	3.0	65
(Rummo) nested, dry .... 2 oz		210	7	41	4	0	1.0	0
FUSILLI								
(Antoine's)								
rainbow, dry .... 2 oz		210	7	41	20	0	1.0	0
tricolor, dry .... 2 oz		210	7	41	20	0	1.0	0
tricolor, vegetable, enriched, dry .... 2 oz		210	7	41	25	2	1.0	0
vegetable, dry .... 2 oz		210	7	41	20	0	1.0	0
(De Cecco)								
enriched, dry .... 2 oz		210	7	41	0	0	1.0	0
spinach, enriched, dry .... 2 oz		210	7	41	5	0	1.0	0
(Pastamania!) tomato and spinach, tre colore, dry .... 2 oz		200	7	40	20	2	1.0	0
GEMELLI								
(Antoine's) macaroni, enriched, dry .... 2 oz		210	7	41	0	0	1.0	0
LASAGNA								
(American Beauty) 100% durum wheat semolina, dry ...... 2 oz		210	7	42	0	0	1.0	0
(Bernardi)								
sheets .... 1 piece		250	9	47	15	2	3.0	5
sheets, wavy .... 1 piece		310	12	60	20	2	2.5	5
(Creamette) 100% semolina, enriched, dry .... 2 oz		210	7	42	0	0	1.0	0
(De Boles)								
Jerusalem artichoke, dry .... 2 oz		210	7	41	0	1	1.0	0
whole wheat, dry.................................. 2 oz		210	9	40	0	0	2.0	0
(De Cecco) 100% semolina, dry .... 2 oz		210	7	41	0	0	1.0	0
(Ener-G Foods) gluten-free, dry .... 2 oz		214	4	42	1	2	0.1	1
(Health Valley)								
whole wheat, dry.................................. 2 oz		170	9	40	10	7	1.0	0
whole wheat, spinach, dry .... 2 oz		170	9	40	15	7	1.0	0
(Hodgson Mill) whole wheat, dry .... 2 oz		190	9	34	10	6	1.0	0
(Mueller's) dry .... 2 oz		210	7	42	0	1	1.0	0
(Ronzoni) curly edge, enriched, dry .... 2 oz		210	7	42	0	0	1.0	0

Food Name	Serv. Size	Total Cal.	Prot. gms	Carbs gms	Sod. mgs	Fiber gms	Fat gms	Chol. mgs
(Westbrae)								
spinach, whole wheat, no egg, dry	2 oz	210	8	40	0	6	2.0	0
whole wheat, no egg, dry	2 oz	210	8	40	0	7	2.0	0
LINGUINE								
(Ancient Harvest) quinoa, wheat-free, dry	2 oz	180	5	35	5	3	2.0	0
(Creamette) enriched, dry	2 oz	210	7	42	0	0	1.0	0
(De Boles) Jerusalem artichoke, dry	2 oz	210	7	41	0	1	1.0	0
(De Cecco) enriched, dry	2 oz	210	7	41	0	0	1.0	0
(DiGiorno)								
dry, approx 1 1/3 cups cooked	3 oz	250	11	46	135	0	3.0	0
refrigerated, uncooked	3 oz	250	11	47	140	0	3.0	0
(Pastamania!) durum wheat, dry	2 oz	200	8	38	20	1	2.0	30
(Quinoa) quinoa, wheat-free, dry	2 oz	180	5	35	5	3	2.0	0
(Ronzoni) enriched, dry	2 oz	210	7	42	0	0	1.0	0
MACARONI								
	2 oz	211	7	43	4	1	0.9	0
elbows, enriched, cooked	1 cup	197	7	40	1	2	0.9	0
elbows, enriched, dry	1 cup	390	13	78	7	3	1.7	0
elbows, unenriched, cooked	1 cup	197	7	40	1	2	0.9	0
elbows, unenriched, dry	1 cup	390	13	78	7	3	1.7	0
elbows, whole wheat, cooked	1 cup elbows	174	7	37	4	4	0.8	0
elbows, whole wheat, dry	1 cup elbows	198	8	43	5	5	0.8	0
small shells, dry	1 cup	345	12	69	7	2	1.5	0
spirals, enriched, cooked	1 cup	189	6	38	1	2	0.9	0
spirals, enriched, dry	1 cup	312	11	63	6	2	1.3	0
spirals, vegetable, enriched, dry	1 cup spirals	209	7	43	25	2	0.6	0
spirals, whole wheat, dry	1 cup spirals	365	15	79	8	9	1.5	0
vegetable, enriched, cooked	1 cup	172	6	36	8	6	0.1	0
vegetable, enriched, dry	1 cup	308	11	63	36	4	0.9	0
(American Beauty)								
elbows, 100% durum wheat semolina, dry	2 oz	210	7	42	0	0	1.0	0
100% durum wheat semolina, dry, 'Curly-Roni'	2 oz	210	7	42	0	0	1.0	0
(Ancient Harvest)								
elbows, quinoa, wheat-free, dry	2 oz	180	5	36	5	3	2.0	0
elbows, wheat-free, gluten-free	2 oz	180	5	35	5	3	2.0	0
(Creamette) elbows, enriched, dry	2 oz	210	7	42	0	0	1.0	0
(De Boles)								
elbows, corn, wheat-free, dry	2 oz	210	5	45	0	1	1.0	0
elbows, dry, 'Primavera'	2 oz	210	9	41	0	0	1.0	0
elbows, Jerusalem artichoke, dry	2 oz	210	7	41	0	1	1.0	0
elbows, whole wheat and Jerusalem artichoke, dry	2 oz	210	7	40	0	5	2.0	0
(Delmonico) dry	2 oz	210	7	42	0	0	1.0	0
(Eden Foods)								
elbows, whole wheat, vegetable	2 oz	210	7	42	10	2	1.0	0
elbows, whole-grain, organic, dry	2 oz	210	10	39	0	6	1.5	0
(Eden Foods) elbows, whole-grain, organic, dry	2 oz	210	10	39	0	6	1.5	0
(Ener-G Foods)								
brown rice, gluten-free, dry	2 oz	212	4	44	1	2	0.1	0
rice, gluten-free, dry	2 oz	214	4	42	1	2	0.1	1
shells, rice, gluten free, dry	2 oz	214	4	42	1	2	0.1	0
(Gioia) dry	2 oz	210	7	41	0	0	1.0	0
(Hodgson Mill) elbows, whole wheat, dry	2 oz	190	9	34	10	6	1.0	na
(Hospitality) elbows, enriched, dry, 'Valu Pack'	1/2 cup	240	8	48	0	2	0.5	0
(P&R) dry	2 oz	210	7	42	0	0	1.0	0
(Prince) dry	2 oz	210	7	43	5	0	1.0	0
(Quinoa) elbows, quinoa, wheat-free, dry	2 oz	180	5	36	5	3	2.0	0
(Ronzoni) dry	2 oz	210	7	41	5	0	1.0	0

Food Name	Serv. Size	Total Cal.	Prot. gms	Carbs gms	Sod. mgs	Fiber gms	Fat gms	Chol. mgs
(San Giorgio) dry, 'Italian/American Style'	2 oz	210	7	42	0	0	1.0	0
(Westbrae) elbows, corn, dry	2 oz	210	4	46	10	0	2.0	0
MANICOTTI *(Ronzoni)* extra fancy, enriched, dry	2 oz	210	7	42	0	0	1.0	0
MOSTACCIOLI								
(American Beauty)								
100% durum wheat semolina, dry	2 oz	210	7	42	0	0	1.0	0
tricolor, 'Italiano' dry	2 oz	210	7	42	0	0	1.0	0
(Creamette) enriched, dry	2 oz	210	7	42	0	2	1.0	0
(Ronzoni) enriched, dry	2 oz	210	9	40	0	2	1.0	0
ORZO *(Ronzoni)* enriched, dry	2 oz	210	7	42	0	0	3.0	0
PAGODAS								
(Ancient Harvest)								
garden	2 oz	180	5	35	5	3	2.0	0
garden, gluten-free	2 oz	180	5	35	5	3	2.0	0
PENNE *(Hodgson Mill)* whole wheat, dry	2 oz	190	9	34	10	6	1.0	0
PENNE RIGATI								
(Antoine's) uncooked	2 oz	210	7	41	0	0	1.0	0
(De Cecco) macaroni, enriched, dry	2 oz	210	7	41	0	0	1.0	0
PENNONI *(De Cecco)* macaroni, enriched, dry	2 oz	210	7	41	0	0	1.0	0
RADIATORE								
(Antoine's) macaroni, enriched, dry	2 oz	210	7	41	0	0	1.0	0
(Hodgson Mill)								
four colors	2 oz	200	8	41	15	1	1.0	0
whole wheat, dry	2 oz	190	9	34	10	6	1.0	0
(Ronzoni) tomato and spinach, tri-color, macaroni, dry	2 oz	210	7	42	30	0	1.0	0
RIBBON								
(Creamette)								
spinach, enriched, dry	2 oz	210	7	42	70	0	1.0	0
yolk-free, dry, 'Dutch'	2 oz	210	7	42	0	0	1.0	0
(De Boles) whole wheat and Jerusalem artichoke, dry	2 oz	210	7	40	0	5	2.0	0
(Eden Foods)								
extra fine, organic, dry	2 oz	220	8	44	0	3	1.0	0
mixed vegetable, dry, 'Herb's'	2 oz	220	10	42	5	2	2.0	60
paella, organic, dry	2 oz	220	8	44	0	3	1.0	0
paella, wheat, w/saffron, organic, dry	2 oz	228	8	44	0	0	1.0	0
parsley garlic, organic, dry	2 oz	220	8	44	0	3	1.0	0
pesto, organic, dry	2 oz	220	8	44	0	3	1.0	0
wheat, parsley garlic, organic, dry	2 oz	228	8	44	0	0	1.0	0
whole grain, dry, 'Herb's' dry	2 oz	200	8	40	10	7	1.5	0
whole grain, spinach, organic, dry	2 oz	200	8	40	10	7	1.5	0
(Hodgson Mill) whole wheat, dry	2 oz	190	10	34	15	5	1.0	0
RIGATONI								
(Creamette) enriched, dry	2 oz	210	7	42	0	0	1.0	0
(De Boles)								
Jerusalem artichoke, dry	2 oz	210	7	41	0	1	1.0	0
Jerusalem artichoke, dry, 'Primavera'	2 oz	210	7	41	0	1	1.0	0
(De Cecco) enriched, dry	2 oz	210	7	41	0	0	1.0	0
(Ronzoni) enriched, dry	2 oz	210	7	42	0	0	1.0	0
ROTELLE								
(American Beauty) 100% durum wheat semolina, dry	2 oz	210	7	42	30	0	1.0	0
(Ancient Harvest) quinoa, wheat-free, dry	2 oz	180	5	35	5	3	2.0	0
(Creamette) enriched, dry	2 oz	210	7	42	0	0	1.0	0
(De Cecco) enriched, dry	2 oz	210	7	41	0	0	1.0	0
(Pastamania!) beet, spinach, and tomato, dry	2 oz	200	8	40	10	1	1.0	0
(Quinoa)								
quinoa, dry	2 oz	210	10	40	11	8	1.0	0
quinoa, wheat-free, dry	2 oz	180	5	35	5	3	2.0	0

Food Name	Serv. Size	Total Cal.	Prot. gms	Carbs gms	Sod. mgs	Fiber gms	Fat gms	Chol. mgs
(Ronzoni) enriched, dry	2 oz	210	9	40	0	2	1.0	0
ROTINI								
(American Beauty)								
100% durum wheat semolina, dry	2 oz	210	7	42	0	0	1.0	0
quinoa, dry	2 oz	210	10	40	11	8	1.0	0
tricolor, 'Italiano' dry	2 oz	210	7	42	0	0	1.0	0
wheat and quinoa, organic, low-salt, no cholesterol	2 oz	210	10	42	8	7	1.0	0
(Bernardi) vegetable	1 1/4 cup	220	9	44	15	2	1.0	0
(Creamette) enriched, dry	2 oz	210	7	42	0	0	1.0	0
(De Boles)								
Jerusalem artichoke, dry	2 oz	210	7	41	0	1	1.0	0
Jerusalem artichoke, garlic and parsley, dry	2 oz	210	7	41	5	2	1.0	0
Jerusalem artichoke, tomato and basil, dry	2 oz	210	7	41	0	2	1.0	0
vegetable, dry, 'Primavera'	2 oz	210	9	41	0	0	1.0	0
(Eden Foods) mixed vegetable	2 oz	210	7	42	10	2	1.0	0
(Hodgson Mill) vegetable, four flavors, dry	2 oz	200	8	na	15	1	1.0	0
(Pasta Perfect)								
....	1 cup	140	5	28	0	1	0.0	0
spinach	1 cup	140	5	27	0	1	0.0	0
RUFFLE								
(Mueller's) trio, dry	2 oz	210	7	42	10	1	1.0	0
SHELLS								
(American Beauty)								
100% durum wheat semolina, dry	2 oz	210	9	40	0	2	1.0	0
100% durum wheat semolina, macaroni, dry	2 oz	210	7	42	0	0	1.0	0
large, durum wheat semolina, dry	2 oz	210	7	42	0	0	1.0	0
medium, durum wheat semolina, dry	2 oz	210	7	42	0	0	1.0	0
tricolor, 'Italiano' dry	2 oz	210	7	42	0	0	1.0	0
(Ancient Harvest) quinoa, wheat-free, dry	2 oz	180	5	35	5	3	2.0	0
(Creamette) medium, enriched, dry	2 oz	210	7	42	0	0	1.0	0
(De Boles)								
....	2 oz	210	7	41	0	1	1.0	0
corn, wheat-free, dry	2 oz	210	5	45	0	0	1.0	0
dry, 'Primavera'	2 oz	210	9	41	0	0	1.0	0
whole wheat and Jerusalem artichoke, dry	2 oz	210	7	40	0	5	2.0	0
(Eden Foods)								
vegetable, organic, dry	2 oz	210	8	42	10	2	1.0	0
w/mixed vegetable, dry, 'Herb's'	2 oz	210	7	42	10	2	1.0	0
wheat, vegetable, no eggs, organic, dry	2 oz	228	8	44	0	0	1.0	0
(Hodgson Mill) whole wheat, medium	2 oz	190	9	34	10	6	1.0	0
(Mueller's)								
dry	2 oz	210	7	42	0	1	1.0	0
jumbo, dry	2 oz	210	7	42	0	1	1.0	0
(Pasta Perfect)	1 cup	140	5	28	0	1	0.0	0
(Pastamania!) tomato and spinach, dry	2 oz	200	8	40	10	1	1.0	0
(Quinoa) quinoa 'Supergrain Wheat-free' dry	2 oz	180	5	35	5	3	2.0	0
(Ronzoni)								
enriched, dry	2 oz	210	7	42	0	0	1.0	0
extra fancy, enriched, dry	2 oz	210	7	42	0	0	1.0	0
jumbo, enriched, dry	2 oz	210	7	42	0	0	1.0	0
(Westbrae) corn, dry	2 oz	210	4	46	10	0	2.0	0
SPAGHETTI								
enriched, cooked	1 cup	197	7	40	1	2	0.9	0
protein-fortified, cooked	1 cup	230	11	44	7	2	0.3	0
unenriched, cooked	1 cup	197	7	40	1	2	0.9	0
(Al Dente) pepper, 'Three Pepper Pasta' dry	2 oz	220	8	40	20	0	2.0	0
(American Beauty) 100% durum wheat semolina, dry	2 oz	210	7	42	0	0	1.0	0

Food Name	Serv. Size	Total Cal.	Prot. gms	Carbs gms	Sod. mgs	Fiber gms	Fat gms	Chol. mgs
(Ancient Harvest) quinoa, wheat-free, dry	2 oz	180	5	35	5	3	2.0	0
(Creamette)								
dry	2 oz	210	7	42	5	0	1.0	0
enriched, thin, dry	2 oz	210	7	42	0	0	1.0	0
spinach, w/egg, uncooked	2 oz	220	8	40	65	1	3.0	70
(De Boles)								
corn, wheat-free, dry	2 oz	210	5	45	0	0	1.0	0
Jerusalem artichoke, dry	2 oz	210	7	41	0	1	1.0	0
Jerusalem artichoke, spinach	2 oz	200	7	41	30	2	1.0	0
whole wheat and Jerusalem artichoke, dry	2 oz	210	7	40	0	5	2.0	0
(DiGiorno) uncooked, approx 1 1/3 cups cooked	3 oz	250	11	47	140	0	3.0	0
(Eden Foods)								
durum wheat, organic, dry	2 oz	210	8	42	10	2	1.0	0
kamut, whole grain, organic, dry	2 oz	210	10	38	0	6	1.5	0
parsley garlic, organic, dry	2 oz	210	7	42	10	2	1.0	0
whole grain, organic, dry	2 oz	210	10	39	0	6	1.5	0
(Ener-G Foods)								
brown rice, gluten-free, dry	2 oz	212	4	44	1	2	0.1	0
rice, gluten-free, dry	2 oz	214	4	42	1	2	0.1	1
(Health Valley)								
amaranth, dry	2 oz	170	7	40	10	9	1.0	0
oat bran, dry	2 oz	120	4	23	2	4	1.0	0
whole wheat, dry	2 oz	170	9	40	10	7	1.0	0
whole wheat, spinach, dry	2 oz	170	9	40	10	7	1.0	0
(Hodgson Mill)								
durum whole wheat, thin, dry	2 oz	190	9	34	25	6	1.0	0
whole wheat, spinach, dry	2 oz	190	9	35	25	5	2.0	0
(Hospitality) enriched, 100% semolina, dry	2 oz	210	7	42	0	2	0.5	0
(Quinoa) quinoa, 'Supergrain'	2 oz	210	10	40	11	8	1.0	0
(Ronzoni)								
enriched, dry	2 oz	210	7	42	0	0	1.0	0
enriched, thin, dry	2 oz	210	7	42	0	0	1.0	0
(Rummo) dry	2 oz	210	7	41	10	0	1.0	0
(Westbrae)								
corn, dry	2 oz	210	4	46	10	0	2.0	0
whole wheat, no egg, dry	2 oz	210	8	40	0	7	2.0	0
whole wheat, spinach, no egg, dry	2 oz	210	8	40	0	6	2.0	0
SPAGHETTINI *(De Cecco)* enriched, dry	2 oz	210	7	41	0	0	1.0	0
SPIRAL								
(American Beauty)								
rainbow, 100% durum wheat semolina, dry	2 oz	210	7	42	30	0	1.0	0
(Antoine's) spicy, uncooked	2 oz	210	7	41	40	0	1.0	0
(Eden Foods)								
kamut, whole grain, organic, dry	2 oz	210	10	38	0	6	1.5	0
sesame rice, whole grain, organic, dry	2 oz	200	10	37	0	6	2.0	0
vegetable, whole grain, organic, dry	2 oz	210	10	39	0	6	1.5	0
wheat, sesame rice, organic, dry	2 oz	212	10	40	0	0	1.0	0
wheat, vegetable, no eggs, organic, dry	2 oz	228	8	44	0	0	1.0	0
(Hodgson Mill) whole wheat, whole grain, dry	2 oz	190	9	34	10	6	1.0	0
(Mueller's) 'Twist Trio' dry	2 oz	210	7	42	10	1	1.0	0
TAGLIATELLE								
(Contadina) spinach	1 1/4 cup	270	12	46	110	4	4.0	105
(Ener-G Foods)								
brown rice, gluten-free, dry	2 oz	212	4	44	1	2	0.1	0
rice, gluten-free, dry	2 oz	214	4	42	1	2	0.1	1
TAGLIERINI *(Pastamania!)* tomato and spinach, dry	2 oz	210	8	40	20	2	2.0	35
TRICOLOR								
(Creamette) dry	2 oz	210	8	42	5	1	1.0	0

Food Name	Serv. Size	Total Cal.	Prot. gms	Carbs gms	Sod. mgs	Fiber gms	Fat gms	Chol. mgs
TRICOLOR PASTA, PRIMAVERA								
(De Boles) tricolor, 'Primavera' dry .... 2 oz	2 oz	200	8	41	8	0	1.0	0
WAGON WHEEL *(Hodgson Mill)* four flavors, dry .... 2 oz	2 oz	200	8	41	15	1	1.0	0
VERMICELLI								
(American Beauty) 100% durum wheat semolina, dry ...... 2 oz	2 oz	210	7	42	0	0	1.0	0
(Creamette) enriched, extra thin, dry .... 2 oz	2 oz	210	7	42	0	0	1.0	0
(Ener-G Foods) rice, gluten-free, dry .... 2 oz	2 oz	214	4	42	1	2	0.1	0
(Ronzoni) enriched, dry .... 2 oz	2 oz	210	7	42	0	0	1.0	0
WHEAT								
(De Boles) whole wheat 'Natural Gourmet' dry .... 2 oz	2 oz	200	7	40	0	6	1.0	0
ZITI								
(De Boles)								
.... 2 oz	2 oz	210	7	41	0	1	1.0	0
Jerusalem artichoke, dry .... 2 oz	2 oz	210	7	41	0	1	1.0	0
(Ronzoni) enriched, dry .... 2 oz	2 oz	210	7	42	0	0	1.0	0
PASTA CHIPS								
(Bachman) pasta snack chip 'Pastapazazz' .... 1 oz	1 oz	150	2	15	340	0	9.0	0
PASTA DISH/ENTRÉE. See also LASAGNA/LASAGNA ENTRÉE; MANICOTTI/MANICOTTI ENTRÉE; RAVIOLI DISH/ENTRÉE; TORTELLINI DISH/ENTRÉE.								
(Budget Gourmet)								
w/chicken, in wine and mushroom sauce w/chicken ... 1 entrée	1 entrée	280	15	40	890	3	7.0	25
(Celentano) and cheese, baked, frozen .... 6 oz	6 oz	290	12	29	350	0	13.0	0
(Chef Boyardee)								
rings and franks, microwave .... 7.5 oz	7.5 oz	190	7	31	980	3	5.0	20
rings and meatballs, microwave .... 7.5 oz	7.5 oz	220	8	33	990	4	8.0	25
(Contadina) chicken, herb, w/tomato sauce, frozen .... 1 oz	1 oz	27	2	4	54	na	0.6	3
(Green Giant)								
Dijon, frozen, 'Microwave Garden Gourmet' .... 1 pkg	1 pkg	300	7	24	560	3	20.0	0
Parmesan, w/sweet peas, frozen, 'One Serving' .... 5.5 oz	5.5 oz	160	9	21	420	3	5.0	10
(Healthy Choice)								
primavera, microwave .... 11 oz	11 oz	280	11	51	360	0	3.0	15
vegetable, Italiano .... 1 entrée	1 entrée	250	9	48	480	6	3.0	10
w/chicken, teriyaki, frozen, 'Classics' .... 12.6 oz	12.6 oz	350	24	58	370	0	3.0	45
w/shrimp, frozen, 'Classics' .... 12.5 oz	12.5 oz	270	16	44	490	0	4.0	50
(Lean Cuisine)								
cheddar bake .... 1 entrée	1 entrée	220	12	29	560	3	6.0	20
w/chicken and herb tomato sauce, frozen .... 9.5 oz	9.5 oz	270	17	38	460	0	6.0	35
w/turkey, Dijon sauce, frozen, 'Lunch Express' .... 9 7/8 oz	9 7/8 oz	290	18	39	540	0	7.0	35
(Lunch Bucket)								
chicken, Italian, lunch cup, 'Light'n Healthy' .... 7.5 oz	7.5 oz	130	7	23	630	0	1.0	10
(Lunch Express)								
and tuna, casserole .... 1 entrée	1 entrée	280	18	39	590	4	6.0	20
and turkey, Dijon .... 1 entrée	1 entrée	270	16	37	570	6	6.0	30
(Marie Callender's)								
frozen, 'Callender's Deluxe' .... 1 cup	1 cup	350	31	4	610	5	23.0	30
primavera, w/chicken, frozen .... 1 cup	1 cup	310	12	22	450	3	19.0	25
w/beef and broccoli .... 15 oz	15 oz	570	35	73	1160	6	15.0	70
(MET-RX) café pasta meal .... 1 cup	1 cup	190	19	27	45	0	1.0	0
(Smart Ones)								
and spinach, Romano .... 1 entrée	1 entrée	260	12	35	510	4	8.0	15
Portafino, in wine sauce, frozen .... 9.5 oz	9.5 oz	160	8	30	220	0	1.0	0
(Tyson) trio, frozen, 'Gourmet Selection' .... 11 oz	11 oz	450	21	53	890	0	17.0	0
(Weight Watchers)								
and spinach, Romano .... 1 entrée	1 entrée	240	11	32	510	4	8.0	5
Italiano, frozen, 'Ultimate 200' .... 8 oz	8 oz	190	17	19	450	0	4.0	5
w/tomato basil sauce .... 1 entrée	1 entrée	260	12	33	360	5	9.0	10

Food Name	Serv. Size	Total Cal.	Prot. gms	Carbs gms	Sod. mgs	Fiber gms	Fat gms	Chol. mgs
ANGEL HAIR								
(Budget Gourmet)	1 entrée	230	8	38	430	3	5.0	10
(Lean Cuisine) frozen	1 entrée	220	8	41	420	6	3.0	0
(Marie Callender's) w/sausage and breadstick, frozen	1 entrée	370	14	43	630	4	15.0	10
(Smart Ones)	1 entrée	170	8	29	520	7	2.0	0
BOW TIES								
(Marie Callender's)								
Alfredo	13 oz	620	20	40	1080	8	42.0	80
and meat sauce	13 oz	480	25	44	970	3	22.0	45
marinara	13 oz	430	18	46	930	6	19.0	30
(Lean Cuisine) and chicken, 'Cafe Classic'	1 entrée	270	19	34	550	5	6.0	60
(Pasta Perfect) w/vegetables	1/2 cup	110	5	19	55	na	1.0	15
(Weight Watchers) Marsala	1 entrée	280	13	36	560	5	9.0	10
CANNELLONI								
(Bernardi) w/beef	1 piece	200	9	19	290	1	10.0	25
(Celentano) Florentine, frozen	12 oz	350	21	48	620	0	8.0	0
(Dining Lite) cheese, frozen	9 oz	310	19	38	650	0	9.0	70
(Lean Cuisine)								
beef, w/tomato sauce, frozen	9 5/8 oz	200	14	28	490	0	3.0	25
cheese	1 entrée	240	19	29	590	4	5.0	22
cheese, w/tomato sauce, frozen	9 1/8 oz	270	23	27	590	0	8.0	25
CAVATELLI *(Celentano)*	2/3 cup	400	16	79	15	9	1.5	15
FETTUCCINE								
(Armour) chicken, frozen, 'Classics'	11 oz	260	17	28	660	0	9.0	50
(Banquet)								
Alfredo	1 entrée	350	11	40	850	4	16.0	25
Alfredo, four cheeses, frozen	1 entrée	480	20	48	1120	3	24.0	55
chicken, frozen, 'Healthy Balance'	11.25 oz	320	17	47	650	0	7.0	35
w/meat sauce, frozen	10 oz	290	16	34	980	0	10.0	25
(Budget Gourmet) primavera, w/chicken	1 entrée	280	14	38	650	3	8.0	30
(Contadina) grilled chicken, frozen, food service product	1 oz	42	2	3	113	0	2.7	10
(Dining Lite) w/broccoli, frozen	9 oz	290	12	33	1020	0	12.0	35
(Green Giant)								
primavera, frozen	1 pkg	230	13	26	610	6	8.0	25
primavera, 'Microwave Garden Gourmet'	1 pkg	260	17	25	640	6	13.0	0
(Hain) Alfredo, 'Pasta & Sauce'	1/4 pkg	180	5	27	420	0	4.0	0
(Healthy Choice)								
Alfredo	1 entrée	250	11	39	480	3	5.0	15
chicken, Alfredo	1 entrée	280	22	35	410	3	7.0	40
chicken, frozen	8.5 oz	240	22	29	370	0	4.0	45
(Kraft) Alfredo, 'Pasta & Cheese' prepared	1/2 cup	180	7	19	590	0	9.0	30
(Lean Cuisine)								
Alfredo, frozen	9 oz	280	14	41	570	0	7.0	15
chicken	1 entrée	270	22	33	580	2	6.0	45
chicken, Alfredo sauce, frozen 'Lunch Express'	10.25 oz	240	16	31	540	0	6.0	35
chicken, frozen	9 oz	280	23	33	500	0	6.0	35
primavera, frozen	10 oz	260	14	32	510	0	8.0	45
(Lunch Express) primavera	1 entrée	420	15	33	690	6	25.0	95
(Marie Callender's)								
Alfredo, frozen	1 cup	190	10	29	400	2	21.0	45
Alfredo, supreme	1 cup	450	15	35	680	4	27.0	80
Alfredo, w/bread	14 oz	800	23	71	1270	5	47.0	95
primavera, w/tortellini	1 cup	430	11	35	670	4	27.0	35
w/broccoli and chicken	13 oz	410	16	32	550	4	24.0	45
(Michelina's) w/creamy pesto sauce 'Lean 'n Tasty'	1 entrée	250	10	38	590	3	6.0	20
(Right Course) chicken, Italiano, w/vegetables, frozen	9 5/8 oz	280	24	29	560	0	8.0	45

Food Name	Serv. Size	Total Cal.	Prot. gms	Carbs gms	Sod. mgs	Fiber gms	Fat gms	Chol. mgs
(Stouffer's)								
Alfredo	1 entrée	580	14	42	810	4	39.0	120
chicken, 'Homestyle'	1 entrée	390	31	32	1250	3	15.0	65
chicken, homestyle, w/vegetable medley, frozen	9.5 oz	350	23	27	780	0	17.0	0
(Ultra Slim Fast)	12 oz	390	31	38	980	0	12.0	65
(Weight Watchers)								
Alfredo, w/broccoli	1 entrée	230	10	34	450	3	6.0	20
chicken	1 entrée	290	19	39	590	4	7.0	50
LINGUINE								
(Banquet) w/meat sauce, frozen, 'Healthy Balance'	11.5 oz	290	11	49	560	0	6.0	25
(Budget Gourmet)								
w/shrimp, frozen	10 oz	330	15	33	1250	0	15.0	75
w/shrimp and clams, 'Light'	1 entrée	280	14	38	800	3	8.0	70
w/tomato sauce, sausage, 'Special Selections'	1 entrée	360	15	43	610	5	14.0	25
(Healthy Choice) w/shrimp, frozen	9.5 oz	230	13	40	420	0	2.0	60
(Lean Cuisine)								
w/clam sauce, frozen	9 5/8 oz	280	17	36	560	0	8.0	30
w/meatballs, frozen, food service product	1 oz	25	2	3	78	1	0.8	3
(Marie Callender's) and Italian sausage	15 oz	710	26	70	1330	8	36.0	30
(Top Shelf) w/clam sauce, packaged	1 serving	330	12	30	1420	0	18.0	85
MACARONI								
(Amy's Kitchen)								
and cheese	1 serving	390	17	50	550	4	14.0	40
and soy cheese	1 serving	360	16	42	500	4	14.0	0
(Banquet)								
and beef, shells, frozen	10 oz	340	20	34	985	0	14.0	35
and cheese	1 entrée	320	11	44	970	4	11.0	20
and cheese, frozen	10 oz	420	14	46	450	0	20.0	30
and cheese, frozen, 'Family Entrées'	8 oz	290	12	32	0	0	13.0	0
(Budget Gourmet)								
and cheese	1 entrée	270	10	45	520	2	6.0	10
and cheese, frozen, 'Side Dish'	5.3 oz	210	9	23	370	0	8.0	25
and cheese, frozen, 'Special Selections'	1 entrée	400	17	38	1320	4	20.0	45
(Chef Boyardee)								
and cheese, canned	7.5 oz	170	7	33	970	2	2.0	25
and cheese, w/shells, canned	7.5 oz	150	6	31	930	0	1.0	0
and chicken, canned	7.5 oz	180	10	30	850	1	2.0	15
canned, 'Roller Coasters'	7.5 oz	230	7	28	1070	3	10.0	19
dinosaurs, in tomato and cheese sauce	1 cup	210	6	45	830	4	0.0	0
dinosaurs, w/mini meatballs, in tomato sauce	1 cup	270	9	38	930	4	9.0	25
elbows w/beef, in sauce, microwave	7.5 oz	210	8	29	1000	0	7.0	15
in cheese sauce, canned, 'ABC's & 123's'	8.6 oz	200	6	42	1020	0	1.0	2
in cheese sauce, canned, 'Sharks'	7.5 oz	170	5	34	780	0	1.0	2
in cheese sauce, canned, 'Smurfs'	7.5 oz	150	6	29	830	3	1.0	2
in cheese sauce, canned, 'Tic Tac Toes'	8.6 oz	190	5	41	1080	0	1.0	0
in cheese sauce, canned, 'Tic Tac Toes'	7.5 oz	160	5	31	870	3	1.0	1
in cheese sauce, microwave, 'ABC's & 123's'	7.5 oz	180	5	37	940	3	1.0	3
in cheese sauce, microwave, 'Dinosaurs'	7.5 oz	180	6	36	880	3	1.0	3
in cheese sauce, microwave, 'Tic Tac Toes'	7.5 oz	170	5	36	930	2	1.0	2
in chicken sauce, canned, 'Pac Man'	7.5 oz	170	6	22	905	0	7.0	0
in sauce, canned 'ABC's & 123's'	7.5 oz	160	5	31	830	3	1.0	2
in sauce, canned 'Turtles'	7.5 oz	150	4	31	830	0	1.0	0
in sauce, microwave, 'Turtles'	7.5 oz	160	5	33	870	2	1.0	3
in tomato and cheese sauce, 'Street Sharks'	1 cup	210	6	47	750	4	0.0	0
in tomato sauce, canned, 'Pac Man'	7.5 oz	150	6	30	830	0	1.0	2
mini bites, canned	7.5 oz	260	8	30	1020	1	12.0	17
shells, in meat sauce, canned	7.5 oz	190	7	31	810	4	6.0	5

Food Name	Serv. Size	Total Cal.	Prot. gms	Carbs gms	Sod. mgs	Fiber gms	Fat gms	Chol. mgs
shells, in meat sauce, microwave	7.5 oz	210	8	32	1090	0	6.0	15
shells, in mushroom sauce, microwave	7.5 oz	170	6	35	1080	0	1.0	2
'Teenage Mutant Ninja Turtles'	1 pkg	227	8	34	840	3	6.8	21
w/beef, canned, 'Beefaroni'	1 cup	260	10	37	870	5	7.0	25
w/beef, microwave, 'Beefaroni'	7.5 oz	220	7	31	1145	2	7.0	18
w/meatballs, canned, 'ABC's & 123's'	8.6 oz	280	9	35	1090	0	11.0	23
w/meatballs, canned, 'Dinosaurs'	8.6 oz	280	9	36	1131	0	11.0	21
w/meatballs, canned, 'Pac Man'	7.5 oz	230	7	32	880	5	9.0	17
w/meatballs, canned, 'Smurfs'	7.5 oz	240	8	31	900	2	9.0	19
w/meatballs, canned, 'Tic Tac Toes'	7.5 oz	240	8	31	1000	0	9.0	18
w/meatballs, canned, 'Tic Tac Toes'	8.6 oz	290	8	39	1045	0	11.0	0
w/meatballs, canned, 'Turtles'	7.5 oz	220	7	30	940	0	8.0	20
w/meatballs, in sauce, canned, 'Zooroni'	7.5 oz	240	8	33	970	0	8.0	17
w/meatballs, 'Street Sharks' (Chef Boyardee)	1 cup	250	8	37	940	4	8.0	25
(Franco-American) and cheese	1 cup	210	8	29	1060	4	7.0	10
(Green Giant)								
and cheese, frozen, 'One Serving'	5.7 oz	230	9	28	590	0	9.0	25
(Healthy Choice)								
and cheese	1 entrée	290	15	50	580	4	7.0	25
and cheese, meatless	1 entrée	320	15	50	580	4	7.0	25
(Heinz)								
and cheese, canned	7.5 oz	190	5	26	1105	0	8.0	0
w/beef, in tomato sauce, canned	7.5 oz	200	8	23	850	0	8.0	0
(Hormel) and cheese, micro cup	7.5 oz	189	7	26	874	0	6.0	17
(Kid Cuisine)								
and cheese, frozen, 'Mega Meal'	12.45 oz	470	14	75	1270	0	13.0	0
and cheese, w/apples, corn, fudge brownie, frozen	1 meal	310	7	54	710	6	7.0	15
and cheese, w/mini franks, frozen	9 oz	380	9	55	1000	0	14.0	40
(Kid's Kitchen)								
beefy, microwave cup	7.5 oz	200	11	25	780	0	6.0	25
and cheese, microwave cup	7.5 oz	260	12	28	650	0	11.0	45
(Lean Cuisine)								
and beef	1 entrée	280	13	40	550	3	8.0	25
and beef, frozen, food service product	1 oz	27	2	3	71	0	0.9	4
and beef, in tomato sauce, frozen	1 pkg	249	14	37	563	3	5.4	23
and cheese	1 entrée	290	13	43	590	4	7.0	20
and cheese, frozen, food service product	1 oz	33	2	4	85	0	1.1	3
(Libby's) and cheese, microwave cup, 'Diner'	7.5 oz	360	14	27	1020	2	22.0	35
(Lipton) and cheese, w/shells, 'Hearty Ones'	11 oz	367	15	60	1406	0	7.4	14
(Lunch Bucket) and cheese, microwave lunch cup	7.5 oz	210	9	24	990	0	9.0	0
(Lunch Express) and cheese, w/broccoli	1 entrée	240	12	35	460	5	6.0	15
(Marie Callender's)								
and beef, w/tomatoes and soft breadstick, frozen	1 entrée	310	12	40	680	5	11.0	15
and cheese	13.5 oz	510	22	65	2020	5	18.0	35
and cheese, frozen, 'Marie's Special'	1 cup	420	20	47	1410	3	17.0	40
(Michelina's)								
and beef, 'Lean 'n Tasty'	1 entrée	230	12	34	830	2	6.0	20
and cheese, 'Lean 'n Tasty'	1 entrée	270	12	41	620	2	6.0	20
(Morton) and cheese casserole, frozen	6.5 oz	290	8	30	760	0	14.0	0
(Myers) and cheese, frozen	3.5 oz	168	7	16	516	0	9.0	0
(Nalley's) w/beef	7.5 oz	180	9	29	900	0	3.0	0
(Nestlé)								
and cheese, canned, 'Chef Mate'	1 pkg	3397	130	425	16105	39	131.9	334
and cheese, canned, 'Chef Mate'	1 cup	283	11	35	1343	3	11.0	28
(Pathmark) w/beef, in tomato sauce, canned, 'No Frills'	7.5 oz	200	9	22	880	0	8.0	0
(Smart Ones) and cheese	1 entrée	220	9	42	640	4	2.0	5
(Stouffer's)								
and beef	1 entrée	420	19	40	1530	5	20.0	50

Food Name	Serv. Size	Total Cal.	Prot. gms	Carbs gms	Sod. mgs	Fiber gms	Fat gms	Chol. mgs
and beef, w/tomato	10 oz	270	15	43	590	4	4.0	25
and cheese	6 oz	330	14	31	940	2	17.0	30
and cheese, frozen, food service product	1 oz	39	2	4	105	0	1.6	3
(Swanson)								
and beef, frozen	12 oz	370	12	48	930	0	15.0	0
and cheese, frozen	12.25 oz	370	13	43	1070	0	15.0	0
and cheese, frozen	7 oz	200	7	24	740	0	8.0	0
and cheese, frozen, 'Homestyle Recipe'	10 oz	390	17	37	1150	0	19.0	0
(Tyson)								
and cheese, frozen, 'Tweety'	8 oz	340	12	49	650	0	10.0	28
frozen, 'Bugs Bunny/Tazmanian Devil'	8 oz	290	13	41	420	0	8.0	0
frozen, 'Daffy Duck & Elmer Fudd'	8 oz	270	11	40	430	0	7.0	0
frozen, 'Foghorn Leghorn/Henry Hawk'	8 oz	230	9	39	320	0	4.0	0
frozen, 'Looney Tunes Sylvester & Tweety'	8 oz	250	13	41	380	0	4.0	0
(Weight Watchers)								
and beef	1 entrée	220	13	32	560	4	4.5	10
in tomato sauce, frozen	1 pkg	282	16	45	492	7	4.6	13
and cheese...................................	1 entrée	280	13	42	590	4	7.0	25
MOSTACCIOLI								
(Banquet) w/meat sauce, frozen, 'Family Entrées'	7 oz	170	7	28	0	0	3.0	0
(Contadina) w/meat sauce, frozen, food service product	1 oz	35	1	5	119	1	1.2	3
PENNE								
(Budget Gourmet)								
w/tomato sauce, Italian sausage, frozen	10 oz	320	12	53	520	0	9.0	5
w/tomato and sausage, 'Special Selections'	1 entrée	330	17	49	530	6	8.0	10
(Healthy Choice) w/roasted tomato sauce	1 entrée	230	9	36	490	5	5.0	10
(Marie Callender's) and pepperoni	15 oz	800	29	74	1780	11	43.0	30
(Michelina's) w/mushrooms, 'Lean 'n Tasty'	1 entrée	250	10	38	650	3	6.0	20
(Weight Watchers)								
and ricotta, spicy	1 entrée	280	12	45	370	5	6.0	5
pollo	1 entrée	290	22	40	620	3	5.0	35
w/sun dried tomatoes	1 entrée	290	13	40	560	5	9.0	10
RIGATONI								
(Chef Boyardee)								
canned, 'Special Recipe' 'Ragatoni'	7.5 oz	210	9	33	1040	4	6.0	20
microwave 'Ragatoni'	7.5 oz	210	8	31	1080	0	6.0	17
(Budget Gourmet)								
tomato sauce, frozen, 'Special Selections'	1 entrée	420	16	41	620	2	22.0	65
w/broccoli and chicken, in cream sauce, frozen	10.8 oz	290	19	44	710	0	7.0	30
w/broccoli, white chicken, in cream sauce	1 entrée	250	10	37	530	1	7.0	20
(Healthy Choice)								
in meat sauce, frozen	9.5 oz	260	16	34	540	0	6.0	30
w/chicken, frozen, 'Classics'	12.5 oz	360	31	50	430	0	4.0	60
(Lean Cuisine)								
....	1 entrée	180	10	25	560	4	4.0	20
jumbo, w/meatballs, 'Hearty Portions'	1 entrée	440	27	62	780	8	9.0	40
(Marie Callender's)								
Parmigiana, family size, frozen	1 cup	320	15	32	670	4	14.0	25
Parmigiana, w/breadstick, frozen	1 cup + bread	300	12	32	650	3	14.0	25
(Stouffer's) w/meat sauce, homestyle, frozen	12 oz	400	21	49	860	0	13.0	0
ROTINI								
(Green Giant)								
cheddar cheese, 'Microwave Garden Gourmet'	1 pkg	230	9	32	570	5	10.0	20
(Mrs. Paul's) seafood, frozen, 'Light'	9 oz	240	12	34	570	0	6.0	25
(Norpac)								
w/spinach rotini and vegetables, 'Pasta Perfect'	1/2 cup	100	4	19	15	na	0.0	0
w/vegetables, vegetarian, 'Pasta Perfect'	1/2 cup	110	5	20	60	3	1.0	0

Food Name	Serv. Size	Total Cal.	Prot. gms	Carbs gms	Sod. mgs	Fiber gms	Fat gms	Chol. mgs
(Weight Watchers) three cheese, w/vegetables, frozen ...... 9 oz		270	14	34	500	0	8.0	5
SHELLS								
(Bernardi)								
cheese stuffed .... 2 pieces		240	12	25	330	1	11.0	60
cheese stuffed, large .... 1 piece		160	8	13	250	1	9.0	50
Florentine .... 1 piece		190	11	17	340	1	8.0	30
(Buitoni) shells, stuffed, frozen, 'Single Serving' .... 9 oz		460	18	46	840	0	13.0	80
(Celentano)								
broccoli stuffed, frozen, 'Great Choice' .... 10 oz		190	12	31	520	0	4.0	0
stuffed, frozen .... 8 oz		330	18	41	680	0	11.0	0
stuffed, lowfat, frozen 'Great Choice' .... 10 oz		250	16	41	675	0	2.0	0
stuffed, w/sauce, frozen .... 10 oz		410	23	51	850	0	14.0	0
stuffed, w/sauce, frozen .... 6.25 oz		340	17	31	420	0	16.0	0
(Healthy Choice)								
stuffed, in tomato sauce, frozen, 'Classics' .... 12 oz		330	24	53	470	0	3.0	35
(Le Menu) stuffed, 3-cheese, frozen 'LightStyle' .... 10 oz		280	17	34	690	0	8.0	25
(Lean Cuisine) cheese stuffed, frozen .... 1 oz		25	1	3	65	0	0.8	3
(Norpac)								
seashells w/vegetables, vegetarian, 'Pasta Perfect' ..... 1/2 cup		130	6	25	65	na	1.0	0
(Stouffer's) cheese, w/tomato sauce, frozen .... 9.25 oz		300	17	28	820	0	13.0	0
SPAGHETTI								
(Banquet)								
w/meat sauce, frozen, 'Casserole' .... 8 oz		270	14	35	1250	0	8.0	0
w/meatballs, frozen .... 10 oz		290	11	44	580	0	10.0	30
(Budget Gourmet)								
marinara .... 1 entrée		290	10	50	790	4	6.0	5
w/tomato and meat sauce, 'Special Selections' .... 1 entrée		320	15	49	470	4	7.0	5
(Buitoni) and meatballs, in sauce, canned .... 7.5 oz		190	9	21	940	0	8.0	20
(Chef Boyardee)								
and beef, in tomato sauce, canned .... 7.5 oz		240	7	30	1120	0	9.0	20
and meatballs .... 1 cup		250	9	32	950	3	10.0	25
and meatballs, in tomato sauce, canned .... 1 pkg		442	16	60	1666	4	15.3	38
and meatballs, in tomato sauce, canned .... 1 serving		250	9	34	941	2	8.6	22
and meatballs, canned, 'Microwave' .... 7.5 oz		230	7	29	1060	0	10.0	20
w/beef, 'Beefagetti' .... 1 cup		250	8	37	990	4	7.0	25
(Dining Lite) w/beef, frozen .... 9 oz		220	12	25	440	0	8.0	20
(Estee) meatballs, canned .... 7.5 oz		240	9	19	130	0	14.0	30
(Featherweight) and meatballs, canned .... 7.5 oz		160	12	23	400	0	3.0	20
(Finast) rings, in tomato sauce, canned .... 7.5 oz		150	4	31	480	0	1.0	0
(Franco-American)								
in tomato and cheese sauce .... 1 cup		210	7	41	1020	3	2.0	5
in tomato and cheese sauce, 'Spaghettio's' .... 1 cup		190	5	36	990	2	2.0	5
in tomato sauce .... 1 cup		270	11	35	1060	4	10.0	30
w/meatballs, 'Spaghettio's' .... 1 cup		260	11	31	1150	5	11.0	20
w/sliced frankfurters, 'Spaghettio's' .... 1 cup		250	10	32	1210	4	11.0	25
(Freezer Queen) w/meat sauce, frozen 'Single Serve' ..... 10 oz		350	14	47	610	0	12.0	0
(Healthy Choice) Bolognese, frozen .... 1 serving		255	14	43	473	5	2.9	17
(Kid Cuisine) w/meat sauce, frozen .... 9.25 oz		310	9	43	690	0	12.0	35
(Le Menu)								
w/beef, sauce, and mushrooms, frozen, 'LightStyle' .... 9 oz		280	12	45	450	0	6.0	15
(Lean Cuisine)								
.... 1 entrée		290	11	50	570	7	5.0	20
w/meat sauce .... 1 entrée		290	14	45	550	4	6.0	20
w/meat sauce, frozen .... 1 entrée		313	14	51	610	6	5.9	13
w/meatballs .... 1 entrée		290	17	40	520	4	7.0	30
w/meatballs and sauce, frozen .... 1 entrée		299	18	40	465	5	7.5	5

Food Name	Serv. Size	Total Cal.	Prot. gms	Carbs gms	Sod. mgs	Fiber gms	Fat gms	Chol. mgs
(Legume)								
and meatballs, vegetarian	1 serving	330	28	46	650	7	4.0	0
w/organic pasta and tofu, vegetarian	1 serving	240	13	23	660	6	11.0	0
w/veggie protein cutlet, vegetarian	1 serving	380	25	47	650	9	10.0	0
(Lunch Express) w/meat sauce	1 entrée	320	15	43	580	5	10.0	30
(Marie Callender's)								
and meat sauce, w/garlic bread	1 cup	380	16	51	700	5	13.0	10
marinara, w/cheese garlic bread	1 cup	410	13	61	680	6	13.0	20
(Michelinas)								
and meatballs, w/Pomodoro sauce, low-fat, frozen	1 pkg	312	14	49	1011	6	7.1	14
and meatballs, w/Pomodoro sauce, low-fat, frozen . . .	1 serving	312	14	49	1011	6	7.1	14
(Morton) w/meatballs, frozen	10 oz	200	6	39	1090	0	3.0	10
(Nalley's) and meatballs, canned	7.5 oz	190	10	29	950	0	4.0	0
(Pathmark)								
w/meatballs, in tomato sauce, canned 'No Frills'	7.5 oz	200	9	22	860	0	8.0	0
(Stouffer's)								
and meatballs	1 entrée	420	19	51	680	5	15.0	45
Parmesan, w/Italian-style green beans, frozen	10.25 oz	240	10	30	810	0	9.0	0
w/meat sauce, frozen	12 7/8 oz	320	16	38	560	0	12.0	0
(Swanson)								
w/Italian meatballs, frozen, 'Homestyle Recipe'	13 oz	490	23	60	940	0	18.0	0
w/meatballs, frozen	12.5 oz	390	14	46	1100	0	17.0	0
(Top Shelf)								
spaghettini, packaged	1 serving	240	13	35	1020	0	5.0	5
w/meat sauce	10 oz	260	14	37	980	0	6.0	20
(Tyson) w/meatballs, frozen, 'Daffy Duck'	8.65 oz	340	11	49	570	0	10.0	20
(Ultra Slim-Fast) w/beef and mushroom sauce	12 oz	370	20	49	990	0	10.0	25
(Van Camp's) w/franks, canned, 'Spaghettee Weenee'	1 cup	243	9	35	1128	1	7.4	0
(Weight Watchers)								
marinara	1 entrée	280	9	46	690	5	7.0	5
w/meat sauce	1 entrée	290	14	45	560	5	6.0	15
SPIRALS *(Chef Boyardee)* canned, spirals, in pizza sauce . . .	7.5 oz	180	5	35	1080	3	3.0	5
ZITI								
(Budget Gourmet) Parmesano	1 entrée	260	11	39	550	4	7.0	10
(Healthy Choice)								
w/zesty tomato sauce, frozen, 'Classics'	12 oz	350	16	59	530	0	5.0	30
(Weight Watchers) w/mozzarella	1 entrée	280	11	45	430	4	6.0	5
PASTA DISH/ENTRÉE MIX. See also NOODLE DISH/ENTRÉE MIX.								
(Fantastic Foods)								
salad, Italian herb, prepared	1 cup	170	7	34	380	2	1.5	0
salad, Oriental, spicy, prepared	1 cup	200	7	37	420	3	3.0	0
(Kraft) salad, Italian, 97% fat free, prepared	3/4 cup	190	8	35	740	2	2.0	3
(Lunch Bucket)								
'Pasta 'n Chicken' microwave lunch cup	7.5 oz	180	9	22	860	0	6.0	45
w/beef, in wine sauce, micro cup, 'Light'n Healthy'	7.5 oz	130	5	21	600	0	3.0	10
(Pasta Roni) Parmesano pasta, 'Tenderthin' prepared . . .	1 serving	226	7	28	536	1	9.6	6
(Suddenly Salad)								
salad, classic, mix only	3/4 cup	190	7	38	910	2	1.5	0
salad, classic, prepared	3/4 cup	250	7	38	910	2	8.0	0
(Ultra Slim-Fast)								
w/beef flavored sauce, prepared	8 oz	230	8	45	1070	4	3.0	0
w/chicken flavored sauce, prep	8 oz	220	8	45	980	4	3.0	0
w/tomato herb sauce, prep	8 oz	220	8	46	1090	5	3.0	0
w/zesty cheese sauce, prepared	8 oz	230	9	44	770	4	4.0	0
ANGEL HAIR								
(Golden Saute)								
w/chicken and broccoli, mix only	1/3 pkg	220	8	44	840	2	1.0	0
w/chicken and broccoli, prepared	1 cup	270	8	44	910	2	7.0	0

Food Name	Serv. Size	Total Cal.	Prot. gms	Carbs gms	Sod. mgs	Fiber gms	Fat gms	Chol. mgs
w/Parmesan, mix only	1/4 pkg	130	5	21	470	0	3.0	0
w/Parmesan, prepared	1/2 cup	160	5	21	500	0	6.0	0
(Pasta Roni)								
w/Parmesan cheese, prepared	1 serving	145	4	18	404	1	6.5	2
w/herb sauce, prepared	1 serving	145	4	19	379	1	6.3	2
CORKSCREW								
(Pasta Roni)								
w/creamy garlic sauce, prepared	1 serving	190	4	18	456	1	11.1	2
w/four cheese sauce, prepared	1 serving	231	7	28	587	1	10.2	6
FETTUCINE								
(Pasta Roni)								
broccoli au gratin, prepared	1 serving	164	6	22	480	1	5.6	23
cheddar, prepared	1 serving	169	6	23	500	1	5.9	6
chicken, prepared	1 serving	181	6	23	576	1	7.6	3
Romanoff, prepared	1 serving	231	7	27	604	1	10.7	6
Stroganoff, prepared	1 serving	209	8	27	6	1	7.9	6
w/Alfredo sauce, prepared	1 serving	265	6	27	627	1	14.1	6
LINGUINE								
(Pasta Roni)								
linguine w/chicken and broccoli sauce, prepared	1 serving	209	6	28	565	2	9.0	3
w/creamy chicken, Parmesan sauce, prepared	1 serving	231	7	26	621	1	10.4	3
MACARONI								
(De Boles)								
and cheddar, w/artichoke pasta shells, mix only	2 oz	210	9	40	160	0	2.0	0
and cheddar, w/artichoke pasta shells, prepared	3/4 cup	220	8	31	140	0	7.0	0
and cheese, w/artichoke pasta elbows, 'Mac & Cheese' mix only	2 oz	210	9	40	160	0	2.0	0
and cheese, w/artichoke pasta elbows, 'Mac & Cheese' prepared	3/4 cup	200	7	27	120	0	8.0	0
and cheese, w/artichoke pasta elbows, mix only	1/2 cup	200	8	33	390	1	3.5	10
and cheese, w/artichoke pasta elbows, prepared	3/4 cup	250	8	33	390	1	8.5	10
and cheese, w/artichoke pasta shells, mix only	1/2 cup	200	8	33	390	1	3.5	10
and cheese, w/artichoke pasta shells, prepared	3/4 cup	250	8	33	390	1	8.5	10
and cheese, w/wheat pasta elbows, mix only	1/2 cup	200	8	32	390	3	4.0	10
and cheese, w/wheat pasta elbows, prepared	3/4 cup	250	8	32	390	3	9.0	10
elbows, w/cheese sauce, mix only	2 oz	210	9	40	160	0	2.0	0
(Fantastic Foods)								
shells, w/curry, 'Tofu Classics' mix only	1/2 cup	200	8	40	500	5	1.5	0
(Hodgson Mill)								
and cheese, w/whole wheat pasta, mix only	1 pkg	774	29	143	1259	16	9.7	16
and cheese, w/whole wheat pasta, mix only	2.5 oz	263	10	48	428	5	3.3	6
(Hormel) and cheese, micro cup	7.5 oz	189	7	26	874	0	6.0	17
(Kraft)								
and cheese, 'Deluxe Dinner' prepared	3/4 cup	260	11	36	590	0	8.0	20
and cheese, 'Dinner' prepared	3/4 cup	290	9	34	530	0	13.0	5
and cheese, 'Dinomac Dinner' prepared	3/4 cup	310	9	36	560	0	14.0	10
and cheese, 'Family Size Dinner' prepared	3/4 cup	290	9	34	490	0	13.0	5
and cheese, original flavor, mix only	1 serving	259	11	48	561	1	2.6	10
and cheese, 'Original' prepared	1 cup	410	12	49	750	1	18.0	10
and cheese, 'Teddy Bears Dinner' prepared	3/4 cup	310	9	36	560	0	14.0	10
and cheese, 'Wild Wheels Dinner' prepared	3/4 cup	310	9	36	560	0	14.0	10
and cheese, w/spirals, 'Dinner' prepared	3/4 cup	340	9	36	600	0	18.0	10
shells w/Velveeta, 'Original'	1 cup	360	16	44	1030	1	13.0	40
(Libby's) and cheese, microwave cup, 'Diner'	7.5 oz	360	14	27	1020	2	22.0	35
(Lipton) and cheese, w/shells, 'Hearty Ones'	11 oz	367	15	60	1406	0	7.4	14
(Lunch Bucket)								
and cheese, microwave lunch cup	7.5 oz	210	9	24	990	0	9.0	0

Food Name	Serv. Size	Total Cal.	Prot. gms	Carbs gms	Sod. mgs	Fiber gms	Fat gms	Chol. mgs
and vegetables, micro cup, 'Light'n Healthy'	7.5 oz	150	4	30	630	0	1.0	0
elbows, in tomato sauce, microwave lunch cup	7.5 oz	190	4	38	860	0	2.0	0
(Nestlé) shells, w/sausage, canned, 'Chef-Mate'	1 cup	382	15	19	987	1	27.6	53
(Pasta Roni) shells w/white cheddar, prepared	1 serving	220	7	27	649	1	9.0	8
(Ultra Slim Fast) and cheese, prepared	1 cup	230	9	46	700	4	3.0	0
PENNE								
(Golden Saute)								
stir-fry, w/chicken, mix only	1/2 cup	220	7	45	850	2	2.0	0
stir fry, w/chicken, prepared	1 cup	270	7	45	920	2	8.0	0
(Pasta Roni) w/herb and butter sauce	1 serving	194	4	19	339	1	11.1	0
RIGATONI								
(Pasta Roni)								
w/tomato basil sauce, prepared	1 serving	81	2	12	237	1	3.0	0
w/white cheddar and broccoli sauce, prepared	1 serving	181	5	22	415	1	8.6	5
ROTINI								
(Golden Saute)								
w/chicken, herbs, and Parmesan, mix only	1 cup	280	8	45	900	3	9.0	5
SPAGHETTI								
(Chef Boyardee)								
w/condensed meat sauce, 'Dinner' prepared	3.25 oz	250	12	37	595	0	6.0	0
w/meat sauce, 'Dinner' prepared	7.9 oz	240	12	42	1155	0	3.0	0
w/mushroom sauce, 'Dinner' prepared	7.9 oz	210	11	41	1085	0	1.0	0
(Fantastic Foods) w/whole wheat noodles, low-fat, 'All-O-Round' prepared	10 oz	211	10	45	275	0	2.0	4
(Hormel) w/meatballs, micro cup	7.5 oz	210	10	27	930	0	7.0	20
(Kid's Kitchen)								
rings, microwave cup, mix only	7.5 oz	180	8	35	930	0	1.0	10
rings and franks, w/tomato sauce, micro cup, mix only	7.5 oz	290	12	33	960	0	12.0	30
w/meatballs, microwave cup	7.5 oz	220	11	26	880	0	8.0	20
(Kraft)								
mild, 'American Style Dinner' prepared	1 cup	300	10	50	630	0	7.0	0
tangy, 'Italian Style Dinner' prepared	1 cup	310	11	49	670	0	8.0	5
w/meat sauce, 'Dinner' prepared	1 cup	360	12	47	880	0	14.0	15
(Libby's) w/meatballs, in sauce, 'Diner' micro cup	7.75 oz	190	10	31	870	2	3.0	15
(Lunch Bucket) and meat sauce' microwave lunch cup	7.5 oz	240	9	39	870	0	5.0	30
(Mountain House)								
w/meat and sauce, freeze-dried, prepared	1 cup	260	12	41	0	0	5.0	0
VERMICELLI								
(Pasta Roni) w/garlic and olive oil sauce, prepared	1 serving	203	5	27	570	1	8.8	0
PASTA SAUCE. See under SAUCE.								
PASTA SEASONING. See under SEASONING MIX.								
PASTRY. See also CAKE, SNACK; PASTRY, TOASTER.								
(Tio Pepe's) churro, original	1 serving	140	2	14	180	0	9.0	10
(Entenmann's) Danish ring	1.5 oz	180	3	18	160	0	10.0	0
APPLE								
(Aunt Fanny's)								
cinnamon roll, old-fashioned, individual	2 oz	180	4	34	125	2	1.0	5
strudel, individual	3 oz	330	4	38	210	0	18.0	0
(Awrey's)								
filled Danish, 2.75 oz, 'Round'	1 piece	270	3	34	310	1	14.0	5
filled Danish, 4.5 oz, 'Round'	1 piece	390	4	50	390	1	20.0	10
filled Danish, 3 oz, 'Square'	1 piece	220	3	34	230	1	8.0	10
filled Danish, 1.7 oz, miniature	1 piece	160	2	21	170	0	8.0	5
(Break Cake)								
roll, sweet, 1.4 oz, multi-pak	1 roll	120	2	24	150	0	2.0	0
roll, sweet, 4.5 oz	2 rolls	380	8	75	460	0	5.0	0

Food Name	Serv. Size	Total Cal.	Prot. gms	Carbs gms	Sod. mgs	Fiber gms	Fat gms	Chol. mgs
(Entenmann's)								
'Apple Puffs'	1 puff	280	4	39	320	0	13.0	0
strudel, old-fashioned	1.5 oz	120	1	17	110	0	5.0	0
(Hormel) 'Apple Dulcita'	4 oz	290	5	44	350	0	10.0	0
(Hostess) filled Danish, fried, 'Breakfast Bake Shop'	1 piece	400	4	46	340	2	22.0	20
(Pepperidge Farm)								
crisp, 'Berkshire'	1 ramekin	250	2	43	130	1	8.0	4
Danish, 2 1/4 oz	1 piece	220	2	35	130	0	8.0	0
fruit square	1 piece	220	2	27	170	0	12.0	0
turnover, frozen	1 piece	300	3	34	210	0	17.0	0
turnover, ready to bake	1 serving	284	4	31	176	2	16.0	na
(Pillsbury)								
cinnamon roll, w/icing, ready to bake	1 roll	140	2	21	310	1	5.0	0
pocket	1 piece	240	4	25	520	0	13.0	0
turnover, refrigerated	1 piece	170	2	23	320	0	8.0	0
(Sara Lee)								
Danish twist	1/8 pkg	190	3	22	200	0	10.0	10
Danish, 'Free & Light'	1/8 pkg	130	2	30	120	0	0.0	0
Danish, 'Individual' 1.3 oz	1 piece	120	2	15	120	0	6.0	0
(Tastykake) pocket	3 oz	323	4	38	222	2	17.6	11
(Tio Pepe's) churro, apple filled, regular size	1 serving	160	2	22	115	1	7.0	15
(Weight Watchers)								
crisp, 'Sweet Celebrations'	1/2 pkg	190	1	40	190	0	5.0	0
roll, sweet 'Microwave'	1/2 pkg	160	3	27	100	0	4.0	5
APRICOT								
(Entenmann's) Danish twist, fat-free, cholesterol-free	1 slice	150	3	34	110	1	0.0	0
(Tio Pepe's) filled churro, regular size	1 serving	170	2	25	130	1	7.0	15
BAVARIAN CREAM								
(Entenmann's)	1.3 oz	80	2	20	90	0	0.0	0
(Rich's) cream puff	1 piece	150	2	17	70	0	8.0	25
(Tio Pepe's) filled churro, regular size	1 serving	160	2	22	120	0	7.0	15
BLACK FOREST *(Entenmann's)* fat-free, cholesterol-free	1 slice	130	3	32	115	2	0.0	0
BLUEBERRY, turnover *(Pepperidge Farm)*	1 piece	310	3	32	230	0	19.0	0
CARAMEL *(Pillsbury)* w/nuts	1 piece	160	2	19	240	0	8.0	0
CHEESE								
(Awrey's)								
filled Danish, 4.5 oz, 'Round'	1 piece	420	5	52	530	1	22.0	15
filled Danish, 2.75 oz, 'Round'	1 piece	280	3	34	350	1	15.0	10
filled Danish, 2.5 oz, 'Square'	1 piece	210	4	25	300	1	11.0	15
filled Danish, miniature 1.7 oz	1 piece	170	2	21	200	4	9.0	5
(Pepperidge Farm) Danish, 2 1/4 oz	1 piece	240	3	25	230	0	14.0	0
(Sara Lee)								
Danish, 'Individual' 1.3 oz	1 piece	130	2	13	130	0	8.0	0
Danish twist	1/8 pkg	200	3	21	270	0	12.0	15
(Tastykake) pocket	3 oz	325	4	41	231	1	16.7	11
CHERRY								
(Aunt Fanny's) strudel, individual	3 oz	320	4	39	190	0	16.0	5
(Hormel) 'Cherry Dulcita'	4 oz	300	5	48	345	0	9.0	0
(Pepperidge Farm) turnover	1 piece	310	3	32	280	0	19.0	0
(Pillsbury) turnover	1 piece	170	2	23	320	0	8.0	0
CHOCOLATE								
Fresh								
churro, creme filled, regular size *(Tio Pepe's)*	1 serving	180	2	28	140	0	7.0	15
fudge tart, frosted *(Toastettes)*	1 serving	190	2	34	280	1	5.0	0
Frozen or refrigerated								
éclair *(Weight Watchers)*	1 serving	150	2	25	160	2	4.0	30
éclair, 'Sweet Celebrations' *(Weight Watchers)*	2.1 oz	150	3	26	110	0	4.0	15

Food Name	Serv. Size	Total Cal.	Prot. gms	Carbs gms	Sod. mgs	Fiber gms	Fat gms	Chol. mgs
éclair, triple chocolate *(Weight Watchers)*	1 serving	160	3	25	190	1	5.0	30
éclair, 2 oz *(Rich's)*	1 piece	210	2	27	110	0	10.0	35
CINNAMON								
(Awrey's) cinnamon-walnut Danish, 'Round' 2.75 oz	1 piece	300	4	31	290	1	18.0	5
(Entenmann's) filbert ring	1.5 oz	190	3	19	160	0	12.0	0
(Tio Pepe's) churro	1 churro	110	1	14	100	2	5.0	15
CINNAMON-RAISIN								
(Awrey's)								
filled Danish, 3 oz, 'Square'	1 piece	290	3	41	280	1	12.0	15
filled Danish, miniature 1.5 oz	1 piece	160	2	21	150	1	8.0	5
(Entenmann's) bun, nonfat, no cholesterol	1 serving	160	3	36	125	1	0.0	0
(Pepperidge Farm) Danish, 2 1/4 oz	1 piece	250	3	35	170	0	11.0	0
(Pillsbury) Danish, w/icing	1 piece	150	2	20	230	0	7.0	0
(Sara Lee) Danish, individual, 1.3 oz	1 piece	150	2	17	140	0	8.0	0
DATE NUT *(Awrey's)* 1 piece	1.6 oz	230	2	35	150	1	10.0	15
ÉCLAIR *(Tasty-Klair)* custard-filled, prepared	1 pie	296	7	27	381	1	17.7	144
LEMON								
(Entenmann's)								
lemon Danish twist	1.2 oz	140	2	17	140	0	7.0	0
twist, fat-free, cholesterol-free	1 slice	130	3	31	140	1	0.0	0
NUT								
(Flanigan Farms)								
and fruit, almond, raisin, date, sunflower seed, no salt	1/4 cup	130	4	12	0	1	8.0	0
peanut, raisin, and sunflower seed, no salt	1/4 cup	130	5	11	4	1	10.0	0
ORANGE *(Pillsbury)* Danish, w/icing	1 piece	150	2	19	250	0	7.0	0
PEACH *(Pepperidge Farm)* turnover	1 piece	310	3	34	260	0	18.0	0
PECAN *(Entenmann's)* Danish ring	1.5 oz	190	3	19	130	0	12.0	0
PINEAPPLE *(Awrey's)* filled Danish, miniature, 1.7 oz	1 piece	157	2	21	180	1	8.0	5
RASPBERRY								
(Awrey's) filled Danish, 3 oz, 'Square'	1 piece	260	3	45	210	1	8.0	10
(Entenmann's)								
cheese, fat-free, cholesterol-free	1 slice	140	3	32	110	1	0.0	0
Danish twist	1.2 oz	140	2	18	120	0	7.0	0
(Hostess) raspberry-filled Danish, fried	1 piece	390	4	49	290	2	20.0	20
(Pepperidge Farm)								
raspberry Danish, 2 1/4 oz	1 piece	220	3	31	140	0	9.0	0
turnover	1 piece	310	4	36	260	0	17.0	0
(Sara Lee) raspberry Danish twist, 1/8 pkg	1/8 pkg	200	3	25	220	0	9.0	15
(Tio Pepe's) churro, regular size	1 serving	160	2	23	125	1	7.0	15
STRAWBERRY								
(Awrey's)								
filled Danish, 4.5 oz, 'Round'	1 piece	400	4	53	410	1	20.0	10
filled Danish, 2.75 oz, 'Round'	1 piece	270	3	34	320	1	14.0	5
filled Danish, miniature, 1.7 oz	1 piece	160	2	21	180	0	8.0	5
WALNUT *(Entenmann's)* Danish ring	1.5 oz	190	3	19	130	0	12.0	0
PASTRY, TOASTER								
APPLE								
(Auburn Farms)								
cinnamon, nonfat	1 pastry	157	2	36	162	1	0.5	0
cinnamon, 'Toast 'n Jammers'	1 pastry	180	3	42	200	4	0.0	0
(Kellogg's)								
cinnamon, frosted, low-fat, 'Pop Tarts'	1 pastry	191	2	40	206	1	2.9	0
cinnamon, 'Pop Tarts'	1 pastry	205	2	37	174	1	5.3	0
cinnamon Danish, 'Pastry Swirls' 'Pop Tarts'	1 pastry	256	3	37	190	1	11.0	0
(Pepperidge Farm)								
cinnamon, 'Croissant Toaster Tarts'	1 pastry	170	3	25	120	0	7.0	0
(Pastry Poppers) fruit juice sweetened, low-sodium	2 oz	212	3	38	115	0	5.4	0

Food Name	Serv. Size	Total Cal.	Prot. gms	Carbs gms	Sod. mgs	Fiber gms	Fat gms	Chol. mgs
(Pillsbury)								
'Danish' 'Toaster Strudel'	1 pastry	197	3	25	188	1	9.8	21
spice, 'Muffins' 'Toaster Strudel'	1 pastry	130	2	21	100	0	5.0	0
'Toaster Strudel'	1 pastry	180	3	9	190	1	7.0	5
(Toastettes)								
'Frosted Tarts'	1 pastry	190	2	35	170	1	5.0	0
'Tarts'	1 pastry	190	2	36	170	1	5.0	0
BANANA NUT								
(Pillsbury)								
'Muffins' 'Toaster Strudel'	1 pastry	130	2	19	85	0	6.0	0
'Strudel Breakfast Pastries' 'Toaster Strudel'	1 pastry	190	2	28	190	0	8.0	0
BERRY *(Kellogg's)* wild, frosted, 'Pop Tarts'	1 pastry	210	2	39	168	1	5.0	0
BLUEBERRY								
(Auburn Farms) nonfat	1 pastry	165	3	38	189	2	0.5	0
(Howard Johnson's) frozen, ready to eat, 'Toasties'	1 serving	235	5	32	408	na	9.7	21
(Kellogg's)								
frosted, 'Pop Tarts'	1 pastry	203	2	37	207	1	5.2	0
low-fat, 'Pop Tarts'	1 pastry	192	2	40	222	1	2.9	0
plain, 'Pop Tarts'	1 pastry	212	2	36	207	1	6.9	0
(Pastry Poppers) fruit juice sweetened, low-sodium	2 oz	212	3	38	115	0	4.5	0
(Pillsbury)								
	1 pastry	180	3	9	200	1	7.0	5
'Strudel Breakfast Pastries' 'Toaster Strudel'	1 pastry	190	2	28	200	0	8.0	0
'Toaster Strudel'	1 pastry	190	3	26	210	0	9.0	5
wild, Maine, 'Toaster Strudel'	1 pastry	120	2	23	135	0	3.0	0
(Toastettes)								
'Frosted Tarts'	1 pastry	190	2	35	190	1	5.0	0
'Tarts'	1 pastry	190	2	35	200	1	5.0	0
BRAN *(Thomas')* 'Toast-r-Cakes'	1 pastry	103	2	18	163	0	2.9	0
BROWN SUGAR CINNAMON								
(Kellogg's)								
frosted, 'Pop Tarts'	1 pastry	211	3	34	185	1	7.4	0
frosted w/cinnamon, low-fat, 'Pop Tarts'	1 pastry	188	2	39	210	1	2.8	0
plain, 'Pop Tarts'	1 pastry	219	3	32	214	1	9.2	0
CHEESE								
(Kellogg's) Danish, 'Pastry Swirls' 'Pop Tarts'	1 pastry	252	3	37	180	0	11.0	1
(Pepperidge Farm) 'Croissant Toaster Tarts'	1 pastry	190	5	22	180	0	10.0	10
(Pillsbury)								
cream cheese	1 pastry	190	3	9	230	0	10.0	15
cream cheese, w/blueberry	1 pastry	190	3	9	220	1	9.0	10
cream cheese, w/strawberry	1 pastry	190	3	9	220	1	9.0	10
CHERRY								
(Kellogg's)								
low-fat, 'Pop Tarts'	1 pastry	192	2	40	222	1	2.9	0
plain, 'Pop Tarts'	1 pastry	204	2	37	220	1	5.4	0
(Pastry Poppers) fruit juice sweetened, low-sodium	2 oz	212	3	38	115	0	4.5	0
(Pillsbury)								
	1 pastry	180	3	9	200	1	7.0	5
'Strudel Breakfast Pastries' 'Toaster Strudel'	1 pastry	190	2	26	200	0	9.0	0
'Toaster Strudel'	1 pastry	190	3	26	200	1	8.0	5
(Toastettes)								
'Frosted Tarts'	1 pastry	190	2	35	180	1	5.0	0
'Tarts'	1 pastry	190	2	35	200	1	5.0	0
CHOCOLATE FUDGE								
(Kellogg's)								
fudge, frosted, 'Pop Tarts'	1 pastry	201	3	37	203	1	4.8	0
fudge, frosted, low-fat, 'Pop Tarts'	1 pastry	190	3	40	249	1	3.0	0

Food Name	Serv. Size	Total Cal.	Prot. gms	Carbs gms	Sod. mgs	Fiber gms	Fat gms	Chol. mgs
milk chocolate, 'Pop Tarts' *(Kellogg's)*	1 pastry	205	3	36	227	1	5.8	0
vanilla creme, frosted, 'Pop Tarts'	1 pastry	203	3	37	229	1	5.3	0
CINNAMON								
(Pillsbury)								
	1 pastry	190	3	9	200	1	8.0	5
'Danish' 'Toaster Strudel'	1 pastry	214	4	24	197	1	11.9	11
'Strudel Breakfast Pastries' 'Toaster Strudel'	1 pastry	190	2	26	200	0	8.0	0
'Toaster Strudel'	1/6 pkg	200	5	23	200	0	10.0	5
(Toastettes) frosted, brown sugar cinnamon	1 pastry	190	2	35	180	1	5.0	0
CORN								
(Pillsbury) old-fashioned, 'Muffins' 'Toaster Strudel'	1 pastry	120	2	17	200	0	5.0	0
(Oroweat) toaster biscuit	1 biscuit	200	5	39	230	1	3.0	5
FRENCH TOAST *(Pillsbury)*	1 pastry	190	3	9	200	1	7.0	5
FRUIT PUNCH *(Toastettes)* 'Frosted Tarts'	1 pastry	190	2	35	200	1	5.0	0
GRAPE *(Kellogg's)* frosted, 'Pop Tarts'	1 pastry	203	2	38	198	1	5.1	0
LEMON *(Pillsbury)* 'Danish' 'Toaster Strudel'	1 pastry	197	3	25	188	1	9.8	21
OAT BRAN *(Awrey's)* w/raisins, 'Toastums'	1 pastry	130	3	17	310	1	5.0	0
PEACH-APRICOT								
(Pastry Poppers) fruit juice sweetened, low-salt	2 oz	212	3	38	115	0	4.5	0
RAISIN								
RAISIN BRAN								
(Pillsbury)								
bran, 'Muffins' 'Toaster Strudel'	1 pastry	120	3	16	220	0	5.0	0
'Danish' 'Toaster Strudel'	1 pastry	197	3	25	188	1	9.8	21
RASPBERRY								
(Auburn Farms)								
nonfat	1 pastry	180	3	42	200	4	0.0	0
'Toast 'n Jammers' *(Auburn Farms)*	1 pastry	180	3	42	200	3	0.0	0
(Kellogg's) frosted, 'Pop Tarts'	1 pastry	205	2	37	211	1	5.5	0
(Pastry Poppers) fruit juice sweetened, low-sodium	2 oz	212	3	38	115	0	4.5	0
(Pillsbury)								
	1 pastry	180	3	9	200	1	7.0	5
'Danish' 'Toaster Strudel'	1 pastry	197	3	25	188	1	9.8	21
'Strudel Breakfast Pastries' 'Toaster Strudel'	1 pastry	190	2	27	200	0	8.0	0
'Toaster Strudel'	1 pastry	180	3	26	200	1	7.0	5
S'MORES *(Kellogg's)* 'Pop Tarts'	1 pastry	204	3	36	199	1	5.5	0
STRAWBERRY								
(Auburn Farms) nonfat	1 pastry	180	3	42	200	4	0.0	0
(Kellogg's)								
frosted, 'Pop Tarts'	1 pastry	203	2	38	169	1	5.0	0
frosted, low-fat, 'Pop Tarts'	1 pastry	191	2	40	201	1	3.0	0
low-fat, 'Pop Tarts'	1 pastry	192	2	40	220	1	2.9	0
'Pastry Swirls' 'Pop Tarts'	1 pastry	254	3	37	170	1	11.0	0
'Pop Tarts'	1 pastry	210	2	37	200	0	6.0	0
(Pastry Poppers) fruit juice sweetened, low-sodium	2 oz	212	3	38	115	0	4.5	0
(Pepperidge Farm) 'Croissant Toaster Tarts'	1 pastry	190	3	28	120	0	7.0	0
(Pillsbury)	1 pastry	180	3	9	200	1	7.0	5
'Danish' 'Toaster Strudel'	1 pastry	197	3	25	188	1	9.8	21
'Strudel Breakfast Pastries' 'Toaster Strudel'	1 pastry	190	2	27	200	0	8.0	0
'Toaster Strudel'	1 pastry	180	3	26	200	1	7.0	5
(Toast N' Jammers) 100% juice sweetened, whole wheat	1 pastry	165	3	38	189	2	0.5	0
(Toastettes) frosted	1 pastry	190	2	35	190	1	5.0	0
PASTRY FLOUR. See under FLOUR.								
PÂTÉ, CANNED								
chicken liver	1 oz	57	4	2	109	0	3.7	111
chicken liver	1 tbsp	26	2	1	50	0	1.7	51

Food Name	Serv. Size	Total Cal.	Prot. gms	Carbs gms	Sod. mgs	Fiber gms	Fat gms	Chol. mgs
goose liver, de foie gras, smoked	1 oz	131	3	1	198	0	12.4	43
goose liver, de foie gras, smoked	1 tbsp	60	1	1	91	0	5.7	20
liver *(Sells)*	2.25 oz	190	8	3	460	0	16.0	0

PATTYPAN SQUASH. See SQUASH, SCALLOP.

PEACH

Canned

extra light, halves or slices, w/liquid	1 cup	104	1	27	12	2	0.2	0
halves *(Hunt's)*	1/2 cup	100	1	24	10	1	0.0	0
in extra heavy syrup, halves or slices, w/liquid	1 cup	252	1	68	21	3	0.1	0
in heavy syrup, halves, w/liquid	1/2 med fruit	73	0	20	6	1	0.1	0
in heavy syrup, slices, w/liquid	1 cup	194	1	52	16	3	0.3	0
in juice, halves, w/liquid	1/2 fruit	43	1	11	4	1	0.0	0
in juice, halves or slices, w/liquid	1 cup	109	2	29	10	3	0.1	0
in light syrup, halves, w/liquid	1/2 fruit	53	0	14	5	1	0.0	0
in light syrup, halves or slices, w/liquid	1 cup	136	1	37	13	3	0.1	0
in water, halves, w/liquid	1/2 fruit	24	0	6	3	1	0.1	0
in water, halves or slices, w/liquid	1 cup	59	1	15	7	3	0.1	0
sliced *(Hunt's)*	1/2 cup	100	1	24	10	1	0.0	0
spiced, in heavy syrup, whole, w/liquid	1 cup	182	1	49	10	3	0.2	0

Dried

sulfured, stewed	1 cup	322	5	83	10	na	1.0	0
sulfured, uncooked	1 cup	377	6	96	12	na	1.2	0
sulfured, uncooked, halves	1 cup	382	6	98	11	13	1.2	0
sulfured, uncooked, halves	1/2 medium	31	0	8	1	1	0.1	0
sulfured, w/added sugar	1 cup	278	3	72	5	6	0.6	0
sulfured, w/o added sugar	1 cup	199	3	51	5	7	0.6	0

Fresh

raw, sliced	1 cup	73	1	19	0	3	0.2	0
raw, whole, large, 2.75 inch diam, 2.5 per lb	1 peach	68	1	17	0	3	0.1	0
raw, whole, medium, 2.5 inch diam, 4 per lb	1 peach	42	1	11	0	2	0.1	0
raw, whole, small, 2 inch diam, 5 per lb	1 peach	34	1	9	0	2	0.1	0

Frozen

in syrup, sliced *(Flav-R-Pac)*	2/3 cup	100	1	25	0	1	0.0	0
sliced *(Flav-R-Pac)*	2/3 cup	50	1	13	0	2	0.0	0
sliced, thawed	1 cup	235	2	60	15	5	0.3	0
sweetened, sliced	10-oz pkg	267	2	68	17	5	0.4	0
sweetened, sliced	10 med slices	146	1	37	9	3	0.2	0

PEACH BUTTER, nonfat *(Smucker's)* | 1 tsp | 15 | 0 | 4 | 0 | 0 | 0.0 | 0 |

PEACH DRINK. See under FRUIT DRINK; FRUIT JUICE BLEND; FRUIT JUICE DRINK; PEACH JUICE.

PEACH JUICE

(Dole) orchard blend, 'Pure & Light'	6 fl oz	90	0	24	10	0	0.0	0
(Mountain Sun) 'Mountain Peach' organic	8 fl oz	112	0	27	0	0	0.0	0
(Smucker's) 'Naturally 100%'	8 fl oz	120	1	30	10	0	0.0	0

PEANUT

ALL TYPES

lightly salted, shelled *(Eagle)*	1 oz	180	7	5	65	2	15.0	0
salted *(Frito-Lay's)*	1 oz	170	6	6	170	0	15.0	0
salted in shell, shelled *(Fisher)*	1/4 cup	170	7	6	170	2	14.0	0
salted, shelled *(Little Debbie)*	1.25 oz	230	10	5	90	0	18.0	1
shelled *(Beer Nuts)*	1 oz	180	7	7	60	0	14.0	0
shelled *(Weight Watchers)*	1 pouch	100	8	4	50	0	7.0	0
shelled, 'Ballpark' *(Eagle)*	1 oz	180	8	5	110	1	15.0	0
shelled, 'Sweet & Crunchy' *(Pathmark)*	1 oz	140	4	15	30	0	8.0	0
shelled, 'Sweet-N-Crunchy' *(Planters)*	1 oz	140	4	15	20	0	8.0	0
spicy, hot, shelled, 'Heat' *(Planters)*	1 oz	170	7	5	190	0	14.0	0
spicy, mild, shelled, 'Heat' *(Planters)*	1 oz	170	7	5	130	0	14.0	0
unsalted, shelled *(Little Debbie)*	1.25 oz	230	10	5	1	0	18.0	0

Food Name	Serv. Size	Total Cal.	Prot. gms	Carbs gms	Sod. mgs	Fiber gms	Fat gms	Chol. mgs
Dry roasted								
lightly salted *(Finast)*	1 oz	160	8	6	120	0	14.0	0
lightly salted *(Fisher)*	1 oz	160	7	6	100	0	14.0	0
lightly salted *(Planters)*	1 oz	170	7	5	110	0	15.0	0
salted *(Fisher)*	1 oz	160	7	6	210	0	14.0	0
salted *(Flavor House)*	1 oz	180	8	5	200	0	14.0	0
salted *(Frito-Lay's)*	1 1/8 oz	190	7	7	300	0	16.0	0
salted *(Guy's)*	1 oz	170	8	3	310	0	14.0	0
salted *(Pathmark)*	1 oz	170	7	5	150	0	14.0	0
salted *(Planters)*	1 oz	160	7	6	250	0	14.0	0
unsalted *(Finast)*	1 oz	160	7	5	15	0	14.0	0
unsalted *(Flavor House)*	1 oz	180	8	5	0	0	14.0	0
unsalted *(Pathmark)*	1 oz	170	7	5	0	0	14.0	0
unsalted *(Planters)*	1 oz	170	7	5	0	0	15.0	0
unsalted, natural *(Flanigan Farms)*	1 oz	170	7	6	1	na	14.0	0
unsalted, 'No Frills' *(Pathmark)*	1 oz	180	8	5	0	0	14.0	0
Golden roasted								
(Fisher)	1/4 cup	160	7	10	220	2	12.0	0
barbecue, crunchy *(Fisher)*	1/4 cup	160	7	10	210	2	11.0	0
Honey roasted								
(Fisher)	1/4 cup	170	6	7	110	1	13.0	0
(Flavor House)	1 oz	160	6	9	120	0	11.0	0
(Little Debbie)	1.13 oz	190	8	9	15	0	13.0	1
(Pathmark)	1 oz	170	6	8	75	0	13.0	0
(Planters)	1 oz	170	6	8	180	0	13.0	0
(Weight Watchers)	1 pouch	100	8	4	50	0	7.0	0
'Honey Roast' *(Eagle)*	1 oz	170	7	7	140	0	13.0	0
unsalted *(Fisher)*	1 oz	150	7	4	0	0	13.0	0
Oil roasted								
(Fisher)	1/4 cup	170	7	5	130	2	15.0	0
(Planters)	1 oz	170	7	5	110	0	14.0	0
lightly salted *(Planters)*	1 oz	170	7	5	80	0	14.0	0
lightly salted	1 oz	160	7	6	65	0	14.0	0
redskin *(Planters)*	1 oz	170	7	5	150	0	15.0	0
salted *(Flavor House)*	1 oz	170	7	5	125	0	15.0	0
salted *(Pathmark)*	1 oz	180	8	5	150	0	14.0	0
salted *(Planters)*	1 oz	170	7	5	160	0	15.0	0
salted, cocktail *(Planters)*	1 oz	170	7	5	160	0	15.0	0
unsalted *(Planters)*	1 oz	170	7	5	0	0	14.0	0
unsalted, cocktail *(Planters)*	1 oz	170	7	5	0	0	15.0	0
Raw								
	1 cup	828	38	24	26	12	71.9	0
	1 oz	161	7	5	5	2	14.0	0
Roasted								
salted, in shell *(Planters)*	1.5 oz	170	7	5	240	0	14.0	0
unsalted, in shell *(Planters)*	1.5 oz	170	7	5	0	0	14.0	0
Yogurt coated *(Harmony)*	17 pieces	210	4	21	30	1	13.0	0
SPANISH								
shelled, salted *(Guy's)*	1 oz	170	8	3	170	0	14.0	0
Dry roasted *(Planters)*	1 oz	160	7	6	200	0	14.0	0
Oil roasted								
(Flavor House)	1 oz	170	7	5	125	0	15.0	0
(Planters)	1 oz	170	7	5	100	0	15.0	0
Raw								
	1 cup	832	38	23	32	14	72.4	0
	1 oz	162	7	4	6	3	14.1	0

Food Name	Serv. Size	Total Cal.	Prot. gms	Carbs gms	Sod. mgs	Fiber gms	Fat gms	Chol. mgs
(Planters)	1 oz	160	7	5	5	0	14.0	0
salted *(Fisher)*	1 oz	160	7	5	0	0	14.0	0
Roasted								
salted *(Eagle)*	1 oz	180	7	5	135	2	15.0	0
salted *(Fisher)*	1/4 cup	180	5	6	130	2	16.0	0
VALENCIA								
Oil roasted								
unsalted	1 cup	848	39	23	1112	13	73.8	0
unsalted	1 oz	167	8	5	219	3	14.5	0
Raw								
unsalted	1 cup	832	37	31	1	13	69.5	0
unsalted	1 oz	162	7	6	0	2	13.5	0
VIRGINIA								
Oil roasted								
unsalted	1 cup	827	37	28	619	13	69.5	0
unsalted	1 oz	164	7	6	123	3	13.8	0
Raw								
unsalted	1 cup	822	37	24	15	12	71.2	0
unsalted	1 oz	160	7	5	3	2	13.8	0
PEANUT BUTTER								
chunky	1 cup	1520	62	56	1254	17	128.8	0
chunky	2 tbsp	188	8	7	156	2	16.0	0
chunky, no salt added	1 cup	1520	62	56	44	17	128.8	0
chunky, no salt added	2 tbsp	188	8	7	5	2	16.0	0
smooth	1 cup	1530	65	50	1205	15	131.7	0
smooth	2 tbsp	190	8	6	149	2	16.3	0
smooth, no salt added	1 cup	1530	65	50	44	15	131.7	0
smooth, no salt added	2 tbsp	190	8	6	5	2	16.3	0
(Arrowhead Mills)								
chunky	2 tbsp	190	9	6	1	5	16.0	0
creamy	2 tbsp	190	9	6	1	5	16.0	0
(Bama)								
chunky	2 tbsp	200	7	6	115	0	17.0	0
creamy	2 tbsp	200	7	6	140	0	17.0	0
crunchy	2 tbsp	200	7	6	115	0	17.0	0
smooth	2 tbsp	200	7	6	140	0	17.0	0
(Estee)								
chunky	2 tbsp	200	8	6	0	0	18.0	0
creamy	2 tbsp	200	8	6	0	0	18.0	0
(Featherweight)								
chunky	1 tbsp	90	4	2	5	0	7.0	0
smooth	1 tbsp	90	4	2	3	0	7.0	0
(Finast)								
chunky, 'Crunchy'	2 tbsp	195	9	6	175	0	17.0	0
smooth	2 tbsp	195	9	6	175	0	17.0	0
(Health Valley)								
chunky, no salt added	2 tbsp	180	8	6	2	3	14.0	0
creamy, no salt added	2 tbsp	180	8	6	2	3	14.0	0
(Hollywood)								
chunky	1 tbsp	35	2	1	25	1	3.0	0
creamy	1 tbsp	35	2	1	25	1	3.0	0
no salt added	1 tbsp	35	2	1	0	1	3.0	0
(JFG)								
creamy	2 tbsp	200	7	8	150	2	16.0	0
creamy, 50% less salt	2 tbsp	200	7	8	75	2	16.0	0
crunchy	2 tbsp	200	7	8	140	2	16.0	0
(Jif)								
creamy	2 tbsp	190	8	7	150	2	16.0	0

Food Name	Serv. Size	Total Cal.	Prot. gms	Carbs gms	Sod. mgs	Fiber gms	Fat gms	Chol. mgs
creamy, 'Simply Jif'	2 tbsp	190	8	6	65	2	16.0	0
crunchy, 'Simply Jif'	2 tbsp	190	8	7	50	2	16.0	0
extra crunchy	2 tbsp	190	8	7	130	2	16.0	0
smooth	2 tbsp	190	9	6	155	0	16.0	0
(Maranatha Natural) crunchy	2 tbsp	190	8	7	5	0	15.0	0
(Pathmark)								
chunky, 'Super Chunky'	2 tbsp	200	7	6	140	0	17.0	0
'Natural'	2 tbsp	200	9	5	130	0	17.0	0
smooth, 'Creamy'	2 tbsp	200	7	6	170	0	17.0	0
smooth, 'No Frills'	2 tbsp	200	7	6	170	0	17.0	0
(Peter Pan)								
creamy	2 tbsp	189	8	7	152	2	16.0	0
creamy, low salt	2 tbsp	197	8	6	10	2	17.5	0
creamy, whipped	2 tbsp	148	6	5	120	2	12.6	0
crunchy	2 tbsp	188	8	6	119	2	15.9	0
crunchy, low salt	2 tbsp	197	8	6	9	2	17.3	0
crunchy, salt-free	2 tbsp	190	9	5	0	2	17.0	0
crunchy, whipped	2 tbsp	148	7	5	94	2	12.5	0
smooth, no salt added	2 tbsp	195	9	5	1	0	17.1	0
(Real Brand)								
creamy	2 tbsp	189	10	5	94	3	16.4	0
crunchy	2 tbsp	189	9	5	92	4	16.3	0
(Reese) creamy	2 tbsp	204	8	6	105	2	16.1	0
(Roaster Fresh) gourmet	1 oz	166	8	5	2	0	14.0	0
(S&W) 'Nutradiet'	1 tbsp	93	3	2	10	0	8.0	0
(Skippy)								
chunky, roasted honey nut	2 tbsp	190	7	6	120	2	17.0	0
chunky, 'Super Chunk'	2 tbsp	190	8	5	140	2	17.0	0
creamy	2 tbsp	190	8	5	150	2	17.0	0
creamy, roasted honey nut	2 tbsp	190	7	6	120	2	17.0	0
(Smucker's)								
chunky, 'Chunky Natural'	2 tbsp	200	8	6	120	0	16.0	0
honey sweetened	2 tbsp	200	7	7	150	0	16.0	0
no salt added, 'Natural'	2 tbsp	200	8	6	10	0	16.0	0
smooth, 'Natural'	2 tbsp	200	8	6	120	0	16.0	0
smooth, no salt added, 'Natural'	2 tbsp	200	8	6	10	0	17.0	0
(Westbrae)								
crunchy, no salt added, 'Natural'	2 tbsp	190	8	7	0	0	16.0	0
crunchy, w/salt, 'Natural'	2 tbsp	190	8	7	5	0	16.0	0
smooth, no salt added, 'Natural'	2 tbsp	190	8	7	0	0	16.0	0
(Woodstock) smooth, unsalted, 'Old Fashioned'	2 tbsp	200	9	6	3	0	16.0	0
PEANUT BUTTER CHIPS								
for baking, 'Reese's' *(Hershey's)*	1.5 oz	230	9	19	90	0	13.0	5
PEANUT BUTTER SPREAD								
(Bama) w/jelly	2 tbsp	150	3	20	75	0	7.0	0
(Bama) w/jelly	2 tbsp	150	3	20	75	0	7.0	0
(Jif) creamy, less fat	2 tbsp	190	8	15	250	2	12.0	0
(Peter Pan) creamy, less fat	2 tbsp	180	8	15	188	2	11.0	0
(Peter Pan) crunchy, less fat	2 tbsp	195	8	15	153	2	11.7	0
(Skippy) chunky, less fat	2 tbsp	180	8	13	170	2	12.4	0
(Skippy) creamy, less fat	2 tbsp	190	9	13	200	1	12.5	0
(Smucker's) w/grape jelly, 'Goober Grape'	2 tbsp	180	5	18	120	0	10.0	0
(Smucker's) w/strawberry jelly, 'Goober Strawberry'	2 tbsp	180	5	18	120	0	10.0	0
PEANUT BUTTER TOPPING, w/caramel *(Smucker's)*	2 tbsp	150	3	29	120	0	2.0	0
PEANUT OIL								
	1 cup	1909	0	0	0	0	216.0	0
	1 tbsp	119	0	0	0	0	13.5	0

Food Name	Serv. Size	Total Cal.	Prot. gms	Carbs gms	Sod. mgs	Fiber gms	Fat gms	Chol. mgs
(Hain)	1 tbsp	120	0	0	0	0	14.0	0
(Wesson)	1 tbsp	122	0	0	0	0	13.6	0
100% pure (Hollywood)	1 tbsp	120	0	0	0	0	14.0	0
100% pure (Planters)	1 tbsp	120	0	0	0	0	14.0	0
pure pressed, organic (Spectrum)	1 tbsp	120	0	0	0	0	14.0	0

PEAR
Canned

Food Name	Serv. Size	Total Cal.	Prot. gms	Carbs gms	Sod. mgs	Fiber gms	Fat gms	Chol. mgs
in extra heavy syrup, halves, w/liquid	1 cup	258	1	67	13	4	0.3	0
in extra heavy syrup, halves, w/1.75 tbsp liquid	1 med half	77	0	20	4	1	0.1	0
in extra light syrup, halves, w/liquid	1 cup	116	1	30	5	4	0.2	0
in extra light syrup, halves, w/liquid	1 med half	36	0	9	2	1	0.1	0
in heavy syrup, w/liquid	1 cup	197	1	51	13	4	0.3	0
in heavy syrup, w/liquid	1 med half	56	0	15	4	1	0.1	0
in juice, halves, w/liquid	1 cup	124	1	32	10	4	0.2	0
in juice, halves, w/liquid	1 med half	38	0	10	3	1	0.1	0
in light syrup, halves, w/liquid	1 cup	143	0	38	13	4	0.1	0
in light syrup, halves, w/liquid	1/2 fruit	43	0	12	4	1	0.0	0
in water, halves, w/liquid	1 cup	71	0	19	5	4	0.1	0
in water, halves, w/liquid	1 med half	22	0	6	2	1	0.0	0

Dried

Food Name	Serv. Size	Total Cal.	Prot. gms	Carbs gms	Sod. mgs	Fiber gms	Fat gms	Chol. mgs
sulfured, stewed, halves	1 cup	324	2	86	8	16	0.8	0
sulfured, uncooked, halves	1 cup	472	3	125	11	14	1.1	0
sulfured, uncooked, halves	1 med half	47	0	13	1	1	0.1	0

Fresh

Food Name	Serv. Size	Total Cal.	Prot. gms	Carbs gms	Sod. mgs	Fiber gms	Fat gms	Chol. mgs
sliced	1 cup	97	1	25	0	4	0.7	0
whole, large, 2 per lb	1 pear	123	1	32	0	5	0.8	0
whole, medium, 2.5 per lb	1 pear	98	1	25	0	4	0.7	0
whole, small, 3 per lb	1 pear	82	1	21	0	3	0.6	0

PEAR JUICE

Food Name	Serv. Size	Total Cal.	Prot. gms	Carbs gms	Sod. mgs	Fiber gms	Fat gms	Chol. mgs
(Knudsen)	8 fl oz	110	1	28	0	0	0.0	0
(Mountain Sun) organic, 'Mountain pear'	8 fl oz	102	0	25	0	0	0.0	0
(Santa Cruz Natural) organic, 'Cruz'	8 fl oz	135	1	32	0	0	1.0	0

PEAR NECTAR. See under FRUIT JUICE DRINK.

PEAS. BLACK-EYED. See BLACK-EYED PEAS.

PEAS, CROWDER. See under BLACK-EYED PEAS.

PEAS, FIELD
Canned

Food Name	Serv. Size	Total Cal.	Prot. gms	Carbs gms	Sod. mgs	Fiber gms	Fat gms	Chol. mgs
'Fresh' (Allens)	1/2 cup	100	7	18	370	0	1.0	0
tiny, w/snaps 'Fresh' (Allens)	1/2 cup	70	6	13	340	0	1.0	0
w/snaps (Bush's Best)	1/2 cup	80	6	16	550	3	0.0	0
w/snaps, 'Fresh' (Allens)	1/2 cup	100	5	20	370	0	1.0	0
w/snaps, seasoned w/pork (Luck's)	1/2 cup	130	7	19	320	4	3.0	3

PEAS, GREEN
Canned

Food Name	Serv. Size	Total Cal.	Prot. gms	Carbs gms	Sod. mgs	Fiber gms	Fat gms	Chol. mgs
dry, early June (Allens)	1/2 cup	80	5	15	320	0	1.0	0
early (A&P)	1/2 cup	70	4	15	350	0	1.0	0
early (Stokely)	1/2 cup	60	4	12	320	0	0.0	0
early, 'LeSueur' (Green Giant)	1/2 cup	60	4	12	380	3	0.0	0
early, 50% less sodium, 'LeSueur' (Green Giant)	1/2 cup	60	4	11	190	4	0.0	0
early June (Green Giant)	1/2 cup	50	3	12	330	3	0.0	0
early June, 'Petit Pois' (S&W)	1/2 cup	70	4	12	330	0	0.0	0
early June (Veg-All)	1/2 cup	50	4	10	370	0	0.0	0
early June, medium (TenderSweet)	1/2 cup	70	4	11	370	3	0.5	0
early June, medium, no salt added (TenderSweet)	1/2 cup	50	4	10	10	4	0.0	0
early June, 'Sun-Vista' (S&W)	1/2 cup	80	6	18	510	5	0.0	0
early June, tiny, party (Stokely)	1/2 cup	60	4	10	360	3	0.0	0
early, very young, small (Green Giant)	1/2 cup	50	3	12	390	3	0.0	0

Food Name	Serv. Size	Total Cal.	Prot. gms	Carbs gms	Sod. mgs	Fiber gms	Fat gms	Chol. mgs
mixed, no salt or sugar added *(IGA)*	1/2 cup	50	4	10	10	0	0.0	0
mixed sizes *(A&P)*	1/2 cup	60	4	12	350	0	1.0	0
no salt added, w/liquid *(Del Monte)*	1/2 cup	60	3	11	10	0	0.0	0
no salt or sugar added *(Stokely)*	1/2 cup	50	4	9	5	0	0.0	0
seasoned, w/liquid *(Del Monte)*	1/2 cup	60	3	11	355	0	0.0	0
small, w/liquid *(Del Monte)*	1/2 cup	50	3	9	355	0	0.0	0
sweet *(Featherweight)*	1/2 cup	70	5	12	10	0	0.0	0
sweet *(Finast)*	1/2 cup	70	4	13	300	0	1.0	0
sweet *(Green Giant)*	1/2 cup	60	4	11	390	4	0.0	0
sweet *(Stokely)*	1/2 cup	70	4	11	370	3	0.5	0
sweet *(Veg-All)*	1/2 cup	50	4	10	370	0	0.0	0
sweet, 50% less sodium *(Green Giant)*	1/2 cup	60	4	11	195	3	0.0	0
sweet, 50% less sodium, 'LeSueur' *(Green Giant)*	1/2 cup	60	4	11	190	4	0.0	0
sweet, garden *(Freshlike)*	1/2 cup	50	4	10	350	0	0.0	0
sweet, garden, no salt added *(Freshlike)*	1/2 cup	50	4	10	10	0	0.0	0
sweet, garden, fancy *(Pathmark)*	1/2 cup	70	4	12	350	0	1.0	0
sweet, large, tender *(Pathmark)*	1/2 cup	70	4	12	350	0	1.0	0
sweet, 'LeSueur' *(Green Giant)*	1/2 cup	60	4	12	380	3	0.0	0
sweet, 'Little Gem' *(Pathmark)*	1/2 cup	70	4	12	350	0	1.0	0
sweet, mini, in brine *(Green Giant)*	1/2 cup	60	4	12	240	4	1.0	0
sweet, mixed sizes *(Veg-All)*	1/2 cup	50	4	10	370	0	0.0	0
sweet, mixed sizes, no salt added *(Pathmark)*	1/2 cup	50	4	10	10	0	0.0	0
sweet, no salt added *(Finast)*	1/2 cup	60	4	12	10	0	0.0	0
sweet, 'No Frills' *(Pathmark)*	1 cup	120	8	25	640	0	1.0	0
sweet, 'Nutradiet' *(S&W)*	1/2 cup	40	3	8	5	0	0.0	0
sweet, 'Perfection' *(S&W)*	1/2 cup	70	4	12	330	0	0.0	0
sweet, small *(Freshlike)*	1/2 cup	50	4	10	350	0	0.0	0
sweet, small *(Pathmark)*	1/2 cup	70	4	12	350	0	1.0	0
sweet, small *(Veg-All)*	1/2 cup	50	4	10	370	0	0.0	0
sweet, tiny, early June *(IGA)*	1/2 cup	70	4	12	340	0	0.0	0
sweet, very young, small *(Green Giant)*	1/2 cup	50	4	12	390	4	0.0	0
sweet, very young, tender *(Green Giant)*	1/2 cup	50	4	11	390	4	0.0	0
sweet, water packed, no sugar or salt added *(Freshlike)*	1/2 cup	50	4	10	10	0	0.0	0
very young, sweet, 'LeSueur' *(Green Giant)*	1/2 cup	50	4	12	390	0	0.0	0
w/liquid *(Del Monte)*	1/2 cup	60	3	10	355	0	0.0	0
Freeze-dried, prepared *(Mountain House)*	1/2 cup	70	4	12	21	0	1.0	0
Fresh								
boiled, drained	1 cup	134	9	25	5	9	0.4	0
boiled, drained	1/2 cup	62	4	11	70	4	0.2	0
raw	1 cup	117	8	21	7	7	0.6	0
Frozen								
(Birds Eye)	3.3 oz	80	5	13	130	4	0.0	0
(Flav-R-Pac)	2/3 cup	70	5	12	105	4	0.5	0
(Freshlike)	3.3 oz	80	5	13	75	0	0.0	0
(Frosty Acres)	3.3 oz	80	5	13	91	2	0.0	0
(Health Valley)	1/2 cup	65	4	11	70	3	0.0	0
(Seabrook)	3.3 oz	80	5	13	91	2	0.0	0
(Southern)	3.5 oz	79	6	14	130	0	0.5	0
(Veg-All)	3.3 oz	80	5	13	75	0	0.0	0
boiled, drained	10-oz pkg	197	13	36	220	14	0.7	0
early, baby, 'LeSueur Select' *(Green Giant)*	1/2 cup	60	4	13	115	4	0.0	0
early, very young, small, 50% less sodium , 'LeSueur' *(Green Giant)*	1/2 cup	60	4	11	190	4	0.0	0
early June, 'Harvest Fresh' *(Green Giant)*	1/2 cup	60	4	12	140	3	1.0	0
LeSueur style, 'Valley Combinations' *(Green Giant)*	1/2 cup	70	4	12	400	2	2.0	0
no salt added *(Flav-R-Pac)*	2/3 cup	70	5	12	15	4	0.5	0

Food Name	Serv. Size	Total Cal.	Prot. gms	Carbs gms	Sod. mgs	Fiber gms	Fat gms	Chol. mgs
petite *(C&W)*	2/3 cup	70	5	12	105	4	0.5	0
petite *(Flav-R-Pac)*	2/3 cup	70	5	12	105	4	0.5	0
petite *(Southern)*	3.5 oz	64	5	11	50	0	0.4	0
petite, no salt added *(C&W)*	2/3 cup	70	5	12	10	4	0.5	0
'Portion Pack' *(Birds Eye)*	3 oz	70	5	12	120	4	0.0	0
'Singles' *(Stokely)*	3 oz	65	4	12	95	0	1.0	0
sweet *(Finast)*	3.3 oz	80	5	13	125	0	0.0	0
sweet *(Green Giant)*	1/2 cup	50	4	11	95	4	0.0	0
sweet, baby, 'LeSueur Select' *(Green Giant)*	2/3 cup	60	5	11	150	5	0.0	0
sweet, 'Harvest Fresh' *(Green Giant)*	1/2 cup	50	4	12	135	3	0.0	0
sweet, no salt added *(Del Monte)*	1/2 cup	60	3	11	10	4	0.0	0
sweet 'Plain Polybag' *(Green Giant)*	2/3 cup	70	4	13	135	4	0.0	0
tender, tiny, 'Deluxe' *(Birds Eye)*	3.3 oz	60	4	11	120	4	0.0	0
tiny *(Freshlike)*	3.3 oz	60	4	11	75	0	0.0	0
tiny *(Frosty Acres)*	3.3 oz	60	4	11	127	2	0.0	0
tiny *(Seabrook)*	3.3 oz	60	4	11	127	2	0.0	0
tiny *(Veg-All)*	3.3 oz	60	4	11	75	0	0.0	0
Sprouted, mature seeds, raw	1 cup	154	11	34	24	na	0.8	0
PEAS, GREEN, DISH/ENTRÉE								
(A&P)								
and carrots, frozen	3.3 oz	60	3	11	75	0	1.0	0
early June, and carrots, canned, no salt added	1/2 cup	60	4	12	10	0	1.0	0
mixed sizes, and carrots, canned	1/2 cup	60	4	12	10	0	1.0	0
sweet, and carrots, frozen	1/2 cup	80	5	13	90	0	1.0	0
(Allens) creamed, 'Fresh'	1/2 cup	90	7	14	440	0	1.0	0
(Birds Eye)								
and pearl onions, frozen, 'Combination Vegetables'	3.3 oz	70	5	13	440	3	0.0	0
(Budget Gourmet)								
w/water chestnuts, Oriental, 'Side Dish'	5 oz	120	5	15	240	0	3.0	5
(Del Monte) and carrots, canned, w/liquid	1/2 cup	50	2	10	355	0	0.0	0
(Finast) and carrots, canned	1/2 cup	55	3	9	315	0	0.0	0
(Flav-R-Pac)								
and carrots, frozen	2/3 cup	50	3	9	75	3	0.0	0
and pearl onions, frozen	2/3 cup	70	4	12	95	4	0.5	0
(Freshlike)								
and carrots, frozen	3.3 oz	60	3	11	60	0	0.0	0
and onions, frozen	3.3 oz	70	4	13	100	0	0.0	0
sweet, and diced carrots, canned, in water, no salt added	1/2 cup	50	3	12	30	0	0.0	0
sweet, and diced carrots, canned, in water, no sugar added	1/2 cup	50	3	12	30	0	0.0	0
sweet, and sliced carrots, canned	1/2 cup	50	3	12	340	0	0.0	0
sweet, and tiny onions, canned	1/2 cup	60	4	12	440	0	0.0	0
(Frosty Acres)								
and carrots, frozen	3.3 oz	60	3	11	75	1	0.0	0
and pearl onions, frozen	3.3 oz	70	4	13	80	0	0.0	0
(Green Giant) and pearl onions, canned, w/liquid	1/2 cup	50	4	11	510	4	0.0	0
(Kohl's) and carrots, canned	1/2 cup	50	3	20	330	0	1.0	0
(Pathmark) and carrots, canned	1/2 cup	60	3	18	330	0	1.0	0
(S&W) and carrots, canned, 'Nutradiet'	1/2 cup	35	2	7	5	0	0.0	0
(Seabrook)								
and carrots, frozen	3.3 oz	60	3	11	75	1	0.0	0
and onions, frozen	3.3 oz	70	4	13	0	0	0.0	0
(Southern) and carrots, frozen	3.5 oz	64	3	12	80	0	0.0	0
(Stokely)								
and carrots, canned	1/2 cup	50	3	9	320	0	0.0	0
and diced carrots, no salt or sugar added	1/2 cup	45	3	8	20	0	0.0	0

Food Name	Serv. Size	Total Cal.	Prot. gms	Carbs gms	Sod. mgs	Fiber gms	Fat gms	Chol. mgs
and sliced carrots, no salt or sugar added .... 1/2 cup		45	3	8	25	0	0.0	0
(Veg-All)								
and carrots, frozen .... 3.3 oz		60	3	11	60	0	0.0	0
and onions, frozen .... 3.3 oz		70	4	13	100	0	0.0	0
sweet, and diced carrots, canned .... 1/2 cup		50	3	12	340	0	0.0	0
sweet, and sliced carrots, canned .... 1/2 cup		50	3	12	340	0	0.0	0
PEAS, PIGEON								
immature seeds, boiled, drained .... 1 cup		170	9	30	8	9	2.1	0
immature seeds, raw .... 1 cup		209	11	37	8	8	2.5	0
immature seeds, raw .... 10 seeds		5	0	1	0	0	0.1	0
red gram, mature seeds, boiled .... 1 cup		203	11	39	8	11	0.6	0
red gram, mature seeds, raw .... 1 cup		703	44	129	35	31	3.1	0
PEAS, PURPLE HULLED								
canned, 'Fresh' *(Allens)* .... 1/2 cup		100	6	16	370	0	1.0	0
frozen *(Frosty Acres)* .... 3.3 oz		130	9	23	6	0	0.0	0
PEAS, SNAP								
sugar snap *(Green Giant)* .... 1/2 cup		30	2	8	0	2	0.0	0
sugar snap, 'Deluxe' *(Birds Eye)* .... 2.6 oz		45	2	9	5	4	0.0	0
sugar snap, frozen *(Flav-R-Pac)* .... 3/4 cup		30	2	7	10	2	0.0	0
sugar snap, 'Harvest Fresh' *(Green Giant)* .... 1/2 cup		30	2	8	100	2	0.0	0
sugar snap, 'Select' *(Green Giant)* .... 1/2 cup		30	2	8	0	2	0.0	0
PEAS, SNOW/Chinese pea pods								
Fresh								
edible-podded, boiled, drained .... 1 cup		67	5	11	6	4	0.4	0
edible-podded, raw, whole .... 10 pods		14	1	3	1	1	0.1	0
edible-podded, raw, chopped .... 1 cup		41	3	7	4	3	0.2	0
edible-podded, raw, whole .... 1 cup		26	2	5	3	2	0.1	0
Frozen								
(Chun King) .... 1.5 oz		20	1	3	10	0	0.0	0
(Flav-R-Pac) .... 1 cup		50	2	6	10	2	0.0	0
(Seabrook) .... 2 oz		20	2	4	0	0	0.0	0
baby, pods *(C&W)* .... 2/3 cup		40	3	7	45	3	0.0	0
'Deluxe' *(Birds Eye)* .... 3 oz		35	2	6	0	3	0.0	0
edible-podded, drained .... 1 cup		83	6	14	8	5	0.6	0
edible-podded, drained .... 1/2 cup		42	3	7	4	2	0.3	0
edible-podded, drained .... 10-oz pkg		132	9	23	13	8	1.0	0
edible-podded, unprepared .... 10-oz pkg		119	8	20	11	9	0.9	0
edible-podded, unprepared .... 1/2 cup		30	2	5	3	2	0.2	0
pods, food service product *(La Choy)* .... 1 cup		41	2	9	9	3	0.0	0
PEAS, SPLIT								
boiled *(A&P)* .... 1 cup		220	16	40	15	0	1.0	0
green, raw *(Arrowhead Mills)* .... 2 oz		200	14	35	14	8	1.0	0
mature seeds, boiled .... 1 cup		231	16	41	4	16	0.8	0
mature seeds, boiled .... 1 tbsp		14	1	3	0	1	0.0	0
mature seeds, raw .... 1 cup		672	48	119	30	50	2.3	0
PEAS AND CARROTS. See under PEAS, GREEN, DISH/ENTRÉE.								
PECAN								
Dried								
chopped .... 1 cup		822	11	16	0	11	85.6	0
halves .... 1 cup		746	10	15	0	10	77.7	0
halves, approx 20 pieces .... 1 oz		196	3	4	0	3	20.4	0
Dry roasted								
unsalted .... 1 oz		201	3	4	0	3	21.1	0
salted .... 1 oz		201	3	4	109	3	21.1	0
Honey roasted *(Planters)* .... 1 oz		200	2	8	80	0	18.0	0
Oil roasted								
salted .... 1 cup		787	10	14	432	10	82.8	0

Food Name	Serv. Size	Total Cal.	Prot. gms	Carbs gms	Sod. mgs	Fiber gms	Fat gms	Chol. mgs
salted, halves, approx 15 pieces	1 oz	203	3	4	111	3	21.3	0
unsalted	1 cup	787	10	14	1	10	82.8	0
unsalted, halves, approx 15 pieces	1 oz	203	3	4	0	3	21.3	0
Raw								
(Fisher)	1 oz	190	2	5	0	0	19.0	0
chips (Planters)	1 oz	190	2	5	0	0	20.0	0
halves (Planters)	1 oz	190	2	5	0	0	20.0	0
pieces (Planters)	1 oz	190	2	5	0	0	20.0	0
Roasted								
chipped pieces, shelled (Azar)	2 oz	370	4	10	4	0	38.0	0
chopped, shelled (Fisher)	1 oz	190	2	5	0	0	19.0	0
ground, shelled (Fisher)	1 oz	190	2	5	0	0	19.0	0
halves, pieces, or chips, shelled (Planters)	1 oz	190	2	5	0	0	20.0	0
halves and pieces, shelled, (Azar)	2 oz	370	4	10	4	0	38.0	0
pieces, shelled (Azar)	2 oz	370	4	10	4	0	38.0	0
pieces, shelled, natural, unsalted (Flanigan Farms)	1 oz	190	3	4	4	na	20.0	0
shelled, natural, unsalted (Flanigan Farms)	1/4 cup	190	2	5	0	2	19.0	0
PECAN BUTTER roasted, organic (Maranatha Natural)	2 tbsp	220	3	7	0	3	21.0	0
PECTIN MIX, unsweetened	1.75 oz	163	0	45	100	4	0.1	0
PENNE. See under PASTA.								
PENNE DISH/ENTRÉE. See under PASTA DISH/ENTRÉE.								
PEPITAS								
dried, in shell	1 lb	1817	82.4	59.8	59	>7.5c	153.9	0
dried, shelled	1 cup	747	33.9	24.6	24	>3.1c	63.3	0
dried, shelled, approx 142 kernels	1 oz	154	7.0	5.1	5	>.6c	13.0	0
natural, unsalted (Flanigan Farms)	1/4 cup	150	7	5	5	4	13.0	0
roasted, shelled	1 cup	1184	74.8	30.5	40	>4.1c	95.6	0
roasted, shelled	1 oz	148	9.4	3.8	5	>.5c	12.0	0
roasted, whole, in shell	1 cup	285	11.9	34.4	12	>23c	12.4	0
roasted, whole, in shell, approx 85 seeds	1 oz	127	5.3	15.3	5	>10c	5.5	0
shelled, salted	1 cup	285	11.9	34.4	368	>23c	12.4	0
shelled, salted	1 lb	2021	84.1	243.8	2608	>163c	88.0	0
shelled, salted	1 oz	127	5.3	15.3	163	>10c	5.5	0
PEPEAO. See CHINESE FUNGUS.								
PEPPER, ANCHO, dried, whole	1 medium	48	2	9	7	4	1.4	0
PEPPER, BANANA								
Canned or jarred, hot (Vlasic)	1 oz	5	0	1	480	0	0.0	0
Fresh								
raw, chopped	1 cup	33	2	7	16	4	0.6	0
raw, whole, small, approx 4-inch long	1 pepper	9	1	2	4	1	0.1	0
raw, whole, medium, approx 4.5-inch long	1 pepper	12	1	2	6	2	0.2	0
raw, whole, large, approx 5-inch long	1 pepper	20	1	4	10	3	0.3	0
PEPPER, BELL/green pepper/red pepper/sweet pepper/yellow pepper								
Canned or jarred								
California roasted (Mezzetta)	1 oz	8	0	0	129	1	0.0	0
fried (Progresso)	1/2 jar	37	1	4	17	1	3.0	0
green, halves, w/liquid	1 cup	25	1	5	1917	2	0.4	0
red, halves, w/liquid	1 cup	25	1	5	1917	2	0.4	0
red, halves, w/liquid	1/2 cup	13	1	3	958	1	0.2	0
roasted (Progresso)	1/2 cup	20	1	5	2	2	1.0	0
'Sweet Pepper Mementos' (Heinz)	1 oz	6	0	1	320	0	0.0	0
Freeze-Dried								
	1/4 cup	5	0	1	3	0	0.0	0
	1 tbsp	1	0	0	1	0	0.0	0
red	1/4 cup	5	0	1	3	0	0.0	0
red	1 tbsp	1	0	0	1	0	0.0	0

Food Name	Serv. Size	Total Cal.	Prot. gms	Carbs gms	Sod. mgs	Fiber gms	Fat gms	Chol. mgs
Fresh								
(Dole) .... 1 medium		25	1	5	0	2	1.0	0
green, boiled, drained, chopped .... 1/2 cup		19	1	5	1	1	0.1	0
green, boiled, drained, minced .... 1 tbsp		3	0	1	0	0	0.0	0
green, boiled, drained, strips .... 1 cup		38	1	9	3	2	0.3	0
green, raw, chopped .... 1 cup		40	1	10	3	3	0.3	0
green, raw, minced .... 1 tbsp		3	0	1	0	0	0.0	0
green, raw, rings, 3-inch diam, 1/4-inch thick .... 1 ring		3	0	1	0	0	0.0	0
green, raw, sliced .... 1 cup		25	1	6	2	2	0.2	0
green, raw, strips .... 10 strips		7	0	2	1	0	0.1	0
green, raw, whole, approx 2.75-inch long, 2.5-inch diam .... 1 pepper		32	1	8	2	2	0.2	0
green, raw, whole, approx 3.75-inch long, 3-inch diam .... 1 pepper		44	1	11	3	3	0.3	0
red, boiled, drained, chopped .... 1/2 cup		19	1	5	1	1	0.1	0
red, boiled, drained, minced .... 1 tbsp		3	0	1	0	0	0.0	0
red, boiled, drained, strips .... 1 cup		38	1	9	3	2	0.3	0
red, raw .... 1 small		20	1	5	1	1	0.1	0
red, raw, chopped .... 1 cup		40	1	10	3	3	0.3	0
red, raw, minced .... 1 tbsp		3	0	1	0	0	0.0	0
red, raw, rings, 3-inch diam, 1/4-inch thick .... 1 ring		3	0	1	0	0	0.0	0
red, raw, sliced .... 1 cup		25	1	6	2	2	0.2	0
red, raw, whole, approx 2.75-inch long, 2.5-inch diam .... 1 medium		32	1	8	2	2	0.2	0
red, raw, whole, approx 3.75-inch long, 3-inch diam .... 1 large		44	1	11	3	3	0.3	0
yellow, raw, strips .... 10 strips		14	1	3	1	0	0.1	0
yellow, whole, approx 3.75-inch long, 30-inch diam ... 1 pepper		50	2	12	4	2	0.4	0
Frozen								
green (Seabrook) .... 1 oz		6	0	1	1	0	0.0	0
green, chopped, unprepared .... 10-oz pkg		57	3	13	14	5	0.6	0
green, diced (Flav-R-Pac) .... 3/4 cup		20	1	4	10	2	0.0	0
red (Seabrook) .... 1 oz		8	0	1	0	0	0.0	0
red, chopped, unprepared .... 10-oz pkg		57	3	13	14	5	0.6	0
red, chopped, unprepared .... 1 oz		6	0	1	1	0	0.1	0
red, diced (Flav-R-Pac) .... 3/4 cup		20	1	4	10	2	0.0	0
red, strips (Flav-R-Pac) .... 3/4 cup		20	1	4	10	2	0.0	0
strips (Flav-R-Pac) .... 3/4 cup		20	1	4	10	2	0.0	0
PEPPER, BELL, DISH/ENTRÉE								
(Celentano) red, sweet, stuffed, frozen .... 13 oz		350	28	28	810	4	20.0	0
(Lean Cuisine) red, stuffed, frozen, 'Salsa'lito' .... 1 oz		26	1	4	80	na	0.6	1
(Stouffer's)								
stuffed, frozen .... 1 entrée		200	9	24	900	1	8.0	25
stuffed, w/beef, in tomato sauce .... 1 pkg		378	16	42	1155	11	16.2	44
stuffed, w/beef, in tomato sauce .... 1 serving		189	8	21	579	5	8.1	22
stuffed, w/sauce, frozen, food service product .... 1 oz		25	1	3	122	0	1.1	3
stuffed, w/o sauce, food service product .... 1 oz		31	2	3	125	1	1.4	5
PEPPER, CHERRY								
Canned or jarred								
diced, drained (Progresso) .... 2 tbsp		30	0	2	30	1	2.0	0
diced, fried (Progresso) .... 2 tbsp		60	0	3	60	1	5.0	0
hot (Progresso) .... 1/2 cup		190	0	3	130	1	20.0	0
hot (Vlasic) .... 1 oz		10	0	2	480	0	0.0	0
hot, pickled (Progresso) .... 1/2 cup		130	0	3	110	1	12.0	0
hot, whole (Progresso) .... 1 med pepper		15	0	3	250	0	0.0	0
hot or mild, rings (Vlasic) .... 1 oz		5	0	1	480	0	0.0	0
mild (Vlasic) .... 1 oz		10	0	2	480	0	0.0	0

Food Name	Serv. Size	Total Cal.	Prot. gms	Carbs gms	Sod. mgs	Fiber gms	Fat gms	Chol. mgs
PEPPER, CHILI/chili								
Canned or jarred								
green *(Santiago)*	2 oz	13	0	3	122	1	0.1	0
green, chopped *(Old El Paso)*	2 tbsp	8	1	2	70	0	1.0	0
green, chopped, no seeds, w/liquid	1/2 cup	14	1	3	798	1	0.1	0
green, diced *(Pancho Villa)*	2 tbsp	5	0	1	110	1	0.0	0
green, diced *(Rosarita)*	2 tbsp	6	0	1	85	1	0.1	0
green, diced, food service product *(Rosarita)*	2 tbsp	6	0	1	85	1	0.1	0
green, diced, w/liquid *(Del Monte)*	1/2 cup	20	0	5	690	0	0.0	0
green, strips, food service product *(Rosarita)*	1/4 cup	4	0	1	74	1	0.1	0
green, whole *(Old El Paso)*	1 med pepper	8	1	1	105	0	1.0	0
green, whole *(Rosarita)*	2 tbsp	4	0	1	74	1	0.1	0
green, whole, diced, sliced, or strips *(Ortega)*	1 oz	10	0	3	20	0	0.0	0
green, whole, food service product *(Rosarita)*	2 tbsp	4	0	1	74	1	0.1	0
green, whole, no seeds, w/liquid	1 med pepper	15	1	4	856	1	0.1	0
green, whole, w/liquid *(Del Monte)*	1/2 cup	20	0	5	690	0	0.0	0
hot, diced *(Ortega)*	1 oz	8	0	2	0	0	0.0	0
hot, whole *(Ortega)*	1 oz	8	0	2	0	0	0.0	0
hot, tiny, Mexican *(Vlasic)*	1 oz	6	0	2	430	0	0.0	0
red, chopped, no seeds, w/liquid	1/2 cup	14	1	3	798	1	0.1	0
red, whole, no seeds, w/liquid	1 med pepper	15	1	4	856	1	0.1	0
Fresh								
green, chopped or diced	1/2 cup	30	2	7	5	1	0.1	0
green, raw, whole	1 med pepper	18	1	4	3	1	0.1	0
red, chopped or diced	1/2 cup	30	2	7	5	1	0.1	0
red, raw, whole	1 med pepper	18	1	4	3	1	0.1	0
Frozen								
green *(Santiago)*	2 oz	15	1	3	13	0	0.2	0
green, chopped *(Old El Paso)*	2 tbsp	5	0	1	110	1	0.0	0
hot, roasted, peeled, chopped *(Baca's)*	2 tbsp	5	0	1	5	0	0.0	0
Sun-dried								
hot, chopped	1 cup	120	4	26	34	11	2.1	0
hot, whole	1 med pepper	2	0	0	0	0	0.0	0
PEPPER, GREEN. See PEPPER, BELL.								
PEPPER, GROUND								
BLACK								
	1 tbsp	16	1	4	3	2	0.2	0
	1 dash	0	0	0	0	0	0.0	0
(Durkee)	1 tsp	8	0	0	0	0	0.0	0
(Laurel Leaf)	1 tsp	8	0	0	0	0	0.0	0
(McCormick/Schilling)	1 tsp	7	0	1	0	0	0.0	0
(Spice Islands)	1 tsp	9	0	2	1	0	0.2	0
coarse grind, 'Mr. Pepper' *(Tone's)*	1 tsp	8	0	2	1	1	0.1	0
fine grind, 'Mr. Pepper' *(Tone's)*	1 tsp	8	0	2	1	0	0.1	0
CAYENNE *(Spice Islands)*	1 tsp	9	0	1	1	1	0.3	0
CHILI								
(Spice Islands)	1 tsp	9	0	1	1	0	0.3	0
fresh ground *(Durkee)*	1 tsp	11	0	0	0	0	0.0	0
fresh ground *(Laurel Leaf)*	1 tsp	11	0	0	0	0	0.0	0
red *(McCormick/Schilling)*	1 tsp	10	0	1	1	1	0.4	0
RED								
(Spice Islands)	1 tsp	9	0	1	1	1	0.3	0
fresh-ground *(Durkee)*	1 tsp	8	0	0	0	0	0.0	0
fresh-ground *(Laurel Leaf)*	1 tsp	8	0	0	0	0	0.0	0
WHITE								
	1 tbsp	21	1	5	0	2	0.2	0

Food Name	Serv. Size	Total Cal.	Prot. gms	Carbs gms	Sod. mgs	Fiber gms	Fat gms	Chol. mgs
.... 1 tsp		7	0	2	0	1	0.1	0
(Durkee) .... 1 tsp		9	0	0	0	0	0.0	0
(Laurel Leaf) .... 1 tsp		9	0	0	0	0	0.0	0
(McCormick/Schilling) .... 1 tsp		8	0	2	0	0	0.0	0
(Spice Islands) .... 1 tsp		9	0	2	1	0	0.2	0
PEPPER, HUNGARIAN, raw .... 1 med pepper		8	0	2	0	na	0.1	0
PEPPER, JALAPEÑO								
Canned or jarred								
(Old El Paso) .... 2 tbsp		16	1	4	100	1	0.0	0
chopped, w/liquid .... 1 cup		37	1	6	2273	4	1.3	0
diced (Ortega) .... 1 oz		10	0	3	20	0	0.0	0
diced (Rosarita) .... 2 tbsp		5	0	1	121	1	0.2	0
for nachos (La Victoria) .... 14 pieces		5	0	1	330	0	0.0	0
for nachos (La Victoria) .... 1 tbsp		2	1	1	335	0	1.0	0
hot (Vlasic) .... 1/4 cup		10	0	2	490	0	0.0	0
marinated (La Victoria) .... 1 tbsp		4	1	1	251	0	1.0	0
marinated (La Victoria) .... 1.5 pieces		10	0	2	300	0	0.0	0
nacho sliced (Rosarita) .... 2 tbsp		4	0	1	448	1	0.1	0
nacho sliced, food service product (Rosarita) .... 2 tbsp		4	0	1	448	1	0.1	0
pickled (Old El Paso) .... 2 peppers		5	0	1	380	0	0.0	0
sliced, w/liquid (Del Monte) .... 1/2 cup		30	1	6	1690	0	1.0	0
sliced, w/liquid .... 1 cup		28	1	5	1738	3	1.0	0
slices, pickled (Old El Paso) .... 2 tbsp		15	0	3	400	1	0.0	0
whole (Old El Paso) .... 2 peppers		14	0	1	480	0	1.0	0
whole (Ortega) .... 1 oz		10	0	3	20	0	0.0	0
whole (Rosarita) .... 2 tbsp		8	1	1	430	1	0.1	0
whole, food service product (Rosarita) .... 2 peppers		6	0	1	568	1	0.1	0
whole, w/escabeche (Rosarita) .... 1.16 oz		8	1	1	430	1	0.2	0
whole, w/liquid .... 1 med pepper		6	0	1	368	1	0.2	0
whole, w/liquid (Del Monte) .... 1/2 cup		30	1	6	1690	0	1.0	0
Fresh								
raw, whole .... 1 pepper		4	0	1	0	0	0.1	0
raw, sliced .... 1 cup		27	1	5	1	3	0.6	0
PEPPER, PEPPERONCINI								
(Progresso) Tuscan .... 1/2 cup		20	0	7	5	1	0.0	0
(Vlasic) .... 1 oz		5	0	1	440	0	0.0	0
PEPPER, PERSIL, dried .... 1 medium		24	1	4	6	2	1.1	0
PEPPER, RED. See PEPPER, BELL.								
PEPPER, SERRANO								
Fresh								
raw, chopped .... 1 cup		34	2	7	11	4	0.5	0
raw, whole .... 1 medium		2	0	0	1	0	0.0	0
PEPPER, SWEET. See PEPPER, BELL.								
PEPPER, TUSCAN, canned or jarred, drained								
(Progresso) .... 3 medium		10	0	1	330	1	0.0	0
PEPPER, YELLOW. See PEPPER, BANANA, PEPPER, BELL.								
PEPPER DISH/ENTRÉE. See PEPPER, BELL, DISH/ENTRÉE.								
PEPPER DILL SEASONING. See under SEASONING MIX.								
PEPPERMINT								
fresh, raw, whole .... 2 leaves		0	0	0	0	0	0.0	0
fresh, raw, chopped .... 2 tbsp		2	0	0	1	0	0.0	0
PEPPERONCINI. See PEPPER, PEPPERONCINI.								
PEPPERONI. See under SAUSAGE.								
PERCH								
Fresh								
mixed species, baked, broiled, grilled, or microwaved ..... 3 oz		99	21	0	67	0	1.0	98
mixed species, raw .... 3 oz		77	16	0	53	0	0.8	77

Food Name	Serv. Size	Total Cal.	Prot. gms	Carbs gms	Sod. mgs	Fiber gms	Fat gms	Chol. mgs
Frozen								
(Booth)	4 oz	100	20	0	90	0	1.0	0
(SeaPak)	4 oz	100	19	0	80	0	2.0	0
fillet, battered *(Van de Kamp's)*	2 pieces	310	12	18	500	0	21.0	30
PERSIL PEPPER. See PEPPER, PERSIL.								
PERSIMMON								
dried, organic *(Flanigan Farms)*	1 pkg	90	1	20	10	1	0.0	0
dried, whole, trimmed, medium, approx 2.5 inch diam	1 fruit	93	0	25	1	5	0.2	0
raw, Japanese, whole, medium, approx 2.5 inch diam	1 fruit	118	1	31	2	6	0.3	0
raw, native, trimmed, medium, approx 2.5 inch diam	1 fruit	32	0	8	0	na	0.1	0
PESTO. See under SAUCE.								
PE-TSAI. See BOK CHOY.								
PHEASANT								
breast, meat only, raw	6.4 oz	242	44	0	60	0	5.9	106
leg, meat only, raw, 1 medium	3.5 oz	133	22	0	45	0	4.3	79
leg, meat only, raw, 1 medium, boneless/skinless	3.3 oz	143	24	0	48	0	4.6	86
PHYLLO DOUGH								
	1 oz	85	2	15	137	1	1.7	0
frozen, ready-to-use *(Apollo)*	1 oz	80	3	18	200	0	0.4	0
PICCALILLI. See under RELISH.								
PICKLE								
BREAD AND BUTTER								
(Claussen)								
chips	4 slices	20	0	4	170	0	0.0	0
sandwich slices	2 slices	25	0	5	210	0	0.0	0
(Heinz) slices 'Cucumber Slices'	1 oz	25	0	6	170	0	0.0	0
(Mrs. Fanning's) slices	2 slices	16	0	3	140	0	0.0	0
(Vlasic)								
chunks, 'Old-Fashion'	1 oz	25	0	6	120	0	0.0	0
'Deli'	1 oz	25	0	6	120	0	0.0	0
'Sandwich Stackers'	1 oz	25	0	6	170	na	0.0	0
sweet, 'Sweet Butter Chips'	1 oz	30	0	7	160	0	0.0	0
sweet, 'Sweet Butter Stix'	1 oz	18	0	5	110	0	0.0	0
DILL								
(Claussen)								
halves, kosher	1 oz	5	0	1	330	0	0.0	0
miniature, kosher	1 piece	5	0	1	300	0	0.0	0
no garlic	1 piece	17	1	3	895	0	0.3	0
sandwich slices, kosher	2 slices	5	0	1	440	0	0.0	0
whole, kosher	1 oz	5	0	1	330	0	0.0	0
(Featherweight) whole	1 piece	4	0	1	5	0	0.0	0
(Heinz)								
baby	1 oz	4	0	1	285	0	0.0	0
chips	1 oz	4	0	1	275	0	0.0	0
halves, 'Deli Style'	1 oz	4	0	1	280	0	0.0	0
hamburger slices	1 oz	2	0	0	405	0	0.0	0
spears, kosher	1 oz	4	0	1	295	0	0.0	0
spears, Polish style	1 oz	4	0	1	285	0	0.0	0
whole, 'Genuine'	1 oz	2	0	0	420	0	0.0	0
whole, kosher	1 oz	4	0	1	295	0	0.0	0
whole, kosher, 'Old Fashioned'	1 oz	4	0	1	280	0	0.0	0
whole, Polish style	1 oz	4	0	1	285	0	0.0	0
whole, processed	1 oz	2	0	0	435	0	0.0	0
(Steinfeld)								
baby, kosher	1 oz	5	0	1	300	0	0.0	0
hamburger chips	1 oz	5	0	1	300	0	0.0	0
(Vlasic)								
baby, whole, kosher	1 oz	5	0	1	220	0	0.0	0

Food Name	Serv. Size	Total Cal.	Prot. gms	Carbs gms	Sod. mgs	Fiber gms	Fat gms	Chol. mgs
chunks, Polish, snack	1 oz	4	0	1	300	0	0.0	0
chunks, zesty, snacks	1 oz	4	0	1	290	0	0.0	0
crunchy	1 oz	4	0	1	210	0	0.0	0
crunchy, half salt	1 oz	4	0	1	125	0	0.0	0
crunchy, zesty	1 oz	4	0	1	250	0	0.0	0
gherkins	1 oz	4	0	1	210	0	0.0	0
hamburger chips, half salt	1 oz	2	0	1	175	0	0.0	0
original	1 oz	5	0	1	390	0	0.0	0
'Sandwich Stackers' kosher	1 oz	5	0	1	210	0	0.0	0
'Sandwich Stackers' Polish	1 oz	5	0	1	280	0	0.0	0
'Sandwich Stackers' zesty	1 oz	5	0	1	280	0	0.0	0
spears, deli style	1 oz	5	0	1	310	0	0.0	0
spears, half salt	1 oz	4	0	1	120	0	0.0	0
spears, kosher	1 oz	4	0	1	175	0	0.0	0
spears, no garlic	1 oz	4	0	1	210	0	0.0	0
spears, Polish	1 oz	5	0	1	280	na	0.0	0
spears, zesty	1 oz	4	0	1	230	0	0.0	0
HOT AND SPICY (Vlasic) garden, mixed	1 oz	4	0	1	380	0	0.0	0
KOSHER. See also DILL.								
(Heinz)								
chips, 'Old Fashioned'	1 oz	4	0	1	270	0	0.0	0
halves, 'Old Fashioned Deli Halves'	1 oz	4	0	1	275	0	0.0	0
(Vlasic) chunks, snack	2 pieces	5	0	1	220	0	0.0	0
SOUR (Claussen) halves, deli style	1 oz	5	0	1	260	0	0.0	0
SWEET								
(Featherweight) sliced	3.5 pieces	24	0	6	5	0	0.0	0
(Heinz)								
cubes, salad,	1 oz	30	0	7	270	0	0.0	0
'Cucumber Stix'	1 oz	25	0	6	145	0	0.0	0
gherkins	1 oz	35	0	8	210	0	0.0	0
mixed, low-sodium	1 oz	40	0	9	200	0	0.0	0
sliced	1 oz	35	0	8	205	0	0.0	0
sliced, 'Cucumber Slices'	1 oz	20	0	5	195	0	0.0	0
(Steinfeld) chips	1 oz	30	0	8	110	0	0.0	0
(Vlasic)	1 oz	35	0	9	170	na	0.0	0
PICKLING SPICE. See under SEASONING MIX.								
PIE								
APPLE								
(Amy's Kitchen) single serving	1 pie	220	2	35	130	2	8.0	25
(Banquet)								
'Family Size'	1/6 pie	250	2	37	290	0	11.0	0
frozen, ready to bake	1 serving	292	3	41	361	1	13.2	9
(Entenmann's)								
beehive, nonfat, cholesterol free	1 piece	270	2	65	330	2	0.0	0
homestyle	2.1 oz	140	1	21	150	0	7.0	0
(McMillin's)	4 oz	430	4	51	340	0	23.0	0
(Mrs. Smith's)								
'Pie In Minutes'	1/8 pie	210	2	29	250	0	9.0	0
less fat, frozen	1 slice	250	2	43	290	1	8.0	0
(Pet-Ritz)	1/16 pie	330	2	53	385	0	12.0	0
(Sara Lee)								
'Homestyle'	1/10 pie	280	2	42	220	0	12.0	0
'Homestyle High'	1/10 pie	400	3	46	450	0	23.0	0
streusel, frozen, 'Free & Light'	1/8 pie	170	1	36	140	0	2.0	0
BANANA CREAM								
(Banquet)	1/6 pie	180	2	21	150	0	10.0	0
(Mrs. Smith's)	1 slice	280	2	37	170	1	14.0	0
(Pet-Ritz)	1/6 pie	170	2	22	155	0	9.0	0

Food Name	Serv. Size	Total Cal.	Prot. gms	Carbs gms	Sod. mgs	Fiber gms	Fat gms	Chol. mgs
BERRY *(McMillin's)*	4 oz	430	3	52	410	0	23.0	0
BLACKBERRY *(Banquet)* frozen, 'Family Size'	1/6 pie	270	3	40	350	0	11.0	0
BLUEBERRY								
(Banquet) 'Family Size'	1/6 pie	270	3	40	350	0	11.0	0
(Mrs. Smith's) 'Pie In Minutes'	1/8 pie	220	2	32	240	0	9.0	0
(Pet-Ritz)	1/6 pie	370	3	50	330	0	12.0	0
(Sara Lee) 'Homestyle'	1/10 pie	300	2	45	210	0	12.0	0
CHERRY								
(Banquet) frozen, 'Family Size'	1/6 pie	250	3	36	260	0	11.0	0
(Entenmann's) beehive, nonfat, cholesterol free	1 piece	270	3	64	310	1	0.0	0
(Mrs. Smith's)								
frozen, 'Pie In Minutes'	1/8 pie	220	2	32	200	0	9.0	0
less fat, frozen	1 slice	250	2	44	310	1	8.0	0
(Pet-Ritz) frozen	1/6 pie	300	3	48	330	0	12.0	0
(Sara Lee)								
frozen, 'Homestyle'	1/10 pie	270	2	37	270	0	13.0	0
streusel, frozen, 'Free & Light'	1/10 pie	160	2	34	140	0	2.0	0
CHOCOLATE								
(Banquet) cream, frozen	1/6 pie	190	2	24	110	0	10.0	0
(McMillin's) pudding	4 oz	420	3	54	350	0	21.0	0
(Pet-Ritz) cream, frozen	1/6 pie	190	1	27	145	0	8.0	0
(Weight Watchers)								
Mississippi mud	1 serving	160	4	24	120	0	5.0	5
mocha	1 serving	170	6	31	125	2	4.0	5
COCONUT								
(Banquet) cream, frozen	1/6 pie	190	2	22	120	0	11.0	0
(Entenmann's) custard	1.8 oz	140	3	16	160	0	8.0	0
(McMillin's) pudding	4 oz	450	4	50	420	0	26.0	0
(Pet-Ritz) cream, frozen	1/6 pie	190	2	27	145	0	8.0	0
EGG CUSTARD *(Pet-Ritz)* frozen	1/6 pie	200	5	28	0	0	8.0	0
KEY LIME *(Mrs. Smith's)*	1 slice	380	5	58	240	0	14.0	15
LEMON								
(Banquet) cream, frozen	1/6 pie	170	2	23	120	0	9.0	0
(McMillin's)	4 oz	450	4	52	330	0	25.0	0
(Mrs. Smith's) meringue, frozen	1/8 pie	210	2	38	130	0	5.0	0
(Pet-Ritz) cream, frozen	1/6 pie	190	2	26	150	0	9.0	0
MINCEMEAT								
(Banquet) frozen, 'Family Size'	1/6 pie	260	3	38	370	0	11.0	0
(Mrs. Smith's) frozen	1 slice	300	2	48	400	2	11.0	0
(Pet-Ritz) frozen	1/6 pie	280	2	48	0	0	9.0	0
(Sara Lee) frozen, 'Homestyle'	1/10 pie	300	3	43	340	0	13.0	0
NEAPOLITAN *(Pet-Ritz)* cream, frozen	1/6 pie	180	1	17	185	0	10.0	0
PEACH								
(Banquet) frozen, 'Family Size'	1/6 pie	245	3	35	280	0	11.0	0
(McMillin's)	4 oz	430	4	52	370	0	24.0	0
(Pet-Ritz) frozen	1/6 pie	320	2	51	320	0	12.0	0
(Sara Lee) frozen, 9-inch, 'Homestyle'	1/10 pie	280	2	41	170	0	12.0	0
PECAN								
(Mrs. Smith's) frozen	1 slice	520	5	73	450	1	23.0	70
(Sara Lee) frozen, 'Homestyle'	1/10 pie	400	4	56	290	0	18.0	55
PUMPKIN								
(Banquet) frozen, 'Family Size'	1/6 pie	200	3	29	350	0	8.0	0
(Mrs. Smith's) frozen	1 slice	270	5	44	350	1	8.0	45
(Pet-Ritz) custard, frozen	1/6 pie	250	4	39	0	0	9.0	0
(Sara Lee) frozen, 'Homestyle'	1/10 pie	240	4	34	250	0	10.0	40
RASPBERRY *(Sara Lee)* frozen, 'Homestyle'	1/10 pie	280	2	39	150	0	13.0	0

Food Name	Serv. Size	Total Cal.	Prot. gms	Carbs gms	Sod. mgs	Fiber gms	Fat gms	Chol. mgs
STRAWBERRY								
(Banquet) cream, frozen	1/6 pie	170	2	22	120	0	9.0	0
(McMillin's)	4 oz	400	3	50	370	0	20.0	0
(Mrs. Smith's) frozen	1 slice	280	2	45	190	1	11.0	0
(Pet-Ritz) cream, frozen	1/6 pie	170	2	20	145	0	9.0	0
STRAWBERRY RHUBARB (Mrs. Smith's) frozen	1 slice	280	2	44	380	0	11.0	0
SWEET POTATO PIE								
(Mrs. Smith's) frozen	1 slice	280	4	43	220	1	11.0	40
(Pet-Ritz) frozen	1/6 pie	150	2	21	110	0	7.0	0
PIE, SNACK								
(Tastykake) 'Klair'	1 piece	402	6	51	315	2	20.1	56
APPLE								
(Break Cake) 'Fried Pie' 4.5 oz	2 pies	430	5	63	370	0	18.0	0
(Drake's)	1 piece	210	2	29	135	0	10.0	0
(Hostess)								
French	1 piece	430	3	60	390	2	20.0	15
'Snack Cake'	1 serving	480	3	67	390	2	22.0	158
(Little Debbie)								
Dutch apple, 2.5 oz	1 piece	270	2	48	170	0	8.0	1
Dutch apple, 2.17 oz	1 piece	230	2	42	150	0	8.0	1
(Tastykake)								
	1 piece	296	3	46	339	3	12.3	0
French, 4.2 oz	1 piece	353	3	63	225	2	10.7	0
(Weight Watchers)	1/2 pkg	200	2	39	280	0	5.0	5
BANANA CREAM (Tastykake) 4.2 oz	1 piece	382	5	54	428	2	16.1	26
BLACKBERRY (Hostess)	1 piece	420	4	59	360	2	18.0	15
BLUEBERRY								
(Drake's) w/apple	1 piece	210	2	30	135	0	10.0	0
(Hostess) 'Snack Cake'	1 serving	480	3	70	460	2	21.0	20
(Tastykake)	1 piece	308	3	55	410	2	9.4	0
CHERRY								
(Break Cake) 'Fried Pie'	2 pies	410	5	64	370	0	16.0	0
(Drake's) w/apple	1 piece	220	2	30	135	0	10.0	0
(Hostess) 'Snack Cake'	1 serving	470	3	65	470	1	22.0	20
(McMillin's)	4 oz	430	3	51	350	0	24.0	0
(Tastykake)	1 piece	298	3	49	306	2	9.7	0
CHOCOLATE								
(Hostess) pudding	1 piece	490	5	76	439	0	19.0	21
(Pepperidge Farm) Mississippi mud,								
'American Collection'	1 ramekin	310	3	23	60	0	23.0	45
(Tastykake) pudding	1 piece	443	6	68	0	0	16.2	0
COCONUT (Tastykake) creme	1 piece	377	5	46	416	2	20.2	65
LEMON								
(Break Cake) 'Fried Pie'	2 pies	490	5	66	370	0	23.0	0
(Drake's)	1 piece	210	2	27	115	0	11.0	0
(Hostess) 'Snack Cake'	1 serving	500	3	66	430	0	24.0	20
(Tastykake)	1 piece	319	4	48	375	2	13.2	39
LEMON-LIME (Tastykake)	1 piece	310	3	54	329	0	8.8	55
OATMEAL								
(Little Debbie)								
cream, 2.75 oz	1 piece	350	4	51	260	0	14.0	1
cream, 1.33 oz	1 piece	160	2	25	125	0	6.0	1
PEACH								
(Hostess) 'Snack Cake'	1 serving	480	3	68	460	1	21.0	25
(Tastykake)	1 piece	310	3	54	329	0	8.8	55
PECAN								
(Little Debbie)								
3 oz	1 piece	280	3	60	340	0	3.0	1

Food Name	Serv. Size	Total Cal.	Prot. gms	Carbs gms	Sod. mgs	Fiber gms	Fat gms	Chol. mgs
1.83 oz .... 1 piece	1 piece	170	2	37	200	0	2.0	1
PINEAPPLE CHEESE *(Tastykake)* .... 1 piece	1 piece	343	5	54	405	2	13.2	19
PUMPKIN *(Tastykake)* .... 1 piece	1 piece	324	5	47	520	2	14.2	28
STRAWBERRY								
(Hostess) .... 1 piece	1 piece	410	4	56	360	2	19.0	15
(Tastykake) .... 1 piece	1 piece	342	3	57	303	1	11.4	0
PIE CRUST								
(Keebler)								
shell, chocolate, food service product, 'Ready Crust' .... 1 slice	1 slice	100	1	13	95	1	4.5	0
tart shell, graham, food service product,								
'Ready Crust' .... 1 serving	1 serving	120	1	15	150	1	6.0	0
(Mrs. Smith's)								
shell, 8-inch .... 1/8 shell	1/8 shell	80	1	8	105	0	5.0	0
shell, 9-inch .... 1/8 shell	1/8 shell	90	1	10	125	0	5.0	0
shell, 9 5/8 inch .... 1/8 shell	1/8 shell	120	2	12	160	0	7.0	0
shell, less fat, frozen, 9-inch .... 1 slice	1 slice	100	1	13	95	0	5.0	0
(Nabisco)								
chocolate cookie crumb, 'Oreo' .... 1 slice	1 slice	140	1	18	180	1	7.0	0
vanilla wafer crumb, 'Nilla' .... 1 slice	1 slice	144	1	18	63	0	7.6	3
(Oronoque)								
deep dish, 9-inch .... 1/8 crust	1/8 crust	100	2	8	95	0	7.0	0
deep dish, 9-inch, frozen .... 1/6 shell	1/6 shell	130	2	11	130	0	9.0	0
deep dish, 10-inch .... 1/8 crust	1/8 crust	130	2	10	120	0	8.0	0
regular, 9-inch .... 1/8 crust	1/8 crust	90	1	7	80	0	6.0	0
regular, 9-inch, frozen .... 1/6 shell	1/6 shell	120	2	9	115	0	8.0	0
regular, 6-inch .... 1/4 crust	1/4 crust	110	2	9	105	0	7.0	0
tart shell, 3-inch .... 1 tart	1 tart	140	2	11	130	0	9.0	0
(Pet-Ritz)								
.... 1/6 shell	1/6 shell	110	1	11	110	0	7.0	7
all vegetable shortening .... 1/6 shell	1/6 shell	110	2	10	60	0	8.0	0
deep dish .... 1/6 shell	1/6 shell	130	1	12	120	0	8.0	7
deep dish, whole grain .... 1/6 shell	1/6 shell	130	1	14	125	0	8.0	0
deep dish, w/vegetable shortening .... 1/6 shell	1/6 shell	140	2	12	75	0	9.0	0
graham cracker .... 1/6 shell	1/6 shell	110	1	8	80	0	6.0	7
9 5/8 inch .... 1/6 shell	1/6 shell	170	2	15	180	0	11.0	7
tart shell, 3-inch .... 1 shell	1 shell	150	3	12	150	0	10.0	7
(Pillsbury) .... 1 slice	1 slice	110	1	12	140	0	7.0	5
PIE CRUST MIX								
(Betty Crocker)								
.... 1 serving	1 serving	110	1	9	150	0	8.0	0
stick .... 1/8 stick	1/8 stick	120	1	10	140	0	8.0	0
(Flako)								
mix only .... 1/4 cup	1/4 cup	130	2	13	170	1	8.0	5
prepared .... 1 serving	1 serving	247	4	24	393	1	15.0	9
(General Mills) mix only .... 1/16 pkg	1/16 pkg	120	1	10	150	0	8.0	0
(Krusteaz) prepared .... 1/8 shell	1/8 shell	90	1	10	120	0	5.0	0
(Nabisco)								
chocolate cookie crumbs, 'Oreo' mix only .... 2 tbsp	2 tbsp	80	1	13	140	0	3.0	0
graham cracker crumbs 'Honey Maid' mix only ...... 2 1/2 tbsp	2 1/2 tbsp	70	1	13	90	0	2.0	0
vanilla wafer crumbs, 'Nilla' mix only .... 2 tbsp	2 tbsp	70	1	12	55	0	2.0	5
(Pillsbury)								
mix only .... 2 tbsp	2 tbsp	100	1	10	150	0	6.0	0
prepared w/water .... 1/8 pkg	1/8 pkg	200	3	20	300	0	13.0	0
PIE FILLING. See also PUDDING PIE FILLING/MIX.								
APPLE PIE FILLING								
(Comstock)								
canned .... 3.5 oz	3.5 oz	120	0	30	15	0	0.0	0

Food Name	Serv. Size	Total Cal.	Prot. gms	Carbs gms	Sod. mgs	Fiber gms	Fat gms	Chol. mgs
canned, 'Lite'	3.5 oz	80	0	20	10	0	0.0	0
(Lucky Leaf)								
canned	4 oz	120	0	30	60	0	0.0	0
canned, 'Deluxe'	4 oz	120	0	35	40	0	0.0	0
canned, 'Plus'	4 oz	121	0	30	24	0	0.0	0
turnover, diced, canned	4 oz	120	0	30	60	0	0.0	0
(Musselman's)								
canned	4 oz	120	0	30	60	0	0.0	0
canned, 'Deluxe'	4 oz	120	0	35	40	0	0.0	0
canned, 'Plus'	4 oz	121	0	30	24	0	0.0	0
turnover, diced, canned	4 oz	120	0	30	60	0	0.0	0
(Pathmark) canned 'No Frills'	4 oz	130	0	33	60	0	0.0	0
(White House) canned	3.5 oz	121	0	29	44	0	1.0	0
APRICOT								
(Comstock) canned	3.5 oz	110	0	29	100	0	0.0	0
(Lucky Leaf) canned	4 oz	150	0	39	90	0	0.0	0
(Musselman's) canned	4 oz	150	0	39	90	0	0.0	0
BANANA *(Comstock)* canned	3.5 oz	110	1	22	300	1	2.0	0
BLACKBERRY								
(Lucky Leaf)								
canned	4 oz	120	1	31	140	0	0.0	0
canned, 'Plus'	4 oz	121	1	30	20	0	0.0	0
(Musselman's)								
canned	4 oz	120	1	31	140	0	0.0	0
canned 'Plus'	4 oz	121	1	30	20	0	0.0	0
BLUEBERRY								
(Comstock)								
canned	3.5 oz	110	0	28	15	1	0.0	0
canned, 'Lite'	3.5 oz	75	0	17	15	1	0.0	0
(Lucky Leaf)								
canned, cultivated	4 oz	120	1	31	150	0	0.0	0
canned, 'Plus'	4 oz	145	0	35	17	0	0.0	0
(Musselman's)								
canned, cultivated	4 oz	120	1	31	150	0	0.0	0
canned 'Plus'	4 oz	145	0	35	17	0	0.0	0
(White House) canned	3.5 oz	118	0	28	48	0	1.0	0
BOYSENBERRY								
(Lucky Leaf) canned	4 oz	120	1	31	140	0	0.0	0
(Musselman's) canned	4 oz	120	1	31	140	0	0.0	0
CHERRY								
(Comstock)								
canned	3.5 oz	110	0	28	15	0	0.0	0
canned, 'Lite'	3.5 oz	75	0	19	15	0	0.0	0
(Lucky Leaf) canned	4 oz	120	1	29	50	0	0.0	0
(Musselman's)								
canned	4 oz	120	1	29	50	0	0.0	0
canned, 'Plus'	4 oz	108	1	26	10	0	0.2	0
(Pathmark) canned 'No Frills'	4 oz	130	0	33	60	0	0.0	0
(White House) canned	3.5 oz	141	0	33	54	0	1.0	0
CHOCOLATE								
(Comstock) canned	3.5 oz	130	1	26	240	0	3.0	0
(Royal) mousse, 'No-Bake'	1/8 pie	130	3	21	190	0	4.0	0
COCONUT *(Comstock)* canned	3.5 oz	120	1	22	290	0	3.0	0
GOOSEBERRY								
(Lucky Leaf) canned	4 oz	180	0	45	30	0	0.0	0
(Musselman's) canned	4 oz	180	0	45	30	0	0.0	0

Food Name	Serv. Size	Total Cal.	Prot. gms	Carbs gms	Sod. mgs	Fiber gms	Fat gms	Chol. mgs
LEMON								
(Comstock) canned	3.5 oz	140	0	34	110	0	1.0	0
(Lucky Leaf) canned	4 oz	200	0	48	235	0	2.0	0
(Lucky Leaf) canned, 'French'	4 oz	180	0	42	140	0	1.0	0
(Musselman's) canned	4 oz	200	0	48	235	0	2.0	0
(Musselman's) canned, 'French'	4 oz	180	0	42	140	0	1.0	0
MINCEMEAT								
(Comstock) canned	3.5 oz	150	0	39	180	1	1.0	0
(Lucky Leaf) canned	4 oz	190	0	48	145	0	1.0	0
(Musselman's) canned	4 oz	190	0	48	145	0	1.0	0
(None Such)								
canned	1/3 cup	200	1	48	280	0	1.0	0
canned, condensed	1/4 pkg	220	1	50	310	0	2.0	0
w/brandy and rum, canned	1/3 cup	220	1	48	260	0	2.0	0
(S&W)	1/4 cup	180	1	43	210	4	2.5	0
PEACH								
(Comstock) canned	3.5 oz	110	0	26	20	0	0.0	0
(Lucky Leaf)								
canned	4 oz	150	0	37	65	0	0.0	0
canned, 'Plus'	4 oz	113	1	27	16	0	0.0	0
(Musselman's)								
canned	4 oz	150	0	37	65	0	0.0	0
canned 'Plus'	4 oz	113	1	27	16	0	0.0	0
(White House) canned	3.5 oz	117	0	28	30	0	1.0	0
PINEAPPLE								
(Comstock) canned	3.5 oz	100	0	28	65	0	0.0	0
(Lucky Leaf) canned	4 oz	110	0	30	65	0	0.0	0
(Musselman's) canned	4 oz	110	0	30	65	0	0.0	0
PUMPKIN								
(Comstock) canned	3.5 oz	100	0	24	180	0	0.0	0
(Libby's)								
canned	1 cup	260	2	64	440	0	0.3	0
canned	1/2 cup	100	1	25	150	2	0.0	0
(Lucky Leaf) canned	4 oz	170	1	33	200	0	4.0	0
(Musselman's) canned	4 oz	170	1	33	200	0	4.0	0
(Stokely) canned	1/2 cup	170	1	44	420	0	0.0	0
RAISIN								
(Comstock) canned	3.5 oz	120	0	32	80	0	0.0	0
(Lucky Leaf) canned	4 oz	130	1	34	120	0	1.0	0
(Musselman's) canned	4 oz	130	1	34	120	0	1.0	0
RASPBERRY								
(Lucky Leaf) black, canned	4 oz	190	0	43	50	0	0.0	0
(Lucky Leaf) red, canned	4 oz	190	0	46	80	0	0.0	0
(Musselman's) black, canned	4 oz	190	0	43	50	0	0.0	0
(Musselman's) red, canned	4 oz	190	0	46	80	0	0.0	0
STRAWBERRY								
(Comstock) canned	3.5 oz	100	0	25	20	1	0.0	0
(Lucky Leaf)								
canned	4 oz	120	0	30	75	0	0.0	0
canned, 'Plus'	4 oz	138	1	34	17	0	0.0	0
(Musselman's)								
canned	4 oz	120	0	30	75	0	0.0	0
canned, 'Plus'	4 oz	138	1	34	17	0	0.0	0
STRAWBERRY-RHUBARB								
(Lucky Leaf) canned	4 oz	120	0	31	95	0	0.0	0
(Musselman's) canned	4 oz	120	0	31	95	0	0.0	0
VANILLA CREME								
(Lucky Leaf)	4 oz	150	0	32	145	0	3.0	0

Food Name	Serv. Size	Total Cal.	Prot. gms	Carbs gms	Sod. mgs	Fiber gms	Fat gms	Chol. mgs
(Musselman's)	4 oz	150	0	32	145	0	3.0	0
PIE MIX								
BANANA CREAM								
(Jell-O)								
'No Bake' prepared	1/8 pie	240	3	27	300	0	14.0	30
'No Bake' mix only	1 pkg	140	1	25	190	0	5.0	0
'No Bake' prepared w/whole milk	1/8 pie	240	3	27	300	0	14.0	30
CHOCOLATE PIE MIX, MOUSSE								
(Jell-O)								
mousse, 'No Bake' mix only	1 pkg	160	2	22	320	0	7.0	0
mousse, 'No Bake' prepared	1/8 pie	260	4	25	430	0	17.0	30
mousse, 'No Bake' prepared w/whole milk	1/8 pie	260	4	25	430	0	17.0	30
(Royal)								
mint, 'No-Bake' prepared	1/8 pie	260	5	25	280	0	15.0	0
mousse, 'No Bake' prepared	1/8 pie	230	4	27	260	0	12.0	0
COCONUT CREAM								
(Jell-O)								
'No Bake' mix only	1 pkg	160	1	25	200	0	7.0	0
'No Bake' prepared	1/8 pie	260	3	27	300	0	16.0	30
'No Bake' prepared w/whole milk	1/8 pie	260	3	27	300	0	16.0	30
LEMON MERINGUE								
(Royal) 'No Bake' prepared	1/8 pie	310	3	50	250	0	11.0	0
PUMPKIN								
(Jell-O)								
'No Bake' mix only	1 pkg	140	1	28	330	0	3.0	0
'No Bake' prepared	1/8 pie	250	4	31	450	0	13.0	30
'No Bake' prepared w/whole milk	1/8 pie	250	4	31	450	0	13.0	30
(Libby's) prepared	1/6 pie	390	7	53	380	0	17.0	70
PIEROGI								
(Mrs. T's)								
potato and American cheese filled	3 pierogies	220	9	32	540	1	6.0	20
potato and onion filled	3 pierogies	180	6	34	340	2	2.0	15
sauerkraut filled	3 pierogies	160	6	32	850	3	1.5	10
PIGEON. See SQUAB.								
PIGEON PEA. See PEAS, PIGEON.								
PIGNOLI NUT. See PINE NUT.								
PIG'S EAR. See under PORK.								
PIG'S FEET. See under PORK.								
PIG'S HEART. See under PORK.								
PIG'S JOWL. See under PORK.								
PIG'S KNUCKLES. See under PORK.								
PIG'S TAIL. See under PORK.								
PIG'S TONGUE. See under PORK.								
PIKE								
NORTHERN								
baked, broiled, grilled, or microwaved	3 oz	96	21	0	42	0	0.7	43
raw	3 oz	75	16	0	33	0	0.6	33
WALLEYE								
baked, broiled, grilled, or microwaved	3 oz	101	21	0	55	0	1.3	94
raw	3 oz	79	16	0	43	0	1.0	73
PILAF ENTRÉE								
(Health Valley)								
oat bran, w/garden vegetables 'Fast Menu'	7.5 oz	210	8	31	445	6	7.0	0
(Weight Watchers) Florentine	1 entrée	290	9	47	550	6	7.0	5
PILI NUT, CANARY TREE								
dried	1 cup	863	13	5	4	na	95.5	0
dried, approx 15 kernels	1 oz	204	3	1	1	na	22.6	0

Food Name	Serv. Size	Total Cal.	Prot. gms	Carbs gms	Sod. mgs	Fiber gms	Fat gms	Chol. mgs
PIMIENTO								
Canned or jarred								
.... 1 cup	1 cup	44	2	10	27	4	0.6	0
all varieties, drained *(Dromedary)* .... 1 oz	1 oz	10	0	2	5	0	0.0	0
chopped .... 1 tbsp	1 tbsp	3	0	1	2	0	0.0	0
sliced .... 1 slice	1 slice	<1	0	0	0	0	0.0	0
whole .... 1 whole pimiento	1 whole pimiento	15	1	3	9	1	0.2	0
PIMIENTO SPREAD *(Price's)* .... 1 oz	1 oz	80	3	2	0	0	6.0	0
PIÑA COLADA. See under COCKTAIL; COCKTAIL MIX.								
PINE NUT/Colorado pinyon/Italian stone pine nut/pignoli/pinnochio/piñon								
(Progresso) .... 1 oz jar	1 oz jar	170	0	2	0	0	13.0	0
dried .... 1 cup	1 cup	770	33	19	5	6	69.0	0
dried .... 1 oz	1 oz	160	7	4	1	1	14.4	0
dried .... 1 tbsp	1 tbsp	49	2	1	0	0	4.4	0
dried .... 10 med nuts	10 med nuts	10	0	0	0	0	0.9	0
natural, unsalted *(Flanigan Farms)* .... 1/4 cup	1/4 cup	150	7	4	0	1	14.0	0
PINEAPPLE								
Canned								
chunks, in extra heavy syrup, w/liquid .... 1 cup	1 cup	216	1	56	3	2	0.3	0
chunks, in heavy syrup, w/liquid .... 1 cup	1 cup	198	1	51	3	2	0.3	0
chunks, in juice, w/liquid .... 1 cup	1 cup	149	1	39	2	2	0.2	0
chunks, in light syrup, w/liquid .... 1 cup	1 cup	131	1	34	3	2	0.3	0
chunks, in water, w/liquid .... 1 cup	1 cup	79	1	20	2	2	0.2	0
crushed, in extra heavy syrup, w/liquid .... 1 cup	1 cup	216	1	56	3	2	0.3	0
crushed, in heavy syrup, w/liquid .... 1 cup	1 cup	198	1	51	3	2	0.3	0
crushed, in juice, w/liquid .... 1 cup	1 cup	149	1	39	2	2	0.2	0
crushed, in light syrup, w/liquid .... 1 cup	1 cup	131	1	34	3	2	0.3	0
crushed, in water, w/liquid .... 1 cup	1 cup	79	1	20	2	2	0.2	0
rings, in heavy syrup, 3-inch diam, w/liquid .... 1 ring	1 ring	38	0	10	0	0	0.1	0
rings, in juice, 3-inch diam, w/liquid .... 1 ring w/liqid	1 ring w/liqid	28	0	7	0	0	0.0	0
rings, in light syrup, 3-inch diam, w/liquid .... 1 ring w/liqid	1 ring w/liqid	25	0	6	0	0	0.1	0
rings, in water, 3-inch diam, w/liquid .... 1 ring w/liqid	1 ring w/liqid	15	0	4	0	0	0.0	0
sliced *(S&W)* .... 1 slice	1 slice	90	0	23	10	1	0.0	0
sliced, in extra heavy syrup, w/liquids .... 1 cup	1 cup	216	1	56	3	2	0.3	0
sliced, in heavy syrup, w/liquid .... 1 cup	1 cup	198	1	51	3	2	0.3	0
sliced, in juice, w/liquid .... 1 cup	1 cup	149	1	39	2	2	0.2	0
sliced, in light syrup, w/liquid .... 1 cup	1 cup	131	1	34	3	2	0.3	0
sliced, in water, w/liquid .... 1 cup	1 cup	79	1	20	2	2	0.2	0
Fresh								
raw, diced .... 1 cup	1 cup	76	1	19	2	2	0.7	0
raw, sliced, 3.5 inch diam, 1/2 inch thick .... 1 slice	1 slice	27	0	7	1	1	0.2	0
raw, sliced, 3.5 inch diam, 3/4 inch thick .... 1 slice	1 slice	41	0	10	1	1	0.4	0
raw, whole, trimmed .... 1 med fruit	1 med fruit	231	2	58	5	6	2.0	0
Frozen								
chunks *(Flav-R-Pac)* .... 2/3 cup	2/3 cup	75	0	19	0	0	0.0	0
chunks, sweetened .... 1 cup	1 cup	208	1	54	5	3	0.2	0
PINEAPPLE DRINK. See under FRUIT DRINK; FRUIT JUICE DRINK.								
PINEAPPLE JUICE. See also under FRUIT JUICE BLEND; FRUIT JUICE DRINK.								
Can, bottle, box, or carton								
unsweetened, w/added ascorbic acid .... 1 cup	1 cup	140	1	34	3	1	0.2	0
unsweetened, w/o added ascorbic acid .... 1 cup	1 cup	140	1	34	3	1	0.2	0
(Del Monte)								
.... 8 fl oz	8 fl oz	110	1	29	15	2	0.0	0
unsweetened .... 6 fl oz	6 fl oz	100	0	25	10	0	0.0	0
(Dole) .... 6 fl oz	6 fl oz	103	1	25	2	0	0.2	0
(IGA) unsweetened .... 6 fl oz	6 fl oz	100	0	25	10	0	0.0	0

Food Name	Serv. Size	Total Cal.	Prot. gms	Carbs gms	Sod. mgs	Fiber gms	Fat gms	Chol. mgs
(J. Hungerford)								
100% juice	9.03 fl oz	124	1	31	9	0	0.0	0
regular	9.03 fl oz	114	0	29	0	0	0.0	0
(Knudsen)	8 fl oz	110	1	25	0	0	0.0	0
(Minute Maid)	6 fl oz	90	1	23	20	0	0.0	0
(Mott's)	9.5 fl oz	169	0	42	0	0	0.0	0
(Pathmark)								
'Hawaiian'	6 fl oz	100	0	25	10	0	0.0	0
unsweetened, 'No Frills'	6 fl oz	100	0	25	0	0	0.0	0
(S&W)								
	8 fl oz	110	0	29	15	2	0.0	0
unsweetened	6 fl oz	90	0	23	10	2	0.0	0
(Veryfine) '100%'	8 fl oz	125	1	31	10	0	0.0	0
Frozen or chilled								
concentrate, prepared	1 cup	130	1	32	3	1	0.1	0
concentrate, unprepared	6 fl oz	387	3	96	6	2	0.2	0
(Minute Maid)	6 fl oz	90	1	23	0	0	0.0	0
PINEAPPLE TOPPING								
(Kraft)	1 tbsp	50	0	13	0	0	0.0	0
(Smucker's)	2 tbsp	130	0	32	0	0	0.0	0
PINK BEAN. See BEAN, PINK.								
PINK GRAPEFRUIT JUICE. See under GRAPEFRUIT JUICE.								
PINK SALMON. See under SALMON.								
PINNOCHIO. See PINE NUT.								
PIÑON. See PINE NUT.								
PINTO BEAN. See BEAN, PINTO.								
PISTACHIO								
in shell *(Dole)*	1 oz	90	3	3	250	0	7.0	0
natural *(Blue Diamond)*	1 oz	140	6	4	210	3	12.0	0
natural, in shell *(Fisher)*	1 oz	170	5	7	85	0	14.0	0
natural, unsalted *(Flanigan Farms)*	1/4 cup	180	6	8	0	3	14.0	0
red *(Blue Diamond)*	1 oz	140	6	3	230	3	12.0	0
red *(Fisher)*	1/4 cup	111	3	4	33	1	9.8	0
Dried								
raw	1 cup	705	26	37	1	13	55.3	0
raw	30 nuts	99	4	5	0	2	7.8	0
raw, approx 47 kernels	1 oz	156	6	8	0	3	12.2	0
Dry roasted								
(Dole)	1 oz	163	6	7	2	0	14.0	0
natural or red *(Planters)*	1 oz	170	6	6	250	0	14.0	0
salted	1 cup	726	27	35	545	13	58.5	0
salted, approx 47 kernels	1 oz	161	6	8	121	3	13.0	0
unsalted	1 cup	730	27	36	13	13	58.5	0
unsalted, approx 47 kernels	1 oz	162	6	8	3	3	13.0	0
Roasted, *(David's)* salted	1 pkg	270	9	11	250	4	21.0	0
PISTACHIO BUTTER, roasted *(Maranatha Natural)*	2 tbsp	170	6	7	5	0	13.0	0
PITA. See under BREAD.								
PITANGA/Surinam cherry								
raw	1 cup	57	1.4	13.0	5	>1.0 c	0.7	0
raw, trimmed	1/2 cup	29	0.7	6.5	3	>.5 c	0.3	0
raw, trimmed	1 oz	9	0.2	2.1	1	>.2 c	0.1	0
raw, trimmed, approx .3 oz	1 medium	2	0.1	0.5	0	tr	0.0	0
raw, untrimmed	1 lb	132	3.2	29.9	11	>2.4 c	1.6	0
PIZZA								
(Banquet)								
cheese, on French bread, frozen, 'Zap'	4.5 oz	310	14	41	800	0	10.0	35
deluxe, on French bread, frozen, 'Zap'	4.8 oz	330	13	39	890	0	13.0	25

Food Name	Serv. Size	Total Cal.	Prot. gms	Carbs gms	Sod. mgs	Fiber gms	Fat gms	Chol. mgs
pepperoni, 'Pizza Pie' .... 1 pizza		470	11	45	970	0	27.0	35
pepperoni, on French bread, 'Zap' .... 4.5 oz		350	15	36	1060	0	16.0	40
sausage, 'Pizza Pie' .... 6 oz		500	11	48	860	0	29.0	35
sausage and pepperoni, 'Pizza Pie' .... 6 oz		470	12	43	930	0	27.0	40
(Celentano)								
cheese, 5.5 oz .... 2 1/4 slices		340	14	46	440	4	11.0	25
thick crust, 6.5 oz .... 1/2 pizza		390	18	62	840	8	12.0	25
(Celeste)								
cheese, individual .... 1 pizza		420	18	42	830	3	20.0	35
cheese, large .... 1 slice		320	14	32	590	3	16.0	25
four cheese, individual, 'Original' .... 1 pizza		480	22	41	920	4	26.0	45
four cheese, zesty, individual .... 1 pizza		470	21	44	970	4	24.0	40
individual, 'Deluxe' .... 1 pizza		470	18	46	1140	5	25.0	25
large, 'Deluxe' .... 1 slice		350	14	35	880	4	18.0	20
pepperoni, individual .... 1 pizza		470	16	41	1100	4	27.0	20
pepperoni, large .... 1 slice		350	13	33	990	3	20.0	20
sausage .... 1/4 pizza		375	16	30	900	3	22.0	15
sausage, individual sized .... 1 pizza		530	23	52	1400	5	27.0	25
sausage, w/green and red peppers, mushrooms, frozen, 'Deluxe' .... 1 pkg		1538	67	133	3050	na	82.6	147
sausage, w/green and red peppers, mushrooms, frozen, 'Deluxe' .... 1 serving		386	17	33	765	na	20.7	37
suprema, individual .... 1 pizza		500	22	49	1290	6	27.0	25
suprema, large .... 1 slice		290	13	27	770	3	16.0	15
vegetable, individual sized .... 1 pizza		420	17	46	1120	5	21.0	5
(Crisp 'N Tasty)								
combination .... 1/2 serving		280	10	27	680	1	15.0	15
pepperoni .... 1/2 serving		280	10	28	710	1	15.0	15
sausage .... 1/2 serving		280	10	27	640	1	15.0	10
(Empire Kosher)								
kosher .... 1 piece		150	7	15	390	0	5.0	15
kosher, on English muffin .... 1 muffin		130	7	15	390	1	5.0	15
kosher, 3 pack .... 1 pizza		210	10	23	630	7	9.0	20
kosher, 10 oz .... 1/2 pizza		340	18	38	970	2	13.0	30
(Graindance Pizza)								
cheese, whole wheat crust, all natural .... 1 slice		200	9	23	400	0	8.0	0
(Healthy Choice)								
cheese, on French bread .... 1 entrée		340	22	51	480	5	5.0	15
deluxe, on French bread, frozen .... 6.25 oz		330	23	41	490	0	8.0	35
pepperoni, on French bread .... 1 entrée		340	24	49	580	6	5.0	20
sausage, on French bread .... 1 entrée		320	21	48	580	5	5.0	25
supreme, on French bread .... 1 entrée		330	21	51	580	6	5.0	20
vegetable, on French bread .... 1 entrée		280	17	45	480	5	4.0	10
(Jack's)								
pepperoni, frozen, 'Jack's Original' .... 1 pkg		1288	60	118	2440	na	64.2	160
pepperoni, frozen, 'Jack's Original' .... 1 serving		323	15	30	612	na	16.1	40
sausage and pepperoni, 'Great Combinations' .... 1 pkg		1389	69	120	2828	na	70.0	175
sausage and pepperoni, 'Great Combinations' .... 1 serving		348	17	30	708	na	17.5	44
(Jeno's)								
cheese, microwave, individual .... 1 serving		240	10	25	530	1	11.0	15
combination, microwave, individual .... 1 serving		310	11	25	720	1	18.0	15
pepperoni, 'Pizza Pocket' .... 1 serving		370	12	35	790	0	20.0	25
pepperoni, frozen, 'Crisp 'n Tasty' .... 1 pkg		516	19	46	1221	3	28.8	23
pepperoni, individual, microwave .... 1 serving		280	10	25	710	1	16.0	15
sausage, individual .... 1 serving		280	10	25	650	1	16.0	10
sausage, 'Pizza Pocket' .... 1 serving		360	11	35	660	0	19.0	15
sausage and pepperoni, 'Crisp 'n Tasty' .... 1 pkg		491	17	52	1239	3	24.2	26

Food Name	Serv. Size	Total Cal.	Prot. gms	Carbs gms	Sod. mgs	Fiber gms	Fat gms	Chol. mgs
sausage and pepperoni, 'Pizza Pocket' .... 1 serving		360	12	35	710	0	20.0	20
supreme, 'Pizza Pocket' .... 1 serving		370	12	36	720	0	19.0	20
(Kashi) spicy Southwest, vegetarian, frozen .... 1 slice		210	9	28	380	11	7.0	9
(Kid Cuisine)								
cheese .... 6.85 oz		380	11	57	390	0	12.0	25
hamburger .... 6.85 oz		330	11	50	700	0	10.0	15
(Lean Cuisine)								
cheese, on French bread .... 1 entrée		350	22	48	400	4	8.0	20
deluxe, on French bread .... 1 entrée		330	23	45	560	5	6.0	30
pepperoni, on French bread .... 1 entrée		330	20	46	590	4	7.0	25
sausage, on French bread, frozen .... 6 oz		350	22	42	600	0	10.0	35
(Mrs. Paterson's)								
supreme, hand held, frozen, 'Aussie Pie' .... 5.5 oz		470	12	44	880	0	27.0	75
(Nature's Hilights)								
Italian cheese .... 1/2 pizza		360	18	46	640	2	12.0	30
soy cheese .... 1/2 pizza		290	16	52	430	2	1.5	0
(Oven Lovin')								
cheese, microwave .... 1/2 pizza		250	11	24	430	0	12.0	10
cheese, on French bread, frozen, microwave .... 1 serving		350	17	40	700	0	14.0	15
combination, microwave .... 1/2 pizza		310	13	26	580	0	18.0	20
combination, on French bread, frozen, microwave .... 1 serving		420	18	41	910	0	21.0	30
pepperoni, microwave .... 1/2 pizza		300	13	25	620	0	17.0	25
pepperoni, on French bread, frozen, microwave ...... 1 serving		410	18	40	980	0	21.0	35
sausage, microwave .... 1/2 pizza		290	12	26	510	0	16.0	15
sausage, on French bread, frozen, microwave .... 1 serving		400	18	41	830	0	20.0	25
supreme, microwave .... 1/2 pizza		310	13	27	570	0	18.0	20
(Pappalo's)								
cheese, on French bread, frozen .... 1 piece		360	16	40	830	0	15.0	0
combination, on French bread, frozen .... 1 piece		430	19	41	1120	0	21.0	0
pepperoni, deep dish .... 1 slice		340	17	37	720	2	14.0	30
pepperoni, deep dish, individual, frozen, 'For One' ..... 1 pizza		525	23	65	983	3	19.5	38
pepperoni, on French bread, frozen .... 1 piece		410	16	41	1130	0	20.0	0
pepperoni, pan pizza .... 1/5 pizza		350	22	40	720	3	11.0	50
pepperoni, pizzeria style, 12 inch .... 1 slice		380	18	38	840	2	17.0	40
pepperoni, traditional crust, 9 inch .... 1/2 pizza		390	23	47	870	4	14.0	45
sausage, deep dish .... 1 slice		330	16	36	600	2	13.0	25
sausage, on French bread, frozen .... 1 piece		410	18	41	1000	0	18.0	0
sausage, pan pizza .... 1/5 pizza		350	22	39	530	3	11.0	40
sausage, pizzeria style crust, 12 inch .... 1 slice		370	18	38	710	2	16.0	30
sausage, traditional crust, 9 inch .... 1/2 pizza		380	22	47	680	4	13.0	40
sausage and pepperoni, deep dish .... 1 slice		330	16	36	650	2	14.0	25
sausage and pepperoni, pan pizza .... 1/5 pizza		360	22	40	630	3	12.0	45
sausage and pepperoni, pizzeria style, 12 inch .... 1 slice		380	18	39	780	2	17.0	35
sausage and pepperoni, traditional crust, 9 inch ..... 1/2 pizza		390	23	45	650	4	15.0	45
supreme, pan pizza .... 1/5 pizza		340	22	37	610	3	12.0	45
supreme, traditional crust, 12 inch .... 1/4 pizza		350	22	38	640	4	12.0	45
supreme, traditional crust, 9 inch .... 1/2 pizza		400	25	46	700	4	16.0	45
three cheese, pan .... 1/5 pizza		310	20	39	490	3	8.0	30
three cheese, traditional crust, 12 inch .... 1/4 pizza		310	20	41	440	4	7.0	30
three cheese, traditional crust, 9 inch .... 1/2 pizza		350	21	47	640	4	11.0	30
(Pepperidge Farm)								
cheese, on croissant pastry .... 1 pizza		430	15	41	640	0	23.0	0
deluxe, on croissant pastry .... 1 pizza		440	16	43	790	0	23.0	0
pepperoni, on croissant pastry .... 1 pizza		420	14	43	690	0	22.0	0
(Pillsbury)								
cheese, on French bread, frozen, 'Microwave' .... 1 piece		370	18	41	680	0	15.0	0
pepperoni, on French bread, frozen, 'Microwave' ...... 1 piece		430	19	45	940	0	19.0	0

Food Name	Serv. Size	Total Cal.	Prot. gms	Carbs gms	Sod. mgs	Fiber gms	Fat gms	Chol. mgs
sausage, on French bread, frozen, 'Microwave' . . . . 1 piece		410	18	48	860	0	16.0	0
sausage combo, w/pepperoni, on French bread, frozen, 'Microwave' . . . . 1 piece		450	19	47	950	0	21.0	0
(Pizsoy)								
cheese, w/tofu mozzarella, whole wheat crust, original . . 1 slice		165	12	28	206	0	5.0	0
(Red Baron)								
cheese . . . . 1/5 pizza		350	16	33	680	2	17.0	30
cheese, 'Deep Dish Singles' . . . . 1 pizza		460	15	41	760	2	23.0	20
cheese, sausage, mushrooms, pepperoni, and vegetable . . . . 1/5 pizza		340	14	31	690	2	18.0	25
pepperoni, 'Deep Dish Singles' . . . . 1 pizza		530	18	47	90	2	31.0	35
pepperoni, frozen, 'Premium Deep Dish Singles' . . . . 1 pkg		961	32	96	1777	na	50.1	57
pepperoni, frozen, 'Premium Deep Dish Singles' . . . . . 1 serving		480	16	48	889	na	25.0	29
pepperoni, frozen . . . . 1 pkg		1788	73	146	4137	na	101.5	150
pepperoni, frozen . . . . 1 serving		442	18	36	1023	na	25.1	37
sausage . . . . 1/5 pizza		340	15	32	700	2	18.0	25
sausage, ham, and pepperoni, 'Deep Dish Singles' . . . . . 1 pizza		490	16	41	970	2	26.0	25
sausage, pepperoni, mushroom, pepper, and onion . . . 1/5 pizza		360	15	33	730	2	19.0	25
supreme, w/sausage, mushrooms, pepperoni, frozen . . . . 1 pkg		1736	69	161	3725	na	91.2	117
supreme, w/sausage, mushrooms, pepperoni, frozen . . . . 1 serving		344	14	32	738	na	18.1	23
two cheese, w/sausage, pepperoni, onions, 'Deluxe' . . . . . 1 pkg		1746	62	166	3653	na	92.3	127
two cheese, w/sausage, pepperoni, onions, 'Deluxe' . . . 1 serving		337	12	32	704	na	17.8	25
(Smart Ones) combo, deluxe, pizza . . . . 1 entrée		380	23	47	550	6	11.0	40
(Soypreme)								
cheese, w/tofu mozzarella, whole wheat crust . . . . 1 slice		209	10	22	300	0	7.0	0
cheese, w/tofu mozzarella, whole wheat crust, 'Garden Patch' . . . . 1 slice		211	10	24	362	0	7.0	0
(Stouffer's)								
bacon cheddar, on French bread . . . . 1 entrée		440	16	44	940	4	22.0	30
Canadian bacon, on French bread . . . . 5.5 oz		370	18	40	1070	0	15.0	0
cheese, on French bread . . . . 1/2 pizza		350	15	42	660	3	14.0	15
cheeseburger, on French bread . . . . 1/2 pizza		440	21	31	1110	5	26.0	55
deluxe, w/sausage, pepperoni, mushroom, on French bread, frozen . . . . 1 pkg		858	32	89	1680	7	41.3	67
deluxe, w/sausage, pepperoni, mushroom, on French bread, frozen . . . . 1 serving		429	16	44	840	4	20.6	33
double cheese, on French bread . . . . 1/2 pizza		420	19	44	790	5	19.0	30
hamburger, on French bread, frozen . . . . 1 pkg		410	23	39	650	0	18.0	0
on French bread, 'Deluxe' . . . . 1/2 pizza		440	19	42	980	5	22.0	35
pepperoni, on French bread . . . . 1/2 pizza		420	18	42	930	3	20.0	35
pepperoni, w/mushrooms, on French bread . . . . 1/2 pizza		430	17	43	1000	3	21.0	30
sausage, on French bread . . . . 1/2 pizza		420	19	41	900	4	20.0	35
sausage and pepperoni, on French bread . . . . 1/2 pizza		490	22	45	1130	4	25.0	4
vegetable, deluxe, on French bread . . . . 1/2 pizza		400	18	43	830	5	17.0	25
w/sausage and pepperoni, on French bread, frozen . . . . . 1 pkg		896	35	87	1720	5	45.0	74
w/sausage and pepperoni, on French bread, frozen . . . 1 serving		448	18	44	860	2	22.5	37
(Tombstone)								
bacon, Canadian style, 12 inch, 'Original' . . . . 3.6 oz		230	12	23	580	0	10.0	25
bacon cheeseburger, 12 inch, 'Special Order' . . . . 4.7 oz		330	17	29	730	0	16.0	40
cheese, microwave, 7 inch . . . . 7.7 oz		500	25	45	940	0	24.0	40
cheese, original, 12 inch . . . . 3.4 oz		230	11	23	460	0	10.0	25
cheese, original, 9 inch . . . . 5.6 oz		380	18	40	730	0	17.0	35
cheese, sausage, and mushroom, original, 12 inch . . . . . . 3.8 oz		240	13	23	570	0	11.0	30
cheese, w/hamburger, original, 12 inch . . . . 3.7 oz		250	13	23	570	0	12.0	30
cheese, w/pepperoni, 'Italian Thincrust' . . . . 3 oz		230	11	15	540	0	14.0	25
cheese, w/sausage, 12' 'Original' . . . . 3.7 oz		240	13	23	590	0	11.0	30

Food Name	Serv. Size	Total Cal.	Prot. gms	Carbs gms	Sod. mgs	Fiber gms	Fat gms	Chol. mgs
cheese and hamburger, original, 9 inch	6.3 oz	440	22	41	960	0	21.0	50
cheese and pepperoni, microwave, 7 inch	7.5 oz	550	27	38	1240	0	32.0	55
cheese and pepperoni, original, 9 inch	6.3 oz	480	21	40	1100	0	26.0	50
cheese and sausage 'Italian Thincrust'	3.2 oz	220	11	15	490	0	13.0	30
cheese and sausage, original, 9 inch	6.3 oz	420	22	41	1000	0	19.0	50
chicken, deluxe, light,	1/2 pizza	180	13	23	440	2	4.0	15
chicken, light, 8 inch	4.5 oz	240	17	28	450	0	8.0	25
deluxe, original, 12 inch	1 slice	310	15	29	690	3	14.0	30
double cheese, w/pepperoni, double top, 12 inch	4.8 oz	360	20	24	920	0	20.0	50
four cheese, 'Special Order'	4.3 oz	300	15	28	630	0	14.0	35
four meat, 'Special Order'	4.6 oz	320	17	28	810	0	15.0	40
four meat, 9 inch, 'Special Order'	3.9 oz	280	14	24	670	0	14.0	35
Italian sausage, 'Special Order'	4.5 oz	300	17	28	740	0	13.0	40
Italian sausage, microwave, 7 inch	8.0 oz	550	28	38	1210	0	32.0	65
pepperoni and sausage, original, 9 inch	6.6 oz	490	24	40	1230	0	26.0	60
pepperoni and sausage, original, frozen	1 pkg	952	40	82	2184	5	51.7	96
pepperoni and sausage, original, frozen	1 serving	317	13	27	728	2	17.2	32
pepperoni, 'Special Order'	4.4 oz	320	16	28	780	0	16.0	40
pepperoni, 8 inch, 'Light'	4.0 oz	250	16	27	630	0	10.0	20
pepperoni, 9 inch, 'Special Order'	3.7 oz	280	13	24	650	0	14.0	30
pepperoni, original, 12 inch	1 slice	400	19	35	930	3	21.0	40
pepperoni, original, frozen, 12 inch	1 pkg	938	44	85	1659	na	47.3	95
pepperoni, original, frozen, 12 inch	1 serving	312	14	28	551	na	15.7	32
pepperoni, original, frozen, 9 inch	1 pkg	1659	71	155	3489	na	83.6	165
pepperoni, original, frozen, 9 inch	1 serving	413	18	39	869	na	20.8	41
pepperoni, thin crust	1 slice	400	18	25	920	2	25.0	50
ranchero, deluxe, 'Mexican Style Thincrust'	3.4 oz	230	11	16	530	0	13.0	40
sausage, double top, w/double cheese, 12 inch	4.8 oz	330	21	24	860	0	16.0	50
sausage and mushroom, original	1 pkg	1496	70	152	3509	na	67.1	129
sausage and mushroom, original	1 serving	306	14	31	718	na	13.7	26
sausage and pepperoni, double top, 12 inch	4.8 oz	340	21	24	910	0	18.0	50
sausage and pepperoni, microwave, 7 inch	8 oz	570	32	39	1430	0	32.0	70
sausage and pepperoni, original	1 pkg	1635	72	153	3944	11	81.7	156
sausage and pepperoni, original	1 serving	328	14	31	790	2	16.4	31
sausage and pepperoni, original, 12 inch	3.7 oz	260	13	23	640	0	13.0	30
supreme, 'Italian Style Thincrust'	3.38 oz	230	11	16	520	0	14.0	30
supreme, 'Special Order'	4.4 oz	320	17	29	800	0	15.0	40
supreme, 9 inch, 'Special Order'	4.0 oz	280	13	24	640	0	14.0	35
supreme, light	1 slice	270	17	30	720	3	9.0	20
supreme, microwave, 7 inch	8.5 oz	550	27	40	1260	0	31.0	55
supreme, original, 12 inch	3.8 oz	270	12	24	630	0	14.0	30
supreme, thin crust	1 slice	380	18	26	840	2	22.0	45
taco, microwave, 7 inch	8.4 oz	590	28	41	1460	0	34.0	100
three sausage, 9 inch, 'Special Order'	3.8 oz	260	14	24	600	0	12.0	35
vegetable, light	1 slice	240	14	31	500	3	7.0	10
(Tony's)								
pepperoni, w/Italian style pastry crust, frozen	1 pkg	1232	45	110	2531	na	67.9	96
pepperoni, w/Italian style pastry crust, frozen	1 serving	406	15	36	834	na	22.4	32
sausage, deep dish, frozen, 'D'Primo'	1 pkg	1576	50	164	3351	na	80.2	63
sausage, deep dish, frozen, 'D'Primo'	1 serving	391	12	41	830	na	19.9	16
sausage and pepperoni, w/Italian style pastry crust	1 pkg	1319	46	126	2186	na	70.2	72
sausage and pepperoni, w/Italian style pastry crust	1 serving	434	15	41	719	na	23.1	24
supreme, w/sausage, pepperoni, mushroom, peppers, onion, Italian crust	1 pkg	1213	48	118	2341	na	60.6	85
supreme, w/sausage, pepperoni, mushroom, peppers, onion, Italian crust	1 serving	400	16	39	772	na	20.0	28
taco style, w/sausage, sauce, corn style crust	1 pkg	1326	43	130	2293	na	70.5	84

Food Name	Serv. Size	Total Cal.	Prot. gms	Carbs gms	Sod. mgs	Fiber gms	Fat gms	Chol. mgs
taco style, w/sausage, sauce, corn style crust .... 1 serving		437	14	43	756	na	23.3	28
(Totino's)								
baconburger, on French bread, 'Party' .... 1/2 pizza		370	15	33	880	2	20.0	15
Canadian bacon, 'Party' .... 1/2 pizza		320	14	33	900	2	15.0	10
cheese, 'Pan Pizza' .... 1/6 pizza		290	15	35	440	0	10.0	20
cheese, family size, 'Party Pizza' .... 1/3 pizza		320	14	43	580	2	11.0	15
cheese, microwaveable, individual .... 1 pizza		240	10	25	530	1	11.0	15
cheese, on French bread, 'Party' .... 1/2 pizza		320	15	33	630	2	14.0	20
combination, 'Party' .... 1/2 pizza		390	15	34	910	2	21.0	20
combination, family size, 'Party Pizza' .... 1/3 pizza		400	17	47	990	3	18.0	20
combination, microwaveable, individual .... 1 pizza		310	11	25	720	1	18.0	15
hamburger, 'Party' .... 1/2 pizza		350	15	33	860	2	18.0	20
Mexican, zesty, 'Party' .... 1/2 pizza		370	15	34	750	2	19.0	15
pepperoni, 'Pan Pizza' .... 1/6 pizza		330	16	35	620	0	15.0	30
pepperoni, 'Party Pizza Family Size' .... 1/3 pizza		410	16	44	1060	3	20.0	20
pepperoni, crisp crust, frozen .... 1 pkg		728	26	69	1946	na	38.9	23
pepperoni, crisp crust, frozen .... 1 serving		364	13	35	973	na	19.4	12
pepperoni, microwaveable, individual .... 1 pizza		280	10	25	710	1	16.0	15
pepperoni, zesty .... 1/2 pizza		380	14	33	920	2	21.0	20
sausage, 'Pan Pizza' .... 1/6 pizza		320	16	35	500	0	13.0	20
sausage, 'Party' .... 1/2 pizza		380	15	34	870	2	20.0	15
sausage, family size, 'Party Pizza' .... 1/3 pizza		410	16	48	870	4	18.0	15
sausage, individual, microwaveable .... 1 pizza		280	10	25	650	1	16.0	10
sausage and pepperoni, 'Pan Pizza' .... 1/6 pizza		330	16	35	560	0	15.0	25
sausage and pepperoni, crisp crust .... 1 pkg		769	28	72	2082	na	40.7	24
sausage and pepperoni, crisp crust .... 1 serving		385	14	36	1041	na	20.4	12
(Tyson)								
hamburger, 'Looney Tunes Wile E. Coyote' .... 6 oz		310	12	40	630	0	11.0	13
pepperoni, 'Looney Tunes Foghorn Leghorn' .... 6.35 oz		400	13	57	610	0	13.0	18
(Weight Watchers)								
cheese .... 6.03 oz		300	24	36	310	0	7.0	10
combination, 'Deluxe' .... 1 serving		380	23	47	550	6	11.0	40
extra cheese .... 1 serving		390	23	49	590	6	12.0	35
pepperoni .... 1 serving		390	23	46	650	4	12.0	45
(Wolfgang Puck's)								
chicken, spicy, 'Pizza California' .... 1/2 pizza		360	19	36	620	5	16.0	45
mushroom and spinach, 'Pizza California' .... 1/2 pizza		270	14	36	380	5	8.0	10
PIZZA CRUST								
(Boboli) cheese, 6 inch .... 1/2 crust		150	6	25	305	na	3.5	1
(Ener-G Foods) gluten-free, 10 inch .... 1 slice		134	1	20	132	1	5.7	0
(Pillsbury) 'All Ready' .... 1/8 crust		90	3	16	170	0	1.0	0
PIZZA CRUST DOUGH *(Rhodes)* frozen .... 1 slice		130	5	23	280	1	2.0	0
PIZZA CRUST MIX								
(Chef Boyardee) 'Quick & Easy' mix only .... 1/6 pkg		150	6	26	300	0	2.0	0
(French Meadow) spelt, organic, yeast-free, prepared ... 1/6 crust		90	3	10	110	2	2.0	0
(Gold Medal)								
just add water, prepared .... 1/4 crust		160	5	32	340	1	2.0	0
'Pouch Mix' mix only .... 1/6 pkg		110	3	22	220	0	1.0	0
(Martha White)								
deep dish, prepared w/water .... 1 slice		110	3	23	110	0	1.0	0
regular, prepared w/water .... 1 slice		100	2	19	125	0	2.0	0
(Robin Hood) 'Pouch Mix' mix only .... 1/6 pkg		110	3	22	220	0	1.0	0
PIZZA DINNER/ENTRÉE								
(Kid Cuisine)								
cheese, 'Mega Meal' .... 9.7 oz		430	17	75	700	0	7.0	0
w/hamburger, apples, corn, chocolate pudding .... 1 meal		330	12	50	440	5	9.0	20

Food Name	Serv. Size	Total Cal.	Prot. gms	Carbs gms	Sod. mgs	Fiber gms	Fat gms	Chol. mgs
PIZZA KIT								
(Chef Boyardee)								
cheese, 'Complete'	1/4 pkg	230	9	36	740	0	6.0	0
cheese, '2 Complete'	1/8 pkg	210	10	31	650	0	5.0	0
pepperoni, 'Complete'	1/4 pkg	250	13	31	870	0	9.0	0
pepperoni, '2 Complete'	1/8 pkg	210	10	31	595	0	7.0	0
plain	1/4 pkg	180	6	32	640	0	3.0	0
sausage	1/4 pkg	270	14	34	930	0	10.0	0
(Contadina)								
cheese	4.94 oz	320	16	41	850	0	10.0	20
pepperoni	4.94 oz	370	18	38	980	0	16.0	30
PIZZA SNACK								
(Jenny's Cuisine) puffs, cheese, w/vegetables, thick crust	1 puff	252	9	34	504	2	8.5	9
(Totino's)								
roll, hamburger, frozen	1 pkg	577	23	66	1041	na	24.4	na
roll, hamburger, frozen	1 serving	231	9	26	417	na	9.8	na
roll, pepperoni, frozen	1 pkg	579	22	59	1302	3	28.4	47
roll, pepperoni, frozen	1 serving	385	14	39	866	2	18.9	31
roll, sausage, frozen	1 pkg	528	21	60	950	4	22.5	36
roll, sausage, frozen	1 serving	351	14	40	632	3	14.9	24
PLANTAIN								
cooked, mashed	1 cup	232	2	62	10	5	0.4	0
cooked, sliced	1 cup	179	1	48	8	4	0.3	0
raw, sliced	1 cup	181	2	47	6	3	0.5	0
raw, whole	1 medium	218	2	57	7	4	0.7	0
PLUM								
Canned								
purple, in heavy syrup, w/liquid	1 medium	41	0	11	9	0	0.0	0
purple, in juice, w/liquid	1 medium	27	0	7	0	0	0.0	0
purple, in light syrup, w/liquid	1 medium	29	0	7	9	0	0.0	0
purple, in water, w/liquid	1 medium	19	0	5	0	0	0.0	0
purple, pitted, in extra heavy syrup, w/liquid	1 cup	264	1	69	50	3	0.3	0
purple, pitted, in heavy syrup, w/liquid	1 cup	230	1	60	49	3	0.3	0
purple, pitted, in juice, w/liquid	1 cup	146	1	38	3	3	0.1	0
purple, pitted, in light syrup, w/liquid	1 cup	159	1	41	50	3	0.3	0
purple, pitted, in water, w/liquid	1 cup	102	1	27	2	2	0.0	0
Fresh								
raw, sliced	1 cup	91	1	21	0	2	1.0	0
raw, whole, approx 2 1/8 inch diam	1 plum	36	1	9	0	1	0.4	0
PLUM, JAPANESE. See UMEBOSHI.								
POI								
	1 cup	269	1	65	29	1	0.3	0
crumbles *(Ener-G Foods)*	1 cup	376	1	75	21	3	8.0	0
POKEBERRY SHOOT								
boiled, drained	1 cup	33	4	5	30	2	0.7	0
boiled, drained	1 tbsp	2	0	0	2	0	0.0	0
raw	1 cup	37	4	6	37	3	0.6	0
POLENTA MIX *(Fantastic Foods)* 'Polenta' prepared	1/2 cup	106	3	18	246	0	2.0	0
POLISH SAUSAGE. See under SAUSAGE.								
POLLACK								
ALASKAN								
baked, broiled, grilled, or microwaved	4 oz	128	26.7	0.0	132	0	1.3	109
raw	1 lb	365	77.9	0.0	449	0	3.6	323
raw	1 oz	23	4.9	0.0	28	0	0.2	20
ATLANTIC								
baked, broiled, grilled, or microwaved	3 oz	100	21	0	94	0	1.1	77
raw	3 oz	78	17	0	73	0	0.8	60

Food Name	Serv. Size	Total Cal.	Prot. gms	Carbs gms	Sod. mgs	Fiber gms	Fat gms	Chol. mgs
WALLEYE								
baked, broiled, grilled, or microwaved	3 oz	96	20	0	99	0	1.0	82
raw	3 oz	69	15	0	84	0	0.7	60
POLLYFISH. See PARROTFISH.								
POMEGRANATE/Chinese apple								
raw, trimmed	1 oz	19	0.3	4.9	1	>.1 c	0.1	0
raw, untrimmed	1 lb	172	2.4	43.6	8	>.5 c	0.8	0
raw, whole, medium, approx 3 3/8 inch diam ...	1 pomegranate	105	1.5	26.4	5	.9	0.5	0
POMEGRANATE JUICE								
(Knudsen)	8 fl oz	85	1	21	0	0	0.0	0
(Knudsen) fruit juice sweetened	8 fl oz	150	1	37	10	0	0.0	0
POMELO/pummelo								
raw, sections	1/2 cup	36	0.7	9.1	1	1.0	<.1	0
raw, trimmed	1 oz	11	0.2	2.7	1	>.1 c	<.1	0
raw, untrimmed	1 lb	95	1.9	24.4	3	>.5 c	0.1	0
raw, whole, medium, approx 5 1/2 inches diam, 2.4 lbs	1 pomelo	228	4.6	58.6	7	6.1	0.2	0
POMFRET								
raw	1 lb	663	78.4	0.0	401	0	36.4	295
raw	1 oz	41	4.9	0.0	25	0	2.3	18
POMPANO, FLORIDA								
baked, broiled, grilled, or microwaved	3 oz	179	20	0	65	0	10.3	54
raw	3 oz	139	16	0	55	0	8.1	43
raw, boneless	1 oz	46	5	0	18	0	2.7	14
POP. See SOFT DRINKS AND MIXERS.								
POPCORN								
(NOTE: All popcorn is popped unless otherwise noted.)								
(Act II)								
artificial butter flavor, 'Butter Lovers' unpopped	3 tbsp	170	3	19	340	4	11.0	0
butter flavor, microwave, unpopped	3 tbsp	170	3	19	400	4	11.0	0
natural, microwave, unpopped	3 tbsp	180	3	19	260	4	12.0	0
(Auburn Farms) caramel, nonfat	2/3 cup	120	0	28	140	1	0.0	0
(Bachman)								
....	0.5 oz	80	1	7	160	0	6.0	0
cheese flavor	0.5 oz	90	1	7	165	0	6.0	0
'Lite'	0.5 oz	50	1	10	35	2	1.0	0
white cheddar cheese flavor	0.5 oz	70	1	7	150	0	4.0	0
(Bearitos)								
buttery	1 cup	60	1	4	47	1	4.0	0
cheese flavor, 'Organic'	1 oz	137	3	13	122	2	8.0	0
herb, lite, organic	3.5 cups	140	3	20	230	1	6.0	0
no salt, no oil	1 cup	30	1	6	3	1	0.5	0
no salt, organic	1 oz	108	4	22	1	1	0.8	0
'Organic Lite'	1 oz	132	3	15	39	3	6.9	0
'Organic Traditional'	1 oz	140	2	12	85	3	9.2	0
(Betty Crocker)								
butter flavor, microwave, 'Pop Secret'	3 cups	100	2	11	170	2	6.0	0
butter flavor, microwave, 'Pop Secret By Request'	3 cups	60	2	12	160	0	1.0	0
butter flavor, microwave, 'Pop Secret Light'	3 cups	70	2	12	115	2	3.0	0
butter flavor, no salt, 'Pop Secret'	3 cups	100	2	11	5	2	6.0	0
butter flavor, original, microwave, 'Pop Secret'	1 cup	35	1	4	50	1	2.5	0
butter flavor, 'Pop Secret'	1/4 bag	120	2	13	250	2	8.0	0
butter flavor, 'Pop Secret Light'	1/4 bag	90	2	13	160	2	4.0	0
butter flavor, 'Pop Secret Pop Qwiz'	1 bag	110	2	11	210	2	7.0	0
butter flavor, 'Pop Secret Pop Qwiz'	2 3/4 cups	80	1	9	130	2	5.0	0
butter flavor, salt-free, 'Pop Secret'	1/4 bag	120	2	13	5	2	7.0	0
butter flavor, singles 'Pop Secret Light'	1 bag	180	4	28	310	4	8.0	0
butter flavor, singles, 'Pop Secret Light'	6 cups	140	3	23	190	4	6.0	0

Food Name	Serv. Size	Total Cal.	Prot. gms	Carbs gms	Sod. mgs	Fiber gms	Fat gms	Chol. mgs
butter flavor, singles, 'Pop Secret' .... 1 bag		250	4	27	460	4	16.0	0
butter flavor, singles, 'Pop Secret' .... 6 cups		200	3	23	310	4	12.0	0
buttery burst, microwave, 'Pop Secret' .... 1 cup		35	1	4	50	1	2.5	0
buttery burst, light, microwave, 'Pop Secret' .... 1 cup		25	1	4	45	1	1.0	0
cheese flavor, microwave, 'Pop Secret' 1/3 pkg .... 3 cups		170	3	15	260	2	11.0	0
natural, 'Pop Secret' .... 1/4 bag		120	2	13	250	2	8.0	0
natural, 'Pop Secret Light' .... 1/4 bag		90	2	13	200	2	4.0	0
natural, 'Pop Secret Pop Qwiz' .... 2 3/4 cups		80	1	9	140	2	5.0	0
natural, 'Pop Secret Pop Qwiz' .... 1 bag		110	2	11	220	2	7.0	0
natural, microwave, 'Pop Secret' .... 3 cups		100	2	11	170	2	6.0	0
natural, microwave, 'Pop Secret By Request' .... 3 cups		60	2	12	170	0	1.0	0
natural, microwave, 'Pop Secret Light' .... 3 cups		70	2	12	160	2	3.0	0
natural, singles, 'Pop Secret Light' .... 1 bag		170	4	26	440	4	7.0	0
natural, singles 'Pop Secret Light' .... 6 cups		150	4	23	320	4	6.0	0
(Bonnie Lee)								
air popped, salted .... 1 qt		109	3	20	1	0	1.0	0
oil popped, salted .... 1 qt		172	3	20	230	0	8.0	0
(Cape Cod)								
all natural .... 3.5 cups		160	3	18	200	3	9.0	0
butter, old fashioned .... 3 cups		170	3	16	220	2	10.0	5
white cheddar cheese flavor .... 0.5 oz		80	2	6	150	0	5.0	0
(Clover Club) white cheddar cheese flavor .... 0.5 oz		70	1	6	140	0	5.0	0
(Country Grown) no added fat or salt, microwave .... 3 cups		85	3	17	0	4	1.0	0
(Cracker Jack)								
butter toffee, w/almonds, pecans, 'Nutty Delux' .... 1 oz		130	1	19	135	1	6.0	5
caramel, w/peanuts .... 1/2 cup		120	2	23	70	1	2.0	0
(Estee) caramel coated, bag .... 1 oz		140	3	25	55	0	3.0	5
(Featherweight)								
butter flavor, low-salt, microwave .... 3 cups		100	3	14	70	0	3.0	0
natural, low-salt, microwave .... 3 cups		80	3	14	0	0	1.0	0
(Frito-Lay's)								
.... 0.5 oz		70	1	9	200	0	3.0	0
cheese flavor .... 0.5 oz		80	1	7	180	0	5.0	0
(Good Health) butterscotch, 100% natural .... 30-g pkg		110	1	24	220	1	0.0	0
(Healthy Choice) natural flavor .... 1 cup		15	1	4	25	1	0.0	0
(Jiffy Pop)								
butter flavor 'Pan Popcorn' .... 4 cups		130	3	16	270	2	6.0	0
butter flavor, microwave .... 4 cups		140	3	17	270	3	7.0	0
microwave .... 4 cups		140	3	17	270	3	7.0	0
'Pan Popcorn' .... 4 cups		130	3	16	270	2	6.0	0
(Jolly Time)								
butter flavored, light, microwave .... 3 cups		60	2	12	105	3	2.0	0
butter flavored, microwave .... 3 cups		90	2	13	95	3	5.0	0
cheddar flavor, microwave .... 3 cups		155	3	17	220	4	10.0	0
natural flavor, light, microwave .... 3 cups		70	2	13	110	3	2.0	0
natural flavor, microwave .... 3 cups		120	2	15	125	3	7.0	0
white, air-popped .... 3 cups		60	2	15	2	4	1.0	0
white, unsalted .... 4 cups		75	3	20	2	5	1.0	0
yellow, air-popped .... 3 cups		60	2	14	2	4	1.0	0
yellow, unsalted .... 4 cups		75	3	19	2	5	1.0	0
(Keebler)								
honey caramel, 'Pop Deluxe' .... 1 oz		120	1	22	180	0	3.0	0
white cheddar cheese flavor .... 1 oz		140	1	13	270	0	10.0	5
(Kettle Poppins)								
brewer's yeast .... 0.5 oz		70	2	8	40	1	2.5	0
lightly salted .... 0.5 oz		70	2	9	40	1	2.5	0
white cheddar .... 0.5 oz		70	2	9	120	1	2.5	1

Food Name	Serv. Size	Total Cal.	Prot. gms	Carbs gms	Sod. mgs	Fiber gms	Fat gms	Chol. mgs
(Lapidus Popcorn Company)								
herb, organic	2 cups	170	3	15	650	4	11.0	0
white cheddar, organic	2 cups	180	3	13	15	2	13.0	5
(Laura Scudder's)								
'Tender Baby White Corn'	0.5 oz	80	1	6	140	0	6.0	0
white cheddar cheese flavor	0.5 oz	70	1	6	140	0	5.0	0
(Louise's)								
nonfat	1 oz	100	1	24	80	1	0.0	0
toffee caramel, buttery, nonfat	1 oz	100	1	24	80	1	0.0	0
(Nature's Choice)								
caramel, original	1 oz	108	1	25	0	0	1.0	0
caramel, w/peanuts	1 oz	114	1	23	0	0	1.0	0
(Orville Redenbacher)								
butter flavored, light, microwave, 'Gourmet'	3 cups	80	2	14	250	3	4.0	0
butter flavored, light, microwave, snack size	3 cups	70	2	11	90	0	3.0	0
butter flavored, microwave, 'Gourmet'	3 cups	110	2	12	300	3	8.0	0
butter flavored, microwave, 'Smart Pop'	3 cups	50	2	11	100	0	1.0	0
butter flavored, microwave, snack size	3 cups	100	2	11	140	0	6.0	0
butter flavored, salt-free, microwave, 'Gourmet'	3 cups	110	2	12	0	3	8.0	0
butter toffee, microwave, 'Gourmet'	2 1/2 cups	210	2	26	85	2	12.0	1
caramel, 'Ready-to-Eat'	1 oz	112	1	22	65	3	3.5	1
caramel, microwave, 'Gourmet'	2 1/2 cups	240	2	29	90	2	14.0	1
cheddar cheese, microwave, 'Gourmet'	3 cups	130	2	14	280	3	8.0	2
cheddar cheese, microwave, 'Gourmet'	3 cups	150	3	13	370	3	10.0	2
hot air, 'Gourmet'	3 cups	40	1	10	0	3	1.0	0
hot air, unpopped	2 tbsp	92	4	24	3	6	0.8	0
natural, light, microwave, 'Gourmet'	3 cups	80	2	14	290	3	4.0	0
natural, microwave, 'Gourmet'	3 cups	110	2	12	550	3	8.0	0
natural, salt-free, microwave 'Gourmet'	3 cups	110	2	12	0	3	8.0	0
original, 'Gourmet'	3 cups	80	1	10	0	3	4.0	0
regular	1 oz	138	3	17	3	5	8.7	0
sour cream and onion, microwave, 'Gourmet'	3 cups	180	3	16	320	3	13.0	1
white cheddar cheese, 'Ready-to-Eat'	1.06 oz	139	3	17	285	4	8.6	1
white, 'Gourmet'	3 cups	80	1	10	0	3	4.0	0
(Painted Desert) microwave	1 cup	27	1	6	0	0	1.0	0
(Pillsbury)								
butter flavor, frozen, microwave	3 cups	210	3	20	480	0	13.0	0
original, frozen, microwave	3 cups	210	3	20	420	0	13.0	0
salt-free, frozen, microwave	3 cups	170	3	23	0	0	7.0	0
(Planters)								
butter flavor, microwave	3 cups	140	2	13	560	0	10.0	0
natural, microwave	3 cups	140	2	14	560	0	9.0	0
(Pop Weaver's)								
butter flavor, microwave	4 cups	140	3	20	230	4	8.0	0
natural, microwave	3 cups	140	3	20	230	4	8.0	0
(Pops-Rite)								
butter flavor, microwave	3 cups	90	2	13	140	0	5.0	0
microwave, 'Natural'	3 cups	90	2	13	190	0	5.0	0
white, air popped, no salt	1 oz	100	3	20	0	1	2.0	0
white, oil popped, unsalted	1 oz	220	3	20	0	1	15.0	0
yellow, air popped, no salt	1 oz	100	2	21	0	1	2.0	0
yellow, oil popped, unsalted	1 oz	220	2	21	0	1	15.0	0
(Smartfood) white cheddar cheese flavor	0.5 oz	80	2	7	150	0	5.0	0
(Tone's)	1 cup	30	1	6	1	2	0.4	0
(Ultra Slim-Fast) butter flavor, 'Lite 'N Tasty'	0.5 oz	60	2	10	150	2	2.0	0
(Vic's)								
caramel, lite, 'Gourmet'	1/2 cup	60	1	10	50	0	2.0	0
white cheddar cheese, lite, 'Gourmet'	2/3 cup	40	1	4	50	0	2.0	1

Food Name	Serv. Size	Total Cal.	Prot. gms	Carbs gms	Sod. mgs	Fiber gms	Fat gms	Chol. mgs
white, lite, 'Gourmet'	1 cup	35	1	6	15	0	2.0	0
yellow cheddar cheese, lite, 'Gourmet'	2/3 cup	40	1	4	60	0	2.0	1
(Weight Watchers)								
butter	0.66 oz	90	2	13	100	0	3.0	0
caramel	1 serving	100	1	22	45	1	1.0	0
'Lightly Salted'	0.66 oz	80	2	12	65	0	4.0	0
microwave	1 oz pkg	100	4	22	5	0	1.0	0
white cheddar cheese flavor	0.66 oz pkg	100	2	10	85	0	6.0	0
(Wise)								
butter flavor	1 cup	80	1	7	140	0	5.0	0
'Tender Baby White Corn'	0.5 oz	80	1	6	140	0	6.0	0
'Tender Eating Baby Popcorn'	0.5 oz	70	1	4	120	0	6.0	0
white cheddar cheese flavor	0.5 oz	70	1	6	140	0	5.0	0
POPCORN OIL								
(Orville Redenbacher) and topping oil	1 tbsp	120	0	0	0	0	13.5	0
(Planters)	1 tbsp	120	0	0	0	0	14.0	0
(Wesson)								
buttery flavor	1 tbsp	120	0	0	0	0	13.5	0
popping and topping oil, food service product	1 tbsp	122	0	0	0	0	13.5	0
POPCORN SEASONING. See under SEASONING MIX.								
POPPY SEED								
	1 tbsp	47	2	2	2	1	3.9	0
	1 tsp	15	1	1	1	0	1.3	0
(McCormick/Schilling)	1 tsp	17	1	1	0	1	1.2	0
(Spice Islands)	1 tsp	13	1	1	1	0	0.9	0
whole (Durkee)	1 tsp	15	0	0	0	0	0.0	0
whole (Laurel Leaf)	1 tsp	15	0	0	0	0	0.0	0
POPPY SEED FILLING (Solo) 'Sokal'	2 tbsp	119	2	21	27	na	3.2	na
POPPY SEED OIL								
	1 cup	1927	0	0	0	0	218.0	0
	1 tbsp	120	0	0	0	0	13.6	0
PORK. See also HAM.								
(NOTE: TRIMMED = Lean; separable fat removed. UNTRIMMED = Separable fat not removed.)								
BACKFAT								
Fresh								
wholesale cuts, raw	1 lb	3683	13.3	0.0	50	0	402.3	259
wholesale cuts, raw	1 oz	230	0.8	0.0	3	0	25.1	16
BACKRIB								
Fresh								
Untrimmed								
raw	1 lb	1279	73.1	0.0	340	0	107.0	367
raw	1 oz	80	4.6	0.0	21	0	6.7	23
raw 'Gourmet' (JM)	5.5 oz	220	15.0	0.0	50	0	18.0	(mq)
roasted	3 oz	315	20.6	0.0	86	0	25.1	100
BELLY								
Fresh								
wholesale cuts, raw	1 lb	2350	42.4	0.0	145	0	240.5	327
wholesale cuts, raw	1 oz	147	2.7	0.0	9	0	15.0	20
BRAIN								
Fresh								
braised	3 oz	117	10.3	0.0	77	0	8.1	2169
in milk gravy (Armour)	2.75 oz	110	7.0	1.0	400	na	8.0	na
raw	1 oz	36	2.9	0.0	34	0	2.6	622
CENTER LOIN								
Fresh								
Trimmed								
chop, bone in, braised	3 oz	172	25	0.0	53	0	7.1	72
chop, bone in, broiled	3 oz	172	26	0.0	51	0	6.9	70

Food Name	Serv. Size	Total Cal.	Prot. gms	Carbs gms	Sod. mgs	Fiber gms	Fat gms	Chol. mgs
chop, bone in, pan fried	3 oz	197	27	0.0	73	0	8.9	78
roast, bone in, roasted	3 oz	169	23	0.0	56	0	7.7	67
Untrimmed								
chop, bone in, braised	3 oz	210	24	0.0	50	0	12.0	73
chop, bone in, broiled	3 oz	204	24	0.0	49	0	11.1	70
chop, bone in, pan fried	3 oz	235	25	0.0	68	0	14.1	78
roast, bone in, roasted	3 oz	199	22	0.0	54	0	11.4	68
CENTER RIB								
Fresh								
Trimmed								
chop, bone in, braised	3 oz	179	24	0.0	35	0	8.6	60
chop, bone in, broiled	3 oz	186	26	0.0	55	0	8.3	69
chop, bone in, pan-fried	3 oz	185	24	0.0	44	0	9.2	60
roast, bone in, roasted	3 oz	182	24	0.0	43	0	8.6	71
Untrimmed								
chop, bone in, braised	3 oz	217	22	0.0	34	0	13.4	62
chop, bone in, broiled	3 oz	224	24	0.0	53	0	13.2	70
chop, bone in, pan-fried	3 oz	225	22	0.0	43	0	14.4	62
roast, bone in, roasted	3 oz	217	23	0.0	39	0	13.0	62
CHITTERLINGS								
Fresh								
raw	1 oz	71	2.8	0.1	10	0	6.5	45
simmered	3 oz	258	8.7	0.0	33	0	24.4	122
CHOP								
Refrigerated or frozen								
boneless, 'America's Cut' *(JM)*	6 oz	330	38.0	0.0	90	0	20.0	(mq)
center cut, 'Always Tender' *(Hormel)*	4 oz	187	21	1.0	424	na	10.8	59
center cut, 'Always Tender' *(Hormel)*	1 oz	47	5	0.0	107	na	2.7	15
COMPOSITE CUTS								
Canned								
(Hormel)	3 oz	240	11.0	2.0	1056	0	21.0	(mq)
chopped *(Hormel)*	3 oz	200	12.0	2.0	1073	0	16.0	(mq)
Fresh								
Trimmed								
leg, loin, and shoulder, cooked	3 oz	180	25	0.0	50	0	8.2	73
leg, loin, and shoulder, raw	1 oz	41	6	0.0	16	0	1.7	17
loin and shoulder, cooked	3 oz	179	25.0	0.0	48	0	8.0	72
loin and shoulder, raw	1 oz	41	6.0	0.0	15	0	1.7	17
retail cuts, cooked	3 oz	232	23.4	0.0	53	0	14.6	77
retail cuts, raw	1 lb	980	86.0	0.0	249	0	67.8	304
retail cuts, raw	1 oz	61	5.4	0.0	16	0	4.2	19
roasted	3 oz	180	24.9	0.0	50	0	8.2	73
Untrimmed								
leg, loin, shoulder, spareribs, cooked	3 oz	232	23	0.0	53	0	14.6	77
leg, loin, shoulder, spareribs, raw	1 oz	64	5	0.0	15	0	4.7	20
loin and shoulder, cooked	3 oz	214	23.6	0.0	48	0	12.6	73
loin and shoulder, raw	1 lb	907	88.6	0.0	231	0	58.5	290
loin and shoulder, raw	1 oz	57	5.5	0.0	14	0	3.7	18
raw	1 lb	1030	82.8	0.0	245	0	74.8	313
raw	1 oz	64	5.2	0.0	15	0	4.7	20
EAR								
Fresh								
raw	1 oz	66	6	0	54	0	4.3	23
simmered	1 medium	184	18	0	185	0	12.0	100
FEET								
Fresh								
raw	1 oz	75	6	0	18	0	5.3	30

Food Name	Serv. Size	Total Cal.	Prot. gms	Carbs gms	Sod. mgs	Fiber gms	Fat gms	Chol. mgs
simmered	3 oz	165	16	0	26	0	10.5	85
Pickled								
approx 6 oz *(Penrose)*	1 piece	220	19	2	2890	0	15.0	0
cured	1 oz	58	4	0	262	0	4.6	26
GROUND								
Fresh								
cooked	3 oz	252	21.8	0.0	62	0	17.6	80
raw	4 oz	297	19	0	63	0	23.9	81
Refrigerated or frozen *(JM)*	3 oz	190	15.0	0.0	40	0	14.0	(mq)
HEART								
Fresh								
braised	1 cup	215	34	1	51	0	7.3	320
braised	1 medium	191	30	1	45	0	6.5	285
raw	1 medium	267	39	3	127	0	9.9	296
raw	1 oz	33	5	0	16	0	1.2	37
HOCKS, refrigerated, hickory smoked *(Cook's)*	3 oz	270	17	5	1150	0	20.0	55
JOWL								
Fresh								
raw	4 oz	740	7	0	28	0	78.7	102
raw	1 oz	186	2	0	7	0	19.7	26
KIDNEYS								
Fresh								
braised	1 cup	211	35.6	0.0	112	0	6.6	672
braised	3 oz	128	21.6	0.0	68	0	4.0	408
raw	1 oz	28	4.7	0.0	34	0	0.9	90
KNUCKLES, jarred, pickled, approx 6 oz *(Penrose)*	1 piece	290	23	1	2380	0	21.0	0
LEG, RUMP HALF								
Fresh								
Trimmed								
raw	1 lb	621	96.3	0.0	313	0	23.5	277
raw	1 oz	39	6.0	0.0	20	0	1.5	17
roasted	3 oz	175	26.3	0.0	55	0	6.9	82
roasted, diced	1 cup	278	41.8	0.0	88	0	11.0	130
Untrimmed								
raw	1 lb	1007	85.0	0.0	277	0	71.2	299
raw	1 oz	63	5.3	0.0	17	0	4.4	19
roasted	3 oz	214	24.5	0.0	53	0	12.1	82
roasted	1.5 oz	117	11.3	0.0	26	0	7.6	40
roasted, diced	1 cup	340	39.0	0.0	84	0	19.3	130
LEG, SHANK HALF								
Fresh								
Trimmed								
raw	1 lb	631	93.5	0.0	304	0	25.5	272
raw	1 oz	39	5.8	0.0	19	0	1.6	17
roasted	3 oz	183	24.0	0.0	54	0	8.9	78
roasted, diced	1 cup	290	38.1	0.0	86	0	14.2	124
Untrimmed								
raw	1 lb	1193	77.5	0.0	249	0	95.4	308
raw	1 oz	75	4.8	0.0	16	0	6.0	19
roasted	3 oz	246	21.5	0.0	50	0	17.0	78
roasted	1.5 oz	129	10.3	0.0	25	0	9.4	39
roasted, diced	1 cup	390	34.2	0.0	80	0	27.1	124
LEG, WHOLE								
Fresh								
Trimmed								
raw	1 lb	617	92.9	0.0	249	0	24.5	308
raw	1 oz	39	5.8	0.0	16	0	1.5	19

Food Name	Serv. Size	Total Cal.	Prot. gms	Carbs gms	Sod. mgs	Fiber gms	Fat gms	Chol. mgs
roasted	3 oz	179	25.0	0.0	54	0	8.0	80
roasted	1.5 oz	94	12.0	0.0	27	0	4.7	40
roasted	1 cup	285	39.7	0.0	86	0	12.7	127
Untrimmed								
raw	1 lb	1111	79.1	0.0	213	0	85.6	331
raw	1 oz	69	4.9	0.0	13	0	5.3	21
roasted	3 oz	232	22.8	0.0	51	0	15.0	80
roasted	1.5 oz	125	10.6	0.0	25	0	8.8	40
roasted, diced	1 cup	369	36.2	0.0	81	0	23.8	127
LIVER								
Fresh								
braised	3 oz	140	22.1	3.2	42	0	3.7	302
fried	3 oz	205	25.4	2.1	94	0	9.8	372
raw	1 oz	38	6.1	0.7	25	0	1.0	85
LOIN								
Fresh								
Trimmed								
blade, braised	3 oz	191	21.3	0.0	53	0	11.1	71
blade, broiled	3 oz	199	21.6	0.0	68	0	11.8	71
blade, pan-fried	3 oz	205	21.0	0.0	66	0	12.8	70
blade, pan-fried in vegetable oil	4 oz	321	27.6	0.0	84	0	22.5	110
blade, roasted	3 oz	210	22.6	0.0	25	0	12.6	79
ribs, country-style, braised	3 oz	199	22.1	0.0	54	0	11.6	73
ribs, country-style, raw	1 oz	45	5.5	0.0	19	0	2.3	18
ribs, country-style, roasted	3 oz	210	22.6	0.0	25	0	12.6	79
whole, braised	3 oz	173	24.3	0.0	43	0	7.8	67
whole, broiled	3 oz	178	24.3	0.0	54	0	8.3	67
whole, chopped, braised	1 cup	382	46.2	0.0	105	0	20.4	147
whole, chopped, broiled	1 cup	360	39.0	0.0	105	0	21.4	133
whole, chopped, roasted	1 cup	336	37.7	0.0	97	0	19.5	126
whole, raw	1 oz	44	5.9	0.0	18	0	2.1	17
whole, roasted	3 oz	178	24.3	0.0	49	0	8.2	69
Untrimmed								
blade, braised	3 oz	275	18.6	0.0	47	0	21.6	72
blade, broiled	3 oz	272	19.1	0.0	59	0	21.1	73
blade, pan-fried	3 oz	291	18.3	0.0	57	0	23.6	72
blade, pan-fried in vegetable oil	4 oz	469	21.3	0.0	69	0	41.9	108
blade, roasted	3 oz	275	20.2	0.0	25	0	20.9	79
ribs, country-style, braised	3 oz	252	20.3	0.0	50	0	18.3	74
ribs, country-style, raw	1 oz	68	4.8	0.0	16	0	5.3	20
ribs, country-style, roasted	3 oz	279	19.9	0.0	44	0	21.5	78
whole, braised	3 oz	203	23	0.0	41	0	11.6	68
whole, broiled	3 oz	206	23.2	0.0	53	0	11.8	68
whole, roasted	3 oz	211	23.0	0.0	50	0	12.4	70
Refrigerated or frozen								
boneless, 'Always Tender' (Hormel)	1 oz	41	5	0.0	100	na	2.0	14
boneless, 'Always Tender' (Hormel)	4 oz	163	21	1.0	400	na	8.0	55
whole or half, center cut, boneless (JM)	3 oz	190	16	0.0	50	0	13.0	0
LUNGS								
Fresh								
braised	3 oz	84	14.1	0.0	69	0	2.6	329
raw	1 oz	24	4.0	0.0	43	0	0.8	91
PANCREAS								
Fresh								
braised	3 oz	186	24.2	0.0	36	0	9.2	268
raw	4 oz	225	21	0.0	50	0	15.0	218

Food Name	Serv. Size	Total Cal.	Prot. gms	Carbs gms	Sod. mgs	Fiber gms	Fat gms	Chol. mgs
SHOULDER								
Fresh								
Trimmed								
arm picnic, braised	3 oz	211	27.4	0.0	87	0	10.4	97
arm picnic, raw	1 oz	40	5.6	0.0	23	0	1.8	18
arm picnic, roasted	3 oz	194	22.7	0.0	68	0	10.7	81
Boston blade, braised	3 oz	232	26.4	0.0	64	0	13.2	99
Boston blade, broiled	3 oz	193	22.7	0.0	63	0	10.7	80
Boston blade, raw	1 oz	47	5.4	0.0	20	0	2.6	19
Boston blade, roasted	3 oz	197	20.6	0.0	75	0	12.2	72
whole, chopped, roasted	1 cup	341	35.5	0.0	107	0	21.0	135
whole, raw	1 lb	671	88.7	0.0	345	0	32.4	304
whole, raw	1 oz	42	5.5	0.0	22	0	2.0	19
whole, roasted	3 oz	195	21.5	0.0	64	0	11.5	77
whole, roasted, diced	1 cup	310	34.2	0.0	101	0	18.3	122
Untrimmed								
arm picnic, braised	3 oz	280	24	0.0	75	0	19.7	93
arm picnic, braised, diced	1 cup	444	38	0.0	119	0	31.3	147
arm picnic, raw	1 oz	72	5	0.0	19	0	5.7	20
arm picnic, roasted	3 oz	269	20.0	0.0	59	0	20.4	80
arm picnic, roasted, diced	1 cup	428	32	0.0	95	0	32.4	127
Boston blade, braised	3 oz	271	24.4	0.0	59	0	18.5	96
Boston blade, broiled	3 oz	220	21.7	0.0	59	0	14.1	81
Boston blade, raw	1 lb	989	80.1	0.0	286	0	71.8	322
Boston blade, roasted	3 oz	229	19.6	0.0	57	0	16.0	73
whole, raw	1 oz	67	4.9	0.0	18	0	5.1	20
whole, roasted	3 oz	248	19.8	0.0	58	0	18.2	77
whole, roasted, diced	1 cup	394	31.4	0.0	92	0	28.9	122
SIRLOIN								
Fresh								
Trimmed								
chop, bone in, braised	3 oz	167	23.0	0.0	45	0	7.7	69
chop, bone in, broiled	3 oz	181	24.2	0.0	61	0	8.6	72
chop, boneless, braised	3 oz	149	23.0	0.0	39	0	5.6	69
chop, boneless, broiled	3 oz	164	26.5	0.0	48	0	5.7	78
chop, boneless, raw	1 lb	581	95.5	0.0	231	0	19.1	286
chop or roast, raw	1 oz	43	6.0	0.0	14	0	1.9	18
roast, bone in, roasted	3 oz	184	24.5	0.0	54	0	8.8	73
roast, boneless, roasted	3 oz	168	24.5	0.0	48	0	7.0	73
Untrimmed								
chop, bone in, braised	3 oz	208	21.6	0.0	43	0	12.8	70
chop, bone in, broiled	3 oz	220	22.6	0.0	58	0	13.7	73
chop, boneless, braised	3 oz	161	22.6	0.0	39	0	7.1	69
chop, boneless, broiled	3 oz	177	25.9	0.0	48	0	7.3	77
chop or roast, raw	1 oz	78	4.9	0.0	12	0	6.3	20
roast, bone in, roasted	3 oz	222	23.1	0.0	51	0	13.6	74
roast, boneless, roasted	3 oz	176	24.2	0.0	48	0	8.0	73
SPARERIBS								
Fresh								
Untrimmed								
braised	3 oz	337	24.7	0.0	79	0	25.8	103
raw	1 oz	81	4.8	0.0	22	0	6.7	22
Refrigerated or frozen, raw, 'Gourmet' *(JM)*	4.5 oz	250	14.0	0.0	70	0	22.0	(mq)
SPLEEN								
Fresh								
braised	3 oz	127	24.0	0.0	91	0	2.7	428
raw	1 oz	28	5.1	0.0	28	0	0.7	103

Food Name	Serv. Size	Total Cal.	Prot. gms	Carbs gms	Sod. mgs	Fiber gms	Fat gms	Chol. mgs
STOMACH								
Fresh								
raw	4 oz	177	19	0.0	59	0	10.8	218
raw	1 oz	45	4.7	0.0	15	0	2.7	55
TAIL								
Fresh								
raw	4 oz	427	20	0	71	0	37.9	110
raw	1 oz	107	5	0	18	0	9.5	28
simmered	3 oz	337	14	0	21	0	30.4	110
TENDERLOIN								
Fresh								
Trimmed								
broiled	3 oz	159	25.9	0.0	55	0	5.4	80
raw	1 lb	544	95.2	0.0	227	0	15.5	295
raw	1 oz	34	5.9	0.0	14	0	1.0	18
roasted	3 oz	139	23.9	0.0	48	0	4.1	67
roasted, chopped or diced	1 cup	232	40.3	0.0	94	0	6.7	130
Untrimmed								
broiled	3 oz	171	25.4	0.0	54	0	6.9	80
raw	1 oz	39	5.8	0.0	14	0	1.5	19
roasted	3 oz	147	23.6	0.0	47	0	5.1	67
Refrigerated, boneless *(JM)*	3 oz	120	17.0	0.0	40	0	5.0	(mq)
TONGUE								
Canned, cured, '8-lb. can' *(Hormel)*	3 oz	190	17	0	966	0	13.0	0
Fresh								
braised	3 oz	230	20	0	93	0	15.8	124
raw	4 oz	254	18	0	124	0	19.4	114
raw	1 oz	64	5	0	31	0	4.9	29
TOP LOIN								
Fresh								
Trimmed								
chop or roast, raw	1 oz	46	6.2	0.0	13	0	2.1	16
chop, boneless, braised	3 oz	172	24.7	0.0	36	0	7.3	62
chop, boneless, broiled	3 oz	173	26.5	0.0	55	0	6.6	68
chop, boneless, pan-fried in vegetable oil	4 oz	291	31.7	0.0	57	0	17.4	92
chop, boneless, pan-fried	3 oz	191	25.9	0.0	48	0	8.9	65
roast, boneless, raw	1 oz	40	6.2	0.0	13	0	1.5	16
roast, boneless, roasted	3 oz	165	25.7	0.0	38	0	6.1	66
roast, boneless, roasted, chopped	1 cup	343	39.5	0.0	64	0	19.3	111
Untrimmed								
chop, boneless, braised	3 oz	198	23.6	0.0	36	0	10.8	64
chop, boneless, broiled	3 oz	195	25.5	0.0	54	0	9.6	69
chop, boneless, pan-fried in vegetable oil	3 oz	337	18.5	0.0	39	0	28.6	72
chop, boneless, pan-fried	3 oz	218	24.7	0.0	47	0	12.6	66
chop or roast, boneless, raw	1 oz	54	5.7	0.0	12	0	3.3	17
roast, boneless, roasted	3 oz	192	24.5	0.0	37	0	9.7	66
roast, boneless, roasted, chopped	1 cup	462	33.9	0.0	62	0	35.2	115
PORK, SALT								
cured *(Hormel)*	2 oz	320	4	0.0	1800	0	33.0	40
cured, raw	8 oz	1698	11	0.0	3232	0	182.7	195
cured, raw	1 oz	212	1	0.0	404	0	22.8	24
PORK AND BEANS. See under BAKED BEANS, CANNED.								
PORK DINNER/ENTRÉE								
(Armour) brain, in milk gravy	2.75 oz	110	7.0	1.0	400	na	8.0	na
(Banquet) cutlet	1 entrée	420	11	38	1060	4	25.0	35
(Bryan Foods) puréed	1/3 cup	140	11	0	30	0	11.0	40
(Chun King) sweet and sour, frozen	13 oz	400	11	78	1460	0	5.0	0

Food Name	Serv. Size	Total Cal.	Prot. gms	Carbs gms	Sod. mgs	Fiber gms	Fat gms	Chol. mgs
(Cook's) picnic, smoked, whole, super trim, water added	3 oz	160	11	1	1570	0	13.0	40
(Healthy Choice) patty, grilled, glazed	1 entrée	300	16	44	380	6	6.0	20
(Hormel)								
loin fillet, lemon garlic, 'Always Tender'	1 oz	33	5	1	165	na	1.2	12
loin fillet, lemon garlic, 'Always Tender'	4 oz	132	20	2	661	na	4.7	47
steak, breaded, frozen	3 oz	220	12	11	0	0	15.0	0
tenderlion, peppercorn, 'Always Tender'	4 oz	123	19	2	666	na	4.3	53
tenderloin, teriyaki, 'Always Tender'	4 oz	134	20	5	462	na	3.4	52
(John Morrell)								
back rib, barbecued, frozen 'Classics'	4.75 oz	240	12	8	480	0	17.0	62
chop, center cut, barbecued, frozen	4.5 oz	230	29	7	410	0	9.0	90
loin, thin sliced, barbecued, frozen	5 slices	150	17	5	440	0	6.0	52
tenderloin, barbecued, frozen, 'Pork Classics'	3 oz	130	18	3	220	0	5.0	53
(La Choy)								
chow mein, bi-pack	1 cup	78	7	9	1183	2	2.2	10
sweet and sour, frozen, food service product	1 cup	241	5	43	1733	4	6.2	7
(Lloyds)								
baby back rib, w/barbecue sauce, fully cooked	3 ribs	350	20	17	770	2	23.0	50
sparerib, w/barbecue sauce, fully cooked	3 ribs	380	22	13	920	1	27.0	60
(Marie Callender's) chop, country fried	15 oz	550	26	50	2240	9	27.0	65
(Pierre)								
nuggets, breaded, frozen, product 1921	1 piece	42	2	2	62	0	2.8	7
patty, country fried, frozen, product 1920	1 piece	279	14	14	432	1	18.7	30
patty, country fried, frozen, product 3701	1 piece	241	14	13	424	1	15.0	30
patty, country fried, frozen, product 3801	1 piece	242	14	13	414	1	15.0	28
steak, country fried, frozen, product 3700	1 piece	293	16	15	483	0	18.7	46
steak, country fried, frozen, product 3800	1 piece	370	19	17	532	0	25.0	57
(Swanson) loin, frozen	10.75 oz	280	20	27	790	0	12.0	0
(Tyson)								
patty, deluxe, frozen, 'Looney Tunes Porky Pig'	6.5 oz	370	14	48	490	0	14.0	35
(Wonderbites)								
and turkey, barbecue, flame broiled, product 9119, 'Lean Magic 30'	1 piece	132	16	8	560	1	4.1	37
barbecue, flame broiled, product 1830	1 piece	207	11	3	383	1	16.2	36
barbecue, flame broiled, product 3734	1 piece	153	15	3	399	1	8.6	44
barbecue, flame broiled, product 3735	1 piece	36	4	1	94	0	2.0	10
barbecue, flame broiled, product 3834	1 piece	152	14	3	394	1	9.0	37
barbecue, flame broiled, product 3835, 'Dippers'	1 piece	41	3	1	95	0	2.9	9
barbecue, flame broiled, product 9800	1 piece	184	16	3	442	1	11.8	43
barbecue, flame broiled, product 9966, 'Dippers'	1 piece	44	4	1	107	0	2.9	10
barbecue, flame broiled, w/100 serving trays, product 9968	1 piece	50	3	1	110	0	3.6	10
barbecue, less fat, flame broiled, product 3730	1 piece	35	4	1	99	0	1.8	9
barbecue, less fat, flame broiled, product 3731	1 piece	140	15	3	401	1	7.4	37
barbecue, ready to cook, product 1190	1 piece	224	10	4	438	1	18.7	39
barbecue, ready to cook, product 1330	1 piece	267	12	5	502	1	22.7	45
Oriental crunch, flame-broiled, frozen, 'Dippers'	1 piece	90	4	5	154	1	6.2	10
Oriental crunch, product 3702	1 piece	87	4	5	143	0	5.9	12
rib, barbecue, flame broiled, frozen, product 3736	1 piece	40	4	2	132	0	1.8	9
rib, barbecue, flame broiled, product 1805, 'Lean Magic'	1 piece	160	17	8	568	1	6.7	38
rib, barbecue, flame broiled, product 1809, 'Lean Magic'	1 piece	47	4	2	142	0	2.6	10
rib, flame broiled, frozen, product 3831, 'Lean Magic' ...	1 piece	132	15	3	402	1	6.3	37
(Rib-B-Q) rib, barbecue, flame broiled, product 3830, 'Lean Magic'	1 piece	39	3	1	102	0	2.5	10
teriyaki, flame broiled, product 3759	1 piece	45	4	2	135	0	2.3	12

Food Name	Serv. Size	Total Cal.	Prot. gms	Carbs gms	Sod. mgs	Fiber gms	Fat gms	Chol. mgs
PORK FAT								
leaf, raw	1 oz	243	0	0.0	1	0	26.7	31
leaf, fresh	4 oz	968	2	0.0	6	0	106.4	124
separable fat from fully cooked ham, roasted	1 oz	167	2.2	0.0	177	0	17.5	24
separable fat from fully cooked ham, unheated	1 oz	164	1.6	<.1	143	0	17.4	19
separable fat from ham and arm picnic, roasted	3 oz	502	6.5	0.0	530	0	52.6	73
separable fat from ham and arm picnic, roasted	1 oz	168	2.2	0.0	177	0	17.5	24
separable fat from ham and arm picnic, unheated	1 oz	164	1.6	0.0	143	0	17.4	19
PORK SEASONING. See under SEASONING MIX.								
PORK SEASONING AND COATING MIX. See under SEASONING AND COATING MIX.								
PORK SKINS								
barbecue	1 oz	153	16	0	756	na	9.0	33
barbecue	1/2 oz	76	8	0	378	na	4.5	16
plain	1 oz	155	17	0	521	0	8.9	27
plain	1/2 oz	77	9	0	261	0	4.4	13
PORK SUBSTITUTE								
(Worthington) vegetarian, 'Choplets'	2 slices	90	17	3	500	2	1.5	0
POT ROAST SEASONING. See under SEASONING MIX, BEEF.								
POTATO								
Canned								
(Stokely)	1/2 cup	50	2	11	360	0	0.0	0
(Veg-All)	1/2 cup	60	1	13	260	0	0.0	0
diced (Bush's Best)	1/2 cup	40	1	8	340	0	0.0	0
diced (Taylor's Brand)	1 cup	90	3	25	292	0	0.0	0
new, extra small, whole (IGA)	1/2 cup	45	2	9	310	0	0.0	0
new, small, whole (IGA)	1/2 cup	45	2	9	300	0	0.0	0
new, whole, drained (Hunt's)	4 oz	70	2	15	230	1	1.0	0
sliced (Bush's Best)	1/2 cup	40	1	8	340	0	0.0	0
sliced (Taylor's Brand)	1 cup	90	3	25	292	0	0.0	0
sliced, w/liquid (Del Monte)	1/2 cup	45	1	10	355	0	0.0	0
white, diced (Allens)	1/2 cup	45	2	10	360	0	1.0	0
white, double diced (Allens)	1/2 cup	45	2	10	540	0	1.0	0
white, sliced (A&P)	1/2 cup	45	2	11	320	0	1.0	0
white, sliced (Allens)	1/2 cup	45	2	10	360	0	1.0	0
white, sliced, no salt added (Pathmark)	1 cup	100	3	20	15	0	0.0	0
white, small, sliced (Finast)	1/2 cup	55	1	13	375	0	0.0	0
white, small, whole (Finast)	1/2 cup	55	1	13	375	0	0.0	0
white, whole (A&P)	1/2 cup	45	2	11	320	0	1.0	0
white, whole, no salt added (Pathmark)	1 cup	100	3	20	15	0	0.0	0
whole (Bush's Best)	1/2 cup	40	1	8	340	0	0.0	0
whole (Stokely)	2/3 cup	70	2	14	450	1	0.0	0
whole, w/liquid (Del Monte)	1/2 cup	45	1	10	355	0	0.0	0
Dried, slices and dices, rehydrated (Basic American)	1/2 cup	72	2	16	240	2	0.1	0
Fresh								
baked, flesh and skin, 2 1/3 x 4 3/4 inch	1 potato	220	5	51	16	5	0.2	0
baked, flesh only	1/2 cup	57	1	13	3	1	0.1	0
baked, flesh only, 2 1/3 x 4 3/4 inch	1 potato	145	3	34	8	2	0.2	0
boiled, cooked in skin, flesh only	1/2 cup	68	1	16	3	1	0.1	0
boiled, cooked in skin, flesh only, 2.5 inch diam	1 potato	118	3	27	5	2	0.1	0
boiled, cooked w/o skin, flesh only	1/2 cup	67	1	16	4	1	0.1	0
boiled, cooked w/o skin, flesh only, 2.5 inch diam	1 potato	116	2	27	7	2	0.1	0
Finnish yellow, raw (Frieda's)	3.5 oz	100	3.3	22.0	na	(mq)	na	0
microwaved, cooked in skin, flesh and skin, 2.5 inch diam	1 potato	212	5	49	16	5	0.2	0
microwaved, cooked in skin, flesh and skin	1/2 cup	78	2	18	5	1	0.1	0

Food Name	Serv. Size	Total Cal.	Prot. gms	Carbs gms	Sod. mgs	Fiber gms	Fat gms	Chol. mgs
microwaved, cooked in skin, flesh/skin,								
2-1/3 x 4.75 inch	1 potato	156	3	36	11	2	0.2	0
raw, diced, flesh and skin	1/2 cup	59	2	13	5	1	0.1	0
raw, sliced	1 cup	142	4	32	46	2	0.3	0
raw, whole, large, 3–4.25 inch diam, flesh and skin	1 potato	145	4	33	11	3	0.2	0
raw, whole, long, 2 1/3 x 4 3/4 inch, flesh and skin	1 potato	160	4	36	12	3	0.2	0
raw, whole, medium, 2.25–3 inch diam, flesh and skin	1 potato	96	3	22	7	2	0.1	0
raw, whole, small, 1.75–2.25 inch diam, flesh and skin	1 potato	73	2	17	6	1	0.1	0
skin, baked	1 skin	115	2	27	12	5	0.1	0
skin, boiled	1 skin	27	1	6	5	1	0.0	0
skin, microwaved	1 skin	77	3	17	9	3	0.1	0
skin, raw	1 skin	22	1	5	4	1	0.0	0
Frozen								
red, whole, 2 to 3 potatoes (C&W)	85 grams	60	1	15	30	1	0.0	0
redskin, diced, frozen (Flav-R-Pac)	3/4 cup	60	1	16	35	1	0.0	0
redskin, tri-cut, frozen (Flav-R-Pac)	2/3 cup	60	1	15	30	1	0.0	0
redskin, wedges, frozen (Flav-R-Pac)	3/4 cup	60	1	15	30	1	0.0	0
skin, baked (Tato Skins)	1 oz	150	1	17	160	0	8.0	0
white, whole (Southern)	3.5 oz	69	2	15	20	0	0.1	0
white, whole, boiled (Seabrook)	3.2 oz	60	2	13	5	0	0.0	0
whole, small (Ore-Ida)	3 oz	70	2	16	45	0	1.0	0
POTATO CHIPS AND SNACKS								
CHIPS								
(Auburn Farms)								
barbecue, nonfat	1 oz	100	3	23	140	1	0.0	0
Cajun, nonfat	1 oz	99	3	23	227	1	0.0	0
cheddar cheese, 96% fat free, 'Spudbakes'	1 oz	100	2	22	105	1	1.0	0
cheddar, nonfat	1 oz	99	3	22	168	1	0.0	0
mesquite barbecue, 98% fat free, 'Spudbakes'	1 oz	110	2	25	75	1	0.5	0
original, nonfat	1 oz	99	3	23	138	1	0.0	0
sour cream and onion, 98% fat free, 'Spudbakes'	1 oz	100	2	21	110	2	0.5	0
sour cream and onion, nonfat	1 oz	99	3	22	138	1	0.0	0
(Bachman)								
barbecue flavor	1 oz	150	2	14	280	0	9.0	0
barbecue flavor, hot	1 oz	150	2	14	200	0	9.0	0
'Kettle Cooked'	1 oz	140	2	16	115	0	8.0	0
plain	1 oz	160	2	14	270	0	10.0	0
'Ridge'	1 oz	160	2	14	260	0	10.0	0
'Ruffled'	1 oz	160	2	14	260	0	10.0	0
Saratoga style, 'Kettle Cooked'	1 oz	140	2	16	115	0	8.0	0
sour cream and onion flavor	1 oz	150	2	14	200	0	9.0	0
unsalted	1 oz	160	2	14	5	0	10.0	0
vinegar flavor	1 oz	150	2	15	610	0	9.0	0
(Barbara's Bakery)								
herb and garlic, 'True Blues'	1 oz	140	2	15	120	0	9.0	0
no salt added	1 1/4 cup	150	2	15	20	1	10.0	0
plain	1 1/4 cup	150	2	15	180	1	10.0	0
rippled	1 1/4 cup	150	2	15	180	1	10.0	0
yogurt and green onion	1 1/4 cup	150	2	15	240	1	9.0	0
yogurt and green onion, no salt added	1 1/4 cup	150	2	15	20	1	9.0	0
(Barrel O'Fun) plain	1 oz	150	2	14	160	0	10.0	0
(Cape Cod)								
dill and sour cream flavor	1 oz	150	2	16	160	0	8.0	0
dill and sour cream flavor, no salt added	1 oz	150	2	16	15	0	8.0	0
no salt added	1 oz	150	2	16	0	0	8.0	0

Food Name	Serv. Size	Total Cal.	Prot. gms	Carbs gms	Sod. mgs	Fiber gms	Fat gms	Chol. mgs
plain	1 oz	150	2	16	120	0	8.0	0
plain, 'Selects'	1 oz *(19 chips)*	130	2	18	110	1	6.0	0
sea salt and vinegar, approx 18 chips	1 oz	150	2	17	130	1	8.0	0
sour cream and chives, approx 18 chips	1 oz	150	2	15	160	1	9.0	0
'Waves'	1 oz	150	2	16	120	0	8.0	0
(Cottage Fries) no salt added	1 oz	160	2	14	5	0	11.0	0
(Eagle)								
barbecue flavor, 'Extra Crunchy'	1 oz	150	2	16	220	0	8.0	0
barbecue flavor, 'Extra Crunchy Louisiana'	1 oz	150	2	16	140	0	8.0	0
barbecue flavor, 'Thins'	1 oz	150	2	15	220	0	10.0	0
cheddar and sour cream, rippled, crispy	1 oz	160	2	14	200	2	11.0	0
'Eagle Thins'	1 oz	150	2	15	220	0	10.0	0
'Extra Crunchy'	1 oz	150	2	16	180	0	8.0	0
extra crunchy, 'Hawaiian Kettle'	1 oz	150	2	17	150	1	8.0	0
Idaho russet	1 oz	150	2	16	180	0	8.0	0
Idaho russet, dark and crunchy	1 oz	140	2	17	150	1	7.0	0
mesquite BBQ, rippled	1 oz	160	2	15	170	1	10.0	0
'Ridged Thins'	1 oz	150	2	15	220	0	10.0	0
ripple chips	1 oz	150	2	14	170	1	10.0	0
sour cream and onion flavor, 'Ridged'	1 oz	150	2	15	280	0	10.0	0
sour cream and onion flavor, thins	1 oz	160	2	14	180	1	10.0	5
spicy, fiesta thins	1 oz	160	2	15	220	1	9.0	0
thins, no salt added	1 oz	150	2	14	0	1	10.0	0
(Featherweight) low salt	1 oz	160	2	14	4	0	11.0	0
(Great Snackers)								
barbecue flavor	1 serving	60	1	8	170	0	3.0	0
cheddar cheese flavor	1 serving	60	1	8	170	0	3.0	0
sour cream and onion	0.5 oz	70	1	10	140	0	3.0	0
toasted onion flavor	1 serving	60	1	8	120	0	3.0	0
(Guiltless Gourmet)								
baked, less salt	1 oz	110	2	22	180	1	1.5	0
baked, seasoned salt	1 oz	110	2	22	230	1	1.5	0
barbecue, baked	1 oz	110	2	22	200	1	1.5	0
sour cream and onion	1 oz	110	2	22	200	1	1.5	0
(Health Valley)								
'Country Dip'	1 oz	160	2	15	60	1	10.0	0
'Country Ripple'	1 oz	160	2	15	60	1	10.0	0
'Country'	1 oz	160	2	15	60	1	10.0	0
'Natural'	1 oz	160	2	15	60	1	10.0	0
no salt added, 'Country Dip'	1 oz	160	2	15	1	1	10.0	0
no salt added, 'Country Natural'	1 oz	160	2	15	1	1	10.0	0
no salt added, 'Country Ripple'	1 oz	160	2	15	1	1	10.0	0
no salt added, 'Country'	1 oz	160	2	15	1	1	10.0	0
(Keebler)								
lightly seasoned	1 oz	140	1	18	190	0	7.0	0
sour cream and onion	1 oz	140	2	17	260	0	7.0	0
(Kettle Chips)								
jalapeño Jack	1 oz	150	2	15	110	0	9.0	0
lightly salted	1 oz	150	2	15	80	0	9.0	0
New York cheddar	1 oz	150	2	15	100	0	9.0	0
no salt added	1 oz	150	2	15	10	0	9.0	0
organically grown, w/sea salt	1 oz	150	2	15	80	0	9.0	0
salsa w/mesquite	1 oz	150	2	15	120	0	9.0	0
sea salt and vinegar	1 oz	150	2	15	120	0	9.0	0
yogurt and green onion	1 oz	150	2	15	120	0	9.0	0
(King Kold)								
'Rip-L'	1 oz	150	2	16	150	0	9.0	0

Food Name	Serv. Size	Total Cal.	Prot. gms	Carbs gms	Sod. mgs	Fiber gms	Fat gms	Chol. mgs
au gratin flavor	1 oz	150	2	15	220	0	8.0	0
barbecue flavor 'BBQ'	1 oz	140	2	16	360	0	8.0	0
dill flavor	1 oz	150	2	16	340	0	8.0	0
onion-garlic flavor	1 oz	150	2	15	420	0	9.0	0
plain	1 oz	150	2	16	160	0	9.0	0
sour cream and onion flavor	1 oz	150	2	15	220	0	10.0	0
(Lay's)								
au gratin, wavy	1 oz	150	2	14	200	1	10.0	3
baked, low-fat	1 oz	110	2	23	150	2	1.5	0
barbecue flavor, approx. 15-20 chips	1 oz	150	1	15	270	1	9.0	0
barbecue flavor, baked, low-fat, 'KC Masterpiece'	1 oz	120	2	22	210	2	3.0	0
barbecue flavor, 'KC Masterpiece'	1 oz	160	2	15	200	1	10.0	0
Cajun flavor, 'Crunch Tators Amazin Cajun'	1 oz	150	2	17	150	1	8.0	0
cheddar cheese flavor, 15–20 chips	1 oz	150	2	14	1	1	10.0	0
cheddar, deli style	1 oz	150	2	16	190	1	10.0	0
chili, deli style	1 oz	150	2	16	210	1	10.0	0
deli style	1 oz	150	1	16	180	1	10.0	0
'Flamin' Hot' 15–20 chips	1 oz	150	2	15	190	1	9.0	0
jalapeño flavor, 'Crunch Tators Hoppin' Jalapeño'	1 oz	140	1	18	200	1	7.0	0
mesquite barbecue flavor 'Crunch Tators Mighty Mesquite'	1 oz	150	2	17	135	1	8.0	0
original	1 oz	150	2	15	180	1	10.0	0
original, 'Crunch Tators' approx 16 chips	1 oz	150	2	17	120	1	8.0	0
ranch flavor, wavy	1 oz	160	2	14	150	1	11.0	0
salt and vinegar flavor	1 oz	150	2	15	340	1	10.0	0
sour cream and onion	1 oz	150	2	15	180	1	9.0	0
sour cream and onion, baked, lowfat	1 oz	120	2	21	210	2	3.0	0
tangy ranch flavor, approx 15–20 chips	1 oz	160	2	15	210	1	10.0	0
unsalted	1 oz	150	2	15	10	0	10.0	0
wavy	1 oz	160	2	15	210	1	10.0	0
(Louise's)								
barbecue, nonfat	1 oz	110	3	23	180	2	0.0	0
Maui onion, nonfat	1 oz	110	3	24	180	2	0.0	0
mesquite barbecue flavor	1 oz	100	2	23	200	0	1.0	0
nonfat, no salt added	1 oz	110	3	24	10	2	0.0	0
original	1 oz	100	2	23	200	0	1.0	0
original, nonfat	1 oz	110	3	23	180	2	0.0	0
vinegar and salt flavor	1 oz	100	2	23	200	0	1.0	0
vinegar and salt, nonfat	1 oz	110	3	23	300	2	0.0	0
(Michael Season's)								
baked, less salt	1 oz	110	3	21	130	1	1.5	0
French onion flavor, baked	1 serving	110	3	21	150	1	1.5	0
hickory barbecue, baked	1 oz	110	3	21	180	1	1.5	0
honey barbecue	1 oz	140	2	20	250	1	6.0	0
honey barbecue, 40% less fat	1 oz	140	2	20	250	1	6.0	0
less fat, rippled	1 oz	140	2	17	120	1	6.7	0
lightly salted, 40% less fat	1 oz	130	2	17	80	1	6.0	0
no salt added, 40% less fat	1 oz	130	2	17	5	1	6.0	0
yogurt and green onion, 40% lower fat	1 oz	130	2	17	105	1	6.0	0
(Mr. Phipps)								
barbecue, tater crisps	0.5 oz	60	1	10	160	0	2.0	0
sour cream 'n onion, tater crisps	0.5 oz	60	1	10	150	0	2.0	0
(Munchos) plain, approx 16 chips	1 oz	160	1	15	230	0	10.0	0
(Nabisco)								
baked, baked, snack chips, 'Zings'	0.5 oz	70	1	10	115	0	3.0	0
cheese, cheddar, baked, cracker chips, 'Zings'	0.5 oz	70	1	9	140	0	3.0	2
cheese, cheddar, cracker chips, 'Zings'	15 pieces	70	1	9	130	0	3.0	0

Food Name	Serv. Size	Total Cal.	Prot. gms	Carbs gms	Sod. mgs	Fiber gms	Fat gms	Chol. mgs
ranch, baked, cracker chips, 'Zings'	0.5 oz	70	1	9	140	0	3.0	2
(O'Boisies)								
plain	1 oz	150	1	16	180	0	9.0	0
sour cream and onion flavor	1 oz	150	2	15	190	0	9.0	0
(Pacific Grain)								
'Rancho-O's'	1 oz	130	2	22	55	0	1.0	0
baked, 100% natural	1 oz	120	2	23	230	0	1.0	0
BBQ, baked, 100% natural	1 oz	120	2	23	150	0	2.0	0
(Poore Brothers)								
barbecue	1 oz	150	2	15	60	2	10.0	0
Cajun	1 oz	140	2	16	55	2	8.0	0
dill pickle	1 oz	140	2	16	95	2	8.0	0
grilled steak and onion	1 oz	140	2	15	110	2	8.0	0
jalapeño	1 oz	140	2	16	100	2	9.0	0
Parmesan and garlic	1 oz	140	2	16	80	2	9.0	0
regular	1 oz	140	2	17	40	2	8.0	0
salt and vinegar	1 oz	140	2	15	125	1	9.0	0
unsalted	1 oz	140	2	17	5	2	8.0	0
(Pringle's)								
barbecue flavor, 'Light'	1 oz	150	2	17	125	0	8.0	0
barbecue flavor, 'Right Crisp'	1 oz	140	2	18	160	1	7.0	0
cheddar and sour cream, 'Ridges'	1 oz	150	1	15	201	1	10.0	0
'Cheez Ums'	1 oz	150	2	14	190	1	10.0	0
French onion flavor, 'Idaho Rippled'	1 oz	170	2	13	175	0	12.0	0
'Idaho Rippled'	1 oz	170	2	13	150	0	12.0	0
'Light'	1 oz	150	2	17	120	0	8.0	0
mesquite barbecue, 'Ridges'	1 oz	150	1	15	150	1	10.0	0
mesquite barbecue, ridged	1 oz	150	1	15	220	1	10.0	0
original flavor, 1/3 less fat	16 chips	140	1	19	135	1	7.0	0
ranch flavor, 'Light'	1 oz	150	2	17	135	0	8.0	0
ranch	1 oz	150	2	15	130	1	10.0	0
ranch, 'Right Crisp'	1 oz	140	2	18	160	1	7.0	0
'Right Crisp'	1 oz	140	2	19	135	1	7.0	0
sour cream and onion	1 oz	160	2	15	135	1	10.0	0
sour cream and onion, 'Right Crisp'	1 oz	140	2	18	120	1	7.0	0
taco and cheddar flavor, 'Idaho Rippled'	1 oz	170	2	13	160	0	12.0	0
(Ruffles)								
barbecue flavor	1 oz	150	1	16	320	0	9.0	0
barbecue, mesequite, 'KC Masterpiece'	1 oz	150	2	15	190	1	9.0	0
Cajun flavor, 'Cajun Spice'	1 oz	150	1	15	240	0	10.0	0
cheddar and sour cream	1 oz	160	2	14	190	1	10.0	0
40% less fat 'Choice' approx 16 chips	1 oz	130	2	18	130	1	6.0	0
French onion flavor	1 oz	150	2	15	180	1	10.0	0
low-fat	1 oz	130	2	18	160	1	6.7	0
mesquite barbecue flavor, 'Mesquite Grille'	1 oz	160	2	14	260	0	10.0	0
1/3 less fat, 'Light Choice'	1 oz	130	2	19	140	0	6.0	0
original	1 serving	150	2	14	180	1	10.0	0
ranch flavor	1 oz	150	2	15	280	1	9.0	0
sour cream and onion flavor	1 oz	150	2	15	240	0	9.0	0
(Snacktime)								
jalapeño flavor, 'Krunchers!'	1 oz	150	2	16	270	0	9.0	0
'Krunchers!'	1 oz	150	2	16	170	0	9.0	0
mesquite barbecue flavor, 'Krunchers!'	1 oz	150	2	16	200	0	9.0	0
(Spicer's)								
barbecue wheat, for weight control	1 oz	100	5	12	75	9	5.0	0
dietetic, natural, for weight control	1 oz	100	4	11	65	9	4.0	0
sour cream and onion, for weight control	1 oz	100	4	12	150	6	4.0	0

Food Name	Serv. Size	Total Cal.	Prot. gms	Carbs gms	Sod. mgs	Fiber gms	Fat gms	Chol. mgs
(Tato Skins)								
cheese and bacon flavor, potato skins	1 oz	150	1	17	180	0	8.0	0
sour cream n' chives flavor, potato skins	1 oz	150	1	17	180	0	8.0	0
(Westbrae)								
potato chips, no salt added	1 oz	150	2	16	10	0	8.0	0
'Ripple'	1 oz	150	2	16	100	0	8.0	0
salted	1 oz	160	2	15	100	0	10.0	0
(Wise)								
barbecue flavor	1 oz	150	2	14	240	0	10.0	0
barbecue flavor, 'Ridgies'	1 oz	150	2	14	240	0	10.0	0
hot	1 oz	160	2	14	290	0	11.0	0
'New York Deli'	1 oz	160	2	14	120	0	11.0	0
onion-garlic flavor	1 oz	150	2	14	250	0	10.0	0
'Plain'	1 oz	150	2	14	190	0	10.0	0
'Ridgies Super Crispy'	1 oz	150	2	14	220	0	10.0	0
'Ridgies'	1 oz	150	2	14	190	0	10.0	0
'Rippled'	1 oz	150	2	14	190	0	10.0	0
sour cream and onion flavor 'Ridgies'	1 oz	160	2	14	240	0	11.0	0
(Zapp's)								
Cajun flavor, 'Lite Kettle'	1 oz	150	2	16	94	0	8.0	0
Cajun flavor, 'Original Kettle'	1 oz	150	2	16	94	0	8.0	0
jalapeño flavor, 'Original Kettle'	1 oz	150	2	16	85	0	8.0	0
'Lite Kettle'	1 oz	150	2	16	45	0	8.0	0
mesquite barbecue flavor, 'Lite Kettle'	1 oz	150	2	16	87	0	8.0	0
mesquite barbecue flavor, 'Original Kettle'	1 oz	150	2	16	87	0	8.0	0
no salt added, 'Lite Kettle'	1 oz	150	2	16	1	0	8.0	0
no salt added, 'Original Kettle'	1 oz	150	2	16	1	0	8.0	0
'Original Kettle'	1 oz	150	2	16	45	0	8.0	0
sour cream and onion flavor 'Lite'	1 oz	150	2	16	79	0	8.0	0
STICKS								
(Allens)								
shoestring, canned	1 oz	140	2	16	190	0	8.0	0
shoestring, no salt added, canned	1 oz	140	1	16	10	0	8.0	0
(Flavor Tree) sour cream and onion	1/4 cup	127	3	13	360	0	8.3	0
(Planters)								
....	1 oz	160	1	15	170	0	10.0	0
barbecue flavor	1 oz	160	1	15	220	0	10.0	0
(S&W)								
fabulous fries, 'Pik-Nik'	2/3 cup	150	2	16	120	1	9.0	0
ketchup and fries, 'Pik-Nik'	2/3 cup	160	2	17	160	1	10.0	0
shoestring, 'Pik-Nik'	2/3 cup	280	2	26	180	2	18.0	0
shoestring, 50% less salt, 'Pik-Nik'	3/4 cup	165	2	16	60	1	12.0	0
shoestring, Sante Fe BBQ, 'Pik-Nik'	2/3 cup	180	2	18	240	2	12.0	0
shoestring, sour cream and cheddar, 'Pik-Nik'	2/3 cup	180	2	17	130	2	13.0	0
POTATO DISH/ENTRÉE								
(A&P)								
fried, crinkle cut	3.5 oz	140	2.0	25.0	25	(mq)	4.0	0
fried, regular	3.5 oz	140	2.0	25.0	25	(mq)	4.0	0
fried, shoestring	3.5 oz	170	2.0	24.0	50	(mq)	6.0	0
fried, steak fries	3.5 oz	140	2.0	24.0	30	(mq)	4.0	0
hash brown	3.5 oz	80	2.0	17.0	20	(mq)	0.0	0
morsels	3.5 oz	140	2.0	23.0	30	(mq)	4.0	0
(Basic American)								
au gratin, 'Classic Casseroles'	3 oz	81	2	13	354	1	2.6	1
hash brown, 'Golden Grill'	1/2 cup	118	1	13	144	1	6.8	0
hash brown, 'ReddiShred'	1/2 cup	134	2	16	161	2	6.8	0
scalloped, 'Classic Casseroles'	3 oz	81	2	13	283	1	2.3	1

Food Name	Serv. Size	Total Cal.	Prot. gms	Carbs gms	Sod. mgs	Fiber gms	Fat gms	Chol. mgs
(Bernardi) gnocchi, uncooked	2/3 cup	281	9	56	601	3	2.0	10
(Budget Gourmet)								
w/broccoli, cheese sauce, frozen, 'Light and Healthy' ...	10.5 oz	300	13	40	740	0	10.0	30
(Crispy Crowns) puffs, frozen, prepared	10 puffs	133	2	18	448	2	6.4	0
(Empire Kosher)								
potato pancake, triangle, latkes w/onions, frozen	2 oz	77	1.0	13.0	108	na	2.4	na
(Healthy Choice)								
casserole, frozen, 'Garden Style'	1 meal	200	11	30	520	6	4.0	10
cheddar broccoli, w/cheese Sauce, frozen	1 pkg	328	13	53	551	6	7.0	27
garden casserole	1 serving	220	11	30	520	6	6.0	10
w/broccoli and cheddar cheese	1 entrée	330	13	53	550	6	7.0	25
(Heinz)								
fried, crinkle cut 'Deep Fries'.........................	3 oz	150	2.0	22.0	30	(mq)	6.0	0
fried 'Deep Fries'	3 oz	160	2.0	23.0	20	(mq)	6.0	0
fried, shoestring 'Deep Fries'	3 oz	200	2.0	25.0	20	(mq)	10.0	0
hash brown, w/butter and onions 'Deep Fries'	3 oz	110	1.0	14.0	80	(mq)	7.0	5
(Hormel) scalloped, w/ham, microwaveable	1 cup	240	7	20	920	2	14.0	35
(Joan of Arc)								
salad, German style, canned	1/2 cup	120	2.0	23.0	550	1.6	3.0	na
salad, homestyle, canned	1/2 cup	340	4.0	32.0	1070	3.0	22.0	na
(Lean Cuisine)								
baked, w/broccoli and cheddar, frozen	10 3/8 oz	290	14	37	590	0	9.0	20
baked, w/sour cream, frozen	10 3/8 oz	230	9	38	570	0	5.0	15
cheddar, 'Deluxe'	1 entrée	230	13	32	570	6	6.0	20
roasted, w/broccoli, cheddar cheese sauce	1 entrée	260	12	39	590	7	6.0	15
scalloped	1 entrée	250	10	38	590	6	6.0	25
(Lunch Bucket) scalloped, microwave cup	7.5 oz	160	4	20	770	0	7.0	35
(MicroMagic)								
fried..	3 oz	290	3.0	40.0	30	(mq)	13.0	na
fried, skinny	3 oz	350	4.0	49.0	40	(mq)	15.0	na
sticks, 'Tater Sticks'	4 oz	390	2.0	43.0	620	(mq)	22.0	na
(Mountain House) hash brown, freeze-dried, prepared	1 cup	150	2.0	36.0	(mq)	(mq)	0.0	na
(Ore-Ida)								
fried, cottage cut	3 oz	120	2.0	19.0	25	(mq)	5.0	0
fried, 'Country Style Dinner Fries'	3 oz	110	2.0	19.0	30	(mq)	3.0	0
fried, crinkle cut, 'Golden Crinkles'	3 oz	120	2.0	19.0	35	(mq)	4.0	0
fried, crinkle cut, 'Lites'	3 oz	90	1.0	16.0	35	(mq)	2.0	0
fried, crinkle cut, microwave	3.5 oz	180	2.0	26.0	35	(mq)	8.0	0
fried, crinkle cut, 'Pixie Crinkles'	3 oz	140	2.0	21.0	40	(mq)	6.0	0
fried, 'Crisp Crowns'	3 oz	160	2.0	20.0	525	(mq)	9.0	0
fried, 'Crispers!'	3 oz	230	2.0	25.0	545	(mq)	15.0	0
fried, French, extra crispy 'Nacho Crispers'	3 oz	180	2.0	21.0	280	na	10.0	0
fried, French, 'Fast Fries'	3 oz	150	2.0	23.0	230	na	7.0	0
fried, 'Golden Fries'	3 oz	120	2.0	19.0	35	(mq)	4.0	0
fried, 'Lites'	3 oz	90	1.0	16.0	30	(mq)	2.0	0
fried, shoestring	3 oz	140	2.0	21.0	30	(mq)	6.0	0
fried, shoestring, 'Lites'	3 oz	90	1.0	15.0	25	(mq)	4.0	0
fried, wedges, 'Home Style Potato Wedges'	3 oz	100	2.0	17.0	45	(mq)	3.0	0
fried, w/onions, 'Crispy Crowns'	3 oz	170	1.0	20.0	570	(mq)	9.0	0
hash brown, 'Golden Patties'	2.5 oz	140	1.0	15.0	295	(mq)	8.0	0
hash brown, microwave	2 oz	130	1.0	12.0	170	(mq)	8.0	0
hash brown, shredded	3 oz	70	1.0	15.0	40	(mq)	<1.0	0
hash brown, 'Southern Style'	3 oz	70	1.0	16.0	35	(mq)	<1.0	0
hashbrown, w/cheddar, 'Cheddar Browns'	3 oz	90	2.0	13.0	415	(mq)	2.0	10
puffs, bacon flavored 'Tater Tots'	3 oz	140	2.0	19.0	625	(mq)	6.0	0
puffs 'Tater Tots'	3 oz	140	1.0	19.0	550	(mq)	7.0	0
puffs, microwave, 'Tater Tots'	4 oz	200	2.0	29.0	670	(mq)	9.0	0

Food Name	Serv. Size	Total Cal.	Prot. gms	Carbs gms	Sod. mgs	Fiber gms	Fat gms	Chol. mgs
puffs, w/onion, 'Tater Tots'	3 oz	140	2.0	19.0	715	(mq)	6.0	0
(Pik-Nik) shoestring	1 oz	160	1	15	103	1	10.3	0
(Quick 'n Crispy)								
fried, crinkle cut	4 oz	370	3.0	44.0	50	(mq)	19.0	na
fried, shoestring	4 oz	390	3.0	48.0	50	(mq)	20.0	na
fried, thin cuts	4 oz	370	3.0	44.0	50	(mq)	19.0	na
wedges	4 oz	280	3.0	36.0	40	(mq)	13.0	na
(Read)								
salad, German style, canned	1/2 cup	120	2.0	23.0	550	1.6	3.0	na
salad, homestyle, canned	1/2 cup	340	4.0	32.0	1070	3.0	22.0	na
(Seabrook)								
fried	3 oz	120	2.0	20.0	25	(mq)	4.0	na
fried, cottage cut	2.8 oz	110	1.0	17.0	14	(mq)	4.0	na
fried, crinkle cut	3 oz	120	2.0	20.0	24	(mq)	4.0	na
fried, shoestring	3 oz	140	2.0	20.0	45	(mq)	6.0	na
(Stouffer's)								
au gratin	1/2 cup	130	4	15	590	1	6.0	15
au gratin, frozen, food service product	1 oz	32	1	4	130	0	1.3	3
scalloped	1/2 cup	140	4	17	450	2	6.0	3
scalloped, frozen, food service product	1 oz	31	1	4	109	0	1.3	1
(Weight Watchers)								
baked, vegetable primavera, frozen	11.15 oz	320	11	49	500	0	9.0	5
baked, w/broccoli and ham, frozen	11.5 oz	240	19	30	520	0	5.0	15
baked, w/turkey, homestyle, frozen	11.25 oz	230	17	27	510	0	7.0	45
w/broccoli and cheese	1 serving	250	12	35	590	6	7.0	10
POTATO DISH/ENTRÉE MIX								
(Arrowhead Mills) Western, flakes	2 oz	140	5.0	44.0	24	na	0.0	0
(Barbara's Bakery)								
mashed, mix only	1/3 cup	70	2	17	10	1	0.0	0
Western, mix only	4 oz	389	7.0	89.0	63	na	1.0	1
(Betty Crocker)								
au gratin, prepared w/margarine and skim milk	1/2 cup	150	4.0	21.0	600	(mq)	5.0	(mq)
hash brown, mix only	1/2 cup	120	3	30	35	3	0.0	0
hash brown, w/onions, prepared w/margarine	1/2 cup	160	2.0	24.0	100	(mq)	6.0	na
hash brown, w/onions, prepared	1/6 pkg	110	2.0	24.0	40	(mq)	1.0	na
mashed, cheddar cheese, 'Potato Buds' mix only	1/12 pkg	110	2.0	20.0	440	na	2.0	na
mashed, cheddar cheese, 'Potato Buds' prepared	1/2 cup	180	3.0	21.0	510	na	9.0	na
mashed, cheddar cheese, 'Potato Buds' reduced fat recipe, mix only	1/12 pkg	140	3.0	21.0	480	na	5.0	na
mashed, 'Potato Buds' mix only	1/3 cup	80	2	18	20	1	0.0	0
mashed, 'Potato Buds' prepared w/o added salt	1/2 cup	130	3.0	17.0	90	(mq)	6.0	(mq)
mashed, 'Potato Buds' prepared	1/2 cup	130	3.0	17.0	360	(mq)	6.0	(mq)
scalloped, cheesy, mix only	1/6 pkg	90	2.0	19.0	500	(mq)	1.0	na
scalloped, cheesy, prepared	1/2 cup	140	3.0	20.0	560	(mq)	5.0	(mq)
scalloped, mix only	1/6 pkg	90	2.0	19.0	520	(mq)	1.0	na
scalloped, prepared	1/2 cup	140	3.0	20.0	580	(mq)	5.0	(mq)
scalloped, sour cream and chives, mix only	1/6 pkg	100	2.0	19.0	460	(mq)	2.0	na
scalloped, sour cream and chives, prepared	1/2 cup	140	3.0	21.0	520	(mq)	5.0	(mq)
scalloped, w/ham, mix only	1/5 cup	100	2.0	20.0	470	(mq)	1.0	(mq)
scalloped, w/ham, prepared	1/2 cup	160	4.0	22.0	540	(mq)	6.0	(mq)
stuffed, butter, herbed, 'Twice Baked' prepared	1/2 cup	220	5.0	20.0	540	(mq)	13.0	(mq)
stuffed, butter, herbed, 'Twice Baked' mix only	1/6 pkg	100	2.0	18.0	440	(mq)	2.0	na
stuffed, cheddar, mild, w/onion, 'Twice Baked' mix only	1/6 pkg	100	2.0	18.0	540	(mq)	2.0	na
stuffed, cheddar, mild, w/onion, 'Twice Baked' prepared	1/2 cup	190	5.0	19.0	640	(mq)	11.0	(mq)

Food Name	Serv. Size	Total Cal.	Prot. gms	Carbs gms	Sod. mgs	Fiber gms	Fat gms	Chol. mgs
stuffed, sour cream and chives, 'Twice Baked,' mix only	1/6 pkg	90	2.0	17.0	480	(mq)	2.0	na
stuffed, sour cream and chives, 'Twice Baked' prepared	1/2 cup	200	5.0	19.0	570	(mq)	11.0	(mq)
stuffed, w/bacon and cheddar, 'Twice Baked' mix only	1/6 pkg	110	3.0	19.0	500	(mq)	2.0	na
stuffed, w/bacon and cheddar, 'Twice Baked' prepared	1/2 cup	210	6.0	21.0	600	(mq)	11.0	(mq)
(Country Store) mashed, prepared	1/3 cup	70	1.0	16.0	10	(mq)	0.0	0
(Ener-G Foods) mix, gluten-free	1 cup	878	0	226	420	0	0.0	0
(Fantastic Foods)								
au gratin, prepared w/whole milk	1/2 cup	156	6.0	25.0	440	(mq)	4.0	(mq)
au gratin, prepared w/whole milk and salted butter	1/2 cup	196	6.0	25.0	495	(mq)	8.0	(mq)
country style, prepared	1/2 cup	85	3.0	19.0	316	(mq)	0.3	na
country style, prepared w/salted butter	1/2 cup	118	3.0	19.0	362	(mq)	4.0	(mq)
(French's)								
au gratin, tangy, prepared	1/2 cup	130	4.0	20.0	480	(mq)	5.0	na
casserole, cheddar and bacon, prepared	1/2 cup	130	4.0	18.0	390	(mq)	5.0	na
scalloped, creamy Italian, prepared	1/2 cup	120	4.0	19.0	430	(mq)	3.0	na
scalloped, crispy top, w/savory onion, prepared	1/2 cup	140	3.0	20.0	430	na	5.0	na
scalloped, real cheese, prepared	1/2 cup	140	4.0	19.0	380	(mq)	5.0	na
scalloped, sour cream and chives, prepared	1/2 cup	150	3.0	19.0	550	(mq)	7.0	na
Western, creamy, prepared	1/2 cup	130	3.0	20.0	520	(mq)	4.0	na
(General Mills)								
au gratin, mix only	1/6 pkg	100	2.0	20.0	520	na	1.0	na
au gratin, prepared w/margarine and 2% milk	1/2 cup	150	3.0	21.0	580	na	6.0	na
au gratin, w/broccoli, homestyle, mix only	1/6 pkg	90	2.0	18.0	490	na	1.0	na
au gratin, w/broccoli, homestyle, prepared w/margarine, 2% milk	1/2 cup	140	3.0	19.0	550	na	6.0	na
hash brown	1/6 pkg	110	2.0	24.0	25	na	<1.0	na
hash brown, prepared w/margarine	1/2 cup	160	2.0	24.0	100	na	6.0	na
julienne, mix only	1/6 pkg	90	2.0	17.0	520	na	1.0	na
julienne, prepared w/margarine and 2% milk	1/2 cup	130	3.0	19.0	580	na	5.0	na
mashed, American cheese, homestyle, mix only	1/6 pkg	100	2.0	20.0	560	na	1.0	na
mashed, American cheese, homestyle, prepared w/margarine, 2% milk	1/2 cup	150	3.0	21.0	620	na	6.0	na
mashed, cheddar and bacon, mix only	1/6 pkg	100	2.0	20.0	480	na	1.0	na
mashed, cheddar and bacon, prepared w/margarine, 2% milk	1/2 cup	150	3.0	21.0	540	na	6.0	na
mashed, cheddar cheese, homestyle, mix only	1/6 pkg	90	2.0	19.0	470	na	1.0	na
mashed, cheddar cheese, homestyle, prepared w/margarine, 2% milk	1/2 cup	150	3.0	21.0	530	na	6.0	na
scalloped, mix only	1/6 pkg	90	2.0	19.0	510	na	1.0	na
scalloped, prepared w/margarine and 2% milk	1/2 cup	140	3.0	20.0	570	na	5.0	na
scalloped, smoky cheddar, mix only	1/6 pkg	100	2.0	20.0	520	na	1.0	na
scalloped, smoky cheddar, prepared w/margarine, 2% milk	1/2 cup	140	3.0	21.0	580	na	5.0	na
scalloped, sour cream and chive	1/6 pkg	100	2.0	19.0	460	na	2.0	na
scalloped, sour cream and chive, prepared w/margarine, 2% milk	1/2 cup	150	3.0	20.0	520	na	6.0	na
scalloped, w/ham, mix only	1/5 pkg	100	2.0	20.0	550	na	1.0	na
scalloped, w/ham, prepared w/margarine and 2% milk	1/2 cup	170	4.0	22.0	620	na	7.0	na
Western, cheesy, homestyle, mix only	1/6 pkg	100	2.0	19.0	500	na	2.0	na
Western, cheesy, homestyle, prepared w/margarine, 2% milk	1/2 cup	150	3.0	20.0	560	na	6.0	na
Western, potato buds, mix only	1/8 pkg	70	2.0	16.0	20	na	0.0	na

Food Name	Serv. Size	Total Cal.	Prot. gms	Carbs gms	Sod. mgs	Fiber gms	Fat gms	Chol. mgs
Western, potato buds, prepared w/o salt	1/2 cup	130	3.0	17.0	90	na	6.0	na
Western, potato buds, prepared	1/2 cup	130	3.0	17.0	360	na	6.0	na
(Hungry Jack)								
mashed, 'Flakes' prepared	1/2 cup	140	3.0	17.0	380	(mq)	7.0	na
Western, flakes	13.3 oz	70	1.0	16.0	25	1.0	0.0	0
Western, flakes, prepared w/margarine, 2% milk, salt, water	1/2 cup	130	2.0	17.0	260	1.0	6.0	0
Western, flakes, prepared w/margarine, 2% milk, water	1/2 cup	130	2.0	17.0	85	1.0	6.0	0
(Idaho) potato pancake, prepared, 3 inch diam	3 pancakes	90	3	16	420	0	2.0	0
(Idaho Spuds)								
potato pancake, prepared, 3 inch diam	3 cakes	90	3.0	16.0	420	(mq)	2.0	na
Western, flakes	13.3 oz	70	1.0	15.0	40	1.0	0.0	0
Western, granules	13.3 oz	60	1.0	14.0	30	1.0	0.0	0
Western, granules, prepared	1/2 cup	130	2.0	16.0	320	(mq)	6.0	na
Western, granules, prepared w/margarine, 2% milk, water	1/2 cup	120	2.0	16.0	85	1.0	5.0	0
Western, granules, prepared w/margarine, 2% milk, salt, water	1/2 cup	120	2.0	16.0	190	1.0	5.0	0
(Idaho Spuds)								
Western, flakes, prepared	1/2 cup	140	3.0	17.0	380	(mq)	7.0	na
Western, flakes, prepared w/margarine, 2% milk, water	1/2 cup	130	3.0	16.0	105	1.0	6.0	0
Western, flakes, prepared w/margarine, 2% milk, salt, water	1/2 cup	130	3.0	16.0	370	1.0	6.0	0
(Idahoan)								
au gratin, prepared	1/2 cup	130	3.0	18.0	475	(mq)	5.0	(mq)
hash brown, herb and butter, mix only	1/6 pkg	90	2.0	16.0	425	(mq)	2.0	na
hash brown, prepared w/unsalted butter	1/2 cup	140	2.0	18.0	50	(mq)	7.0	na
hash brown, 'Quick One-Pan' prepared	1/2 cup	140	2.0	18.0	400	(mq)	7.0	na
mashed, cheddar, spicy, mix only	1/6 pkg	90	2.0	17.0	450	(mq)	1.0	na
mashed, cheddar, spicy, prepared	1/2 cup	140	3.0	21.0	500	(mq)	5.0	(mq)
scalloped, prepared	1/2 cup	140	3.0	20.0	425	(mq)	5.0	(mq)
scalloped, prepared w/o added salt, w/unsalted butter . . .	1/2 cup	140	3.0	16.0	55	(mq)	7.0	(mq)
scalloped, sour cream and chives, mix only	1/6 pkg	90	2.0	15.0	340	(mq)	2.0	na
scalloped, sour cream and chives, prepared	1/2 cup	130	2.0	18.0	400	(mq)	5.0	(mq)
Western, 'Complete' mix only	1/3 cup	100	2.0	19.0	310	2.0	2.0	0
Western, mix only	1/3 cup	80	2.0	18.0	15	2.0	0.0	0
(Ore-Ida)								
mashed, natural butter flavor, prepared w/2% milk	1/2 cup	170	4.0	23.0	230	na	5.0	5
mashed, natural butter flavor, unprepared	2.25 oz	100	1.0	14.0	140	na	3.0	5
(Pillsbury)								
au gratin, tangy, 'Specially' mix only	1/6 pkg	90	2.0	19.0	470	1.0	1.0	0
au gratin, tangy, prepared w/butter and whole milk	1/2 cup	140	3.0	20.0	520	1.0	6.0	15
mashed, cheddar and bacon, 'Specialty' mix only	1/6 pkg	90	2.0	18.0	430	1.0	1.0	0
mashed, cheddar and bacon, 'Specialty' prepared w/butter, whole milk	1/2 cup	140	3.0	19.0	480	1.0	6.0	15
potato pancake, 'Specialty'	1/8 pkg	70	2.0	16.0	400	1.0	0.0	0
potato pancake, 'Specialty' prepared w/water and egg, 3 inch diam each	3 cakes	90	3.0	16.0	420	1.0	2.0	55
scalloped, sour cream and chives, 'Specialty,' mix only . .	1/6 pkg	100	2.0	18.0	450	1.0	2.0	0
scalloped, sour cream and chives, 'Specialty,' prepared w/butter, whole milk	1/2 cup	150	3.0	20.0	500	1.0	6.0	15
Western, cheesy, 'Specialty' mix only	1/6 pkg	100	2.0	19.0	490	1.0	2.0	0
Western, cheesy, 'Specialty,' prepared w/butter, whole milk	1/2 cup	150	3.0	20.0	540	1.0	6.0	15
Western, creamy white sauce, 'Specialty,' mix only	1/6 pkg	100	2.0	19.0	410	1.0	2.0	0

Food Name	Serv. Size	Total Cal.	Prot. gms	Carbs gms	Sod. mgs	Fiber gms	Fat gms	Chol. mgs
POTATO JUICE, bottled *(Biotta)*	6 fl oz	144	2	31	222	0	0.1	0
POTATO SALAD. See under POTATO DISH/ENTRÉE.								
POTATO SALAD DRESSING. See under SALAD DRESSING.								
POTATO SALAD SEASONING. See under SEASONING MIX.								
POTATO SEASONING. See under SEASONING MIX.								
POTATO STARCH *(Featherweight)*	1 cup	620	0	154	51	0	1.0	0
POTATO STICKS. See under POTATO CHIPS AND SNACKS.								
POTTED MEAT SPREAD								
(Armour)	1.83 oz	100	7	1	550	0	7.0	0
(Hormel)	1 oz	53	4	2	280	0	4.0	23
(Libby's)	1/4 cup	110	10	0	440	0	7.0	30
POULTRY SEASONING. See under SEASONING MIX, CHICKEN and TURKEY.								
POWER BAR. See under SPORTS AND DIET/NUTRITION BARS.								
PRESERVES. See JAM AND PRESERVES.								
PRETZEL								
(A & Eagle)	1 oz	110	3	22	570	0	2.0	0
(Bachman)								
hard	1 oz	110	3	23	290	0	1.0	0
hard, unsalted	1 oz	110	3	23	50	0	1.0	0
logs	1 oz	110	3	21	470	0	2.0	0
'Nutzels'	1 oz	110	3	21	470	0	2.0	0
'Petite'	1 oz	110	3	21	410	0	2.0	0
rings	1 oz	110	3	21	410	0	2.0	0
rod	1 oz	110	3	21	240	0	2.0	0
sodium-free, 'Petite'	1 oz	110	3	21	2	0	2.0	0
thin	1 oz	110	3	21	410	0	2.0	0
thin, 'Thin'n Light'	1 oz	110	3	21	410	0	2.0	0
treats	1 oz	110	3	21	410	0	2.0	0
twist	1 oz	110	3	21	410	0	2.0	0
(Barbara's Bakery)								
Bavarian	2 pretzels	100	5	20	170	3	1.5	0
Bavarian, no salt added	2 pretzels	100	5	20	20	3	1.5	0
mini, no salt added	18 pretzels	100	5	21	30	4	1.5	0
mini, no salt added, 17 pretzels	1 oz	110	4	21	10	0	1.0	0
none-grain	2 pretzels	100	4	20	180	3	1.5	0
(Bearitos) stick, thin, organic	30 grams	110	3	24	350	1	0.5	0
(Benzel's Bretzles) tiny, thin	1 oz	104	3	23	470	1	0.0	0
(Cape Cod) multigrain, no fat	30 pretzels	110	3	25	310	3	0.0	0
(Delicious)								
party	1 oz	110	3	23	500	0	1.0	0
stick	1 oz	110	3	23	500	0	1.0	1
twist	1 oz	110	3	23	500	0	1.0	0
(Eagle)								
Bavarian, sourdough, no fat	1 oz	110	3	24	430	1	0.0	0
Bavarian, sourdough, no fat, no salt added	1 oz	110	3	24	60	1	0.0	0
mini bites, low-fat	1 oz	110	3	22	470	1	10.0	0
stick, low-fat	1 oz	110	3	24	470	1	1.0	0
twist, thin, low-fat	1 oz	110	3	22	470	1	10.0	0
twist, thin, no fat	1 oz	100	3	22	470	1	0.0	0
(Estee)								
Dutch style, unsalted	2 pretzels	110	3	23	30	0	1.0	0
unsalted	15 pretzels	75	2	16	5	0	1.0	0
unsalted	5 pretzels	25	1	5	5	1	1.0	0
(Featherweight) low-salt	20 pieces	110	3	23	30	0	1.0	0
(Harmony) yogurt coated	1/3 cup	140	2	21	210	0	5.0	0
(J&J Snack Foods)								
Bavarian, soft	1 pretzel	180	6	34	360	1	2.5	0

Food Name	Serv. Size	Total Cal.	Prot. gms	Carbs gms	Sod. mgs	Fiber gms	Fat gms	Chol. mgs
Bavarian, twist, soft .... 1 pretzel		210	8	41	430	2	3.0	0
cheese-filled, soft, 'Superpretzel' .... 1 pretzel		380	14	61	937	4	7.0	3
cinnamon-raisin, soft, king size, 'Superpretzel' .... 1 pretzel		390	12	76	570	3	4.0	0
cinnamon-raisin, soft, regular size, 'Superpretzel' ..... 1 pretzel		190	6	38	290	2	2.0	0
cinnamon-raisin, w/icing, soft, king size, 'Superpretzel' .... 1 pretzel		420	12	85	580	3	4.0	0
cinnamon-raisin, w/icing, soft, regular size, 'Superpretzel' .... 1 pretzel		210	6	43	290	2	2.0	0
jalapeño, soft, 'Superpretzel' .... 1 pretzel		360	13	78	460	4	0.0	0
rod, sweet dough, soft .... 1 pretzel		300	8	60	230	2	3.0	0
soft, all natural, regular size .... 1 pretzel		190	8	41	160	2	0.0	0
soft, king size, 'Superpretzel' .... 1 pretzel		390	14	83	320	4	0.0	0
soft, no salt, frozen, 'Superpretzel' .... 1 pretzel		170	6	37	140	2	0.0	0
stick, cheese-filled, nacho, 'Superpretzel' .... 2 softstix		140	5	24	270	1	2.5	10
stick, cheese-filled, pizza, 'Superpretzel' .... 2 softstix		140	5	24	250	1	2.5	10
stick, sweet dough, soft .... 1 pretzel		170	5	34	130	1	1.5	0
(Keebler)								
braids, 'Butter Pretzels' .... 1 oz		110	3	21	620	0	1.0	0
knots, 'Butter Pretzels' .... 1 oz		110	3	21	530	0	1.0	0
(Louise's) sourdough, nonfat .... 1 oz		90	1	19	470	1	0.0	0
(M&M Mars) w/cheddar, 'Combos' .... 10 combos		139	3	20	335	na	5.1	2
(Michael Season's) mini .... 18 pretzels		120	3	21	30	1	1.0	na
(Mister Salty)								
Dutch style .... 2 pretzels		120	3	25	580	1	1.0	0
'Juniors' .... 1 oz		110	2	22	500	0	2.0	0
rings .... 1 oz		110	3	21	510	0	2.0	0
rings, butter flavor .... 1 oz		110	3	21	570	0	2.0	0
stick .... 1 oz		110	3	23	380	1	1.0	5
stick, butter flavor .... 1 oz		110	3	22	620	0	1.0	0
stick, nonfat .... 47 stick		110	3	23	370	1	0.0	0
stick, very thin, approx 92 pieces .... 1 oz		110	3	22	600	1	3.0	0
twist, nonfat .... 9 pieces		110	3	23	380	1	0.0	0
(Mr. Phipps)								
less salt .... 16 pretzels		120	2	21	410	1	2.5	0
original, nonfat .... 16 pretzels		100	2	22	630	1	0.0	0
(Mr. Salty)								
30% less sodium .... 88 stick		110	3	25	400	1	0.0	0
nonfat .... 16 pretzels		100	2	22	621	1	0.0	0
(Nabisco) chips, sesame .... 8 pieces		60	1	10	250	0	2.0	0
(Pepperidge Farm) 'Snack Stick' .... 8 pieces		120	3	23	430	1	3.0	0
(Quinlan)								
beer .... 1 oz		110	3	22	446	0	1.4	0
logs .... 1 oz		103	3	22	388	0	0.8	0
oat bran .... 1 oz		115	4	22	156	0	1.5	0
rice bran, no salt .... 1 oz		101	3	20	52	2	2.3	0
stick .... 1 oz		105	3	22	538	0	0.6	0
thin .... 1 oz		104	3	22	765	0	0.6	0
thin, 'Ultra Thin' .... 1 oz		106	3	23	618	0	0.6	0
tiny, thin .... 1 oz		109	3	21	601	0	1.5	0
tiny, thin, no salt .... 1 oz		115	3	22	10	0	1.6	0
(Rokeach)								
Dutch style .... 1 oz		110	3	24	0	0	0.0	0
Dutch style, unsalted .... 1 oz		110	2	20	30	0	0.0	0
'Party' .... 1 oz		110	2	23	0	0	1.0	0
unsalted, 'Baldies' .... 1 oz		110	2	20	30	0	0.0	0
(Rold Gold)								
baked, 33% less sodium .... 10 pretzels		110	3	23	340	1	0.0	0

Food Name	Serv. Size	Total Cal.	Prot. gms	Carbs gms	Sod. mgs	Fiber gms	Fat gms	Chol. mgs
Bavarian, 3 pretzels	1 oz	120	3	22	430	0	2.0	0
rod	1 oz	110	3	22	370	1	1.0	0
stick	1 oz	110	2	23	760	0	1.0	0
stick, nonfat	1 oz	110	3	23	530	1	0.0	0
thin twist	1 oz	110	3	23	420	1	1.0	0
thin, baked, 33% less sodium, fat-free'	1 oz	110	3	23	340	1	0.0	0
tiny, twist, nonfat	1 oz	100	3	23	420	1	0.0	0
'Tiny Tim'	1 oz	110	2	23	610	0	1.0	0
twist, thin, 10 twists	1 oz	110	2	23	470	0	1.0	0
(Seyfert's) rod, butter flavor	1 oz	110	3	21	530	0	1.0	0
(Snyder's) pieces, buttermilk ranch, sourdough	1 oz	130	2	19	250	0	5.0	0
(Ultra Slim Fast) twist	1 oz	100	2	21	460	3	1.0	0
PRICKLY PEAR								
raw, sliced	1 cup	61	1	14	7	5	0.8	0
raw, whole, trimmed	1 medium	42	1	10	5	4	0.5	0
PROTEIN BAR. See under SPORTS AND DIET/NUTRITION BARS.								
PRUNE								
Canned								
in heavy syrup, w/liquid	1 cup	246	2	65	7	9	0.5	0
in heavy syrup, w/liquid	5 medium	90	1	24	3	3	0.2	0
Dried								
low-moisture, stewed	1 cup	316	3	83	6	na	0.7	0
low-moisture, uncooked	1 cup	447	5	118	7	na	1.0	0
pitted, stewed	1 cup	265	3	70	5	16	0.6	0
pitted, uncooked	1 cup	406	4	107	7	12	0.9	0
uncooked	1 medium	20	0	5	0	1	0.0	0
PRUNE JUICE								
Canned or bottled								
	1 cup	182	2	45	10	3	0.1	0
	1 fl oz	23	0	6	1	0	0.0	0
(Del Monte) unsweetened	6 fl oz	120	1	33	10	0	0.0	0
(J. Hungerford) 100% juice	9.03 fl oz	178	2	44	10	3	0.0	0
(Knudsen) organic	8 fl oz	170	1	42	0	0	0.0	0
(Lucky Leaf)	6 fl oz	150	0	36	0	0	0.0	0
(Mott's)								
	6 fl oz	130	1	32	8	0	0.0	0
country style	6 fl oz	130	1	32	7	0	0.0	0
(Pathmark)								
'All Natural'	6 fl oz	120	1	30	10	0	0.0	0
w/prune pulp, 'Homestyle'	6 fl oz	130	1	32	10	0	0.0	0
(S&W) unsweetened	6 fl oz	120	1	31	20	0	0.0	0
(SunSweet)	6 fl oz	130	1	33	20	0	0.0	0
PSYLLIUM FIBER, smooth texture (Metamucil)	1 heaping tsp	20	0	5	na	3	0.0	na
PUDDING. See also PUDDING MIX; PUDDING/PIE FILLING MIX.								
ALMOND								
(Imagine Foods) nondairy, low-fat, 'Dream Pudding'	4 oz	150	1	31	30	0	2.0	0
BANANA								
(Del Monte) 'Pudding Cup'	5 oz	180	3	30	285	0	5.0	0
(Hunt's) 'Snack Pack'	1/2 cup	158	2	25	163	0	5.8	0
(Imagine Foods) nondairy, 'Dream Pudding'	4 oz	120	1	30	5	0	0.0	0
(Lucky Leaf)	4 oz	150	2	24	110	0	5.0	0
(Musselman's)	4 oz	150	2	24	110	0	5.0	0
BUTTERSCOTCH								
(Crowley)	4.5 oz	150	3	27	210	0	3.0	10
(Del Monte) 'Pudding Cup'	5 oz	180	3	31	285	0	5.0	0
(Featherweight)	1/2 cup	100	0	21	160	0	1.0	0

Food Name	Serv. Size	Total Cal.	Prot. gms	Carbs gms	Sod. mgs	Fiber gms	Fat gms	Chol. mgs
(Hunt's) 'Snack Pack' .... 4 oz		153	2	24	211	0	5.7	1
(Imagine Foods) nondairy .... 1 cup		150	1	31	45	0	3.0	0
(Lucky Leaf) .... 4 oz		170	2	26	135	0	7.0	0
(Musselman's) .... 4 oz		170	2	26	135	0	7.0	0
(Rich's) frozen .... 3 oz		130	2	18	130	0	6.0	0
(Ultra Slim-Fast) 'Lite 'N Tasty' .... 4 oz		100	2	21	230	2	1.0	0
(White House) .... 3.5 oz		113	1	20	195	0	3.0	0
BUTTERSCOTCH-CHOCOLATE-VANILLA								
(Jell-O) swirl .... 4 oz		180	3	28	140	0	5.0	0
CARAMEL *(Hershey's)* caramello .... 4 oz		180	3	28	170	0	6.0	0
CAROB								
(Imagine Foods) nondairy, nonfat, 'Dream Pudding' .... 4 oz		130	1	31	30	0	0.0	0
CHOCOLATE								
(Crowley) .... 4.5 oz		190	4	29	100	0	3.0	10
(Del Monte)								
'Pudding Cup' .... 5 oz		190	4	31	280	0	6.0	0
'Pudding Snack Light' .... 4.25 oz		100	2	19	85	0	1.0	0
fudge, 'Pudding Cup' .... 5 oz		190	4	31	260	0	6.0	0
(Estee) .... 1/2 cup		70	5	12	85	0	1.0	2
(Featherweight) .... 1/2 cup		100	1	21	110	0	1.0	0
(Hershey's)								
.... 4 oz		180	3	29	260	0	5.0	0
fudge, 'Snack Pack' .... 4 oz		158	2	24	178	0	5.9	0
'Hershey's Special Dark' .... 4 oz		180	4	30	135	0	5.0	0
'Light' 'Snack Pack' .... 4 oz		100	3	20	120	0	2.0	0
milk chocolate variety, 'Snack Pack' .... 4 oz		166	2	26	166	0	5.9	1
nonfat, 'Snack Pack' .... 4 oz		96	2	21	212	0	0.4	0
'Snack Pack' .... 4 oz		161	2	25	178	0	5.9	0
(Imagine Foods) nondairy .... 1 cup		170	1	36	65	1	3.0	0
(Jell-O)								
.... 4 oz		170	3	28	130	0	6.0	0
fat free .... 1 serving		102	3	23	192	1	0.5	2
fudge .... 4 oz		170	3	28	130	0	6.0	0
fudge, 'Light Pudding Snacks' .... 4 oz		100	3	22	125	0	1.0	5
fudge, 'Pudding Snacks' .... 4 oz		170	3	28	130	0	6.0	0
fudge-milk chocolate swirl .... 4 oz		170	3	28	135	0	6.0	0
'Light Pudding Snacks' .... 4 oz		100	3	21	125	0	2.0	5
milk chocolate 'Pudding Snacks' .... 4 oz		170	4	29	135	0	6.0	0
nonfat .... 1 serving		100	3	23	190	1	0.0	0
nonfat, 'Free' .... 4 oz		100	3	24	200	0	0.0	0
(Lucky Leaf)								
.... 4 oz		180	2	27	100	0	7.0	0
fudge .... 4 oz		180	2	25	105	0	8.0	0
(Musselman's)								
.... 4 oz		180	2	27	100	0	7.0	0
fudge .... 4 oz		180	2	25	105	0	8.0	0
(Pathmark) 'No Frills' .... 5 oz		200	2	30	140	0	8.0	0
(Rich's) frozen .... 3 oz		140	2	18	135	0	7.0	0
(Swiss Miss)								
fudge .... 4 oz		175	3	28	207	0	5.6	1
fudge, 'Light' .... 4 oz		100	3	20	120	0	1.0	0
fudge, nonfat .... 1/2 cup		103	2	23	151	0	0.3	1
milk chocolate variety .... 4 oz		166	2	26	166	0	2.9	1
nonfat .... 1/2 cup		100	2	22	154	0	0.4	1
sundae .... 4 oz		220	2	36	140	0	7.0	5
(Ultra Slim-Fast) chocolate .... 4 oz		100	2	21	240	2	1.0	0
(White House) chocolate .... 3.5 oz		120	2	22	130	0	4.0	0

Food Name	Serv. Size	Total Cal.	Prot. gms	Carbs gms	Sod. mgs	Fiber gms	Fat gms	Chol. mgs
CHOCOLATE ALMOND (Hershey's) .... 4 oz		180	3	29	210	0	6.0	0
CHOCOLATE AND VANILLA								
(Hershey's)								
'Kisses' .... 4 oz		180	3	29	210	0	6.0	0
'Kisses-Free' .... 4 oz		100	2	22	180	0	0.0	0
(Jell-O)								
'Light Pudding Snacks' .... 4 oz		100	3	21	125	0	2.0	5
nonfat .... 1 serving		100	3	23	210	1	0.0	0
swirl .... 4 oz		170	3	28	135	0	6.0	0
swirl, 'Free' .... 4 oz		100	3	24	220	0	0.0	0
swirl, 'Pudding Snacks' .... 4 oz		180	3	28	140	0	6.0	0
swirl, variety pack .... 1 snack		100	3	23	190	0	0.0	0
(Swiss Miss)								
parfait, 'Light' .... 4 oz		100	2	20	110	0	1.0	0
nonfat .... 1/2 cup		104	2	23	171	0	0.3	1
chocolate-vanilla-chocolate swirl .... 4 oz		172	3	27	163	0	6.0	1
variety .... 4 oz		171	2	27	162	0	6.0	1
CHOCOLATE-CARAMEL								
(Hunt's) swirl, 'Snack Pack' .... 4 oz		165	3	25	178	0	5.9	1
(Jell-O) swirl, 'Pudding Snacks' .... 4 oz		170	3	28	130	0	6.0	0
CHOCOLATE MARSHMALLOW								
(Hunt's)								
'Snack Pack' .... 4 oz		155	2	23	124	0	5.9	0
s'mores, 'Snack Pack' .... 4 oz		154	1	25	129	0	5.6	1
CHOCOLATE MINT								
(Hershey's) 'York Peppermint Pattie' .... 4 oz		180	3	29	210	0	6.0	0
(Jell-O) swirl, 'Free' .... 4 oz		100	3	24	220	0	0.0	0
CHOCOLATE PEANUT BUTTER								
(Hunt's) chocolate peanut butter swirl, 'Snack Pack' .... 4 oz		169	2	26	173	0	6.3	1
CHOCOLATE RASPBERRY (Healthy Choice) .... 1 cup		110	2	22	125	0	2.0	0
COCONUT								
(Imagine Foods) nondairy, low-fat, 'Dream Pudding' .... 4 oz		150	1	32	10	0	2.0	0
LEMON								
(Imagine Foods) nondairy .... 1 cup		150	1	33	50	1	3.0	0
(Hunt's) 'Snack Pack' .... 4 oz		138	0	28	85	0	2.8	0
(White House) .... 3.5 oz		152	0	37	65	0	1.0	0
RICE								
(Crowley) .... 4.5 oz		125	4	22	80	0	2.0	10
(Lucky Leaf) .... 4 oz		120	3	20	95	0	3.0	0
(Musselman's) .... 4 oz		120	3	20	95	0	3.0	0
(White House) .... 3.5 oz		111	1	20	135	0	3.0	0
TAPIOCA								
(Crowley) .... 4.5 oz		135	4	27	70	0	1.0	5
(Del Monte) 'Pudding Cup' .... 5 oz		180	3	30	250	0	4.0	0
(Healthy Choice) French creme .... 1 cup		110	1	21	125	0	2.0	0
(Hunt's)								
nonfat, 'Snack Pack' .... 1/2 cup		95	2	21	185	0	0.3	0
'Snack Pack' .... 4 oz		151	2	23	134	0	5.7	1
'Snack Pack Light' .... 4 oz		100	2	18	105	0	2.0	0
(Jell-O) .... 4 oz		170	3	27	140	0	4.0	0
(Lucky Leaf) .... 4 oz		140	1	20	95	0	6.0	0
(Musselman's) .... 4 oz		140	1	20	95	0	6.0	0
(Swiss Miss)								
'Light' .... 4 oz		100	2	18	105	0	2.0	0
nonfat .... 1/2 cup		99	2	22	151	0	0.3	1
(White House) .... 3.5 oz		131	1	19	105	0	6.0	0

Food Name	Serv. Size	Total Cal.	Prot. gms	Carbs gms	Sod. mgs	Fiber gms	Fat gms	Chol. mgs
VANILLA								
(Crowley)	4.5 oz	140	3	26	130	0	3.0	10
(Del Monte)								
'Pudding Cup'	5 oz	180	3	32	285	0	5.0	0
'Pudding Snack Light'	4.25 oz	100	1	19	200	0	1.0	0
(Estee)	1/2 cup	70	4	12	65	0	1.0	2
(Featherweight)	1/2 cup	100	0	20	150	0	2.0	0
(Healthy Choice) French	1 cup	110	2	20	125	0	2.0	0
(Hunt's)								
'Snack Pack'	4 oz	158	2	25	141	0	5.7	0
'Snack Pack Light'	4 oz	93	2	21	167	0	0.4	1
(Jell-O)								
	4 oz	180	3	28	140	0	7.0	0
fat free	1 serving	104	2	23	241	0	0.2	2
'Free'	4 oz	100	3	23	250	0	0.0	0
'Light Pudding Snacks'	4 oz	100	3	20	130	0	2.0	5
pudding snack	1 serving	100	2	23	240	0	0.0	0
(Lucky Leaf)	4 oz	170	2	25	135	0	7.0	0
(Musselman's)	4 oz	170	2	25	135	0	7.0	0
(Pathmark) 'No Frills'	5 oz	200	2	28	150	0	8.0	0
(Rich's) frozen	3 oz	130	2	18	160	0	6.0	0
(Swiss Miss)								
'Light'	4 oz	100	2	18	110	0	2.0	0
nonfat	1/2 cup	99	2	22	162	0	0.4	1
sundae	4 oz	175	2	27	174	0	6.8	1
(Ultra Slim-Fast) 'Lite 'N Tasty'	4 oz	100	2	21	230	2	1.0	0
(White House)	3.5 oz	111	1	20	135	0	3.0	0
PUDDING BAR, FROZEN								
(Jell-O)								
chocolate fudge, 'Pudding Pops'	1 bar	80	2	13	90	0	2.0	0
chocolate-peanut butter swirl 'Pudding Pops'	1 bar	80	2	12	75	0	3.0	0
chocolate-vanilla swirl, 'Pudding Pops'	1 bar	80	2	13	70	0	2.0	0
double chocolate swirl, 'Pudding Pops'	1 bar	80	2	13	90	0	2.0	0
milk chocolate, 'Pudding Pops'	1 bar	80	2	13	90	0	2.0	0
PUDDING MIX. See also PUDDING/PIE FILLING MIX.								
BANANA								
(Jell-O)								
cream, instant, prepared w/whole milk	1/2 cup	160	4	28	410	0	4.0	15
cream, microwave, prepared w/whole milk	1/2 cup	150	4	25	220	0	4.0	15
instant, sugar-free, prepared w/2% milk	1/2 cup	80	4	11	390	0	2.0	10
(Royal)								
cream, instant, prepared w/whole milk	1/2 cup	180	4	29	390	0	5.0	0
cream, prepared w/whole milk	1/2 cup	160	4	27	210	0	4.0	0
BUTTER ALMOND								
(Royal) toasted, instant, prepared w/whole milk	1/2 cup	170	4	30	350	0	4.0	0
BUTTER PECAN *(Jell-O)* instant, prepared w/whole milk	1/2 cup	170	4	28	410	0	5.0	15
BUTTERSCOTCH								
(D-Zerta) low-calorie, prepared w/nonfat milk	1/2 cup	70	4	12	65	0	0.0	0
(Featherweight)								
instant, prepared w/whole milk	1/2 cup	100	4	19	190	0	0.0	5
prepared as directed	1/2 cup	12	0	3	6	0	0.0	0
(Jell-O)								
cook and serve	1 serving	80	0	20	5	0	0.0	0
instant, prepared w/whole milk	1/2 cup	160	4	28	450	0	4.0	15
instant, sugar-free, prepared w/2% milk	1/2 cup	90	4	12	390	0	2.0	10
microwave, prepared w/whole milk	1/2 cup	170	4	28	180	0	4.0	15
prepared, w/whole milk	1/2 cup	170	4	30	190	0	4.0	15

Food Name	Serv. Size	Total Cal.	Prot. gms	Carbs gms	Sod. mgs	Fiber gms	Fat gms	Chol. mgs
(Royal)								
instant, prepared w/whole milk	1/2 cup	180	4	29	390	0	5.0	0
instant, sugar-free, prepared w/2% milk	1/2 cup	100	4	16	470	0	2.0	0
prepared, w/whole milk	1/2 cup	160	4	27	210	0	4.0	0
CHOCOLATE								
(D-Zerta) lower calorie	1 serving	20	0	5	0	1	0.0	0
(Featherweight)								
instant, prepared	1/2 cup	110	5	22	190	0	0.0	5
prepared	1/2 cup	12	0	3	0	0	0.0	15
(Jell-O)								
cook and serve, sugar-free, mix only	1/2 cup	30	1	7	100	0	0.0	0
cook and serve, sugar-free, prepared w/nonfat milk	1/2 cup	70	5	13	160	0	3.0	0
cook and serve, sugar-free, prepared w/2% milk	1/2 cup	90	5	13	160	0	3.0	10
fudge, instant, sugar-free, prepared w/2% milk	1/2 cup	100	5	14	330	0	3.0	10
fudge, instant, sugar-free, prepared w/whole milk	1/2 cup	180	5	31	440	0	5.0	15
fudge, prepared w/whole milk	1/2 cup	160	5	28	170	0	4.0	15
instant, prepared w/whole milk	1/2 cup	180	4	31	480	0	4.0	15
instant, sugar-free, prepared w/2% milk	1/2 cup	90	4	13	380	0	3.0	10
microwave, prepared w/whole milk	1/2 cup	170	5	28	190	0	5.0	15
milk chocolate, instant, prepared w/whole milk	1/2 cup	180	5	31	470	0	5.0	15
milk chocolate, microwave, prepared w/whole milk	1/2 cup	160	4	27	190	0	5.0	15
milk chocolate, prepared w/whole milk	1/2 cup	160	4	28	170	0	4.0	15
prepared w/whole milk	1/2 cup	160	5	28	170	0	4.0	15
(Royal)								
chocolate chip, prepared w/whole milk	1/2 cup	190	4	35	390	0	4.0	0
dark and sweet, prepared w/whole milk	1/2 cup	190	4	35	390	0	4.0	0
instant, prepared w/whole milk	1/2 cup	190	4	35	390	0	4.0	0
instant, sugar-free, prepared w/2% milk	1/2 cup	110	5	17	480	0	3.0	0
prepared w/whole milk	1/2 cup	180	5	33	150	0	4.0	0
(Weight Watchers) instant, prepared w/nonfat milk	1/2 cup	90	6	18	420	0	1.0	0
CHOCOLATE MINT								
(Royal) instant, prepared w/whole milk	1/2 cup	190	4	35	390	0	4.0	0
COCONUT								
(Jell-O) cream, instant, prepared w/whole milk	1/2 cup	180	4	27	320	0	6.0	15
(Royal) toasted, instant, prepared w/whole milk	1/2 cup	170	4	30	350	0	4.0	0
CUSTARD								
(Jell-O)								
egg, golden, 'Americana' prepared w/whole milk	1/2 cup	160	5	23	200	0	5.0	80
(Royal) prepared w/whole milk	1/2 cup	150	4	22	115	0	5.0	0
FLAN								
(Jell-O) prepared w/whole milk	1/2 cup	150	4	26	65	0	4.0	15
(Royal) w/caramel sauce, prepared w/whole milk	1/2 cup	150	4	22	115	0	5.0	0
KEY LIME *(Royal)* prepared w/whole milk	1/2 cup	160	1	30	120	0	3.0	0
LEMON								
(Featherweight) custard, prepared w/whole milk	1/2 cup	40	1	8	40	0	0.0	0
(French's) prepared	1/2 cup	110	1	22	110	0	1.0	0
(Jell-O) instant, prepared w/whole milk	1/2 cup	170	4	29	360	0	4.0	15
(Royal)								
instant, prepared w/whole milk	1/2 cup	180	1	29	350	0	5.0	0
lemon, prepared w/whole milk	1/2 cup	160	1	30	120	0	3.0	0
PISTACHIO								
(Jell-O)								
instant, prepared w/whole milk	1/2 cup	170	4	28	410	0	5.0	15
instant, sugar-free, prepared w/2% milk	1/2 cup	90	4	12	390	0	3.0	10
(Royal) instant, prepared w/whole milk	1/2 cup	170	4	30	350	0	4.0	0
RASPBERRY								
(Salada) and pie glaze, prepared w/whole milk	1/2 cup	130	0	32	5	0	0.0	0

Food Name	Serv. Size	Total Cal.	Prot. gms	Carbs gms	Sod. mgs	Fiber gms	Fat gms	Chol. mgs
RICE *(Jell-O)* rice 'Americana' prepared w/whole milk	1/2 cup	170	5	30	160	0	4.0	15
STRAWBERRY								
(Salada) and pie glaze, prepared w/whole milk	1/2 cup	130	0	32	5	0	0.0	0
TAPIOCA								
(Jell-O) vanilla, 'Americana' prepared w/whole milk	1/2 cup	160	4	27	170	0	4.0	15
(Minute) mix only	1 1/2 tsp	20	0	5	0	0	0.0	0
(Royal) vanilla, prepared w/whole milk	1/2 cup	160	4	27	150	0	4.0	0
VANILLA								
(D-Zerta) low-calorie, prepared w/nonfat milk	1/2 cup	70	4	12	65	0	0.0	0
(Featherweight)								
instant, prepared	1/2 cup	100	4	19	190	0	0.0	5
custard, prepared w/whole milk	1/2 cup	40	1	8	40	0	0.0	0
(Jell-O)								
cook and serve, sugar-free, prepared w/skim milk	1/2 cup	60	4	11	200	0	2.0	0
cook and serve, sugar-free, prepared w/2% milk	1/2 cup	80	4	11	200	0	2.0	10
cook and serve, sugar-free, mix only	1/2 cup	20	0	5	140	0	0.0	0
French, instant, prepared w/whole milk	1/2 cup	160	4	28	400	0	4.0	15
instant, prepared w/whole milk	1/2 cup	170	4	29	410	0	4.0	15
instant, sugar-free, prepared w/2% milk	1/2 cup	90	4	12	390	0	2.0	10
microwave, prepared w/whole milk	1/2 cup	160	4	26	180	0	4.0	15
prepared w/whole milk	1/2 cup	160	4	26	200	0	4.0	15
(Royal)								
instant, prepared w/whole milk	1/2 cup	180	4	29	390	0	5.0	0
instant, sugar-free, prepared w/2% milk	1/2 cup	100	4	16	470	0	2.0	0
prepared w/whole milk	1/2 cup	160	4	27	210	0	4.0	0
PUDDING/PIE FILLING MIX. See also PUDDING MIX.								
BANANA								
(Jell-O)								
cream, instant, prepared w/whole milk	1/2 cup	160	4	28	410	0	4.0	15
cream, mix only	1 pkg	50	0	14	120	0	0.0	0
cream, prepared w/whole milk	1/6 pkg	100	3	17	160	0	3.0	10
instant, sugar-free, mix only	1 pkg	25	0	6	330	0	0.0	0
instant, sugar-free, prepared w/2% milk	1/2 cup	80	4	11	390	0	2.0	10
microwave, cream, mix only	1 pkg	80	0	19	160	0	0.0	0
microwave, cream, prepared w/whole milk	1/2 cup	150	4	25	220	0	4.0	15
(Royal)								
cream, instant, mix only	1 serving	90	0	22	390	0	0.0	0
cream, mix only	1 serving	80	0	20	110	0	0.0	0
BUTTER PECAN *(Jell-O)* instant, prepared w/whole milk	1/2 cup	170	4	28	410	0	5.0	15
BUTTERSCOTCH								
(D-Zerta)								
lower calorie, mix only	1 pkg	25	0	6	0	0	0.0	0
lower calorie, prepared	1/2 cup	70	4	12	65	0	0.0	0
(Jell-O)								
instant, sugar-free, mix only	1 pkg	25	0	6	330	0	0.0	0
instant, sugar-free, prepared w/2% milk	1/2 cup	90	4	12	390	0	2.0	10
instant, prepared w/whole milk	1/2 cup	160	4	28	450	0	4.0	15
microwave, mix only	1 pkg	90	0	23	120	0	0.0	0
microwave, prepared w/whole milk	1/2 cup	170	4	28	180	0	4.0	15
regular, mix only	1 pkg	90	0	24	130	0	0.0	0
regular, prepared w/whole milk	1/2 cup	170	4	30	190	0	4.0	15
(My-T-Fine) prepared	1/2 cup	90	0	22	190	0	0.0	0
(Royal)								
instant, mix only	1 serving	90	0	22	400	0	0.0	0
prepared	1/2 cup	90	0	23	180	0	0.0	0
CHERRY VANILLA *(Royal)* instant, mix only	1 serving	90	0	23	300	0	0.0	0

Food Name	Serv. Size	Total Cal.	Prot. gms	Carbs gms	Sod. mgs	Fiber gms	Fat gms	Chol. mgs
CHOCOLATE								
(D-Zerta)								
lower calorie, mix only	1 pkg	20	0	5	0	0	0.0	0
lower calorie, prepared	1/2 cup	60	5	11	70	0	0.0	0
(Jell-O)								
cook and serve, nonfat, lower calorie	1 serving	90	0	23	107	0	0.3	0
cook and serve, sugar-free, prepared	1 serving	31	1	7	109	1	0.3	0
fat-free, sugar-free, prepared	1 serving	34	1	8	318	1	0.3	0
fudge, instant, mix only	1 pkg	100	1	25	380	0	1.0	0
fudge, instant, prepared w/whole milk	1/2 cup	180	5	31	440	0	5.0	15
fudge, instant, sugar-free, mix only	1 pkg	35	1	8	270	0	1.0	0
fudge, mix only	1 pkg	90	1	22	110	0	0.0	0
instant, mix only	1 pkg	100	0	25	420	0	0.0	0
instant, mix only	1 serving	99	0	25	414	1	0.3	0
instant, prepared w/whole milk	1/2 cup	180	4	31	480	0	4.0	15
instant, sugar-free, mix only	1 pkg	30	0	7	320	0	0.0	0
instant, sugar-free, prepared w/2% milk	1/2 cup	100	5	14	330	0	3.0	10
instant, sugar-free, prepared w/2% milk	1/2 cup	90	4	13	380	0	3.0	10
microwave, mix only	1 pkg	90	1	22	130	0	1.0	0
microwave, prepared w/whole milk	1/2 cup	170	5	28	190	0	5.0	15
milk chocolate, instant, mix only	1 pkg	100	1	25	410	0	1.0	0
milk chocolate, instant, prepared w/whole milk	1/2 cup	180	5	31	470	0	5.0	15
milk chocolate, microwave, mix only	1 pkg	90	0	21	130	0	1.0	0
milk chocolate, microwave, prepared w/whole milk	1/2 cup	160	4	27	190	0	5.0	15
milk chocolate, mix only	1 pkg	90	0	22	110	0	0.0	0
milk chocolate, prepared w/whole milk	1/2 cup	160	4	28	170	0	4.0	15
sugar-free, mix only,	1 pkg	30	1	7	100	0	0.0	0
prepared w/whole milk	1/2 cup	160	5	28	170	0	4.0	15
sugar-free, prepared w/2% milk	1/2 cup	90	5	13	160	0	3.0	10
(My-T-Fine)								
fudge, prepared	1/2 cup	100	1	24	140	1	0.0	0
prepared	1/2 cup	100	1	23	135	0	0.0	0
(Royal)								
chocolate chip, instant, mix only	1 serving	110	1	26	390	0	1.0	0
dark and sweet, prepared	1/2 cup	90	1	22	95	1	0.0	0
instant, mix only	1 serving	110	1	27	450	0	0.0	0
instant, sugar-free, prepared	1/2 cup	50	0	11	420	0	0.0	0
prepared	1/2 cup	90	1	22	90	0	0.0	0
CHOCOLATE ALMOND								
(My-T-Fine) prepared	1/2 cup	100	1	23	135	0	1.0	0
(Royal) instant, prepared	1/2 cup	120	0	26	440	0	1.0	0
CHOCOLATE PEANUT BUTTER CHIP								
(Royal) instant, mix only	1 serving	110	1	26	480	0	1.0	0
COCONUT								
(Jell-O)								
cream, mix only	1 pkg	60	0	12	100	0	2.0	0
cream, prepared w/whole milk	1/6 pkg	110	3	16	140	0	4.0	10
cream, instant, prepared w/whole milk	1/2 cup	180	4	27	320	0	6.0	15
(Royal) toasted, instant	1/2 cup	100	0	20	450	0	2.0	0
CUSTARD *(Royal)*	1/2 cup	60	0	16	75	0	0.0	0
FLAN								
(Jell-O)								
flan, mix only	1 pkg	80	0	20	5	0	0.0	0
flan, prepared w/whole milk	1/2 cup	150	4	26	65	0	4.0	15
(Royal) caramel, prepared	1/2 cup	60	0	15	55	0	0.0	0
KEY LIME *(Royal)* mix only	1 serving	50	0	13	120	0	0.0	0

Food Name	Serv. Size	Total Cal.	Prot. gms	Carbs gms	Sod. mgs	Fiber gms	Fat gms	Chol. mgs
LEMON								
(Jell-O)								
instant, mix only	1 pkg	90	0	23	300	0	0.0	0
instant, prepared w/whole milk	1/2 cup	170	4	29	360	0	4.0	15
mix only	1 pkg	50	0	13	70	0	0.0	0
prepared	1/6 pkg	170	2	38	95	0	2.0	90
(My-T-Fine) mix only	1 serving	90	0	22	170	0	0.0	0
(Royal)								
instant, mix only	1 serving	90	0	23	320	0	0.0	0
meringue, 'No-Bake'	1/8 pie	210	3	38	170	0	5.0	0
mix only	1 serving	50	0	13	120	0	0.0	0
PISTACHIO								
(Jell-O)								
instant, mix only	1 pkg	100	0	22	350	0	1.0	0
instant, prepared w/whole milk	1/2 cup	170	4	28	410	0	5.0	15
instant, sugar-free, mix only	1 pkg	30	0	6	330	0	1.0	0
instant, sugar-free, prepared w/2% milk	1/2 cup	90	4	12	390	0	3.0	10
(Royal) instant, mix only	1 serving	90	0	22	360	0	1.0	0
STRAWBERRY *(Royal)* instant, mix only	1 serving	100	0	24	330	0	0.0	0
TAPIOCA *(My-T-Fine)* mix only	1 serving	80	0	19	160	0	0.0	0
VANILLA								
(D-Zerta)								
lower calorie, mix only	1 pkg	25	0	6	0	0	0.0	0
lower calorie, prepared	1/2 cup	70	4	12	65	0	0.0	0
(Jell-O)								
cook and serve, nonfat, lower calorie	1 serving	86	0	22	138	0	0.0	0
cook and serve, sugar-free, prepared	1 serving	21	0	5	113	0	0.0	0
fat-free, sugar-free, prepared	1 serving	26	0	6	332	0	0.1	0
French, instant, mix only	1 pkg	90	0	23	350	0	0.0	0
French, instant, prepared w/whole milk	1/2 cup	160	4	28	400	0	4.0	15
French, mix only	1 pkg	90	0	24	125	0	0.0	0
French, prepared w/whole milk	1/2 cup	170	4	30	190	0	4.0	15
instant, mix only	1 pkg	94	0	23	353	0	0.2	0
instant, prepared w/whole milk	1/2 cup	170	4	29	410	0	4.0	15
instant, sugar-free, mix only	1 pkg	25	0	6	330	0	0.0	0
instant, sugar-free, prepared w/2% milk	1/2 cup	90	4	12	390	0	2.0	10
microwave, mix only	1 pkg	80	0	21	120	0	0.0	0
microwave, prepared w/whole milk	1/2 cup	160	4	26	180	0	4.0	15
mix only	1 pkg	80	0	21	140	0	0.0	0
prepared w/whole milk	1/2 cup	160	4	26	200	0	4.0	15
sugar-free, mix only	1 pkg	20	0	5	140	0	0.0	0
sugar-free, prepared w/2% milk	1/2 cup	80	4	11	200	0	2.0	10
(My-T-Fine)								
mix only	1 serving	80	0	20	160	0	0.0	0
prepared	1/2 cup	90	0	22	120	0	0.0	0
(Nutra/Balance) low-lactose	1 serving	242	8	36	94	0	7.5	3
(Royal)								
chocolate chip, instant, mix only	1 serving	90	0	22	350	0	1.0	0
(Royal) instant, mix only	1 serving	90	0	23	325	0	0.0	0
PUERTO RICAN CHERRY. See ACEROLA.								
PUFF PASTRY								
ready-to-bake, frozen, baked	1 oz	158	2	13	72	0	10.9	0
ready-to-bake, frozen, unprepared	1 oz	156	2	13	71	0	10.8	0
(Pepperidge Farm)								
sheet, frozen	1/4 sheet	260	4	22	290	0	17.0	0
shell, mini, frozen	1 shell	50	1	4	40	0	4.0	0
shell, patty, frozen	1 shell	210	3	16	180	0	15.0	0

Food Name	Serv. Size	Total Cal.	Prot. gms	Carbs gms	Sod. mgs	Fiber gms	Fat gms	Chol. mgs
PUMMELO, RAW. See POMELO.								
PUMPKIN								
Fresh								
boiled, drained, mashed	1 cup	49	2	12	2	3	0.2	0
raw, cubed, 1-inch cubes	1 cup	30	1	8	1	1	0.1	0
Canned								
	1 cup	83	3	20	590	7	0.7	0
(Del Monte)	1/2 cup	35	1	9	10	0	0.0	0
solid pack *(Libby's)*	1/2 cup	40	2	9	5	5	0.5	0
(Stokely)	1/2 cup	40	2	10	15	0	0.0	0
PUMPKIN FLOWER								
boiled, drained	1 cup	20	1	4	8	1	0.1	0
raw	1 cup	5	0	1	2	na	0.0	0
raw, whole	1 medium	<1	0	0	0	na	0.0	0
PUMPKIN LEAF								
boiled, drained	1 cup	15	2	2	6	2	0.2	0
raw	1 cup	7	1	1	4	na	0.2	0
PUMPKIN PIE SPICE. See under SEASONING MIX.								
PUMPKIN SEED								
dried, kernels	1 cup	747	34	25	25	5	63.3	0
dried, kernels, hulled, approx 142 seeds	1 oz	153	7	5	5	1	13.0	0
dry roasted, w/tamari, garlic, and cayenne *(Eden Foods)*	1 oz	170	11	5	80	3	11.0	0
roasted, kernels	1 cup	1185	75	30	41	9	95.6	0
roasted, kernels	1 oz	148	9	4	5	1	11.9	0
roasted, salted *(David's)*	1 pkg	320	15	6	17	2	25.0	0
roasted, whole	1 cup	285	12	34	12	na	12.4	0
roasted, whole, approx 85 seeds	1 oz	126	5	15	5	na	5.5	0
PUMPKINFISH. See SUNFISH.								
PUNCH. See under FRUIT DRINK; FRUIT DRINK MIX; FRUIT JUICE DRINK.								
PURPLE HULLED PEAS. See PEAS, PURPLE HULLED.								
PURSLANE/pussley								
boiled, drained	1 cup	21	2	4	51	na	0.2	0
boiled, drained	1/2 cup	10	0.9	2.1	26	>.5 c	0.1	0
raw	1 cup	7	0.6	1.5	19	>.3 c	0.0	0
raw	1/2 cup	4	0.3	0.7	10	>.2 c	<.1	0
PUSSLEY. See PURSLANE.								

Q

Food Name	Serv. Size	Total Cal.	Prot. gms	Carbs gms	Sod. mgs	Fiber gms	Fat gms	Chol. mgs
QUAIL/bobwhite								
breast, meat only, raw	1 oz	35	6.4	0.0	16	0	0.8	(mq)
giblets, raw	3.5 oz	176	21.8	6.7	70	0	6.2	350
meat and skin, raw	1 oz	54	5.6	0.0	15	0	3.4	(mq)
meat only, raw	1 oz	34	6.0	0.0	29	0	0.9	24
QUEEN CRAB. See under CRAB.								
QUICHE								
(Nancy's)								
broccoli-cheddar, frozen, microwave, 'French Baked'	1 quiche	490	17	33	750	2	33.0	165
Monterey Jack, w/Swiss and bacon, 'Classic French'	1 quiche	520	21	30	670	1	37.0	210
(Stilwell)								
bacon and onion	1/6 carton	210	12	4	480	1	16.0	185
broccoli and cheese	1/6 carton	180	10	4	270	1	14.0	180
ham	1/6 carton	190	12	4	330	0	15.0	200
spinach and onion	1/6 carton	190	10	7	280	1	13.0	200

Food Name	Serv. Size	Total Cal.	Prot. gms	Carbs gms	Sod. mgs	Fiber gms	Fat gms	Chol. mgs
three cheese	1/6 carton	200	13	4	310	1	16.0	190
QUINCE								
raw, trimmed	1 medium	52	0.4	14.1	4	1.8	0.1	0
raw, trimmed	1 oz	16	0.1	4.3	1	>.5 c	<.1	0
raw, untrimmed	1 lb	158	1.1	42.3	11	>4.7 c	0.3	0
QUINOA								
flakes, steam-rolled, uncooked *(Ancient Harvest)*	1/3 cup	105	3	23	5	3	1.0	0
flakes, steam-rolled, uncooked *(Quinoa)*	1/3 cup	105	3	23	5	3	1.0	0
organic, uncooked *(Arrowhead Mills)*	1/4 cup	140	5	25	0	4	2.0	0
uncooked *(Eden Foods)*	2 oz	200	8	38	30	4	4.0	0
uncooked	1 cup	636	22	117	36	10	9.9	0
whole grain, uncooked *(Ancient Harvest)*	1/4 cup	159	5	28	8	6	2.0	0
whole grain, uncooked *(Quinoa)*	1/4 cup	159	5	28	8	6	2.0	0
QUINOA FLOUR. See under FLOUR.								
QUINOA SEED								
(Arrowhead Mills)	2 oz	200	9	35	3	5	3.0	0
wild, uncooked *(Eden Foods)*	1/4 cup	170	7	31	0	3	2.5	0

R

Food Name	Serv. Size	Total Cal.	Prot. gms	Carbs gms	Sod. mgs	Fiber gms	Fat gms	Chol. mgs
RABBIT								
domesticated, composite cuts, raw	1 oz	39	6	0	12	0	1.6	16
domesticated, composite cuts, roasted	3 oz	167	25	0	40	0	6.8	70
domesticated, composite cuts, stewed	3 oz	175	26	0	31	0	7.1	73
wild, raw	1 oz	32	6	0	14	0	0.7	23
wild, stewed	3 oz	147	28	0	38	0	3.0	105
RACCOON, roasted	3 oz	217	25	0	67	0	12.3	82
RADICCHIO								
fresh, raw, leaf	1 med leaf	2	0	0	2	0	0.0	0
fresh, raw, shredded	1 cup	9	1	2	9	0	0.1	0
RADISH								
fresh, raw, sliced	1 cup	23	1	4	28	2	0.6	0
fresh, raw, sliced	1/2 cup	12	0	2	14	1	0.3	0
fresh, raw, whole *(Dole)*	7 med radishes	20	0	3	35	0	0.0	0
fresh, raw, whole, large, 1–1.25-inch diam	1 radish	2	0	0	2	0	0.0	0
fresh, raw, whole, medium, 3/4–1-inch diam	1 radish	1	0	0	1	0	0.0	0
fresh, raw, whole, small, under 3/4-inch diam	1 radish	<1	0	0	0	0	0.0	0
BLACK/winter radish								
raw, trimmed	1 lb	77	4.5	16.3	82	(mq)	0.5	0
raw, trimmed	1 oz	5	0.3	1.0	5	(mq)	<.1	0
ORIENTAL. See DAIKON.								
RED								
fresh, raw, sliced	1 cup	23	1	4	28	2	0.6	0
fresh, raw, sliced	1/2 cup	12	0	2	14	1	0.3	0
fresh, raw, whole *(Dole)*	7 med radishes	20	0	3	35	0	0.0	0
fresh, raw, whole, large, 1–1.25-inch diam	1 radish	2	0	0	2	0	0.0	0
fresh, raw, whole, medium, 3/4–1-inch diam	1 radish	1	0	0	1	0	0.0	0
fresh, raw, whole, small, under 3/4-inch diam	1 radish	<1	0	0	0	0	0.0	0
WHITE ICICLE								
raw, sliced	1/2 cup	7	0.6	1.3	8	>.4 c	0.1	0
raw, trimmed	1 oz	4	0.3	0.7	5	>.2 c	<.1	0
raw, untrimmed	1 lb	41	3.2	7.7	47	>2.1 c	0.3	0
raw, whole, approx 7-inch long	1 medium	2	0.2	0.5	3	>.1 c	0.0	0
RADISH JUICE, bottled *(Biotta)*	6 fl oz	39	2	8	101	0	0.1	0

Food Name	Serv. Size	Total Cal.	Prot. gms	Carbs gms	Sod. mgs	Fiber gms	Fat gms	Chol. mgs
RADISH LEAVES, trimmed	1 oz	15	0.8	2.8	(mq)	>.4 c	0.1	0
RADISH SEED								
sprouted	1 lb	186	17.3	13.9	28	(mq)	11.5	0
sprouted	1 oz	12	1.1	0.9	2	(mq)	0.7	0
sprouted, raw	1 cup	16	1	1	2	na	1.0	0
sprouted, raw	1/2 cup	8	0.7	0.7	1	>.4 c	0.5	0
RAG GOURD. See GOURD, DISHCLOTH.								
RAINBOW SMELT. See SMELT, RAINBOW.								
RAISIN								
Golden								
seedless	1 cup packed	498	6	131	20	7	0.8	0
seedless	1 cup	438	5	115	17	6	0.7	0
seedless *(S&W)*	1/4 cup	130	1	31	10	2	0.0	0
seedless *(Sun-Maid)*	1/4 cup	130	1	31	10	3	0.0	0
Dark								
seeded	1 cup packed	488	4	129	46	11	0.9	0
seeded	1 cup	429	4	114	41	10	0.8	0
seedless	1 cup packed	495	5	131	20	7	0.8	0
seedless	1 cup	435	5	115	17	6	0.7	0
seedless	50 medium	78	1	21	3	1	0.1	0
seedless *(S&W)*	1/4 cup	130	1	31	10	2	0.0	0
seedless, for baking *(Sun-Maid)*	1/4 cup	124	1	30	7	2	0.0	0
seedless, mini-box	0.5 oz	42	0	11	2	1	0.1	0
seedless, natural *(Sun-Maid)*	1/4 cup	130	1	31	10	3	0.0	0
RAMBUTAN								
canned, in syrup	1 cup	175	1	45	24	2	0.4	0
canned, in syrup	1 medium	7	0	2	1	0	0.0	0
canned, in syrup, drained	1 cup	123	1	31	17	1	0.3	0
RASPBERRY/bramble								
Canned, in heavy syrup, w/liquid	1 cup	233	2	60	8	8	0.3	0
Fresh								
raw	1 pint	153	3	36	0	21	1.7	0
raw	1 cup	60	1	14	0	8	0.7	0
raw	10 medium	9	0	2	0	1	0.1	0
Frozen								
(Flav-R-Pac)	1 cup	50	1	11	0	2	0.0	0
in syrup *(Flav-R-Pac)*	2/3 cup	230	1	57	40	4	0.0	0
red, sweetened	10-oz pkg	293	2	74	3	12	0.5	0
red, sweetened, unthawed	1 cup	258	2	65	3	11	0.4	0
RASPBERRY JUICE *(Smucker's)* red, 'Naturally 100%'	8 fl oz	120	0	30	10	0	0.0	0
RASPBERRY SYRUP. See under SYRUP.								
RASPBERRY TOPPING								
(Flav-R-Pac)	2 tbsp	45	0	11	0	2	0.0	0
(Knudsen) pourable	1 oz	75	0	18	0	0	1.0	0
(Smucker's) nonfat, 'Light'	2 tbsp	55	0	14	0	0	0.0	0
RAVIOLI DISH/ENTRÉE								
(Amy's Kitchen)								
cheese, in sauce, organic, frozen	8-oz entrée	340	15	44	580	6	12.0	20
cheese, organic, frozen	1 cup	215	12	26	346	3	5.0	7
(Bernardi)								
beef, breaded	1 cup	270	11	43	660	2	6.0	25
beef, jumbo, round	1 cup	450	22	48	930	3	19.0	135
beef, square	1 cup	280	14	37	530	2	9.0	65
beef ravioletti, square	1 cup	330	13	47	540	2	10.0	30
cheese, jumbo	1 cup	380	26	47	400	2	9.0	210
cheese, round, jumbo	1 cup	410	21	48	570	2	15.0	50
cheese, square	1 cup	260	14	36	320	2	7.0	40

Food Name	Serv. Size	Total Cal.	Prot. gms	Carbs gms	Sod. mgs	Fiber gms	Fat gms	Chol. mgs
cheese ravioletti	1 cup	280	13	40	360	2	8.0	15
chicken, jumbo, round	1 cup	450	21	52	420	2	17.0	115
Espanol, breaded	1 cup	290	13	43	840	2	6.0	25
Florentine, round, jumbo	1 cup	370	21	53	440	3	10.0	60
pesto, round, jumbo	1 cup	480	21	57	510	4	19.0	110
seafood, round, jumbo	1 cup	440	18	57	790	3	15.0	120
vegetable, jumbo, round	1 cup	430	15	59	440	2	15.0	90
(Buitoni)								
cheese, frozen	4 oz	360	12	31	220	0	8.0	65
cheese, in sauce, canned	7.5 oz	190	7	27	790	0	6.0	5
meat, in sauce, canned	7.5 oz	180	7	28	890	0	4.0	5
(Celentano)								
cheese, mini	12 ravioli	270	13	42	150	2	6.0	30
cheese, round	6 raviolis	400	21	61	390	11	9.0	100
frozen	6.5 oz	380	21	50	510	0	11.0	0
frozen, 'Great Choice'	6 ravioli	360	12	69	700	1	4.0	35
mini, frozen	4 oz	250	13	39	210	0	5.0	0
(Chef Boyardee)								
beef, canned, microwave	7.5 oz	190	7	31	1160	2	4.0	11
beef, canned 'Sir Chomps'	7.5 oz	170	7	32	690	4	3.0	15
beef, in tomato and meat sauce, canned	1 pkg	400	15	64	2044	6	9.4	26
beef, in tomato and meat sauce, canned	1 cup	230	9	37	1150	4	5.0	20
beef, microwave cup, 'Main Meals'	10.5 oz	290	12	52	0	0	4.0	0
beef, mini, in tomato and meat sauce	1 pkg	404	15	69	2019	6	8.0	30
beef, mini, in tomato and beef sauce	1 cup	240	8	37	1180	3	6.0	20
beef, w/meat sauce, canned, 'Smurfs'	7.5 oz	230	9	38	1160	0	5.0	11
beef and cheese, in tomato sauce	1 cup	220	9	38	1110	4	3.0	15
cheese, canned 'Sir Chomps'	7.5 oz	170	6	38	740	6	1.0	5
cheese, in meat sauce, canned, microwave	7.5 oz	200	6	37	1010	0	3.0	10
cheese, in tomato sauce	1 cup	210	7	44	860	4	0.0	0
chicken, canned	7.5 oz	180	7	29	1100	0	4.0	13
chicken, mini, canned	7.5 oz	220	7	29	1090	0	8.0	0
(Contadina)								
beef, refrigerated, 'Fresh'	3 oz	270	13	30	250	0	11.0	75
beef and garlic	1 1/4 cup	350	17	39	350	3	14.0	110
cheese	1 cup	280	13	31	350	2	12.0	31
cheese, light	1 cup	240	13	35	340	2	5.0	60
chicken, refrigerated, 'Fresh'	3 oz	260	11	32	310	0	10.0	80
chicken and rosemary	1 1/4 cup	330	13	43	420	3	12.0	85
garden vegetable, light	1 1/4 cup	290	15	43	370	3	6.0	65
(DiGiorno)								
cheese, w/herb, Italian, refrigerated, cooked	1 cup	280	12	35	490	0	10.0	35
sausage, Italian, refrigerated, cooked	1 cup	270	13	34	520	0	9.0	40
(Estee) beef, canned	7.5 oz	230	8	25	100	0	11.0	10
(Finast) beef, in sauce, canned	7.5 oz	250	7	33	1165	0	10.0	0
(Franco-American) beef, in meat sauce	1 cup	280	11	38	1160	2	9.0	20
(Healthy Choice) cheese, Parmigiana	1 entrée	260	11	44	200	6	5.0	20
(Hormel) beef, in tomato sauce, micro cup	7.5 oz	247	8	28	951	0	11.0	21
(Kid Cuisine)								
cheese, mini, frozen	8.75 oz	250	6	52	730	0	2.0	20
cheese, mini, w/applesauce, corn, and brownie, frozen	1 meal	310	7	61	750	5	4.0	10
(Kid's Kitchen)								
mini, microwave cup	7.5 oz	230	10	34	870	0	6.0	15
(Lean Cuisine) cheese	1 entrée	270	11	40	580	5	7.0	45
(Libby's) beef, in sauce, microwave cup, 'Diner'	7.75 oz	240	13	35	890	2	5.0	15

Food Name	Serv. Size	Total Cal.	Prot. gms	Carbs gms	Sod. mgs	Fiber gms	Fat gms	Chol. mgs
(Lucca)								
beef	1 cup	190	9	28	370	4	5.0	45
chicken, w/savory herbs	1 cup	180	11	26	450	4	4.0	55
Italian sausage, w/herbs and seasonings	1 cup	200	9	29	520	4	6.0	55
(Lunch Express) cheese	1 entrée	360	15	43	700	7	14.0	60
(Marie Callender's)								
w/marinara sauce and 1 oz								
garlic bread, frozen	1 serving	370	14	47	520	4	14.0	35
(Nalley's) beef, canned	7.5 oz	180	8	30	1040	0	3.0	0
(Pathmark)								
beef, bite size, in tomato sauce, 'No Frills'	7.5 oz	180	7	28	890	0	4.0	0
cheese in tomato sauce, canned, 'No Frills'	7.5 oz	185	7	27	790	0	6.0	0
(Progresso)								
beef, frozen	1 cup	260	9	45	940	4	5.0	5
cheese, frozen	1 cup	220	9	43	930	4	2.0	5
(Smart Ones) Florentine	1 entrée	220	9	43	490	4	2.0	5
(Weight Watchers) cheese, baked, frozen	9 oz	240	18	27	370	0	6.0	30

RED BEAN. See BEAN, RED.
RED CABBAGE. See CABBAGE, RED.
RED CURRANT. See under CURRANT.
RED CURRY BASE. See under SEASONING MIX, CURRY.
RED PEPPER. See PEPPER, BELL. See also under PEPPER, CHILI; PEPPER, GROUND.
RED PERCH. See OCEAN PERCH, ATLANTIC.
RED SALMON. See under SALMON.
REFRIED BEANS. See under BEAN DISH/ENTRÉE.
RELISH

Food Name	Serv. Size	Total Cal.	Prot. gms	Carbs gms	Sod. mgs	Fiber gms	Fat gms	Chol. mgs
CORN, canned *(Green Giant)*	1 tbsp	20	0	5	40	0	0.0	0
CRANBERRY-ORANGE, for chicken, canned								
(Ocean Spray)	1/4 cup	120	0	29	35	1	0.0	0
DILL, nonfat *(Vlasic)*	1 oz	2	0	1	415	0	0.0	0
HAMBURGER *(Heinz)*	1 oz	40	0	9	255	0	0.0	0
HOT DOG *(Vlasic)*	1 oz	40	0	8	255	0	1.0	0
INDIA *(Heinz)*	1 oz	35	0	9	215	0	0.0	0
PICCALILLI								
(Heinz)	1 oz	30	0	7	145	0	0.0	0
(Progresso)	1/2 cup	190	1	4	220	1	20.0	0
not *(Vlasic)*	1 oz	35	0	8	165	0	0.0	0
PICKLE								
dill *(Vlasic)*	1 tbsp	5	0	1	240	1	0.0	0
hot dog *(Heinz)*	1 tbsp	15	0	4	105	0	0.0	0
India *(Vlasic)*	1 tbsp	15	0	4	140	0	0.0	0
sweet *(Claussen)*	1 tbsp	15	0	3	85	0	0.0	0
sweet *(Heinz)*	1 tbsp	15	0	4	110	0	0.0	0
sweet *(Vlasic)*	1 tbsp	15	0	4	140	0	0.0	0
RENNIN, emzyme tablet, unsweetened	0.35 oz	8	0	2	2579	0	0.0	0
RHUBARB								
Fresh								
raw, whole	1 med stalk	11	0	2	2	1	0.1	0
raw, diced	1 cup	26	1	6	5	2	0.2	0
Frozen								
(Flav-R-Pac)	1 cup	30	1	5	0	2	0.5	0
w/sugar, cooked	1 cup	278	1	75	2	5	0.1	0
uncooked, diced	1 cup	29	1	7	3	2	0.2	0
RICE								
ARBORIO								
(Colavita) dry	1 oz	100	2	22	5	0	0.0	0
(Fantastic Foods) dry, 'Elegant Grains'	1/4 cup	210	4	45	0	1	0.0	0

Food Name	Serv. Size	Total Cal.	Prot. gms	Carbs gms	Sod. mgs	Fiber gms	Fat gms	Chol. mgs
BASMATI								
(Arrowhead Mills)								
brown, long-grain, dry	2 oz	200	4	44	3	3	1.0	0
white, long grain, dry	1/4 cup	150	3	33	0	2	1.0	0
(Fantastic Foods)								
brown, cooked, w/1 tbsp salted butter	1/2 cup	115	3	22	20	0	2.0	0
brown, dry, 'Elegant Grains'	1/4 cup	170	3	36	0	1	1.5	0
white, cooked, prep w/1 tbsp salted butter	1/2 cup	116	2	23	18	0	1.0	0
white, dry, 'Elegant Grains'	1/4 cup	180	3	38	0	1	0.0	0
(Texmati) white, long-grain, cooked w/o salt or butter	1/2 cup	82	3	31	0	0	0.0	0
BROWN								
long grain, cooked	1 cup	216	5	45	10	4	1.8	0
long grain, raw	1 cup	685	15	143	13	6	5.4	0
medium grain, cooked	1 cup	218	5	46	2	4	1.6	0
medium grain, raw	1 cup	688	14	145	8	6	5.1	0
(Arrowhead Mills)								
long grain, raw	2 oz	200	4	44	3	3	1.0	0
medium grain, raw	2 oz	200	4	44	3	3	1.0	0
short grain, raw	2 oz	200	4	44	3	3	1.0	0
Spanish, quick, dry	1/3 cup	150	4	30	250	2	1.0	0
vegetable, quick, dry	1/3 cup	150	4	30	160	3	1.0	0
wild, dry	1/3 cup	140	4	28	220	3	1.0	0
(Carolina) long grain, cooked, no salt or butter	1/2 cup	110	2	23	0	0	0.0	0
(Eden Foods)								
traditional	1/2 cup	200	8	38	80	3	2.0	0
udon, organic, traditional, dry	1/2 cup	200	8	38	80	3	2.0	0
(Fantastic Foods)								
cooked	1 cup	240	7	55	650	2	2.0	0
w/miso, dry	1/2 cup	250	7	55	570	1	3.0	0
(Lundberg Family)								
golden rose, organic	1/4 cup	160	3	34	0	1	2.0	0
long grain, cooked	1 cup	232	5	50	0	3	1.2	0
(Mahatma) long grain, cooked, no salt or butter	1/2 cup	110	2	23	10	0	0.0	0
(Minute) instant	1/2 cup	120	3	25	5	0	1.0	0
(River) long grain, cooked, no salt or butter	1/2 cup	110	2	23	0	0	0.0	0
(S&W)								
long grain, cooked, no salt or butter	3.5 oz	110	2	25	0	0	0.0	0
long grain, dry	1/4 cup	150	3	32	0	1	1.0	0
(Uncle Ben's)								
instant, original, dry	1/4 cup	170	4	37	0	1	1.5	0
long grain, cooked, no salt or butter	2/3 cup	130	3	27	0	0	1.0	0
precooked, prepared, no salt or butter	1/2 cup	90	2	21	11	1	1.0	0
GLUTINOUS								
white, cooked	1 cup	169	4	37	9	2	0.3	0
white, raw	1 cup	685	13	151	13	5	1.0	0
JASMINE *(Fantastic Foods)* uncooked, 'Elegant Grains'	1/4 cup	170	3	38	0	1	0.0	0
WHITE								
long grain, cooked	1 cup	205	4	45	2	1	0.4	0
long grain, dry	1 cup	675	13	148	9	2	1.2	0
long grain, parboiled, cooked	1 cup	200	4	43	5	1	0.5	0
long grain, parboiled, dry	1 cup	686	13	151	9	3	1.0	0
long grain, precooked or instant, enriched, dry	1 cup	360	7	79	6	2	0.3	0
long grain, precooked or instant, enriched, prepared	1 cup	162	3	35	5	1	0.3	0
medium grain, cooked	1 cup	242	4	53	0	1	0.4	0
medium grain, dry	1 cup	702	13	155	2	3	1.1	0
short grain, cooked	1 cup	242	4	53	0	na	0.4	0
short grain, dry	1 cup	716	13	158	2	6	1.0	0

Food Name	Serv. Size	Total Cal.	Prot. gms	Carbs gms	Sod. mgs	Fiber gms	Fat gms	Chol. mgs
(Botan) long grain, Calrose	1/4 cup	150	3	33	0	0	0.0	0
(Carolina)								
long grain, cooked, w/o salt, butter	1/2 cup	100	2	22	10	0	0.0	0
long grain, instant, cooked, w/o salt, butter	1/2 cup	110	2	23	0	0	0.0	0
(Dynasty) long grain, enriched	1 oz	118	2	26	0	0	0.0	0
(Finast) long grain, cooked, w/o salt, butter	1/2 cup	115	2	26	0	0	0.0	0
(Mahatma) long grain, cooked, w/o salt, butter	1/2 cup	110	2	23	0	0	0.0	0
(Minute)								
long grain, cooked, w/o salt, butter	2/3 cup	120	3	27	0	0	0.0	0
long grain, cooked, w/o salt, butter	1/2 cup	90	2	20	0	0	0.0	0
long grain, 'Premium' cooked, w/o salt, butter	2/3 cup	120	3	27	0	0	0.0	0
'Original'	2/3 cup	120	3	27	5	0	0.0	0
(River) long grain, cooked, w/o salt, butter	1/2 cup	100	2	22	10	0	0.0	0
(S&W) long grain, cooked, w/o salt, butter	3.5 oz	106	2	23	0	0	0.0	0
(Success) long grain, enriched, cooked, w/o salt, butter	1/2 cup	100	2	21	0	0	0.0	0
(Uncle Ben's)								
long grain, cooked, w/o salt and butter	2/3 cup	130	3	28	0	0	1.0	0
long grain, cooked, w/o salt, butter	1/2 cup	90	2	20	10	0	1.0	0
long grain, instant, cooked, w/salt and butter	2/3 cup	130	3	27	310	0	2.0	0
long grain, instant, cooked, w/o salt, butter	2/3 cup	120	3	27	10	0	1.0	0
long grain, 'Natural' cooked, w/salt, butter	2/3 cup	150	3	28	420	0	3.0	0
long grain, parboiled, cooked, w/salt, butter	2/3 cup	140	2	28	410	0	2.0	0
long grain, parboiled, cooked, w/o salt, butter	2/3 cup	120	2	28	0	0	1.0	0
(Water Maid) long grain, cooked, w/o salt, butter	1/2 cup	100	2	22	10	0	0.0	0
RICE, WILD								
cooked *(Fantastic Foods)*	1/2 cup	83	3	18	0	0	0.0	0
cooked	1 cup	166	7	35	5	3	0.6	0
extra fancy, prepared *(Gourmet House)*	1 oz	107	4	22	8	1	0.3	0
giant, prepared *(Gourmet House)*	1 oz	106	4	22	3	1	0.3	0
raw	1 cup	571	24	120	11	10	1.7	0
select, prepared *(Gourmet House)*	1 oz	106	4	22	14	1	0.3	0
RICE AND BEANS. See under RICE DISH/ENTRÉE.								
RICE BEVERAGE								
(Amazake Light) nondairy, original flavor	1 cup	90	2	20	75	2	0.0	0
(Don Jose)								
original flavor, 'Horchata'	8 fl oz	70	1	6	95	0	4.0	0
strawberry flavor, 'Horchata'	8 fl oz	70	1	7	95	0	3.5	0
(Eden Foods) original flavor, organic, w/soy	8 fl oz	120	7	16	85	0	3.0	0
(Grainaissance)								
almond flavor, sweet brown rice, 'Amazake'	8 fl oz	198	4	37	20	0	4.0	0
apricot flavor, sweet brown rice, 'Amazake'	8 fl oz	158	3	36	20	0	0.0	0
cocoa-almond flavor, brown rice, 'Amazake'	8 fl oz	198	4	36	20	0	4.0	0
mocha java flavor, sweet brown rice, 'Amazake'	8 fl oz	178	3	37	20	0	2.0	0
original flavor, brown rice, 'Amazake'	8 fl oz	148	2	34	20	0	0.0	0
sesame flavor, sweet brown rice, 'Amazake'	8 fl oz	198	4	37	20	0	1.0	0
vanilla pecan flavor, brown rice, 'Amazake'	8 fl oz	198	4	37	20	0	4.0	0
(Imagine Foods)								
carob flavor, brown rice, nondairy, 'Rice Dream Lite'	8 fl oz	150	1	32	80	0	3.0	0
carob flavor, nondairy, 'Rice Dream'	8 fl oz	150	1	32	100	0	2.5	0
chocolate flavor, brown rice, nondairy, 'Rice Dream'	8 fl oz	190	1	44	80	0	3.0	0
chocolate flavor, enriched, nondairy, 'Rice Dream'	8 fl oz	170	1	36	115	0	3.0	0
chocolate flavor, nondairy, 'Rice Dream'	8 fl oz	160	1	35	100	0	2.5	0
nondairy, 'Rice Dream'	8 fl oz	130	1	28	90	0	2.0	0
original flavor, enriched, nondairy, 'Rice Dream'	8 fl oz	120	1	25	90	0	2.0	0
vanilla flavor, brown rice, nondairy, 'Rice Dream Lite'	8 fl oz	120	1	28	80	0	2.0	0
vanilla flavor, enriched, nondairy, 'Rice Dream'	8 fl oz	130	1	28	90	0	2.0	0
(Sovex) original vanilla flavor, 'Better Than Milk'	2 tbsp	72	1	17	90	0	0.0	0

Food Name	Serv. Size	Total Cal.	Prot. gms	Carbs gms	Sod. mgs	Fiber gms	Fat gms	Chol. mgs
(Westbrae Naturals)								
plain	8 fl oz	100	1	18	70	0	3.0	0
vanilla flavor	8 fl oz	120	1	22	70	0	3.0	0
RICE BEVERAGE MIX								
Devan Sweet) made from organic brown rice	1 1/2 tsp	25	0	2	0	0	0.0	0
RICE BRAN, crude	1 cup	373	16	59	6	25	24.6	0
RICE BRAN OIL								
	1 cup	1927	0	0	0	0	218.0	0
	1 tbsp	120	0	0	0	0	13.6	0
(Hain)	1 tbsp	120	0	0	0	0	14.0	0
RICE CAKE								
(Lundberg Family)								
all flavors, sodium-free	1 cake	60	1	14	3	0	0.5	0
all flavors, very low sodium	1 cake	60	1	14	30	0	0.5	0
APPLE CINNAMON								
(Hain)	1 serving	50	1	11	10	0	0.0	0
(Quaker) nonfat	1 cake	40	1	9	0	0	0.0	0
BROWN RICE								
	1 cake	35	1	7	29	0	0.3	0
buckwheat	1 cake	34	1	7	10	0	0.3	0
buckwheat, unsalted	1 cake	34	1	7	0	na	0.3	0
corn	1 cake	35	1	7	26	0	0.3	0
multigrain	1 cake	35	1	7	23	0	0.3	0
multigrain, unsalted	1 cake	35	1	7	0	na	0.3	0
unsalted	1 cake	35	1	7	2	0	0.3	0
rye	1 cake	35	1	7	10	0	0.3	0
w/sesame seed	1 cake	35	1	7	20	0	0.3	0
w/sesame seed, unsalted	1 cake	35	1	7	0	na	0.3	0
(Lundberg) unsalted	1 cake	70	1	16	0	2	0.0	0
HONEY NUT *(Hain)*	1 serving	50	1	11	25	0	0.0	0
BARBECUE *(Hain)* mini	0.5 oz	70	1	10	50	0	3.0	0
CARAWAY RYE *(Lundberg)*	1 cake	60	1	14	120	2	0.0	0
CAROB COATED								
(Carafection)								
'Mint Rice Crisps'	1 oz	139	2	17	26	0	7.0	0
'Rice Crisps'	1 oz	139	2	17	26	0	7.0	0
CHEESE								
(Hain)								
mini	0.5 oz	60	1	10	80	0	2.0	0
nacho, mini	0.5 oz	70	1	10	90	0	2.0	5
(Lundberg Family)								
mini	5 cakes	57	1	13	116	0	1.0	1
mini	5 cakes	57	1	13	116	0	1.0	1
CINNAMON								
(Quaker) crunch	1 serving	50	1	11	25	0	0.0	0
(Chico-San) sugar, mini	5 cakes	50	1	12	0	0	0.0	0
CORN *(Quaker)*	1 cake	35	1	7	53	0	0.2	0
DILL *(Lundberg Family)* creamy, mini	5 cakes	60	1	13	57	0	1.0	2
HONEY NUT *(Chico-San)* unglazed, mini	4 cakes	60	1	2	35	0	1.0	0
MUGWORT *(Grainaissance)* bake and serve, 'Mochi'	2 oz	140	3	29	2	0	1.3	0
MULTIGRAIN								
(Chico-San) very low sodium	1 cake	35	1	8	30	0	0.0	0
(Hain) five grain	1 cake	40	1	8	10	0	1.0	0
(Pritikin)								
sodium-free *(Pritikin)*	1 cake	35	1	7	0	0	0.0	0
very low sodium	1 cake	35	1	7	30	0	0.0	0
(Quaker)	0.32 oz	34	1	7	29	0	0.4	0

Food Name	Serv. Size	Total Cal.	Prot. gms	Carbs gms	Sod. mgs	Fiber gms	Fat gms	Chol. mgs
PLAIN								
(Chico-San) nonfat, original	1 cake	35	1	8	30	0	0.0	0
(Grainaissance) organic, bake and serve, 'Mochi'	2 oz	140	3	29	2	0	1.3	0
(Hain)								
	1 cake	40	1	8	10	0	1.0	0
mini	0.5 oz	60	1	12	20	0	1.0	0
mini, unsalted	0.5 oz	60	1	12	5	0	1.0	0
unsalted	1 cake	40	1	8	5	0	1.0	0
unsalted, mini	0.5 oz	60	1	12	5	0	1.0	0
(Konriko) unsalted, original	1 cake	30	0	7	1	0	0.0	0
(Koyo)								
organic, lightly salted	1 cake	40	1	8	80	0	0.0	0
organic, no added salt	1 cake	40	1	8	0	0	0.0	0
(Lundberg Family) organic, lightly salted	1 cake	60	1	14	140	0	0.5	0
(Pritikin)								
sodium-free	1 cake	35	1	7	0	0	0.0	0
very low sodium	1 cake	35	1	7	35	0	0.0	0
(Quaker)								
	0.32 oz	35	1	7	36	0	0.3	0
lightly salted	1 cake	35	1	7	35	0	0.0	0
unsalted	1 cake	35	1	7	0	0	0.3	0
RAISIN								
(Grainaissance) cinnamon, bake and serve, 'Mochi'	2 oz	143	3	30	77	0	1.2	0
RYE *(Quaker)*	1 cake	34	1	7	12	0	0.4	0
SESAME								
(Chico-San) original	1 cake	35	1	8	0	0	0.0	0
(Grainaissance) garlic, bake and serve, 'Mochi'	2 oz	143	3	28	25	0	1.9	0
(Hain)								
unsalted	1 cake	40	1	8	5	0	1.0	0
	1 cake	40	1	8	10	0	1.0	0
(Pritikin)								
nonfat, sodium-free	1 cake	35	1	7	0	0	0.0	0
nonfat, very low sodium	1 cake	35	1	7	35	0	0.0	0
(Quaker)	0.32 oz	35	1	7	36	0	0.3	0
(Westbrae)								
double sesame	0.28 oz	30	1	6	65	0	1.0	0
garlic	0.28 oz	30	1	6	55	0	1.0	0
TERIYAKI								
(Hain) mini	0.5 oz	50	1	12	75	0	1.0	0
(Westbrae)	0.28 oz	30	1	6	45	0	1.0	0
WHEAT *(Quaker)*	1 cake	34	1	7	52	1	0.3	0
WHOLE GRAIN, herb and garlic *(American Grains)*	0.5 oz	60	1	11	92	0	1.7	0
RICE CHIPS, brown rice *(Eden Foods)*	1-oz bag	130	2	19	197	0	5.0	0
RICE DISH/ENTRÉE								
(Bearitos)								
rice and beans, Cajun style	1 cup	140	7	26	490	5	1.0	0
rice and beans, Cuban style	1 cup	150	7	27	490	5	1.0	0
rice and beans, Mexican style	1 cup	160	7	30	490	4	1.0	0
(Lean Cuisine)								
Mexican style, w/chicken, frozen, 'Lunch Express'	9 1/8 oz	270	12	43	580	0	5.0	20
(Lunch Express) stir-fry, w/chicken	1 entrée	280	11	39	590	3	9.0	15
(Marie Callender's) w/chicken and broccoli, cheesy	12 oz	390	24	44	1220	6	13.0	55
(Smart Ones) Santa Fe style rice and beans	1 entrée	290	12	43	590	6	8.0	20
(Suzi Wan) sweet and sour	1 cup	268	5	46	754	1	6.9	0
(Weight Watchers)								
and vegetables, Hunan style	1 entrée	250	7	39	630	8	7.0	5
and vegetables, Peking style	1 entrée	270	7	48	640	3	6.0	5

Food Name	Serv. Size	Total Cal.	Prot. gms	Carbs gms	Sod. mgs	Fiber gms	Fat gms	Chol. mgs
paella	1 entrée	280	7	48	680	5	7.0	5
rice and beans, Santa Fe style, 'Smart Ones'	1 entrée	290	12	41	670	10	9.0	5
risotto, w/cheese and mushrooms	1 entrée	290	11	44	540	4	8.0	20
RICE DISH/ENTRÉE MIX								
(Casbah)								
pilaf, nutted, prepared	3/4 cup	190	5	35	500	1	2.0	0
pilaf, prepared	3/4 cup	210	9	38	390	1	0.5	0
Spanish pilaf *(Casbah)* prepared	3/4 cup	200	4	40	430	1	0.5	0
tabbouleh rice, mix only	1 oz	90	3	20	350	1	1.0	0
(Ener-G Foods)								
brown rice pilaf, 'Old World' prepared	1 cup	364	9	76	418	6	3.0	0
gluten-free, low-sodium, mixonly	1 cup	507	9	111	6	3	2.0	0
gluten-free, mix only	1 cup	528	9	97	283	3	1.8	0
(Fantastic Foods)								
rice and beans, Caribbean, mix only	1 serving	230	10	44	480	6	1.5	0
rice and beans, northern Italian, mix only	1 serving	240	8	49	460	4	1.5	0
rice and beans, Szechuan, mix only	1 serving	210	7	41	480	3	2.0	0
rice and pinto beans, Tex-Mex, mix only	2.3 oz	240	8	48	590	6	2.5	0
rice and red beans, Cajun, mix only	2.3 oz	230	10	46	480	8	3.0	0
(La Choy) fried, prepared	1 cup	236	5	53	1024	2	1.1	0
(Lundberg Family)								
blend, brown and white, mix only	1/4 cup	150	4	35	0	3	1.5	0
brown rice picante, prepared, 'Spanish Fiesta' 'Quick'	1 cup	260	6	53	670	5	2.5	na
brown rice, exotic wild rice, and mushrooms, prepared, 'Quick'	1 cup	260	6	53	800	4	3.0	na
(Minute)								
long grain and wild, mix only	1/2 cup	120	3	25	530	0	0.0	0
long grain and wild, prepared w/salted butter	1/2 cup	150	3	25	570	0	4.0	10
(Rice A Roni)								
beef flavored, 1/3 less sodium, prepared	2.5 oz	158	4	30	423	1	2.8	0
beef flavored, prepared	2.5 oz	169	5	27	598	na	4.5	na
chicken flavored, 'Fast Cook' prepared	2.5 oz	141	3	23	519	1	3.7	3
chicken flavored, 1/3 less sodium, prepared	2.5 oz	158	4	30	390	1	2.8	0
chicken flavored, prepared	2.5 oz	181	4	29	618	1	5.4	0
fried, 1/3 less sodium, prepared	2.5 oz	147	3	29	525	1	2.0	0
fried, prepared	2.5 oz	181	3	29	900	1	6.2	0
herb and butter, prepared	2.5 oz	175	3	30	655	1	5.1	3
long grain and wild, original, prepared	2.5 oz	164	4	28	700	2	4.8	0
long grain and wild, w/chicken, almond, prepared	2.5 oz	164	4	28	700	2	4.8	0
pilaf, long grain and wild, prepared	2.5 oz	135	3	24	514	1	3.1	0
pilaf, prepared	2.5 oz	175	3	30	621	1	5.1	0
Spanish, 'Fast Cook' prepared	2.5 oz	141	3	25	567	1	3.1	0
Spanish, prepared	2 oz	122	3	21	546	1	3.6	0
Stroganoff, prepared	2.5 oz	203	5	28	587	1	8.2	3
w/chicken, broccoli, prepared	2.5 oz	164	4	29	793	1	4.2	0
white cheddar and herb, prepared	2.5 oz	192	4	28	553	1	7.9	3
RICE FLOUR. See under FLOUR.								
RICE SEASONING. See under SEASONING MIX.								
RICE STICK, wild rice *(Golden Flavor)* wild	1 oz	150	5	17	170	2	7.0	0
RICE SYRUP. See under SYRUP.								
RISOTTO. See under RICE DISH/ENTRÉE.								
ROAST BEEF HASH. See under HASH.								
ROCKFISH, PACIFIC								
baked, broiled, grilled, or microwaved	3 oz	103	20	0	65	0	1.7	37
raw	3 oz	80	16	0	51	0	1.3	30
ROE								
mixed species, cooked	3 oz	173	24	2	99	0	7.0	407

Food Name	Serv. Size	Total Cal.	Prot. gms	Carbs gms	Sod. mgs	Fiber gms	Fat gms	Chol. mgs
mixed species, cooked	1 oz	58	8	1	33	0	2.3	136
mixed species, raw	3 oz	119	19	1	77	0	5.5	318
mixed species, raw	1 oz	40	6	0	26	0	1.8	106
ROLL. See also BREAD; BUN; CROISSANT; ENGLISH MUFFIN; ROLL, SWEET.								
(Brownberry) assorted, 'Hearth'	1 roll	124	4	24	247	2	2.3	7
(Country Oven) enriched, brown and serve	1 roll	80	2	13	140	0	2.0	0
(King's Hawaiian Bread) ready-to-eat	1 roll	90	3	15	80	1	2.0	10
(Pepperidge Farm) brown and serve, 'Hearth'	1 roll	50	2	10	100	0	1.0	0
(Wonder)								
gem style, brown and serve	1 roll	80	2	13	140	1	2.0	0
plain pan	1 roll	80	2	14	140	1	1.0	0
CLUB *(Pepperidge Farm)* brown and serve, 'Deli Classic'	1 roll	100	3	19	190	1	1.0	0
CRESCENT *(Pepperidge Farm)* butter, 'Deli Classic'	1 roll	110	2	13	150	0	6.0	15
DINNER								
(Arnold) '24 Dinner Party'	1 roll	51	2	9	81	1	1.2	1
(Awrey's)								
'Black Forest'	1 roll	50	2	10	110	0	1.0	0
cracked wheat	1 roll	50	2	10	120	0	1.0	0
crusty	1 roll	70	2	12	150	0	1.0	0
plain	1 roll	60	2	11	115	0	1.0	0
w/poppy seed	1 roll	59	2	11	115	0	1.0	0
w/sesame seed	1 roll	60	2	11	115	0	1.0	0
(Ener-G Foods) tapioca, gluten-free	1 serving	151	2	24	6	1	5.7	0
(Home Pride)								
wheat	1 roll	70	3	12	140	1	1.0	0
white	1 roll	80	2	14	170	1	2.0	0
(Pepperidge Farm)								
country style, 'Classic'	1 roll	50	2	9	90	0	1.0	0
'Old Fashioned'	1 roll	50	2	7	85	0	2.0	5
'Party'	1 roll	30	1	5	50	0	1.0	0
(Pillsbury)								
butterflake	1 serving	130	3	19	530	1	5.0	0
hot	1 serving	130	4	21	220	1	3.0	15
(Roman Meal)	1 roll	69	3	13	140	1	1.2	0
(Wonder)								
	1 roll	80	2	14	140	1	1.0	0
brown and serve	1 serving	80	2	13	150	0	2.0	0
EGG *(Levy's)* 'Old Country Deli'	1 roll	146	5	28	431	2	2.8	11
FINGER w/poppy seeds	1 roll	50	2	8	80	0	2.0	5
FRENCH								
(Du Jour) petite, brown and serve	1 roll	230	9	45	490	2	2.0	0
(Francisco) 'International'	1 roll	108	4	21	285	1	1.5	0
(Pepperidge Farm)								
brown and serve, 'Deli Classic'	1/2 roll	120	4	24	250	1	1.0	0
'Deli Classic' 4 per pkg	1/2 piece	120	4	22	250	1	2.0	0
'Deli Classic' 9 per pkg	1 roll	100	4	20	230	1	1.0	0
sourdough	1 piece	100	4	19	240	1	1.0	0
HARD, including Kaiser	1 oz	83	3	15	154	1	1.2	0
HOAGIE								
(Wonder)	1 roll	400	13	73	800	3	7.0	0
(Pepperidge Farm) soft, 'Deli Classic'	1 roll	210	8	34	320	1	5.0	0
ITALIAN *(Du Jour)* crusty, brown and serve	1 roll	80	3	16	200	1	1.0	0
KAISER								
(Arnold) 'Francisco'	1 roll	184	7	35	338	2	2.9	5
(Brownberry) 'Hearth'	1 roll	152	5	29	318	2	2.8	9
(Holsum) 'Big'	1 bun	200	5	38	320	0	3.0	0
LUIGI 'Twin Pack' *(Colombo Brand)*	2 oz piece	146	8	25	334	0	1.6	0

Food Name	Serv. Size	Total Cal.	Prot. gms	Carbs gms	Sod. mgs	Fiber gms	Fat gms	Chol. mgs
ONION								
(Holsum) 'Big'	1 bun	190	6	32	190	0	4.0	0
(Levy's) 'Old Country Deli'	1 roll	153	6	31	380	2	1.9	11
(Pepperidge Farm) w/poppy seeds, sandwich	1 roll	150	5	26	260	1	3.0	0
PARKER HOUSE								
(Bridgford)	1 roll	85	3	16	172	0	1.3	0
(Pepperidge Farm)	1 roll	60	2	9	80	0	1.0	5
POTATO								
(Mrs. Wright's) Dutch style, long	1 roll	150	4	27	250	1	2.5	0
(Pepperidge Farm)								
....	1 roll	160	4	28	260	1	4.0	0
'Hearty Classic'	1 roll	90	2	14	125	0	3.0	0
SANDWICH								
(Arnold) w/egg, 'Dutch'	1 roll	123	5	22	203	2	3.3	1
(Awrey's) oat bran	1 roll	120	4	22	250	1	2.0	0
(Pepperidge Farm)								
'Deli Classic'	1 roll	110	4	16	150	0	4.0	10
w/sesame seeds	1 roll	140	5	23	230	1	3.0	0
SOFT *(Pepperidge Farm)* 'Family'	1 roll	100	4	18	190	1	2.0	0
SOUR *(Colombo Brand)* 'Sour '49er'	1.2-oz roll	90	5	16	189	0	0.6	0
SWEET *(Colombo Brand)* 'Sweet '49er'	1.2-oz roll	96	5	15	196	0	1.8	0
STEAK								
(Colombo Brand)								
sour	2.6-oz roll	200	10	35	413	0	2.2	0
sweet	2.6-oz roll	206	10	34	439	0	3.3	0
TWIST *(Pepperidge Farm)* golden, 'Heat 'n Serve'	1 piece	110	2	14	150	0	5.0	5
WHEAT								
(Country Oven) w/honey, brown and serve	1 roll	70	2	13	240	0	2.0	0
(King's Hawaiian Bread) w/honey, ready-to-eat	1 roll	90	3	15	80	1	2.0	8
ROLL, SWEET. See also BUN, SWEET; PASTRY.								
CARAMEL NUT *(Aunt Fanny's)* individual	2 oz	190	4	33	125	1	6.0	5
CHEESE *(Weight Watchers)* frozen, microwave	1/2 pkg	180	5	32	210	0	4.0	5
CHERRY								
(Break Cake)								
4.5 oz	2 rolls	400	8	79	390	0	3.0	0
multi-pak, 1.4 oz	1 roll	130	2	25	125	0	2.0	0
CINNAMON								
(Aunt Fanny's)								
11-oz size, rectangular	2 oz	181	4	34	83	0	3.0	8
individual	1.9 oz	180	4	32	150	1	5.0	5
(Awrey's)								
homestyle	1 piece	240	4	40	200	1	7.0	5
swirl, 'Grande'	1 piece	340	4	46	370	1	16.0	10
(Break Cake)								
4.5 oz	2 rolls	420	9	73	430	0	10.0	0
multi pak, 1.3 oz	1 roll	120	3	22	125	0	3.0	0
nut, 3 oz	2 rolls	330	5	52	220	0	11.0	0
(Hostess Snack Cake)	1 serving	210	3	34	190	0	7.0	10
(Hungry Jack) iced, refrigerated	2 pieces	290	3	37	570	0	14.0	0
(Pillsbury)								
iced, refrigerated	1 piece	110	1	17	260	0	5.0	0
raisin, w/icing	1 serving	180	2	26	310	1	7.0	0
w/icing	1 serving	140	2	21	330	0	5.0	0
(Sara Lee) all butter	2 oz piece	230	3	31	220	0	11.0	0
(Weight Watchers) glazed	1 serving	200	4	33	200	2	5.0	5
FRUIT *(Aunt Fanny's)* Dixie, individual	2 oz	180	3	34	120	1	4.0	5
ORANGE *(Hostess)* swirl, 'Breakfast Bake Shop'	1 piece	230	3	26	150	1	12.0	10

Food Name	Serv. Size	Total Cal.	Prot. gms	Carbs gms	Sod. mgs	Fiber gms	Fat gms	Chol. mgs
PECAN								
(Aunt Fanny's) 11-oz size, rectangular	2 oz	184	4	32	79	0	4.0	8
(Break Cake) multi pak, 1.3 oz	1 roll	120	2	22	120	0	3.0	0
(Hostess) caramel swirl, 'Breakfast Bake Shop'	1 piece	240	3	23	160	2	15.0	10
(Hostess) spinner, 'Breakfast Bake Shop'	1 piece	220	3	30	135	1	10.0	5
RAISIN (Break Cake) cinnamon, multi pak, 1.25 oz	1 roll	120	2	21	110	0	3.0	0
STRAWBERRY								
(Aunt Fanny's) 11-oz size, rectangular	2 oz	190	4	35	140	0	4.0	5
(Weight Watchers) frozen, microwave	1/2 pkg	170	3	29	90	0	5.0	20
ROLL, SWEET, DOUGH								
(Pillsbury)								
apple cinnamon, w/icing, refrigerated, prepared	1 roll	140	2	21	310	1.0	5.0	0
cinnamon raisin, w/icing, refrigerated, prepared	1 roll	180	2	26	310	1.0	7.0	0
cinnamon, w/icing, refrigerated, prepared	1 roll	150	2	24	334	na	5.0	na
ROLL DOUGH								
(Mrs. Wright's) crescent, refrigerated	1 roll	80	2	13	250	1	3.0	0
(Pillsbury)								
butterflake, refrigerated	1 roll	140	3	20	530	0	5.0	0
crescent, cheese, refrigerated	2 rolls	210	4	21	600	1	12.0	5
(Rhodes)								
cinnamon, frozen	1 roll	236	4	35	238	1	9.6	12
nonfat, no preservatives, 'Lite'	1 roll	89	3	18	135	1	0.4	0
Parker House style, frozen	1 oz	90	2	14	156	0	2.0	0
wheat, flaked, frozen	1 roll	140	6	24	210	3	3.0	0
white, frozen	1 roll	98	3	17	141	1	2.1	0
white, Texas style, frozen	1 roll	156	5	28	224	1	3.3	0
whole wheat, Texas style, frozen	1 roll	140	7	24	210	4	3.0	0
ROLL MIX								
(Dromedary)								
hot, mix only	1/8 pkg	209	6	41	363	0	2.0	0
hot, prepared	2 pieces	239	6	41	410	0	5.0	0
(Krusteaz) hot, prepared	1 roll	150	3	28	190	0	3.0	0
(Pillsbury)								
hot	1/4 cup	110	3	21	200	1	1.0	0
'Hot Roll Mix' prepared	1/16 pkg	120	4	21	210	0	2.0	15
ROMAN BEAN. See BEAN, CRANBERRY.								
ROOT BEER. See under SOFT DRINKS and MIXERS.								
ROSE COCO BEAN. See BEAN, CRANBERRY.								
ROSE PERCH. See OCEAN PERCH, ATLANTIC.								
ROSELLE								
raw, trimmed	1 cup	28	0.6	6.4	3	>.7 c	0.4	0
trimmed	1 oz	14	0.3	3.2	2	>.3 c	0.2	0
untrimmed	1 lb	136	2.7	31.3	16	>3.2 c	1.8	0
ROSEMARY								
Dried								
	1 tbsp	11	0	2	2	1	0.5	0
	1 tsp	4	0	1	1	1	0.2	0
(McCormick/Schilling)	1 tsp	6	0	1	0	1	0.0	0
(Spice Islands)	1 tsp	5	0	1	1	0	0.2	0
Fresh								
	1 tbsp	2	0	0	0	0	0.1	0
	1 tsp	1	0	0	0	0	0.0	0
Ground								
(Durkee)	1 tsp	5	0	0	0	0	0.0	0
(Laurel Leaf)	1 tsp	5	0	0	0	0	0.0	0
ROTINI. See under PASTA.								
ROTINI DISH/ENTRÉE. See under PASTA DISH/ENTRÉE.								

Food Name	Serv. Size	Total Cal.	Prot. gms	Carbs gms	Sod. mgs	Fiber gms	Fat gms	Chol. mgs
ROTINI DISH/ENTRÉE MIX. See under PASTA DISH/ENTRÉE MIX.								
RUCOLA. See ARUGULA.								
RUGULA. See ARUGULA.								
RUM								
80 proof	1 fl oz	64	0	0	0	0	0.0	0
86 proof	1 fl oz	70	0	0	0	0	0.0	0
90 proof	1 fl oz	73	0	0	0	0	0.0	0
94 proof	1 fl oz	76	0	0	0	0	0.0	0
100 proof	1 fl oz	82	0	0	0	0	0.0	0
RUM RUNNER. See under COCKTAIL MIX.								
RUTABAGA								
Fresh								
boiled, drained, cubed	1 cup	66	2	15	34	3	0.4	0
boiled, drained, mashed	1 cup	94	3	21	48	4	0.5	0
raw, cubed	1 cup	50	2	11	28	4	0.3	0
raw, whole	1 medium	139	5	31	77	10	0.8	0
Canned, diced (Allens)	1/2 cup	20	1	4	260	0	1.0	0
RYE								
	1 cup	566	25	118	10	25	4.2	0
flakes, rolled (Arrowhead Mills)	1/3 cup	110	4	24	0	4	0.5	0
whole-grain (Arrowhead Mills)	2 oz	190	7	42	1	8	1.0	0
RYE CAKE (Quaker) 'Grain Cakes'	.32 oz piece	35	1	7	52	1	0.3	0
RYE FLOUR. See under FLOUR.								
RYE WHISKEY. See WHISKEY.								

S

Food Name	Serv. Size	Total Cal.	Prot. gms	Carbs gms	Sod. mgs	Fiber gms	Fat gms	Chol. mgs
SABLEFISH. See COD, ALASKAN.								
SACCHARIN. See under SUGAR SUBSTITUTE.								
SAFFLOWER OIL								
expeller pressed (Hollywood)	1 tbsp	120	0	0	0	0	14.0	0
'Hi-Oleic' (Hain)	1 tbsp	120	0	0	0	0	14.0	0
100% pure pressed (Loriva')	1 tbsp	120	0	0	0	0	12.0	0
over 70% oleic	1 cup	1927	0	0	0	0	218.0	0
over 70% oleic	1 tbsp	124	0	0	0	0	14.0	0
pure pressed, organic (Spectrum)	1 tbsp	120	0	0	0	0	14.0	0
salad or cooking, over 70% linoleic	1 cup	1927	0	0	0	0	218.0	0
salad or cooking, over 70% linoleic	1 tbsp	120	0	0	0	0	13.6	0
salad or cooking, over 70% oleic	1 cup	1927	0	0	0	0	218.0	0
salad or cooking, over 70% oleic	1 tbsp	120	0	0	0	0	13.6	0
SAFFLOWER SEED, kernels, dried	1 oz	147	5	10	1	na	10.9	0
SAFFLOWER SEED MEAL, partially defatted	1 oz	97	10	14	1	na	0.7	0
SAFFRON								
dried	1 tbsp	7	0	1	3	0	0.1	0
dried	1 tsp	2	0	0	1	0	0.0	0
SAGE								
ground	1 tbsp	6	0	1	0	1	0.3	0
ground	1 tsp	2	0	0	0	0	0.1	0
ground (Durkee)	1 tbsp	9	0	0	0	0	0.0	0
ground (Durkee)	1 tsp	3	0	0	0	0	0.0	0
ground (Laurel Leaf)	1 tbsp	9	0	0	0	0	0.0	0
ground (Laurel Leaf)	1 tsp	3	0	0	0	0	0.0	0
ground (McCormick/Schilling)	1 tsp	4	0	0	0	0	0.0	0
ground (Spice Islands)	1 tsp	4	0	1	1	0	0.1	0

Food Name	Serv. Size	Total Cal.	Prot. gms	Carbs gms	Sod. mgs	Fiber gms	Fat gms	Chol. mgs
SALAD DRESSING								
(Estee) regular	1 tbsp	4	0	1	13	0	0.0	0
(Johnny's) lite	2 tbsp	70	0	14	380	0	2.0	0
(Ott's) lower calorie, 'Famous'	1 tbsp	26	0	4	60	0	1.3	0
BACON								
(Estee) and tomato	1 tbsp	8	1	1	35	0	1.0	5
(Kraft)								
and tomato	2 tbsp	140	1	2	280	0	14.0	3
and tomato, reduced calorie	1 tbsp	30	0	2	150	0	2.0	0
creamy, lower calorie	1 tbsp	30	0	2	150	0	2.0	0
(T. Marzetti) buttermilk, refrigerated	1 tbsp	93	0	0	127	0	10.0	2
BLUE CHEESE								
(Estee)	1 tbsp	8	1	1	50	0	1.0	0
(Featherweight) 'Neu Bleu'	1 tbsp	4	0	1	110	0	0.0	0
(Hidden Valley Ranch)								
	2 tbsp	20	0	4	270	0	0.0	0
low-fat	1 tbsp	10	0	3	140	0	0.0	0
(Kraft)								
	2 tbsp	45	0	11	360	1	0.0	0
chunky	1 tbsp	60	1	2	230	0	6.0	5
chunky, lower calorie	1 tbsp	30	0	2	240	0	2.0	5
(La Martinique) vinaigrette	2 tbsp	160	2	0	450	0	17.0	5
(Lawry's) 'Classic' 1 oz	1 tbsp	186	0	2	385	0	2.0	0
(Litehouse)								
and dip, refrigerated, 'Lite'	1 tbsp	33	1	1	86	0	3.0	0
and dip, refrigerated, 'Original'	1 tbsp	77	1	0	82	0	8.0	0
country, and dip, refrigerated	1 tbsp	76	1	0	84	0	8.0	0
(Roka)								
	1 tbsp	60	1	1	170	0	6.0	10
lower calorie	1 tbsp	16	1	1	280	0	1.0	5
(S&W) 'Nutradiet'	1 tbsp	25	0	2	200	0	2.0	0
(T. Marzetti)								
	1 tbsp	90	1	1	180	0	9.0	2
buttermilk, refrigerated	1 tbsp	90	1	1	161	0	10.0	5
chunky, refrigerated	1 tbsp	78	1	1	159	0	8.0	14
'Light'	1 tbsp	90	1	1	180	0	9.0	2
refrigerated, 'Lite'	1 tbsp	45	0	0	150	0	5.0	5
(Walden Farms) calorie-free	2 tbsp	0	0	0	260	0	0.0	0
(Wish-Bone)								
chunky	1 tbsp	75	0	1	149	0	7.9	1
chunky, light	2 tbsp	80	1	2	410	0	8.0	0
BUTTERMILK								
(Hain) buttermilk, 'Old Fashioned'	1 tbsp	70	0	0	100	0	7.0	0
(Hollywood) 'Old Fashioned'	1 tbsp	75	0	1	40	0	8.0	0
(Kraft)								
creamy	1 tbsp	80	0	1	120	0	8.0	5
creamy, lower calorie	1 tbsp	30	0	1	125	0	3.0	5
(Seven Seas) 'Buttermilk Recipe'	1 tbsp	80	0	1	130	0	8.0	5
(T. Marzetti) and herbs	1 tbsp	95	0	0	150	0	10.0	3
CAESAR								
(Cardini's)	2 tbsp	80	0	1	100	1	8.0	9
(Cook's Classics)	1 tbsp	50	1	1	30	0	5.0	0
(Estee)	2 tbsp	8	1	1	130	0	1.0	2
(Hain)								
creamy	1 tbsp	60	0	1	220	0	6.0	5
creamy, low-salt	1 tbsp	60	0	1	15	0	6.0	5
(Hollywood)	1 tbsp	70	1	2	65	0	7.0	0

Food Name	Serv. Size	Total Cal.	Prot. gms	Carbs gms	Sod. mgs	Fiber gms	Fat gms	Chol. mgs
(Johnny's) 'Great Caesar'	2 tbsp	170	1	1	260	0	18.0	1
(Kraft) golden	1 tbsp	70	0	1	180	0	7.0	0
(Lawry's) 'Classic'	1 tbsp	130	1	1	337	0	13.5	0
(Litehouse) and dip, refrigerated	1 tbsp	57	0	0	84	0	6.0	0
(T. Marzetti)								
....	1 tbsp	80	0	1	170	0	8.0	2
light, 50% less fat	2 tbsp	80	1	1	370	0	7.0	10
refrigerated	1 tbsp	75	0	0	178	0	8.0	0
house	1 tbsp	75	1	1	180	0	8.0	1
(Walden Farms) calorie-free	2 tbsp	0	0	0	360	0	0.0	0
(Weight Watchers)								
nonfat	1 tbsp	5	0	1	195	0	0.0	0
(Weight Watchers) nonfat, 'Single Serve'	1 tbsp	6	0	1	270	0	0.0	0
(Wish-Bone)								
....	1 tbsp	77	0	1	248	0	8.0	1
w/olive oil	2 tbsp	100	0	2	400	0	10.0	0
w/olive oil, 'Lite'	2 tbsp	60	1	3	410	0	5.0	0
CATALINA *(Kraft)* Catalina, nonfat	2 tbsp	35	0	8	320	1	0.0	0
CELERY SEED								
(T. Marzetti)								
and onion	1 tbsp	75	0	9	90	0	6.0	0
refrigerated	1 tbsp	72	0	5	101	0	5.0	0
CHEESE								
(Bernstein's) 'Cheese Fantastico Parmesan'	2 tbsp	30	1	5	360	0	1.0	0
(Featherweight)	1 tbsp	20	0	1	70	0	2.0	0
(Hollywood)	1 tbsp	80	0	2	60	0	8.0	0
(Lawry's) creamy, w/Parmesan, 'Classic'	1 oz	156	0	5	178	0	15.1	0
(Wish-Bone)	1 tbsp	89	0	1	170	0	9.2	1
CILANTRO *(Paula's)* and tomato, 'Herb Garden'	0.5 oz	54	0	1	26	0	6.0	0
CITRUS *(Hain)* tangy, 'Canola'	1 tbsp	50	0	1	75	0	5.0	0
COLESLAW								
(Best Foods) 'One Step'	2 tbsp	160	0	4	180	0	16.0	5
(Hellmann's) 'One Step'	2 tbsp	160	0	4	180	0	16.0	5
(Blue Plate)	2 tbsp	140	0	5	240	0	13.0	15
(JFG)	2 tbsp	140	0	5	240	0	13.0	15
(Kraft)	1 tbsp	70	0	4	200	0	6.0	10
(Litehouse) refrigerated	1 tbsp	80	0	2	41	0	8.0	0
(T. Marzetti)								
light	1 tbsp	50	0	6	240	0	3.0	0
original	1 tbsp	79	1	3	180	0	7.0	14
'South Recipe'	1 tbsp	66	0	6	93	0	5.0	9
(Hidden Valley Ranch) coleslaw, nonfat	2 tbsp	35	0	9	200	1	0.0	0
CREAMY								
(Estee) nonfat	1 tbsp	4	0	1	13	0	0.0	0
(Hain)								
....	1 tbsp	80	0	0	100	0	8.0	0
no salt added	1 tbsp	80	0	1	25	0	8.0	0
(Hollywood) creamy	1 tbsp	90	0	2	140	0	9.0	0
(Kraft)								
house, ...	1 tbsp	60	0	1	115	0	6.0	0
house, lower calorie	1 tbsp	30	0	1	115	0	2.0	0
lower calorie	1 tbsp	25	0	1	120	0	2.0	0
nonfat, no oil, lower calorie	1 tbsp	4	0	1	220	0	0.0	0
w/real sour cream	1 tbsp	50	0	1	120	0	5.0	0
zesty	1 tbsp	50	0	1	260	0	5.0	0
zesty, lower calorie	1 tbsp	20	0	1	230	0	2.0	0
(Life) creamy, egg-free, 'All Natural'	1 tbsp	39	1	2	4	0	4.0	0

Food Name	Serv. Size	Total Cal.	Prot. gms	Carbs gms	Sod. mgs	Fiber gms	Fat gms	Chol. mgs
(Pathmark)								
....	1 tbsp	70	0	1	260	0	7.0	0
zesty	1 tbsp	70	0	1	370	0	8.0	0
zesty, nonfat, lower calorie	1 tbsp	6	0	1	190	0	0.0	0
(Rancher's Choice)								
....	1 tbsp	90	0	1	140	0	10.0	5
lower calorie	1 tbsp	30	0	1	150	0	3.0	5
(S&W)								
nonfat, no oil	1 tbsp	2	0	0	290	0	0.0	0
'Nutradiet'	1 tbsp	10	0	1	180	0	1.0	0
(Seven Seas) creamy	1 tbsp	70	0	1	240	0	7.0	0
(Weight Watchers) creamy, nonfat, 'Single Serve'	1 tbsp	9	0	2	430	0	0.0	0
(Wish-Bone)								
....	1 tbsp	56	0	2	149	0	5.5	1
herbal, 'Classics'	1 tbsp	70	0	1	228	0	7.3	0
'Lite'	1 tbsp	26	0	2	148	0	2.0	1
CUCUMBER								
(Featherweight) creamy, nonfat	1 tbsp	4	0	1	80	0	0.0	0
(Hain) dill, creamy	1 tbsp	80	0	0	210	0	8.0	5
(Herb Magic) creamy, no oil	2 tbsp	15	0	4	270	na	0.0	0
(Kraft)								
creamy	1 tbsp	70	0	1	190	0	8.0	0
creamy, less fat, lower calorie	1 tbsp	25	0	1	220	0	2.0	0
DIJON								
(Estee) creamy	1 tbsp	8	1	1	100	0	1.0	5
(Featherweight) creamy	1 tbsp	20	0	1	80	0	2.0	0
(Great Impressions) mustard	1 tbsp	57	0	0	103	0	6.1	18
(Cook's Classics) oil-free	1 tbsp	8	0	2	100	0	0.0	0
(Pritikin) w/balsamic vinegar, nonfat	2 tbsp	30	0	6	125	0	0.0	0
DILL								
(Nasoya) creamy	2 tbsp	63	1	3	145	0	5.4	0
(Hain) cucumber, creamy	1 tbsp	80	0	0	210	0	8.0	5
(Paula's) and garlic, 'Herb Garden'	0.5 oz	54	0	1	28	0	6.0	0
FRENCH								
(Catalina)								
....	1 tbsp	60	0	4	180	0	5.0	0
reduced calorie	1 tbsp	18	0	3	120	0	1.0	0
(Cook's Classics) 'Country French'	1 tbsp	10	0	3	80	0	0.0	0
(Estee)								
....	1 tbsp	4	0	1	10	0	0.0	0
creamy..	2 tbsp	10	0	2	130	0	0.0	0
(Featherweight)	1 tbsp	14	0	3	15	0	0.0	0
(Great Impressions) w/green pepper, low-calorie	1 tbsp	64	0	4	188	0	5.2	0
(Hain)								
creamy..	1 tbsp	60	0	1	80	0	6.0	0
spicy mustard, 'Canola'	1 tbsp	50	1	1	190	0	5.0	5
(Hollywood) creamy	1 tbsp	70	0	2	45	0	7.0	0
(Kraft)								
....	1 tbsp	60	0	2	125	0	6.0	0
'Miracle'	1 tbsp	70	0	3	240	0	6.0	0
reduced calorie	1 tbsp	20	0	3	120	0	1.0	0
(Litehouse) country herb, and marinade, refrigerated	1 tbsp	54	0	2	196	0	5.0	0
(Pathmark)								
creamy..	1 tbsp	60	0	2	90	0	5.0	0
reduced calorie	1 tbsp	20	0	3	160	0	1.0	0
(Pritikin)	2 tbsp	35	0	8	130	0	0.0	0
sodium-free	1 tbsp	10	0	3	0	0	0.0	0

Food Name	Serv. Size	Total Cal.	Prot. gms	Carbs gms	Sod. mgs	Fiber gms	Fat gms	Chol. mgs
(S&W) 'Nutradiet'	1 tbsp	18	0	3	120	0	0.0	0
(Seven Seas)								
creamy	1 tbsp	60	0	2	240	0	6.0	0
'French! Light'	1 tbsp	35	0	2	210	0	3.0	0
(T. Marzetti)								
California French	1 tbsp	90	1	5	100	0	6.0	4
California, 'Light'	1 tbsp	40	0	3	180	0	3.0	2
country	1 tbsp	72	0	4	110	0	6.0	6
fat-free, 'California French'	1 tbsp	16	1	4	140	0	0.0	0
'Frenchette'	1 tbsp	10	0	3	140	0	0.0	0
honey, blue, refrigerated	1 tbsp	70	0	5	122	0	6.0	1
honey, refrigerated	1 tbsp	74	0	5	115	0	6.0	0
honey, refrigerated, 'Lite'	1 tbsp	48	0	5	118	0	3.0	0
'Light'	1 tbsp	16	0	3	160	0	1.0	0
(Ultra Slim-Fast) cholesterol-free	1 tbsp	20	0	4	105	0	1.0	0
(Weight Watchers) low-calorie	1 tbsp	10	0	2	170	0	0.0	0
(Wish-Bone)								
'Deluxe Food Service'	1 tbsp	61	0	2	86	0	5.6	0
'Deluxe'	1 tbsp	60	0	2	83	0	5.4	0
garlic, creamy	1 tbsp	55	0	2	158	0	5.3	0
'Lite'	1 tbsp	31	0	2	70	0	2.5	0
'Lite Sweet 'n Spicy'	1 tbsp	18	0	3	110	0	0.5	0
low-calorie, 'Lite'	1 tbsp	30	0	2	67	0	2.5	0
red, low-calorie, 'Lite'	1 tbsp	17	0	3	155	0	0.4	0
'Sweet'n Spicy'	1 tbsp	63	0	3	156	0	5.7	0
FRUIT SALAD								
(Knott's Berry Farm)	1 tbsp	50	2	3	75	0	5.0	0
(Great Impressions) orange marmalade	1 tbsp	87	0	5	48	0	7.1	11
GARLIC								
(Cook's Classics) 'Garlic Lover's'	1 tbsp	50	0	1	95	0	5.0	0
(Estee) creamy, nonfat	1 tbsp	2	0	0	10	0	0.0	0
(Hain) and sour cream	1 tbsp	70	0	0	100	0	7.0	0
(Kraft)								
creamy	2 tbsp	110	0	2	360	0	11.0	0
creamy	1 tbsp	50	0	1	170	0	5.0	0
(Life) w/tofu, and dip, 'All Natural'	1 tbsp	70	1	1	0	0	7.1	75
(Pritikin) herb, nonfat, sodium-free	1 tbsp	6	0	2	0	0	0.0	0
(Wish-Bone) creamy	1 tbsp	74	0	1	158	1	8.0	0
HERB								
(Featherweight)								
	1 tbsp	25	0	2	65	0	2.0	0
nonfat	1 tbsp	6	0	1	5	0	0.0	0
(Hain) savory, 'No Salt Added'	1 tbsp	90	0	0	25	0	10.0	0
(Nasoya)								
garden	2 tbsp	62	1	3	149	0	5.4	0
garlic, 'Vegi-Dressing'	1 tbsp	40	1	1	50	0	3.0	0
(Pritikin) garlic and, nonfat, sodium-free	1 tbsp	6	0	2	0	0	0.0	0
(Seven Seas)								
and spice, 'Viva'	1 tbsp	60	0	1	170	0	6.0	0
'Viva Herbs and Spices! Light'	1 tbsp	30	0	1	200	0	3.0	0
HOMESTYLE								
(Dorothy Lynch)								
	1 tbsp	55	0	5	85	0	3.8	0
lower calorie	1 tbsp	30	0	7	80	0	1.0	0
HONEY (Hain) and sesame	1 tbsp	60	0	2	210	0	5.0	0
HONEY MUSTARD								
(Cook's Classics) apple	1 tbsp	50	0	2	80	0	6.0	0

Food Name	Serv. Size	Total Cal.	Prot. gms	Carbs gms	Sod. mgs	Fiber gms	Fat gms	Chol. mgs
(Knott's Berry Farm) 'Peggy Jane's'	1 tbsp	60	0	2	40	0	6.0	0
(Kraft) Dijon, nonfat	2 tbsp	45	0	10	330	1	0.0	0
(Litehouse) and dip, refrigerated	1 tbsp	67	0	2	55	0	7.0	0
(Marzetti) Dijon, peppercorn	2 tbsp	150	0	7	250	0	13.0	20
(Pritikin) Dijon	2 tbsp	45	0	11	130	1	0.0	0
(T. Marzetti)								
Dijon	1 tbsp	67	0	3	51	0	6.0	7
Dijon, light	1 tbsp	24	0	6	69	0	0.0	0
Dijon, refrigerated	1 tbsp	68	0	3	103	0	6.0	9
Dijon ranch	1 tbsp	89	1	1	100	0	9.0	14
(Weight Watchers) Dijon, nonfat	1 tbsp	23	0	6	75	0	0.0	0
(Wish-Bone) Dijon, 'Healthy Sensation!'	1 tbsp	25	0	5	140	0	0.0	0
ITALIAN								
(Bernstein's) herb and garlic, creamy	1 tbsp	60	0	1	135	0	6.0	5
(Best Foods) creamy, homestyle	2 tsp	60	0	0	80	0	7.0	5
(Cardini's)	2 tbsp	130	0	1	195	0	14.0	0
(Cook's Classics) garlic gusto, oil free	1 tbsp	6	0	1	90	0	0.0	0
(Estee)								
creamy	2 tbsp	14	1	2	130	0	1.0	0
nonfat	2 tbsp	4	0	1	130	0	0.0	0
(Featherweight) nonfat	1 tbsp	4	0	1	120	0	0.0	0
(Hain)								
'Canola'	1 tbsp	50	0	1	150	0	5.0	0
no oil	1 tbsp	2	0	1	170	0	0.0	0
no salt added, 'Traditional'	1 tbsp	60	0	1	20	0	6.0	0
Thousand Island, no oil	1 tbsp	12	0	3	150	0	0.0	1
'Traditional'	1 tbsp	80	0	0	330	0	8.0	0
(Herb Magic) no oil	2 tbsp	10	0	2	260	na	0.0	na
(Hidden Valley Ranch) Parmesan, lowfat	1 tbsp	16	0	3	140	0	1.0	0
(Hollywood)	1 tbsp	90	0	1	300	0	9.0	0
(Kraft)								
creamy, 'Deliciously Light'	1 tbsp	25	0	1	120	0	2.0	0
creamy, 'Reduce-Calorie'	1 tbsp	25	0	1	120	0	2.0	0
creamy, w/real sour cream	1 tbsp	50	0	1	120	0	5.0	0
'Deliciously Light'	1 tbsp	35	0	1	115	0	3.0	0
house	1 tbsp	60	0	1	115	0	6.0	0
house, reduced calorie	1 tbsp	30	0	1	115	0	2.0	0
nonfat	2 tbsp	20	0	4	430	0	0.0	0
nonfat, 'Free'	2 tbsp	20	0	4	430	0	0.3	1
nonfat, 'Healthy Sensation'	2 tbsp	15	0	2	280	0	0.0	0
nonfat, oil-free 'Reduce-Calorie'	1 tbsp	4	0	1	220	0	0.0	0
'Presto'	1 tbsp	70	0	1	150	0	7.0	0
zesty	2 tbsp	109	0	2	505	0	11.1	0
zesty	1 tbsp	50	0	1	260	0	5.0	0
zesty, reduced calorie	1 tbsp	20	0	1	230	0	2.0	0
(Litehouse) creamy, and dip, refrigerated	1 tbsp	60	0	0	76	0	6.0	0
(Nasoya)								
creamy	2 tbsp	61	1	3	188	0	5.2	0
'Vegi-Dressing'	1 tbsp	40	1	1	50	0	3.0	0
(Ott's)	1 tbsp	80	0	0	87	0	9.1	1
(Pritikin)								
sodium-free, nonfat	1 tbsp	8	0	2	0	0	0.0	0
zesty, nonfat	2 tbsp	20	0	5	115	0	0.0	0
(Seven Seas)								
creamy	2 tbsp	120	0	1	510	0	12.0	0
nonfat	2 tbsp	50	0	12	330	1	0.0	0
nonfat, 'Free Viva'	1 tbsp	4	0	1	220	0	0.0	0

Food Name	Serv. Size	Total Cal.	Prot. gms	Carbs gms	Sod. mgs	Fiber gms	Fat gms	Chol. mgs
'Viva Creamy Italian! Light'	1 tbsp	45	0	1	230	0	4.0	0
'Viva Italian! Light'	1 tbsp	30	0	1	230	0	3.0	0
'Viva'	1 tbsp	50	0	1	240	0	5.0	0
(T. Marzetti)								
creamy	1 tbsp	80	0	1	100	0	8.0	4
garlic, refrigerated	1 tbsp	81	0	1	73	0	9.0	9
gusto	1 tbsp	58	0	0	204	0	8.0	0
'Light'	1 tbsp	35	0	1	300	0	3.0	0
nonfat, 'Fat-Free'	1 tbsp	5	0	1	270	0	0.0	0
nonfat, 'Frenchette'	1 tbsp	6	0	2	280	0	0.0	0
'Olde Venice'	2 tbsp	130	0	2	490	0	13.0	0
Romano cheese, refrigerated	1 tbsp	77	1	1	183	0	8.0	3
Romano	1 tbsp	80	0	0	135	0	8.0	2
w/olive oil	1 tbsp	60	0	1	220	0	7.0	0
(Ultra Slim-Fast) cholesterol-free	1 tbsp	6	0	1	105	0	1.0	0
(Walden Farms)								
calorie-free	2 tbsp	0	0	0	350	0	0.0	0
country, calorie-free	2 tbsp	0	0	0	260	1	0.0	0
w/sun-dried tomatoes, calorie-free	2 tbsp	0	0	0	390	0	0.0	0
(Weight Watchers)								
	1 tbsp	2	0	0	140	0	0.0	0
creamy	1 tbsp	3	0	1	180	0	0.0	0
creamy, nonfat	1 tbsp	12	0	3	85	0	0.0	0
creamy, whipped	1 tbsp	50	0	2	80	0	5.0	5
nonfat	1 tbsp	6	0	1	200	0	0.0	0
nonfat, 'Single Serve'	0.75 oz	8	0	2	270	0	0.0	0
(Wish-Bone)								
	1 tbsp	46	0	2	280	0	4.5	0
'Lite'	1 tbsp	7	0	1	212	0	0.3	0
nonfat, 'Healthy Sensation!'	1 tbsp	6	0	1	140	0	0.0	0
olive oil, 'Classic'	1 tbsp	34	0	2	190	0	3.0	0
'Robusto'	1 tbsp	47	0	2	288	0	4.5	0
MAYONNAISE TYPE								
(A&P)	1 tbsp	70	1	2	100	0	7.0	0
(Bama)	1 tbsp	50	0	3	105	0	4.0	0
(Blue Plate)	1 tbsp	70	0	2	105	0	7.0	5
(Finast)	1 tbsp	70	0	2	90	0	7.0	0
(Hain) eggless, no salt added	1 tbsp	110	0	0	0	0	12.0	0
(JFG)	1 tbsp	50	0	2	125	0	5.0	5
(Kraft)								
light	1 tbsp	50	0	1	120	0	4.9	5
'Miracle Whip'	1 tbsp	70	0	2	85	0	7.0	5
'Miracle Whip Light'	1 tbsp	45	0	2	125	0	4.0	0
nonfat	1 tbsp	11	0	2	120	0	0.4	2
nonfat, 'Miracle Whip-Free'	1 tbsp	20	0	5	210	0	0.0	0
(Ott's) 'Famous'	1 tbsp	40	0	4	195	0	2.7	1
(P&Q)	1 tbsp	50	1	3	110	0	5.0	8
(Pathmark) 'No Frills'	1 tbsp	50	0	3	120	0	5.0	5
(Spin Blend)								
	1 tbsp	60	0	3	110	0	5.0	10
cholesterol-free	1 tbsp	40	0	2	110	0	4.0	0
(Weight Watchers)								
whipped	1 tbsp	45	0	3	100	0	4.0	0
whipped, low-sodium	1 tbsp	50	0	1	45	0	5.0	5
whipped, nonfat	1 tbsp	12	0	4	125	0	0.0	0
ONION								
(Kraft) and chives, creamy	1 tbsp	70	0	1	150	0	7.0	0

Food Name	Serv. Size	Total Cal.	Prot. gms	Carbs gms	Sod. mgs	Fiber gms	Fat gms	Chol. mgs
(Paula's) toasted, nonfat	2 tbsp	10	0	3	80	0	0.0	0
(Wish-Bone) and chives, 'Lite'	1 tbsp	37	0	2	164	0	3.3	0
ORIENTAL STYLE *(Featherweight)*	1 tbsp	20	0	1	75	0	2.0	0
PARMESAN *(T. Marzetti)* peppercorn, refrigerated	1 tbsp	81	1	1	129	0	9.0	6
PEANUT *(A Taste of Thai)* spicy	1 tbsp	40	1	6	360	1	1.5	0
PEPPERCORN								
(Litehouse) and dip, refrigerated	1 tbsp	67	0	0	66	0	7.0	0
(T. Marzetti) cracked, refrigerated	1 tbsp	62	0	0	135	0	7.0	13
(Weight Watchers) creamy, nonfat	1 tbsp	8	0	2	85	0	0.0	0
PESTO *(Cardini's)* pasta, w/basil	2 tbsp	140	0	0	195	0	14.0	0
POPPYSEED								
(Great Impressions)	2 tbsp	131	0	8	130	0	11.0	0
(Hain) Natural Classics	2 tbsp	140	1	3	250	0	14.0	5
(Knott's Berry Farm)								
	2 tbsp	120	0	10	190	0	9.0	0
Peggy Jane's'	1 tbsp	60	0	4	90	0	5.0	0
(La Martinique)	2 tbsp	170	0	8	330	0	15.0	na
(Litehouse) and dip, refrigerated	1 tbsp	65	0	3	83	0	6.0	0
(T. Marzetti) refrigerated	1 tbsp	72	1	5	146	0	6.0	8
POTATO SALAD								
(Best Foods) One Step	2 tbsp	160	0	2	370	0	17.0	5
(Blue Plate)	2 tbsp	130	0	1	380	0	14.0	15
(Hellmann's) One Step	2 tbsp	160	0	2	370	0	17.0	5
(JFG)	2 tbsp	130	0	1	380	0	14.0	15
(T. Marzetti)	1 tbsp	80	0	3	170	0	7.0	9
RANCH								
(Bernstein's) Parmesan garlic	2 tbsp	45	2	7	280	0	1.0	5
(Best Foods)								
homestyle	2 tsp	70	0	1	120	0	7.0	0
homestyle, light,	1 1/3 tbsp	70	0	2	200	0	7.0	0
(Hellmann's)								
homestyle	2 tsp	70	0	1	120	0	7.0	0
light, homestyle	1 1/3 tbsp	70	0	2	200	0	7.0	0
(Herb Magic) no oil	2 tbsp	15	1	4	270	na	0.0	0
(Hidden Valley Ranch)								
94% fat-free	2 tbsp	40	0	5	320	0	2.0	0
honey Dijon	2 tbsp	35	1	7	270	0	0.0	0
honey Dijon, low-fat	1 tbsp	20	0	3	140	0	1.0	0
original, 'Light'	1 tbsp	40	0	2	140	0	4.0	5
(Kraft)								
	2 tbsp	148	0	1	287	0	15.6	8
buttermilk	2 tbsp	150	0	1	240	0	16.0	3
cucumber	2 tbsp	140	0	2	220	0	15.0	0
light, 'Light Done Right!'	2 tbsp	77	0	3	303	0	6.8	8
nonfat	2 tbsp	48	0	11	354	0	0.3	0
nonfat, 'Healthy Sensation'	2 tbsp	40	0	9	280	0	0.0	0
peppercorn, nonfat	2 tbsp	45	0	11	330	1	0.0	0
w/salsa	2 tbsp	130	0	1	320	0	13.0	10
(Litehouse)								
and dip, refrigerated	1 tbsp	59	0	1	67	0	6.0	0
and dip, refrigerated, 'Lite	1 tbsp	35	1	1	80	0	3.0	0
country, and dip, refrigerated	1 tbsp	61	0	1	75	0	7.0	0
jalapeño, and dip, refrigerated	1 tbsp	60	0	1	80	0	6.0	0
(Pritikin) sodium-free, nonfat	1 tbsp	16	0	4	0	0	0.0	0
(Seven Seas)								
'Buttermilk Recipe Ranch! Light'	1 tbsp	50	0	1	135	0	5.0	0
nonfat	2 tbsp	45	0	11	330	1	0.0	0

Food Name	Serv. Size	Total Cal.	Prot. gms	Carbs gms	Sod. mgs	Fiber gms	Fat gms	Chol. mgs
'Viva Ranch! Light'	1 tbsp	50	0	2	125	0	5.0	5
'Viva'	1 tbsp	80	0	1	135	0	8.0	5
(T. Marzetti)								
(T. Marzetti)	1 tbsp	90	0	0	92	0	2.0	3
buttermilk, refrigerated	1 tbsp	93	0	0	127	0	10.0	2
buttermilk, refrigerated, 'Lite'	1 tbsp	45	0	1	135	0	5.0	3
Caesar	1 tbsp	95	1	1	150	0	10.0	3
fat-free	1 tbsp	12	1	3	220	0	0.0	0
garden	1 tbsp	100	0	1	165	0	10.0	2
honey Dijon	1 tbsp	89	1	1	100	0	9.0	14
'Light'	1 tbsp	40	0	2	166	0	4.0	2
Parmesan, refrigerated	1 tbsp	86	0	1	120	0	9.0	6
peppercorn	1 tbsp	85	0	1	13	0	9.0	4
peppercorn, fat-free	1 tbsp	14	0	3	173	0	0.0	0
(Walden Farms) calorie-free	2 tbsp	0	0	0	360	1	0.0	0
(Weight Watchers)								
creamy, nonfat	1 tbsp	25	0	6	100	0	0.0	0
creamy, nonfat, 'Single Serve'	1 pkt	35	0	8	140	0	0.0	0
(Wish-Bone)								
	1 tbsp	78	0	1	156	0	8.3	4
and salsa, 'Santa Fe'	2 tbsp	150	0	3	220	0	15.0	5
lite	2 tbsp	100	0	5	300	0	9.0	5
nonfat, 'Healthy Sensation!'	1 tbsp	16	0	3	140	0	0.0	0
RASPBERRY								
(Walden Farms) diet	2 tbsp	<1	0	0	380	0	0.0	0
(Pritikin) vinaigrette, w/olive oil	2 tbsp	45	0	11	70	0	0.0	0
RUSSIAN								
(Kraft)								
	1 tbsp	60	0	4	130	0	5.0	0
creamy	1 tbsp	60	0	2	150	0	5.0	5
reduced calorie	1 tbsp	30	0	4	130	0	1.0	0
w/pure honey, low-calorie	1 tbsp	60	0	4	130	0	5.0	0
(Featherweight) nonfat	1 tbsp	6	0	1	125	0	0.0	0
(S&W) Russian, 'Nutradiet'	1 tbsp	25	0	4	120	0	1.0	0
(Weight Watchers) whipped	1 tbsp	50	0	2	80	0	5.0	5
(Wish-Bone)								
	1 tbsp	46	0	6	147	0	2.5	0
'Food Service'	1 tbsp	47	0	6	147	0	2.5	0
'Lite'	1 tbsp	22	0	4	126	0	0.6	0
SAN FRANCISCO (Lawry's) w/Romano cheese, 'Classic'	1 oz	136	1	2	547	0	14.0	0
SESAME								
(Hain) honey	1 tbsp	60	0	2	210	0	5.0	0
(Nasoya) garlic	2 tbsp	63	1	3	137	0	5.4	0
SOUR CREAM								
(Crowley) nondairy	1 oz	40	1	1	5	0	4.0	0
(Friendship) 'Sour Treat'	1 oz	36	1	2	15	0	3.0	0
SPINACH SALAD (T. Marzetti) refrigerated	1 tbsp	35	0	2	100	0	10.0	0
SWEET AND SOUR								
(Herb Magic) no oil	2 tbsp	35	0	9	240	na	0.0	0
(Old Dutch) oil-, fat-, and cholesterol-free	2 tbsp	50	0	13	480	na	0.0	0
(T. Marzetti)								
'Fat-Free'	1 tbsp	20	0	5	130	0	0.0	0
'Light'	1 tbsp	45	0	5	105	0	3.0	0
refrigerated	1 tbsp	72	0	5	99	0	6.0	0
THOUSAND ISLAND								
(Best Foods) homestyle	1 1/3 tbsp	80	0	3	200	0	8.0	0
(Estee)	1 tbsp	8	0	2	30	0	0.0	0

Food Name	Serv. Size	Total Cal.	Prot. gms	Carbs gms	Sod. mgs	Fiber gms	Fat gms	Chol. mgs
(Featherweight)	1 tbsp	18	0	3	70	0	0.0	0
(Hain)	1 tbsp	50	0	0	85	0	5.0	0
(Hollywood)	1 tbsp	60	0	3	15	0	6.0	5
(Kraft)								
....	1 tbsp	60	0	2	150	0	5.0	5
'Free'	1 tbsp	20	0	5	135	0	0.0	0
reduced calorie	1 tbsp	20	0	3	135	0	1.0	0
w/bacon	1 tbsp	60	0	2	100	0	6.0	0
(Litehouse) and dip, refrigerated	1 tbsp	65	0	1	99	0	7.0	0
(S&W) 'Nutradiet'	1 tbsp	25	0	2	105	0	2.0	0
(Seven Seas)								
creamy	1 tbsp	50	0	2	150	0	5.0	5
'Thousand Island! Light'	1 tbsp	30	0	3	160	0	2.0	5
(T. Marzetti)								
....	1 tbsp	74	0	2	120	0	7.0	5
fat-free	1 tbsp	17	0	4	172	0	0.0	0
'Frenchette'	1 tbsp	20	0	3	155	0	0.0	4
light	1 tbsp	35	0	3	155	0	3.0	4
refrigerated	1 tbsp	82	0	6	93	0	5.0	0
(Ultra Slim-Fast) cholesterol-free	1 tbsp	18	0	4	95	0	1.0	0
(Walden Farms)	2 tbsp	0	0	0	290	1	0.0	0
(Weight Watchers) whipped	1 tbsp	50	0	2	80	0	5.0	5
(Wish-Bone)								
....	1 tbsp	63	0	3	158	0	5.6	7
'Lite'	1 tbsp	36	0	2	99	0	3.0	9
TOMATO								
(Cook's Classics) basil	1 tbsp	12	1	1	115	0	1.0	0
(Featherweight) zesty, nonfat	1 tbsp	2	0	0	5	0	0.0	0
TUNA SALAD								
(Best Foods) 'One Step'	2 tbsp	140	0	4	270	0	14.0	5
(Blue Plate)	2 tbsp	130	0	1	290	0	13.0	10
(Hellmann's) 'One Step'	2 tbsp	140	0	4	270	0	14.0	5
(JFG)	2 tbsp	130	0	1	290	0	13.0	10
VINAIGRETTE								
(Great Impressions) balsamic vinegar and oil	1 tbsp	67	1	2	367	0	6.5	0
(Hain)								
cheese	1 tbsp	55	0	0	130	0	6.0	5
Dijon	1 tbsp	50	0	0	180	0	5.0	5
Dijon, creamy, 'Natural Classics'	2 tbsp	130	0	3	280	0	13.0	3
Swiss cheese	1 tbsp	60	0	0	160	0	7.0	5
tomato, garden, 'Canola'	1 tbsp	60	0	1	150	0	6.0	0
(Herb Magic) no oil	2 tbsp	10	0	3	270	na	0.0	0
(Hollywood) Dijon	1 tbsp	60	0	2	40	0	6.0	0
(Knott's Berry Farm) w/sun dried tomato	1 tbsp	45	0	1	100	0	4.0	0
(Kraft) oil and vinegar	1 tbsp	70	0	1	210	0	8.0	0
(La Martinique) French	2 tbsp	170	0	0	430	na	19.0	na
(Lawry's)								
Chinese vinegar, w/sesame and ginger, 'Classic'	1 tbsp	145	0	2	325	0	15.0	0
(Litehouse) sour cream and chives, refrigerated	1 tbsp	63	0	1	72	0	7.0	0
(Marie's)								
herb, 'Lite and Zesty'	1 tbsp	16	0	4	130	0	0.0	0
Italian, 'Lite and Zesty'	1 tbsp	16	0	4	135	0	0.0	0
(Newman's Own) olive oil and vinegar	2 tbsp	150	0	1	150	0	16.0	0
(Pritikin)								
herb, sodium-free	1 tbsp	8	0	2	0	0	0.0	0
olive oil, raspberry	2 tbsp	45	0	11	70	0	0.0	0

Food Name	Serv. Size	Total Cal.	Prot. gms	Carbs gms	Sod. mgs	Fiber gms	Fat gms	Chol. mgs
(S&W)								
balsamic wine, 'Vintage Lites'	2 tbsp	35	0	8	460	0	0.0	0
mango key lime, 'Vintage Lites'	2 tbsp	30	0	7	390	0	0.0	0
Oriental rice wine, 'Vintage Lites'	2 tbsp	30	0	8	280	0	0.0	0
raspberry blush, 'Vintage Lites'	2 tbsp	40	0	10	410	0	0.0	0
red wine w/herb, 'Vintage Lites'	2 tbsp	40	0	11	440	0	0.0	0
white wine w/herb, 'Vintage Lites'	2 tbsp	40	0	10	450	0	0.0	0
(Seven Seas) red wine vinegar	2 tbsp	15	0	3	410	0	0.0	0
(Simply Delicious)								
ginger plum, 'Un-Dressing'	1 tbsp	36	0	1	199	0	4.0	0
herb garlic, 'Un-Dressing'	1 tbsp	43	0	1	132	0	4.0	0
honey mustard, 'Un-Dressing'	1 tbsp	41	0	2	122	0	4.0	0
lemon tahini, 'Un-Dressing'	1 tbsp	43	0	1	170	0	4.0	9
lime cilantro, 'Un-Dressing'	1 tbsp	41	0	1	116	0	4.0	0
pink peppercorn, 'Un-Dressing'	1 tbsp	40	0	1	148	0	4.0	0
(Walden Farms)								
balsamic, diet	2 tbsp	0	0	0	380	0	0.0	0
honey Dijon	2 tbsp	0	0	0	270	1	0.0	0
(Weight Watchers) tomato	1 tbsp	8	0	2	150	0	0.0	0
(Wish-Bone)								
Dijon, 'Classic'	1 tbsp	60	0	1	171	0	6.1	1
Dijon, lite	2 tbsp	60	0	3	410	0	5.0	0
olive oil	1 tbsp	28	0	2	111	0	2.3	0
olive oil, 'Lite'	1 tbsp	16	0	2	111	0	0.9	0
red wine	1 tbsp	51	0	4	216	0	3.8	0
VEGETABLE *(T. Marzetti)* and dip, refrigerated	1 tbsp	88	0	1	120	0	10.0	2
WINE VINEGAR								
(Estee) red wine, nonfat	1 tbsp	2	0	0	10	0	0.0	0
(Featherweight) red wine, nonfat	1 tbsp	6	0	1	100	0	0.0	0
(Great Impressions)								
red wine, and oil	1 tbsp	64	1	3	277	0	6.1	0
white wine, and oil	1 tbsp	63	1	1	242	0	6.6	0
(Kraft)								
red wine, and oil	1 tbsp	60	0	4	200	0	4.0	0
red wine, nonfat	2 tbsp	15	0	3	400	0	0.0	0
(Lawry's)								
red wine, w/Cabernet, 'Classics'	1 tbsp	138	0	5	178	0	13.7	0
vintage, w/sherry wine, 'Classics'	1 tbsp	110	4	3	415	0	10.5	0
white wine, w/Chardonnay, 'Classic'	1 tbsp	153	0	3	178	0	15.7	0
(Marie's) white wine, nonfat, 'Lite and Zesty'	1 tbsp	20	0	5	135	0	0.0	0
(Pathmark) red wine, and oil	1 tbsp	70	0	2	235	0	7.0	0
(Seven Seas)								
red wine, and oil, 'Viva Red Wine!'	1 tbsp	45	0	1	190	0	4.0	0
red wine, and oil, 'Viva'	1 tbsp	70	0	1	290	0	7.0	0
SALAD DRESSING MIX								
BACON *(Lawry's)* mix only	1 pkg	65	5	9	1820	1	0.8	0
BLUE CHEESE								
(Best Foods) blue cheese, homestyle, mix only	2 tsp	45	0	1	130	0	4.5	10
(Good Seasons)								
and herbs, mix only	1 pkg	4	0	1	150	0	0.0	0
and herbs, prepared	1 tbsp	70	0	1	150	0	8.0	0
(Hain) 'No Oil' prepared	1 tbsp	14	1	1	180	0	1.0	5
(Hidden Valley Ranch)								
mix only	1.1 oz	112	4	19	1931	0	2.0	0
prepared	1 tbsp	58	0	1	95	0	6.0	2
(Tone's) blue cheese, mix only	1 tsp	13	0	2	146	0	0.2	0
(Weight Watchers) mix only	1 tbsp	8	0	1	110	0	0.0	0

Food Name	Serv. Size	Total Cal.	Prot. gms	Carbs gms	Sod. mgs	Fiber gms	Fat gms	Chol. mgs
BUTTERMILK								
(Good Seasons)								
'Farm Style' prepared	1 tbsp	60	1	1	135	0	6.0	5
nonfat, 'Farm Style' mix only	1 pkg	4	0	1	95	0	0.0	0
(Hain) 'No Oil' prepared	1 tbsp	11	1	1	150	0	1.0	0
(Hidden Valley Ranch) original recipe, prepared	1 tbsp	58	0	1	110	0	3.0	4
(Tone's) mix only	1 tsp	10	0	2	389	1	0.2	1
CAESAR								
(Good Seasons) gourmet, prepared	2 tbsp	150	0	3	300	0	16.0	0
(Hain) 'No Oil' prepared	1 tbsp	6	0	1	200	0	1.0	0
(Lawry's) mix only	1 pkg	75	3	9	1962	0	3.1	0
CHEESE								
(Good Seasons)								
garlic, mix only	1 serving	40	0	8	2640	0	0.0	0
garlic, prepared	2 tbsp	140	0	1	330	0	16.0	0
Italian, mix only	1 pkg	4	0	1	130	0	0.0	0
CHICKEN SALAD *(Kikkoman)* Chinese, mix only	1 tbsp	30	1	6	500	0	0.0	0
DILL								
(Good Seasons)								
'Classic' mix only	1 tbsp	2	0	0	150	0	0.0	0
'Classic' prepared	1 tbsp	70	0	1	150	0	8.0	0
(Knorr) and dip, mix only	1 tbsp	2	1	1	65	0	1.0	0
FRENCH								
(Hain) 'No Oil' prepared	1 tbsp	12	0	3	340	0	0.0	0
(Weight Watchers) mix only	1 tbsp	3	0	1	150	0	0.0	0
GARLIC								
(Good Seasons)								
and herb, mix only	1 serving	40	0	8	2720	0	0.0	0
and herb, prepared	1 tbsp	70	0	1	190	0	8.0	0
(Hain) and cheese, 'No Oil' prepared	1 tbsp	6	1	1	180	0	1.0	0
HERB								
(Good Seasons)								
'Classic' mix only	1 pkg	2	0	0	150	0	0.0	0
'Classic' prepared	1 tbsp	70	0	1	150	0	8.0	0
zesty, lowfat recipe, prepared	1 tbsp	12	0	1	150	0	1.0	0
zesty, mix only	1 tbsp	6	0	1	130	0	0.0	0
zesty, nonfat recipe, prepared	1 tbsp	6	0	1	150	0	0.0	0
(Hain) 'No Oil' prepared	1 tbsp	2	0	1	140	0	0.0	0
(Hidden Valley Ranch)								
creamy, mix only	0.9 oz	76	3	16	1931	0	0.0	0
creamy, prepared	1 tbsp	58	0	1	100	0	6.0	5
HONEY MUSTARD								
(Good Seasons)								
low-fat recipe, prepared	1 tbsp	18	0	2	130	0	1.0	0
nonfat recipe, mix only	1 serving	160	0	40	2240	0	0.0	0
nonfat recipe, prepared	1 tbsp	10	0	2	130	0	0.0	0
prepared	1 tbsp	80	0	2	125	0	8.0	0
ITALIAN								
(Good Seasons)								
cheese, 'Lite' mix only	1 tbsp	25	0	1	135	0	3.0	0
cheese, mix only	1 pkg	4	0	1	130	0	0.0	0
cheese, prepared	1 tbsp	70	0	1	130	0	8.0	0
creamy, fat-free recipe, prepared	1 tbsp	8	0	2	140	0	0.0	0
creamy, low-fat recipe, prepared	1 tbsp	16	0	2	150	0	1.0	0
creamy, nonfat, mix only	1 serving	80	0	24	2160	0	0.0	0
lemon and herbs, mix only	1 tbsp	70	0	1	140	0	8.0	0
lemon and herbs, prepared	1 tbsp	70	0	1	140	0	8.0	0

Food Name	Serv. Size	Total Cal.	Prot. gms	Carbs gms	Sod. mgs	Fiber gms	Fat gms	Chol. mgs
'Lite' mix only .... 1 tbsp		25	0	1	180	0	3.0	0
mild, mix only .... 1 serving		80	0	16	2960	0	0.0	0
mild, prepared .... 1 tbsp		70	0	1	190	0	8.0	0
mix only .... 1 serving		40	0	8	2560	0	0.0	0
mix only .... 1 tbsp		6	0	1	170	0	0.0	0
'No Oil' mix only .... 1 tbsp		6	0	2	30	0	0.0	0
nonfat, mix only .... 1 serving		80	0	24	2320	0	0.0	0
nonfat, prepared .... 2 tbsp		10	0	3	290	0	0.0	0
prepared w/o oil .... 1 tbsp		6	0	2	30	0	0.0	0
prepared .... 1 tbsp		70	0	1	170	0	8.0	0
prepared .... 2 tbsp		140	0	1	320	0	15.0	0
zesty, 'Lite' mix only .... 1 tbsp		25	0	1	135	0	3.0	0
zesty, 'Lite' prepared .... 1 tbsp		25	0	1	135	0	3.0	0
zesty, mix only .... 1 pkg		2	0	1	120	0	0.0	0
zesty, mix only .... 1 serving		40	0	8	1760	0	0.0	0
zesty, prepared .... 1 tbsp		70	0	1	120	0	8.0	0
(Lawry's)								
mix only .... 1 pkg		45	2	9	2255	0	0.2	0
w/cheese, mix only .... 1 pkg		74	2	12	1624	0	2.1	0
(Tone's)								
creamy, mix only .... 1 tsp		13	0	3	251	0	0.1	0
mix only .... 1 tsp		12	0	3	323	0	0.1	0
LEMON								
(Good Seasons)								
and herbs, Italian, prepared .... 1 tbsp		70	0	1	140	0	8.0	0
and herbs, Italian, mix only .... 1 pkg		2	0	1	140	0	0.0	0
RANCH								
(Good Seasons)								
'Lite' prepared .... 1 tbsp		30	1	2	115	0	2.0	5
Italian, 'Lite' prepared .... 1 tbsp		30	1	2	115	0	2.0	5
Italian, prepared .... 1 tbsp		60	0	1	110	0	6.0	5
lower calorie, mix only .... 1 serving		160	0	32	3202	0	0.0	0
mix only .... 1 serving		80	0	16	2243	0	0.0	0
prepared .... 1 tbsp		60	0	1	110	0	6.0	5
(Hidden Valley Ranch)								
lower calorie, mix only .... 1.1 oz		98	3	17	2301	0	2.0	0
lower calorie, prepared .... 1 tbsp		35	0	2	120	0	3.0	4
original, mix only .... 1 oz		93	3	18	2211	0	1.0	0
original, prepared .... 1 tbsp		58	0	1	105	0	6.0	5
w/bacon, mix only .... 1.2 oz		118	7	1	1953	0	2.0	0
w/bacon, prepared .... 1 tbsp		58	0	1	135	0	6.0	5
RUSSIAN *(Weight Watchers)* mix only .... 1 tbsp		4	0	1	120	0	0.0	0
SESAME, Oriental *(Good Seasons)* mix only .... 1/8 envelope		15	0	3	360	0	0.0	0
SOY SESAME *(Kikkoman)* mix only .... 2 tsp		15	1	3	270	0	1.0	0
THOUSAND ISLAND								
(Best Foods) homestyle, mix only .... 2 tsp		40	0	1	110	0	4.0	0
(Weight Watchers) nonfat, mix only .... 1 tbsp		4	0	1	140	0	0.0	0
VINAIGRETTE Oriental *(Kikkoman)* mix only .... 2 tsp		20	0	3	230	0	0.0	0
SALAD MIX								
(Suddenly Salad)								
Caesar, mix only .... 2/3 cup		150	5	30	580	1	1.0	0
Caesar, prepared .... 3/4 cup		220	5	30	580	1	9.0	0
ranch, and bacon, prepared .... 3/4 cup		330	7	30	480	1	20.0	15
ranch, and bacon, low-fat, prepared .... 3/4 cup		180	7	30	530	1	2.0	3
SALAD SEASONING. See under SEASONING MIX.								
SALAD TOPPING								
(Produce Partners) seasoned .... 1 tbsp		30	2	3	40	0	1.0	0

Food Name	Serv. Size	Total Cal.	Prot. gms	Carbs gms	Sod. mgs	Fiber gms	Fat gms	Chol. mgs
(Salad Crispins)								
bacon and onion, 'American Style'	1 tbsp	35	1	4	125	0	1.0	0
cheddar and onion	1 tbsp	35	1	4	115	0	1.0	0
Italian style, w/Parmesan cheese	1 tbsp	35	1	4	95	0	1.0	0
ranch	1 tbsp	35	1	4	125	0	1.0	0
(Salad Nibbler)								
buttermilk ranch, crouton topping	1 oz	128	7	13	241	0	5.0	2
cheddar, seasoned, crouton topping	1 oz	129	6	13	224	0	6.0	2
(Schilling) seasoned	1 tbsp	35	1	2	95	0	1.5	0
(Special Edition)								
garlic and cheese, sesame, nuggets	1 tbsp	40	1	3	130	0	2.5	0
sesame, nuggets	1 tbsp	35	1	3	115	0	2.5	0
(Tone's) 'American'	1 tsp	7	1	1	34	0	0.3	1

SALISBURY STEAK. See under BEEF DINNER/ENTRÉE.

SALMON

ATLANTIC

Fresh

farmed, baked, broiled, grilled, or microwaved	3 oz	175	19	0	52	0	10.5	54
farmed, raw	3 oz	156	17	0	50	0	9.2	50
wild, baked, broiled, grilled, or microwaved	3 oz	155	22	0	48	0	6.9	60
wild, raw	3 oz	121	17	0	37	0	5.4	47

BLUEBACK. See under SOCKEYE.

CHINOOK/king

Fresh

baked, broiled, grilled, or microwaved	3 oz	196	22	0	51	0	11.4	72
raw	3 oz	153	17	0	40	0	8.9	56

Smoked

	3 oz	99	16	0	666	0	3.7	20
boneless	1 oz	33	5	0	222	0	1.2	7
flaked	1 cup	159	25	0	1066	0	5.9	31
lox	3 oz	99	16	0	1700	0	3.7	20
lox	1 oz	33	5	0	567	0	1.2	7

CHUM/keta

Canned

(Bumble Bee)	1 cup	306	47	0	0	0	11.4	0
(Libby's)	3.7 oz	130	20	0	450	0	6.0	40
drained, w/bone	3 oz	120	18	0	414	0	4.7	33
drained, w/bone, no salt added	3 oz	120	18	0	64	0	4.7	33
w/liquid *(Bumble Bee)*	3.5 oz	160	20	0	490	0	8.0	60

Fresh

baked, broiled, grilled, or microwaved	3 oz	131	22	0	54	0	4.1	81
raw	3 oz	102	17	0	43	0	3.2	63

Frozen

(Peter Pan Seafoods) fillet portion, raw	3.5 oz	120	20	0	50	0	3.8	74
(Peter Pan Seafoods) side, pinbone in, raw	3.5 oz	120	20	0	50	0	3.8	74
(Peter Pan Seafoods) steak, raw	3.5 oz	120	20	0	50	0	3.8	74

COHO/silver

Canned

meat only *(Deming's)*	1/2 cup	140	22	0	450	0	5.0	0

Fresh

farmed, baked, broiled, grilled, or microwaved	3 oz	151	21	0	44	0	7.0	54
farmed, raw	3 oz	136	18	0	40	0	6.5	43
wild, baked, broiled, grilled, or microwaved	3 oz	118	20	0	49	0	3.7	47
wild, boiled or poached	3 oz	156	23	0	45	0	6.4	48
wild, raw	3 oz	124	18	0	39	0	5.0	38

HUMPBACK. See PINK.

KETA. See COHO.

Food Name	Serv. Size	Total Cal.	Prot. gms	Carbs gms	Sod. mgs	Fiber gms	Fat gms	Chol. mgs
KING. See CHINOOK.								
MIXED SPECIES								
Canned, boneless, skinless *(Libby's)*	3.25 oz	110	16	1	420	0	4.0	50
Frozen, steak, w/o seasoning mix *(SeaPak)*	8-oz pkg	270	46	0	115	0	9.0	170
Smoked, Nova, sliced *(Lascco)*	3 oz	120	18	0	1070	0	6.0	35
PINK/humpback								
Canned								
(Captains Choice)	3 oz	110	16	0	420	0	5.0	55
Alaska, w/liquid *(Deming's)*	1/2 cup	140	20	0	450	0	6.0	65
Alaskan, fancy *(Crown Prince)*	3.5 oz	140	20	0	450	0	6.0	40
Alaskan, fresh packed *(Libby's)*	3.7 oz	130	20	0	450	0	6.0	40
boneless, skinless *(Chicken of the Sea)*	2 oz	60	10	0	280	0	2.0	20
boneless, skinless, w/liquid *(Bumble Bee)*	3.5 oz	120	17	0	420	0	5.0	25
chunk, boneless, skinless, w/liquid *(Deming's)*	3.25 oz	120	17	0	420	0	5.0	0
drained, w/bones	3 oz	118	17	0	64	0	5.1	47
w/bones and liquid	3 oz	118	17	0	471	0	5.1	47
w/liquid *(Bumble Bee)*	1 cup	310	45	0	851	0	13.0	0
w/liquid *(Bumble Bee)*	3.5 oz	160	20	0	490	0	8.0	50
w/liquid *(Del Monte)*	1/2 cup	160	22	0	660	0	7.0	0
w/liquid *(Featherweight)*	2 oz	70	11	0	45	0	3.0	20
w/liquid *(Libby's)*	7.75 oz	310	45	0	790	0	13.0	0
Fresh								
baked, broiled, grilled, or microwaved	3 oz	127	22	0	73	0	3.8	57
raw	3 oz	99	17	0	57	0	2.9	44
RED. See SOCKEYE.								
SILVER. See COHO.								
SOCKEYE/red								
Canned								
(Bumble Bee)	1 cup	376	45	0	1148	0	20.5	0
(Libby's)	7.75 oz	380	45	0	760	0	21.0	0
(S&W)	3 oz	152	18	0	369	0	8.8	56
Alaska *(Deming's)*	1/2 cup	170	20	0	450	0	9.0	65
Alaska, medium *(Deming's)*	1/2 cup	150	21	0	450	0	7.0	65
blueback *(Rubinstein's)*	1/2 cup	170	20	0	450	0	9.0	0
blueback, 'Fancy' *(S&W)*	1/2 cup	190	25	0	590	0	10.0	0
boneless, skinless, w/liquid *(Bumble Bee)*	3.5 oz	130	17	0	420	0	6.0	30
drained, w/bone	3 oz	130	17	0	457	0	6.2	37
drained, w/bone, no salt added	3 oz	130	17	0	64	0	6.2	37
'Nutradiet' *(S&W)*	1/2 cup	188	22	0	47	0	11.0	0
w/liquid *(Bumble Bee)*	3.5 oz	180	20	0	490	0	10.0	60
w/liquid *(Del Monte)*	1/2 cup	180	23	0	660	0	9.0	0
Fresh								
baked, broiled, grilled, or microwaved	3 oz	184	23	0	56	0	9.3	74
raw	3 oz	143	18	0	40	0	7.3	53
SALMON OIL. See under FISH OIL.								
SALMON SUBSTITUTE *(Mox Lox)* smoked	1.5 oz	25	2	3	380	0	1.0	5
SALSA. See also under SAUCE.								
(Arizona Cactus Ranch)								
cactus fruit or prickly pear, organic	2 tbsp	15	1	4	120	0	0.0	0
(Chi-Chi's)								
hot	1 oz	8	2	2	153	0	2.0	2
medium	1 oz	7	2	2	135	0	2.0	2
mild	1 oz	7	2	2	116	0	2.0	2
(Del Monte)								
burrito, can or jar	1/4 cup	20	0	4	355	0	0.0	0
green chili, mild	1/4 cup	20	0	3	590	0	0.0	0
roja, mild	1/4 cup	20	0	4	510	0	0.0	0

Food Name	Serv. Size	Total Cal.	Prot. gms	Carbs gms	Sod. mgs	Fiber gms	Fat gms	Chol. mgs
(Eagle)								
medium	2 tbsp	10	3	2	250	1	0.0	0
mild	2 tbsp	10	3	2	250	1	0.0	0
w/cheese, medium	2 tbsp	40	1	3	300	0	3.0	5
(Enrico's)								
hot, chunky style	2 tbsp	8	1	2	34	0	0.0	0
hot, chunky style, no salt added	2 tbsp	8	1	2	10	0	0.0	0
mild, chunky style	2 tbsp	8	1	2	34	0	0.0	0
mild, chunky style, no salt added	2 tbsp	8	1	2	10	0	0.0	0
(Garden of Eden)								
nonfat, organic, 'Great Garlic/Hot Habenero'	2 tbsp	10	0	2	95	0	0.0	0
(Guiltless Gourmet)								
medium	2 tbsp	10	0	2	140	0	0.0	0
red pepper, roasted	2 tbsp	10	0	2	120	0	0.0	0
Southwestern grill	2 tbsp	10	0	2	150	0	0.0	0
tomatillo	2 tbsp	10	0	2	160	1	0.0	0
(Hain)								
green chili, hot	1/4 cup	22	1	4	480	0	0.0	0
mild	1/2 cup	20	1	4	410	0	0.0	0
(Heluva Good)								
hot	2 tbsp	10	0	2	180	0	0.0	0
mild	2 tbsp	10	0	2	180	0	0.0	0
(Hot Cha Cha) 'Texas'	1 oz	6	0	3	2	0	0.0	0
(Kaukauna)								
Mexican, medium	2 tbsp	15	0	3	170	0	0.0	0
Mexican, mild	2 tbsp	15	0	3	170	0	0.0	0
(La Victoria)								
'Brava'	1 tbsp	6	1	1	100	0	1.0	0
'Casera'	1 tbsp	4	1	1	80	0	1.0	0
chili dip, chunky	2 tbsp	9	0	2	148	0	0.0	na
green chili	2 tbsp	10	0	2	150	0	0.0	0
green chili, mild	2 tbsp	8	0	1	175	0	0.1	na
green jalapeño	1 tbsp	4	1	1	105	0	1.0	0
green jalapeño	2 tbsp	10	0	1	181	0	0.3	0
hot	1 tbsp	2	0	0	33	0	0.1	0
hot	2 tbsp	9	0	2	171	0	0.1	0
hot, 'Victoria'	2 tbsp	7	0	1	163	0	0.1	0
hot, thick and chunky	2 tbsp	9	0	1	133	0	0.1	0
jalapeña	2 tbsp	12	0	2	148	0	0.2	0
medium	2 tbsp	8	0	1	150	0	0.1	0
medium, 'Suprema'	2 tbsp	8	0	1	166	0	0.1	0
medium, thick and chunky	2 tbsp	8	0	1	160	0	0.1	0
mild	2 tbsp	8	0	1	182	0	0.1	0
mild, 'Suprema'	2 tbsp	8	0	2	179	0	0.1	0
mild, thick and chunky	2 tbsp	8	0	1	157	0	0.1	0
omelet	1 tbsp	6	1	1	95	0	1.0	0
'Ranchera'	1 tbsp	6	1	1	85	0	1.0	0
red jalapeño	1 tbsp	6	1	1	95	0	1.0	0
'Suprema'	2 tbsp	10	0	2	220	0	0.0	0
'Victoria'	1 tbsp	4	1	1	80	0	1.0	0
(Litehouse) medium, 'Zesty'	1 tbsp	4	0	1	110	0	0.0	0
(Mi Ranchito)								
hot, restaurant style	2 tbsp	10	0	2	120	0	0.0	0
mild, fat-free, restaurant style	2 tbsp	10	0	2	120	0	0.0	0
(Millina's Finest) hot, mild or garlic, fat-free, organic	2 tbsp	10	0	2	60	0	0.0	0
(Mission)								
hot	2 tbsp	5	0	2	70	0	0.0	0

Food Name	Serv. Size	Total Cal.	Prot. gms	Carbs gms	Sod. mgs	Fiber gms	Fat gms	Chol. mgs
mild	2 tbsp	5	0	2	70	0	0.0	0
'Poco Picante'	2 tbsp	5	0	2	70	0	0.0	0
(Nabisco)								
green chili, hot	1 tbsp	6	0	2	190	0	0.0	0
green chili, medium	1 tbsp	6	0	1	190	0	0.0	0
green chili, mild	1 tbsp	8	0	2	190	0	0.0	0
taco, hot, can or jar, 'Thick & Smooth'	1 tbsp	8	0	2	105	0	0.0	0
taco, medium, can or jar, 'Thick & Smooth'	1 tbsp	8	0	2	105	0	0.0	0
taco, mild, can or jar, 'Thick & Smooth'	1 tbsp	8	0	2	115	0	0.0	0
(Old El Paso)								
green chili, medium	2 tbsp	10	0	2	110	1	0.0	0
green chili, 'Thick 'n Chunky'	2 tbsp	3	0	1	270	0	0.0	0
homestyle, medium	2 tbsp	5	0	1	110	0	0.0	0
homestyle, mild	2 tbsp	5	0	1	110	0	0.0	0
hot, 'Pico de Gallo'	2 tbsp	5	0	2	260	1	0.0	0
hot, 'Thick n' Chunky'	2 tbsp	10	0	2	130	0	0.0	0
medium, 'Pico de Gallo'	2 tbsp	5	0	2	260	1	0.0	0
medium, 'Salsa Verde'	2 tbsp	10	0	2	95	0	0.0	0
medium, 'Thick n'Chunky'	2 tbsp	10	0	2	140	0	0.0	0
mild or medium, chunky	2 tbsp	15	1	3	230	1	0.0	0
mild, 'Thick n' Chunky'	2 tbsp	10	0	2	140	0	0.0	0
taco, hot	1 tbsp	5	0	1	90	0	0.0	0
taco, medium	1 tbsp	5	0	1	70	0	0.0	0
taco, mild	1 tbsp	5	0	1	85	0	0.0	0
taco, mild, extra chunky	1 tbsp	5	0	1	80	0	0.0	0
verde, 'Thick 'n Chunky'	2 tbsp	10	1	2	135	0	1.0	0
(Ortega)								
green chili, hot	1 oz	10	0	2	180	0	0.0	0
green chili, medium	1 oz	8	0	2	180	0	0.0	0
green chili, mild	1 oz	8	0	2	180	0	0.0	0
medium, thick and chunky	1 tbsp	4	0	1	150	0	0.0	0
ranchera	1 oz	12	0	3	250	0	0.0	0
taco, hot, can or jar	1 oz	10	0	2	300	0	0.0	0
taco, mild, can or jar	1 oz	10	0	2	290	0	0.0	0
(Pablo's)								
hot, 'Deli Style'	1 oz	10	1	2	250	0	0.0	0
mild, 'Deli Style'	1 oz	10	1	2	250	0	0.0	0
(Pace)								
medium, thick and chunky	2 tbsp	4	1	1	101	0	1.0	0
mild, thick and chunky	2 tbsp	4	1	1	101	0	1.0	0
salsa dip, medium, 'Chunky'	2 tbsp	4	1	1	102	0	1.0	0
salsa dip, mild, 'Chunky'	2 tbsp	4	1	1	101	0	1.0	0
(Parrot Brand)								
black bean, medium, organic, nonfat	2 tbsp	10	0	2	115	1	0.0	0
hot, fat-free, organic	2 tbsp	10	1	2	72	1	0.0	0
pinto bean, medium, fat-free, organic	2 tbsp	9	0	2	64	10	0.0	0
tomatillo, spicy, all natural, 'Green Verde'	2 tbsp	17	0	2	91	1	0.0	0
(Pritikin) very low-sodium	1/4 cup	25	1	5	15	0	0.0	0
(Progresso)								
Italian, hot	2 tbsp	10	1	2	170	1	0.0	0
Italian, medium	2 tbsp	10	1	2	170	1	0.0	0
Italian, mild	2 tbsp	10	1	2	170	1	0.0	0
(Rosarita)								
green chili, mild, food service product	2 tbsp	7	0	2	167	0	0.1	0
green chili, extra chunky, 'de Mexico Style'	2 tbsp	30	1	7	280	0	1.0	0
green chili, mild	1.09 oz	7	0	2	167	0	0.1	0
green tomatillo, 'de Mexico Style'	2 tbsp	20	1	4	190	0	1.0	0

Food Name	Serv. Size	Total Cal.	Prot. gms	Carbs gms	Sod. mgs	Fiber gms	Fat gms	Chol. mgs
green tomatillo, medium	2 tbsp	8	0	2	188	1	0.2	0
hot, chunky	3 tbsp	25	1	6	300	1	1.0	0
jalapeño picante, hot	2 tbsp	8	0	2	240	0	0.1	0
jalapeño picante, medium	2 tbsp	8	0	2	240	0	0.1	0
jalapeño picante, mild	2 tbsp	8	0	2	239	0	0.1	0
medium, chunky	3 tbsp	25	1	6	350	1	1.0	0
medium, extra chunky	2 tbsp	7	0	1	228	0	0.2	0
mild, 'Casa Mamita'	1.13 oz	7	0	1	170	0	0.1	0
mild, chunky	3 tbsp	25	1	6	340	1	1.0	0
picante, food service product	2 tbsp	26	0	6	342	0	0.1	0
roasted, mild	2 tbsp	10	0	2	232	1	0.3	0
taco, medium, chunky	3 tbsp	25	1	6	310	1	1.0	0
taco, mild	2 oz	27	1	6	304	0	0.1	1
taco, mild, chunky	3 tbsp	25	1	6	300	1	1.0	0
traditional, 'de Mexico Style'	2 tbsp	12	1	3	350	0	0.0	0
traditional, medium	2 tbsp	7	0	2	234	1	0.1	0
traditional, mild	2 tbsp	7	1	1	248	1	0.1	0
(S&W)								
hot, 'Sun-Vista'	2 tbsp	5	0	2	170	1	0.0	0
medium, 'Ready Cut'	1/4 cup	20	1	4	190	1	0.0	0
mild, 'Ready Cut'	1/4 cup	20	1	4	190	1	0.0	0
w/chipotle, 'Ready Cut'	1/4 cup	20	1	4	190	1	0.0	0
w/cilantro, 'Ready Cut'	1/4 cup	20	1	4	190	1	0.0	0
(Santiago) chunky	1 fl oz	10	0	2	232	0	0.1	0
(Sun Vista) hot	2 tbsp	5	0	2	170	1	0.0	0
(Territorial House) green chili	0.5 oz	4	1	1	80	0	1.0	0
(Timpone's) tomato, fresh roasted, 'Salsa Muy Rica'	2 tbsp	10	0	2	110	0	0.0	0
(Tostitos)								
con queso	4 tbsp	80	2	10	560	1	5.0	5
con queso, low-fat	4 tbsp	80	2	8	560	1	3.0	5
medium or hot	4 tbsp	30	2	6	520	2	0.0	0
mild	4 tbsp	30	2	6	520	2	0.0	0
'Ultimate Garden'	4 tbsp	30	2	6	460	2	0.0	0
SALSIFY/oyster plant/vegetable oyster								
boiled, drained, sliced	1 cup	92	4	21	22	4	0.2	0
boiled, drained, sliced	1/2 cup	46	1.9	10.5	11	2.1	0.1	0
raw, sliced	1 cup	109	4	25	27	4	0.3	0
raw, sliced	1/2 cup	55	2.2	12.5	13	2.2	0.1	0
SALSIFY, BLACK/scorzonera								
raw	1 lb	372	15.0	84.4	91	(mq)	0.1	0
raw	1 oz	23	0.9	5.3	6	(mq)	tr	0
SALT								
iodized *(Morton)*	1 tsp	0	0	0	2300	0	0.0	0
kosher *(Morton)*	1 tsp	0	0	0	1880	0	0.0	0
'Nature's Seasons' *(Morton)*	1 tsp	3	0	1	1400	0	0.1	0
non-iodized *(Morton)*	1 tsp	0	0	0	2300	0	0.0	0
sea *(Hain)*	1 tsp	0	0	0	2255	0	0.0	0
sea *(Tone's)*	1 tsp	0	0	0	2132	0	0.0	0
table	1 cup	0	0	0	113173	0	0.0	0
table	1 dash	0	0	0	155	0	0.0	0
table	1 tbsp	0	0	0	6976	0	0.0	0
table	1 tsp	0	0	0	2325	0	0.0	0
SALT PORK. See PORK, SALT.								
SALT SEASONING. See under SEASONING MIX.								
SALT SUBSTITUTE								
(Featherweight)	1/4 tsp	0	0	0	0	0	0.0	0
(Morton)	1 tsp	1	0	0	1	0	0.0	0

Food Name	Serv. Size	Total Cal.	Prot. gms	Carbs gms	Sod. mgs	Fiber gms	Fat gms	Chol. mgs
'Chef Shaker' *(Diamond Crystal)*	1/2 tsp	0	0	0	0	na	0.0	0
extra spicy *(Mrs. Dash)*	0.13 tsp	2	0	0	1	na	0.0	0
'Lite' *(Lawry's)*	1 tsp	8	0	2	357	0	0.1	0
lite, 1/2 the salt of regular salt *(Morton)*	1/4 tsp	0	0	0	290	0	0.0	0
'Lite Salt' *(Morton)*	1 tsp	1	0	0	1100	0	0.0	0
'Salt-Free' *(Lawry's)*	1 tsp	10	0	2	2	0	0.2	0
'Salt-It' *(Estee)*	1/8 tsp	0	0	0	0	0	0.0	0
seasoned *(Adolph's)*	1/4 tsp	0	0	0	0	0	0.0	0
seasoned *(Featherweight)*	1/4 tsp	0	0	0	0	0	0.0	0
seasoned *(Morton)*	1 tsp	2	0	1	1	0	0.1	0
seasoned *(Mrs. Dash)*	0.13 tsp	2	0	0	1	na	0.0	0
seasoned, 'Instead of Salt' *(Health Valley)*	1 tsp	11	1	2	3	0	0.5	0
seasoned, 'Salt-Free' *(Lawry's)*	1 tsp	3	0	1	7	0	0.1	0
SAND PEAR. See ASIAN PEAR.								
SANDWICH								
BEEF								
(Healthy Choice) Philly beef steak, 'Hearty Handfuls'	1 entrée	290	16	47	550	5	5.0	15
(Hot Pockets)								
beef and cheddar stuffed sandwich, frozen	1 pkg	403	16	39	906	na	20.2	53
pocket, w/cheddar, frozen	5 oz	370	17	36	1390	0	17.0	60
pocket, w/cheese, no gravy, 'Beef & Cheddar'	1 pocket	524	17	36	620	1	34.8	42
(Igor's Piroshki) pocket, w/cheddar	1 sandwich	370	15	31	630	2	20.0	45
(Kid Cuisine)								
double patty w/cheese, frozen, 'Mega Meal'	9.1 oz	480	20	55	1040	0	20.0	0
patty w/cheese, frozen	6.25 oz	400	12	47	550	0	19.0	40
(Lean Pockets) pocket, w/broccoli, frozen	1 pkg	250	11	30	760	0	8.0	0
(Manwich)								
'Chili Fixin's'	1 cup	290	20	20	980	5	14.0	65
extra thick and chunky, prepared	1 sandwich	330	17	36	870	3	13.0	50
Mexican, prepared	1 sandwich	310	17	30	690	2	13.0	50
'sloppy Joe', prepared	1 sandwich	310	17	31	620	1	13.0	50
(MicroMagic)								
burger, w/cheese, frozen	4.75 oz	450	17	29	790	0	25.0	80
hamburger, frozen	4 oz	350	13	26	500	0	18.0	55
(Mrs. Paterson's)								
steak, w/mushroom, pocket, hand held, 'Aussie Pie'	5.5 oz	410	14	43	820	0	20.0	80
(Pierre)								
submarine, flame-broiled	1 piece	152	16	2	294	1	8.9	41
submarine, flame-broiled, 'Hot Diggity Sub'	1 piece	158	16	2	291	1	9.5	41
(Tyson) barbecue, no bone, frozen, microwave	1 sandwich	200	15	29	600	0	2.7	30
CALZONE								
(Amy's Kitchen) cheese, pocket, organic, frozen	1 sandwich	290	14	38	390	3	9.0	20
CANADIAN BACON								
(Quick Meal)								
Canadian bacon, w/egg and cheese, on muffin	4.5 oz	250	16	29	680	0	8.0	115
CHICKEN								
(Banquet) breast patty, bun, microwave	4 oz	310	16	31	664	0	14.0	0
(BestFresh)								
breast, teriyaki, charbroiled	1 sandwich	490	34	45	1030	6	20.0	60
w/cucumber yogurt dressing	1 sandwich	390	24	38	960	1	15.0	70
(Hot Pockets)								
w/broccoli, cheese, stuffed, 'Croissant Pockets'	1 pkg	602	23	78	1303	3	22.0	74
chicken, w/cheddar, pocket, frozen	5 oz	310	16	38	720	0	11.0	0
(Kid Cuisine) chicken, dinner	8.2 oz	470	16	61	830	0	17.0	40
(Lean Pockets)								
fajita, pocket, frozen	1 pocket	250	13	36	810	0	6.0	30
Oriental, pocket, frozen	1 pkg	250	14	35	840	0	6.0	0

Food Name	Serv. Size	Total Cal.	Prot. gms	Carbs gms	Sod. mgs	Fiber gms	Fat gms	Chol. mgs
supreme, glazed, frozen	1 pkg	464	20	68	1119	na	12.5	46
supreme, glazed, frozen	1 serving	233	10	34	562	na	6.3	23
w/Parmesan, pocket, frozen	1 pkg	270	19	35	750	0	6.0	0
(MicroMagic) frozen	4.5 oz	390	13	42	650	0	16.0	35
(Quick Meal)								
. . . .	4.3 oz	320	16	40	640	0	11.0	65
biscuit	4.2 oz	310	13	36	900	0	13.0	50
grilled	4.7 oz	300	21	35	620	0	9.0	60
(Tyson)								
barbecue, frozen, microwave	4 oz	230	16	27	510	0	6.0	0
breast, frozen, microwave	3.5 oz	275	14	27	0	0	12.0	0
breast, grilled, boneless	3.5 oz	150	17	2	400	0	8.0	44
breast, grilled, microwave	1 entrée	210	13	25	460	2	6.0	25
grilled, boneless	3.5 oz	200	15	25	470	0	5.0	32
mini, frozen, microwave	3.5 oz	230	12	39	0	0	5.0	0
(Weight Watchers)								
grilled, 'Ultimate 200'	4 oz	200	18	22	420	0	5.0	20
w/broccoli, cheese, pocket sandwich, 'On-The-Go'	1 pkg	266	13	40	388	na	6.1	14
EGG *(Great Starts)* w/bacon and cheese, muffin	1 sandwich	290	14	25	750	2	15.0	95
ENGLISH MUFFIN *(Weight Watchers)*	1 sandwich	210	13	28	420	2	5.0	20
FISH								
(Fisher Boy) burger, crunchy	1 burger	180	15	18	870	0	6.0	0
(Quick Meal)	5.2 oz	430	16	56	910	0	16.0	68
HAM								
(Hot Pockets)								
and cheese, pocket, frozen	5 oz	360	19	36	1320	0	16.0	90
and cheese, stuffed	1 pkg	681	30	77	1331	na	28.4	100
and cheese, stuffed	1 serving	340	15	38	666	na	14.2	50
w/cheese, no gravy, pocket, 'Ham 'n Cheese'	1 pocket	524	17	36	620	1	34.8	42
(Igor's Piroshki) and cheese, pocket	1 sandwich	370	14	46	880	3	15.0	35
(Owens) and cheese, refrigerated, 'Border Breakfasts'	2 oz	150	7	14	600	0	6.0	0
(Red Baron)								
and cheese, 'Premium Pockets'	1 pkg	721	30	73	2128	na	34.2	83
and cheese, 'Premium Pockets'	1 serving	356	15	36	1052	na	16.9	41
(Swanson)								
and cheese, on bagel, refrigerated, 'Great Starts'	3 oz	240	12	28	600	0	8.0	0
(Weight Watchers)								
and cheese, on bagel	3 oz	210	13	28	460	0	6.0	15
and cheese, pocket, frozen, 'Ultimate 200'	4 oz	200	14	24	490	0	6.0	5
HOT DOG								
(Kid Cuisine) w/bun	6.7 oz	450	13	27	880	0	19.0	40
(Kid Cuisine) w/bun, 'Mega Meal'	8.25 oz	500	16	52	1260	0	25.0	0
PIZZA								
(Hot Pockets)								
pepperoni, pocket, frozen	5 oz	380	17	40	1240	0	17.0	45
pepperoni, stuffed, frozen	1 pkg	735	27	77	1352	na	35.3	82
pepperoni, stuffed, frozen	1 serving	367	14	39	676	na	17.7	41
sausage, pocket, frozen	5 oz	360	15	40	590	0	16.0	65
(Igor's Piroshki) pepperoni and sausage, pocket	1 sandwich	400	18	39	590	3	19.0	40
(Lean Pockets)								
pocket, frozen, 'Deluxe'	1 pkg	280	14	34	500	0	9.0	0
sausage and pepperoni, pocket, frozen, 'Deluxe'	1 pocket	300	13	37	670	0	11.0	35
(Weight Watchers) pocket, 'Deluxe' 'Ultimate 200'	4 oz	200	15	25	400	0	5.0	5
PORK								
(Quick Meal) barbecue	4.3 oz	350	16	40	550	0	14.0	65
(Swanson) rib, hot, smothered	10.25 oz	340	13	50	690	0	10.0	25
SUBMARINE *(BestFresh)* 'Deluxe'	1 sandwich	790	39	59	2070	8	44.0	105

Food Name	Serv. Size	Total Cal.	Prot. gms	Carbs gms	Sod. mgs	Fiber gms	Fat gms	Chol. mgs
TURKEY								
(BestFresh) smoked	1 sandwich	580	39	49	1770	7	26.0	80
(Healthy Deli)								
w/corned beef, 'Doubledecker'	1 oz	30	5	1	195	0	0.7	12
w/ham, 'Doubledecker'	1 oz	30	5	1	185	0	0.9	11
(Hot Pockets) w/ham and cheese, frozen	5 oz	320	17	37	780	0	11.0	0
(Igor's Piroshki) and Swiss, w/broccoli, frozen	1 sandwich	320	15	41	580	3	11.0	20
(Lean Pockets) w/broccoli and cheese, frozen	1 pocket	260	13	32	680	0	9.0	30
VEGGIE								
(Ken & Robert's)								
barbecue style, 'Truly Amazing'	5 oz	320	11	50	560	2	10.0	0
broccoli cheddar, 'Truly Amazing'	5 oz	275	11	37	540	0	9.0	0
Greek style, 'Truly Amazing'	5 oz	270	11	35	500	0	10.0	0
Indian style, 'Truly Amazing'	5 oz	300	10	41	500	1	12.0	0
Oriental style, 'Truly Amazing'	5 oz	295	10	41	572	1	12.0	0
pizza style, 'Truly Amazing'	5 oz	315	12	42	620	1	12.0	0
Tex Mex style, 'Truly Amazing'	5 oz	310	11	43	595	0	11.0	0
(Morningstar Farms)								
burger and cheese style, 'Stuffed Sandwiches'	1 sandwich	290	14	10	400	2	8.0	10
ham and cheese style, 'Stuffed Sandwiches'	1 sandwich	300	15	45	520	1	7.0	10
pepperoni pizza style, 'Stuffed Sandwiches'	1 sandwich	280	12	42	420	5	7.0	5
SANDWICH FILLING MIX								
(French's) sloppy Joe, mix only	1/8 pkg	16	0	4	390	0	0.0	0
(Hunt's)								
sloppy Joe, barbecue, 'Manwich' mix only	1/4 cup	57	1	14	887	1	0.2	0
sloppy Joe, bold, 'Manwich' mix only	1/4 cup	63	1	13	802	na	1.1	0
sloppy Joe, Mexican, 'Manwich' mix only	1/4 cup	27	1	5	552	1	0.2	0
sloppy Joe, original, 'Manwich' mix only	1/4 cup	32	1	6	365	1	0.4	0
sloppy Joe, thick and chunky, 'Manwich'	1/4 cup	44	1	9	737	1	0.5	0
(McCormick/Schilling) sloppy Joe, mix only	1 tsp	15	0	3	360	0	0.0	0
(Schilling) sloppy Joe, mix only	1/4 pkg	26	1	6	750	0	0.5	0
(Tone's) sloppy Joe, mix only	1 tsp	14	0	3	347	0	0.1	0
SANDWICH SPREAD. See also LUNCHEON MEAT SPREAD; POTTED MEAT SPREAD.								
(Best Foods)	1 tbsp	50	0	3	170	0	5.0	3
(Blue Plate)	1 tbsp	75	0	3	105	0	7.0	5
(Hellmann's)	1 tbsp	50	0	3	170	0	5.0	3
(JFG)	1 tbsp	60	0	3	150	0	5.0	7
(Oscar Mayer)								
	2 oz	130	4	8	460	0	10.0	25
pork, chicken, and beef	1 serving	71	2	5	246	0	5.0	14
SAPODILLA								
fresh, raw, pulp	1 cup	200	1	48	29	13	2.7	0
fresh, raw, whole	1 medium	141	1	34	20	9	1.9	0
SAPOTE/marmalade plum								
fresh, raw, trimmed	1 oz	38	0.6	9.6	3	>.5 c	0.2	0
fresh, raw, trimmed, whole, approx 11.2 oz	1 medium	302	5	76	23	6	1.4	0
fresh, raw, untrimmed	1 lb	431	6.8	108.7	31	>6.1 c	1.9	0
SARDINE								
ATLANTIC								
Canned								
in oil, drained, w/bone	1 oz	59	7	0	143	0	3.2	40
in oil, drained, w/bone	2 medium	50	6	0	121	0	2.7	34
in oil, drained, w/bone	1 cup	310	37	0	752	0	17.1	212
BRISLING/Norwegian								
Canned								
(S&W)	3 oz	257	16	0	306	0	20.9	96
in mild sardine oil, drained *(Empress)*	3.75 oz	260	19	1	0	0	20.0	0

Food Name	Serv. Size	Total Cal.	Prot. gms	Carbs gms	Sod. mgs	Fiber gms	Fat gms	Chol. mgs
in mustard sauce *(Crown Prince)*	3.75 oz	240	18	2	450	0	18.0	0
smoked, in oil *(Crown Prince)*	3.75 oz	260	19	1	120	0	42.0	0
w/liquid *(Underwood)*	3.75 oz	260	19	1	450	0	20.0	0
MAINE								
Canned								
in mustard, drained *(Beach Cliff)*	3 oz	227	13	4	350	0	18.0	0
in soybean oil, drained *(Beach Cliff)*	3 oz	240	16	0	20	0	20.0	0
in tomato sauce, drained *(Beach Cliff)*	3 oz	210	15	0	350	0	17.0	0
in water, drained *(Beach Cliff)*	3 oz	230	17	1	350	0	18.0	0
MIXED SPECIES								
Canned								
boneless, skinless *(S&W)*	3 oz	177	21	0	443	0	10.6	35
in mustard sauce *(Underwood)*	3.75 oz	220	16	2	650	0	16.0	0
in oil *(Featherweight)*	1 1/8 oz	130	19	1	65	0	10.0	45
in olive oil, boneless, skinless *(Crown Prince)*	1 pkg	230	24	0	300	1	15.0	40
in soya oil, drained *(Underwood)*	3.75 oz	230	16	1	400	0	18.0	0
in Tabasco sauce, drained *(Underwood)*	3 oz	220	16	1	400	0	16.0	0
in tomato sauce *(Del Monte)*	1/2 cup	360	19	45	540	0	12.0	0
in tomato sauce *(Underwood)*	3.75 oz	220	16	2	500	0	16.0	0
in tomato sauce, drained, w/bone	1 cup	158	15	0	368	0	10.7	54
in tomato sauce, drained, w/bone	1 medium	68	6	0	157	0	4.6	23
in water *(Featherweight)*	1 1/8 oz	95	9	1	65	0	7.0	20
kippered, 'Kippered Snacks' *(Brunswick)*	3.5 oz	185	16	1	610	0	14.0	0
NORWEGIAN. See BRISLING.								
SARDINE OIL. See under FISH OIL.								
SAUCE								
ALFREDO SAUCE								
(Bernardi)	1/2 cup	180	6	10	500	1	13.0	35
(Contadina)								
	1/2 cup	400	7	8	510	0	38.0	80
frozen, food service product	1 oz	67	1	3	142	0	5.7	11
light	1/2 cup	190	3	10	550	0	13.0	40
pouch, food service product	1 oz	70	1	2	181	0	6.1	10
refrigerated 'Fresh'	6 oz	540	9	10	620	0	53.0	85
(DiGiorno)								
light	1/4 cup	140	5	9	600	0	9.0	30
reduced-fat, 'Lighter Varieties'	1/4 cup	180	5	15	580	0	11.0	35
refrigerated	2 oz	200	4	2	490	0	20.0	55
(Five Brothers)								
	1/4 cup	120	2	2	430	0	11.0	40
w/mushrooms	1/4 cup	80	2	3	490	0	7.0	30
(Progresso) canned, 'Authentic Pasta Sauces'	1/2 cup	340	13	6	1080	0	30.0	95
APPLE-APRICOT								
(Lucky Leaf) 'Fruit n' Sauce'	4 oz	90	0	22	20	0	0.0	0
(Musselman's) 'Fruit n' Sauce'	4 oz	90	0	22	20	0	0.0	0
APPLE-CHERRY								
(Lucky Leaf) 'Fruit n' Sauce'	4 oz	100	0	24	20	0	0.0	0
(Musselman's) 'Fruit n' Sauce'	4 oz	100	0	24	20	0	0.0	0
APPLE-CRANBERRY *(Lucky Leaf)*	4 oz	80	0	19	15	0	0.0	0
APPLE-PEACH								
(Lucky Leaf) 'Fruit n' Sauce'	4 oz	90	0	22	20	0	0.0	0
(Musselman's) 'Fruit n' Sauce'	4 oz	90	0	22	20	0	0.0	0
APPLE-PINEAPPLE								
(Lucky Leaf) 'Fruit n' Sauce'	4 oz	110	0	26	20	0	0.0	0
(Musselman's) 'Fruit n' Sauce'	4 oz	110	0	26	20	0	0.0	0
APPLE-STRAWBERRY								
(Lucky Leaf) 'Fruit n' Sauce'	4 oz	100	0	24	20	0	0.0	0

Food Name	Serv. Size	Total Cal.	Prot. gms	Carbs gms	Sod. mgs	Fiber gms	Fat gms	Chol. mgs
(Musselman's) 'Fruit n' Sauce'	4 oz	100	0	24	20	0	0.0	0
BARBECUE								
(Bull's Eye)								
regular	0.5 oz	22	0	5	47	0	0.0	0
Ridge's	2 tbsp	63	0	15	302	na	0.1	na
(Cattleman's)								
classic	2 tbsp	70	0	15	410	0	0.0	0
mild	1 tbsp	25	0	5	260	0	0.0	0
smoky	1 tbsp	25	0	5	300	0	0.0	0
(Enrico's)								
'Original'	1 tbsp	18	1	3	4	0	1.0	0
mesquite	1 tbsp	18	1	3	4	0	1.0	0
(Estee) regular	1 tbsp	18	1	3	5	0	1.0	0
(Golden Dipt) Cajun style	1 oz	90	0	5	360	0	8.0	0
(Hain) honey	1 tbsp	14	0	1	120	0	1.0	0
(Healthy Choice)								
hickory	1.13 oz	26	0	6	229	1	0.2	0
hot and spicy	1.13 oz	25	0	6	229	1	0.2	0
original	1.13 oz	25	0	6	229	1	0.2	0
(Heinz)								
Cajun style	1 tbsp	15	0	3	108	0	0.1	0
chunky, 'Thick & Rich'	1 tbsp	24	0	5	230	0	0.0	0
Hawaiian style	1 tbsp	19	0	4	108	0	0.1	0
Hawaiian style, 'Thick & Rich'	1 oz	40	0	10	210	0	0.0	0
hickory smoke	1 tbsp	19	0	4	56	0	0.1	0
hickory smoke, 'Thick & Rich'	1 tbsp	20	0	5	220	0	0.0	0
hickory, 'Select'	1 oz	35	0	8	260	0	0.0	0
hot, 'Thick & Rich'	1 tbsp	20	0	5	220	0	0.0	0
mesquite smoke, 'Thick & Rich'	1 oz	30	0	7	380	0	0.0	0
mushroom	1 tbsp	14	0	3	219	0	0.1	0
mushroom, 'Thick & Rich'	1 tbsp	20	0	5	220	0	0.0	0
'Old Fashioned'	1 tbsp	18	0	4	180	0	0.1	0
old fashioned, 'Thick & Rich'	1 oz	35	0	8	350	0	0.0	0
onion	1 tbsp	15	0	3	255	0	0.1	0
onion, 'Thick & Rich'	1 tbsp	20	0	5	200	0	0.0	0
original, 'Thick & Rich'	1 tbsp	20	0	5	230	0	0.0	0
'Select'	1 tbsp	18	0	4	60	0	0.1	0
Texas style, hot, 'Thick & Rich'	1 tbsp	15	0	3	210	0	0.2	0
(Hunt's)								
'Chicken Sensations'	1 tbsp	35	0	3	308	0	2.7	0
country style	1.2 oz	39	0	9	399	0	0.3	0
hickory	1 tbsp	20	1	5	160	1	1.0	0
hickory, 'Light'	1.13 oz	27	1	6	245	1	0.2	0
homestyle	1.23 oz	41	1	10	381	1	0.1	0
Kansas City style	1.23 oz	43	0	10	220	1	0.2	0
New Orleans style	1.23 oz	41	1	9	383	1	0.2	0
original recipe	2 tbsp	40	0	9	410	1	0.0	0
Southern style	1.2 oz	40	1	9	361	1	0.4	0
Texas style	1.23 oz	42	0	10	305	1	0.1	0
western style	1.23 oz	41	0	10	394	1	0.2	0
(Kraft)								
chunky, 'Thick 'n Spicy'	2 tbsp	60	0	13	420	0	1.0	0
hickory smoke	2 tbsp	39	0	9	418	0	0.1	0
hickory smoke, 'Thick 'N Spicy'	2 tbsp	50	0	12	450	0	0.0	0
hickory smoke, w/onion bits	2 tbsp	50	0	11	340	0	1.0	0
honey, 'Thick 'N Spicy'	2 tbsp	60	0	13	360	0	0.0	0
hot	2 tbsp	40	0	9	520	0	0.0	0

Food Name	Serv. Size	Total Cal.	Prot. gms	Carbs gms	Sod. mgs	Fiber gms	Fat gms	Chol. mgs
Kansas City style	2 tbsp	50	0	11	310	0	0.0	0
Kansas City style, 'Thick 'N Spicy'	2 tbsp	60	0	14	310	0	0.0	0
mesquite smoke	2 tbsp	40	0	9	420	0	0.0	0
mesquite smoke, 'Thick 'N Spicy'	2 tbsp	50	0	12	440	0	0.0	0
original	2 tbsp	39	0	9	424	0	0.1	0
original, 'Thick 'N Spicy'	2 tbsp	50	0	12	440	0	0.0	0
roasted garlic	2 tbsp	50	0	12	360	0	0.0	0
salsa style	2 tbsp	45	0	9	420	0	0.0	0
w/Italian seasonings	2 tbsp	50	0	10	280	0	1.0	0
w/onion bits	2 tbsp	45	0	11	360	0	0.0	0
(LaChoy) Oriental	1 tbsp	16	1	4	304	1	0.1	0
(Lawry's)								
Dijon and honey	1/2 cup	203	5	27	1768	0	1.2	0
orange juice, 'California Grill'	1/4 cup	34	4	3	3846	0	0.7	0
(Libby's) w/beef, 'Sloppy Joe'	1/3 cup	110	5	7	190	0	7.0	0
(Luzianne) mustard base, 'Cajun'	2 tbsp	110	0	19	350	0	4.0	0
(Marzetti) original, 'Texas Best'	2 tbsp	42	1	4	315	na	2.7	0
(Maull's) smoky	1 tbsp	20	1	4	139	1	1.0	1
(Open Pit)								
hickory	2 tbsp	50	0	11	430	0	0.5	0
original	2 tbsp	50	0	11	415	0	0.5	0
(Open Range)								
hickory	1.2 oz	37	1	9	423	1	0.2	0
hickory, food service product	2 tbsp	37	0	9	424	1	0.2	0
original	1.2 oz	38	1	9	333	1	0.2	0
original, food service product	2 tbsp	38	1	9	332	1	0.2	0
(Ott's)								
regular	1 tbsp	14	0	3	147	0	0.1	1
smoky	1 tbsp	14	0	3	149	0	0.1	1
(Woodys) sweet and sour	2 tbsp	70	0	17	610	1	0.0	0
BASIL-HERB								
(Golden Dipt) 'Nature Bay'	2 grams	8	0	1	36	0	0.0	0
(Nature Bay)	2 grams	8	0	1	36	0	0.0	0
BEARNAISE (Great Impressions)	2 tbsp	192	1	0	148	0	21.0	48
BEEF								
(Ragu)								
barbecue, 'Beef Tonight'	4 oz	70	2	15	580	0	1.0	0
skillet lasagna, 'Beef Tonight'	4 oz	60	3	9	630	0	1.0	5
stroganoff, 'Beef Tonight'	4 oz	130	1	6	770	0	12.0	10
(Simmer Chef) Stroganoff, family style	1/2 cup	110	2	8	760	1	7.0	5
BOLOGNESE								
(Contadina)								
	5 oz	130	8	0	500	0	7.0	25
refrigerated, 'Fresh'	7.5 oz	230	22	12	600	0	11.0	50
(Progresso) canned, 'Authentic Pasta Sauces'	1/2 cup	150	10	12	520	3	8.0	20
BROCCOLI (Simmer Chef) creamy	1/2 cup	110	1	9	670	2	8.0	5
BROWNING (Gravymaster)	1 tsp	12	1	2	1	0	0.0	0
CACCIATORE								
(Recipe Sauces)	3.9 oz	40	1	9	570	0	1.0	0
(Simmer Chef) old country	1/2 cup	110	2	15	540	2	4.0	0
CARBONARA (DiGiorno) refrigerated	2 oz	200	4	3	380	0	19.0	40
CHARDONNAY (Golden Dipt)	1 oz	60	0	1	160	0	6.0	0
CHEESE								
(Contadina)								
four cheese, refrigerated 'Fresh'	6 oz	470	12	8	500	0	45.0	147
four cheese, w/white wine & shallots	1/2 cup	320	8	8	240	0	28.0	70
(DiGiorno) four cheese	1/4 cup	160	5	3	410	0	15.0	30

Food Name	Serv. Size	Total Cal.	Prot. gms	Carbs gms	Sod. mgs	Fiber gms	Fat gms	Chol. mgs
(J. Hungerford)								
cheddar, 'Stadium'	2 oz	80	1	6	500	0	5.0	4
nacho	2.01 oz	120	2	7	440	0	9.0	5
nacho, 'Stadium'	2.01 oz	80	1	6	410	0	5.0	4
(Kaukauna)								
nacho	1 oz	80	3	4	330	0	6.0	8
nacho, medium, microwaveable	2 tbsp	90	3	4	330	0	7.0	10
nacho, mild, microwaveable	2 tbsp	90	3	4	330	0	7.0	10
(Kraft)								
jalapeño pepper, pasteurized process, 'Cheez Whiz'	2 tbsp	90	4	3	510	0	7.0	25
pasteurized process, 'Cheez Whiz'	2 tbsp	90	4	3	540	0	7.0	20
salsa, mild, pasteurized process, 'Cheez Whiz'	2 tbsp	100	4	3	530	0	7.0	25
(La Victoria)								
cheddar	1/4 cup	105	1	6	633	0	8.5	2
nacho, w/jalapeño peppers	1/4 cup	122	1	7	547	0	9.7	4
(Lucky Leaf)								
cheddar	4 oz	220	3	12	1000	0	18.0	0
cheddar, aged	4 oz	240	5	11	920	0	20.0	0
cheddar, mild, aged	4 oz	200	5	9	790	0	18.0	0
cheddar, sharp, aged	4 oz	230	9	6	850	0	17.0	0
nacho	4 oz	220	4	11	1010	0	18.0	0
(Musselman's)								
cheddar	4 oz	220	3	12	1000	0	18.0	0
cheddar, aged	4 oz	240	5	11	920	0	20.0	0
cheddar, mild, aged	4 oz	200	5	9	790	0	18.0	0
cheddar, sharp, aged	4 oz	230	9	6	850	0	17.0	0
nacho	4 oz	220	4	11	1010	0	18.0	0
(Nestlé)								
cheddar, 'Chef Mate'	1 cup	327	7	32	1885	0	18.8	25
cheddar, 'Chef Mate'	1/4 cup	82	2	8	471	0	4.7	6
cheddar, sharp, 'Chef Mate'	1 cup	532	22	7	1893	3	46.0	91
cheddar, sharp, 'Chef Mate'	1/4 cup	133	5	2	473	1	11.5	23
con queso, 'Que Bueno'	1 cup	335	15	14	2220	0	24.1	63
con queso, 'Que Bueno'	1/4 cup	84	4	4	555	0	6.0	16
golden, 'Chef-Mate'	1 cup	554	27	9	2006	3	45.5	116
golden, 'Chef-Mate'	1/4 cup	139	7	2	501	1	11.4	29
jalapeño, 'Que Bueno'	1 pkg	3876	96	370	27255	0	224.2	301
jalapeño, 'Que Bueno'	1/4 cup	81	2	8	571	0	4.7	6
nacho, mild, 'Que Bueno'	1 cup	476	18	10	1968	2	40.5	81
nacho, mild, 'Que Bueno'	1/4 cup	119	5	3	492	1	10.1	20
nacho, 'Que Bueno'	1 cup	512	21	16	2318	2	40.4	116
nacho, 'Que Bueno'	1/4 cup	128	5	4	580	0	10.1	29
(Pablo's)								
jalapeño, 'Deli Style'	1 oz	59	2	4	470	0	4.0	5
nacho, 'Deli Style'	1 oz	59	2	4	470	0	4.0	5
(Snow's) Welsh rarebit	1/2 cup	170	9	10	460	0	11.0	0
(Weight Watchers) cheddar, sharp	2 tbsp	70	4	7	190	0	3.0	10
(White House)								
cheddar, aged	3.5 oz	213	4	10	810	0	18.0	0
jalapeño	3.5 oz	193	3	10	890	0	16.0	0
nacho	3.5 oz	193	3	10	890	0	16.0	0
CHICKEN								
(Hunt's) Southwestern, 'Chicken Sensations'	1 tbsp	27	0	1	281	0	2.6	0
(Ragu)								
cacciatore, 'Chicken Tonight'	4 oz	70	1	12	490	0	2.0	0
French, country, 'Chicken Tonight'	4 oz	140	1	6	730	0	12.0	5
herbed, w/wine, 'Chicken Tonight'	4 oz	100	2	13	610	0	4.0	5

Food Name	Serv. Size	Total Cal.	Prot. gms	Carbs gms	Sod. mgs	Fiber gms	Fat gms	Chol. mgs
honey mustard, light, 'Chicken Tonight'	4 oz	50	1	12	420	0	1.0	0
Italian, primavera, 'Light'	4 oz	50	2	9	540	0	1.0	0
primavera, creamy, 'Chicken Tonight'	4 oz	90	1	9	650	0	6.0	5
sweet and sour, 'Chicken Tonight'	4 oz	80	0	19	280	0	0.0	0
sweet and spicy, light, 'Chicken Tonight'	4 oz	50	2	10	390	0	1.0	0
w/mushrooms, creamy, 'Chicken Tonight'	4 oz	110	1	5	650	0	10.0	5
CHILI								
(Chef Boyardee) hot dog, w/beef	1 oz	30	1	4	140	0	1.0	0
(Del Monte)	1 tbsp	20	0	5	480	0	0.0	0
(El Molino) green, mild	2 tbsp	10	0	2	210	0	0.0	0
(Featherweight)	1 tbsp	8	0	2	10	0	0.0	0
(Gebhardt) hot dog	2 tbsp	20	1	2	150	0	1.0	0
(Heinz)	1 oz	30	0	7	430	0	0.0	0
(Just Rite) hot dog sauce	2.19 oz	50	2	5	265	2	2.9	2
(Las Palmas) red	1/2 cup	25	1	3	670	0	1.0	0
(Manwich) 'Chili Fixin's'	5.3 oz	110	6	20	900	5	1.0	0
(Open Range) hot dog	2.22 oz	61	3	6	255	2	3.5	4
(S&W)								
'Chili Makin's'	1/2 cup	100	5	20	782	0	1.0	0
steakhouse	1 tbsp	15	0	4	180	0	0.0	0
(Wolf Brand) hot dog	1.25 oz	44	2	4	199	0	2.3	0
CHOCOLATE (Chocolate Mountain)	2 tbsp	120	1	20	80	0	4.0	4
CLAM								
(Buitoni) red, canned	5 oz	190	8	28	560	0	6.0	20
(Contadina)								
red, refrigerated, 'Fresh'	7.5 oz	120	7	15	800	0	4.0	35
white, refrigerated, 'Fresh'	6 oz	290	8	13	800	0	23.0	94
(Ferrara)								
red, canned	4 oz	70	5	8	320	0	2.0	10
white, canned	4 oz	80	5	4	570	0	5.0	10
(Progresso)								
red, canned	1/2 cup	70	5	7	560	0	3.0	0
white, canned	1/2 cup	110	9	1	280	0	8.0	0
COCKTAIL								
(Del Monte)	1/4 cup	100	1	24	910	0	0.0	0
(Estee)	1 tbsp	10	1	2	35	0	1.0	0
(Golden Dipt)								
extra hot	1 tbsp	20	0	5	210	0	0.0	0
regular	1 tbsp	20	0	5	210	0	0.0	0
(Great Impressions)								
	1 tbsp	21	0	5	182	0	0.1	0
'Brandy Glow'	1 tbsp	68	0	2	106	0	6.7	10
low-salt	1 tbsp	21	0	5	6	0	0.1	0
(Heinz)	1/4 cup	60	1	14	680	1	0.0	0
(S&W)	1 tsp	20	0	5	220	0	0.0	0
(Sauceworks)	1 tbsp	14	0	3	170	0	0.0	0
(Stokely)	1 tbsp	18	0	5	90	0	0.0	0
CRANBERRY-ORANGE								
(Ocean Spray) crushed, for chicken, 'CranFruit'	2 oz	90	0	23	10	0	0.0	0
CRANBERRY-RASPBERRY								
(Ocean Spray) crushed, for chicken, 'CranFruit'	2 oz	90	0	23	10	0	0.0	0
CRANBERRY-STRAWBERRY								
(Ocean Spray) crushed, for chicken, 'CranFruit'	2 oz	90	0	22	10	0	0.0	0
CREOLE								
(Enrico's) Cajun, 'Light'	4 oz	76	2	9	284	0	2.8	0
(Golden Dipt) cooking sauce	1 oz	20	0	2	190	0	1.0	0
(Nestlé)								
'Chef Mate'	1 cup	99	4	15	1357	3	2.8	0

Food Name	Serv. Size	Total Cal.	Prot. gms	Carbs gms	Sod. mgs	Fiber gms	Fat gms	Chol. mgs
'Chef Mate'	1/4 cup	25	1	4	339	1	0.7	0
CURRY								
(Flavor of the Rain Forest) ginger, stir-fry	1 tbsp	15	1	2	173	0	1.0	0
(TAJ Cuisine of India) Bombay	4 oz	90	2	10	470	2	5.0	0
DIABLE *(Escoffier)* nonat	1 tbsp	20	0	4	160	0	0.0	0
DIJONAISSE *(Golden Dipt)*	1 oz	52	0	2	130	0	4.0	0
ENCHILADA								
(Del Monte)								
hot	1/2 cup	45	1	11	1090	0	0.0	0
mild	1/2 cup	45	1	11	1150	0	0.0	0
(El Molino) hot	2 tbsp	16	0	2	100	0	1.0	0
(Gebhardt)	1/4 cup	35	1	4	218	1	2.0	0
(La Victoria)								
	1 cup	80	1	10	1520	0	5.0	0
	1/4 cup	20	0	3	397	0	0.9	0
(Las Palmas) hot	1/2 cup	25	1	3	670	0	1.0	0
(Nestlé)								
'Que Bueno'	1 pkg	1928	56	259	9946	39	76.3	0
'Que Bueno'	2 tbsp	15	0	2	77	0	0.6	0
(Old El Paso)								
green	2 tbsp	11	1	3	200	0	0.0	0
green chili	1/4 cup	30	1	3	330	0	1.5	0
hot	1/4 cup	30	1	4	250	0	1.0	0
mild	1/4 cup	25	0	4	160	0	1.0	0
(Ortega)								
hot	1 oz	12	0	3	280	0	0.0	0
mild	1 oz	12	0	3	280	0	0.0	0
(Rosarita)								
	1/4 cup	23	1	3	409	0	1.1	0
food service product	1/4 cup	23	1	3	5	0	1.1	0
mild	2.5 oz	25	1	3	230	1	1.0	0
(Santiago)	1 fl oz	11	0	2	138	0	0.1	0
FAJITA								
(S&W) Southwestern	1 tbsp	10	0	2	230	1	0.0	0
(Tio Sancho) 'Skillet Sauce'	1 oz	14	1	2	590	0	0.5	0
FORESTIERA *(Contadina)* refrigerated, 'Fresh'	7.5 oz	270	6	15	830	0	9.0	15
GARLIC								
(A Taste of Thai) chili pepper	1 tbsp	10	0	2	220	0	0.0	0
(Golden Dipt) herb, nonfat, 'Nature Bay'	2 grams	8	0	1	87	0	0.0	0
(Hunt's) Italian, 'Chicken Sensations'	1 tbsp	30	0	1	326	1	2.7	0
GINGER								
(Flavor of the Rain Forest) curry, stir-fry	1 tbsp	15	1	2	173	0	1.0	0
(Mr. Spice) stir fry, fat-free, salt-free	1 tbsp	11	1	3	0	0	0.0	0
HERB *(Lawry's)* and garlic, w/lemon juice	1/4 cup	36	4	4	3688	0	0.4	0
HOISIN *(Dynasty)*	2 tbsp	80	1	15	540	1	1.5	0
HOLLANDAISE *(Great Impressions)*	2 tbsp	192	1	0	107	0	21.0	48
HONEY MUSTARD								
(Ragu) light, Chicken Tonight'	4 oz	50	1	12	420	0	0.5	0
(Simmer Chef)	1/2 cup	150	1	30	400	1	2.0	0
HORSERADISH								
(Great Impressions)	1 tbsp	74	0	1	199	0	7.6	1
(Heinz)	1 tbsp	74	0	2	113	0	7.4	0
(Life) strong, 'All Natural'	1/2 tbsp	7	1	1	2	0	1.0	0
(Sauceworks)	1 tbsp	50	0	2	105	0	5.0	5
HOT DOG								
(Chili Bowl) chili, w/beef	1/4 cup	100	3	6	260	3	7.0	10

Food Name	Serv. Size	Total Cal.	Prot. gms	Carbs gms	Sod. mgs	Fiber gms	Fat gms	Chol. mgs
(Gebhardt)								
chili, food service product	1/4 cup	61	3	6	255	2	3.5	4
chili, w/beef	1/4 cup	57	3	6	262	2	3.2	12
(Hunt's) chili, w/beef	1/4 cup	61	3	6	255	2	3.5	4
(Just Rite)	1/4 cup	50	2	5	265	2	2.9	2
(Nestlé)								
chili, w/beef, 'Chef-Mate'	1 pkg	3368	131	449	19382	83	115.7	214
chili, w/beef, 'Chef-Mate'	1/4 cup	69	3	9	399	2	2.4	4
Coney Island, 'Chef-Mate'	1 cup	303	9	23	1533	6	19.7	7
Coney Island, 'Chef-Mate'	1/4 cup	76	2	6	383	1	4.9	2
HOT SAUCE								
(Gebhardt) pepper, 'Louisiana Style'	1/2 tsp	0	0	0	45	0	0.0	0
(Tabasco) pepper	1 tsp	1	0	0	30	0	0.0	0
(Tabasco) pepper	1/4 tsp	1	0	1	9	0	0.0	0
(Gebhardt)	1 tsp	1	0	0	89	0	0.0	0
HUNTER *(McCormick/Schilling)*	1 tbsp	25	1	4	270	0	0.0	0
ITALIAN								
(Nestlé) 'Chef-Mate'	1 cup	125	2	24	627	2	2.4	0
(Nestlé) 'Chef-Mate'	1/4 cup	61	1	11	304	1	1.2	0
JALAPEÑO *(Tabasco)*	1 tsp	0	0	0	70	0	0.0	0
KUNG PAO *(Dynasty)* spicy hot	2 tbsp	50	1	6	600	1	2.5	0
LEMON								
(Nestlé) 'Chef-Mate'	1 pkg	2849	5	679	170	0	12.5	0
(Nestlé) 'Chef-Mate'	2 tbsp	43	0	10	3	0	0.2	0
LEMON BUTTER DILL *(Golden Dipt)*	1 oz	100	0	4	190	0	9.0	0
LEMON DILL *(Golden Dipt)* 'Nature Bay'	1 oz	110	0	3	150	0	11.0	0
LEMON HERB *(Hunt's)* 'Chicken Sensations'	1 tbsp	31	0	2	378	0	2.7	0
LOBSTER SAUCE *(Progresso)* rock	1/2 cup	120	4	11	430	2	8.0	10
MARINARA. See also SAUCE, PASTA.								
(Angela Mia) food service product	1/2 cup	47	2	9	503	4	0.3	0
(Bernardi)	1/2 cup	120	2	20	480	2	4.0	0
(Buitoni)	1/2 cup	70	1	11	570	0	3.0	0
(Contadina)								
	1 cup	145	3	17	938	3	7.0	0
	1/2 cup	73	2	9	469	2	3.5	0
frozen, food service product	1 oz	18	0	2	88	1	0.9	0
(Five Brothers) w/burgundy wine	1/2 cup	80	2	9	480	2	4.0	0
(Hunt's) chunky	1/2 cup	60	1	12	526	2	1.6	5
(Millina's Finest)								
organic	4 oz	48	2	9	210	0	0.5	0
Zinfandel, organic	4 oz	44	2	9	215	0	0.5	0
(Pathmark)								
'All Natural'	1/2 cup	80	2	12	710	0	2.0	0
'No Frills'	1/2 cup	80	1	12	620	0	3.0	0
(Prego)	1/2 cup	110	2	12	670	3	6.0	0
(Progresso)								
	1/2 cup	90	4	9	520	0	5.0	1
'Authentic Pasta Sauces'	1/2 cup	110	4	10	250	2	6.0	4
(Ragu) 'Old World Style'	1/2 cup	90	2	9	820	3	5.0	0
(Rokeach)	3 oz	60	1	9	257	0	2.0	0
(Westbrae)								
	4 oz	40	2	7	370	0	1.0	0
w/mushrooms	4 oz	50	2	7	380	0	29.0	0
MESQUITE								
(Lawry's) w/lime juice	1/4 cup	24	3	3	4142	0	0.4	0
(S&W) and marinade	1 tbsp	10	0	3	400	0	0.0	0
MEXICAN *(S&W)* mild, 'Tomato Garden'	1/4 cup	20	1	4	190	1	0.0	0

Food Name	Serv. Size	Total Cal.	Prot. gms	Carbs gms	Sod. mgs	Fiber gms	Fat gms	Chol. mgs
MOLE POBLANO *(La Victoria)*	2 oz	240	8	28	1847	9	10.3	0
MUSHROOM *(Simmer Chef)* and herb, creamy	1/2 cup	110	0	7	580	0	9.0	5
NEWBURG *(Snow's)* canned, w/sherry	1/3 cup	120	3	10	520	0	8.0	0
ONION *(Simmer Chef)* and mushroom, hearty	1/2 cup	50	1	9	670	1	1.0	0
ORANGE DIJON *(Golden Dipt)* 'Nature Bay'	1 oz	110	0	6	200	0	9.0	0
ORANGE *(LaChoy)* Mandarin	1 tbsp	24	0	6	38	0	0.0	0
OREGANO HERB *(Golden Dipt)* 'Nature Bay'	2 grams	6	0	1	88	0	0.0	0
PARMIGIANA *(Betty Crocker)* 'Recipe Sauces'	3.9 oz	50	2	9	430	0	1.0	0
PASTA/spaghetti. See also SAUCE, MARINARA; SAUCE, TOMATO.								
(Angela Mia)	1/2 cup	49	2	11	607	3	0.5	0
(Campbell's)								
extra garlic and onion	4 oz	50	2	12	320	2	1.0	0
'Homestyle'	4 oz	40	2	10	360	2	0.0	0
Italian style	4 oz	50	2	12	360	2	0.0	0
mushroom	4 oz	50	2	11	330	2	1.0	0
traditional, 'Healthy Request'	4 oz	50	2	12	360	2	0.0	0
w/fresh mushrooms, 'Healthy Request'	4 oz	50	2	11	330	2	1.0	0
(Chef Boyardee)								
meat flavor	3.75 oz	80	2	11	650	0	3.0	0
meat flavor, 'Original'	3.75 oz	120	3	13	650	0	6.0	0
meatless, 'Jars'	4 oz	60	1	11	790	0	1.0	0
mushroom flavor	3.75 oz	60	1	11	790	0	1.0	0
mushroom flavor, 'Jars'	4 oz	70	1	11	655	0	2.0	0
mushroom flavor, 'Original'	3.75 oz	80	1	13	680	0	3.0	0
w/ground beef, 'Jars'	4 oz	90	2	14	605	0	3.0	0
(Classico) sun-dried tomato, 'Di Capri'	1/2 cup	80	2	8	430	2	4.5	0
(Contadina)								
meat flavored, 'Original Recipe'	1/2 cup	100	3	17	430	0	3.2	2
mushroom, 'Original Recipe'	1/2 cup	90	2	18	430	0	2.3	0
traditional, 'Original Recipe'	1/2 cup	90	2	17	440	0	2.3	0
(Del Monte) flavored w/meat	1/2 cup	70	2	9	440	0	2.0	0
traditional	1/2 cup	70	1	11	430	0	2.0	0
w/garlic and onion	1/2 cup	70	1	10	430	0	2.0	0
w/mushrooms	1/2 cup	70	1	11	440	0	2.0	0
(DiGiorno) plum tomato and mushroom, refrigerated	5 oz	100	3	20	240	0	1.0	0
(Eden Foods)								
and pizza sauce, organic	4 oz	80	3	10	320	0	3.0	0
organic, no salt added	4 oz	80	3	14	0	0	2.0	0
(Enrico's)								
all natural, no salt added	4 oz	60	2	9	30	0	1.0	0
garlic and sun-dried tomatoes, all natural	3.5 oz	62	2	9	474	2	2.0	2
Italian style, all natural	3.5 oz	53	2	11	333	1	1.0	9
mushroom and green pepper, all natural	4 oz	60	2	9	345	0	1.0	0
mushroom and green pepper, no salt added	4 oz	60	2	9	30	0	1.0	0
mushroom flavor	4 oz	60	2	9	0	0	1.0	0
organic tomatoes, 'Hot & Spicy Arabiati'	3.5 oz	60	2	9	464	3	1.8	0
original, all natural	4 oz	60	2	9	345	0	1.0	0
peppers and mushrooms, all natural	4 oz	60	2	9	345	0	1.0	0
w/fresh mushrooms	4 oz	60	2	9	336	0	1.0	0
(Featherweight) mushroom flavor	4 oz	60	2	11	310	0	1.0	0
(Five Brothers)								
garden vegetable primavera	1/2 cup	70	2	9	500	2	3.0	0
tomato basil	1/2 cup	60	2	8	470	2	2.0	0
w/sautéed mushrooms	1/2 cup	90	2	10	460	3	4.0	0
(Healthy Choice)								
garlic and herb	4 oz	40	2	9	390	0	1.0	0
garlic and herb, original	1/2 cup	50	2	10	390	2	0.0	0

Food Name	Serv. Size	Total Cal.	Prot. gms	Carbs gms	Sod. mgs	Fiber gms	Fat gms	Chol. mgs
garlic and onion	1/2 cup	40	2	9	390	2	0.0	0
garlic and onion, chunky	4 oz	40	2	10	350	0	0.0	0
Italian vegetable, chunky	4.41 oz	50	2	11	331	3	0.6	0
mushroom and green pepper, super chunky	1/2 cup	45	2	9	390	2	0.0	0
mushroom, chunky	4 oz	45	2	10	350	0	0.0	0
mushroom, super chunky	1/2 cup	40	2	9	390	2	0.0	0
traditional	4 oz	40	2	9	380	0	1.0	0
vegetable primavera, super chunky	1/2 cup	45	2	9	390	2	0.0	0
w/chunky mushrooms, nonfat	4 oz	45	2	10	350	0	0.0	0
w/mushrooms	4 oz	40	2	9	390	0	1.0	0
w/vegetables, Italian style, chunky	4 oz	40	1	9	350	0	0.0	0
(Hunt's)								
'Homestyle'	4 oz	60	2	10	530	2	2.0	0
'Traditional'	4 oz	70	2	12	530	0	2.0	0
100% natural, 'Old Country'	4 oz	60	2	8	560	0	2.0	0
garlic and herb, 'Classic'	4.41 oz	58	2	10	598	2	2.1	0
garlic and herb, 'Light'	4.41 oz	39	2	7	379	3	0.8	0
garlic and herb, 'Old Country'	1/2 cup	63	2	9	522	3	2.7	0
garlic and onion, 'Classic Italian'	1/2 cup	58	2	10	598	2	2.1	0
Italian sausage	1/2 cup	77	2	12	596	2	2.7	2
Italian style vegetable, chunky	1/2 cup	63	2	13	528	2	1.0	0
Italian vegetable, 'Old Country'	1/2 cup	64	2	9	616	3	2.6	0
light meat	4.41 oz	45	2	8	437	3	1.2	2
meat flavor	4 oz	70	2	12	570	0	2.0	0
meat flavored, 'Home Style'	1/2 cup	57	2	7	596	2	2.6	2
meat flavored, 'Old Country'	1/2 cup	56	2	7	474	3	2.6	0
meat flavored, 'Original'	1/2 cup	65	2	11	604	2	2.3	3
meat	4.44 oz	65	2	11	604	2	2.3	3
meat, 'Homestyle'	4.41 oz	56	2	7	596	2	2.6	2
mushroom flavor	4 oz	70	2	12	560	0	2.0	0
mushroom	4.44 oz	65	2	11	604	2	2.3	0
mushroom, 'Home Style'	1/2 cup	57	2	7	586	2	2.6	0
mushroom, light	4.41 oz	39	2	7	379	3	0.8	0
mushroom, 'Old Country'	1/2 cup	53	2	7	542	3	2.7	0
mushroom, 'Original'	1/2 cup	65	2	11	604	2	2.3	0
Parmesan, 'Classic Italian'	1/2 cup	50	2	8	634	2	2.1	0
spaghetti, cheese and garlic, Italian style	1/2 cup	65	3	9	690	2	2.4	1
spaghetti, chunky	4 oz	50	1	12	470	2	1.0	0
spaghetti, tomato basil, 'Classic'	4.41 oz	48	2	8	613	4	2.1	0
spaghetti, tomato, garlic, and onion, chunky	1/2 cup	61	1	13	526	2	1.0	0
spaghetti, w/tomato chunks, 'Chunky Style'	4 oz	50	1	12	470	0	1.0	0
tomato and basil, 'Classic Italian'	1/2 cup	48	2	8	613	4	2.1	0
traditional, 'Light'	4 oz	40	2	9	360	0	0.0	0
traditional, 'Home Style'	1/2 cup	57	2	7	596	2	2.6	0
traditional, 'Old Country'	1/2 cup	53	2	7	542	3	2.7	0
traditional, 'Original'	1/2 cup	65	2	11	621	4	2.3	0
w/meat	4 oz	70	2	12	570	2	2.0	2
w/mushrooms	4 oz	70	2	12	560	2	2.0	0
w/mushrooms, 'Light'	4 oz	40	2	9	330	0	0.0	0
(McCormick/Schilling) herb and garlic	1 tbsp	20	1	2	500	0	0.0	0
(Millina's Finest)								
sweet pepper and onion, nonfat organic	4 oz	41	2	7	305	0	0.5	0
tomato and mushroom, nonfat, organic	4 oz	45	2	9	200	0	0.0	0
tomato basil, nonfat, organic	4 oz	46	2	9	232	0	0.5	0
(Nestlé)	1/2 cup	70	2	12	563	2	1.6	0
(P&Q)								
meat flavor	1/2 cup	70	1	11	510	0	2.0	0

Food Name	Serv. Size	Total Cal.	Prot. gms	Carbs gms	Sod. mgs	Fiber gms	Fat gms	Chol. mgs
meatless	1/2 cup	70	1	14	540	0	1.0	0
mushroom flavor	1/2 cup	70	1	14	580	0	1.0	0
(Pastorelli) 'Italian Chef'	4 oz	81	3	11	430	1	3.0	0
(Pathmark)								
meat flavor, 'All Natural'	1/2 cup	80	2	11	790	0	3.0	0
meat flavor, 'No Frills'	1/2 cup	90	2	11	620	0	5.0	0
meatless, 'All Natural'	1/2 cup	70	2	11	710	0	2.0	0
meatless, 'No Frills'	1/2 cup	80	1	11	583	0	3.0	0
mushroom flavor, 'All Natural'	1/2 cup	70	2	11	730	0	2.0	0
(Prego)								
....	1/2 cup	110	2	19	420	3	3.0	0
garden combination	4 oz	80	2	14	420	0	2.0	0
garden combination, chunky	1/2 cup	100	2	19	480	3	2.0	0
garlic and cheese, extra chunky	1/2 cup	130	3	22	610	3	3.5	0
low-salt	1/2 cup	110	2	11	25	3	6.0	0
meat flavored	1/2 cup	140	3	21	500	3	6.0	5
mushroom	1/2 cup	150	2	23	670	3	5.0	0
mushroom, extra chunky, extra spicy	1/2 cup	120	2	19	510	3	4.0	0
mushroom, w/onion, extra chunky	1/2 cup	110	2	18	500	3	3.0	5
mushroom, w/tomato, chunky	1/2 cup	110	2	19	510	3	3.0	0
mushroom and green pepper, chunky	1/2 cup	120	2	18	430	6	4.5	5
mushroom flavor	4 oz	130	2	20	630	0	5.0	0
onion, tomato-based, 'Extra Chunky'	4 oz	110	2	14	490	0	5.0	0
onion, w/garlic	1/2 cup	110	2	19	420	3	3.0	0
sausage, w/peppers, extra chunky	1/2 cup	180	4	22	570	3	9.0	10
spaghetti, traditional, '100% Natural'	2 tbsp	136	2	21	557	4	5.0	0
three cheese	1/2 cup	100	3	18	460	3	2.0	5
tomato and onion, w/garlic, extra chunky	1/2 cup	110	2	19	480	3	3.5	0
traditional	1/2 cup	140	2	23	610	2	4.5	0
(Pritikin)								
garden style, chunky	1/2 cup	50	2	11	30	0	0.0	0
original	1/2 cup	60	2	14	35	0	1.0	0
(Progresso)								
meat flavor	1/2 cup	110	4	13	660	0	5.0	5
mushroom flavor	1/2 cup	110	3	13	630	0	5.0	5
primavera, creamy, 'Authentic Pasta Sauces'	1/2 cup	190	5	8	410	1	17.0	54
Sicilian, 'Authentic Pasta Sauces'	1/2 cup	30	1	2	660	1	2.5	0
spaghetti	1/2 cup	110	3	13	660	0	5.0	2
(Ragu)								
beef flavored, 'Hearty'	1/2 cup	130	4	19	580	3	4.5	3
'Fresh Italian'	4 oz	90	2	13	490	0	3.0	0
garden, 'Light'	1/2 cup	50	2	11	390	3	0.0	0
garden harvest, 'Today's Recipe'	4 oz	50	2	8	370	0	1.0	0
'Gardenstyle Chunky'	1/2 cup	120	2	18	540	3	4.0	0
green and red pepper, 'Gardenstyle Chunky'	1/2 cup	120	2	19	570	2	4.0	0
'Homestyle'	4 oz	50	2	6	390	0	2.0	0
Italian garden combination, 'Chunky Gardenstyle'	4 oz	110	2	15	500	0	5.0	0
Italian tomato, 'Hearty'	1/2 cup	120	3	19	580	3	3.0	0
meat flavored, 'Old World Style'	1/2 cup	90	3	9	820	3	5.0	3
mushroom, 'Old World Style'	1/2 cup	80	2	10	820	3	3.5	0
mushroom, chunky, 'Light'	1/2 cup	50	3	11	390	2	0.0	0
mushroom, chunky, 'Today's Recipe'	4 oz	50	2	8	370	0	1.0	0
no sugar added, 'Light'	1/2 cup	60	3	9	390	3	1.5	0
Parmesan, 'Hearty'	1/2 cup	120	4	18	630	2	4.0	3
smooth, traditional 'Old World'	1/2 cup	80	2	12	756	3	2.6	na
spaghetti, 'Chunky Gardenstyle'	4 oz	70	2	10	440	0	3.0	0
spaghetti, 'Slow Cooked Homestyle'	4 oz	110	2	15	510	0	5.0	0

Food Name	Serv. Size	Total Cal.	Prot. gms	Carbs gms	Sod. mgs	Fiber gms	Fat gms	Chol. mgs
'Thick & Hearty'	4 oz	100	2	15	460	0	3.0	0
tomato, garlic, and onion, 'Gardenstyle Chunky'	1/2 cup	120	2	19	550	3	4.0	0
tomato, Italian, 100% natural,	1/2 cup	120	3	19	580	3	3.0	0
tomato and herbs, 'Today's Recipe'	4 oz	50	2	8	370	0	1.0	0
traditional, 'Old World Style'	1/2 cup	80	2	10	820	3	3.5	0
vegetable primavera, 'Gardenstyle Super'	1/2 cup	110	2	17	480	4	4.0	0
w/meat, 'Homestyle'	4 oz	110	2	15	510	0	5.0	2
w/mushrooms, 'Gardenstyle Super'	1/2 cup	120	3	19	540	3	4.0	0
w/mushrooms, 'Homestyle'	4 oz	110	2	15	530	0	2.0	0
w/mushrooms, 'Thick & Hearty'	4 oz	100	2	15	460	0	3.0	0
w/mushrooms and green peppers, 'Gardenstyle Chunky'	1/2 cup	120	2	18	570	3	4.0	0
w/mushrooms and onions, 'Gardenstyle Chunky'	1/2 cup	120	2	19	560	3	4.0	0
w/sautéed onion and garlic, 100% natural, 'Hearty'	1/2 cup	130	3	19	530	3	5.0	0
w/sautéed onion and mushroom, 'Hearty'	1/2 cup	110	3	17	550	3	4.0	0
w/tomato and herbs, 'Homestyle'	4 oz	110	2	15	510	0	5.0	0
w/tomato and herbs, 'Ragu Fine Italian'	4 oz	90	2	13	490	0	3.0	0
(S&W) 'Ready Cut'	1/4 cup	20	1	4	210	1	0.0	0
(Sutter Home) Zinfandel wine	1/2 cup	100	2	11	520	0	5.0	0
(Timpone's) fresh garlic and basil, 'Mom's Sauce'	4.5 oz	70	2	7	490	1	4.0	0
(Weight Watchers)								
meat flavor	1/3 cup	50	2	9	440	0	1.0	0
mushroom flavor, nonfat	1/3 cup	40	1	9	430	0	0.0	0
(Westbrae)								
primavera	4 oz	60	2	7	490	0	3.0	0
primavera, nonfat, no salt added	4 oz	40	2	7	105	0	0.0	0
PEANUT								
(Mr. Spice) Thai, nonfat, salt-free	1 tbsp	19	1	3	0	0	1.0	0
(San-J) Thai	1 tbsp	30	1	3	311	1	1.3	0
PEPPER DILL (Golden Dipt) 'Nature Bay'	2 grams	8	0	1	96	0	0.0	0
PEPPER								
(Hunt's) homestyle, hot	1 tsp	1	0	0	205	0	0.0	0
(Hunt's) orignal homestyle, original	1 tsp	1	0	0	205	0	0.0	0
PEPPER STEAK (Betty Crocker) 'Recipe Sauces'	3.8 oz	50	1	8	270	0	2.0	0
PEPPERCORN (McCormick/Schilling) green, blend	2 tsp	20	1	3	360	0	0.0	0
PESTO								
(Christopher Ranch) basil and garlic	1/4 cup	230	4	4	325	3	23.0	0
(Contadina)								
frozen, food service product	1 oz	66	3	2	109	1	5.4	7
refrigerated, 'Fresh'	2.33 oz	350	6	6	420	0	34.0	10
w/basil	1/4 cup	310	6	5	440	0	30.0	10
w/sun-dried tomatoes	1/4 cup	250	3	6	520	3	24.0	0
(DiGiorno) refrigerated	2.3 oz	340	8	5	430	0	32.0	20
PICANTE								
(Azteca) mild	1 tbsp	4	0	1	85	0	0.0	0
(Chi-Chi's)								
hot	1 oz	10	2	2	268	0	2.0	2
medium	1 oz	8	2	2	192	0	2.0	2
mild	1 oz	9	2	2	198	0	2.0	2
(Del Monte)								
hot	1/2 cup	20	0	4	385	0	0.0	0
hot, chunky	1/4 cup	15	0	3	405	0	0.0	0
(Estee)	2 tbsp	8	1	2	60	0	0.0	0
(Gebhardt)	1 tbsp	4	0	1	120	0	0.0	0
(Guiltless Gourmet)								
hot	2 tbsp	8	0	1	133	1	0.0	0
medium	2 tbsp	8	0	1	133	1	0.0	0

Food Name	Serv. Size	Total Cal.	Prot. gms	Carbs gms	Sod. mgs	Fiber gms	Fat gms	Chol. mgs
mild	2 tbsp	8	0	1	133	1	0.0	0
(Hunt's) mild, 'Homestyle'	1.09 oz	11	1	2	256	1	0.2	0
(La Victoria)								
medium	2 tbsp	5	0	1	180	0	0.0	0
mild	2 tbsp	10	1	2	230	0	0.0	0
(LaCasita) mild, chunky	2 oz	16	1	4	226	0	0.0	0
(Nestlé)								
'Que Bueno'	1 pkg	1311	47	257	32382	0	8.9	0
'Que Bueno'	2 tbsp	10	0	2	252	0	0.1	0
(Old El Paso)								
'Thick 'n Chunky'	2 tbsp	6	1	1	310	1	0.0	0
all varieties, 'Chunky'	2 tbsp	7	0	2	270	0	0.0	0
all varieties	2 tbsp	8	1	2	310	0	1.0	0
hot	2 tbsp	10	0	2	230	0	0.0	0
hot, 'Thick n' Chunky'	2 tbsp	10	0	2	160	0	0.0	0
medium	2 tbsp	10	0	2	230	0	0.0	0
medium, 'Thick n' Chunky'	2 tbsp	10	0	2	140	0	0.0	0
mild	2 tbsp	10	0	2	230	0	0.0	0
mild, 'Thick n' Chunky'	2 tbsp	10	0	2	130	0	0.0	0
(Ortega) picante, can or jar	1 oz	10	0	2	300	0	0.0	0
(Pace)								
extra mild, 'Thick & Chunky'	2 tsp	3	0	1	111	0	0.1	0
hot, 'Thick & Chunky'	2 tsp	3	0	1	111	0	0.1	0
medium, 'Thick & Chunky'	2 tsp	3	0	1	111	0	0.1	0
mild, 'Thick & Chunky'	2 tsp	3	0	1	111	0	0.1	0
(Rosarita)								
	1.09 oz	7	0	1	247	0	0.1	0
hot, chunky	3 tbsp	18	1	4	515	1	1.0	0
jalapeño, hot, zesty	1.09 oz	8	0	2	246	1	0.2	0
jalapeño, medium, zesty	1.09 oz	9	0	2	254	1	0.2	0
jalapeño, mild, zesty	1.09 oz	8	1	2	239	1	0.1	0
jalapeño, zesty, 'de Mexico Style'	2 tbsp	12	1	3	370	0	0.0	0
mild	3.5 oz	45	2	9	1015	0	1.0	0
mild, chunky	3 tbsp	25	1	5	630	1	1.0	0
(S&W) hot, 'Sun-Vista'	2 tbsp	10	0	2	260	0	0.0	0
(Santiago)	1 fl oz	10	0	2	216	0	0.1	0
(Sun Vista) hot	2 tbsp	10	0	2	260	0	0.0	0
(Sun Vista) mild	2 tbsp	5	0	2	200	0	0.0	0
(Wise)	2 tbsp	12	0	3	130	0	0.0	0
PIZZA								
(Angela Mia)								
food service product	1/4 cup	63	1	4	251	2	0.5	0
super heavy, food service product	1/4 cup	29	2	6	36	3	0.5	0
super heavy, 'Premium Choice'	2.26 oz	28	3	6	36	3	0.5	0
(Chef Boyardee)								
w/cheese	2.63 oz	70	1	7	385	0	4.0	0
w/cheese, 'Jars'	3.88 oz	90	1	10	565	0	6.0	0
(Contadina)								
	1/4 cup	25	1	4	30	1	0.5	0
deluxe	1/4 cup	34	1	5	117	1	0.7	2
original, 'Quick & Easy'	1/4 cup	30	1	5	330	0	1.0	0
pepperoni flavor	1/4 cup	30	1	4	360	1	1.0	0
'Pizza Squeeze'	1/4 cup	30	1	5	330	0	1.0	0
w/Italian cheese	1/4 cup	30	1	4	350	1	1.0	0
(Eden Foods) and pasta sauce, organic	4 oz	80	3	10	320	0	3.0	0
(Enrico's) all natural, no salt added, 'Homemade Style'	4 oz	60	2	9	30	0	1.0	0
(Hunt's)	2.36 oz	32	2	5	416	2	1.1	0

Food Name	Serv. Size	Total Cal.	Prot. gms	Carbs gms	Sod. mgs	Fiber gms	Fat gms	Chol. mgs
fully prepared	2.22 oz	21	1	4	251	2	0.5	0
(Nestlé) deluxe	1 pkg	1623	66	261	5559	60	34.6	90
(Pastorelli) 'Italian Chef'	4 oz	90	3	12	430	0	3.0	0
(Pizza Quick) traditional	3 tbsp	35	1	3	330	0	2.0	0
PLUM								
(Dynasty) nonfat	2 tbsp	80	1	18	210	0	0.0	0
(La Choy)								
	1 tbsp	25	0	6	4	0	0.1	0
food service product	1 tbsp	25	0	6	5	0	0.0	0
PRIMAVERA								
(McCormick/Schilling) blend	1 tbsp	30	0	4	490	0	1.0	3
(Ragu) Italian, light, 'Chicken Tonight'	4 oz	50	2	9	540	0	1.0	0
RIB (Dip n'Joy) 'Saucy Rib'	1 oz	60	0	14	250	0	0.0	0
RIGOLETTO (DiGiorno) refrigerated	5 oz	110	2	9	660	0	8.0	0
ROBERT (Escoffier) 'Sauce Robert'	1 tbsp	20	0	5	70	0	0.0	0
SANDWICH								
(Hunt's)								
barbecue flavored, 'Manwich'	1/4 cup	60	1	14	890	1	0.0	0
bold flavor, 'Manwich'	2.22 oz	62	1	13	802	1	1.1	0
extra thick and chunky, 'Manwich'	2.5 oz	60	1	15	640	0	1.0	0
'Manwich'	2.26 oz	32	1	6	365	1	0.4	0
Mexican, 'Manwich'	2.26 oz	26	1	5	552	1	0.2	0
nonfat, 'Manwich'	2.5 oz	40	1	10	390	0	0.0	0
thick and chunky, 'Manwich'	2.29 oz	44	1	9	737	1	0.5	0
SAUSAGE AND BELL PEPPER Contadina)								
spicy Italian	1/2 cup	100	4	9	540	3	5.0	40
SEAFOOD								
(Great Impressions)								
Creole	1 tbsp	21	0	5	182	0	0.1	0
dipping	1 tbsp	17	1	2	129	0	0.7	0
Polynesian, dipping	1 tbsp	38	1	10	127	0	1.0	0
(Progresso) mixed	1/2 cup	110	5	12	445	2	6.0	11
SEASONING								
(A Taste of Thai)	1 tbsp	15	2	1	1760	0	0.0	0
(Cajun Sunshine) hot pepper	1 tsp	0	0	0	160	na	0.0	na
(Dragon Sauce) rice, vegetables, and stir fry	1 tsp	5	1	1	260	na	0.0	na
(Eden Foods)								
carob, 'EdenBlend'	8 oz	150	6	23	105	0	4.0	0
original, 'EdenBlend'	8 oz	120	7	16	85	0	3.0	0
original, 'Edensoy'	8 oz	130	10	13	105	0	4.0	0
original extra, 'EdenBlend'	8 oz	130	10	13	105	0	4.0	0
(Maggi) Asian	1 tsp	0	1	0	410	0	0.0	0
(Tennessee Sunshine)	1 tsp	0	0	0	160	na	0.0	na
(Tiger Sauce) meat, seafood, and poultry	1 tsp	10	0	2	140	na	0.0	na
(Yucatan Sunshine) habañero pepper	1 tsp	0	0	0	125	na	0.0	na
SHRIMP (Tone's) 'Craboil'	1 tsp	10	0	1	1	0	0.6	1
SHOYU. See under Soy Sauce, below.								
SLOPPY JOE								
(Del Monte)								
hickory flavor	1/4 cup	70	1	18	700	0	0.0	0
Italian recipe	2.5 oz	60	1	14	650	0	0.0	0
original recipe	1/4 cup	70	1	16	680	0	0.0	0
(Hormel) 'Not-so-Sloppy-Sloppy Joe'	2.24 oz	70	1	16	730	0	1.0	5
(Libby's)	1/3 cup	45	1	10	430	1	0.0	0
SOY								
from hydrolyzed vegetable protein	1/4 cup	24	1	4	3300	0	0.0	0
from hydrolyzed vegetable protein	1 tbsp	7	0	1	1024	0	0.0	0

Food Name	Serv. Size	Total Cal.	Prot. gms	Carbs gms	Sod. mgs	Fiber gms	Fat gms	Chol. mgs
from hydrolyzed vegetable protein	1 tsp	2	0	0	341	0	0.0	0
shoyu, from soy and wheat	1 cup	150	20	20	13885	2	0.1	0
shoyu, from soy and wheat	1 tbsp	9	1	1	871	0	0.0	0
shoyu, from soy and wheat	1 tsp	3	0	0	289	0	0.0	0
shoyu, from soy and wheat, low-sodium	1 cup	135	13	22	8499	2	0.2	0
shoyu, from soy and wheat, low-sodium	1 tbsp	10	1	2	600	0	0.0	0
shoyu, from soy and wheat, low-sodium	1 tsp	3	0	0	177	0	0.0	0
tamari, from soy	1 tbsp	11	2	1	1005	0	0.0	0
tamari, from soy	1 tsp	4	1	0	335	0	0.0	0
(Angostura)	1 tbsp	10	1	1	390	na	0.0	0
(Eden Foods)								
shoyu, from soy and wheat, organic	1/2 tsp	2	0	0	140	0	0.0	0
shoyu, naturally brewed	1/2 tsp	2	0	0	140	0	0.0	0
shoyu, reduced-sodium, organic	1/2 tsp	2	0	0	80	0	0.0	0
tamari, wheat-free, organic	1/2 tsp	2	0	0	160	0	0.0	0
(Golden Dipt) honey, 'Nature Bay'	1 oz	90	0	5	250	0	8.0	0
(Kikkoman)								
'Lite'	1 tbsp	10	1	1	605	0	0.0	0
naturally brewed	1 tbsp	10	2	0	920	0	0.0	0
(La Choy)								
	1 tbsp	11	2	1	1227	0	0.0	0
food service product	1 tbsp	11	1	1	1315	0	0.0	0
light	1 tbsp	15	2	2	542	0	0.0	0
light, food service product	1 tbsp	15	1	2	505	0	0.0	0
shoyu	1 tsp	1	0	0	429	0	0.0	0
shoyu, 'Lite'	1 tsp	1	0	0	220	0	0.0	0
(San-J) tamari, less salt	1 tbsp	16	2	1	607	0	0.0	0
(Westbrae)								
low-salt	1/2 tsp	2	1	1	170	0	0.0	0
mild	1/2 tsp	2	1	1	85	0	0.0	0
organic	1/2 tsp	2	1	1	105	0	0.0	0
wheat-free	1/2 tsp	3	1	1	140	0	0.0	0
STEAK								
(A.1.)								
bold	1 tbsp	18	0	4	160	0	0.0	0
regular	1 tbsp	18	0	4	160	0	0.0	0
(Adolph's) '100% Natural'	1/4 tsp	0	0	0	310	0	0.0	0
(Angostura)								
regular	1 tbsp	12	0	3	90	na	0.0	0
salsa flavor	1 tbsp	8	0	2	85	na	0.0	0
(Bullfighter) and burger	1 tbsp	15	0	4	220	na	0.0	na
(Heinz 57)								
hickory smoke, '57'	1 tbsp	16	0	4	180	0	0.0	0
traditional	1 tbsp	12	0	3	200	0	0.0	0
(Hunt's)	1 tbsp	10	0	2	256	0	0.1	0
(Kikkoman)	1 tbsp	20	0	5	290	0	0.0	0
(Lea & Perrins)	1 oz	40	1	10	220	0	1.0	0
STIR-FRY								
(Dynasty) Chinese	2 tbsp	60	1	5	1000	0	3.0	0
(Flavor of the Rain Forest)								
ginger, curry	1 tbsp	15	1	2	173	0	1.0	0
honey hibiscus	1 tbsp	45	0	2	106	0	4.0	0
lime coconut, for seafood	1 tbsp	49	0	1	121	0	5.0	3
'Mango Grille'	1 tbsp	13	0	2	136	0	1.0	0
papaya pepper	1 tsp	3	0	1	50	0	0.0	0
savory	1 tsp	4	0	1	90	0	0.0	0
(Kikkoman)	1 tbsp	15	1	3	530	0	0.0	0

Food Name	Serv. Size	Total Cal.	Prot. gms	Carbs gms	Sod. mgs	Fiber gms	Fat gms	Chol. mgs
(La Choy)								
and marinade, food service product	1 tbsp	25	1	5	672	0	0.1	0
Mandarin soy	1/4 cup	35	1	8	426	1	0.1	0
Szechwan	1/4 cup	42	1	9	312	0	0.1	0
(Lawry's)	1/4 cup	120	2	20	1128	0	3.8	0
(Mr. Spice) ginger, fat-free, salt-free	1 tbsp	11	1	3	0	0	0.0	0
(Nestlé) all-purpose, 'Chef-Mate'	1 tbsp	16	0	2	233	0	0.6	0
(S&W) Oriental	1 tbsp	20	1	5	390	0	0.0	0
STROGANOFF *(Betty Crocker)* 'Recipe Sauces'	4 oz	60	1	6	540	0	4.0	10
SUKIYAKI *(Kikkoman)*	1 tbsp	20	1	4	460	0	0.0	0
SWEET AND SOUR								
(A Taste of Thai) tangy, hot	2 tbsp	30	0	8	95	0	0.0	0
(Betty Crocker) 'Recipe Sauces'	4.1 oz	130	1	32	360	0	0.0	0
(Contadina)	2 tbsp	40	0	8	110	0	1.0	0
(Dynasty)	2 tbsp	70	0	14	125	0	1.0	0
(Great Impressions)								
Hawaiian	2 tbsp	102	0	26	1	0	0.0	0
hot	2 tbsp	102	0	26	1	0	0.0	0
regular	2 tbsp	102	0	26	1	0	0.0	0
(Hickory Farms)								
Hawaiian	2 tbsp	102	0	26	2	0	0.0	0
regular	2 tbsp	102	0	26	1	0	0.0	0
(Kikkoman)	2 tbsp	35	0	9	190	0	0.0	0
(La Choy)								
	1/4 cup	69	1	18	377	1	0.0	0
	1 tbsp	29	0	7	52	0	0.1	0
duck sauce	1 tbsp	31	0	7	64	0	0.1	0
food service product	2 tbsp	58	0	14	121	0	0.1	0
(Lawry's)	1/4 cup	549	3	12	4056	0	7.5	0
(Nestlé) glaze, 'Chef-Mate'	2 tbsp	51	0	12	229	0	0.0	0
(Ragu) 'Chicken Tonight'	4 oz	80	0	19	280	0	0.0	0
(Sauceworks)	1 tbsp	25	0	5	50	0	0.0	0
(Simmer Chef) Oriental	1/2 cup	110	0	23	280	0	1.0	0
SZECHUAN								
(LaChoy) hot and spicy	1 oz	48	0	12	141	0	0.2	0
(Nestlé) 'Chef-Mate'	2 tbsp	42	0	6	436	0	1.8	0
(San-J)	1 tbsp	15	1	2	473	0	0.1	0
TACO								
(Chi-Chi's)								
hot	1 oz	18	2	4	254	0	2.0	1
thick, chunky	1 oz	12	2	3	140	0	2.0	2
(Del Monte)								
hot	1/4 cup	15	0	4	440	0	0.0	0
mild	1/2 cup	15	0	4	480	0	0.0	0
(El Molino) red, mild	2 tbsp	10	0	2	170	0	0.0	0
(Enrico's) mild, no salt added	2 tbsp	14	1	3	25	0	0.0	0
(Estee)	2 tbsp	14	1	3	25	0	0.0	0
(Hain) and dip	4 tbsp	25	1	5	350	0	1.0	5
(Heinz)								
medium	1 tbsp	6	0	1	0	0	0.0	0
mild	1 tbsp	6	0	1	0	0	0.0	0
(La Victoria)								
green	1 tbsp	0	0	1	90	0	0.0	0
green, medium	1 tbsp	5	0	1	96	0	0.1	0
green, mild	1 tbsp	5	0	1	96	0	0.1	0
mild	1 tbsp	7	0	1	103	0	0.1	0
red	1 tbsp	5	0	1	80	0	0.0	0

Food Name	Serv. Size	Total Cal.	Prot. gms	Carbs gms	Sod. mgs	Fiber gms	Fat gms	Chol. mgs
red, medium .... 1 tbsp		7	0	1	103	0	0.1	0
(Lawry's)								
chunky .... 1/4 cup		22	1	4	549	0	0.4	0
'Sauce'n Seasoner' .... 1/4 cup		40	1	8	636	0	0.6	0
(Manwich) seasoning .... 1/4 cup		30	1	6	620	1	0.0	0
(Old El Paso)								
canned .... 2 tbsp		15	1	3	300	1	0.0	0
hot .... 2 tbsp		10	1	2	130	0	1.0	0
medium .... 2 tbsp		10	1	2	130	0	1.0	0
mild or medium, extra chunky .... 1 tbsp		5	0	1	80	0	0.0	0
mild .... 2 tbsp		10	1	2	130	0	1.0	0
(Ortega)								
hot .... 1 oz		12	0	3	210	0	0.0	0
mild .... 1 oz		12	0	3	220	0	0.0	0
Western style .... 1 oz		8	0	2	180	0	0.0	0
(Pancho Villa) mild .... 2 tbsp		15	0	3	170	0	0.0	0
(Rosarita)								
.... 0.18 oz		2	0	0	40	0	0.0	0
food service product .... 1 tbsp		2	0	0	40	0	0.0	0
(Santiago) .... 1 fl oz		13	0	3	164	0	0.2	0
TAMARI. See under Soy Sauce, above.								
TANGY, nonfat, salt-free *(Mr. Spice)* .... 1 tsp		4	1	1	0	0	0.0	0
TARTAR								
(Best Foods)								
.... 2 tbsp		140	0	1	260	na	16.0	10
low-fat .... 2 tbsp		40	0	7	360	na	1.5	0
(Golden Dipt)								
.... 1 tbsp		70	0	2	100	0	7.0	10
'Lite' .... 1 tbsp		50	0	4	40	0	4.0	5
(Great Impressions) .... 1 tbsp		86	0	1	76	0	9.0	10
(Heinz) .... 1 tbsp		71	0	2	124	0	7.2	0
(Hellmann's)								
.... 1 tbsp		70	0	0	220	0	8.0	5
low-fat .... 2 tbsp		40	0	7	360	na	1.5	0
(Kraft) nonfat, 'Free' .... 1 tbsp		10	0	3	120	0	0.0	0
(Life) egg-free, all-natural .... 1 tbsp		38	1	1	2	0	4.0	0
(Sauceworks)								
.... 1 tbsp		50	0	2	85	0	5.0	5
lemon and herb flavor, natural .... 1 tbsp		70	0	0	85	0	8.0	5
(Weight Watchers) .... 1 tbsp		35	0	3	80	0	3.0	5
TEMPURA, dipping sauce *(Kikkoman)* .... 1 tsp		5	0	1	340	0	0.0	0
TERIYAKI								
(Angostura) .... 1 tbsp		10	0	2	260	na	0.0	0
(Betty Crocker) 'Recipe Sauces' .... 3.9 oz		60	2	13	860	0	1.0	0
(Golden Dipt) ginger .... 1 oz		120	1	12	920	0	7.0	0
(Kikkoman)								
baste and glaze .... 2 tbsp		50	1	11	810	0	0.0	0
baste and glaze, w/honey and pineapple .... 2 tbsp		80	1	18	770	0	0.0	0
(La Choy)								
.... 1/4 cup		47	1	11	577	1	0.1	0
.... 1 tbsp		17	1	3	917	1	0.1	0
basting .... 1.23 oz		37	1	8	1524	0	0.0	0
hot .... 1 tbsp		17	2	3	994	0	0.4	0
light .... 1 tbsp		18	1	4	439	0	0.0	0
'Sauce & Marinade' .... 1 oz		30	1	5	1640	0	0.0	0
thick and rich .... 1 oz		41	1	9	509	0	0.1	1

Food Name	Serv. Size	Total Cal.	Prot. gms	Carbs gms	Sod. mgs	Fiber gms	Fat gms	Chol. mgs
(Lawry's)								
barbecue	1/8 cup	82	4	14	6115	0	1.1	0
w/pineapple juice	1/4 cup	72	6	11	7100	0	0.4	0
(Nestlé) 'Chef-Mate'	1 tbsp	21	0	4	159	0	0.6	0
(S&W)								
and marinade	1 tbsp	25	1	5	480	0	0.0	0
and marinade, light	1 tbsp	25	1	5	220	0	0.0	0
TOMATO								
(S&W)								
herb and garlic, Italian	1 tbsp	15	0	2	150	0	1.0	0
original, 'Tomato Garden'	1/4 cup	20	0	4	200	1	0.0	0
(Simmer Chef) Mexicali, zesty	1/2 cup	90	2	16	400	1	3.0	5
TONKATSU *(Kikkoman)*	1 tbsp	20	0	5	290	0	0.0	0
VEGETABLE *(Contadina)* garden, 'Light'	0.5 oz	50	2	10	620	0	0.0	0
WHITE *(Golden Dipt)* French	1 oz	55	0	3	210	0	4.0	0
WORCESTERSHIRE								
(Angostura)	1 tsp	5	0	1	20	0	0.0	0
(French's)								
regular	1 tsp	0	0	1	55	0	0.0	0
smoky	1 tsp	0	0	1	55	0	0.0	0
(Heinz)	1 tbsp	6	0	1	170	0	0.0	0
(Lea & Perrins)								
	1 tsp	5	1	1	55	0	1.0	0
white wine	1 tsp	3	1	1	42	0	1.0	0
(Life) 'All Natural'	1/2 tbsp	5	1	1	2	0	1.0	0
(Wine & Pepper) w/sherry, hot pepper	1 tsp	0	0	1	90	na	0.0	na
SAUCE MIX								
ALFREDO								
(French's) 'Pasta Toss' mix only	2 tsp	25	1	2	310	0	2.0	0
(Lawry's) 'Pasta Alfredo' mix only	1 pkg	226	8	19	3222	1	13.3	0
(Schilling) 'Pasta Prima' mix only	1/4 envelope	40	2	3	410	0	2.5	10
(Knorr) CPC, mix only	2 tbsp	62	2	7	730	na	2.7	5
BARBECUE								
(Blue Plate) concentrate	2 tbsp	110	0	19	350	0	4.0	0
(Woody's) concentrate, 'Cook-in' Sauce'	2 tbsp	50	1	4	490	1	4.0	0
BEEF SAUCE								
(Lipton) sauté, golden, mix only	1/6 pkg	120	3	24	520	0	2.0	0
(Lipton) sauté, golden, prepared w/2 tsp butter	1/2 cup	180	3	24	570	0	8.0	0
CHEESE								
(Custom Foods)								
cheddar, 'Superb' mix only	1 serving	60	1	8	685	1	2.6	4
nacho, 'Superb' mix only	1 serving	60	1	8	733	0	2.6	3
(Durkee) mix only	1/4 cup	25	1	4	260	0	1.5	2
(French's) prepared w/whole milk	1/4 cup	80	3	7	430	0	4.0	0
(McCormick/Schilling)								
mix only	1/4 pkg	35	2	4	477	0	1.5	0
nacho, mix only	1/4 pkg	42	3	5	409	0	1.5	0
(Nestlé)								
nacho, 'Trio' mix only	2 tbsp	51	1	8	338	0	1.9	2
supreme, 'Trio' mix only	2 tbsp	54	1	7	361	0	2.4	4
'Trio' mix only	2 tbsp	54	1	7	310	0	2.3	2
CHICKEN								
(McCormick/Schilling)								
cacciatore 'Sauce Blends' mix only	1 pkg	132	4	28	1092	0	4.8	0
Creole 'Sauce Blends' mix only	1 pkg	140	2	24	1084	0	4.8	0
curry 'Sauce Blends' mix only	1 pkg	152	2	24	1288	0	5.6	0
Dijon 'Sauce Blends' mix only	1 pkg	156	3	20	1414	0	6.8	0

Food Name	Serv. Size	Total Cal.	Prot. gms	Carbs gms	Sod. mgs	Fiber gms	Fat gms	Chol. mgs
mesquite marinade, 'Sauce Blends' mix only .... 1 pkg		132	2	24	2068	0	3.0	0
teriyaki, 'Sauce Blends' mix only .... 1 pkg		172	7	28	1380	0	3.6	0
CURRY								
(S&B)								
golden, hot, mix only .... 1/5 pkt		120	1	11	810	1	7.0	5
golden, medium hot, mix only .... 1/5 pkt		120	1	10	790	1	7.0	5
ENCHILADA								
(Old El Paso) mix only .... 2 tsp		10	0	2	540	1	0.0	0
(Tio Sancho) 'Dinner Kit' mix only .... 3 oz		278	5	62	4058	2	1.5	0
HOLLANDAISE								
(McCormick/Schilling) mix only .... 1/4 pkg		51	1	4	170	0	3.8	0
(Tone's) mix only .... 1 tsp		15	0	1	60	0	1.0	0
ITALIAN								
(Custom Foods) all purpose, 'Red Label' mix only ..... 1 serving		19	0	4	359	0	0.2	0
LEMON BUTTER Weight Watchers) mix only .... 1 tbsp		6	1	1	90	0	0.0	0
PASTA/spaghetti								
(Estee) prepared w/margarine and nonfat milk .... 4 oz		60	2	9	30	0	1.0	0
(Featherweight) prepared w/margarine and nonfat milk ..... 4 oz		60	2	11	310	0	1.0	0
(French's)								
cheese and garlic, 'Pasta Toss' mix only .... 2 tsp		25	1	2	320	0	2.0	0
Italian, 'Pasta Toss' mix only .... 2 tsp		25	1	2	340	0	2.0	0
Romanoff 'Pasta Toss' mix only .... 2 tsp		30	1	1	310	0	2.0	0
w/mushrooms, prepared .... 5/8 cup		100	2	13	1050	0	4.0	0
(Lawry's)								
'Rich & Thick' mix only .... 1 pkg		147	4	28	2172	1	2.2	0
w/importted mushrooms, mix only .... 1 pkg		143	5	26	2015	2	1.5	0
(McCormick/Schilling) mix only .... 1/4 pkg		32	1	6	615	0	0.3	0
(Prego) prepared w/margarine and nonfat milk .... 4 oz		130	2	20	630	0	5.0	0
(Ragu) prepared w/margarine and nonfat milk .... 4 oz		80	2	9	740	0	4.0	0
PEANUT (A Taste of Thai) mix only .... 2 tbsp		25	1	4	115	0	0.5	0
PESTO (French's) 'Pasta Toss' mix only .... 2 tsp		20	1	1	280	0	1.0	0
SANDWICH (Manwich) mix only .... 0.25 oz		22	0	5	351	0	0.1	0
SEAFOOD (Old Bay) 'Old Bay Seas'n' mix only .... 1/5 pkg		30	0	4	160	0	0.0	0
SOUR CREAM (McCormick/Schilling) mix only .... 1/4 pkg		44	1	4	272	0	2.8	0
SPAGHETTI. See SAUCE, PASTA.								
STROGANOFF								
(Lawry's) mix only .... 1 pkg		123	5	26	2814	1	0.3	0
(McCormick/Schilling) mix only .... 2 tsp		15	1	3	350	0	0.0	0
(Natural Touch) prepared as directed .... 4 oz		90	4	10	0	0	3.0	0
SWEET AND SOUR								
(Kikkoman) mix only .... 1 1/2 tbsp		60	0	14	220	0	0.0	0
(Sun Bird) Oriental, mix only .... 1/2 tbsp		15	0	4	110	0	0.0	0
TACO (Tio Sancho) 'Dinner Kit' prepared .... 2 oz		62	2	13	750	1	0.2	0
TAHINI (Casbah) prepared .... 1/4 cup		160	5	10	160	1	13.0	0
TERIYAKI (Kikkoman) mix only .... 2 tsp		20	0	5	640	0	0.0	0
SAUERKRAUT								
Canned								
(A&P) w/liquid .... 1/2 cup		20	1	5	800	0	1.0	0
(Allens) shredded, w/liquid .... 1/2 cup		21	1	5	880	0	1.0	0
(Bush's Best)								
'Bavarian Kraut' .... 1/2 cup		60	1	15	400	3	0.0	0
chopped, 'Kraut' .... 1/2 cup		20	1	5	680	0	0.0	0
kosher, deli-style, 'Kraut' .... 1/2 cup		20	1	5	680	0	0.0	0
shredded, 'Kraut' .... 1/2 cup		20	1	5	680	0	0.0	0
(Del Monte)								
.... 2 tbsp		0	0	1	180	1	0.0	0
w/liquid .... 1/2 cup		25	1	6	775	0	0.0	0

Food Name	Serv. Size	Total Cal.	Prot. gms	Carbs gms	Sod. mgs	Fiber gms	Fat gms	Chol. mgs
(Eden Foods) organic	1/2 cup	25	2	4	580	3	1.0	0
(Finast) w/liquid	1/2 cup	30	1	6	800	0	0.0	0
(Libby's)								
Bavarian style, w/caraway seeds	2 tbsp	15	0	3	180	1	0.0	0
crispy	2 tbsp	5	0	1	190	1	0.0	0
(Pathmark) w/liquid	1/2 cup	20	0	4	880	0	0.0	0
(S&W)	2 tbsp	5	0	2	180	0	0.0	0
(Silver Floss) Bavarian style	1/2 cup	35	1	7	500	0	0.0	0
(Snow Floss) w/liquid	1/2 cup	28	1	4	780	1	0.0	0
(Stokely)								
Bavarian style, w/caraway seeds, mild	1/2 cup	35	0	7	860	3	0.0	0
Bavarian style, w/liquid	1/2 cup	30	1	7	780	0	0.0	0
shredded and chopped, w/liquid	1/2 cup	20	1	4	810	0	0.0	0
shredded, traditional	2 tbsp	5	0	1	190	1	0.0	0
extra mild	1/2 cup	80	0	18	850	3	0.0	0
(Vlasic) w/liquid, 'Old Fashioned'	1/2 cup	4	0	1	280	0	0.0	0
Frozen or refrigerated								
(Claussen)	1/4 cup	5	0	1	210	1	0.0	0
(S&W)	2 tbsp	5	0	1	220	0	0.0	0
SAUERKRAUT JUICE, canned or bottled *(Biotta)*	6 fl oz	21	1	4	1482	0	0.1	0
SAUSAGE								
(Armour) links, 'Premium Smokee'	2 links	150	6	2	480	0	13.0	40
(Eckrich) minced, roll	1 oz slice	80	4	1	300	0	7.0	0
(Hickory Farms) 'Safari'	1 oz	98	5	1	343	0	9.0	14
(JM)								
patty, cooked	1 patty	70	2	1	170	0	6.0	0
patty, raw	1 oz	130	3	1	180	0	14.0	0
raw, 'Tasty Link'	2 links	220	6	1	340	0	21.0	0
(Jones Dairy Farm)								
patty	1 patty	155	6	0	281	0	14.4	36
patty, 'Golden Brown'	1 patty	155	5	0	250	0	14.7	29
patty, spicy, 'Golden Brown'	1 link	100	3	0	159	0	9.5	18
roll, 'Cello Roll'	1 slice	105	4	0	200	0	9.6	24
(Oscar Mayer) link, 'Smokie Links'	1 serving	130	5	1	433	0	11.7	27
BEEF								
(Eckrich)								
	1 oz	100	3	1	270	0	9.0	0
'Lean Supreme'	1 oz	80	4	1	230	0	7.0	0
'Smok-Y-Links'	2 links	160	6	2	350	0	14.0	0
(Hillshire Farm)								
'Flavorseal'	2 oz	180	7	2	490	0	16.0	0
hot links	1 serving	260	10	2	650	0	24.0	60
(Jones Dairy Farm) 'Golden Brown'	1 link	75	4	0	159	0	6.1	18
(Oscar Mayer) 'Smokies'	1 serving	128	5	1	425	0	11.5	28
(Pemmican) Tabasco	1.1 oz	120	5	2	410	0	10.0	0
BEERWURST								
beef, 4-inch diam, 1/8 inch slice	1 slice	76	3	0	236	0	6.9	14
beef, 2.5-inch diam, 1/4 inch slice	1 slice	20	1	0	62	0	1.8	4
pork, 4-inch diam, 1/8 inch slice	1 slice	55	3	0	285	0	4.3	14
pork, 2.5-inch diam, 1/4 inch slice	1 slice	14	1	0	74	0	1.1	4
BERLINER								
pork and beef	1 oz	65	4	1	368	0	4.9	13
pork and beef, 2.5-inch diam, 1/4 inch slice	1 slice	53	4	1	298	0	4.0	11
BLOOD SAUSAGE								
	1 oz	107	4	0	193	0	9.8	34
5 x 4 5/8 x 1/16 inch slice	1 slice	95	4	0	170	0	8.6	30
BOCKWURST								
pork, veal, milk, and eggs	1 oz	87	4	0	313	0	7.8	17

Food Name	Serv. Size	Total Cal.	Prot. gms	Carbs gms	Sod. mgs	Fiber gms	Fat gms	Chol. mgs
pork, veal, milk, and eggs, 7 links per lb	1 link	200	9	0	718	0	17.9	38
BRATWURST								
pork, cooked	1 oz	85	4	1	158	0	7.3	17
pork, cooked, 4 per 12 oz pkg	1 link	256	12	2	473	0	22.0	51
(Eckrich)	1 link	310	11	1	820	0	30.0	0
(Hickory Farms)								
'Brotwurst'	1 oz	90	4	1	277	0	8.0	8
cheddar, 'Cheddy Brots'	1 oz	98	4	1	259	0	9.0	7
hot, 'Hot Brots'	1 oz	96	4	1	269	0	9.0	8
(Johnsonville) w/real Wisconsin beef	1 link	300	14	1	800	0	27.0	70
(Kahn's)	1 link	190	7	2	490	0	17.0	0
BRAUNSCHWEIGER								
	1 oz	102	4	1	324	0	9.1	44
2.5-inch diam, 1/4-inch slice	1 slice	65	2	1	206	0	5.8	28
(Hormel)	1 oz	80	4	0	322	0	7.0	0
(JM)	1 oz	80	3	2	260	0	6.0	0
(Oscar Mayer)								
	1 oz	100	4	1	230	0	9.0	50
	1 slice	100	4	1	320	0	9.0	50
'German Brand'	1 oz	96	4	1	329	0	8.7	45
'Tube'	1 oz	97	4	1	301	0	8.7	47
BREAKFAST								
(Green Giant)								
links, frozen	3 links	110	12	5	340	4	5.0	0
patties, frozen	2 patties	100	10	5	280	3	4.0	0
(Healthy Choice)								
links	2 links	50	7	3	300	0	1.5	15
patties	2 patties	50	7	3	300	0	1.5	15
(Hudson) turkey, ground	1 oz	65	4	0	180	0	5.3	0
(Louis Rich)								
turkey, 85% fat-free	1 oz	55	6	1	230	0	3.0	25
turkey, ground, cooked	1 oz	56	6	0	215	0	3.5	22
(Mr. Turkey) turkey	2.5 oz	190	17	0	665	0	13.4	92
(The Turkey Store) links, mild	2 oz	140	8	1	360	0	11.0	45
BROWN AND SERVE								
(Eckrich) 'Lean Supreme'	2 links	120	7	1	440	0	10.0	0
(Hormel)								
link, uncooked	2 links	180	7	0	411	0	17.0	0
link, cooked	2 links	140	6	0	430	0	13.0	0
(Jones Dairy Farm) link, 'Light'	1 link	60	4	1	150	0	4.1	16
(Swift)								
link, 'Country Recipe'	1 link	130	4	1	240	0	12.0	0
link, 'Premium Original'	1 link	130	3	1	260	0	12.0	0
link, beef, 'Premium Brown 'N Serve'	1 link	120	4	1	250	0	12.0	0
link, maple flavored	1 link	120	3	1	260	0	12.0	0
link, microwave	1 link	120	4	1	270	0	12.0	0
link, smoked flavor	1 link	120	4	1	280	0	11.0	0
link, w/bacon	1 link	120	4	1	270	0	11.0	0
link, w/ham	1 link	130	3	1	260	0	13.0	0
patty, 'Country Recipe'	1 patty	130	4	1	240	0	12.0	0
patty, 'Premium Original'	1 patty	120	4	1	270	0	12.0	0
CAPOCOLLO *(Hormel)*	1 oz	80	5	0	273	0	6.0	0
CERVELAT								
(Hillshire Farm) Thuringer	2 oz	180	9	1	650	0	15.0	0
(Hormel)								
Thuringer, 'Old Smokehouse Chub'	1 oz	100	5	0	332	0	9.0	0
Thuringer, 'Old Smokehouse Sliced'	1 oz	100	5	0	321	0	9.0	0

Food Name	Serv. Size	Total Cal.	Prot. gms	Carbs gms	Sod. mgs	Fiber gms	Fat gms	Chol. mgs
Thuringer, 'Old Smokehouse'	1 oz	90	4	1	328	0	8.0	0
Thuringer, 'Viking Club Cervelat'	1 oz	90	5	0	325	0	8.0	0
(JM)								
Thuringer, beef	1 oz slice	80	5	1	340	0	7.0	0
Thuringer, 'Cervalot'	1 oz slice	70	4	1	260	0	6.0	0
(Oscar Mayer)								
Thuringer, beef	1 serving	142	7	1	655	0	12.4	37
Thuringer, beef, sliced	1 slice	71	3	0	328	0	6.2	18
Thuringer, beef and pork	1 oz	95	4	0	352	0	8.4	21
Thuringer, beef and pork, 4-inch diam, 1/8-inch slice	1 slice	77	4	0	286	0	6.8	17
CHEESE								
(Eckrich)								
'Smok-Y-Links'	2 links	160	6	2	360	0	14.0	0
hot, 'Smok-Y-Links'	2 links	150	6	1	360	0	14.0	0
maple flavored, 'Smok-Y-Links'	2 links	160	6	2	390	0	14.0	0
original, 'Smok-Y-Links'	2 links	160	6	2	340	0	14.0	0
w/ham, 'Smok-Y-Links'	2 links	160	6	2	500	0	15.0	0
(Hillshire Farm)								
bun size, 'Cheddarwurst'	2 oz	200	8	1	480	0	18.0	0
hot, 'Flavorseal'	2 oz	180	7	2	510	0	16.0	0
links, 'Cheddarwurst'	2 oz	190	8	1	480	0	17.0	0
smoked, 'Cheddarwurst'	1 serving	260	11	3	900	0	23.0	50
(Hormel) 'Smokie Cheezers'	2 links	168	9	1	623	0	15.0	0
(Louis Rich)								
turkey, and cheddar, smoked, 90% fat-free	1 oz	45	5	1	270	0	3.0	20
turkey, w/cheese, smoked	1 oz	47	5	1	269	0	2.8	18
(Oscar Mayer)								
pork and turkey, little, 'Smokies'	1 link	28	1	0	93	0	2.5	6
'Smokies'	1 serving	130	6	1	450	0	11.7	30
CHORIZO								
pork and beef	1 oz	129	7	1	350	0	10.8	25
pork and beef, 4-inch link	1 link	273	14	1	741	0	23.0	53
(Carmelita)								
beef	2.5 oz	250	8	5	510	0	23.0	80
pork	2.5 oz	250	8	3	500	0	23.0	110
GERMAN STYLE *(Hickory Farms)*	1 oz	100	5	1	385	0	8.0	20
HEAD CHEESE *(Oscar Mayer)*	1 slice	50	5	0	360	0	4.0	25
HONEY ROLL								
beef	1 oz	52	5	1	375	0	3.0	14
beef, 4-inch diam, 1/8-inch slice	1 slice	42	4	1	304	0	2.4	12
HOT								
(JM)								
patty, cooked	1 patty	70	2	1	170	0	6.0	0
patty, raw	1 oz	130	3	1	180	0	14.0	0
(OHSE) 'Hot Links'	1 oz	80	4	4	310	0	3.0	0
JALAPEÑO *(Bar-S)* smoked	2 oz	180	7	2	630	0	16.0	40
ITALIAN STYLE								
pork, cooked, 5 links per lb	1 link	216	13	1	618	0	17.2	52
pork, cooked, 4 links per lb	1 link	268	17	1	765	0	21.3	65
pork, raw, 7 links per lb	1 link	315	13	1	665	0	28.5	69
pork, raw, 4 links per lb	1 link	391	16	1	826	0	35.4	86
(Hillshire Farm) smoked, 'Flavorseal'	2 oz	200	7	1	500	0	18.0	0
(Johnsonville)								
hot	1 link	300	14	1	800	0	27.0	70
mild	1 link	300	14	1	800	0	27.0	70
(Shelton's) turkey	1 serving	160	7	0	310	0	16.0	30
(The Turkey Store) turkey, hot	3 oz	140	15	2	681	0	9.0	45

Food Name	Serv. Size	Total Cal.	Prot. gms	Carbs gms	Sod. mgs	Fiber gms	Fat gms	Chol. mgs
KIELBASA								
pork and beef	1 oz	88	4	1	305	0	7.7	19
(Eckrich)								
light, 'Lean Supreme Polska'	1 oz	72	4	1	224	0	6.0	0
w/o skin, 'Polska'	1 link	180	7	2	420	0	16.0	0
(Healthy Choice) low-fat	2 oz	70	7	6	480	0	1.5	20
(Hillshire Farm) bun size	1 serving	180	7	2	660	0	16.0	40
(Hormel)								
'Kolbase'	3 oz	220	12	1	904	0	19.0	0
w/o skin	1/2 link	180	12	1	826	0	14.0	0
(Louis Rich) turkey, smoked, 90% fat-free	1 oz	40	5	1	250	0	2.0	20
(Mr. Turkey) 'Polska Kielbasa'	1 oz	59	4	1	264	0	4.4	15
KNOCKWURST								
pork and beef	1 oz	87	3	0	286	0	7.9	16
pork and beef, 4-inch x 1 1/8 inch diam	1 link	209	8	1	687	0	18.9	39
(Hebrew National) beef, 1 link	3 oz	263	10	1	877	0	25.0	26
LIVER. See SAUSAGE, BRAUNSCHWEIGER.								
LUNCHEON								
pork and beef	1 oz	74	4	0	335	0	5.9	18
pork and beef, 4-inch diam, 1/8-inch slice	1 slice	60	4	0	272	0	4.8	15
MILD *(Jones Dairy Farm)* 'Golden Brown'	1 link	100	3	0	150	0	9.8	18
MORTADELLA								
beef and pork	1 oz	88	5	1	353	0	7.2	16
beef and pork, 15 per 8-oz pkg	1 slice	47	2	0	187	0	3.8	8
NEW ENGLAND STYLE								
pork and beef	1 oz	46	5	1	346	0	2.1	14
pork and beef, 4-inch diam, 1/8-inch slice	1 slice	37	4	1	281	0	1.7	11
(Eckrich) New England brand	1 oz slice	35	5	1	370	0	1.0	0
(Light & Lean) New England brand	2 slices	90	10	0	0	0	6.0	0
(Oscar Mayer)	1 slice	60	8	1	570	0	2.5	25
PEPPERONI								
pork and beef, 10 1/4 inch long x 1 3/8 inch diam	1 sausage	1247	53	7	5120	0	110.4	198
pork and beef, 1 3/8 inch diam, 1/8-inch slice	1 slice	27	1	0	112	0	2.4	4
(Gallo Salame)								
deli style	11 slices	160	7	0	610	0	14.0	30
pizza style	9 slices	140	6	0	550	0	13.0	30
(Hickory Farms)	1 oz	140	6	1	578	0	13.0	23
(Hormel)								
	1 oz	140	6	0	462	0	13.0	0
bits	1 tbsp	35	2	0	0	0	3.0	0
'Chunk'	1 oz	140	6	0	423	0	12.0	0
'Leoni Brand'	1 oz	130	6	0	508	0	12.0	0
'Perma-Fresh'	2 slices	80	3	0	281	0	7.0	0
'Rosa'	1 oz	140	6	0	626	0	13.0	0
'Rosa Grande'	1 oz	140	6	0	512	0	13.0	0
turkey, 'Pillow Pak'	1 serving	74	9	1	557	na	3.5	37
(JM) sliced	8 slices	70	3	1	290	0	6.0	0
(Oscar Mayer)	15 slices	140	6	0	550	0	13.0	25
PICKLED								
(Penrose)								
beer	1 link	40	2	1	220	0	3.0	0
firecracker	1 link	40	2	1	220	0	3.0	0
firecracker, giant	1 link	170	9	1	870	0	14.0	0
hot	1 link	40	2	1	220	0	3.0	0
red hot	1 link	40	2	1	220	0	3.0	0
POLISH STYLE. See also KIELBASA.								
pork	1 oz	92	4	0	248	0	8.1	20

Food Name	Serv. Size	Total Cal.	Prot. gms	Carbs gms	Sod. mgs	Fiber gms	Fat gms	Chol. mgs
pork, 10-inch long x 1.25-inch diam .... 1 sausage		740	32	4	1989	0	65.2	159
(Hormel) .... 2 links		170	9	0	574	0	14.0	0
(OHSE)								
hot .... 1 oz		70	4	3	270	0	5.0	0
.... 1 oz		80	4	1	290	0	7.0	0
(Penrose) pickled .... 1 link		40	2	1	220	0	3.0	0
(Pilgrim's Pride) .... 3 oz		131	13	2	780	0	7.7	72
PORK								
link, 4-inch long x 1 1/8 inch diam .... 1 link		265	15	1	1020	0	21.6	46
link, fresh, cooked, 4-inch long x 7/8-inch diam								
before cooking .... 1 link		48	3	0	168	0	4.1	11
link, fresh, raw, 7/8-inch diam x 4-inch long .... 1 link		117	3	0	187	0	11.3	19
link, 2-inch long x 3/4-inch diam .... 1 link		62	4	0	240	0	5.1	11
patty, fresh, cooked, 3 7/8 inch diam x 1/4-inch								
thick before cooking .... 1 patty		100	5	0	349	0	8.4	2.9
patty, fresh, raw 3 7/8 inch diam x 1/4-inch thick .... 1 patty		238	7	1	380	0	23.0	39
(Hormel)								
links, 'Midget Links' .... 2 links		143	7	0	327	0	13.0	0
links, 'Little Sizzlers' .... 2 links		103	6	0	172	0	9.0	0
(Jimmy Dean)								
hot .... 2 oz		250	10	0	540	0	24.0	50
'Light' .... 1.2 oz		80	6	1	230	0	7.0	25
links .... 2 links		180	7	1	380	0	17.0	0
patties .... 1 patty		140	5	1	300	0	13.0	0
regular, cooked .... 1 oz		120	4	1	240	0	11.0	0
sage .... 2 oz		250	10	0	540	0	24.0	50
(JM)								
and bacon, cooked, 'Tasty Link' .... 2 links		100	6	1	240	0	9.0	0
cooked, 'Tasty Link' .... 2 links		190	6	1	290	0	18.0	0
raw, 'Tasty Link' .... 2 links		260	6	1	380	0	26.0	0
(Jones Dairy Farm)								
.... 1 link		140	3	0	176	0	13.7	24
'Golden Brown Light' .... 1 link		55	3	1	132	0	4.2	16
'Light' .... 1 link		70	4	1	232	0	5.0	21
(Oscar Mayer)								
link .... 2 links		170	9	1	410	0	15.0	40
link, cooked .... 1 link		82	4	0	201	0	7.3	18
link, 'Little Friers' cooked .... 1 link		82	3	0	219	0	7.5	17
(Owens)								
country style .... 2 oz		290	10	0	420	0	27.0	20
country style, hot .... 2 oz		290	10	0	460	0	27.0	15
country style, sage .... 2 oz		250	11	1	310	0	23.0	20
(Pierre)								
link, all meat, product 3755 .... 1 piece		85	8	0	232	0	5.3	27
patty, all meat, product 3750 .... 1 piece		85	8	0	232	0	5.3	27
patty, all meat, product 3751 .... 1 piece		174	17	1	473	0	10.8	55
patty, all meat, product 3850 .... 1 piece		95	8	1	231	0	6.6	27
patty, all meat, product 3851 .... 1 piece		193	16	1	469	0	13.4	55
(Tyson) country, whole hog .... 3.5 oz		320	13	1	905	0	29.0	49
PORK AND BEEF								
link, 4-inch long x 1 1/8 inch diam .... 1 link		228	9	1	643	0	20.6	48
link, fresh, cooked, 4-inch long x 7/8-inch diam								
before cooking .... 1 link		51	2	0	105	0	4.7	9
link, 2-inch long x 3/4-inch diam .... 1 link		54	2	0	151	0	4.9	11
patty, fresh, cooked, 3 7/8 inch diam x 1/4-inch								
thick before cooking .... 1 patty		107	4	1	217	0	9.8	19
PORK AND TURKEY *(Oscar Mayer)* little, 'Smokies' .... 1 link		27	1	0	92	0	2.4	6

Food Name	Serv. Size	Total Cal.	Prot. gms	Carbs gms	Sod. mgs	Fiber gms	Fat gms	Chol. mgs
SAGE *(Jimmy Dean)* cooked	1 oz	120	4	1	240	0	11.0	0
SALAMI. See also under LUNCHEON MEAT.								
beef and pork, cooked	1 oz	71	4	1	302	0	5.7	18
beef and pork, cooked, 4-inch diam, 1/8 inch slice	1 slice	58	3	1	245	0	4.6	15
beef, cooked	1 oz	74	4	1	333	0	5.9	18
beef, cooked, 4-inch diam, 1/8 inch slice	1 slice	60	3	1	270	0	4.8	15
pork, dry or hard, 3 1/8 inch diam, 1/16-inch slice	1 slice	41	2	0	226	0	3.4	8
pork and beef, dry or hard, 3 1/8 inch diam, 1/16-inch slice	1 slice	42	2	0	186	0	3.4	8
SCRAPPLE *(Jones Dairy Farm)*	1 slice	65	3	4	165	0	3.7	24
SMOKED								
(Eckrich)								
'Lean Supreme'	1 oz	70	4	1	230	0	6.0	0
'No skin'	1 link	180	7	2	420	0	16.0	0
(Healthy Choice) low-fat	2 oz	70	7	6	480	0	1.5	20
(Hillshire Farm)								
'Flavorseal'	2 oz	190	7	1	500	0	17.0	0
original, bun size	1 serving	180	7	2	660	0	16.0	40
(Hormel) 'Smokies'	2 links	160	9	2	597	0	14.0	0
(OHSE)	1 oz	80	4	1	320	0	7.0	0
(Oscar Mayer) link 'Big & Juicy'	2.7 oz	227	9	1	757	0	20.5	48
(Pilgrim's Pride)	3 oz	144	13	3	890	0	9.1	64
SUMMER								
(Eckrich)	1 oz slice	80	4	1	320	0	7.0	0
(Hormel)								
beef, 'Beefy'	1 oz	100	5	0	313	0	9.0	0
'Perma-Fresh'	2 slices	140	10	0	706	0	11.0	0
'Tangy, Chub'	1 oz	90	5	0	317	0	7.0	0
'Thuringer'	1 oz	90	4	0	332	0	9.0	0
(Lean & Lite)	1 oz	43	6	1	0	0	2.3	18
(Light & Lean)	2 slices	100	6	0	0	0	8.0	0
(Louis Rich)								
turkey	1 oz slice	55	5	0	326	0	3.9	21
turkey, 85% fat-free	1 oz slice	55	5	1	325	0	4.0	25
(OHSE)								
	1 oz	75	5	2	340	0	5.0	0
beef	1 oz	80	5	1	330	0	6.0	0
(Oscar Mayer) sliced	1 slice	69	4	0	331	0	6.1	19
SWEDISH STYLE *(Hickory Farms)*	1 oz	100	5	0	380	0	9.0	20
TURKEY								
(Butterball)	1 oz	50	4	1	250	0	4.0	0
(Jimmy Dean) 'Light'	1.2 oz	80	6	1	230	0	7.0	25
(Louis Rich)								
link, cooked	1 link	46	5	0	234	0	2.7	18
link, cooked, 85% fat-free	0.84 oz	45	6	1	235	0	3.0	20
original or hot	2.5 oz	120	12	1	430	0	8.0	55
smoked	1 serving	90	8	2	515	0	5.4	36
(Norbest) 'Tasti-Lean, Chub or Links'	1 oz	53	5	0	179	0	2.8	0
(Shelton's)								
links	1 serving	140	6	0	260	0	14.0	30
patty	1 serving	140	10	0	370	0	11.0	45
VEGETARIAN								
(Boca) breakfast patty, vegetarian	1 patty	70	9	4	300	2	3.0	0
(Garden Sausage) garden sausage, meatless, soy-free	1 oz	95	4	18	65	4	1.0	0
(Heartline)								
Italian style, cooked	2 oz	176	19	9	680	0	7.0	0
pepperoni style, lite	0.5 oz	22	5	1	135	3	0.0	0

Food Name	Serv. Size	Total Cal.	Prot. gms	Carbs gms	Sod. mgs	Fiber gms	Fat gms	Chol. mgs
(Loma Linda)								
breakfast links, vegetarian	2 links	93	8	3	226	1	5.6	1
'Linketts'	1 link	70	7	1	160	1	4.5	0
'Little Links'	2 links	90	8	1	230	2	6.0	0
(Morningstar Farms)								
'Breakfast Links'	2 links	60	8	2	340	2	2.0	0
'Breakfast Patties'	1 patty	80	10	3	270	2	3.0	0
'Sausage Style Recipe Crumbles'	2/3 cup	90	11	5	370	2	3.0	0
(Worthington)								
breakfast links, vegetarian	2 links	63	8	2	338	2	2.4	1
breakfast patty, vegetarian	1 pkg	8531	1065	399	27839	212	297.6	82
breakfast patty, vegetarian	1 patty	79	10	4	259	2	2.8	1
'Leanies'	1 link	100	7	2	430	1	7.0	0
'Low Fat Veja-Links'	1 link	40	5	1	190	0	1.5	0
'Prosage Links'	2 links	63	8	2	338	2	2.4	1
'Prosage Patties'	1 patty	96	10	3	296	2	3.2	1
'Prosage' roll, frozen	5/8-inch slice	142	10	2	392	2	10.4	1
'Saucettes'	2 slices	86	6	1	205	1	6.5	1
'Super Links'	1 link	110	7	2	350	1	8.0	0
'Veja-Links'	1 link	49	5	1	192	0	3.0	1
VIENNA								
beef and pork, canned, 7/8-inch diam x 2-inch long . . .	1 sausage	45	2	0	152	0	4.0	8
(Armour)								
chicken, in beef stock, lite, canned, 'Premium'	2 oz	150	6	1	400	0	13.0	0
hot and spicy, canned	2.5 oz	190	6	3	860	0	17.0	0
in barbecue sauce, canned	2.5 oz	190	6	4	760	0	17.0	0
in beef stock, canned	2 oz	180	5	1	530	0	17.0	0
in beef stock, lite, canned	2 oz	150	6	1	400	0	13.0	0
smoked, canned	2 oz	180	5	1	530	0	17.0	0
(Hormel)								
canned	1 oz	69	3	2	225	0	7.0	15
chicken, canned	1 oz	56	3	1	220	0	5.0	27
no broth, canned	4 links	200	7	1	479	0	18.0	0
(Libby's)								
chicken, in beef broth, canned	2 oz	130	7	3	560	0	10.0	0
in barbecue sauce, canned	2.5 oz	180	8	2	420	0	15.0	0
in beef broth, canned, approx. 3 1/2 links	2 oz	160	6	1	330	0	15.0	0
SAUSAGE STICK								
(Hickory Farms) stick, 'Sportsman Stick'	1 oz	138	9	4	1075	0	10.0	40
(Slim Jim) smoked, 'Giant Slim'	1.1 oz	180	7	2	470	0	16.0	0
(Slim Jim) Tabasco, 'Handi-Paks'	0.31 oz	50	2	1	130	0	4.0	0
(Slim Jim) smoked, 'Jumbo Jim'	1 oz	150	8	2	430	0	12.0	0
(Slim Jim) smoked, pepperoni 'Handi-Paks'	0.31 oz	50	2	1	130	0	4.0	0
(Slim Jim) smoked, spicy 'Handi-Paks'	0.31 oz	50	2	1	130	0	4.0	0
SAVORY								
ground	1 tbsp	12	0	3	1	2	0.3	0
ground	1 tsp	4	0	1	0	1	0.1	0
ground *(Durkee)*	1 tsp	5	0	0	0	0	0.0	0
ground *(Laurel Leaf)*	1 tsp	5	0	0	0	0	0.0	0
ground *(McCormick/Schilling)*	1 tsp	7	0	2	0	1	0.0	0
ground *(Spice Islands)*	1 tsp	5	0	1	1	0	0.1	0
summer, ground *(Tone's)*	1 tsp	4	0	1	1	0	0.1	0
SAVOY CABBAGE. See CABBAGE, SAVOY.								
SCALLION								
Fresh								
raw, chopped *(Dole)*	1 tbsp	2	0	0	0	0	0.1	0
raw, tops and bulb, chopped	1 cup	32	2	7	16	3	0.2	0

Food Name	Serv. Size	Total Cal.	Prot. gms	Carbs gms	Sod. mgs	Fiber gms	Fat gms	Chol. mgs
raw, tops and bulb, chopped	1 tbsp	2	0	0	1	0	0.0	0
raw, tops and bulb, whole, large, 5 1/4 inch long	1 scallion	8	0	2	4	1	0.0	0
raw, tops and bulb, whole, medium, 4 1/8 inch long	1 scallion	5	0	1	2	0	0.0	0
raw, tops and bulb, whole, small, 3-inch long	1 scallion	2	0	0	1	0	0.0	0
Freeze dried								
(McCormick/Schilling)	1 tsp	4	0	1	3	0	0.0	0
SCALLOP								
mixed species, breaded and fried	2 large	67	6	3	144	na	3.4	19
mixed species, raw	2 large	26	5	1	48	0	0.2	10
mixed species, raw	3 oz	75	14	2	137	0	0.6	28
SCALLOP SQUASH. See SQUASH, SCALLOP.								
SCALLOP SUBSTITUTE								
made from Surimi	3 oz	84	11	9	676	0	0.3	19
vegetarian, 'Skallops' (Worthington)	1/2 cup	86	15	3	412	3	1.4	0
SCORZONERA. See SALSIFY, BLACK.								
SCOTCH KALE. See KALE, SCOTCH.								
SCRAPPLE. See under SAUSAGE.								
SCROD ENTRÉE								
(Gorton's) frozen, baked 'Microwave Entrées'	1 pkg	320	22	17	420	0	18.0	80
SCUP/sea bream								
baked, broiled, grilled, or microwaved	3 oz	115	21	0	46	0	3.0	57
raw	1 cup	174	31	0	70	0	4.5	86
raw	3 oz	89	16	0	36	0	2.3	44
raw, boneless	1 oz	30	5	0	12	0	0.8	15
SEA BASS. See BASS, SEA.								
SEA BREAM. See SCUP.								
SEA DEVIL. See MONKFISH.								
SEA PERCH. See OCEAN PERCH, ATLANTIC.								
SEA TROUT. See under TROUT.								
SEA VEGETABLE								
AGAR, raw	2 tbsp	3	0	1	1	0	0.0	0
ALARIA, dry (Maine Coast)	1/3 cup	18	1	3	301	3	0.0	0
DULSE								
dry (Maine Coast)	1/3 cup	18	2	3	122	2	0.0	0
raw	3.5 oz	<1	0.0	0.0	2085	>1.2 c	3.2	0
HIZIKI, dry (Eden Foods)	1/2 cup	30	0	6	160	6	0.0	0
IRISH MOSS, raw	2 tbsp	5	0	1	7	0	0.0	0
KELP								
dry (Maine Coast)	1/3 cup	17	1	3	312	3	0.0	0
raw	2 tbsp	4	0	1	23	0	0.1	0
KOMBU, wild, 7-inch pieces (Eden Foods)	1/2 piece	10	0	2	90	1	0.0	0
LAVER								
raw	10 sheets	9	2	1	12	1	0.1	0
raw	2 tbsp	4	1	1	5	0	0.0	0
NORI								
dry (Maine Coast)	1/3 cup	22	2	3	113	3	0.0	0
dry (Eden Foods)	1 piece	10	1	1	5	1	0.0	0
dry, for sushi (Eden Foods)	1 sheet	10	1	1	5	1	0.0	0
WAKAME								
dry (Eden Foods)	1/2 cup	25	2	4	660	4	0.0	0
flakes, instant (Eden Foods)	1 tsp	3	0	0	72	0	0.0	0
raw	2 tbsp	5	0	1	87	0	0.1	0
SEA VEGETABLE CHIP (Eden Foods)	1 oz	130	1	22	200	0	5.0	0
SEAFOOD DINNER/ENTRÉE. See also individual listings.								
(Armour) w/natural herbs, frozen, 'Classics Lite'	10 oz	190	13	29	1020	0	2.0	35
(Budget Gourmet)								
Newburg, frozen	10 oz	350	17	43	660	0	12.0	70

Food Name	Serv. Size	Total Cal.	Prot. gms	Carbs gms	Sod. mgs	Fiber gms	Fat gms	Chol. mgs
shrimp w/scallops, frozen, 'Mariner'	11.5 oz	320	16	43	690	0	9.0	70
(Cajun Cookin') gumbo, frozen	17 oz	330	16	51	1330	0	7.0	0
(Mrs. Paul's)								
shrimp and clams, w/linguini, frozen, 'Light'	10 oz	240	12	36	750	0	5.0	40
(Pillsbury) casserole, frozen, 'Microwave Classic'	1 pkg	420	15	37	950	0	24.0	0
(Swanson) Creole, w/rice, frozen, 'Homestyle Recipe'	9 oz	240	7	40	810	0	6.0	0

SEAFOOD SEASONING. See under SEASONING MIX.

SEASONING AND COATING MIX. See also MARINADE; MARINADE MIX.

ALL-PURPOSE

Food Name	Serv. Size	Total Cal.	Prot. gms	Carbs gms	Sod. mgs	Fiber gms	Fat gms	Chol. mgs
(Golden Dipt) breading	1 oz	90	3	20	630	0	0.0	0
(Shake 'N Bake) country mild recipe	1/4 pkt	80	1	10	500	0	4.0	0

CHICKEN

Food Name	Serv. Size	Total Cal.	Prot. gms	Carbs gms	Sod. mgs	Fiber gms	Fat gms	Chol. mgs
(Don's Chuck Wagon) frying mix, super crispy	1/4 cup	95	3	21	850	1	0.0	0
(Golden Dipt)								
	1 oz	90	2	20	1430	0	0.0	0
frying mix	1 oz	90	2.0	20.0	1430	(mg)	0.0	0
(Luzianne) Cajun coating, bake, fry, or microwave	2 tbsp	100	3	20	1260	1	0.5	0
(Oven Fry)								
extra crispy recipe	1 serving	60	2	10	420	0	1.0	0
home style flour recipe	1 serving	40	1	7	470	0	1.0	0
(Shake 'N Bake)								
barbecue	1 serving	45	0	9	410	0	1.0	0
hot and spicy	1/4 pkt	80	2	15	380	0	2.0	0
original	1 serving	40	1	7	220	0	1.0	0
'Original Barbecue Recipe'	1/4 pkt	90	1	18	840	0	2.0	0
(Tone's) Cajun, batter seasoning	1 tsp	12	0	3	75	0	0.1	0

FISH

Food Name	Serv. Size	Total Cal.	Prot. gms	Carbs gms	Sod. mgs	Fiber gms	Fat gms	Chol. mgs
(Tone's) Cajun	1 tsp	12	0	3	49	0	0.1	0
(Don's Chuck Wagon) no MSG	1/4 cup	95	4	21	940	1	0.0	0
(Shake 'N Bake) original	1 serving	70	1	14	420	1	1.5	0

Food Name	Serv. Size	Total Cal.	Prot. gms	Carbs gms	Sod. mgs	Fiber gms	Fat gms	Chol. mgs
FLOUR, seasoned, all-purpose, dry (Kentucky Kernel)	1/4 cup	90	3	20	1360	0	0.0	0

PORK

Food Name	Serv. Size	Total Cal.	Prot. gms	Carbs gms	Sod. mgs	Fiber gms	Fat gms	Chol. mgs
(Oven Fry) extra crispy recipe	1 serving	60	2	11	340	0	1.5	0
(Shake 'N Bake)								
	1 serving	45	0	9	410	0	1.0	0
hot and spicy	1/8 pkt	45	1	8	220	0	1.0	0
'Original Recipe'	1/8 pkt	40	1	8	310	0	1.0	0

SEAFOOD

Food Name	Serv. Size	Total Cal.	Prot. gms	Carbs gms	Sod. mgs	Fiber gms	Fat gms	Chol. mgs
(Don's Chuck Wagon) seasoned, no MSG	1/4 cup	95	2	21	990	1	0.0	0
(Golden Dipt)								
fish fry, Cajun style, mix only	2/3 oz	60	2	14	470	0	0.0	0
fish fry, mix only	2/3 oz	60	2	14	430	0	0.0	0
mix only	2/3 oz	60	1	14	600	0	0.0	0
(Luzianne) bake, fry, or microwave, Cajun, mix only	2 tbsp	100	2	22	1200	1	0.5	0

SEASONING MIX

ALL-PURPOSE

Food Name	Serv. Size	Total Cal.	Prot. gms	Carbs gms	Sod. mgs	Fiber gms	Fat gms	Chol. mgs
(Knorr)	1 gram	5	0	0	240	0	0.0	0
(Mrs. Dash) table blend	0.13 tsp	2	0	0	1	na	0.0	0
(Praise Allah) for steak, meats, stews, and gravies	1/4 tsp	0	0	0	105	na	0.0	na
(Spike All Purpose) all natural	1/4 tsp	1	0	0	161	0	0.0	0
(Trader Joe's) salt-free, '21 Seasoning Salute'	1/4 tsp	0	0	0	0	0	0.0	0
APPLE PIE SPICE (Tone's)	1 tsp	9	0	2	1	1	0.2	0
BARBECUE SPICE (Tone's)	1 tsp	9	0	1	713	0	0.4	0

BEEF

Food Name	Serv. Size	Total Cal.	Prot. gms	Carbs gms	Sod. mgs	Fiber gms	Fat gms	Chol. mgs
(Adolph's) stew, 'Meal Makers'	1 tbsp	20	1	4	750	0	0.0	0
(Bag 'n Season)								
pot roast	1 tsp	10	1	1	390	na	0.0	0

Food Name	Serv. Size	Total Cal.	Prot. gms	Carbs gms	Sod. mgs	Fiber gms	Fat gms	Chol. mgs
Swiss steak	1 tsp	15	0	2	430	na	0.0	0
(French's) w/onions, ground	1/4 pkg	25	1	6	440	0	0.0	0
(Kikkoman) broccoli beef stir-fry	2 tsp	15	1	3	480	0	0.0	0
(Lawry's)								
pot roast, 'Seasoning Blends'	1 pkg	122	4	25	4008	1	0.7	0
stew, 'Seasoning Blends'	1 pkg	131	5	26	3181	1	0.7	0
(McCormick/Schilling) stew	2 tsp	15	1	3	410	0	0.0	0
(Schilling)								
pot roast, 'Bag'n Season'	1 pkg	55	4	9	3030	0	0.6	0
steak, 'Montreal LaGrille'	1/4 tsp	0	0	0	150	0	0.0	0
steak, broiled, 'Spice Blends'	1/4 tsp	1	0	0	273	0	0.0	0
stew	1/2 pkg	33	1	6	806	0	0.3	0
stew, 'Bag'n Season'	1 pkg	87	8	11	4320	0	1.0	1
stew, 'Bag'n Season'	1 tsp	15	1	1	670	na	0.0	0
Stroganoff	1/4 pkg	32	1	6	1078	0	0.3	0
Swiss steak, 'Bag'n Season'	1 pkg	81	2	17	2651	0	0.4	1
(Sun Bird) beef and broccoli, Oriental	3/4 tbsp	20	0	5	140	0	0.0	0
(Tone's) steak, blackened	1 tsp	9	0	2	486	0	0.3	0
BURRITO								
(Lawry's) 'Seasoning Blends'	1 pkg	132	6	23	2516	1	1.7	0
(Old El Paso)	2 tsp	20	1	3	290	1	0.0	0
(Tio Sancho) 'Dinner Kit'	3.25 oz	265	12	49	5031	6	2.1	0
CAJUN								
(Luzianne)	1/4 tsp	0	0	0	260	0	0.0	0
(Tone's)	1 tsp	9	0	2	215	1	0.2	0
CHICKEN								
(Featherweight)	1/4 pkg	18	1	8	30	0	0.0	0
(Kikkoman) roast	1 tbsp	25	1	4	1980	0	0.0	0
(Lawry's) Southwest, 'Seasoning Blends'	1 pkg	71	1	16	3947	0	0.3	0
(Schilling)								
'Bag'n Season'	1 pkg	134	3	19	4771	0	5.0	1
barbecue, tangy	2 tsp	20	0	3	400	0	0.0	0
fried chicken	1/4 tsp	1	0	0	132	0	0.1	0
rotisserie style	3/4 tsp	0	0	1	340	0	0.0	0
CHILI								
(Carroll Shelby's) Texas brand, original	3 tbsp	80	2	14	1600	0	1.5	0
(Gebhardt)								
'Chili Quik'	1 tbsp	14	0	3	204	0	0.3	0
'Chili Quik' food service product	1 tbsp	18	1	4	407	1	0.4	0
(Hain)								
hot	1/4 pkg	30	1	5	370	0	1.0	0
medium	1/4 pkg	30	1	5	300	0	1.0	0
mild	1/2 pkg	30	1	5	330	0	1.0	0
(Lawry's) 'Seasoning Blends'	1 pkg	143	5	27	2291	2	1.8	0
(McCormick/Schilling) original	1 tbsp	25	1	4	240	2	0.5	0
(Old El Paso)	1 tbsp	25	1	4	770	1	0.5	0
(Schilling)	1/4 pkg	27	1	5	290	0	0.5	0
(Tio Sancho)	1.23 oz	109	4	6	832	4	2.2	0
(Tone's)	1 tsp	12	0	2	231	0	0.3	0
(Wick Fowler's)								
mild, 'False Alarm'	2 tbsp	50	2	9	980	0	1.5	0
'2 Alarm'	3 tbsp	60	2	10	980	0	1.5	0
CHILI POWDER								
	1 tbsp	24	1	4	76	3	1.3	0
	1 tsp	8	0	1	26	1	0.4	0
(Gebhardt)	1 tbsp	3	0	1	1	0	0.2	0

Food Name	Serv. Size	Total Cal.	Prot. gms	Carbs gms	Sod. mgs	Fiber gms	Fat gms	Chol. mgs
(Tone's)								
hot	1 tsp	8	0	1	25	1	0.4	0
mild	1 tsp	8	0	1	25	1	0.4	0
CHOP SUEY *(Sun Bird)* Oriental	1 tbsp	20	0	5	550	0	0.0	0
CHOW MEIN *(Kikkoman)*	1 tbsp	20	1	3	570	0	0.0	0
CREOLE, no MSG *(Tony Chachere's)*	1/4 tsp	0	0	0	310	0	0.0	0
CURRY								
(A Taste of Thai)								
panang curry base	1 tbsp	25	0	2	180	0	2.0	0
red curry base	1 tbsp	20	0	1	430	0	1.5	0
CURRY POWDER								
	1 tbsp	20	1	4	3	2	0.9	0
	1 tsp	7	0	1	1	1	0.3	0
(Tone's)	1 tsp	6	0	1	1000	0	0.3	0
DILL *(Schilling)* 'Parsley Patch It's a Dilly'	1 tsp	11	0	2	5	0	0.4	0
ENCHILADA								
(Lawry's) 'Seasoning Blends'	1 pkg	152	5	30	1723	1	1.2	0
(Old El Paso)	1/8 pkg	6	0	1	80	0	0.0	0
FAJITA								
(Crown Colony)	1/2 tsp	5	0	1	95	0	0.0	0
(Lawry's) 'Seasoning Blends'	1 pkg	63	2	14	2118	1	0.4	0
FISH *(Featherweight)*	1/4 pkg	18	1	8	10	0	0.0	0
FIVE-SPICE *(Tone's)* Oriental	1 tsp	9	0	2	2	1	0.3	0
FRENCH FRY *(Tone's)*	1 tsp	5	0	1	1551	0	0.1	0
GARLIC								
(Golden Dipt)	2 grams	8	0	1	87	0	0.0	0
(Lawry's) concentrate	1 tbsp	15	0	0	21	0	1.6	0
(Schilling)								
'Parsley Patch'	1 tsp	13	1	2	1	0	0.5	0
'Season All'	1/4 tsp	2	0	0	163	0	0.0	0
spread	1/2 tbsp	45	0	1	140	0	4.0	0
GARLIC AND HERB								
(Cook's Classics) spread	1 tbsp	100	1	0	90	0	11.0	na
(Mrs. Dash) seasoning	0.13 tsp	2	0	0	0	na	0.0	0
(Schilling) spread	1/2 tbsp	45	0	1	125	0	4.5	0
GARLIC BREAD								
(Gran' Mere's) spread, all-purpose	1 oz	90	0	2	135	0	9.0	0
(Lawry's) spread	1/2 tbsp	47	0	1	15	0	4.6	0
(Molly McButter) garlic butter flavored	1/2 tsp	3	0	1	37	0	0.0	0
(Schilling) 'Garlic Bread Sprinkle'	1/4 tsp	5	0	0	25	0	0.4	0
(Tone's) 'Garlic Bread Sprinkle'	1 tsp	17	0	1	167	0	1.6	1
GARLIC PEPPER *(Lawry's)*	1/4 tsp	0	0	0	70	0	0.0	0
GARLIC SALT								
(Good Day)	1/4 tsp	0	0	0	520	0	0.0	0
(Lawry's)	1/4 tsp	0	0	0	240	0	0.0	0
(Morton)	1 tsp	3	1	1	1300	0	0.1	0
(Schilling)	1/4 tsp	0	0	0	490	0	0.0	0
(Tone's)	1 tsp	2	0	0	1706	0	0.0	0
GREEK *(Cavender's)* all purpose	1/4 tsp	0	0	0	241	0	0.0	0
GUACAMOLE								
(Lawry's) 'Seasoning Blend'	1 pkg	60	2	13	1495	1	0.4	0
(Old El Paso)	1/7 pkg	7	0	2	240	0	0.0	0
GUMBO *(Tone's)* file powder	1 tsp	8	0	2	1	1	0.2	0
HERB								
(Lawry's) mixed, 'Pinch of Herbs'	1 tsp	9	0	1	259	0	0.5	0
(Schilling) Italian, 'Bag'n Season'	1 pkg	94	2	21	1367	0	0.2	0

Food Name	Serv. Size	Total Cal.	Prot. gms	Carbs gms	Sod. mgs	Fiber gms	Fat gms	Chol. mgs
ITALIAN								
(Tone's)	1 tsp	3	0	1	1	0	0.1	0
(Trader Joe's) salt-free	1/4 tsp	0	0	0	0	0	0.0	0
LEMON DILL *(Schilling)* 'Bag'n Season'	1 pkg	161	3	15	2035	0	11.0	0
LEMON HERB								
(Mrs. Dash)	0.13 tsp	2	0	0	1	na	0.0	0
(Schilling) 'Spice Blends'	1/4 tsp	1	0	0	154	0	0.1	0
LEMON PEPPER								
(Lawry's)								
	1/4 tsp	<1	0	0	80	0	0.0	0
'Spice Blends'	1 tsp	6	0	1	340	0	0.1	0
(Schilling)								
'Parsley Patch'	1 tsp	13	0	1	2	0	0.6	0
salt-free	1/4 tsp	0	0	0	0	0	0.0	0
'Spice Blends'	1 tsp	7	0	1	618	0	0.0	0
(Tone's)								
	1 tsp	6	0	1	1086	1	0.2	0
coarse ground, 'Mr. Pepper'	1 tsp	12	0	3	1	0	0.1	0
fine ground, 'Mr. Pepper'	1 tsp	12	0	3	1	0	0.1	0
(Trader Joe's) salt-free	1/4 tsp	0	0	0	0	0	0.0	0
KOTTERIN MIRIN *(Kikkoman)* sweet	1 tbsp	40	0	10	15	0	0.0	0
MEAT LOAF								
(Adolph's) 'Meal Makers'	1 tbsp	30	1	7	360	1	0.0	0
(Bag 'n Season)	2 tsp	15	1	2	390	1	0.0	0
(French's)	1/8 pkg	20	1	5	620	0	0.0	0
(Lawry's) 'Seasoning Blends'	1 pkg	355	16	65	6547	2	1.2	0
(Schilling) 'Bag'n Season'	1 pkg	111	1	26	3090	0	0.7	1
MEATBALL								
(French's)	1/4 pkg	35	1	7	830	0	0.0	0
(Schilling) Swedish	1/6 pkg	45	1	4	790	0	1.0	0
MENUDO *(Gebhardt)*	1 tsp	4	0	1	182	0	0.2	0
MESQUITE *(Tone's)*	1 tsp	13	0	3	467	0	0.1	0
MEXICAN *(Tone's)*	1 tsp	6	0	1	4185	0	0.1	0
NACHO *(Lawry's)* 'Seasoning Blends'	1 pkg	141	7	15	2168	2	6.8	0
ORIENTAL *(Schilling)* 'Bag'n Season'	1 pkg	152	5	31	1912	0	8.0	0
PAD THAI *(Kikkoman)*	2 tsp	20	0	4	430	0	0.0	0
PARSLEY *(Schilling)* all purpose 'Parsley Patch'	1 tsp	6	0	1	3	0	0.0	0
PASTA								
(Tone's) spaghetti	1 tsp	11	0	3	469	0	0.1	0
(Trader Joe's) salt-free	1/4 tsp	0	0	0	0	0	0.0	0
PEPPER								
(Lawry's)	1/4 tsp	0	0	1	0	na	0.0	0
(Schilling) seasoned, 'All Pepper'	1/4 tsp	1	0	0	106	0	0.0	0
PEPPER DILL *(Golden Dipt)*	2 grams	8	0	1	96	0	0.0	0
PICKLING SPICE *(Tone's)*	1 tsp	10	0	1	1	0	0.6	0
POPCORN								
(Tone's)	1 tsp	0	0	0	2455	0	0.0	0
(McCormick/Schilling) 'Parsley Patch'	1 tsp	10	1	3	4	0	0.1	0
PORK								
(Bag 'n Season)								
chop	2 tsp	15	0	4	590	na	0.0	0
spare rib	1 tbsp	30	1	6	590	1	0.0	0
(Schilling)								
chop, 'Bag'n Season'	1 pkg	103	1	24	3126	0	0.4	0
spare rib, 'Bag'n Season'	1 pkg	185	0	42	3690	0	1.5	2
POTATO								
(Perfect Potatoes) herb and garlic	1/6 pkt	20	0	5	370	0	0.0	0

Food Name	Serv. Size	Total Cal.	Prot. gms	Carbs gms	Sod. mgs	Fiber gms	Fat gms	Chol. mgs
(Potato Shakers)								
cheddar, zesty	8 grams	30	1	5	500	0	1.0	0
Parmesan and herb	8 grams	25	1	5	740	0	0.5	0
(Shake 'N Bake) herb and garlic	1/8 pkt	20	0	5	370	0	0.0	0
POTATO SALAD *(Tone's)*	1 tsp	5	0	0	1498	0	0.2	0
PROTEIN *(Bragg)* liquid aminos	1/2 tsp	2	0.265	0	121	0	0.0	0
PUMPKIN PIE								
	1 tbsp	19	0	4	3	1	0.7	0
	1 tsp	6	0	1	1	0	0.2	0
RICE								
(Kikkoman) fried	1 1/3 tbsp	30	1	6	490	0	0.0	0
(Lawry's) Mexican, 'Seasoning Blends'	1 pkg	94	4	17	3246	2	2.0	0
(McCormick/Schilling) fried, w/chicken	1 tbsp	35	1	6	780	1	0.0	0
(Sun Bird) fried	1/2 tbsp	12	0	3	380	0	0.0	0
SALAD								
(Lawry's) taco, 'Seasoning Blends'	1 pkg	124	4	25	1451	2	0.9	0
(Schilling) 'Salad Supreme'	1 tsp	11	1	1	2807	0	0.1	0
SALT								
(Estee) 'Seasoned Salt-It'	1/8 tsp	0	0	0	0	0	0.0	0
(Good Day)	1/4 tsp	0	0	0	400	0	0.0	0
(Lawry's)								
	1/4 tsp	0	0	0	380	0	0.0	0
'Hot n' Spicy'	1 tsp	3	0	2	79	0	0.1	0
no MSG	1/4 tsp	0	0	0	380	0	0.0	0
(Morton) seasoned	1 tsp	4	1	1	1300	0	0.1	0
(Schilling)								
'California style'	1/4 tsp	0	0	0	250	0	0.0	0
no MSG, 'Home Style'	1/4 tsp	0	0	0	370	0	0.0	0
no MSG, 'Season All'	1/4 tsp	0	0	0	340	0	0.0	0
SAUSAGE *(Tone's)* pork	1 tsp	12	0	3	1	1	0.3	0
SEAFOOD								
(Golden Dipt)								
all purpose	1/4 tsp	2	0	0	85	0	0.0	0
blackened redfish	1/4 tsp	2	0	0	140	0	0.0	0
broiled fish	1/4 tsp	2	0	0	125	0	0.0	0
lemon pepper	1/4 tsp	8	1	1	115	0	0.0	0
shrimp and crab, Cajun style	1/4 tsp	2	0	0	200	0	0.0	0
(Old Bay) seafood, poultry, meat seasoning	1/2 tsp	0	0	0	330	0	0.0	0
(Schilling) Chesapeake Bay	1/2 tsp	2	0	0	202	0	0.1	0
(Tone's)								
	1 tsp	10	1	1	1	0	0.7	0
Chesapeake	1 tsp	8	0	1	1032	0	0.3	0
SESAME								
(Eden Foods)								
garlic, shake, organic	1/2 tsp	10	0	0	35	1	1.5	0
shake, organic	1/2 tsp	10	0	0	40	1	0.5	0
seaweed, shake, organic	1/2 tsp	10	0	0	35	1	0.5	0
(Maranatha Natural) sesame salt	7 grams	200	7	7	460	0	16.0	0
(Schilling) all-purpose, 'Parsley Patch'	1 tsp	15	1	1	2	0	1.0	0
SLOPPY JOE *(Lawry's)* 'Seasoning Blends'	1 pkg	126	3	28	3442	1	0.4	0
SOUR CREAM FLAVORED *(Molly McButter)*	1/2 tsp	4	0	1	65	0	0.1	0
STIR-FRY								
(Adolph's) teriyaki flavor, 'Meal Makers'	1 tbsp	30	1	7	1170	0	0.0	0
(Gilroy)	1 tsp	6	0	1	5	0	0.0	0
(Kikkoman)								
	1 tbsp	30	1	6	680	0	0.0	0
shrimp, Szechwan	1 1/3 tbsp	30	1	5	640	0	0.5	0

Food Name	Serv. Size	Total Cal.	Prot. gms	Carbs gms	Sod. mgs	Fiber gms	Fat gms	Chol. mgs
tomato beef	2 tsp	20	0	4	400	0	0.0	0
(McCormick/Schilling)	2 tsp	20	1	3	490	0	0.0	0
(Sun Bird) Oriental	1/2 tbsp	15	0	3	310	0	0.0	0
TACO								
(Hain)	1/10 pkg	10	1	2	200	0	0.0	0
(Lawry's) 'Seasoning Blends'	1 pkg	118	3	24	1441	1	1.1	0
(McCormick/Schilling) mild	2 tsp	20	1	4	460	1	0.0	0
(Nabisco) mild, mix for one taco	1 serving	90	2	18	999	0	1.0	0
(Old El Paso)								
	2 tsp	20	0	5	550	0	0.0	0
40% less sodium	2 tsp	20	0	4	330	0	0.0	0
(Ortega) meat	1 oz	90	2	18	1970	0	1.0	0
(Pancho Villa)	2 tsp	20	0	5	550	0	0.0	0
(Schilling)	1/4 pkg	31	1	6	675	0	0.5	0
(Tio Sancho)								
	1.25 oz	104	2	21	2500	2	1.4	0
'Dinner Kit'	1.51 oz	132	3	26	2623	2	1.7	0
TURKEY (Schilling) roast, 'Bag'n Season'	1 pkg	146	6	20	1935	0	5.0	0
TERIYAKI (Golden Dipt) ginger	1 oz	120	1	12	920	0	7.0	0
SEAWEED. See SEA VEGETABLE.								
SEITAN								
Philly steak slices, vegetarian (White Wave)	3 slices	60	14	2	105	0	0.0	0
traditional, vegetarian (White Wave)	1 piece	140	31	4	240	1	0.0	0
turkey style, vegetarian, sandwich sliced (White Wave)	1 slice	80	13	7	400	1	0.0	0
SEITAN MIX								
quick, flavored (Arrowhead Mills) mix only	1/3 cup	150	21	14	20	2	1.0	0
SELTZER. See under SOFT DRINKS AND MIXERS.								
SEMOLINA								
enriched	1 cup	601	21	122	2	7	1.8	0
unenriched	1 cup	601	21	122	2	7	1.8	0
whole grain	1 cup	602	21.2	121.6	2	6.5	1.8	0
whole grain	1 oz	102	3.6	20.6	<1	1.1	0.3	0
SERRANO PEPPER. See PEPPER, SERRANO.								
SESAME BUTTER/tahini. See also TAHINI MIX.								
	1 tbsp	95	3	4	2	1	8.1	0
made from raw and stone ground kernels	1 oz	162	5	7	21	3	13.6	0
made from raw and stone ground kernels	1 tbsp	86	3	4	11	1	7.2	0
made from roasted and toasted kernels	1 oz	169	5	6	33	3	15.2	0
made from roasted and toasted kernels	1 tbsp	89	3	3	17	1	8.1	0
made from unroasted kernels, hulls removed	1 oz	172	5	5	0	3	16.0	0
made from unroasted kernels, hulls removed	1 tbsp	85	3	3	0	1	7.9	0
(Arrowhead Mills) organic	1 oz	170	6	4	5	0	17.0	0
(Erewhon) 'Sesame Tahini'	2 tbsp	200	6	3	65	0	18.0	0
(Maranatha Natural)								
raw, 'Sesame Tahini'	2 tbsp	210	8	3	5	0	19.0	0
roasted, 'Sesame Tahini'	2 tbsp	210	8	3	20	0	19.0	0
(Roaster Fresh)								
gourmet	1 oz	168	5	6	3	0	15.0	0
roasted, w/o salt, creamy	1 oz	168	5	6	3	0	15.0	0
(Westbrae)								
Mid-Eastern, organic, no salt added	2 tbsp	220	9	3	0	0	20.0	0
organic, 'Natural'	2 tbsp	220	6	6	35	0	19.0	0
original, no salt added	2 tbsp	210	8	1	0	na	19.0	0
raw, organic	2 tbsp	210	8	1	0	0	19.0	0
toasted, organic, no salt added	2 tbsp	220	8	3	0	0	19.0	0
SESAME MEAL, partially defatted	1 oz	161	5	7	11	na	13.6	0

Food Name	Serv. Size	Total Cal.	Prot. gms	Carbs gms	Sod. mgs	Fiber gms	Fat gms	Chol. mgs
SESAME OIL								
....	1 cup	1927	0	0	0	0	218.0	0
....	1 tbsp	120	0	0	0	0	13.6	0
(Hain)	1 tbsp	120	0	0	0	0	14.0	0
100% pure *(Dynasty)*	1 tbsp	130	0	0	0	0	14.0	0
100% pure, extra virgin *(Loriva')*	1 tbsp	120	0	0	0	0	14.0	0
hot pepper *(Eden Foods)*	1 tbsp	120	0	0	0	0	14.0	0
pure pressed, organic *(Spectrum)*	1 tbsp	120	0	0	0	0	14.0	0
toasted *(Eden Foods)*	1 tbsp	130	0	0	0	0	14.0	0
toasted *(International Collection)*	1 tbsp	120	0	0	0	0	14.0	0
toasted, pure pressed, organic *(Spectrum)*	1 tbsp	120	0	0	0	0	14.0	0
unrefined *(Eden Foods)*	1 tbsp	120	0	0	0	0	14.0	0
SESAME SEED/sim sim								
Dried								
hulled	1 cup	882	40	14	60	17	82.2	0
hulled	1 tbsp	47	2	1	3	1	4.4	0
hulled	1 tsp	16	1	0	1	0	1.5	0
hulled *(Arrowhead Mills)*	1 oz	160	6	4	3	4	14.0	0
whole	1 cup	825	26	34	16	17	71.5	0
whole	1 tbsp	52	2	2	1	1	4.5	0
whole *(Arrowhead Mills)*	1 oz	160	5	6	4	3	14.0	0
Raw								
(McCormick/Schilling)	1 tsp	21	1	0	7	0	1.6	0
hulled, natural, unsalted *(Flanigan Farms)*	1/4 cup	160	5	7	0	3	14.0	0
whole *(Durkee)*	1 tsp	13	0	0	0	0	0.0	0
whole *(Laurel Leaf)*	1 tsp	13	0	0	0	0	0.0	0
whole *(Spice Islands)*	1 tsp	9	1	1	1	1	0.4	0
Roasted and toasted, whole	1 oz	160	5	7	3	4	13.6	0
Toasted								
hulled, salted	1 cup	726	22	33	753	22	61.4	0
hulled, salted	1 oz	161	5	7	167	5	13.6	0
hulled, unsalted	1 cup	726	22	33	50	22	61.4	0
hulled, unsalted	1 oz	161	5	7	11	5	13.6	0
SESAME STICKS								
wheat-based, unsalted	1 oz	153	3	13	8	na	10.4	0
wheat-based, unsalted	2 oz	307	6	26	16	na	20.8	0
wheat-based, unsalted	1 oz	153	3	13	422	1	10.4	0
wheat-based, unsalted	2 oz	307	6	26	844	2	20.8	0
SESBANIA FLOWER. See KATURAY.								
SHAD, AMERICAN								
baked, broiled, grilled, or microwaved	3 oz	214	18	0	55	0	15.0	82
raw	3 oz	167	14	0	43	0	11.7	64
SHALLOT								
Freeze-dried								
chopped	1/4 cup	13	0	3	2	na	0.0	0
chopped	1 tbsp	3	0	1	1	na	0.0	0
chopped *(McCormick/Schilling)*	1 tsp	2	0	0	0	0	0.0	0
Fresh								
raw	3.5 oz	72	2.5	16.8	12	>.7 c	0.1	0
raw, chopped	1 tbsp	7	0	2	1	na	0.0	0
raw, trimmed	1 oz	20	0.7	4.8	3	>.2 c	<.1	0
raw, untrimmed	1 lb	287	10.0	67.1	48	>2.8 c	0.4	0
SHARK								
MAKO, frozen, steak, boneless, raw *(Peter Pan Seafoods)* ...	3.5 oz	87	19	0	79	0	1.2	51
MIXED SPECIES, fresh								
batter dipped, fried	3 oz	194	16	5	104	0	11.7	50
raw	3 oz	110	17.8	0.0	67	0	3.8	43

Food Name	Serv. Size	Total Cal.	Prot. gms	Carbs gms	Sod. mgs	Fiber gms	Fat gms	Chol. mgs
SHEA NUT OIL								
....	1 cup	1927	0	0	0	0	218.0	0
....	1 tbsp	120	0	0	0	0	13.6	0
SHEEPSHEAD/fathead								
baked, broiled, grilled, or microwaved	3 oz	107	22	0	62	0	1.4	54
raw	3 oz	92	17	0	60	0	2.0	43
SHELLIE BEAN. See BEAN, SHELLY.								
SHELLY BEAN. See BEAN, SHELLY.								
SHERBET. See also FRUIT BAR, FROZEN; ICE BAR/DESSERT; SHERBET BAR, FROZEN; SORBET.								
(Borden) orange	1/2 cup	110	1	25	40	0	1.0	0
(Darigold) orange	1/2 cup	120	1	26	25	0	1.0	0
(Dreyers)								
strawberry kiwi	1/2 cup	120	1	27	30	na	1.0	5
Swiss orange	1/2 cup	150	1	30	45	na	2.5	5
(Edys)								
strawberry kiwi	1/2 cup	120	1	27	30	na	1.0	5
Swiss orange	1/2 cup	150	1	30	45	na	2.5	5
(Sealtest) all flavors	1/2 cup	130	1	28	30	0	1.0	5
SHERBET BAR, FROZEN								
(Creamsicle) all flavors, w/cream, sugar-free	1 bar	25	1	5	20	0	1.0	0
(Fudgsicle)								
all flavors, fat-free	1 bar	70	2	14	45	0	0.0	0
all flavors, sugar-free	1 bar	35	2	6	50	0	1.0	5
chocolate	1 bar	70	2	12	70	0	1.0	0
chocolate, w/nuts, no sugar, 'Fudge Nut Dip'	1 bar	130	2	12	40	0	8.0	5
SHERRY								
(Gallo)								
....	2 fl oz	64	0	2	0	0	0.0	0
cream, 'Livingston Cellars'	2 fl oz	78	0	6	0	0	0.0	0
very dry, 'Livingston Cellars'	2 fl oz	60	0	1	0	0	0.0	0
(Italian Swiss Colony)								
cream	2 fl oz	85	0	7	4	0	0.0	0
dry	2 fl oz	63	0	1	4	0	0.0	0
straight	2 fl oz	67	0	2	4	0	0.0	0
SHIITAKE. See MUSHROOM, SHIITAKE.								
SHIMEJI. See MUSHROOM, OYSTER.								
SHORTENING								
For baking								
hydrogenated soybean oil w/palm and cottonseed oils ...	1 cup	1812	0	0	0	0	205.0	0
hydrogenated soybean oil w/palm and cottonseed oils ...	1 tbsp	113	0	0	0	0	12.8	0
For bread								
hydrogenated soybean oil w/cottonseed oil	1 cup	1812	0	0	0	0	205.0	0
hydrogenated soybean oil w/cottonseed oil	1 tbsp	113	0	0	0	0	12.8	0
For cake and frosting								
hydrogenated soybean oil	1 cup	1812	0	0	0	0	205.0	0
hydrogenated soybean oil	1 tbsp	113	0	0	0	0	12.8	0
For cake mix								
hydrogenated soybean and cottonseed oils	1 cup	1812	0	0	0	0	205.0	0
hydrogenated soybean and cottonseed oils	1 tbsp	113	0	0	0	0	12.8	0
For confectionery								
fractionated palm oil	1 cup	1927	0	0	0	0	218.0	0
fractionated palm oil	1 tbsp	120	0	0	0	0	13.6	0
hydrogenated coconut and/or palm kernel oil	1 cup	1812	0	0	0	0	205.0	0
hydrogenated coconut and/or palm kernel oil	1 tbsp	113	0	0	0	0	12.8	0
For frying								
heavy-duty, beef tallow and cottonseed oil	1 cup	1845	0	0	0	0	205.0	205
heavy-duty, beef tallow and cottonseed oil	1 tbsp	115	0	0	0	0	12.8	13

Food Name	Serv. Size	Total Cal.	Prot. gms	Carbs gms	Sod. mgs	Fiber gms	Fat gms	Chol. mgs
heavy-duty, hydrogenated palm oil	1 cup	1812	0	0	0	0	205.0	0
heavy-duty, hydrogenated palm oil	1 tbsp	113	0	0	0	0	12.8	0
heavy-duty, hydrogenated soybean (under 1% linoleic)	1 cup	1812	0	0	0	0	205.0	0
heavy-duty, hydrogenated soybean (under 1% linoleic)	1 tbsp	113	0	0	0	0	12.8	0
heavy-duty, hydrogenated soybean (30% linoleic), w/stabilizers	1 cup	1812	0	0	0	0	205.0	0
heavy-duty, hydrogenated soybean (30% linoleic), w/stabilizers	1 tbsp	113	0	0	0	0	12.8	0
hydrogenated soybean and cottonseed oils	1 cup	1812	0	0	0	0	205.0	0
hydrogenated soybean and cottonseed oils	1 tbsp	113	0	0	0	0	12.8	0
Household								
hydrogenated soybean and cottonseed oils	1 cup	1812	0	0	0	0	205.0	0
hydrogenated soybean and cottonseed oils	1 tbsp	113	0	0	0	0	12.8	0
hydrogenated soybean oil w/palm oil	1 cup	1812	0	0	0	0	205.0	0
hydrogenated soybean oil w/palm oil	1 tbsp	113	0	0	0	0	12.8	0
lard and vegetable oil	1 cup	1845	0	0	0	0	205.0	115
lard and vegetable oil	1 tbsp	115	0	0	0	0	12.8	7
(Crisco)								
vegetable oil	1 tbsp	110	0	0	0	0	12.0	0
(Finast)								
vegetable oil	1 tbsp	110	0	0	0	0	13.0	0
vegetable oil, butter flavor	1 tbsp	110	0	0	0	0	12.0	0
(Wesson) vegetable oil	1 tbsp	109	0	0	0	0	12.1	0
Industrial								
hydrogenated soybean oil w/cottonseed oil	1 cup	1812	0	0	0	0	205.0	0
hydrogenated soybean oil w/cottonseed oil	1 tbsp	113	0	0	0	0	12.8	0
lard and vegetable oil	1 cup	1845	0	0	0	0	205.0	115
lard and vegetable oil	1 tbsp	115	0	0	0	0	12.8	7
(Wesson)								
'Crystal'	1 tbsp	122	0	0	0	0	13.5	0
low-melt	1 tbsp	122	0	0	0	0	13.5	0
'Super'	1 tbsp	122	0	0	0	0	13.5	0
'Wesgold'	1 tbsp	122	0	0	0	0	13.5	0
'Wespour'	1 tbsp	122	0	0	0	0	13.5	0
Multipurpose								
hydrogenated soybean and palm oils	1 cup	1812	0	0	0	0	205.0	0
hydrogenated soybean and palm oils	1 tbsp	113	0	0	0	0	12.8	0
(Quest)								
'Cirol'	1 oz	256	0	2	0	na	28.4	0
'Durola Select'	1 oz	256	0	0	0	0	28.4	0
'Duromel'	1 oz	256	0	0	0	0	28.4	0
SHOYU. See under SAUCE.								
SHRIMP. See also SHRIMP DISH/ENTRÉE.								
Canned								
medium, deveined, in water and salt (S&W)	1/4 cup	45	10	0	650	0	0.0	115
mixed species	1 cup	154	30	1	216	0	2.5	221
mixed species	10 medium	38	7	0	54	0	0.6	55
mixed species	3 oz	102	20	1	144	0	1.7	147
mixed species, cooked	1 oz	34	7	0	48	0	0.6	49
mixed species, drained (Louisiana Brand)	2 oz	58	12	0	0	0	1.0	0
mixed species, large, drained (ShopRite)	2 oz	50	10	0	720	0	1.0	0
peeled, broken (Crown Prince)	1/2 can	60	13	1	360	0	0.5	145
small, deveined, in water and salt (S&W)	1/4 cup	45	10	0	650	0	0.0	115
tiny, peeled (Crown Prince)	1/2 can	60	13	1	360	0	0.5	145
Fresh								
mixed species, boiled, poached, or steamed	3 oz	84	18	0	190	0	0.9	166

Food Name	Serv. Size	Total Cal.	Prot. gms	Carbs gms	Sod. mgs	Fiber gms	Fat gms	Chol. mgs
mixed species, large, boiled, poached, or steamed	4 shrimp	22	5	0	49	0	0.2	43
mixed species, raw	3 oz	90	17	1	126	0	1.5	129
mixed species, raw, large	4 shrimp	30	6	0	41	0	0.5	43
mixed species, raw, medium	1 shrimp	6	1	0	9	0	0.1	9
mixed species, raw, small	1 shrimp	5	1	0	7	0	0.1	8
Frozen								
butterfly, 'Specialty' (Gorton's)	4 oz	160	19	16	540	0	1.0	0
cooked, peeled, deveined, tail off, 250/300 count								
(Contessa)	3 oz	40	10	0	420	0	0.0	95
w/tails (Harvest Of The Sea)	3 oz	70	17	0	280	0	0.0	0

SHRIMP COCKTAIL. See under SHRIMP DISH/ENTRÉE.

SHRIMP DISH/ENTRÉE

Food Name	Serv. Size	Total Cal.	Prot. gms	Carbs gms	Sod. mgs	Fiber gms	Fat gms	Chol. mgs
(Armour)								
baby bay, frozen, 'Classics Lite'	9.75 oz	220	12	31	890	0	6.0	105
Creole, frozen, 'Classics Lite'	11.25 oz	260	6	53	900	0	2.0	45
(Booth)								
Alfredo, w/fettucini, frozen	10 oz	260	19	28	620	0	8.0	0
cocktail, w/garlic butter sauce and vegetable rice	10 oz	400	13	40	750	(mq)	25.0	(mq)
New Orleans, w/wild rice, frozen	10 oz	230	13	35	950	0	5.0	0
Oriental, w/pineapple rice, frozen	10 oz	190	11	30	950	0	3.0	0
primavera, w/fettuccini, frozen	10 oz	200	16	28	760	0	3.0	0
w/garlic butter sauce and vegetable rice, frozen	10 oz	400	13	40	750	0	25.0	0
(Budget Gourmet)								
cocktail, w/fettuccine, frozen	9.5 oz	375	10	38	660	(mq)	20.0	145
mariner, frozen, 'Light & Healthy'	1 dinner	230	11	40	550	0	6.0	55
(Cajun Cookin')								
Creole, frozen	12 oz	390	17	55	1130	0	11.0	0
etouffée, frozen	17 oz	360	19	52	1170	0	9.0	0
jambalaya, frozen	12 oz	450	20	43	800	0	20.0	0
(Gorton's)								
breaded, w/original seasoning	6 shrimp	229	10	18	549	1	13.0	80
crisps, frozen, 'Specialty'	4 oz	280	9	26	740	0	15.0	0
crunchy, frozen, microwave, 'Crunchy Shrimp'	1/2 pkg	160	7	12	380	0	9.0	40
crunchy, whole, frozen, 'Microwave Specialty'	5 oz	380	14	35	870	0	20.0	65
popcorn	1 cup	260	9	21	600	1	16.0	60
scampi, baked	6 shrimp	250	9	18	409	1	16.0	70
scampi, frozen, 'Microwave Entrées'	1 pkg	390	10	21	470	0	30.0	0
(Healthy Choice)								
Creole, frozen	11.25 oz	210	8	42	560	0	1.0	65
marinara	1 entrée	250	10	44	360	5	4.0	55
w/vegetables	1 entrée	270	15	39	580	6	6.0	50
(Hudson) stir-fry, complete meal kit, frozen	1 3/4 cup	210	15	35	990	3	2.0	83
(LaChoy)								
chow mein	1 cup	53	3	10	948	2	0.9	9
chow mein, canned	3/4 cup	35	4	4	940	2	1.0	50
cocktail, w/lobster sauce, 'Fresh & Lite'	10 oz	240	12	36.4	946	2.8	6.2	118
(Longacre)								
salad, 'Saladfest'	1 oz	45	2.0	2.0	150	na	3.0	25
salad, w/seafood, 'Saladfest'	1 oz	42	2.0	2.0	160	na	3.0	15
(Marie Callender's) over angel hair pasta, frozen	1 cup	300	11	37	470	3	12.0	30
(Mrs. Paul's)								
breaded, fried, frozen	3 oz	200	9	16	430	0	11.0	0
Cajun style, frozen, 'Light'	9 oz	230	9	37	740	0	5.0	60
cocktail, w/clams and linguini, 'Light'	10 oz	240	12	36	750	(mq)	5.0	40
primavera, frozen 'Light'	9.5 oz	180	11	28	840	0	3.0	125
(Right Course) primavera, frozen	9 5/8 oz	240	12	32	590	0	7.0	50
(Sau-Sea) cocktail	4 oz	113	7	19	1020	na	1.0	102

Food Name	Serv. Size	Total Cal.	Prot. gms	Carbs gms	Sod. mgs	Fiber gms	Fat gms	Chol. mgs
(SeaPak)								
battered, frozen, 'Shrimp 'n Batter'	4 oz	260	11	20	470	0	15.0	20
breaded, butterfly, frozen, 'Mikado'	4 oz	160	12	26	170	0	1.0	110
breaded, butterfly/round, frozen	4 oz	150	14	20	0	0	1.0	0
cocktail, 'Super Valu' heat and serve	4 oz	210	12	30	730	(mq)	4.0	80
w/crab meat stuffing, battered, frozen	4 oz	260	8	27	780	0	13.0	0
(Shanghai) stir-fry, frozen	10.3 oz	170	18	19	1200	0	2.0	55
(Smart Ones)								
marinara	1 entrée	200	8	37	590	4	2.0	40
marinara, w/linguini, frozen	8 oz	150	8	26	390	0	1.0	60
(Ultra Slim-Fast)								
Creole, frozen	12 oz	240	12	45	730	0	4.0	80
marinara, frozen	12 oz	290	17	53	880	0	3.0	70
SHRIMP PASTE, canned	1 tsp	13	1.5	0.1	10	0	0.7	12
SHRIMP SALAD. See under SHRIMP DISH/ENTRÉE.								
SHRIMP SUBSTITUTE, made from surimi	3 oz	86	11	8	599	0	1.3	31
SICAMA. See JICAMA								
SILVER HAKE. See WHITING.								
SILVER SALMON. See under SALMON.								
SIM SIM. See SESAME SEED.								
SISYMBRIUM SEED								
dried, whole	1 cup	235	9	43	68	na	3.4	0
dried, whole	1 oz	90	3	17	26	na	1.3	0
SKIL. See COD, ALASKAN.								
SKIPJACK. See under TUNA.								
SKUNK CABBAGE. See CABBAGE, SKUNK.								
SLIMEHEAD. See ORANGE ROUGHY.								
SLOPPY JOE MIX. See under SANDWICH FILLING MIX.								
SLOPPY JOE SEASONING. See under SEASONING MIX.								
SMELT, RAINBOW								
baked, broiled, grilled, or microwaved	3 oz	105	19	0	65	0	2.6	77
raw	3 oz	82	15	0	51	0	2.1	60
SNACK BAR. See also BREAKFAST BAR; CAKE, SNACK; FRUIT BAR; GRANOLA/CEREAL BAR; SPORTS AND DIET/NUTRITION BARS.								
(Barbara's Bakery)								
apple-filled, whole grain, organic	1.3 oz bar	120	1	29	55	2	0.0	0
blueberry-filled, whole grain, organic	1.3 oz bar	120	1	29	55	2	0.0	0
raspberry-filled, whole grain, organic, nonfat	1 bar	110	1	28	26	2	0.0	0
strawberry-filled, whole grain, organic, nonfat	1.3 oz bar	120	1	29	55	2	0.0	0
(Bear Valley)								
carob cocoa, food bar, 'Pemmican'	3.75 oz	440	16	68	80	7	12.0	0
coconut almond, food bar, 'Meal Pack'	3.75 oz	400	13	56	80	6	12.0	0
fruit and nut, food bar, 'Pemmican'	3.75 oz	420	17	59	90	9	13.0	0
sesame lemon, food bar, 'Meal Pack'	3.75 oz	410	17	57	85	4	13.0	0
(Clif)								
chocolate chip, '100% Natural Endurance'	2.4 oz	250	4	51	45	3	3.0	0
dark chocolate, '100% Natural Endurance'	2.4 oz	250	5	52	20	2	2.0	0
(Earth Grains)								
banana apple walnut, 'Bagel Power Bar'	1 bar	270	12	45	280	0	6.0	0
citrus almond, w/mixed fruit 'Bagel Power Bar'	1 bar	260	12	45	280	0	4.0	0
fruit and nut, 'Bagel Power Bar'	1 bar	240	9	48	280	0	3.0	0
(Edgebar) chocolate crunch	1 bar	234	11	46	95	0	2.0	5
(Fruit Boosters)								
apple, low-fat	1 bar	130	1	27	0	1	2.0	0
blueberry, low-fat	1 bar	130	1	27	0	1	2.0	0
(General Mills) date	1/32 pkg	60	1	9	35	0	2.0	0

Food Name	Serv. Size	Total Cal.	Prot. gms	Carbs gms	Sod. mgs	Fiber gms	Fat gms	Chol. mgs
(Glenny's)								
apple-cinnamon	1.25 oz	120	1	28	15	0	1.0	0
caramel	1.25 oz	120	1	29	65	0	1.0	0
chocolate	1.25 oz	120	1	28	20	0	1.0	0
raspberry	1.25 oz	120	1	29	15	0	1.0	0
(Golden Temple)								
original, 100% natural, 'Wha Guru Chew'	1.13 oz	166	5	14	0	0	9.0	0
sesame almond, 100% natural, 'Wha Guru Chew'	1.13 oz	162	4	11	0	0	11.0	0
(Great Cakes)								
all natural 'Summer Fruits'	3 oz	190	7	35	7	16	2.5	0
all natural 'Tropical Fruits'	3 oz	185	7	35	4	16	2.0	0
(Health Valley)								
apple, 'Bakes'	1 serving	100	2	16	27	3	3.0	0
'Date Bakes'	1 serving	100	3	16	25	3	3.0	0
fruit, 'Fruit & Fitness'	2 bars	200	4	39	234	5	3.0	0
fruit-nut, 'Oat Bran Jumbo Fruit Bars'	1 serving	150	4	29	11	8	4.0	0
oat bran, 'Fig & Nut Bakes'	1 serving	110	2	19	18	3	3.0	0
oat bran, 'Oat Bran Jumbo Fruit Bars'	1 serving	170	4	28	9	7	5.0	0
oat bran, raisin and cinnamon	1 serving	140	3	32	12	6	2.0	0
'Oat Bran Apricot Bakes'	1 serving	100	2	19	18	3	2.0	0
'Raisin Bakes'	1 serving	100	2	16	19	3	3.0	0
rice bran, almond, and date	1 serving	190	4	29	6	6	6.0	0
(Kellogg's)								
apple-cinnamon, wheat, whole-grain oats, fruit	1 bar	140	2	26	65	1	4.0	0
wheat, whole-grain oats, fruit	1 bar	140	2	26	65	1	4.0	0
(Kudos)								
peaches and cream, 'Pan Squares'	1 sq.	150	2	22	105	2	6.0	0
peanut butter and chocolate chip, 'Pan Squares'	1 sq.	170	3	20	105	2	9.0	0
strawberry and cream cheese, 'Pan Squares'	1 sq.	150	2	22	105	2	6.0	0
(Marin)								
fig, honey sweetened, organic	1 bar	120	2	21	100	3	3.0	0
fig, organic	1 bar	70	1	16	100	2	0.0	0
(Natural Nectar)								
almond, 'Treat Yourself Right'	1 bar	150	3	22	40	5	5.0	0
apple, 'Original Fruit Bar'	1 bar	100	2	15	15	4	3.0	0
apple-cinnamon, low-fat, 'Fi-Bar'	1 bar	90	1	22	65	2	1.0	0
apple-oatmeal spice 'Fi-Bar A.M.'	1 bar	150	3	27	25	5	3.0	0
banana nut, 'Fi-Bar A.M.'	1 bar	150	2	26	20	5	4.0	0
chocolate, 'Fi-Bar Lite'	2.5 oz	190	4	29	140	0	6.0	5
cocoa-almond crunch, 'Fi-Bar'	1 bar	130	3	21	20	4	4.0	0
cocoa-almond, whole grain, 'Fi-Bar Chewy & Nutty'	1 bar	140	3	23	25	2	4.5	0
cocoa peanut butter crunch, 'Chewy & Nutty'	1 bar	130	3	20	20	2	4.0	0
cocoa peanut, 'Fi-Bar Chewy & Nutty'	1 bar	130	3	20	20	4	1.0	0
coconut	1 bar	120	2	20	30	6	4.0	0
cranberry, w/wild berries, 'Original Fruit Bar'	1 bar	120	2	23	15	4	2.0	0
lemon, 'Original Fruit Bar'	1 bar	100	2	15	15	4	3.0	0
Mandarin orange 'Original Fruit Bar'	1 bar	100	2	15	15	4	3.0	0
peanut butter	1 bar	130	3	20	30	6	4.0	0
peanut butter, 'Treat Yourself Right'	1 bar	150	4	18	55	5	5.0	0
raisin nut bran, 'Fi-Bar A.M.'	1 bar	150	3	26	30	5	4.0	0
raspberry, 'Canadian'	1 bar	120	2	21	15	3	3.0	0
raspberry, 'Original Fruit Bar'	1 bar	120	2	23	15	4	2.0	0
strawberry, 'Canadian'	1 bar	120	2	21	15	3	3.0	0
strawberry, 'Original Fruit Bar'	1 bar	120	2	23	15	4	2.0	0
strawberry-oatmeal, w/almonds, 'Fi-Bar A.M.'	1 bar	150	3	24	30	5	4.0	0
vanilla almond, 'Fi-Bar Chewy & Nutty'	1 bar	130	3	21	20	4	4.0	0
vanilla almond crunch, 'Canadian Chewy & Nutty'	1 bar	130	3	21	20	2	4.0	0

Food Name	Serv. Size	Total Cal.	Prot. gms	Carbs gms	Sod. mgs	Fiber gms	Fat gms	Chol. mgs
vanilla peanut, 'Fi-Bar Chewy & Nutty'	1 bar	130	3	20	20	4	4.0	0
(Pemmican) carob cocoa, meatless	1 pkg	440	16	68	80	7	12.0	0

SNACK BAR MIX. See also CAKE, SNACK, MIX.

(Betty Crocker)								
caramel oatmeal, 'Supreme Dessert' mix only	1/32 pkg	90	1	15	50	0	3.0	0
caramel oatmeal, 'Supreme Dessert' prepared w/margarine	1 bar	110	1	15	65	0	5.0	0
chocolate and toffee, 'Supreme Dessert' mix only	1/32 pkg	90	1	17	55	0	2.0	0
chocolate and toffee, 'Supreme Dessert' prepared	1 bar	110	1	17	55	0	4.0	10
chocolate peanut butter 'Supreme Dessert' prepared	1 bar	110	1	14	100	0	5.0	10
chocolate peanut butter, 'Supreme Dessert' mix only	1/32 pkg	100	1	14	85	0	4.0	0
date, 'Classic' prepared	1 bar	60	1	9	35	0	2.0	0
M&M's cookie bars, 'Supreme Dessert' mix only	1/32 pkg	100	1	16	60	0	3.0	0
M&M's cookie bars, 'Supreme Dessert' prepared	1 bar	110	1	16	80	0	5.0	10
raspberry, 'Supreme Dessert' mix only	1/32 pkg	100	1	16	80	0	3.0	0
raspberry, 'Supreme Dessert' prepared	1/32 pkg	100	1	16	95	0	4.0	0
Sunkist lemon, 'Supreme Dessert' mix only	1/32 pkg	100	1	17	55	0	3.0	0
Sunkist lemon, 'Supreme Dessert' prepared w/4 eggs	1 bar	110	1	17	65	0	4.0	30

SNACK CHIP. See also BAGEL CHIPS, BANANA CHIPS; CARROT CHIPS; CORN CHIPS AND SNACKS; PASTA CHIPS; POTATO CHIPS AND SNACKS; RICE CHIPS; SEA VEGETABLE CHIPS; SNACK MIX; TARO CHIPS; TORTILLA CHIPS; VEGETABLE CHIPS; WASABI CHIPS.

(Bake-Itos) pico de gallo	1 oz	110	3	23	59	0	0.9	0
(Bugles)								
nacho flavor	1 1/3 cup	160	2	18	300	0	9.0	0
original flavor	1 1/3 cup	160	1	18	310	1	9.0	0
ranch flavor	1 1/3 cup	160	2	18	310	1	9.0	0
(Frito-Lay's)								
'Funyuns'	1 oz	140	2	18	270	1	7.0	0
'Munchos'	1 oz	160	1	16	260	1	10.0	0
(Sun Chips)								
French onion	1 oz	140	2	19	115	2	6.0	0
harvest cheddar	1 oz	140	2	19	115	2	6.0	0
original	1 oz	140	2	19	115	2	6.0	0

SNACK MIX

(Burns & Ricker) nonfat, 'Party Mix'	3/4 cup	120	4	23	210	1	0.0	0
(Eagle) 'Snack Mix'	1/2 cup	150	4	17	270	1	7.0	0
(Flavor Tree)								
no salt, 'Party Mix'	1 1/2 cups	163	4	13	8	0	10.8	0
original, 'Party Mix'	1/4 cup	163	3	12	407	0	11.0	0
(General Mills)								
barbecue flavor, 'Chex'	1 oz	130	3	18	380	0	5.0	0
cheese, 'Chex'	2/3 cup	120	3	18	288	2	4.9	0
cool sour cream and onion flavor,'Chex'	2/3 cup	130	3	19	300	0	5.0	0
golden cheddar, 'Chex'	2/3 cup	130	3	19	300	0	5.0	0
nacho cheese, 'Chex'	2/3 cup	130	3	19	430	0	5.0	0
(Harmony)								
Oriental, party mix	1/4 cup	150	5	11	270	2	10.0	0
'Swiss Mix'	1/4 cup	190	4	27	15	2	8.0	0
(Nabisco)								
original flavor, 'Doo Dads'	1/2 cup	129	3	18	360	2	5.2	0
traditional, baked, 'Ritz'	1 oz	130	2	18	310	0	6.0	0
(Pepperidge Farm)								
'Classic'	1 oz	140	4	14	360	1	8.0	0
lightly smoked	1 oz	150	4	13	350	1	9.0	0
spicy	1 oz	140	4	14	340	1	8.0	5
super cheddar, 'Goldfish Party Mix'	1 oz	140	4	15	330	0	7.0	15
w/cashews and almonds, 'Nutty Deluxe' 'Goldfish'	1/2 cup	180	5	20	330	2	9.0	25

Food Name	Serv. Size	Total Cal.	Prot. gms	Carbs gms	Sod. mgs	Fiber gms	Fat gms	Chol. mgs
w/honey roasted peanuts, original, 'Goldfish'	1/2 cup	170	5	21	360	2	8.0	5
(Super Snax)	1 oz	137	3	17	207	0	6.5	0
SNACK STICKS, sesame and cheese, 'Twigs'								
(Nabisco)	15 sticks	150	4	17	300	1	7.0	0
SNAP BEAN. See BEAN, GREEN.								
SNAP PEAS. See PEAS, SNAP.								
SNAPPER								
mixed species, baked, broiled, grilled, or microwaved	3 oz	109	22	0	48	0	1.5	40
mixed species, raw	3 oz	85	17	0	54	0	1.1	31
SOBA NOODLE. See under NOODLE, JAPANESE.								
SOCKEYE SALMON. See under SALMON.								
SODA. See under SOFT DRINKS AND MIXERS.								
SOFT DRINKS AND MIXERS. See also WATER, FLAVORED.								
(A&W)								
cream	1 fl oz	14	0	4	2	0	0.0	0
cream, diet	1 fl oz	1	0	0	4	0	0.1	0
root beer	1 fl oz	15	0	4	5	0	0.1	0
root beer, diet	1 fl oz	1	0	0	4	0	0.0	0
(Canada Dry)								
Collins mixer	8 fl oz	80	0	20	17	0	0.0	0
ginger ale	8 fl oz	90	0	21	7	0	0.0	0
ginger ale, 'Golden'	8 fl oz	100	0	24	24	0	0.0	0
grape, 'Concord'	8 fl oz	130	0	32	21	0	0.0	0
tonic water	8 fl oz	90	0	22	7	0	0.0	0
whiskey sour mixer	8 fl oz	90	0	22	17	0	0.0	0
(Coca-Cola)								
'Caffeine-Free Coke'	12 fl oz	145	0	41	13	0	0.0	0
'Caffeine-Free Diet Coke'	12 fl oz	2	0	0	6	0	0.0	0
'Classic Coke'	12 fl oz	145	0	41	13	0	0.0	0
'Coke'	6 fl oz	77	0	20	4	0	0.0	0
'Diet Cherry Coke'	6 fl oz	1	0	0	4	0	0.0	0
'Diet Coke'	12 fl oz	2	0	0	6	0	0.0	0
'Tab'	6 fl oz	1	0	0	4	0	0.0	0
(Dr Diablo) cola	12 fl oz	140	0	38	14	0	0.0	0
(Dr Pepper)								
'Caffeine-Free Diet Dr Pepper'	12 fl oz	3	0	0	18	0	0.0	0
cola	12 fl oz	150	0	38	18	0	0.0	0
cola, caffeine-free	12 fl oz	150	0	38	18	0	0.0	0
'Diet Dr Pepper'	12 fl oz	3	0	0	18	0	0.0	0
(Fresca) citrus	6 fl oz	2	0	0	0	0	0.0	0
(Health Valley)								
ginger ale	12 fl oz	153	1	35	30	0	1.0	0
root beer, 'Old Fashioned'	12 fl oz	120	1	26	12	0	1.0	0
root beer, sarsaparilla	12 fl oz	153	1	35	27	0	1.0	0
wild berry	12 fl oz	142	1	33	27	0	1.0	0
(Hires)								
cream, caffeine-free	6 fl oz	90	1	24	40	0	1.0	0
cream, diet, caffeine-free	6 fl oz	2	1	1	45	0	1.0	0
root beer, caffeine-free	6 fl oz	90	1	23	55	0	1.0	0
root beer, caffeine-free, diet, w/NutraSweet	6 fl oz	2	1	1	70	0	1.0	0
(Jolt) cola	6 fl oz	85	0	21	10	0	0.0	0
(Mello Yello)								
citrus	6 fl oz	87	0	22	14	0	0.0	0
citrus, diet	6 fl oz	3	0	0	1	0	0.0	0
(Mug) root beer, diet	12 fl oz	4	0	1	39	0	0.0	0
(Natural 90 Diet) all flavors	6 fl oz	2	0	1	10	0	0.0	0
(Pathmark) cola, sugar-free, 'No Frills'	8 fl oz	0	0	0	0	0	0.0	0

Food Name	Serv. Size	Total Cal.	Prot. gms	Carbs gms	Sod. mgs	Fiber gms	Fat gms	Chol. mgs
(Pepsi-Cola)								
'Light'	12 fl oz	1	0	0	2	0	0.0	0
'Wild Cherry'	12 fl oz	163	0	43	2	0	0.0	0
'Diet Crystal'	6 fl oz	0	0	0	35	0	0.0	0
'Caffeine-Free Diet Pepsi'	12 fl oz	1	0	0	2	0	0.0	0
(Santa Cruz Natural) ginger ale, organic, 'Sparkling'	8 fl oz	155	1	36	0	0	1.0	0
(Schweppes)								
bitter lemon	6 fl oz	82	0	20	13	0	0.0	0
blackberry, 'Royal'	6 fl oz	35	0	8	5	0	0.0	0
citrus, tropical, 'Royal'	6 fl oz	35	0	8	5	0	0.0	0
club soda	6 fl oz	0	0	0	25	0	0.0	0
Collins mixer	6 fl oz	75	0	18	51	0	0.0	0
ginger ale	6 fl oz	65	0	16	10	0	0.0	0
ginger ale, sugar-free	6 fl oz	2	0	1	39	0	0.0	0
grape	6 fl oz	95	0	23	15	0	0.0	0
grapefruit	6 fl oz	80	0	20	28	0	0.0	0
kiwi-passionfruit, 'Royal'	6 fl oz	35	0	8	5	0	0.0	0
lemon-lime	6 fl oz	72	0	18	30	0	0.0	0
orange, sparkling	6 fl oz	88	0	22	17	0	0.0	0
peaches and cream, 'Royal'	6 fl oz	35	0	8	5	0	0.0	0
raspberry ginger ale, diet	6 fl oz	2	0	1	55	0	0.0	0
root beer	6 fl oz	76	0	19	17	0	0.0	0
seltzer, all flavors	6 fl oz	0	0	0	5	0	0.0	0
seltzer, low-sodium	6 fl oz	0	0	0	7	0	0.0	0
sour lemon	6 fl oz	79	0	19	12	0	0.0	0
strawberry-banana, 'Royal'	6 fl oz	35	0	8	5	0	0.0	0
tonic water	6 fl oz	64	0	16	8	0	0.0	0
tonic water, diet	6 fl oz	2	0	1	45	0	0.0	0
vanilla bean, 'Royal'	6 fl oz	35	0	8	5	0	0.0	0
Vichy water	6 fl oz	0	0	0	76	0	0.0	0
wild cherry, 'Royal'	6 fl oz	35	0	8	5	0	0.0	0
wild raspberry, 'Royal'	6 fl oz	35	0	8	5	0	0.0	0
(7UP)								
cherry citrus	12 fl oz	148	0	39	32	0	0.0	0
cherry citrus, diet	12 fl oz	4	0	0	32	0	0.0	0
lemon-lime	12 fl oz	144	0	36	32	0	0.0	0
lemon-lime, diet	12 fl oz	4	0	0	32	0	0.0	0
(Shasta)								
black cherry	12 fl oz	162	0	44	29	0	0.0	0
cherry cola	12 fl oz	140	0	38	22	0	0.0	0
citrus mist	12 fl oz	170	0	46	19	0	0.0	0
club soda	12 fl oz	0	0	0	46	0	0.0	0
cola	12 fl oz	147	0	40	3	0	0.0	0
Collins mixer	12 fl oz	118	0	32	23	0	0.0	0
'Creme'	12 fl oz	154	0	42	23	0	0.0	0
fruit punch	12 fl oz	173	0	47	32	0	0.0	0
ginger ale	12 fl oz	120	0	33	23	0	0.0	0
grape	12 fl oz	177	0	48	34	0	0.0	0
lemon-lime	12 fl oz	146	0	39	19	0	0.0	0
'Luigi Berry'	8 fl oz	130	0	32	30	0	0.0	0
'Mario Punch'	8 fl oz	130	0	31	40	0	0.0	0
orange	12 fl oz	177	0	48	28	0	0.0	0
'Princess Toadstool Cherry'	8 fl oz	130	0	31	30	0	0.0	0
red berry	12 fl oz	158	0	43	20	0	0.0	0
root beer	12 fl oz	154	0	42	31	0	0.0	0
strawberry	12 fl oz	147	0	40	36	0	0.0	0
tonic water	12 fl oz	121	0	33	17	0	0.0	0

Food Name	Serv. Size	Total Cal.	Prot. gms	Carbs gms	Sod. mgs	Fiber gms	Fat gms	Chol. mgs
'Yoshi Apple'	8 fl oz	130	0	31	30	0	0.0	0
(Slice) orange, 'Diet'	12 fl oz	12	0	2	2	0	0.0	0
(Soda-Licious)								
cherry cola	1 pouch	100	1	22	20	0	1.0	0
fruit punch, red	1 pouch	100	1	22	20	0	1.0	0
grape	1 pouch	100	1	22	20	0	1.0	0
lemon-lime	1 pouch	100	1	22	20	0	1.0	0
orange	1 pouch	100	1	22	20	0	1.0	0
root beer	1 pouch	100	1	22	20	0	1.0	0
(Spree)								
cherry-lime	12 fl oz	158	0	43	2	0	0.0	0
cola	12 fl oz	147	0	40	1	0	0.0	0
ginger ale	12 fl oz	120	0	33	1	0	0.0	0
grapefruit	12 fl oz	154	0	42	1	0	0.0	0
lemon-lime	12 fl oz	154	0	42	1	0	0.0	0
lemon-tangerine	12 fl oz	165	0	45	1	0	0.0	0
lime, Mandarin	12 fl oz	154	0	42	1	0	0.0	0
root beer	12 fl oz	154	0	42	2	0	0.0	0
tropical blend	12 fl oz	146	0	41	2	0	0.0	0
(Squirt)								
citrus	1 fl oz	13	0	3	2	0	0.0	0
citrus, 'Diet'	1 fl oz	1	0	0	1	0	0.0	0
citrus berry, 'Ruby Red'	8 fl oz	120	0	30	25	0	0.0	0
(Vernors)								
ginger ale	3.5 fl oz	40	0	10	4	0	0.1	0
ginger ale, 'Diet'	3.5 fl oz	1	0	0	7	0	0.1	0
(Wink) grapefruit	8 fl oz	120	0	30	19	0	0.0	0
SOLE								
Fresh								
baked, broiled, grilled, or microwaved	3 oz	99	20.5	0.0	89	0	1.3	58
raw	3 oz	77	16.0	0.0	69	0	1.0	41
Frozen								
Atlantic *(Booth)*	4 oz	90	19	0	180	0	1.0	0
fillet *(SeaPak)*	4 oz	90	20	0	135	0	1.0	0
fillet, lightly breaded *(Van de Kamp's)*	1 serving	220	14	17	410	0	11.0	40
fillet, 'Natural' *(Van de Kamp's)*	4 oz	100	22	0	105	0	2.0	35
'Fishmarket Fresh' *(Gorton's)*	5 oz	110	24	1	140	0	1.0	0
SOLE DISH/ENTRÉE								
(Gorton's)								
fillet, stuffed, frozen, 'Select' approx 5 oz	1 fillet	160	16	18	730	0	3.0	50
in lemon butter, frozen, 'Microwave Entrées'	1 pkg	380	25	17	560	0	24.0	120
(Healthy Choice)								
au gratin, frozen	11 oz	270	16	40	470	0	5.0	55
w/lemon butter sauce, frozen	8.25 oz	230	16	33	430	0	4.0	45
SOMEN NOODLE. See under NOODLE, JAPANESE.								
SORBET. See also SHERBET.								
(Cascadian Farm)								
blackberry sorbet, all-fruit, organic, nonfat	1/2 cup	90	0	22	76	1	0.0	0
blackberry, nonfat	1 oz	25	1	21	0	0	0.1	0
blackberry, w/vanilla ice cream, organic	1/2 cup	110	2	21	30	1	2.0	10
orange, w/vanilla ice cream, organic	1/2 cup	110	2	21	30	0	2.0	10
raspberry, all-fruit, organic, nonfat	1/2 cup	90	0	21	55	1	0.0	0
raspberry, nonfat	1 oz	28	1	21	0	0	0.2	0
raspberry, w/vanilla ice cream, organic	1/2 cup	110	2	21	30	1	2.0	10
strawberry, all-fruit, organic, nonfat	1/2 cup	70	1	17	41	1	0.0	0
strawberry, nonfat	1 oz	26	1	22	0	0	0.1	0
(Diamond Crystal) lower calorie, all flavors	1 serving	30	0	7	30	na	0.0	0

Food Name	Serv. Size	Total Cal.	Prot. gms	Carbs gms	Sod. mgs	Fiber gms	Fat gms	Chol. mgs
(Dole)								
Mandarin orange, nonfat	4 oz	110	1	28	9	0	0.1	0
peach, nonfat	4 oz	120	1	28	11	0	0.6	0
pineapple, nonfat	4 oz	120	1	28	11	0	0.1	0
raspberry, nonfat	4 oz	110	0	28	12	0	0.1	0
strawberry, nonfat	4 oz	110	1	28	1	0	0.1	0
(Frusen Gladje) raspberry, nonfat	1/2 cup	140	0	36	15	0	0.0	0
(Haagen-Dazs)								
blueberry, w/vanilla ice cream	1/2 cup	190	3	25	35	0	8.0	0
key lime, w/vanilla ice cream	1/2 cup	200	2	29	30	0	7.0	0
lemon, 'Ice Cream Shop'	4 oz	140	1	34	5	0	0.0	0
orange, 'Ice Cream Shop'	4 oz	113	1	30	7	0	0.0	0
raspberry	1/2 cup	120	0	29	5	1	0.0	0
raspberry, nonfat, 'Ice Cream Shop'	4 oz	93	0	22	7	0	0.0	0
strawberry	1/2 cup	130	0	33	0	1	0.0	0
(Real Fruit)								
red raspberry, chunky, nonfat	1/2 cup	100	0	25	5	0	0.0	0
tropical blend, chunky, nonfat	1/2 cup	100	0	26	5	1	0.0	0
wildberry, chunky, nonfat	1/2 cup	100	0	25	10	1	0.0	0
(TCBY Treats) all flavors, soft serve, nonfat	1/2 cup	100	0	24	30	0	0.0	0
SORGHUM								
broomcorn, whole grain	3.5 oz	327	9.9	72.9	1	>3.2 c	2.9	0
whole grain	1 cup	651	21.7	143.3	na	>4.6 c	6.3	0
whole grain	1 oz	96	3.2	21.2	na	>.7 c	0.9	0
SORGHUM SYRUP. See under SYRUP.								
SORREL								
boiled, drained	4 oz	23	2.1	3.3	3	>.8 c	0.7	0
raw, trimmed	1 oz	6	0.6	0.9	1	>.2 c	0.2	0
raw, trimmed, chopped	1/2 cup	15	1.3	2.1	3	1.9	0.5	0
raw, untrimmed	1 lb	70	6.4	10.2	13	>2.5 c	2.2	0
SOUP. See also SOUP MIX.								
ASPARAGUS, CREAM OF								
Canned, condensed								
prepared w/milk	1 cup	161	6	16	1042	1	8.2	22
prepared w/water	1 cup	85	2	11	981	0	4.1	5
unprepared	10.75-oz can	210	6	26	2385	1	9.9	12
unprepared	1 cup	173	5	21	1963	1	8.2	10
Frozen								
(Kettle Ready)	3/4 cup	62	1	5	406	0	4.3	0
(Myers)	9.75 oz	152	11	10	992	0	8.0	0
(Soup Supreme)	1 cup	160	4	17	920	1	9.0	0
BARLEY W/MUSHROOM								
Canned, condensed *(Rokeach)* prepared	1 cup	85	3	17	904	0	0.2	0
BARLEY BEAN, frozen *(Tabatchnick)*	7.5 oz	130	6	22	217	0	2.0	0
BEAN								
Canned, condensed								
w/frankfurter, prepared	1 cup	188	10	22	1093	na	7.0	13
w/frankfurter, unprepared	11.25-oz can	453	24	53	2651	15	16.9	29
w/frankfurter, unprepared	1 cup	373	20	44	2186	12	14.0	24
w/pork, prepared	1 cup	172	8	23	951	9	5.9	3
w/pork, unprepared	11.5-oz can	421	19	55	2311	19	14.4	7
w/pork, unprepared	1 cup	347	16	46	1907	16	11.9	5
(Campbell's)								
'Homestyle' prepared	1 cup	130	6	25	700	0	1.0	0
w/bacon, 'Healthy Request' unprepared	1/2 cup	150	7	26	480	7	2.0	5
(Stouffer's) navy bean, classic, food service product,								
prepared	1 cup	128	6	18	951	4	3.2	7

Food Name	Serv. Size	Total Cal.	Prot. gms	Carbs gms	Sod. mgs	Fiber gms	Fat gms	Chol. mgs
Canned, ready to use								
w/ham, chunky, commercial product . . . . 19.25-oz can		519	28	61	2184	25	19.1	49
w/ham, chunky, commercial product . . . . 1 cup		231	13	27	972	11	8.5	22
(Grandma Brown's) . . . . 1 cup		190	9	31	700	10	3.4	1
(Health Valley) five bean vegetable, nonfat . . . . 7.5 oz		100	8	14	260	3	0.0	0
(Hormel) w/ham, 'Hearty Soups' . . . . 7.5 oz		190	9	29	640	0	4.0	23
Frozen								
(Kettle Ready)								
w/beef, vegetable . . . . 3/4 cup		85	4	11	448	0	3.0	0
w/ham . . . . 3/4 cup		113	7	20	459	0	3.6	0
(Soup Supreme)								
royal navy, food service product . . . . 1 cup		140	7	24	1110	5	2.0	0
w/ham, food service product . . . . 1 cup		140	8	23	910	5	2.0	10
(Tabatchnick) Northern bean . . . . 7.5 oz		164	8	29	240	0	2.0	0
BEAN AND HAM, heat and serve (Healthy Choice) . . . . 1 cup		160	12	29	480	5	1.5	2
BEEF								
Canned, condensed								
(Campbell's)								
prepared . . . . 1 cup		80	5	10	830	0	2.0	10
w/bouillon, prepared . . . . 1 cup		16	3	1	820	0	0.0	0
w/broth, prepared . . . . 1 cup		16	3	1	820	0	0.0	0
Canned, ready to use								
chunky . . . . 19-oz can		383	26	44	1946	3	11.5	32
chunky . . . . 1 cup		170	12	20	866	1	5.1	14
(Campbell's)								
'Chunky' . . . . 10 3/4-oz can		200	15	24	1100	0	5.0	0
Stroganoff style, 'Chunky' . . . . 10 3/4-oz can		320	15	28	1230	0	16.0	0
w/vegetables and pasta, 'Home Cookin' . . . . 10 3/4-oz can		140	12	18	1060	0	2.0	0
(College Inn) w/broth, ready to serve . . . . 1 cup		18	2	1	1280	0	0.0	0
(Health Valley) w/broth, no salt added . . . . 7.5 oz		17	1	2	0	0	1.0	1
(Healthy Choice) 'Hearty Beef' . . . . 7.5 oz		120	9	17	580	0	2.0	20
(Progresso)								
. . . . 10.5-oz can		180	15	17	840	0	6.0	35
hearty . . . . 9.5 oz		160	15	15	820	0	4.0	35
w/broth, seasoned . . . . 1/2 cup		10	2	1	380	0	1.0	0
w/minestrone . . . . 10.5-oz can		180	15	18	1000	0	6.0	35
(Swanson) w/broth, ready to serve . . . . 7.25 oz		18	2	0	750	0	1.0	0
BEEF AND POTATO								
Canned, ready to use (Healthy Choice) . . . . 1 cup		110	10	17	450	5	1.0	5
BEEF BARLEY								
Canned, ready to use								
(Progresso)								
. . . . 10.5-oz can		150	13	16	870	3	5.0	30
low-fat, 'Healthy Classics' . . . . 1 cup		142	11	20	470	3	1.9	19
BEEF BROTH/BOUILLON								
Canned, condensed								
prepared . . . . 1 cup		23	3	0	969	na	1.3	1
unprepared . . . . 10.5-oz can		72	13	4	1550	0	0.0	0
unprepared . . . . 1 cup		59	11	4	1279	0	0.0	0
Canned, ready to use								
. . . . 14-oz can		28	5	0	1294	0	0.9	0
. . . . 10.5-oz can		41	7	0	1910	0	1.3	0
. . . . 1 cup		17	3	0	782	0	0.5	0
and tomato juice . . . . 5.5-oz can		62	1	14	220	0	0.2	0
and tomato juice . . . . 1 oz		11	0	3	40	0	0.0	0
(College Inn) . . . . 7 oz		16	3	1	960	0	0.0	0

Food Name	Serv. Size	Total Cal.	Prot. gms	Carbs gms	Sod. mgs	Fiber gms	Fat gms	Chol. mgs
(Health Valley)								
no salt added	6.9 oz	10	1	2	5	0	0.0	0
nonfat	1 cup	20	5	0	160	0	0.0	0
regular	6.9 oz	10	1	2	290	0	0.0	0
(Swanson) clear	1 cup	20	2	1	820	0	1.0	0
BEEF MUSHROOM								
Canned, condensed								
prepared	1 cup	73	6	6	942	0	3.0	7
unprepared	10.75-oz can	186	14	16	2358	1	7.3	15
unprepared	1 cup	153	12	13	1940	1	6.0	13
BEEF NOODLE								
Canned, condensed								
prepared	1 cup	83	5	9	952	1	3.1	5
unprepared	10.75-oz can	204	12	22	2315	2	7.5	12
unprepared	1 cup	168	10	18	1905	2	6.2	10
(Campbell's) 'Homestyle' prepared	1 cup	80	5	7	810	0	4.0	20
Canned, ready to use *(Progresso)*	9.5 oz	170	15	18	1030	0	4.0	40
BEEF VEGETABLE								
Canned, condensed								
(Campbell's) 'Healthy Request' unprepared	1/2 cup	70	5	9	490	0	2.0	5
(Progresso) and rotini, prepared	1 cup	120	11	10	830	3	3.5	20
Canned, ready to use								
country, chunky	1 cup	153	12	16	868	na	4.4	24
w/barley, prepared	1 cup	77	5	10	898	na	1.8	8
(Healthy Choice) 'Vegetable Beef'	7.5 oz	130	8	21	530	0	1.0	15
(Hormel)								
'Hearty Soups'	7.5 oz	90	6	15	730	0	1.0	5
micro cup, 'Hearty Soups'	1 container	71	5	12	811	0	1.0	9
(Lipton) 'Hearty Ones'	11-oz container	229	10	40	921	0	3.0	29
(Progresso)	10.5-oz can	170	17	18	880	0	3.0	40
BERRY								
Canned, ready to use *(Great Impressions)* 'Three Berry'	3/4 cup	107	1	26	90	0	0.2	0
BLACK BEAN								
Canned, condensed								
prepared	1 cup	116	6	20	1198	4	1.5	0
unprepared	11-oz can	284	15	48	3026	21	4.1	0
unprepared	1 cup	234	12	40	2493	17	3.4	0
(Stouffer's) prepared	1 cup	192	9	30	847	14	3.2	7
Canned, ready to use								
(Health Valley)								
	7.5 oz	160	7	24	285	17	3.0	0
and vegetable, nonfat	1 cup	110	11	24	280	12	0.0	0
no salt added	7.5 oz	160	7	24	20	17	3.0	0
Frozen								
(Kettle Ready) w/ham	3/4 cup	154	8	23	613	0	6.2	0
(Soup Supreme) Southern style, food service product	1 cup	150	9	23	1450	7	3.0	5
BLUEBERRY, canned, ready to use *(Great Impressions)*	3/4 cup	95	0	23	92	0	0.3	0
BORSCHT								
Canned, ready to use								
(Gold's)								
	1 cup	100	4	21	1280	0	0.0	0
low-calorie	1 cup	20	1	5	1160	0	1.0	0
(Manischewitz)								
low-calorie	1 cup	20	1	4	725	0	0.0	0
w/beets	1 cup	80	1	20	660	0	0.0	0
(Rokeach)								
	1 cup	96	1	23	985	0	0.3	0

Food Name	Serv. Size	Total Cal.	Prot. gms	Carbs gms	Sod. mgs	Fiber gms	Fat gms	Chol. mgs
'Diet'	1 cup	29	1	6	897	1	0.2	0
'Unsalted'	1 cup	103	1	23	50	1	0.3	0
BROCCOLI								
Canned, ready to use *(Health Valley)* carotene, nonfat	1 cup	70	6	16	240	7	0.0	0
BROCCOLI, CREAM OF								
Canned, condensed								
(Campbell's)								
'Healthy Request' unprepared	1/2 cup	70	2	9	480	1	2.0	5
prepared w/whole milk	1 cup	140	5	14	850	0	7.0	0
unprepared	1/2 cup	80	2	12	730	1	3.0	3
(Stouffer's) prepared w/whole milk	1 cup	272	9	17	783	2	19.2	48
Canned, ready to use								
(Andersen's)	.5 oz	170	5	20	670	0	8.0	0
(Stouffer's) food service product	1 cup	288	10	13	903	2	21.6	43
(Progresso) 'Healthy Classics'	1 cup	88	2	13	578	2	2.8	5
Frozen								
(Kettle Ready)	6 oz	94	1	6	417	0	7.2	0
(Myers)	9.75 oz	174	8	11	905	0	11.0	0
(Soup Supreme)								
food service product	1 cup	180	6	16	760	2	11.0	5
w/cheese, food service product	1 cup	190	6	16	890	1	12.0	15
(Tabatchnick)	7.5 oz	90	4	10	285	0	4.0	4
CABBAGE SOUP, frozen *(Tabatchnick)*	7.5 oz	110	2	21	185	0	2.0	0
CAULIFLOWER, CREAM OF, frozen *(Kettle Ready)*	3/4 cup	93	2	6	445	0	7.0	0
CELERY, CREAM OF								
Canned, condensed								
unprepared	10.75-oz can	220	4	21	2309	2	13.6	34
unprepared	1 cup	181	3	18	1900	2	11.2	28
prepared w/milk	1 cup	164	6	15	1009	1	9.7	32
prepared w/water	1 cup	90	2	9	949	1	5.6	15
(Campbell's)								
'Healthy Request' unprepared	1/2 cup	70	2	11	480	1	2.0	5
prepared w/water	1 cup	100	2	8	820	0	7.0	5
CHEDDAR CAULIFLOWER								
Frozen *(Soup Supreme)* food service product	1 cup	130	4	13	1100	2	8.0	5
CHEDDAR VEGETABLE								
Frozen, *(Soup Supreme)* food service product	1 cup	140	4	14	1110	2	8.0	5
CHEESE								
Canned, condensed								
prepared w/milk	1 cup	231	9	16	1019	1	14.6	48
prepared w/water	1 cup	156	5	11	958	1	10.5	30
unprepared	11-oz can	378	13	26	2331	2	25.4	72
unprepared	1 cup	311	11	21	1920	2	20.9	59
(Campbell's)								
nacho, prepared w/water	1 cup	110	4	8	740	0	8.0	0
nacho, prepared w/whole milk	1 cup	180	8	13	800	0	12.0	0
Frozen								
(Kettle Ready)								
cheddar, cream of	3/4 cup	158	4	7	616	0	12.5	0
cheddar, cream of, w/broccoli	3/4 cup	137	4	5	533	0	11.3	0
(Myers) and broccoli	9.75 oz	325	12	19	1257	0	23.0	0
(Soup Supreme) cheddar, club, food service product	1 cup	240	8	17	1280	1	16.0	20
CHERRY, canned, ready to use *(Great Impressions)*	3/4 cup	123	1	30	88	0	0.2	0
CHICKEN								
Canned, condensed								
w/dumplings, prepared	10.5-oz can	234	14	15	2092	1	13.4	82
w/dumplings, prepared	1 cup	96	6	6	860	0	5.5	34

Food Name	Serv. Size	Total Cal.	Prot. gms	Carbs gms	Sod. mgs	Fiber gms	Fat gms	Chol. mgs
w/dumplings, unprepared	10.5-oz can	235	14	15	2095	1	13.4	80
w/dumplings, unprepared	1 cup	194	11	12	1729	1	11.1	66
(Stouffer's) prepared	1 cup	104	2	12	1111	1	4.8	16
Canned, ready to use								
chunky	19-oz can	383	27	37	1908	3	14.2	65
chunky	10.75-oz can	217	15	21	1080	2	8.1	37
chunky	1 cup	178	13	17	889	2	6.6	30
(Campbell's) 'Chunky Old Fashioned'	10 3/4 oz	180	12	21	1220	0	5.0	0
(Healthy Choice) hearty	1 cup	130	9	18	460	3	2.5	10
(Progresso)								
'Homestyle'	9.5 oz	110	11	12	740	0	3.0	20
spicy, w/penne	1 cup	120	8	13	680	0	4.0	20
w/meatballs, 'Chickarina'	9.5 oz	130	8	13	820	0	5.0	20
Frozen (Tabatchnick)	7.5 oz	65	2	10	255	0	2.0	0
CHICKEN, CREAM OF								
Canned, condensed								
prepared w/milk	10.75-oz can	464	18	36	2540	1	27.8	66
prepared w/milk	1 cup	191	7	15	1047	0	11.5	27
prepared w/water	10.75-oz can	285	8	23	2396	1	17.9	24
prepared w/water	1 cup	117	3	9	986	0	7.4	10
unprepared	10.75-ox can	284	8	23	2397	1	17.9	24
unprepared	1 cup	233	7	19	1973	1	14.7	20
(Campbell's)								
'Healthy Request' prepared w/water	1 cup	70	2	11	490	0	2.0	10
'Healthy Request' unprepared	1/2 cup	80	2	12	480	0	2.0	10
98% nonfat, unprepared	1/2 cup	80	3	9	910	0	3.0	10
Canned, ready to use (Progresso)	9.5 oz	190	10	12	970	0	11.0	35
Frozen								
(Kettle Ready)	3/4 cup	98	6	5	668	0	6.2	0
(Soup Supreme)	1 cup	160	8	14	910	2	8.0	15
CHICKEN AND BROCCOLI, CREAM OF								
Canned, condensed								
(Campbell's)								
'Healthy Request' unprepared	1/2 cup	80	3	10	480	1	2.5	5
prepared	1 cup	110	3	9	710	0	7.0	10
CHICKEN BARLEY								
Canned, condensed (Campbell's) prepared	1 cup	70	3	10	850	0	2.0	0
Canned, ready to use (Progresso)	9.25 oz	100	10	12	740	4	2.0	20
CHICKEN BROTH/BOUILLON								
Canned, condensed								
prepared	1 cup	38	5	1	763	0	1.4	0
unprepared	10.75-oz can	95	13	2	1909	0	3.2	3
unprepared	1 cup	78	11	2	1571	0	2.6	3
(Campbell's) prepared	1 cup	30	1	2	710	0	2.0	0
Canned, ready to use								
(Campbell's)								
'Healthy Request'	1 cup	16	3	1	470	0	0.0	0
low-salt	1 cup	40	4	2	140	0	2.0	5
nonfat, 'Healthy Request'	1 cup	16	3	1	470	0	0.0	0
(College Inn)								
	1 cup	35	1	0	1320	0	3.0	0
lower salt	7 oz	20	1	0	550	0	2.0	5
(Hain)								
	8.75 oz	70	2	0	870	0	6.0	5
'No Salt Added'	8.75 oz	60	3	0	75	0	5.0	5
(Health Valley)								
	7.5 oz	35	4	1	410	0	2.0	2

Food Name	Serv. Size	Total Cal.	Prot. gms	Carbs gms	Sod. mgs	Fiber gms	Fat gms	Chol. mgs
no salt added	7.5 oz	35	4	1	0	0	2.0	2
nonfat	1 cup	30	6	0	170	0	0.0	0
(Pritikin) defatted	1 cup	18	3	1	160	0	1.0	0
(Progresso) nonfat	1/2 cup	8	2	0	360	0	0.0	5
(Shelton's)								
nonfat	1 cup	10	2	0	60	0	0.0	0
w/salt and pepper	1 cup	35	2	0	580	0	2.5	2
(Swanson) clear	1 cup	30	2	1	1000	0	2.0	0
CHICKEN CORN CHOWDER								
Canned, ready to use *(Healthy Choice)*	1 cup	160	8	26	470	4	2.5	5
CHICKEN GUMBO								
Canned, condensed								
prepared	1 cup	56	3	8	954	2	1.4	5
unprepared	10.75-oz can	137	6	20	2321	5	3.5	9
unprepared	1 cup	113	5	17	1910	4	2.9	8
Frozen								
(Kettle Ready)	3/4 cup	94	4	12	473	0	3.5	0
(Soup Supreme)								
food service product	1 cup	90	5	11	1300	1	2.5	10
spicy, Southern style, food service product	1 cup	110	6	14	960	1	3.0	15
Canned, ready to use								
(Campbell's) w/sausage, 'Home Cookin'	10.75-oz can	140	11	15	1090	0	4.0	0
CHICKEN MINESTRONE								
Canned, ready to use								
(Campbell's) 'Home Cookin'	10 3/4 oz	180	15	17	950	0	6.0	0
(Progresso)	10.5 oz	140	12	14	1060	0	4.0	20
CHICKEN MUSHROOM								
Canned, condensed								
prepared	1 cup	132	4	9	942	0	9.2	10
unprepared	10.75-oz can	332	11	23	2358	1	22.3	24
unprepared	1 cup	274	9	19	1940	1	18.3	20
Canned, ready to use								
chowder, chunky	1 cup	192	7	17	814	3	10.6	14
(Campbell's) creamy, 'Chunky'	10.5 oz	270	12	13	1280	0	19.0	0
CHICKEN NOODLE								
Canned, condensed								
prepared	1 cup	75	4	9	1106	1	2.5	7
unprepared	10.5-oz can	182	10	23	2256	2	5.5	15
unprepared	1 cup	150	8	19	1862	1	4.6	12
(Campbell's)								
creamy, prepared w/2% milk	1 cup	180	8	16	850	0	9.0	0
creamy, prepared w/water	1/2 cup	120	4	10	800	0	7.0	0
'Healthy Request' unprepared	1/2 cup	70	3	9	480	0	2.0	15
Teddy bear pasta in chicken broth, prepared	1 cup	60	2	11	770	0	1.0	5
unprepared	10.75-oz can	156	8	21	2291	2	4.6	27
(Progresso) prepared	1 cup	80	9	8	730	1	2.0	20
Canned, ready to use								
chunky	19-oz can	393	29	38	1908	9	13.5	43
chunky	1 cup	175	13	17	850	4	6.0	19
w/celery and carrots, homestyle	1 cup	95	6	9	985	na	3.4	21
w/meatballs, chunky	20-oz can	227	19	19	2376	na	8.2	23
w/meatballs, chunky	1 cup	99	8	8	1039	na	3.6	10
(Campbell's)								
'Chunky'	10 3/4 oz	200	14	20	1140	0	7.0	0
hearty, 'Healthy Request'	1 cup	100	5	14	480	1	3.0	15
'Home Cookin'	10 3/4 oz	140	13	12	1150	0	4.0	0
low-salt	1 cup	170	11	18	120	2	5.0	50

Food Name	Serv. Size	Total Cal.	Prot. gms	Carbs gms	Sod. mgs	Fiber gms	Fat gms	Chol. mgs
(Hain)								
....	9.5 oz	120	9	11	980	0	4.0	20
low-salt, low-fat, 'Homestyle Naturals'	1 cup	80	7	8	100	1	2.0	15
(Healthy Choice)								
old-fashioned	1 cup	150	8	23	480	1	2.5	15
w/pasta	1 cup	120	8	17	470	1	2.5	5
(Hormel)								
'Hearty Soups'	7.5 oz	110	7	14	690	0	3.0	18
micro cup, 'Hearty Soups'	1 container	108	7	14	686	0	3.0	22
(Lipton) 'Hearty Ones Homestyle'	11 oz	227	10	37	989	0	4.0	37
(Lunch Bucket) microwave cup	7.25 oz	90	4	13	810	0	2.0	25
(Pritikin) w/ribbon pasta	1 cup	80	6	13	180	1	1.0	5
(Progresso)								
'Healthy Classics'	1 cup	76	6	9	460	1	1.6	19
w/rotini, hearty	1 cup	90	10	8	860	1	2.0	20
(Weight Watchers)								
....	10.5 oz	80	6	9	1230	0	2.0	0
microwave cup	7.5 oz	90	8	13	450	0	1.0	15
Frozen								
(Kettle Ready)	3/4 cup	94	5	12	569	0	3.0	0
(Myers)	9.75 oz	87	8	5	1046	0	5.0	0
(Soup Supreme)								
food service product	1 cup	120	7	15	1050	1	3.0	20
seasoned, food service product	1 cup	100	3	16	1120	1	2.5	10
CHICKEN RICE								
Canned, condensed								
prepared	10.5-oz can	147	9	17	1981	2	4.6	18
prepared	1 cup	60	4	7	815	1	1.9	7
unprepared	10.5-oz can	146	9	17	1982	1	4.6	15
unprepared	1 cup	121	7	14	1636	1	3.8	12
(Campbell's)								
'Healthy Request' unprepared	1/2 cup	60	2	10	480	1	2.5	15
'Healthy Request' prepared	1 cup	60	2	7	480	0	3.0	10
(Progresso) and vegetable, prepared	1 cup	110	7	12	790	1	3.0	15
Canned, ready to use								
chunky	19-oz can	286	28	29	1994	2	7.2	27
chunky	1 cup	127	12	13	888	1	3.2	12
(Campbell's)								
hearty, 'Healthy Request'	1 cup	110	5	15	480	0	3.0	10
microwave	10.5 oz	120	5	20	1130	2	2.5	10
(Healthy Choice)	7.5 oz	140	5	18	510	0	4.0	15
(Hormel) 'Hearty Soup'	7.5 oz	110	5	17	890	0	2.0	6
(Progresso)								
....	10.5 oz	120	9	12	990	0	4.0	25
....	9.5 oz	130	9	16	750	0	3.0	25
wild rice	9.5 oz	120	6	17	850	0	3.0	20
wild rice, w/vegetables	1 cup	93	6	12	784	na	2.2	14
w/vegetables, 'Healthy Classics'	1 cup	88	6	13	459	1	1.5	17
Frozen								
(Soup Supreme)								
w/white and wild rice, food service product	1 cup	210	8	17	1230	0	12.0	20
CHICKEN VEGETABLE								
Canned, condensed								
prepared	10.5-oz can	182	9	21	2297	2	6.9	23
prepared	1 cup	75	4	9	945	1	2.8	10
unprepared	10.5-oz can	182	9	21	2298	2	6.9	21
unprepared	1 cup	150	7	17	1897	2	5.7	17

Food Name	Serv. Size	Total Cal.	Prot. gms	Carbs gms	Sod. mgs	Fiber gms	Fat gms	Chol. mgs
(Campbell's) 'Healthy Request' unprepared . . . . 1/2 cup		80	3	12	480	1	2.0	5
Canned, ready to use								
chunky . . . . 19-oz can		372	28	42	2399	na	10.8	38
chunky . . . . 1 cup		166	12	19	1068	na	4.8	17
(Campbell's)								
'Chunky' . . . . 9.5 oz		170	10	19	1080	0	6.0	25
hearty, 'Healthy Request' . . . . 1 cup		120	7	16	420	0	3.0	10
'Home Cookin' . . . . 10 3/4 oz		180	11	25	970	0	4.0	0
low-sodium, 'Chunky' . . . . 10 3/4 oz		240	15	21	95	0	11.0	10
(Hain)								
. . . . 9.5 oz		120	8	14	930	0	4.0	15
no salt added . . . . 9.5 oz		130	8	14	100	0	4.0	20
(Health Valley)								
chunky . . . . 7.5 oz		125	7	20	425	4	2.0	11
chunky, no salt added . . . . 7.5 oz		125	7	20	60	4	2.0	11
(Hormel) and rice, micro cup, 'Hearty Soups' . . . . 1 container		114	5	16	1025	0	3.0	7
(Pritikin) . . . . 1 cup		70	5	12	150	2	1.0	5
(Progresso) . . . . 9.5 oz		140	9	17	800	0	4.0	25
CHILI BEEF								
Canned, condensed								
unprepared . . . . 11.25-oz can		412	16	52	2514	23	16.0	32
unprepared . . . . 1 cup		339	13	43	2072	19	13.2	26
prepared . . . . 1 cup		170	7	21	1035	10	6.6	13
(Campbell's) prepared . . . . 1 cup		140	5	20	840	0	5.0	10
(Stouffer's) w/beans, food service product, prepared . . . . . . 1 cup		144	8	19	583	6	3.2	10
Canned, ready to use								
(Campbell's)								
'Chunky' . . . . 11 oz		290	21	37	1120	0	7.0	0
'Microwave' . . . . 7.5 oz		190	7	32	870	0	4.0	0
(Healthy Choice) . . . . 1 cup		170	15	29	440	6	1.5	3
Frozen								
(Kettle Ready)								
jalapeño . . . . 3/4 cup		173	11	15	531	0	8.0	0
traditional . . . . 3/4 cup		161	12	14	454	0	6.5	0
(Soup Supreme)								
panhandle, food service product . . . . 1 cup		200	14	16	1100	4	10.0	35
w/beans, classic, food service product . . . . 1 cup		250	19	23	1020	7	10.0	45
w/beans, grande, food service product . . . . 1 cup		250	18	23	1080	6	10.0	45
CLAM CHOWDER								
Canned, condensed								
Manhattan, prepared . . . . 10.75-oz can		190	5	30	1405	4	5.4	6
Manhattan, prepared . . . . 1 cup		78	2	12	578	1	2.2	2
Manhattan, unprepared . . . . 10.75-oz can		186	5	30	1394	4	5.4	6
Manhattan, unprepared . . . . 1 cup		153	4	24	1147	3	4.4	5
New England, prepared w/milk . . . . 10.75-oz can		397	23	40	2408	4	16.0	54
New England, prepared w/milk . . . . 1 cup		164	9	17	992	1	6.6	22
New England, prepared w/water . . . . 10.75-oz can		231	12	30	2224	4	7.0	12
New England, prepared w/water . . . . 1 cup		95	5	12	915	1	2.9	5
New England, unprepared . . . . 10.75-oz can		214	13	27	2266	2	6.1	12
New England, unprepared . . . . 1 cup		176	11	22	1865	2	5.0	10
(Campbell's)								
Manhattan style, 'Seashore Soups' unprepared . . . . 1/2 cup		70	2	10	820	0	2.0	5
New England, prepared w/whole milk . . . . 1 cup		150	7	17	930	0	7.0	0
New England, 'Seashore Soups' unprepared . . . . 1/2 cup		80	3	12	870	0	3.0	5
(Doxsee) Manhattan, prepared . . . . 7.5 oz		70	3	11	780	0	2.0	0
(Gorton's)								
New England, prepared w/whole milk . . . . 1/4 can		140	7	17	740	0	5.0	15

Food Name	Serv. Size	Total Cal.	Prot. gms	Carbs gms	Sod. mgs	Fiber gms	Fat gms	Chol. mgs
New England, unprepared	3.75 oz	70	3	12	670	0	1.0	5
(Snow's)								
Manhattan, prepared	7.5 oz	70	3	11	780	0	2.0	0
Manhattan, unprepared	3.75 oz	70	3	9	630	0	2.0	0
New England, prepared w/whole milk	7.5 oz	140	8	13	670	0	6.0	0
New England, unprepared	3.75 oz	70	5	8	620	0	2.0	0
(Stouffer's)								
Boston, food service product, prepared w/milk	1 cup	208	9	20	919	2	10.4	32
Manhattan, food service product, prepared	1 cup	80	4	10	823	2	2.4	8
New England, food service product, prepared w/whole milk	1 cup	248	11	21	999	2	13.6	40
Canned, ready to use								
Manhattan, chunky	19-oz can	302	16	42	2248	6	7.6	32
Manhattan, chunky	1 cup	134	7	19	1001	3	3.4	14
(Campbell's)								
New England, 'Healthy Request'	1 cup	100	4	14	490	0	3.0	10
New England, 'Home Cookin''	10 3/4 oz	260	8	15	1240	0	18.0	0
(Gorton's)	7.5 oz	140	7	17	720	0	5.0	20
(Hain) New England, ready to serve	9.25 oz	180	8	26	780	0	4.0	25
(Health Valley)								
Manhattan	7.5 oz	110	6	15	510	13	2.0	15
Manhattan, no salt added	7.5 oz	110	6	15	60	13	2.0	15
(Healthy Choice) New England	1 cup	120	7	22	480	3	1.0	5
(Hormel)								
New England, 'Hearty Soup'	7.5 oz	130	5	16	790	0	5.0	30
New England, micro cup, 'Hearty Soups'	1 container	118	5	15	882	0	5.0	30
(Progresso)								
Manhattan	1 cup	110	12	11	710	3	2.0	10
New England	1 cup	180	6	17	850	2	10.0	15
New England, 'Healthy Classics'	1 cup	117	5	20	529	1	2.0	5
(Stouffer's)								
Boston, food service product, 'Heat 'N Serve'	1 cup	192	10	20	975	2	8.0	34
New England, food service product, 'Heat 'N Serve'	1 cup	184	10	23	871	2	5.6	25
(Weight Watchers) New England	7.5 oz	90	5	16	450	0	0.0	5
Frozen								
(Kettle Ready)								
Boston	3/4 cup	131	4	13	417	0	7.3	0
Manhattan	3/4 cup	69	4	8	549	0	2.6	0
New England	3/4 cup	116	3	11	373	0	6.5	0
(Myers) New England	9.75 oz	152	7	21	910	0	5.0	0
(Soup Supreme)								
Boston, food service product	1 cup	200	11	17	940	1	10.0	30
New England, food service product	1 cup	180	9	22	730	1	6.0	15
(Stouffer's) New England	1 cup	180	8	16	790	0	9.0	0
(Tabatchnick) New England	3/4 cup	98	6	14	255	0	2.0	0
CONSOMMÉ								
Canned, condensed *(Campbell's)* beef, w/gelatin, prepared	1 cup	25	4	2	750	0	0.0	0
CORN								
Canned, condensed								
(Campbell's)								
golden, cream, prepared w/2% milk	1 cup	160	6	23	760	0	5.0	10
golden, cream, prepared w/water	1 cup	110	2	18	700	0	3.0	5
golden, cream, unprepared	1/2 cup	110	2	18	700	0	3.0	5
Canned, ready to use								
(Health Valley)								
country, and vegetable	7.5 oz	70	4	13	290	3	0.0	0
country, and vegetable, nonfat	1 cup	70	5	17	135	7	0.0	0

Food Name	Serv. Size	Total Cal.	Prot. gms	Carbs gms	Sod. mgs	Fiber gms	Fat gms	Chol. mgs
CORN AND BROCCOLI CHOWDER								
Frozen *(Kettle Ready)* .... 3/4 cup		102	1	13	323	0	5.0	0
CORN CHOWDER								
Canned, condensed								
(Snow's)								
New England, prepared w/milk .... 7.5 oz		150	5	18	640	0	6.0	0
New England, unprepared .... 3.75 oz		80	2	13	590	0	2.0	0
(Stouffer's) food service product, prepared w/whole milk ... 1 cup		264	7	28	1055	2	13.6	16
Canned, ready to use								
(Progresso) .... 9.25 oz		200	5	22	840	0	10.0	10
(Stouffer's) 'Heat 'N Serve' .... 1 cup		280	6	21	791	2	20.0	5
Frozen *(Soup Supreme)* Captain's .... 1 cup		200	6	29	770	2	7.0	5
CRAB								
Canned, condensed								
(Stouffer's) Maryland, food service product, prepared ..... 1 cup		80	3	10	735	3	2.4	18
Canned, ready to use								
.... 13-oz can		114	8	16	1867	1	2.3	15
.... 1 cup		76	5	10	1235	1	1.5	10
CREOLE								
Canned, ready to use *(Campbell's)* 'Chunky' .... 10-3/4 oz		240	11	31	910	0	8.0	0
Frozen *(Soup Supreme)* Southern style .... 1 cup		110	4	20	1660	2	3.0	5
ESCAROLE								
Canned, ready to use								
.... 19.5-oz can		61	3	4	8616	na	4.0	6
.... 1 cup		27	2	2	3864	na	1.8	2
(Progresso) in chicken broth .... 9.25 oz		30	2	2	1100	0	1.0	5
FISH CHOWDER								
Canned, condensed								
(Snow's)								
New England, prepared w/whole milk .... 7.5 oz		130	9	11	620	0	6.0	0
New England, unprepared .... 3.75 oz		60	5	6	560	0	2.0	0
GARLIC AND PASTA								
Canned, ready to use *(Progresso)* 'Healthy Classics' .... 1 cup		100	4	18	450	3	1.3	5
GAZPACHO								
Canned, ready to use								
.... 13-oz can		70	11	7	1118	1	0.4	0
.... 1 cup		46	7	4	739	0	0.2	0
GREEN PEA								
Canned, condensed								
prepared w/milk .... 11.25-oz can		579	31	78	2353	7	17.1	43
prepared w/milk .... 1 cup		239	13	32	970	3	7.0	18
prepared w/water .... 1 cup		165	9	27	918	3	2.9	0
unprepared .... 11.25-oz can		399	21	64	2227	7	7.1	0
unprepared .... 1 cup		329	17	53	1836	6	5.9	0
HAM AND BEAN								
Canned, ready to use								
(Campbell's) w/butter beans, 'Chunky' .... 10 3/4 oz		280	12	34	1180	0	10.0	0
(Progresso) .... 9.5 oz		140	11	28	950	8	2.0	10
ITALIAN STYLE WEDDING								
Canned, condensed								
(Stouffer's) food service product, prepared .... 1 cup		216	10	25	1790	na	8.0	29
LEMON, canned, ready to use *(Great Impressions)* ...... 3/4 cup		90	0	22	109	0	1.0	0
LENTIL								
Canned, ready to use								
w/ham .... 20-oz can		318	21	46	3016	na	6.3	17
w/ham .... 1 cup		139	9	20	1319	na	2.8	7
(Hain)								
.... 9.5 oz		160	9	25	690	0	3.0	5

Food Name	Serv. Size	Total Cal.	Prot. gms	Carbs gms	Sod. mgs	Fiber gms	Fat gms	Chol. mgs
no salt added .... 9.5 oz	9.5 oz	160	9	24	65	0	3.0	5
(Health Valley)								
.... 7.5 oz	7.5 oz	170	9	28	435	17	2.0	0
and carrot, nonfat .... 1 cup	1 cup	90	10	25	220	14	0.0	0
no salt added .... 7.5 oz	7.5 oz	170	9	28	25	17	2.0	0
(Healthy Choice) .... 1 cup	1 cup	140	9	28	470	4	1.0	0
(Progresso)								
.... 1 cup	1 cup	140	9	22	750	7	2.0	0
'Healthy Classics' .... 1 cup	1 cup	126	8	20	443	6	1.5	0
w/sausage .... 9.5 oz	9.5 oz	170	8	21	840	5	8.0	20
Frozen *(Tabatchnick)* .... 7.5 oz	7.5 oz	170	11	27	240	0	2.0	0
MACARONI AND BEAN								
Canned, ready to use *(Progresso)* .... 10 1/2 oz	10 1/2 oz	150	9	27	1020	8	4.0	0
MENUDO, canned, ready to use *(Old El Paso)* .... 1/2 can	1/2 can	476	15	14	770	2	52.0	176
MINESTRONE								
Canned, condensed								
prepared .... 10.5-oz can	10.5-oz can	199	10	27	2215	2	6.1	6
prepared .... 1 cup	1 cup	82	4	11	911	1	2.5	2
unprepared .... 10.5-oz can	10.5-oz can	203	10	27	2217	2	6.1	3
unprepared .... 1 cup	1 cup	167	9	23	1830	2	5.0	2
(Campbell's) 'Healthy Request' unprepared .... 1/2 cup	1/2 cup	90	4	17	480	2	1.0	0
(Stouffer's) food service product, prepared .... 1 cup	1 cup	104	4	16	959	2	2.4	4
Canned, ready to use								
chunky .... 19-oz can	19-oz can	286	11	47	1940	13	6.3	11
chunky .... 1 cup	1 cup	127	5	21	864	6	2.8	5
(Campbell's) hearty, 'Healthy Request' .... 1 cup	1 cup	120	4	24	480	3	2.0	3
(Hain)								
.... 9.5 oz	9.5 oz	170	8	27	1060	0	2.0	0
no salt added .... 9.5 oz	9.5 oz	160	7	28	35	0	4.0	0
(Health Valley)								
.... 7.5 oz	7.5 oz	130	6	19	637	13	3.0	0
no salt added .... 7.5 oz	7.5 oz	130	6	19	80	13	3.0	0
nonfat .... 1 cup	1 cup	80	8	21	210	11	0.0	0
(Healthy Choice) .... 1 cup	1 cup	110	4	24	480	5	1.0	0
(Hormel)								
'Hearty Soups' .... 7.5 oz	7.5 oz	100	5	17	460	0	1.0	5
micro cup, 'Hearty Soups' .... 1 container	1 container	104	7	15	903	0	2.0	10
(Lipton) 'Hearty Ones' .... 11 oz	11 oz	189	8	36	821	0	3.2	6
(Progresso)								
.... 1 cup	1 cup	130	6	22	960	5	2.5	0
chunky, hearty .... 9.25 oz	9.25 oz	110	7	16	740	0	2.0	5
chunky, zesty .... 9.5 oz	9.5 oz	150	7	19	1130	4	8.0	10
'Healthy Classics' .... 1 cup	1 cup	123	5	20	470	1	2.5	0
(Stouffer's) food service product, 'Heat 'N Serve' .... 1 cup	1 cup	80	3	10	871	2	2.4	5
Frozen								
(Kettle Ready) hearty .... 3/4 cup	3/4 cup	104	3	15	577	0	4.4	0
(Soup Supreme) food service product .... 1 cup	1 cup	70	3	11	1030	2	2.5	0
(Tabatchnick) .... 7.5 oz	7.5 oz	137	8	24	265	0	2.0	0
MUSHROOM								
Canned, condensed								
w/beef stock, prepared .... 10.75-oz can	10.75-oz can	208	8	23	2354	2	9.8	18
w/beef stock, prepared .... 1 cup	1 cup	85	3	9	969	1	4.0	7
w/beef stock, unprepared .... 10.75-oz can	10.75-oz can	207	8	23	2358	0	9.8	18
w/beef stock, unprepared .... 1 cup	1 cup	171	6	19	1940	0	8.1	15
(Campbell's)								
beefy, prepared .... 1 cup	1 cup	60	4	5	960	0	3.0	10

Food Name	Serv. Size	Total Cal.	Prot. gms	Carbs gms	Sod. mgs	Fiber gms	Fat gms	Chol. mgs
w/ground beef, prepared . . . . 1 cup		90	4	10	820	0	4.0	25
MUSHROOM BARLEY								
Canned, condensed								
prepared . . . . 10.75-oz can		178	5	28	2164	2	5.5	0
prepared . . . . 1 cup		73	2	12	891	1	2.3	0
unprepared . . . . 10.75-oz can		186	5	29	2227	na	5.5	0
unprepared . . . . 1 cup		153	4	24	1832	na	4.5	0
Canned, ready to use								
(Hain) . . . . 9.5 oz		100	4	17	600	0	2.0	10
(Health Valley)								
. . . . 7.5 oz		100	5	16	394	9	2.0	0
no salt added . . . . 7.5 oz		100	5	16	20	9	2.0	0
Frozen								
(Tabatchnick)								
. . . . 7.5 oz		92	2	16	234	0	2.0	0
'No Salt' . . . . 7.5 oz		97	4	18	77	0	1.0	0
MUSHROOM, CREAM OF								
Canned, condensed								
prepared w/milk . . . . 10.75-oz can		494	15	36	2227	1	33.0	48
prepared w/milk . . . . 1 cup		203	6	15	918	0	13.6	20
prepared w/water . . . . 10.75-oz can		314	6	23	2141	1	21.8	6
prepared w/water . . . . 1 cup		129	2	9	881	0	9.0	2
unprepared . . . . 10.75-oz can		314	5	23	2111	1	23.1	3
unprepared . . . . 1 cup		259	4	19	1737	1	19.0	3
(Campbell's)								
'Healthy Request' unprepared . . . . 1/2 cup		70	1	10	480	0	2.5	10
98% nonfat, unprepared . . . . 1/2 cup		70	1	9	830	0	3.0	3
Canned, ready to use								
(Campbell's) low-sodium . . . . 10 1/2 oz		210	3	18	55	0	14.0	0
(Hain) creamy . . . . 9.25 oz		110	4	16	740	0	4.0	15
(Progresso) . . . . 9.25 oz		160	4	14	1120	0	10.0	15
(Weight Watchers) . . . . 10 1/2 oz		90	3	14	1250	0	2.0	0
Frozen								
(Kettle Ready) . . . . 3/4 cup		85	1	6	371	0	6.4	0
(Soup Supreme) food service product . . . . 1 cup		200	4	13	940	1	15.0	10
(Tabatchnick) . . . . 3/4 cup		75	3	11	325	0	2.0	3
ONION								
Canned, condensed								
prepared . . . . 10.5-oz can		141	9	20	2561	2	4.2	0
prepared . . . . 1 cup		58	4	8	1053	1	1.7	0
unprepared . . . . 10.5-oz can		137	9	20	2563	2	4.2	0
unprepared . . . . 1 cup		113	8	16	2116	2	3.5	0
(Stouffer's) French, food service product, prepared . . . . 1 cup		72	1	9	1551	2	2.4	4
Frozen								
(Kettle Ready) French . . . . 3/4 cup		42	1	5	562	0	2.2	0
(Soup Supreme) French, food service product . . . . 1 cup		80	2	11	1110	1	4.0	0
ONION, CREAM OF								
Canned, condensed								
prepared w/milk . . . . 10.75-oz can		452	16	45	2438	2	22.8	78
prepared w/milk . . . . 1 cup		186	7	18	1004	1	9.4	32
prepared w/water . . . . 10.75-oz can		261	7	31	2253	2	12.8	36
prepared w/water . . . . 1 cup		107	3	13	927	1	5.3	15
unprepared . . . . 10.75-oz can		268	7	32	2318	1	12.8	37
unprepared . . . . 1 cup		221	6	26	1908	1	10.5	30
(Campbell's)								
prepared w/4 oz soup, 2 oz whole milk, 2 oz water . . . . . . 1 cup		140	4	15	860	0	7.0	0

Food Name	Serv. Size	Total Cal.	Prot. gms	Carbs gms	Sod. mgs	Fiber gms	Fat gms	Chol. mgs
PEA								
Frozen								
(Kettle Ready) tortellini, in tomato	3/4 cup	122	4	15	447	0	5.4	0
(Tabatchnick)								
	7.5 oz	175	10	31	290	0	1.0	0
'No Salt'	7.5 oz	175	10	31	79	0	1.0	0
PEPPER POT								
Canned, condensed								
prepared	1 cup	104	6	9	971	0	4.6	10
prepared	10.5-oz can	252	15	23	2362	1	11.3	23
unprepared	10.5-oz can	250	15	23	2360	1	11.3	24
unprepared	1 cup	207	13	19	1948	1	9.3	20
POT ROAST								
Frozen (Soup Supreme) Yankee, food service product	1 cup	90	6	13	730	2	1.5	15
POTATO, CREAM OF								
Canned, condensed								
prepared w/milk	10.75-oz can	361	14	42	2577	1	15.7	54
prepared w/milk	1 cup	149	6	17	1061	0	6.4	22
prepared w/water	10.75-oz can	178	4	28	2431	1	5.8	12
prepared w/water	1 cup	73	2	11	1000	0	2.4	5
unprepared	10.75-oz can	180	4	28	2431	1	5.7	15
unprepared	1 cup	148	3	23	2000	1	4.7	13
(Campbell's) prepared w/tofu, 1 tbsp oil	1 cup	120	3	15	900	0	4.0	0
(Stouffer's) food service product, prepared w/whole milk	1 cup	264	9	28	1127	2	12.8	32
Frozen (Soup Supreme) food service product	1 cup	190	5	22	750	1	9.0	5
Canned, ready to use								
(Andersen's)	7.5 oz	200	4	25	630	0	10.0	0
(Stouffer's) food service product, 'Heat 'N Serve'	1 cup	240	10	28	1031	2	9.6	22
POTATO-LEEK								
Canned, ready to use								
(Health Valley)								
	7.5 oz	130	4	23	360	7	2.0	0
no salt added	7.5 oz	130	4	23	20	7	2.0	0
RED BEAN AND RICE, (Norpac) lowfat, 'Soup Supreme'	1 cup	130	5	26	770	5	1.5	0
SCHAV, canned, ready to serve (Gold's)	1 cup	25	2	4	1380	0	0.0	15
SCOTCH BROTH								
Canned, condensed								
prepared	10.5-oz can	193	12	23	2461	3	6.4	12
prepared	1 cup	80	5	9	1012	1	2.6	5
unprepared	10.5-oz can	197	12	23	2461	3	6.4	12
unprepared	1 cup	162	10	19	2032	2	5.3	10
(Campbell's) prepared	1 cup	80	4	9	870	0	3.0	10
SEAFOOD BISQUE, frozen (Myers)	9.75 oz	163	9	13	1393	0	8.0	0
SEAFOOD CHOWDER								
Canned, condensed								
(Snow's)								
New England, prepared w/whole milk	7.5 oz	140	8	14	670	0	6.0	0
New England, unprepared	3.75 oz	60	4	6	640	0	2.0	0
SEAFOOD GUMBO								
Frozen (Soup Supreme) food service product	1 cup	90	5	14	900	1	1.5	20
SHRIMP AND OKRA GUMBO								
Frozen								
(Soup Supreme) Southern style, food service product	1 cup	110	5	16	1660	1	3.0	20
SHRIMP, CREAM OF								
Canned, condensed								
prepared w/milk	10.75-oz can	397	17	34	2516	1	22.6	84
prepared w/milk	1 cup	164	7	14	1037	0	9.3	35

Food Name	Serv. Size	Total Cal.	Prot. gms	Carbs gms	Sod. mgs	Fiber gms	Fat gms	Chol. mgs
unprepared	10.75-oz can	220	7	20	2373	1	12.6	40
unprepared	1 cup	181	6	16	1953	1	10.4	33
(Campbell's)								
'Seashore Soups' prepared w/2% milk	1/2 cup	140	5	13	810	0	10.0	20
'Seashore Soups' prepared w/whole milk	1 cup	160	5	13	860	0	10.0	0
'Seashore Soups' unprepared	1/2 cup	90	2	8	810	0	6.0	20
SIRLOIN BURGER								
Canned, ready to use *(Campbell's)* 'Chunky'	10 3/4 oz	220	12	23	1240	0	9.0	0
SPINACH, CREAM OF								
Frozen								
(Myers)	9.75 oz	174	9	10	905	0	11.0	0
(Stouffer's)	3/4 cup	210	7	12	1020	0	15.0	0
(Tabatchnick)	3/4 cup	85	5	12	200	0	2.0	4
SPLIT PEA								
Canned, condensed								
w/ham, prepared w/milk	11.5-oz can	461	25	68	2444	6	10.7	18
w/ham, prepared w/water	1 cup	190	10	28	1007	2	4.4	8
w/ham, unprepared	11.5-oz can	460	25	68	2445	6	10.7	20
w/ham, unprepared	1 cup	379	21	56	2018	5	8.8	16
(Campbell's) w/ham and bacon, prepared w/water	1 cup	160	9	24	780	0	4.0	5
(Rokeach) w/egg barley, prepared w/water	1 cup	132	8	24	757	0	0.5	0
(Stouffer's) w/ham, food service product, prepared								
w/water	1 cup	176	11	29	1103	6	1.6	7
Canned, ready to use								
w/ham, chunky	19-oz can	415	25	60	2167	9	8.9	16
w/ham, chunky	1 cup	185	11	27	965	4	4.0	7
(Andersen's) nonfat	7.5 oz	130	9	24	770	0	0.0	0
(Campbell's) low-salt	1 cup	240	12	38	50	5	4.0	5
(Grandma Brown's)	1 cup	208	12	31	522	6	4.1	1
(Hain)								
	9.5 oz	170	11	28	970	0	1.0	0
no salt added	9.5 oz	170	11	29	40	0	1.0	0
(Health Valley)								
and carrot, nonfat	1 cup	110	8	17	230	4	0.0	0
green	7.5 oz	190	11	34	276	15	0.3	0
no salt added	7.5 oz	190	11	34	25	15	0.3	0
(Healthy Choice) and ham	1 cup	160	13	25	480	3	1.5	3
(Progresso)								
green	10 1/2 oz	201	12	31	920	0	3.0	0
'Healthy Classics'	1 cup	180	10	30	420	5	2.3	5
w/ham	1 cup	160	9	20	830	5	4.0	15
Frozen								
(Kettle Ready) w/ham	3/4 cup	155	11	25	483	0	4.4	0
(Soup Supreme) w/ham, food service product	1 cup	120	9	18	1030	6	1.5	5
STOCKPOT								
Canned, condensed								
prepared	11-oz can	240	12	28	2544	na	9.5	12
prepared	1 cup	99	5	11	1047	na	3.9	5
unprepared	11-oz can	243	12	28	2546	na	9.5	9
unprepared	1 cup	200	10	23	2097	na	7.8	8
TOMATO								
Canned, condensed								
prepared w/milk	10.75-oz can	391	15	54	1806	7	14.6	42
prepared w/milk	1 cup	161	6	22	744	3	6.0	17
prepared w/water	10.75-oz can	208	5	40	1690	1	4.7	0
prepared w/water	1 cup	85	2	17	695	0	1.9	0
unprepared	10.75-oz can	207	5	40	1690	1	4.7	0

Food Name	Serv. Size	Total Cal.	Prot. gms	Carbs gms	Sod. mgs	Fiber gms	Fat gms	Chol. mgs
unprepared	1 cup	171	4	33	1391	1	3.8	0
(Campbell's)								
'Healthy Request' unprepared	1/2 cup	90	1	18	460	1	1.5	0
'Healthy Request' prepared w/1/2 cup 2% milk	1 cup	140	5	22	490	0	3.0	5
'Healthy Request' prepared w/water	1 cup	90	1	17	430	0	2.0	0
'Healthy Request' prepared w/whole milk	1 cup	150	5	22	490	0	4.0	10
(Stouffer's)								
hearty, food service product, prepared w/water	1 cup	96	3	13	1031	2	3.2	4
Canned, ready to use								
(Campbell's) w/tomato pieces, low-salt	1 cup	170	4	28	60	2	6.0	10
(Health Valley)								
	7.5 oz	100	2	17	450	1	3.0	0
no salt added	7.5 oz	100	2	17	40	1	3.0	0
(Healthy Choice) garden	1 cup	100	5	19	420	5	1.5	0
(Progresso)								
	9.5 oz	120	4	20	1100	0	3.0	0
garden, 'Healthy Classics'	1 cup	99	3	19	480	4	1.0	0
(Stouffer's)								
garden, food service product, 'Heat 'N Serve'	1 cup	112	2	10	863	3	7.2	14
Frozen								
(Soup Supreme)								
basil, vegetarian, low-fat, food service product	1 cup	100	3	15	690	1	3.0	5
Florentine, food service product	1 cup	90	3	16	1000	2	1.5	0
TOMATO, CREAM OF								
Canned, condensed								
(Campbell's)								
'Healthy Request' prepared w/nonfat milk	1/2 cup	130	5	22	490	0	2.0	5
'Homestyle' prepared w/water	1 cup	110	1	20	810	0	3.0	5
'Homestyle' prepared w/whole milk	1 cup	180	5	25	860	0	7.0	0
prepared w/whole milk	1 cup	150	5	22	740	0	4.0	0
zesty, prepared w/water	1 cup	100	1	20	760	0	2.0	0
TOMATO BEEF								
Canned, condensed								
w/noodles, prepared	10.75-oz can	338	11	51	2230	4	10.4	12
w/noodles, prepared	1 cup	139	4	21	917	1	4.3	5
w/noodles, unprepared	10.75-oz can	342	11	51	2230	4	10.4	9
w/noodles, unprepared	1 cup	281	9	42	1835	3	8.6	8
Canned, ready to use *(Progresso)* w/rotini	9.5 oz	170	12	18	930	0	6.0	30
TOMATO BISQUE								
Canned, condensed								
prepared w/milk	11-oz can	481	15	71	2692	1	16.0	55
prepared w/milk	1 cup	198	6	29	1109	1	6.6	23
unprepared	11-oz can	300	5	58	2546	2	6.1	12
unprepared	1 cup	247	5	47	2097	2	5.0	10
TOMATO RICE								
Canned, condensed								
prepared	11-oz can	288	5	53	1980	4	6.6	6
prepared	1 cup	119	2	22	815	1	2.7	2
unprepared	1 cup	239	4	44	1632	3	5.4	3
unprepared	11-oz can	290	5	53	1981	4	6.6	3
Frozen *(Tabatchnick)*	3/4 cup	73	2	14	300	0	1.0	0
TOMATO TORTELLINI, canned, ready to use *(Progresso)*	1 cup	120	5	13	910	2	5.0	10
TOMATO VEGETABLE								
Canned, ready to use *(Health Valley)* nonfat	1 cup	80	6	17	240	5	0.0	0
TORTELLINI								
Canned, ready to use								
(Progresso)								
	9.5 oz	90	5	11	930	0	3.0	10

Food Name	Serv. Size	Total Cal.	Prot. gms	Carbs gms	Sod. mgs	Fiber gms	Fat gms	Chol. mgs
creamy	9.25 oz	240	5	17	910	0	16.0	35
TURKEY								
Canned, condensed								
prepared	10.75-oz can	166	9	21	1981	2	4.9	12
prepared	1 cup	68	4	9	815	1	2.0	5
unprepared	10.75-oz can	168	9	21	1983	2	4.8	12
unprepared	1 cup	138	8	17	1632	2	4.0	10
Canned, ready to use								
chunky	18.75-oz can	303	23	32	2080	na	9.9	21
chunky	1 cup	135	10	14	923	na	4.4	9
TURKEY RICE								
Canned, ready to use								
(Hain)								
	9.5 oz	100	8	10	970	0	3.0	20
no salt added	9.5 oz	120	7	13	85	0	4.0	15
(Healthy Choice) white and wild rice	1 cup	90	7	14	415	2	2.0	3
TURKEY VEGETABLE								
Canned, condensed								
prepared	10.5-oz can	176	8	21	2203	1	7.4	6
prepared	1 cup	72	3	9	906	0	3.0	2
unprepared	10.5-oz can	179	8	21	2202	1	7.4	3
unprepared	1 cup	148	6	17	1818	1	6.1	2
Canned, ready to use								
(Campbell's) 'Chunky'	9 1/3 cup	150	9	16	1060	0	6.0	0
(Weight Watchers)	10 1/2 oz	70	4	10	1020	0	2.0	0
VEGETABLE								
Canned, condensed								
(Campbell's)								
'Healthy Request' unprepared	1/2 cup	90	3	16	480	2	1.0	5
'Homestyle' prepared	1 cup	60	2	9	880	0	2.0	0
vegetarian	1/2 cup	60	2	14	720	2	0.0	0
w/pasta, 'Healthy Request' unprepared	1/2 cup	90	2	18	830	2	1.0	0
w/pasta, hearty, prepared	1 cup	70	3	15	800	0	1.0	0
(Stouffer's) vegetarian, food service product, prepared	1 cup	96	2	14	783	3	2.4	0
Canned, ready to use								
chunky	19-oz can	275	8	43	2269	3	8.3	0
chunky	1 cup	122	4	19	1010	1	3.7	0
(Campbell's)								
hearty, 'Healthy Request'	1 cup	100	3	20	470	2	1.0	0
Mediterranean, 'Chunky' ready to serve	9.5 oz	170	4	24	1010	0	6.0	0
(Hain)								
Italian, w/pasta	9.5 oz	160	4	25	910	0	5.0	20
Italian, w/pasta, low-sodium	9.5 oz	140	4	22	90	0	6.0	20
vegetarian	9.5 oz	140	4	22	920	0	4.0	0
vegetarian, no salt added	9.5 oz	150	5	23	45	0	5.0	0
(Health Valley)								
	7.5 oz	110	4	20	296	4	1.0	0
5-bean, chunky, no salt added	7.5 oz	110	4	21	56	11	2.0	0
5-bean, nonfat	1 cup	140	10	32	250	13	0.0	0
no salt added	7.5 oz	110	4	20	40	4	1.0	0
power carotene	1 cup	70	5	17	240	6	0.0	0
(Healthy Choice)								
country	1 cup	100	5	22	430	5	0.5	0
garden	1 cup	120	6	24	480	3	1.0	0
(Hormel)								
country, 'Hearty Soups'	7.5 oz	90	4	14	730	0	2.0	2
country, micro cup, ' Hearty Soups'	1 container	89	5	13	865	0	2.0	1

Food Name	Serv. Size	Total Cal.	Prot. gms	Carbs gms	Sod. mgs	Fiber gms	Fat gms	Chol. mgs
(Lunch Bucket) country, microwave cup	7.25 oz	70	1	15	740	0	1.0	0
(Norpac) vegerarian, low-fat, 'Soup Supreme'	1 cup	70	3	13	560	3	1.5	0
(Progresso)								
. . . .	9.5 oz	80	4	15	1190	4	2.0	5
'Healthy Classics'	1 cup	81	4	13	466	1	1.3	5
(Stouffer's)								
vegetarian, food service product, 'Heat 'N Serve'	1 cup	96	3	16	823	4	2.4	0
(Westbrae)								
Sante Fe, nonfat	1 cup	115	6	23	570	4	0.0	0
Southwest, spicy, nonfat	1 cup	70	4	15	500	2	0.0	0
(Weight Watchers)								
vegetarian, chunky	10 1/2 oz	100	3	18	1250	0	2.0	0
w/beef stock	10 1/2 oz	90	4	13	1370	0	2.0	0
Frozen								
(Kettle Ready) garden	3/4 cup	85	3	12	296	0	3.0	0
(Soup Supreme)								
harvest, food service product	1 cup	90	3	17	960	3	1.5	0
Italian, zesty, food service product	1 cup	70	3	14	720	2	1.0	0
(Tabatchnick)								
. . . .	7.5 oz	97	4	18	190	0	1.0	0
no salt	7.5 oz	92	2	16	77	0	2.0	0
VEGETABLE BARLEY								
Canned, ready to use *(Health Valley)* nonfat	1 cup	90	6	19	210	4	0.0	0
VEGETABLE BEEF								
Canned, condensed								
prepared	10.5-oz can	199	7	32	1969	1	4.6	6
prepared	1 cup	82	3	13	810	0	1.9	2
unprepared	10.5-oz can	197	7	32	1970	4	4.6	3
unprepared	1 cup	162	6	26	1626	3	3.8	2
(Campbell's)								
'Healthy Request' prepared	1 cup	70	4	10	470	0	2.0	10
'Healthy Request' unprepared	1/2 cup	80	5	11	480	2	2.0	5
(Stouffer's) w/barley, food service product, prepared	1 cup	144	4	12	1103	2	8.8	11
Canned, ready to use								
(Campbell's)								
hearty, 'Healthy Request'	1 cup	140	9	20	480	3	2.5	20
low-salt, 'Chunky'	1 cup	160	13	11	95	4	4.5	80
old-fashioned, 'Chunky'	10 3/4 oz	190	13	20	1100	0	6.0	25
(Stouffer's) w/barley, 'Heat 'N Serve'	1 cup	144	6	11	943	2	8.8	9
(Weight Watchers) microwave cup	7.5 oz	90	8	13	450	0	1.0	10
Frozen								
(Myers)	9.75 oz	120	9	8	1030	0	6.0	0
(Soup Supreme)								
food service product	1 cup	80	5	14	1020	2	1.5	10
w/barley, food service product	1 cup	90	5	14	830	2	2.0	10
VEGETABLE BROTH								
Canned, ready to use								
(Hain)								
. . . .	9.5 oz	45	1	10	1180	0	0.0	0
low-sodium	9.5 oz	40	1	8	85	0	1.0	0
(Swanson) canned	1 cup	20	2	3	1000	0	1.0	0
WILD RICE								
Canned, ready to use								
(Hain) 99% fat free, 'Healthy Naturals'	1 cup	80	2	15	480	1	2.0	0
ZUCCHINI, frozen *(Tabatchnick)*	3/4 cup	80	3	12	285	0	2.0	3
SOUP MIX								
ASPARAGUS, CREAM OF, prepared	1 cup	58	2	9	800	na	1.7	0

Food Name	Serv. Size	Total Cal.	Prot. gms	Carbs gms	Sod. mgs	Fiber gms	Fat gms	Chol. mgs
BEAN								
w/bacon, prepared .... 1 cup	1 cup	106	5	16	927	9	2.1	3
(Bean Cuisine)								
'Island Black Bean' bag, prepared .... 1 cup	1 cup	160	9	29	15	9	1.0	0
'Island Black Bean' box, prepared .... 1 cup	1 cup	126	7	24	7	8	1.0	0
'Mesa Maise & Bean' prepared .... 1 cup	1 cup	180	10	32	20	10	1.5	0
'Rocky Mountain Red Bean' prepared .... 1 cup	1 cup	190	11	35	15	12	1.5	0
13-bean bouillabaisse, bag, prepared .... 1 cup	1 cup	110	7	19	15	7	0.5	0
13-bean bouillabaisse, box, prepared .... 1 cup	1 cup	99	6	18	5	5	1.0	0
'White Bean Provencal' bag, prepared .... 1 cup	1 cup	180	10	32	15	11	1.0	0
'White Bean Provencal' box, prepared .... 1 cup	1 cup	103	6	19	7	6	1.0	0
(Fantastic Foods) 5-bean, 'Hearty Soups' mix only .... 2.3 oz	2.3 oz	230	12	43	480	10	1.0	0
(Hodgson Mill) choice, no barley, mix only .... 1/4 cup	1/4 cup	150	9	27	5	11	0.0	0
(Hormel) w/ham, chowder 'Micro-Cup Hearty Soups' prepared .... 1 container	1 container	191	10	31	664	0	3.0	30
BEEF								
broth, cubed, mix only .... 1 cube	1 cube	9	1	1	611	0	0.3	0
broth, dried, prepared .... 1 cup	1 cup	19	1	2	1359	0	0.7	1
(American Institutional) stock, concentrated, mix only ...... 2 tsp	2 tsp	20	2	2	570	0	0.0	0
(Soup Starter) hearty, 'Homestyle' mix only .... 27 grams	27 grams	90	2	20	740	0	1.0	0
(Tone's) base, mix only .... 1 tsp	1 tsp	11	0	1	1	0	0.6	0
(Ultra Slim-Fast) w/noodles, prepared .... 6 oz	6 oz	45	5	7	700	2	1.0	5
BEEF NOODLE								
prepared .... 1 cup	1 cup	40	2	6	1042	1	0.8	3
(Campbell's)								
w/vegetables, prepared .... 6 oz	6 oz	220	7	44	1600	0	2.0	0
microwave cup, prepared .... 1.35 oz	1.35 oz	130	6	23	1270	0	2.0	0
'Ramen Noodle' prepared .... 6 oz	6 oz	160	5	32	890	0	1.0	0
(Estee) prepared .... 6 oz	6 oz	20	1	3	140	0	1.0	1
(Lipton)								
'Cup-A-Soup' prepared .... 6 oz	6 oz	44	2	8	746	0	0.7	0
hearty, prepared .... 6 oz	6 oz	107	4	20	698	0	1.4	0
BEEF VEGETABLE *(Soup Starter)* 'Homestyle' mix only .... 26 grams	26 grams	90	3	18	790	0	1.0	0
BOUILLON								
Beef flavor								
(Diamond Crystal) dried, instant, low-salt, mix only .... 1 serving	1 serving	10	0	2	10	0	0.0	0
(Featherweight) dried, instant, mix only .... 1 tsp	1 tsp	18	0	2	10	0	1.0	5
(Herb-Ox)								
cubed, mix only .... 1 cube	1 cube	5	0	1	900	0	0.0	0
cubed, low-salt, mix only .... 1 cube	1 cube	10	0	2	5	0	0.0	0
granulated, mix only .... 1 tsp	1 tsp	5	0	1	1020	0	0.0	0
(Lite-Line) dried, instant, low-sodium, mix only .... 1 tsp	1 tsp	12	1	2	5	0	1.0	0
(Steero)								
cubed, mix only .... 1 cube	1 cube	6	1	1	930	0	1.0	0
dried, instant, mix only .... 1 tsp	1 tsp	6	1	1	930	0	1.0	0
(Weight Watchers) dried, instant, 'Broth Mix' mix only ...... 1 pkt	1 pkt	8	1	1	930	0	0.0	0
(Wyler's)								
cubed, mix only .... 1 cube	1 cube	6	1	1	930	0	1.0	0
dried, mix only .... 1 tsp	1 tsp	5	0	1	900	0	0.0	0
dried, instant, mix only .... 1 tsp	1 tsp	6	1	1	930	0	1.0	0
dried, low-salt, mix only .... 1 tsp	1 tsp	10	0	2	10	0	0.0	0
Brown								
(G. Washington's) dried, 'Seasoning & Broth' mix only ... 0.14 oz	0.14 oz	6	0	1	1015	0	0.0	0
Chicken flavor								
(Diamond Crystal) dried, instant, low-salt, mix only .... 1 serving	1 serving	10	0	2	20	0	0.0	0
(Featherweight) dried, instant, mix only .... 1 tsp	1 tsp	18	0	2	5	0	1.0	5

Food Name	Serv. Size	Total Cal.	Prot. gms	Carbs gms	Sod. mgs	Fiber gms	Fat gms	Chol. mgs
(Herb-Ox)								
cubed, mix only	1 cube	5	0	1	1100	0	0.0	0
cubed, low-salt	1 cube	10	0	2	5	0	0.0	0
granulated, mix only	1 tsp	5	0	1	1100	0	0.0	0
(Lite-Line) dried, instant, low-sodium, mix only	1 tsp	12	1	2	5	0	1.0	0
(Steero)								
cubed, mix only	1 cube	8	1	1	990	0	1.0	0
dried, instant, mix only	1 tsp	8	1	1	990	0	1.0	0
(Weight Watchers) dried, instant 'Broth Mix' mix only	1 pkt	8	1	1	990	0	0.0	0
(Wyler's)								
cubed, mix only	1 cube	8	1	1	900	0	1.0	0
dried, instant, mix only	1 tsp	8	1	1	900	0	1.0	0
dried, low-salt, mix only	1 tsp	10	0	2	0	0	0.0	0
Golden								
(G. Washington's)								
dried, kosher, 'Seasoning & Broth' mix only	0.13 oz	6	0	1	1015	0	0.0	0
dried, 'Seasoning & Broth' mix only	0.13 oz	6	0	1	935	0	0.0	0
Onion flavor								
(G. Washington's) dried, 'Seasoning & Broth' mix only	0.11 cup	12	1	2	695	0	0.0	0
(Wyler's) dried, instant, mix only	1 tsp	10	1	1	670	0	1.0	0
Vegetable								
(G. Washington's) dried, 'Seasoning & Broth' mix only	0.11 cup	12	1	2	715	0	0.0	0
(Herb-Ox) cubed, mix only	1 cube	5	0	1	980	0	0.0	0
(Wyler's) dried, instant, mix only	1 tsp	6	1	1	910	0	1.0	0
BROCCOLI								
(Fantastic Foods) and cheddary, creamy, mix only	1.4 oz	160	7	26	590	2	3.0	10
(Lipton)								
and cheese, 'Cup-A-Soup' mix only	1 serving	67	2	9	545	1	2.9	3
creamy, 'Cup-A-Soup Food Service' prepared	6 oz	62	2	9	658	0	2.3	0
creamy, 'Cup-A-Soup' prepared	6 oz	62	1	9	610	0	2.4	0
golden, 'Cup-A-Soup Lite' prepared	6 oz	42	1	16	427	0	1.2	1
(Ultra Slim-Fast) creamy, prepared	6 oz	75	5	14	800	2	1.0	0
CAULIFLOWER, prepared	1 cup	69	3	11	843	na	1.7	0
CELERY, prepared	1 cup	64	3	10	838	na	1.6	0
CHEESE								
(Fantastic Noodles) cheddar, creamy, w/noodles, prepared	6 oz	178	7	21	578	0	8.0	0
(Hain)								
'Savory Soup & Sauce Mix' prepared	6 oz	250	6	20	890	0	16.0	0
and broccoli, prepared	6 oz	310	7	19	980	0	22.0	0
CHICKEN								
broth, cubed, mix only	1 cube	11	1	1	743	0	0.6	1
broth, dried, mix only	1 tsp	5	0	0	372	0	0.3	0
broth, dried, prepared	6 fl oz	16	1	1	1115	0	0.8	1
(American Institutional) stock, concentrated, mix only	2 tsp	15	1	1	620	0	0.0	0
(Campbell's) w/white meat, creamy, prepared	6 oz	90	3	12	1020	0	4.0	0
(Lipton)								
broth, 'Cup-A-Soup' prepared	1 serving	18	1	3	442	0	0.1	0
Florentine, 'Lite' prepared	6 oz	42	10	8	481	0	0.5	6
lemon, 'Cup-A-Soup Lite' prepared	6 oz	48	2	9	419	0	0.4	4
w/pasta, fat-free, 'Cup-A-Soup' prepared	1 serving	44	2	8	449	0	0.3	0
w/pasta, beans, 'Kettle Creations' prepared	1 serving	106	5	19	699	3	1.3	6
w/corn, 'Country' prepared	6 oz	133	3	18	704	0	5.5	0
hearty, supreme, 'Cup-A-Soup' prepared	1 serving	90	1	14	635	1	3.8	1
CHICKEN, CREAM OF								
(Lipton)								
'Cup-A-Soup' mix only	1 envelope	68	1	12	636	1	2.2	1
'Food Service' prepared	6 oz	84	2	9	840	0	4.4	0

Food Name	Serv. Size	Total Cal.	Prot. gms	Carbs gms	Sod. mgs	Fiber gms	Fat gms	Chol. mgs
w/vegetables, prepared	6 oz	93	2	14	708	0	3.1	0
hearty, 'Country Style' prepared	6 oz	69	4	11	688	0	1.1	0
CHICKEN LEEK *(Ultra Slim Fast)* creamy, prepared	6 oz	50	5	7	1070	2	1.0	2
CHICKEN NOODLE								
prepared	1 cup	58	2	9	578	0	1.4	10
(Campbell's)								
'Lowfat Block' prepared	1 cup	160	5	32	940	0	1.0	0
microwave cup, mix only	1.35 oz	140	7	22	1340	0	3.0	0
'Ramen Noodle' prepared	1 cup	190	5	26	970	0	8.0	0
w/vegetables, prepared	1 cup	270	6	38	1470	0	10.0	0
w/vegetables, low-fat, prepared	1 cup	220	7	44	1500	0	2.0	0
w/white meat, prepared	6 oz	90	6	12	770	0	2.0	0
(Estee) 'Instant' prepared	6 oz	25	1	4	135	0	1.0	1
(Lipton)								
and rice, prepared	6 oz	47	2	8	667	0	0.8	0
'Cup-A-Soup' prepared	6 oz	48	3	7	635	0	1.1	0
hearty, 'Cup-A-Soup' mix only	1 envelope	61	3	10	591	0	1.2	14
prepared w/water	1 cup	81	4	12	792	0	1.8	0
real chicken broth, 'Soup Secrets' prepared	1 serving	62	2	9	724	0	1.9	14
'Soup Secrets' prepared	1 serving	77	3	11	690	0	2.0	15
supreme, prepared	6 oz	107	2	12	757	0	5.9	0
w/diced white meat, prepared	1 cup	81	4	12	795	0	1.8	0
w/meat, 'Cup-A-Soup' prepared	1 serving	381	16	62	4177	2	8.0	88
w/vegetables, 'Cup' prepared	6 oz	47	3	8	566	0	0.6	8
w/vegetable, hearty, prepared	1 cup	75	3	12	687	0	1.6	0
(Mrs. Grass) 'Chickeny Rich' mix only	1/4 pkg	70	2	10	900	0	2.0	0
(Soup Starter) 'Homestyle' mix only	21 grams	70	2	15	770	0	1.0	10
(Ultra Slim-Fast) prepared	6 oz	45	5	6	970	2	1.0	5
CHICKEN RICE, prepared w/water	1 cup	58	2	9	931	1	1.4	2
CHICKEN VEGETABLE, prepared w/water	1 cup	49	3	8	803	0	0.8	3
CHILI *(Fantastic Foods)* 'Cha Cha Chili' 'Hearty Soups'								
mix only	2.4 oz	220	18	37	470	13	1.0	0
CHILI PEPPER *(A Taste of Thai)* hot and sour, prepared	1 cup	40	0	5	1330	0	2.0	0
CLAM CHOWDER								
(Golden Dipt)								
Manhattan, mix only	1/4 pkg	80	2	13	700	0	2.0	3
Manhattan, prepared	1 cup	95	3	13	745	1	3.7	1
New England, mix only	1/4 pkg	70	2	12	680	0	2.0	2
CONSOMMÉ w/gelatin, prepared	1 cup	17	2	2	3301	0	0.0	0
CORN CHOWDER								
(Bean Cuisine) 'Sante Fe' prepared	1 cup	112	6	21	9	6	1.0	0
(Fantastic Foods) and potato, creamy, mix only	1.6 oz	170	6	34	440	3	2.0	5
COUSCOUS-LENTIL								
(Fantastic Foods) 'Hearty Soups' mix only	2.3 oz	230	12	44	480	7	1.0	0
CRAB *(Kikkoman)* Chinese style, mix only	1 tbsp	25	1	5	920	0	0.0	0
EGG FLOWER								
(Kikkoman)								
corn, Chinese style, mix only	1 tbsp	50	2	11	850	0	0.0	0
hot and sour, Chinese style, mix only	2 tsp	30	1	6	880	0	0.0	0
vegetable, Chinese style, mix only	1 1/2 tbsp	45	1	7	920	0	2.0	0
GINGER *(A Taste of Thai)* tangy coconut, prepared	1 cup	250	3	3	1050	0	1.5	0
GREEN PEA								
prepared w/water	1 cup	133	8	23	1220	3	1.6	3
(Hain) 'Savory Soup Mix' prepared	6 oz	310	4	16	940	0	10.0	0
(Lipton)								
'Cup-A-Soup' prepared	6 oz	113	4	14	553	0	4.2	0
'Cup-A-Soup Food Service' prepared	6 oz	115	4	15	635	1	4.5	0

Food Name	Serv. Size	Total Cal.	Prot. gms	Carbs gms	Sod. mgs	Fiber gms	Fat gms	Chol. mgs
Virginia, 'Country Style' prepared	6 oz	148	5	17	828	1	6.4	0
Virginia, prepared	6 oz	113	5	15	664	0	4.1	1
HERB								
(Lipton)								
Fiesta, 'Recipe Secrets' prepared	1 serving	29	1	6	559	0	0.3	1
savory, w/garlic 'Recipe Secrets' prepared	1 serving	31	1	6	477	0	0.4	1
LEEK								
prepared	1 cup	71	2	11	965	3	2.1	3
(Ultra Slim-Fast) creamy, prepared	6 oz	80	5	15	780	2	1.0	0
LENTIL								
(Bean Cuisine) 'Lots of Lentil' prepared	1 cup	230	9	20	0	10	0.0	0
(Fantastic Foods) country, 'Hearty Soups' mix only	2.3 oz	230	15	41	480	12	1.0	0
(Hain) 'Savory Soup Mix' prepared w/water	6 oz	130	4	20	810	0	2.0	0
(Legumes Plus)								
Cajun, w/brown rice, mix only	1/5 cup	190	10	34	170	3	1.0	0
meatless, mix only	1/4 cup	190	15	31	460	15	1.0	0
minestrone style, mix only	1/3 cup	150	9	28	530	2	0.5	0
pasta-pasta, mix only	1/3 cup	180	11	33	420	4	1.0	0
red curry, mix only	1/5 cup	200	13	34	410	2	1.0	0
robust bacon flavor, mix only	1/4 cup	170	12	26	450	11	2.0	0
subtly seasoned, mix only	1/3 cup	190	14	31	470	15	1.0	0
w/barley, hearty, mix only	1/4 cup	140	8	26	390	8	1.0	0
w/country vegetable, mix only	1/3 cup	180	12	34	470	6	0.0	0
w/herbs and rice, mix only	1/6 cup	150	7	29	470	2	1.0	0
w/wagon wheel pasta, mix only	1/3 cup	190	13	34	450	5	0.5	0
w/wild rice and herbs, mix only	1/4 cup	160	6	31	440	10	1.0	0
zesty tomato, mix only	1/4 cup	180	13	29	250	12	1.0	0
(Lipton) homestyle, 'Kettle Creations' prepared	1 serving	127	7	22	753	5	1.2	0
LOBSTER BISQUE *(Golden Dipt)* mix only	1/4 pkg	30	1	5	560	0	1.0	2
MINESTRONE								
(Cous-cous) tomato, prepared	10 oz	200	9	41	590	0	0.0	0
(Fantastic Foods) hearty, mix only	1.5 oz	150	6	29	480	4	1.0	0
(Hain) 'Savory Soup Mix' prepared	6 oz	110	4	20	870	0	1.0	0
(Manischewitz) prepared	6 oz	50	3	9	160	0	1.0	0
MISO								
(Kikkoman)								
red, prepared	1 serving	35	2	4	790	0	1.0	0
shiro, white, prepared	1 serving	35	3	4	820	0	1.0	0
tofu, prepared	1 serving	35	3	4	740	0	1.0	0
tofu-spinach	1 serving	35	3	4	790	0	1.0	0
MUSHROOM								
(Estee) 'Instant' prepared	6 oz	40	1	3	115	0	2.0	10
(Fantastic Foods) garlic, creamy, mix only	1.5 oz	160	7	28	480	2	3.0	10
(Hain)								
no salt added, 'Savory Soup & Recipe Mix' prepared	6 oz	250	5	15	180	0	20.0	0
'Savory Soup & Recipe Mix' prepared	6 oz	210	4	11	710	0	15.0	0
(Lipton)								
beef flavor, prepared	1 cup	38	2	7	763	0	0.5	0
beefy, 'Recipe Secrets' prepared	1 serving	33	1	7	645	0	0.4	0
MUSHROOM, CREAM OF								
(Lipton) 'Cup-A-Soup' prepared	6 oz	71	1	9	756	0	3.2	0
NOODLE								
(Campbell's)								
double noodle, in chicken broth, mix only	1.71 oz	200	8	36	770	0	2.0	0
hearty, 'Quality Soup & Recipe' prepared	1 cup	90	4	15	840	0	1.0	0
Oriental, 'Ramen Noodle Lowfat Block' prepared	1 cup	150	5	31	940	0	1.0	0
Oriental, 'Ramen Noodle' prepared	1 cup	190	5	26	930	0	8.0	0

Food Name	Serv. Size	Total Cal.	Prot. gms	Carbs gms	Sod. mgs	Fiber gms	Fat gms	Chol. mgs
'Quality Soup & Recipe' prepared . . . . 1 cup		110	5	19	700	0	2.0	0
w/chicken broth, microwave cup, mix only . . . . 1.35 oz		130	6	23	1360	0	2.0	0
w/vegetables, Oriental, 'Cup-A-Ramen Lowfat' prepared . . . . 1 cup		220	7	44	1400	0	2.0	0
w/vegetables, Oriental, 'Cup-A-Ramen' prepared . . . . 1 cup		270	6	38	1210	0	10.0	0
(Fantastic Foods)								
curry ramen, mix only . . . . 1.5 oz		140	6	28	490	3	1.0	0
vegetable miso ramen, mix only . . . . 1.3 oz		130	5	25	540	2	1.0	0
(Kikkoman) memmi, noodle soup base, mix only . . . . 2 tbsp		40	2	7	2020	0	0.0	0
(Lipton)								
giggle noodle, 'Soup Secrets' prepared . . . . 1 serving		74	3	11	736	0	2.1	18
ring noodle, 'Cup-A-Soup' prepared . . . . 1 serving		53	2	9	557	0	1.1	12
ring noodle, 'Soup Secrets' prepared . . . . 1 serving		66	2	10	724	0	2.0	16
w/extra noodle, 'Soup Secrets' prepared . . . . 1 serving		86	3	15	681	1	1.6	23
(Oodles of Noodles) Oriental, prepared . . . . 1 cup		390	10	49	1660	0	18.0	0
(Top Ramen) Oriental, mix only . . . . 1 serving		190	4	28	487	na	7.2	na
Beef flavor								
(Cup O'Noodles) prepared . . . . 1 cup		290	8	33	1490	0	14.0	0
(Oodles of Noodles) prepared . . . . 1 cup		390	9	49	1810	0	18.0	0
(Top Ramen) prepared . . . . 1 cup		390	9	49	1810	0	18.0	0
Chicken flavor								
(Campbell's)								
'Cup 2 Minute Soup' prepared . . . . 6 oz		90	4	15	910	0	2.0	0
double noodle, prepared . . . . 1 cup		200	8	36	770	0	2.0	0
(Cup O'Noodles)								
country, 'Hearty' prepared . . . . 1 cup		300	8	35	1210	0	14.0	0
prepared . . . . 1 cup		300	9	32	1790	0	16.0	0
(Oodles of Noodles) prepared . . . . 1 cup		400	10	48	1910	0	18.0	0
(Top Ramen) individual package, mix only . . . . 1 container		296	6	37	1434	na	14.1	na
Pork flavor								
(Campbell's)								
'Ramen Noodle' prepared . . . . 1 cup		200	5	26	860	0	8.0	0
'Ramen Noodle Lowfat Block' prepared . . . . 1 cup		150	4	31	1140	0	1.0	0
w/vegetables, microwave, mix only . . . . 1.7 oz		180	7	32	1320	0	2.0	0
(Cup O'Noodles)								
vegetable beef, 'Hearty' prepared . . . . 1 cup		290	8	36	1150	0	15.0	0
w/old fashioned vegetables, 'Hearty' prepared . . . . 6 oz		290	6	34	1250	0	15.0	0
w/seafood, savory, 'Hearty' prepared . . . . 1 cup		300	7	34	1170	0	15.0	0
w/shrimp, prepared . . . . 1 cup		300	10	32	1480	0	14.0	0
(Oodles of Noodles) prepared . . . . 1 cup		390	10	51	2060	0	20.0	0
(Top Ramen) prepared . . . . 1 cup		390	10	51	2060	0	20.0	0
ONION								
prepared . . . . 1 cup		27	1	5	849	1	0.6	0
(Estee) prepared . . . . 6 oz		25	1	4	140	0	1.0	0
(Hain)								
'Savory Soup, Dip & Recipe Mix' no salt, prepared . . . . 6 oz		50	1	9	470	0	1.0	0
'Savory Soup, Dip & Recipe Mix' prepared . . . . 6 oz		50	2	6	900	0	2.0	0
(Lipton)								
'Recipe Secrets' prepared . . . . 1 serving		18	0	4	610	0	0.1	0
beefy, 'Recipe Secrets' prepared . . . . 1 serving		25	1	5	607	0	0.6	0
(Mrs. Grass) 'Soup & Dip Mix' mix only . . . . 1/4 pkg		35	1	6	1070	0	1.0	0
(Ultra Slim-Fast) creamy, prepared . . . . 6 oz		45	5	7	1180	2	1.0	0
ONION MUSHROOM *(Lipton)* 'Recipe Secrets' prepared . . . . 1 serving		32	1	6	626	0	0.8	0
ORIENTAL *(Lipton)* 'Cup-A-Soup Lite' prepared . . . . 6 oz		45	2	6	457	0	1.7	3
OSUIMONO *(Kikkoman)* Japanese clear broth, prepared . . . . 1 serving		0	0	1	660	0	0.0	0

Food Name	Serv. Size	Total Cal.	Prot. gms	Carbs gms	Sod. mgs	Fiber gms	Fat gms	Chol. mgs
OXTAIL, prepared	1 cup	71	3	9	1210	1	2.6	3
PASTA *(Lipton)* spirals, 'Soup Secrets' prepared	1 serving	64	2	11	657	0	0.9	2
PASTA AND BEAN								
(Bean Cuisine)								
'Ultima Pasta E Fagioli' bag, prepared	1 cup	190	11	34	15	10	1.0	5
'Ultima Pasta E Fagioli' box, prepared	1 cup	117	7	22	8	4	1.0	0
(Lipton) homestyle, 'Kettle Creations' prepared	1 serving	125	6	23	693	4	1.4	0
POTATO LEEK *(Hain)* 'Savory Soup Mix' prepared	6 oz	260	4	20	690	0	18.0	0
SCALLOP *(Kikkoman)* Chinese style, mix only	1 tbsp	35	1	7	1020	0	0.0	0
SEAFOOD CHOWDER *(Golden Dipt)* mix only	1/4 pkg	70	2	12	730	0	2.0	2
SHRIMP								
(Campbell's)								
w/vegetables 'Cup-A-Ramen' prepared	1 cup	280	6	40	1190	0	10.0	0
w/vegetables, low-fat, prepared	1 cup	230	7	45	1290	0	2.0	0
(Kikkoman) Chinese style, mix only	1 tbsp	30	1	5	830	0	0.5	3
SHRIMP BISQUE *(Golden Dipt)* mix only	1/4 pkg	30	1	5	570	0	1.0	2
SPLIT PEA								
(Bean Cuisine)								
'Thick As Fog Split Pea' bag, prepared	1 cup	140	9	24	10	10	0.5	0
'Thick As Fog Split Pea' box, prepared	1 cup	116	8	21	13	1	1.0	0
(Legumes Plus)								
green, traditional, mix only	1/4 cup	180	11	32	490	12	1.0	0
yellow, mix only	1/4 cup	170	16	30	740	10	2.5	0
(Manischewitz) green, prepared w/water	6 oz	45	3	9	320	0	1.0	0
TOMATO								
prepared	1 cup	103	2	19	943	1	2.4	0
(Estee) 'Instant' prepared	6 oz	40	1	5	95	0	1.0	0
(Hain) 'Savory Soup & Recipe Mix' prepared	6 oz	220	3	19	770	0	14.0	0
(Lipton) 'Cup-A-Soup' mix only	1 envelope	95	2	20	506	1	0.9	2
(Ultra Slim-Fast) creamy, prepared	6 oz	60	5	10	990	2	1.0	0
TOMATO RICE PARMESANO								
(Fantastic Foods) creamy, mix only	1 serving	200	6	41	550	2	2.0	0
TOMATO VEGETABLE								
prepared	1 cup	56	2	10	1146	1	0.9	0
(Fantastic Foods)								
ramen noodle, mix only	1.5 oz	150	5	31	490	3	1.0	0
w/noodles, prepared	7 oz	158	5	20	434	0	8.0	0
VEGETABLE								
(American Institutional) stock, concentrated, mix only	2 tsp	15	0	3	510	0	0.0	0
(Campbell's) nonfat, 'Quality Soup & Recipe' prepared	1 cup	40	1	8	710	0	0.0	0
(Cous-cous) Parmesan, prepared	10 oz	200	9	35	550	0	3.0	0
(Hain)								
no salt added, 'Savory Soup Mix' prepared	6 oz	80	2	13	330	0	1.0	0
'Savory Soup Mix' prepared	6 oz	80	2	13	730	0	1.0	0
(Lipton)								
'Cup-A-Soup' mix only	1 serving	52	1	10	518	0	1.0	10
'Recipe Secrets' mix only	1 serving	28	1	6	603	1	0.2	0
spring, 'Cup-A-Soup' mix only	1 envelope	47	2	8	497	1	1.0	8
(Manischewitz) prepared	6 oz	50	3	9	65	0	1.0	0
(Ultra Slim-Fast) hearty, prepared	6 oz	45	5	5	850	2	1.0	0
VEGETABLE, CREAM OF, prepared	1 cup	107	2	12	1170	1	5.7	0
VEGETABLE BARLEY								
(Fantastic Foods) hearty, mix only	1.5 oz	150	6	29	470	6	0.5	0
VEGETABLE BEEF, prepared	1 cup	57	3	9	1066	0	1.2	1
WAKAME *(Kikkoman)* prepared	1 serving	15	1	3	700	0	0.0	0
SOUR CREAM								
cultured	1 cup	493	7	10	123	0	48.2	102
cultured	1 tbsp	26	0	1	6	0	2.5	5

Food Name	Serv. Size	Total Cal.	Prot. gms	Carbs gms	Sod. mgs	Fiber gms	Fat gms	Chol. mgs
half and half, less fat, cultured	1 cup	326	7	10	98	0	29.0	93
half and half, less fat, cultured	1 tbsp	20	0	1	6	0	1.8	6
(Alta Dena) pasteurized, 100% natural	1 oz	60	1	1	15	0	6.0	0
(Bison)	2 tbsp	50	1	1	15	0	5.0	20
(Breakstone's)								
half and half, 'Light Choice'	1 tbsp	25	1	1	10	0	2.0	5
less fat	2 tbsp	47	1	2	18	0	3.7	16
nonfat	2 tbsp	29	2	5	23	0	0.4	3
regular	1 tbsp	30	0	1	5	0	3.0	10
(Crowley)								
French onion	2 tbsp	50	1	1	130	0	5.0	20
light	2 tbsp	30	1	2	25	0	2.0	5
regular	2 tbsp	50	1	1	15	0	5.0	20
(Darigold)	1 tbsp	23	1	1	5	0	2.8	5
(Friendship)								
low-fat, 'Lite Delite'	2 tbsp	35	1	2	25	0	2.0	8
regular	2 tbsp	55	1	1	15	0	5.0	42
(Knudsen)								
light	2 tbsp	40	1	2	20	0	3.0	10
nonfat	2 tbsp	35	2	6	25	0	0.0	0
regular, 'Hampshire'	2 tbsp	60	1	1	10	0	6.0	20
(Land O'Lakes)								
'Light'	2 tbsp	40	2	4	35	0	2.0	5
nonfat	2 tbsp	30	1	5	35	0	0.0	0
w/chives, 'Light'	2 tbsp	40	2	4	150	0	2.0	5
(Naturally Yours) no fat, 'Real Dairy'	2 tbsp	15	3	1	15	0	0.0	0
(Sealtest)								
half and half, 'Light'	1 tbsp	25	1	1	10	0	2.0	5
regular	1 tbsp	30	0	1	5	0	3.0	10
(Tone's) w/chives, topping	1 tsp	16	0	1	1	0	1.2	57
(Weight Watchers) light	2 tbsp	35	2	2	40	0	2.0	0
SOUR CREAM SUBSTITUTE								
cultured	1 cup	479	6	15	235	0	44.9	0
cultured	1 oz	59	1	2	29	0	5.5	0
(Crowley) nondairy	1 oz	40	1	1	5	0	4.0	0
(IMO)	1 tbsp	30	0	0	15	0	3.0	0
(Light n' Lively) nonfat, cultured	1 tbsp	10	1	1	30	0	0.0	10
(Pet)	1 tbsp	25	1	1	25	0	2.0	1
(Tofutti) no cholesterol, 'Sour Supreme'	1 tbsp	25	1	1	60	na	2.5	0
SOURSOP. See GUANABANA.								
SOY BEVERAGE								
(Ah Soy)								
carob	6 fl oz	160	4	30	120	0	3.0	0
chocolate	6 fl oz	160	4	29	120	0	3.0	0
vanilla	6 fl oz	160	5	23	140	0	5.0	0
(Eden Foods)								
'Edensoy'	8 fl oz	150	6	23	90	0	3.0	0
'Edensoy' carob, natural	8.45 fl oz	160	6	30	125	0	5.0	0
'Edensoy' original, natural, organic, dairy-free	8.45 fl oz	140	10	14	120	0	4.0	0
'Edensoy' vanilla, natural	8.45 fl oz	150	8	25	140	0	3.0	0
'Edensoy Extra'	8 fl oz	150	6	24	95	0	3.0	0
'Edensoy Extra' vanilla, dairy-free	8.45 fl oz	150	8	25	95	3	3.0	0
(Health Valley) nonfat, 'Soy Moo'	8 fl oz	110	6	22	60	1	0.0	0
(Pacific Foods)								
'Pacific Lite' plain	8 fl oz	100	4	14	115	0	2.5	0
'Pacific Lite' vanilla	8 fl oz	110	4	18	115	0	2.0	0
'Pacific Select' plain	8 fl oz	100	4	14	115	0	3.0	0

Food Name	Serv. Size	Total Cal.	Prot. gms	Carbs gms	Sod. mgs	Fiber gms	Fat gms	Chol. mgs
'Pacific Select' vanilla	8 fl oz	120	4	17	115	0	3.0	0
(Sovex) 'Better Than Milk' original, premixed	8 fl oz	90	2	15	85	0	2.0	0
(Vitasoy)								
carob supreme	8 fl oz	210	8	32	160	1	6.0	0
cocoa, light	8 fl oz	130	4	25	130	1	2.0	0
cocoa, rich	8 fl oz	210	8	32	180	1	6.0	0
original, creamy	8 fl oz	160	9	14	180	1	7.0	0
original, light	8 fl oz	90	4	15	95	1	2.0	0
vanilla delite	8 fl oz	190	7	27	130	1	6.0	0
vanilla, light	8 fl oz	110	4	20	95	1	2.0	0
(Westbrae Natural Foods)								
'WestSoy' almond malted, lite	6 fl oz	160	5	26	140	0	4.0	0
'WestSoy' almond malted, natural	6 fl oz	250	7	31	140	0	11.0	0
'WestSoy' banana, creamy, lite	6 fl oz	160	5	26	140	0	3.0	0
'WestSoy' carob malted, natural	6 fl oz	270	7	37	120	0	11.0	0
'WestSoy' carob, malted, lite	6 fl oz	160	5	27	140	0	3.0	0
'WestSoy' cocoa, lite	8 fl oz	140	3	27	95	0	2.0	10
'WestSoy' cocoa-mint malted, nondairy, frozen	6 fl oz	270	6	37	140	0	11.0	0
'WestSoy' cocoa-mint, lite	6 fl oz	160	5	26	140	0	3.0	0
'WestSoy' java malted, natural	6 fl oz	270	7	37	140	0	11.0	0
'WestSoy' original, natural	8 fl oz	150	7	18	115	0	5.0	0
'WestSoy' plain, lite	8 fl oz	100	4	16	100	0	2.0	0
'WestSoy' unsweetened, natural	8 fl oz	100	7	5	40	0	5.0	0
'WestSoy' vanilla malted, natural	6 fl oz	250	7	31	140	0	11.0	0
'WestSoy' vanilla royale, lite	6 fl oz	160	5	26	140	0	3.0	0
'WestSoy' vanilla, lite	8 fl oz	110	3	20	80	0	2.0	0
'WestSoy' vanilla, natural	8 fl oz	120	4	22	140	0	2.5	0
'WestSoy Plus' carob	8 fl oz	160	6	21	80	0	5.0	0
'WestSoy Plus' plain	8 fl oz	150	6	18	140	0	5.0	0
'WestSoy Plus' vanilla	8 fl oz	150	6	20	120	0	5.0	0

SOY BEVERAGE MIX

Food Name	Serv. Size	Total Cal.	Prot. gms	Carbs gms	Sod. mgs	Fiber gms	Fat gms	Chol. mgs
(Better Than Milk)								
(Darifree) fat free	3 tbsp	90	0	21	115	0	0.0	0
(Snoe Tofu) lactose & cholesterol free	3 tbsp	90	2	10	160	0	5.0	0
(Solait)								
chocolate	2 tbsp	114	5	18	120	2	3.0	0
original	3 tbsp	90	4	13	80	2	2.0	0
vanilla bean	3 tbsp	98	3	16	60	1	2.0	0
(Sovex)								
'Better Than Milk'	2 tbsp	98	1	19	173	0	2.0	0
'Better Than Milk' carob, nondairy	1 fl oz	130	2	20	175	0	5.0	0
'Better Than Milk' light	2 tbsp	70	2	14	105	0	0.5	0
'Better Than Milk' natural, light, nondairy	2 tbsp	80	2	15	120	0	1.0	0
'Better Than Milk' original	2 tbsp	100	2	16	100	0	2.5	0
(Soy Moo)	8 fl oz	125	9	11	55	0	5.0	0

SOY CHEESE. See under CHEESE SUBSTITUTE.

SOY MEAL

Food Name	Serv. Size	Total Cal.	Prot. gms	Carbs gms	Sod. mgs	Fiber gms	Fat gms	Chol. mgs
defatted, raw	1 cup	414	55	49	4	na	2.9	0
defatted, raw, crude protein basis Nx 6.25	1 cup	411	60	44	4	na	2.9	0

SOY PROTEIN CONCENTRATE

Food Name	Serv. Size	Total Cal.	Prot. gms	Carbs gms	Sod. mgs	Fiber gms	Fat gms	Chol. mgs
produced by acid wash	1 oz	94	16	9	255	2	0.1	0
produced by alcohol extraction	1 oz	94	16	9	1	2	0.1	0

SOY PROTEIN ISOLATE

Food Name	Serv. Size	Total Cal.	Prot. gms	Carbs gms	Sod. mgs	Fiber gms	Fat gms	Chol. mgs
	1 oz	96	23	2	285	2	1.0	0
K type	1 oz	92	23	3	14	2	0.1	0
K type, crude protein basis Nx 6.25	1 oz	91	25	1	14	1	0.1	0

Food Name	Serv. Size	Total Cal.	Prot. gms	Carbs gms	Sod. mgs	Fiber gms	Fat gms	Chol. mgs
(Protein Technologies)								
'ProPlus'	1 oz	108	24	0	11	na	1.1	0
'Supro'	1 oz	110	25	0	337	na	1.1	0
SOY SAUCE. See under SAUCE.								
SOYBEAN								
Dried								
mature, boiled	1 cup	298	29	17	2	10	15.4	0
mature, boiled	1 tbsp	19	2	1	0	1	1.0	0
mature, dry-roasted	1 cup	774	68	56	3	14	37.2	0
mature, raw	1 cup	774	68	56	4	17	37.1	0
mature, roasted	1 cup	810	61	58	7	30	43.7	0
mature, sprouted, raw	1/2 cup	43	5	3	5	0	2.3	0
mature, sprouted, raw	10 sprouts	12	1	1	1	0	0.7	0
mature, sprouted, steamed	1 cup	76	8	6	9	1	4.2	0
raw *(Arrowhead Mills)*	2 oz	230	19	19	2	13	10.0	0
roasted halves *(Solnuts)*	1 oz	146	13	8	10	3	6.8	0
Green								
boiled, drained	1 cup	254	22	20	25	8	11.5	0
raw	1 cup	376	33	28	38	11	17.4	0
SOYBEAN, FERMENTED/natto	1 cup	371	31	25	12	9	19.3	0
SOYBEAN CURD. See TOFU.								
SOYBEAN FLAKES *(Arrowhead Mills)*	2 oz	250	20	18	2	8	11.0	0
SOYBEAN OIL								
salad or cooking	1 cup	1927	0	0	0	0	218.0	0
salad or cooking	1 tbsp	120	0	0	0	0	13.6	0
salad or cooking, hydrogenated	1 cup	1927	0	0	0	0	218.0	0
salad or cooking, hydrogenated	1 tbsp	120	0	0	0	0	13.6	0
(Crisco)	1 tbsp	120	0	0	0	0	14.0	0
(Hain) salad or cooking	1 tbsp	120	0	0	0	0	14.0	0
(IGA) salad or cooking	1 tbsp	120	0	0	0	0	14.0	0
SOYBEAN-COTTONSEED OIL								
salad or cooking, hydrogenated	1 cup	1927	0	0	0	0	218.0	0
salad or cooking, hydrogenated	1 tbsp	120	0	0	0	0	13.6	0
SOYBEAN-LECITHIN OIL								
	1 cup	1663	0	0	0	0	218.0	0
	1 tbsp	104	0	0	0	0	13.6	0
SOYMILK								
	1 cup	81	7	4	29	3	4.7	0
	1 fl oz	10	1	1	4	0	0.6	0
SOYMILK MIX, powder *(Soyamel)*	8 oz	130	7	10	210	0	7.0	0
SOYNUT								
dry-roasted *(Karen's Kitchen)*	1 oz	90	12	7	200	8	4.0	0
dry-roasted, honey-coated *(Nature's Select)*	1 oz	130	12	13	180	8	4.0	0
SPAGHETTI. See under PASTA								
SPAGHETTI DISH/ENTRÉE. See under PASTA DISH/ENTRÉE.								
SPAGHETTI SQUASH. See SQUASH, SPAGHETTI.								
SPANISH MACKEREL. See under MACKEREL.								
SPANISH PEANUT. See under PEANUT.								
SPEARMINT								
dried	1 tbsp	5	0	1	6	0	0.1	0
dried	1 tsp	1	0	0	2	0	0.0	0
dried *(McCormick/Schilling)*	1 tsp	2	0	0	2	0	0.0	0
fresh	2 tbsp	5	0	1	3	1	0.1	0
SPINACH. See also SPINACH DISH/ENTRÉE.								
Canned								
(Allens)	1/2 cup	28	2	3	35	0	1.0	0
(Finast)	1/2 cup	25	3	4	360	0	0.0	0

Food Name	Serv. Size	Total Cal.	Prot. gms	Carbs gms	Sod. mgs	Fiber gms	Fat gms	Chol. mgs
(Stokely)	1/2 cup	30	2	3	420	0	0.0	0
chopped *(Allens)*	1/2 cup	28	2	3	330	0	1.0	0
chopped *(Bush's Best)*	1/2 cup	25	2	4	330	0	0.0	0
chopped, w/liquid *(Del Monte)*	1/2 cup	25	2	4	355	0	0.0	0
cut *(Freshlike)*	1/2 cup	20	2	4	340	0	0.0	0
cut *(Veg-All)*	1/2 cup	20	2	4	340	0	0.0	0
cut, w/butter sauce *(Green Giant)*	1/2 cup	40	2	5	280	2	1.5	3
cut, water packed, no salt added *(Freshlike)*	1/2 cup	20	2	4	20	0	0.0	0
cut, water packed, no sugar or salt added *(Freshlike)*	1/2 cup	20	2	4	20	0	0.0	0
drained	1 cup	49	6	7	58	5	1.1	0
no salt, w/liquid	1 cup	44	5	7	176	5	0.9	0
no salt added *(Finast)*	1/2 cup	25	3	4	110	0	0.0	0
no salt added *(Pathmark)*	1/2 cup	30	2	4	35	0	1.0	0
'Premium Northwest' *(S&W)*	1/2 cup	25	2	3	395	0	0.0	0
regular pack, w/liquid	1 cup	44	5	7	746	4	0.9	0
sliced *(Allens)*	1/2 cup	28	2	3	330	0	1.0	0
whole leaf *(Allens)*	1/2 cup	28	2	3	330	0	1.0	0
whole leaf *(Featherweight)*	1/2 cup	35	2	4	30	0	1.0	0
whole leaf *(Pathmark)*	1/2 cup	30	2	4	370	0	1.0	0
whole leaf, 'No Frills' *(Pathmark)*	1 cup	45	5	8	700	0	1.0	0
whole leaf, w/liquid *(Del Monte)*	1/2 cup	25	2	4	355	0	0.0	0
whole leaf, w/liquid, no salt added *(Del Monte)*	1/2 cup	25	2	4	35	0	0.0	0
Fresh								
raw	1 cup	7	1	1	24	1	0.1	0
raw	1 med leaf	2	0	0	8	0	0.0	0
raw *(Dole)*	3 oz	9	3	0	107	8	0.3	0
Frozen								
chopped *(A&P)*	3.3 oz	20	3	4	90	0	1.0	0
chopped *(Birds Eye)*	3.3 oz	20	3	3	90	3	0.0	0
chopped *(C&W)*	1/3 cup	20	2	2	115	2	0.0	0
chopped *(Finast)*	3.3 oz	20	3	3	70	0	0.0	0
chopped *(Flav-R-Pac)*	1/3 cup	20	2	2	115	2	0.0	0
chopped *(Frosty Acres)*	3.3 oz	20	3	3	70	1	0.0	0
chopped *(Seabrook)*	3.3 oz	20	3	3	70	1	0.0	0
chopped *(Southern)*	3.5 oz	25	3	4	100	0	0.3	0
chopped or leaf, boiled, drained	10-oz pkg	62	7	12	708	7	0.5	0
chopped or leaf, boiled, drained	1/2 cup	27	3	5	306	3	0.2	0
chopped or leaf, no salt added, drained	10-oz pkg	62	7	12	189	7	0.5	0
chopped or leaf, no salt added, drained	1/2 cup	27	3	5	82	3	0.2	0
chopped or leaf, unprepared	10-oz pkg	68	8	11	210	9	0.9	0
chopped or leaf, unprepared	1 cup	37	5	6	115	5	0.5	0
cut *(Freshlike)*	3.3 oz	20	3	4	75	0	0.0	0
cut *(Green Giant)*	3/4 cup	25	3	3	65	3	0.0	0
cut *(Seabrook)*	3.3 oz	20	3	4	77	1	0.0	0
cut *(Veg-All)*	3.3 oz	20	3	4	75	0	0.0	0
'Harvest Fresh' *(Green Giant)*	1/2 cup	25	3	3	240	2	0.0	0
'Plain Polybag' *(Green Giant)*	1/2 cup	25	3	6	100	5	0.0	0
whole leaf *(A&P)*	3.3 oz	25	3	4	100	0	1.0	0
whole leaf *(Birds Eye)*	3.3 oz	20	3	4	90	3	0.0	0
whole leaf *(Finast)*	3.3 oz	20	3	4	75	0	0.0	0
whole leaf *(Flav-R-Pac)*	1/3 cup	20	2	2	115	2	0.0	0
whole leaf *(Frosty Acres)*	3.3 oz	20	3	4	75	1	0.0	0
whole leaf *(Southern)*	3.5 oz	25	3	4	100	0	0.3	0
whole leaf, 'Portion Pack' *(Birds Eye)*	3.2 oz	20	3	3	70	2	0.0	0
SPINACH, MALABAR								
cooked	1 med bunch	4	1	0	9	0	0.1	0
cooked	1 cup	10	1	1	24	1	0.3	0

Food Name	Serv. Size	Total Cal.	Prot. gms	Carbs gms	Sod. mgs	Fiber gms	Fat gms	Chol. mgs
SPINACH, NEW ZEALAND								
boiled, drained, chopped	1 cup	22	2	4	193	na	0.3	0
raw, chopped	1 cup	8	1	1	73	na	0.1	0
SPINACH, VINE/basella								
raw	1 lb	86	8.2	15.4	(mq)	>3.2	1.4	0
raw	3.5 oz	19	1.8	3.4	24	>0.7	0.3	0
SPINACH DISH/ENTRÉE								
(Birds Eye) creamed, 'Combination Vegetables'	3 oz	60	2	5	310	1	4.0	0
(Budget Gourmet) au gratin, frozen	1 pkg	222	7	11	654	2	16.6	42
(Green Giant) creamed	1/2 cup	80	4	10	520	2	3.0	0
(Stouffer's)								
cream of, side dish	1/2 cup	160	4	8	380	2	12.0	15
creamed	1 pkg	336	7	18	670	5	26.3	32
creamed, food service product	1 oz	46	1	2	102	1	3.8	7
soufflé, side dish	1/2 cup	150	6	9	480	0	10.0	120
SPINY LOBSTER. See under LOBSTER.								
SPIRULINA. See under ALGAE.								
SPLIT PEAS. See PEAS, SPLIT.								
SPONGE GOURD. See GOURD, DISHCLOTH.								
SPORTS AND DIET/NUTRITION BARS								
(Advantage Bar)								
almond brownie, 'Atkins Diet Food Bar'	1 bar	230	20	3	223	2	10.0	3
chocolate coconut, 'Atkins Diet Food Bar'	1 bar	250	18	2	197	1	13.0	5
chocolate peanut butter, 'Atkins Diet Food Bar'	1 bar	218	19	3	124	1	13.0	1
praline crunch, 'Atkins Diet Food Bar'	1 bar	221	21	3	180	na	13.0	1
(Bally BFIT)								
chocolate covered chocolate energy bar	1 bar	240	12	37	144	2	5.0	10
chocolate covered peanut energy bar	1 bar	240	12	37	220	2	5.0	10
wafer snack, 'Trim Fat'	2 wafers	25	na	5	0	1	0.0	na
(Bear Valley)								
coconut almond food bar, 'Meal Pack'	1 pkg	400	16	56	80	6	12.0	0
sesame lemon food bar, 'Meal Pack'	1 pkg	410	17	57	85	4	13.0	0
(Biochem Ultimate)								
chocolate brownie nut food bar, low-carbohydrate	1 bar	240	23	2	260	na	7.0	na
chocolate chip protein bar	1 bar	290	30	19	35	na	5.0	na
honey almond food bar, low-carbohydrate	1 bar	240	25	2	230	na	7.0	na
(BIOX)								
chocolate and peanut butter protein bar	1 bar	300	21	37	160	1	7.0	15
chocolate chip protein bar	1 bar	330	27	48	120	3	3.0	21
chocolate protein bar	1 bar	290	21	40	140	2	5.0	15
triple chocolate chip protein bar	1 bar	330	27	48	120	3	4.0	20
(Biozone) 'Food Bar'	1 bar	180	15	20	na	na	4.0	na
(Boulder Bar)								
apple cinnamon energy bar	1 bar	190	8	37	70	4	2.0	0
berry energy bar	1 bar	190	8	37	70	4	2.0	0
chocolate energy bar	1 bar	200	8	40	60	4	3.0	0
peanut butter energy bar	1 bar	210	8	37	45	3	4.0	0
(Clif)								
apple cherry, '100% Natural Endurance'	2.4 oz	250	4	52	100	2	2.0	0
apricot, '100% Natural Endurance'	2.4 oz	250	6	50	55	2	2.0	0
(Clif Bar)								
apple cherry energy bar	1 bar	250	4	52	100	5	2.0	0
apricot energy bar	1 bar	250	6	50	55	5	2.0	0
carrot cake energy bar	1 bar	240	9	42	50	5	4.0	0
chocolate almond fudge energy bar	1 bar	250	10	39	40	6	5.0	0
chocolate chip energy bar	1 bar	250	4	51	45	3	3.0	0
chocolate chip peanut energy bar	1 bar	250	12	40	110	5	6.0	0

Food Name	Serv. Size	Total Cal.	Prot. gms	Carbs gms	Sod. mgs	Fiber gms	Fat gms	Chol. mgs
chocolate espresso energy bar	1 bar	250	4	51	100	5	3.0	0
chocolate pecan nutrition bar, for women, 'Luna'	1 bar	180	10	24	125	1	5.0	0
cookies 'n cream energy bar	1 bar	250	9	42	80	5	5.0	0
lemon zest nutrition bar, for women, 'Luna'	1 bar	180	10	26	50	1	4.0	0
peanut butter energy bar, crunchy	1 bar	250	10	45	150	4	4.0	0
real berry energy bar	1 bar	250	4	52	100	5	2.0	0
(Complete Bar)								
chocolate, '40/30/30 Bar'	1 bar	190	14	21	160	0	6.0	0
graham, '40/30/30 bar'	1 bar	190	14	21	160	0	6.0	0
peanut butter, '40/30/30 Bar'	1 bar	190	14	21	160	0	6.0	0
(Complete Protein Diet) 'Complete Protein Diet Bar'	1 bar	190	22	2	120	1	5.0	0
(Energx)								
chocolate protein cookie, all natural	2 cookies	200	15	28	150	5	3.0	0
oatmeal raisin protein cookie, all natural	2 cookies	200	15	31	180	4	2.0	0
peanut butter protein cookie, all natural	2 cookies	200	15	31	190	4	3.0	0
(Fi-Bar) strawberry, oatmeal, almond 'A.M. snack bar'	1 bar	150	3	24	30	5	4.0	0
(Figurines)								
chocolate caramel, '100'	1 bar	100	2	10	55	0	6.0	0
chocolate caramel, w/8 oz nonfat milk	2 bars	280	13	33	250	2	12.0	5
chocolate peanut butter, w/8 oz nonfat milk	2 bars	290	14	31	230	2	12.0	5
chocolate, w/8 oz nonfat milk	2 bars	280	12	34	230	2	11.0	5
S'mores, w/8 oz nonfat milk	2 bars	290	12	34	230	2	11.0	5
vanilla, w/8 oz nonfat milk	2 bars	290	13	33	230	2	12.0	5
(Gatorade Bar) peanut butter energy bar	1 bar	260	7	47	180	1	5.0	0
(Genisoy)								
apple spice protein bar, yogurt-coated, soy	1 bar	220	14	32	130	1	4.0	0
café mocha protein bar, soy	1 bar	220	14	34	150	1	3.5	0
café mocha protein bar, soy	1 bar	220	14	34	150	1	4.0	0
chocolate coated protein bar, soy	1 bar	220	14	33	190	1	3.5	0
chocolate mint protein bar, soy	1 bar	220	14	33	150	2	4.0	0
chocolate protein bar, uncoated, soy	1 bar	210	14	36	160	2	0.0	0
peanut butter fudge protein bar, soy	1 bar	230	14	31	160	2	5.0	0
(Jenny Craig)								
chocolate peanut nutrition meal	1 bar	220	10	33	240	1	5.0	na
lemon meringue nutrition meal	1 bar	210	10	31	130	na	5.0	na
oatmeal raisin nutrition meal	1 bar	210	10	35	75	3	3.0	0
(Jog Mate) muscle recovery protein supplement	1 tube	100	10	8	230	na	3.0	10
(Kashi) chocolate and peanut butter high-protein bar, 'Golean'	1 bar	280	13	50	150	7	6.0	0
(Lean Body)								
coconut cream meal replacement	1 bar	300	30	19	35	0	7.0	5
mint chocolate chip meal replacement	1 bar	300	30	19	35	1	7.0	5
(Maxxbar) chocolate chip energy bar	1 bar	170	10	25	75	1	4.0	0
(MET-RX)								
apple caramel energy bar, 'Sourceone'	1 bar	190	15	30	80	1	3.0	0
apple cinnamon oatmeal cereal bar, 'Caffe'	1 pkt	290	25	43	35	4	3.0	0
chocolate cheesecake energy bar, 'Sourceone'	1 bar	190	15	30	40	1	3.0	0
chocolate chip cookie dough energy bar	1 bar	340	27	50	110	0	4.0	0
chocolate chip graham cracker energy bar	1 bar	320	27	48	95	1	3.0	0
chocolate peanut energy bar, 'Sourceone'	1 bar	190	15	30	95	1	3.0	0
chocolate raspberry energy bar, 'Sourceone'	1 bar	180	15	31	65	1	3.0	0
devil's food energy bar, 'Sourceone'	1 bar	190	15	30	90	1	3.0	0
extreme chocolate nutrition bar	1 bar	240	38	18	384	3	8.0	24
extreme vanilla nutrition bar	1 bar	320	27	48	110	0	3.0	0
fudge brownie nutrition bar	1 bar	320	26	52	110	2	3.0	0
high-protein bar, 'Protein Plus'	1 bar	290	32	15	85	1	8.0	5
oatmeal raisin energy bar, iced, 'Sourceone'	1 bar	180	15	33	60	0	3.0	0

Food Name	Serv. Size	Total Cal.	Prot. gms	Carbs gms	Sod. mgs	Fiber gms	Fat gms	Chol. mgs
peanut butter cookie dough energy bar	1 bar	340	27	50	110	0	4.0	0
traditional flavor oatmeal cereal bar, 'Caffe'	1 pkt	280	27	35	15	5	4.0	0
(MLO Hardbody)								
chocolate truffle energy bar, 'Vita-Ox Formula'	1 bar	280	11	41	140	3	7.0	0
honey almond energy bar, 'Vita-Ox Formula'	1 bar	280	7	46	100	3	7.0	0
peanut butter energy bar, 'Vita-Ox Formula'	1 bar	290	7	46	120	3	7.0	0
pineapple coconut energy bar, 'Vita-Ox Formula'	1 bar	280	9	46	120	2	7.0	0
(Myoplex)								
chocolate fudge food bar	1 bar	340	24	44	140	2	7.0	5
chocolate nutrition bar, deluxe, 'Plus'	1 bar	340	24	42	144	2	7.0	6
chocolate peanut butter nutrition bar, deluxe, 'Plus'	1 bar	340	12	45	240	0	7.0	6
chocolate peanut butter precision nutrition bar, deluxe, 'Plus'	1 bar	340	24	44	230	0	7.0	4
chocolate precision nutrition bar, deluxe	1 bar	340	24	43	150	2	7.0	5
(Nature's Plus) high-protein wafers, all flavors								
'Spirutein'	6 wafers	99	14	9	0	2	1.0	0
(Nextra) apple protein crunch energy bar	1 pkg	140	17	14	180	2	2.0	10
(Nutrablast) 'Nutrablast Her for Women'	1 bar	190	11	27	240	1	6.0	na
(Odwalla Bar)								
'C Monster Food Bar'	1 bar	230	4	52	35	4	2.0	0
carrot raisin food bar, organic	1 bar	230	6	51	55	5	2.0	0
chocolate raspberry food bar	1 bar	240	7	45	40	5	5.0	0
cranberry citrus food bar	1 bar	240	5	52	55	4	2.0	0
peanut crunch food bar	1 bar	260	9	44	220	4	7.0	0
'Super Protein Food Bar'	1 bar	260	9	44	220	4	7.0	0
(Peak Bar)								
chocolate chip energy bar	1 bar	314	5	58	202	3	6.0	23
chocolate malt energy bar	1 bar	290	6	62	200	2	4.0	20
fruit mania energy bar	1 bar	284	5	58	202	3	5.0	23
peanut chocolate chunk energy bar	1 bar	295	7	56	200	3	7.0	10
(PowerBar)								
apple crisp, 'Harvest'	1 bar	240	7	45	80	4	4.0	0
apple-cinnamon	1 bar	230	10	45	96	3	3.0	0
banana	1 bar	230	9	45	96	3	2.0	0
blueberry, 'Harvest'	1 bar	240	7	45	80	4	4.0	0
cherry crunch, 'Harvest'	1 bar	240	7	45	80	4	4.0	0
chocolate energy gel	1 pack	120	0	28	50	0	2.0	0
chocolate	1 bar	230	10	45	90	3	2.0	0
chocolate, 'Essentials'	1 bar	180	10	28	105	3	4.0	0
chocolate, 'Harvest'	1 bar	240	7	45	80	4	4.0	0
chocolate, 'Protein Plus'	1 bar	290	24	38	290	3	5.0	5
lemon lime energy gel	1 pack	110	0	28	50	0	0.0	0
malt nut	1 bar	230	10	45	90	3	3.0	0
mocha	1 bar	230	10	45	90	3	3.0	0
oatmeal raisin	1 bar	230	10	45	120	3	3.0	0
peanut butter	1 bar	230	10	45	110	3	3.0	0
peanut butter w/chocolate chips, 'Harvest'	1 bar	240	7	45	72	4	5.0	0
strawberry, 'Harvest'	1 bar	240	7	45	80	4	4.0	0
tropical fruit energy gel	1 pack	110	0	28	50	0	0.0	0
vanilla energy gel	1 pack	110	0	28	50	0	0.0	0
vanilla yogurt, 'Protein Plus'	1 bar	290	24	38	190	2	5.0	5
wild berry	1 bar	230	10	45	90	3	3.0	0
(PR Bar)								
Bavarian mint nutrition bar, '40-30-30'	1 bar	190	13	21	144	2	7.0	0
carrot cake food bar	1 bar	200	13	23	105	na	6.0	na
chocolate peanut nutrition bar	1 bar	190	14	19	130	na	6.0	0
granola food bar	1 bar	180	14	21	125	2	6.0	0

Food Name	Serv. Size	Total Cal.	Prot. gms	Carbs gms	Sod. mgs	Fiber gms	Fat gms	Chol. mgs
iced brownie food bar	1 bar	200	13	22	170	1	6.0	0
strawberry yogurt food bar	1 bar	200	13	23	100	na	6.0	na
(Pure Protein Bar)								
chocolate chip protein bar	1 bar	190	20	11	25	1	4.0	3
white chocolate protein bar	1 bar	180	21	11	25	0	3.0	3
(Sci Fit)								
chocolate protein bar	1 bar	334	35	22	70	1	5.0	5
cinnamon protein bar	1 bar	334	35	22	40	1	6.0	5
oatmeal protein bar	1 bar	330	35	24	35	1	6.0	5
(Shaklee)								
'Carbo Crunch'	1 bar	180	9	27	85	0	4.0	0
'Fiber Blend Tablets'	5 tablets	6	1	1	10	3	0.5	0
(Slim-Fast)								
chocolate chip crunch	1 bar	120	2	16	25	2	4.0	0
Dutch chocolate	1 bar	140	5	20	80	2	5.0	3
peanut butter	1 bar	150	6	19	80	2	5.0	3
(Sportpharma Promax)								
double fudge brownie protein bar	1 bar	270	20	34	190	2	5.0	14
Dutch chocolate protein bar	2 scoops	270	50	2	220	na	2.0	85
lemon chiffon protein bar	1 bar	270	20	41	125	1	4.0	5
(Sweet Success) oatmeal raisin, chewy	1 bar	120	2	23	30	3	4.0	3
(Tiger's Milk)								
peanut butter and honey snack, carob coated	1 bar	160	6	23	90	0	5.0	0
(Trek Barr)								
apple raisin cinnamon energy bar	1 bar	130	3	29	25	2	1.0	0
chocolate extreme energy bar	1 bar	130	3	29	20	3	2.0	0
java express energy bar	1 bar	130	3	29	20	3	2.0	0
mountain berry energy bar	1 bar	130	3	29	20	3	2.0	0
peach apricot energy bar	1 bar	130	3	29	20	2	1.0	0
peanut butter chocolate chip energy bar	1 bar	130	3	26	50	2	2.0	0
(Twinlab)								
apple sports bar, 'Protein Fuel'	1 bar	340	35	12	250	0	5.0	0
chocolate food bar, 'Soy Sensations'	1 bar	180	15	22	200	5	6.0	0
chocolate sports bar, 'Protein Fuel'	1 bar	320	35	12	250	2	5.0	0
lemon food bar, 'Soy Sensations'	1 bar	180	15	23	200	5	5.0	0
peanut butter sports bar, 'Protein Fuel'	1 bar	340	35	12	280	0	5.0	0
peanut food bar, 'Soy Sensations'	1 bar	170	15	23	230	7	5.0	0
peanut nutrition bar, creamy, 'Ironman'	1 bar	230	16	23	280	0	8.0	0
(Ultra Slim-Fast)								
apple breakfast	1 bar	160	2	38	250	1	0.0	0
blueberry breakfast	1 bar	170	1	39	170	2	0.0	0
brownie	1 bar	120	2	20	45	1	4.0	0
caramel crunch, chewy	1 bar	120	1	22	45	2	3.5	3
choco almond crunch	1 bar	120	2	20	35	1	4.0	0
chocolate chip crunch snack	1 bar	120	2	19	30	3	4.0	0
fig breakfast	1 bar	160	2	37	270	2	0.0	0
peanut butter crunch	1 bar	120	2	19	45	2	4.0	0
peanut caramel crunch	1 bar	120	1	22	35	2	4.0	3
strawberry breakfast	1 bar	170	2	39	190	2	0.0	0
vanilla crunch	1 bar	120	2	20	30	1	4.0	0
(Viactiv) apple crunch, 'Energy Bar for Women'	1 bar	180	6	29	90	na	5.0	na
(Weider)								
'Sportsfood Enerquench Bar'	1 bar	200	6	44	80	0	1.0	0
chewable, 'Victory Explosive Workout'	6 wafers	30	1	6	60	0	0.0	0
protein bar, 'Sportsfood'	1 bar	160	10	21	140	0	4.0	0
(Weight Watchers)								
chocolate brownie, chewy, 'Sweet Success'	1 bar	120	2	23	45	3	4.0	3

Food Name	Serv. Size	Total Cal.	Prot. gms	Carbs gms	Sod. mgs	Fiber gms	Fat gms	Chol. mgs
chocolate chip, chewy 'Sweet Success'	1 bar	120	2	23	40	3	4.0	3
chocolate peanut butter, chewy 'Sweet Success'	1 bar	120	2	23	35	3	4.0	3
(Zone Perfect)								
apple cinnamon crunch nutrition bar, '40-30-30'	1 bar	210	14	23	340	1	7.0	0
strawberry yogurt nutrition bar, '40-30-30'	1 bar	210	14	24	320	1	7.0	na

SPORTS AND DIET/NUTRITION DRINKS. See SPORTS AND DIET/NUTRITION DRINK MIX.

Food Name	Serv. Size	Total Cal.	Prot. gms	Carbs gms	Sod. mgs	Fiber gms	Fat gms	Chol. mgs
(All Sport)								
fruit punch	8 fl oz	70	0	20	55	na	0.0	0
grape, caffeine-free, 'Thirst Quencher'	8 fl oz	70	0	20	55	0	0.0	0
lemon-lime, 'Thirst quencher, caffeine-free	8 fl oz	70	0	19	55	0	0.0	0
orange, caffeine-free, 'Thirst Quencher'	8 fl oz	70	0	19	55	0	0.0	0
(Clinical Resource) yogurt, flavored	8 fl oz	250	9	44	65	na	4.2	na
(Dannon) yogurt drink, all flavors, 'Dan'up'	8 fl oz	190	6	32	110	0	4.0	10
(Endurox) 'Endurox R4'	12 fl oz	280	14	53	230	na	2.0	10
(Ensure)								
black walnut flavor liquid nutrition	8 fl oz	250	9	34	0	0	8.8	0
chocolate liquid nutrition	8 fl oz	250	9	34	200	0	8.8	5
chocolate liquid nutrition, 'Plus'	8 fl oz	355	14	47	250	0	12.6	5
chocolate liquid nutrition, w/fiber	8 fl oz	260	10	38	200	0	8.8	5
eggnog flavor liquid nutrition	8 fl oz	250	9	34	0	0	8.8	0
strawberry flavor liquid nutrition	8 fl oz	250	9	34	200	0	8.8	5
strawberry flavor liquid nutrition, 'Plus'	8 fl oz	355	13	47	250	0	12.6	5
vanilla liquid nutrition	8 fl oz	250	9	34	200	0	8.8	5
vanilla liquid nutrition, 'Plus'	8 fl oz	355	13	47	250	0	12.6	5
vanilla liquid nutrition, w/fiber	8 fl oz	260	9	38	200	0	8.8	5
(Gatorade)								
fruit punch, low-sodium, no caffeine	8 fl oz	50	0	14	110	0	0.0	0
grape, low-sodium, no caffeine	8 fl oz	50	0	14	110	0	0.0	0
lemon and tea	8 fl oz	50	0	14	110	0	0.0	0
lemon-lime, 'Thirst Quencher'	8 fl oz	50	0	14	110	0	0.0	0
lemon-lime, 'Thirst Quencher Light'	8 fl oz	25	0	7	80	0	0.0	0
orange, 'Thirst Quencher'	8 fl oz	50	0	14	110	0	0.0	0
original, 'Thirst Quencher'	8 fl oz	50	0	14	110	0	0.0	0
pineapple-citrus, 'Thirst Quencher Light'	8 fl oz	25	0	7	80	0	0.0	0
tropical fruit, 'Thirst Quencher'	8 fl oz	50	0	14	110	0	0.0	0
(Genesis Nutrition)								
'Super Carbo Charge'	1 serving	348	0	87	0	na	0.0	0
'Super Metabolic Optimizer'	1 serving	260	15	48	65	na	1.0	0
'Super Weight Gain 1800'	1 serving	1800	40	284	na	na	24.0	na
'Super Workout Pak'	1 serving	0	0	0	na	0	0.0	0
(Go Healthy)								
chocolate nutrition drink	8 fl oz	235	14	40	210	na	3.0	na
mocha nutrition drink	8 fl oz	235	14	40	210	na	3.0	na
orange cream nutrition drink	8 fl oz	220	14	36	200	na	3.0	na
strawberry-banana nutrition drink	8 fl oz	220	14	36	200	na	3.0	na
vanilla nutrition drink	8 fl oz	220	14	36	200	na	3.0	na
(Knudsen)								
fruit juice sweetened, all flavors	8 fl oz	70	1	18	25	0	0.0	0
'Lemon Recharge'	1 cup	70	0	18	25	na	0.0	0
'Orange Recharge'	1 cup	70	0	18	25	na	0.0	0
'Tropical Recharge'	1 cup	70	0	18	25	na	0.0	0
'Vita Juice Fortified Blend'	8 fl oz	120	2	29	35	na	0.0	0
(Nutra/Balance)								
'Nutra/Shake Free'	4 fl oz	200	7	25	75	na	8.0	18
'Nutra/Shake with Fiber'	4 fl oz	200	7	40	73	3	1.3	0
'Nutra/Shake'	4 fl oz	229	7	35	63	na	6.9	21

Food Name	Serv. Size	Total Cal.	Prot. gms	Carbs gms	Sod. mgs	Fiber gms	Fat gms	Chol. mgs
(Nutrament)								
chocolate shake, meal replacement	12 fl oz	360	16	52	250	0	10.0	0
vanilla shake, meal replacement	12 fl oz	360	16	52	250	0	10.0	0
(Opti-Carb 140)								
grape	16 fl oz	140	0	35	9	0	0.0	0
orange	16 fl oz	140	0	35	9	0	0.0	0
(Power Burst)								
lemonade, advanced performance beverage	8 fl oz	50	0	14	25	0	0.0	0
(Powerade)								
fruit punch	16 fl oz	144	0	38	56	0	0.0	0
grape	16 fl oz	146	0	38	56	0	0.0	0
lemon-lime	16 fl oz	144	0	38	56	0	0.0	0
'Mountain Blast'	16 fl oz	146	0	38	56	0	0.0	0
orange	16 fl oz	144	0	38	56	0	0.0	0
(Pro-formance)								
fruit punch	8 fl oz	99	0	26	0	0	0.0	0
grape	8 fl oz	99	0	26	0	0	0.0	0
lemon-lime	8 fl oz	99	0	26	0	0	0.0	0
orange	8 fl oz	99	0	26	0	0	0.0	0
(Resource)								
chocolate health shake	4 fl oz	190	6	32	110	0	4.0	5
vanilla health shake	4 fl oz	190	6	32	100	0	4.0	5
(Sego)								
chocolate, 'Lite'	10 fl oz	150	11	20	480	0	3.0	5
chocolate, 'Very Chocolate'	10 fl oz	225	11	43	450	0	1.0	5
chocolate malt, 'Very Chocolate'	10 fl oz	225	11	43	450	0	1.0	5
Dutch chocolate, 'Lite'	10 fl oz	150	11	20	480	0	3.0	5
French vanilla, 'Lite'	10 fl oz	150	11	17	390	0	4.0	5
strawberry, 'Lite'	10 fl oz	150	11	17	390	0	4.0	5
strawberry, 'Very Strawberry'	10 fl oz	225	11	34	360	0	5.0	5
vanilla, plain, 'Lite'	10 fl oz	150	11	17	390	0	4.0	5
vanilla, 'Very Vanilla'	10 fl oz	225	11	34	360	0	5.0	5
(Shasta)								
lemon-lime, caffeine-free, 'Body Works'	8 fl oz	60	0	15	95	0	0.0	0
orange, caffeine-free, 'Body Works'	8 fl oz	60	0	15	95	0	0.0	0
(Slim Fast)								
chocolate shake	8 fl oz	190	13	33	240	2	1.3	9
chocolate shake, 'Nutra Start'	1 shake	210	10	40	370	5	2.5	0
strawberry shake	8 fl oz	190	13	33	264	2	0.7	9
vanilla shake, 'Nutra Start'	1 shake	210	10	38	350	5	2.5	3
(Sustacal)								
chocolate, liquid food, nutritionally complete	8 fl oz	240	15	33	220	0	5.5	0
vanilla, liquid food, nutritionally complete	8 fl oz	240	15	33	220	0	5.5	0
(Weight Watchers)								
chocolate mocha, w/phenylalanine, 'Sweet Success'	10 fl oz	200	11	32	230	6	3.0	0
chocolate, w/phenylalanine, 'Sweet Success'	10 fl oz	200	12	38	240	6	3.0	5
dark chocolate fudge, 'Sweet Success'	10 fl oz	200	11	32	210	6	3.0	0
milk chocolate, creamy, 'Sweet Success'	10 fl oz	200	11	32	230	6	3.0	0
vanilla, w/phenylalanine, 'Sweet Success'	10 fl oz	200	11	32	230	6	3.0	0
(Ultra Slim-Fast)								
'Chocolate Fantasy'	8 fl oz	270	11	51	288	8	1.9	9
chocolate fudge shake	1 shake	220	10	42	180	5	3.0	10
chocolate royale shake	1 shake	220	10	38	330	5	3.0	5
coffee shake	1 shake	220	10	38	300	5	3.0	5
French vanilla	12 fl oz	220	13	38	240	5	1.0	0
milk chocolate shake	1 shake	220	10	42	330	5	3.0	5
strawberry shake	1 shake	220	10	42	460	5	3.0	10
vanilla shake	1 shake	220	10	38	460	5	3.0	10

Food Name	Serv. Size	Total Cal.	Prot. gms	Carbs gms	Sod. mgs	Fiber gms	Fat gms	Chol. mgs
(Yogloo)								
yogurt, fruit basket, nonfat	10 fl oz	170	3	40	80	0	0.0	0
yogurt, original, nonfat	10 fl oz	170	3	40	80	0	0.0	0
yogurt, peach, nonfat	10 fl oz	170	3	40	80	0	0.0	0
yogurt, strawberry, nonfat	10 fl oz	170	3	40	80	0	0.0	0
SPORTS AND DIET/NUTRITION DRINK MIX								
(Alba)								
milkshake mix, double fudge, sugar-free, mix only	0.75 oz	60	6	10	135	0	0.0	0
milkshake mix, strawberry, sugar-free, mix only	0.75 oz	60	5	11	130	0	0.0	0
milkshake mix, vanilla flavor, no sugar, mix only	0.75 oz	70	6	11	160	0	0.0	0
(Alba '77)								
'Fit'N' chocolate marshmallow, prepared	6 fl oz	346	28	52	690	1	3.6	0
'Fit'N' chocolate, prepared	6 fl oz	346	26	56	709	1	2.5	0
'Fit'N' frosty double fudge, prepared	6 fl oz	346	28	52	728	1	3.3	0
'Fit'N' strawberry, prepared	6 fl oz	333	25	55	805	0	1.7	0
'Fit'N' vanilla, prepared	6 fl oz	333	26	55	810	0	1.4	0
(Amerifit) 'Heavy Weight Bulk Up' prepared	12 fl oz	71	4	14	71	0	0.3	8
(Balance Drink) meal replacement, '40-30-30'								
mix only	2 scoops	180	14	19	300	na	6.0	5
(Bally)								
muscle growth supplement, whey, mix only	1 scoop	100	19	3	55	na	2.0	15
protein supplement, soy	2 scoops	80	16	1	150	na	1.0	na
'Mass Builder' vanilla	4 scoops	750	25	163	420	2	1.0	10
(BFIT-RX)								
meal replacement, chocolate, light, mix only	1 pkt	190	20	26	290	1	1.0	5
meal replacement, vanilla, mix only	1 pkt	290	40	27	430	1	2.0	10
meal replacement for women, mix only	1 pkt	220	20	33	288	0	1.0	6
(Bio-Design X) vanilla, whey, mix only	20 grams	77	16	1	45	na	1.0	15
(BIOX) protein drink, chocolate, mix only	1 pkg	130	19	12	180	2	1.0	15
(Champion Nutrition)								
'Heavyweight Gainer 900' prepared	1 serving	650	30	105	120	na	12.0	na
(Complete Protein Diet)								
complete protein diet, chocolate, mix only	1 pkt	200	35	3	70	0	5.0	20
(EAS Precision)								
whey protein, 'Muscle Builder' mix only	3 tbsp	100	20	3	50	1	1.0	15
(Gatorade)								
'Thirst Quencher' fruit punch, prepared	8 fl oz	60	0	15	110	0	0.0	0
'Thirst Quencher' lemonade, prepared	8 fl oz	60	0	15	110	0	0.0	0
'Thirst Quencher' lemon-lime, mix only	3/4 scoop	58	0	15	96	na	0.0	na
(Genesis Nutrition)								
milk and egg protein drink, mix only	1 tbsp	39	8	2	na	na	0.0	0
'Super Trim Fast' mix only	1 serving	90	7	15	na	3	0.5	na
'Super Trim Fast' prepared	1 serving	198	17	27	na	3	2.0	na
(Genisoy)								
protein shake, chocolate, ultra soy protein, mix only	1 scoop	120	14	16	150	2	0.0	0
(Knox)								
gelatin drink, orange flavor, mix only	1 envelope	39	6	4	17	0	0.1	0
gelatin drink, orange flavor, w/aspartame, mix only	1 envelope	41	7	3	18	na	0.1	0
(Labrada)								
'Kwik Size XXXL' mix only	5 scoops	740	30	150	130	3	2.0	30
'Proplex+' mix only	1 scoop	90	17	3	35	0	1.0	30
(Lean Body)								
chocolate peanut butter, mix only	1 pkt	300	45	28	250	1	2.0	25
vanilla, mix only	1 pkt	300	45	28	200	1	2.0	25
(MET-RX)								
apple pie à la mode, mix only	1 pkt	250	37	22	370	1	2.0	15
extreme chocolate, mix only	1 pkt	240	38	18	384	3	1.0	0

Food Name	Serv. Size	Total Cal.	Prot. gms	Carbs gms	Sod. mgs	Fiber gms	Fat gms	Chol. mgs
milk chocolate, w/protein, mix only	3 scoops	220	46	7	120	1	2.0	15
original flavor, mix only	1 pkt	250	37	22	370	1	2.0	15
peach, mix only	1 pkt	250	37	22	370	1	2.0	15
strawberry cream, w/protein, mix only	3 scoops	210	46	3	115	0	1.0	15
vanilla butter cream, w/protein, mix only	3 scoops	210	46	3	115	0	1.0	15
white chocolate mocha, mix only	1 pkt	250	37	22	370	1	2.0	15
(MLO)								
'MUS-L Blast 2000' chocolate, mix only	4 scoops	580	20	118	350	3	3.0	51
'MUS-L Blast 2000' strawberry and banana, mix only ...	4 scoops	570	20	118	370	na	3.0	50
'MUS-L Blast 2000' vanilla, mix only	4 scoops	570	20	118	370	na	3.0	50
(Myoplex)								
'Mass Drink' chocolate cream, mix only	1 pkt	500	33	75	570	2	7.0	10
'Mass Drink' strawberry cream, light, mix only	1 pkt	280	42	24	330	1	2.0	15
'Mass Drink' strawberry cream, mix only	1 pkt	500	33	76	570	1	7.0	10
'Mass Drink' vanilla cream, light, mix only	1 pkt	280	42	24	330	1	2.0	15
'Mass Drink' vanilla cream, mix only	1 pkt	500	33	75	570	1	7.0	10
nutrition drink, chocolate cream, light, mix only	1 pkt	190	25	20	450	0	2.0	5
nutrition drink, chocolate cream, mix only	1 pkt	280	42	24	330	1	2.0	15
nutrition drink, chocolate, deluxe, mix only	1 pkt	280	42	24	336	1	2.0	15
(Nature's Plus)								
'Carrot-tein' mix only	1 scoop	97	14	11	120	0	0.0	0
'Fruitein' mix only	1 scoop	96	10	14	120	0	0.0	0
high-protein drink, banana, mix only	1 scoop	94	14	10	120	2	0.0	0
high-protein drink, cappuccino, mix only	1 scoop	100	14	11	120	2	0.0	0
high-protein drink, chocolate, vanilla, mix only	1 scoop	87	14	8	120	2	0.0	0
'Oxy-Nectar' mix only	1 scoop	107	10	17	0	0	0.0	0
(Olympian Labs)								
carbohydrate loading recovery drink, mix only	3 scoops	336	1	80	0	3	1.0	0
100% egg white w/complex carbs, vanilla, mix only ...	2 scoops	120	15	15	240	0	1.0	0
(Opti-Lean)								
chocolate, mix only	1 pkt	170	20	20	60	0	1.0	10
vanilla, mix only	1 pkt	170	20	20	60	0	1.0	10
(Scandishake)								
chocolate shake, instant, mix only	3 oz	440	4	58	120	2	21.0	0
chocolate shake, instant, lactose-free, mix only	3 oz	190	7	55	70	3	21.0	0
weight-gain shake, instant, lactose-free, mix only	3 oz	440	7	55	116	0	21.0	0
weight-gain shake, instant, sweetened w/aspartame, mix only	3 oz	440	7	55	100	0	21.0	0
weight-gain shake, instant, vanilla or strawberry, mix only ...	3 oz	440	4	58	90	0	21.0	0
(Shaklee)								
'After Exercise Energizer'	1/3 cup	180	12	33	90	0	0.5	3
'Daily Blend' mix only	1 1/2 tbsp	40	1	13	0	5	0.0	0
'Fiber Blend' 25% soluble/75% insoluble, mix only	1 tbsp	20	1	5	0	3	1.0	0
'Fiber Plan' fruit-flavored, mix only	2 tbsp	90	0	22	5	5	0.0	0
'Fiber Plan' unflavored, mix only	2 tsp	20	0	5	0	4	0.0	0
'Meal Shake' Bavarian cocoa, mix only	1/4 cup	120	7	23	70	3	0.5	3
'Meal Shake' Bavarian cocoa, prepared w/low-fat milk	8 fl oz prep	230	15	32	200	3	5.0	20
'Meal Shake' French vanilla, mix only	1/4 cup	120	7	23	80	3	0.5	3
'Meal Shake' French vanilla, prepared w/low-fat milk	8 fl oz	230	15	32	200	3	5.0	20
'Physique' mix only	1/2 cup	210	14	38	80	0	0.5	3
'Physique' prepared w/2 oz mix, 8 oz nonfat milk	1 serving	300	22	50	205	0	1.0	6
'Physique' prepared w/3 oz mix, 8 oz water	1 serving	320	21	57	120	0	1.0	3
protein drink, cocoa flavor, mix only	1/2 cup	110	16	8	140	0	1.0	0
protein drink, instant, mix only	1/4 cup	100	16	8	140	0	0.5	0
'Slim Plan' high fiber, low-fat, low-sodium, mix only	1/2 cup	210	15	33	370	4	3.0	3
(Slim-Fast)								
chocolate malt shake, prepared w/skim milk	8 fl oz	190	13	33	240	2	1.0	9

Food Name	Serv. Size	Total Cal.	Prot. gms	Carbs gms	Sod. mgs	Fiber gms	Fat gms	Chol. mgs
vanilla shake, prepared w/skim milk	1 cup	190	14	33	264	2	0.7	9
(Sportpharma)								
'Actisyn' strawberry flavor, mix only	1 pkt	150	27	8	220	1	1.0	10
'Just Whey' vanilla cream, mix only	1 oz	110	23	2	105	2	1.0	10
'Musclemax' chocolate, mix only	3 scoops	450	25	85	100	1	1.0	10
'Nutriforce' chocolate royale, mix only	1 pkt	250	40	21	210	2	2.0	0
'Nutriforce' French vanilla, mix only	1 pkt	260	40	21	230	0	2.0	0
(Strength Systems) 'USA Diet Octane' prepared	8 fl oz	127	21	9	50	2	1.0	0
(Weight Watchers)								
'Sweet Success' chocolate almond, mix only	1 scoop	90	7	12	150	6	2.0	0
'Sweet Success' chocolate almond, prepared	8 fl oz	180	15	24	280	6	2.0	0
'Sweet Success' chocolate, mix only	1 scoop	90	7	19	210	6	1.5	5
'Sweet Success' dark chocolate fudge, mix only	1 scoop	90	7	11	150	6	2.0	0
'Sweet Success' dark chocolate fudge, prepared	8 fl oz	180	15	23	280	6	2.0	0
(Tiger's Milk)								
'Breakfast Booster' mix only	2 tbsp	70	2	14	20	0	1.0	0
'Energy Booster' mix only	3 round tbsp	120	0	28	10	0	1.0	0
'Energy Booster' prepared w/8 oz nonfat milk	8 fl oz	200	8	40	135	0	1.0	0
'Protein Booster' Dutch chocolate, mix only	3 round tbsp	90	8	12	140	0	1.0	0
'Protein Booster' Dutch chocolate, prepared w/skim milk	8 fl oz	200	20	28	270	0	1.0	0
'Protein Booster' vanilla-orange creme, mix only	3 round tbsp	90	8	12	140	0	1.0	0
'Protein Booxter' vanilla-orange creme, prepared w/nonfat milk	8 fl oz	200	20	28	270	0	1.0	0
(Turbo Nutrition)								
protein powder, chocolate, prepared w/low-fat milk	8 fl oz	330	36	34	450	0	6.0	0
protein powder, strawberry flavored, mix only	2 oz	210	28	22	300	0	1.0	0
protein powder, strawberry flavored, prepared w/whole milk	8 fl oz	360	36	33	420	0	9.0	0
weight gain protein powder, chocolate, mix only	2 oz	210	28	22	320	0	1.0	0
(Twinlab)								
'Fuel Plex' whey protein, chocolate, mix only	1 pkt	300	45	25	310	0	2.0	40
'Fuel Plex' whey protein, strawberry, mix only	1 pkt	300	45	25	310	0	2.0	40
'Fuel Plex' whey protein, vanilla, mix only	1 pkt	300	45	25	310	0	2.0	40
(Ultra Slim-Fast)								
'Cafe Mocha' mix only	1 scoop	100	5	24	130	6	1.0	0
'Cafe Mocha' prepared w/nonfat milk	8 fl oz	200	15	38	280	6	1.0	0
'Chocolate Fantasy' 'Plus' mix only	1.41 oz	120	3	33	140	8	1.0	0
chocolate fudge shake, prepared w/skim milk	8 fl oz	200	13	36	216	5	2.6	9
chocolate malt shake, prepared w/skim milk	8 fl oz	200	13	36	216	5	1.3	9
'Chocolate Royale' shake, prepared w/skim milk	8 fl oz	200	13	36	264	6	1.3	9
French vanilla, mix only	1 scoop	100	5	24	120	4	1.0	0
French vanilla, prepared w/8 oz nonfat milk	1 serving	190	14	36	250	4	1.0	0
milk chocolate shake, prepared w/skim milk	8 fl oz	210	13	36	240	6	1.3	9
'Mixes w/Fruit Juice' mix only	1 scoop	90	10	17	75	6	0.0	0
'Mixes w/Fruit Juice' prepared w/orange juice	8 fl oz	200	11	43	80	6	1.0	0
'Plus' chocolate, mix only	1 scoop	120	3	33	140	8	1.0	0
'Plus' chocolate, prepared w/nonfat milk	12 fl oz	250	15	50	330	8	2.0	0
'Plus' piña colada flavor, mix only	1.16 oz	90	5	24	120	8	1.0	0
'Plus' piña colada flavor, prepared w/nonfat milk	8 fl oz	190	15	38	260	6	1.0	0
'Plus' strawberry jubilee, mix only	1 scoop	110	3	32	140	8	1.0	0
'Plus' strawberry jubilee, prepared w/nonfat milk	12 fl oz	240	15	50	330	8	2.0	0
strawberry shake, prepared w/skim milk	8 fl oz	200	13	36	264	4	1.3	9
vanilla shake, prepared w/skim milk	8 fl oz	200	13	33	264	6	0.7	9
(Weider)								
beef protein drink, mix only	1 cup	420	66	39	781	0	0.0	0
beef protein drink, prepared w/nonfat milk	8 fl oz	165	23	19	293	0	0.0	0

Food Name	Serv. Size	Total Cal.	Prot. gms	Carbs gms	Sod. mgs	Fiber gms	Fat gms	Chol. mgs
'Big' chocolate malt, sugar-free, mix only .... 4 scoops		320	18	58	370	0	2.0	0
'Big' chocolate malt, sugar-free, prepared w/milk ...... 16 fl oz		620	34	81	610	0	18.0	0
'Carbo Energizer' orange flavor, mix only .... 4 scoops		230	0	58	40	0	0.0	0
'Crash Weight Gain No. 7' vanilla, mix only .... 4 round tbsp		300	6	61	84	0	3.0	0
'Crash Weight Gain No. 7' vanilla, prepared w/milk ..... 16 fl oz		610	22	83	0	0	21.0	0
'Dynamic Body Shaper' Dutch chocolate, mix only .... 2 scoops		110	13	12	170	0	1.0	0
'Dynamic Body Shaper' Dutch chocolate, mix only .... 2 scoops		190	21	24	320	0	1.0	0
'Dynamic Body Shaper' mix only .... 1 cup		420	39	66	631	3	1.5	0
'Dynamic Body Shaper' prepared w/nonfat milk .... 8 fl oz		173	16	26	251	1	0.7	3
'Dynamic Muscle Builder' chocolate, mix only .... 2 scoops		200	26	21	300	0	1.0	0
'Dynamic Muscle Builder' chocolate, natural, mix only..................................... 2 scoops		120	18	9	170	0	1.0	0
'Dynamic Muscle Builder' chocolate, prepared .... 11 fl oz		220	18	36	260	0	1.0	0
'Dynamic Muscle Builder' mix only .... 1/3 cup		190	18	27	160	1	0.0	0
'Dynamic Muscle Builder' mix only .... 3 heaping tbsp		100	18	6	116	0	0.0	0
'Dynamic Muscle Builder' prepared w/whole milk .... 8 fl oz		250	26	17	116	0	9.0	0
'Dynamic Muscle Builder' prepared w/skim milk .... 8 fl oz		206	20	29	214	1	0.3	3
'Dynamic Muscle Builder' vanilla, natural, mix only .... 2 scoops		120	18	9	180	0	1.0	0
'Dynamic Protein' vanilla, mix only .... 2 scoops		100	16	10	150	0	0.0	0
'Dynamic Protein' vanilla, prepared w/skim milk .... 8 fl oz		190	24	22	280	0	1.0	0
'Dynamic Weight Gainer 1250' milkshake, prepared w/water .... 16 fl oz		330	18	61	400	0	1.0	0
'Dynamic Weight Gainer 1250' milkshake, prepared w/whole milk .... 16 fl oz		630	34	84	640	0	17.0	0
'Dynamic Weight Gainer 1250' milkshake, prepared w/whole milk .... 32 fl oz		1250	68	168	1280	0	34.0	0
'Dynamic Weight Gainer' chocolate, prepared .... 11 fl oz		280	18	48	320	0	2.0	0
'Dynamic Weight Gainer' Dutch chocolate, mix only ... 4 scoops		320	18	61	400	0	1.0	0
'Dynamic Weight Gainer' mix only .... 1 cup		660	36	124	820	0	1.0	0
'Dynamic Weight Gainer' peanut butter, mix only ..... 4 scoops		330	18	61	390	0	2.0	0
'Dynamic Weight Gainer' prepared w/whole milk .... 1 cup		252	14	34	260	0	6.6	26
'Dynamic Weight Gainer' vanilla, mix only .... 4 tbsp		310	20	54	183	0	2.0	0
'Dynamic Weight Gainer' vanilla, prepared w/milk ...... 16 fl oz		630	36	76	0	0	20.0	0
'Dynamic' vanilla, natural, prepared w/skim milk .... 16 fl oz		200	26	21	310	0	1.0	0
egg protein drink, mix only .... 1 cup		360	60	27	931	0	0.0	0
egg protein drink, prepared w/nonfat milk .... 8 fl oz		150	21	16	330	0	0.0	0
'Fat Burner System' mix only .... 1/3 cup		110	13	11	170	3	1.0	0
'Fat Burner System' prepared w/skim milk .... 8 fl oz		146	16	17	221	2	1.1	3
'Giant Mega Mass 4000' mix only .... 1 cup		547	27	106	400	0	1.3	16
'Giant Mega Mass 4000' prepared w/low-fat milk .... 8 fl oz		336	18	59	260	0	3.0	17
'Mass 1000' mix only .... 1 cup		513	23	104	340	2	0.7	27
'Mass 1000' prepared w/low-fat milk .... 8 fl oz		290	15	51	215	1	2.9	22
'90% Plus Protein' chocolate malt, mix only ..... 3 heaping tbsp		180	33	12	0	0	1.0	0
'90% Plus Protein' chocolate malt, sugar-free, mix only .... 3 heaping tbsp		100	24	0	293	0	0.0	0
'90-Plus Protein' vanilla, sugar-free, mix only .... 2 scoops		100	25	1	150	0	0.0	0
'90-Plus Protein' vanilla, sugar-free, prepared w/skim milk .... 8 fl oz		190	33	13	280	0	1.0	0
'Nitro-Fire' protein blend, mix only .... 2 tbsp		110	8	17	100	0	1.0	0
'Nitro-Fire' protein blend, prepared w/skim milk .... 8 fl oz		190	16	29	230	0	1.0	0
'Performance Builder' mix only .... 1 cup		601	54	93	751	3	3.0	0
'Performance Builder' prepared w/skim milk .... 8 fl oz		218	20	32	281	na	1.1	3
'Performance Shaper' mix only .... 1 cup		450	45	66	721	3	1.5	0
'Performance Shaper' prepared w/skim milk .... 1 cup		180	17	26	274	1	0.7	3
'Performance Weight Gainer' mix only .... 1 cup		585	27	117	375	0	1.5	0
'Performance Weight Gainer' prepared w/low-fat milk .... 8 fl oz		306	16	54	223	0	0.9	11
'Protein Blast' chocolate, prepared .... 11.5 fl oz		270	22	44	240	0	1.0	0

Food Name	Serv. Size	Total Cal.	Prot. gms	Carbs gms	Sod. mgs	Fiber gms	Fat gms	Chol. mgs
'Signature Line Dynamic Muscle Builder' mix only .... 2 scoops		120	18	9	180	0	1.0	0
'Sports Food Enerquench' lemon-lime, prepared .... 8 fl oz		60	0	15	0	0	0.0	0
'Sports Food Enerquench' orange flavor, prepared ...... 8 fl oz		60	0	15	0	0	0.0	0
'Sports Foods Gainer' chocolate supreme, prepared w/water .... 1 serving		300	14	53	110	0	3.0	0
'Sports Foods Gainer' chocolate, prepared w/skim milk .... 1 serving		460	30	77	390	0	3.0	0
'Sports Foods Gainer' vanilla frost, prepared w/water .... 1 serving		300	14	53	150	0	3.0	0
'Sports Foods Gainer' vanilla, prepared w/skim milk .... 1 serving		460	30	77	430	0	3.0	0
'Sports Foods Gainer' wild strawberry, prepared w/skim milk .... 1 serving		460	30	77	430	0	3.0	0
'Sports Foods Gainer' wild strawberry, prepared w/water .... 1 serving		300	14	53	150	0	3.0	0
'Sports Gainer' French vanilla, prepared w/skim milk ... 12 fl oz		460	30	77	390	0	3.0	0
'Sports Gainer' French vanilla, prepared w/water ...... 12 fl oz		300	14	53	110	0	3.0	0
'Sports Gainer' strawberry, prepared w/skim milk ...... 16 fl oz		460	30	77	430	0	3.0	0
'Sports Gainer' strawberry, prepared w/water .... 12 fl oz		300	14	53	150	0	3.0	0
'Sports Line Power Shake' Dutch chocolate, prepared .. 11 fl oz		220	15	37	150	0	1.0	0
'Super Mega Mass 2000' banana, mix only .... 1 cup		547	27	106	400	0	1.5	15
'Super Mega Mass 2000' banana, prepared w/low-fat milk .... 8 fl oz		334	18	59	261	0	3.1	17
'Super Mega Mass 2000' chocolate, mix only .... 1 cup		547	27	106	400	0	1.5	15
'Super Mega Mass 2000' chocolate, prepared w/low-fat milk .... 8 fl oz		334	18	59	261	0	3.1	17
'Super Mega Mass 2000' strawberry, mix only .... 1 cup		547	27	106	400	0	1.5	15
'Super Mega Mass 2000' strawberry, prepared w/low-fat milk .... 8 fl oz		334	18	59	261	0	3.1	17
'Super Mega Mass 2000' vanilla, mix only .... 1 cup		547	27	106	400	0	1.5	15
'Super Mega Mass 2000' vanilla, prepared w/low-fat milk .... 8 fl oz		334	18	59	261	0	3.1	17
vegetable protein drink, mix only .... 1 cup		390	45	42	721	0	0.0	0
vegetable protein drink, prepared w/nonfat milk .... 8 fl oz		158	17	20	278	0	0.0	0
'Victory CarboFire' prepared w/water .... 8 fl oz		250	0	62	50	0	0.0	0
'Victory Explosive Workout' citrus, mix only .... 4 tbsp		190	0	48	50	0	0.0	0
'Victory Mass 1000' vanilla, prepared w/low-fat milk .... 16 fl oz		1020	51	180	760	0	11.0	0
'Victory Mass 1000' vanilla, prepared w/water .... 16 fl oz		770	35	156	520	0	1.0	0
'Victory Mega Mass 2000' prepared w/low-fat milk .... 24 fl oz		2000	106	351	1510	0	19.0	0
'Victory Mega Mass 2000' prepared w/water .... 16 fl oz		1090	55	211	800	0	3.0	0
'Victory Mega Mass 2000' prepared w/water .... 24 fl oz		1640	82	317	1200	0	5.0	0
'Victory Mega Mass 2000' prepared w/water .... 8 fl oz		550	27	106	400	0	2.0	0
(Weight Watchers)								
'Sweet Success' chocolate raspberry, mix only .... 1 scoop		90	7	11	150	6	2.0	5
'Sweet Success' vanilla flavor, mix only .... 1 scoop		90	7	20	180	6	0.5	5
SPOT								
baked, broiled, grilled, or microwaved .... 3 oz		134	20	0	31	0	5.3	65
raw .... 3 oz		105	16	0	25	0	4.2	51
SPRING ONION. See SCALLION.								
SQUAB								
average of all parts, meat and skin, raw .... 3 oz		252	16	0	46	0	20.4	81
average of all parts, meat only, raw .... 3 oz		122	15	0	44	0	6.4	77
light meat, meat only, raw .... 3 oz		115	19	0	47	0	3.9	77
SQUASH. See also ZUCCHINI.								
ACORN								
baked, cubed .... 1 cup		115	2	30	8	9	0.3	0
boiled, mashed .... 1 cup		83	2	22	7	6	0.2	0

Food Name	Serv. Size	Total Cal.	Prot. gms	Carbs gms	Sod. mgs	Fiber gms	Fat gms	Chol. mgs
raw, approx 4-inch diam	1 squash	172	3	45	13	6	0.4	0
raw, cubed	1 cup	56	1	15	4	2	0.1	0
raw, cubed *(Frieda of California)*	1 oz	16	1	4	3	0	0.1	0
BANANA, baked *(Frieda of California)*	1 oz	18	1	4	3	0	0.1	0
BUTTERNUT								
Fresh								
baked, cubed	1 cup	82	2	22	8	na	0.2	0
raw, cubed	1 cup	63	1	16	6	na	0.1	0
Frozen								
boiled, mashed	1 cup	94	3	24	5	na	0.2	0
unprepared	12-oz pkg	194	6	49	7	4	0.3	0
unprepared	4-lb pkg	1034	32	261	36	24	1.8	0
unprepared *(Flav-R-Pac)*	1/3 cup	30	1	8	5	2	0.0	0
CROOKNECK								
Canned, yellow *(Allens)*	1/2 cup	16	1	3	230	0	1.0	0
Frozen								
cooked *(Kohl's)*	4 oz	45	1	11	0	0	1.0	0
yellow *(Seabrook)*	3.3 oz	18	1	4	1	1	0.0	0
yellow *(Southern)*	3.5 oz	21	2	4	20	0	0.1	0
HUBBARD								
Fresh								
baked, cubed	1 cup	103	5	22	16	na	1.3	0
boiled, mashed	1 cup	71	3	15	12	7	0.9	0
raw, cubed	1 cup	46	2	10	8	na	0.6	0
MARROW/vegetable marrow								
raw, trimmed	1 oz	4	0.2	1.0	na	>.1 c	<.1	0
SCALLOP								
boiled, mashed	1 cup	38	2	8	2	5	0.4	0
boiled, sliced	1 cup	29	2	6	2	3	0.3	0
raw, sliced	1 cup	23	2	5	1	na	0.3	0
SPAGHETTI								
boiled or baked, drained	1 cup	42	1	10	28	2	0.4	0
raw, cubed	1 cup	31	1	7	17	na	0.6	0
SUMMER. See also ZUCCHINI.								
Canned								
crookneck or straightneck, no salt added, mashed, drained	1 cup	31	1	7	12	3	0.2	0
crookneck or straightneck, no salt added, diced, drained	1 cup	27	1	6	11	3	0.1	0
crookneck or straightneck, no salt added, drained	1 cup	28	1	6	11	3	0.2	0
Fresh								
all varieties, boiled, drained, sliced	1 cup	36	2	8	2	3	0.6	0
all varieties, raw, sliced	1 cup	23	1	5	2	2	0.2	0
all varieties, raw, whole	1 large	65	4	14	6	6	0.7	0
all varieties, raw, whole	1 medium	39	2	9	4	4	0.4	0
all varieties, raw, whole	1 small	24	1	5	2	2	0.2	0
crookneck or straightneck, boiled, drained, sliced	1 cup	36	2	8	2	3	0.6	0
crookneck or straightneck, drained, solid, sliced	1/2 cup	18	1	4	1	1	0.3	0
crookneck or straightneck, raw, sliced	1 cup	25	1	5	3	2	0.3	0
Frozen								
crookneck or straightneck, drained, sliced	1 cup	48	2	11	12	3	0.4	0
crookneck or straightneck, sliced, unprepared	1 cup	26	1	6	7	2	0.2	0
WINTER								
Fresh								
all varieties, baked, cubed	1 cup	80	2	18	2	6	1.3	0
all varieties, raw, cubed	1 cup	43	2	10	5	2	0.3	0

Food Name	Serv. Size	Total Cal.	Prot. gms	Carbs gms	Sod. mgs	Fiber gms	Fat gms	Chol. mgs
Frozen								
cooked *(Birds Eye)*	4 oz	45	1	11	0	2	0.0	0
cooked *(Seabrook)*	4 oz	45	1	11	2	1	0.0	0
YELLOW, frozen, sliced *(Flav-R-Pac)* sliced	2/3 cup	15	1	2	15	1	0.0	0
SQUASH DISH/ENTRÉE								
(Stouffer's) casserole, frozen, food service product	1 oz	35	2	2	91	0	2.1	7
SQUASH SEED								
dried, kernels	1 cup	747	34	25	25	5	63.3	0
dried, kernels, hulled, approx 142 seeds	1 oz	153	7	5	5	1	13.0	0
roasted, kernels	1 cup	1185	75	30	41	9	95.6	0
roasted, kernels	1 oz	148	9	4	5	1	11.9	0
roasted, whole	1 cup	285	12	34	12	na	12.4	0
roasted, whole, approx 85 seeds	1 oz	126	5	15	5	na	5.5	0
SQUID/calamari								
mixed species, fried	3 oz	149	15	7	260	0	6.4	221
mixed species, raw	3 oz	78	13	3	37	0	1.2	198
mixed species, raw, boneless	1 oz	26	4	1	12	0	0.4	66
SQUIRREL								
raw	1 oz	34	6	0	29	0	0.9	24
roasted	3 oz	147	26	0	101	0	4.0	103
STAR FRUIT/carambola								
raw, cubed	1 cup	45	1	11	3	4	0.5	0
raw, sliced	1 cup	36	1	8	2	3	0.4	0
raw, whole, large, approx 4.5-inch long	1 fruit	42	1	10	3	3	0.4	0
raw, whole, medium, approx 3 5/8 inch long	1 fruit	30	0	7	2	2	0.3	0
raw, whole, small, approx 3-inch long	1 fruit	23	0	5	1	2	0.2	0
STEAK SAUCE. See under SAUCE.								
STEW. See also under individual types of dinner/entrée listings.								
(Stouffer's) Cajun seasoned, frozen, food service product	1 oz	24	1	2	99	1	1.4	6
STIR-FRY ENTRÉE KIT								
(Tyson)								
	9 oz	230	22	15	480	0	9.0	80
'Yoshida Oriental Sauce'	1.6 oz	100	2	22	1260	0	1.0	0
STIR-FRY SEASONING. See under SEASONING MIX.								
STRAW MUSHROOM. See MUSHROOM, STRAW.								
STRAWBERRY								
Canned, in heavy syrup, w/liquid	1 cup	234	1	60	10	4	0.7	0
Fresh								
raw, halved	1 cup	46	1	11	2	3	0.6	0
raw, puréed	1 cup	70	1	16	2	5	0.9	0
raw, sliced	1 cup	50	1	12	2	4	0.6	0
raw, trimmed	1 pint	107	2	25	4	8	1.3	0
raw, whole	1 cup	43	1	10	1	3	0.5	0
raw, whole, extra large, approx 1 5/8 inch diam	1 berry	8	0	2	0	1	0.1	0
raw, whole, large, approx 1 3/8 inch diam	1 berry	5	0	1	0	0	0.1	0
raw, whole, medium, approx 1 1/4 inch diam	1 berry	4	0	1	0	0	0.0	0
raw, whole, small, approx 1 inch diam	1 berry	2	0	0	0	0	0.0	0
Frozen								
sliced *(Flav-R-Pac)*	1/2 cup	150	1	33	0	2	1.5	0
sliced, sweetened	10-oz pkg	273	2	74	9	5	0.4	0
sliced, sweetened, thawed	1 cup	245	1	66	8	5	0.3	0
whole *(Flav-R-Pac)*	1 cup	50	1	13	5	2	1.0	0
whole, sweetened	10-oz pkg	222	1	60	3	5	0.4	0
whole, sweetened, thawed	1 cup	199	1	54	3	5	0.4	0
whole, unsweetened	1 med berry	4	0	1	0	0	0.0	0
whole, unsweetened	20 oz pkg	198	2	52	11	12	0.6	0
whole, unsweetened, thawed	1 cup	77	1	20	4	5	0.2	0
whole, unsweetened, unthawed	1 cup	52	1	14	3	3	0.2	0

Food Name	Serv. Size	Total Cal.	Prot. gms	Carbs gms	Sod. mgs	Fiber gms	Fat gms	Chol. mgs

STRAWBERRY COLADA. See under COCKTAIL MIX.
STRAWBERRY DRINK. See under FRUIT DRINK; FRUIT JUICE BLEND; FRUIT JUICE DRINK.
STRAWBERRY GUAVA. See GUAVA, STRAWBERRY.
STRAWBERRY TOPPING

Food Name	Serv. Size	Total Cal.	Prot. gms	Carbs gms	Sod. mgs	Fiber gms	Fat gms	Chol. mgs
....	1 cup	864	1	225	71	3	0.3	0
....	2 tbsp	107	0	28	9	0	0.0	0
(Flav-R-Pac)	2 tbsp	40	0	10	0	0	0.0	0
(Kraft) nonfat	1 tbsp	50	0	14	5	0	0.0	0
(Smucker's)								
nonfat...	2 tbsp	120	0	30	0	0	0.0	0
nonfat, 'Light'	2 tbsp	55	0	14	0	0	0.0	0
STRAWBERRY TOPPING, pourable (Knudsen)	1 oz	75	0	18	0	0	1.0	0

STRING BEAN. See BEAN, GREEN.
STRIPED BASS. See BASS, STRIPED.
STRIPED MULLET. See MULLET, STRIPED.
STROGANOFF ENTRÉE. See under BEEF DINNER/ENTRÉE; BEEF SUBSTITUTE DINNER/ENTRÉE MIX.
STUFFING

Food Name	Serv. Size	Total Cal.	Prot. gms	Carbs gms	Sod. mgs	Fiber gms	Fat gms	Chol. mgs
(Stouffer's) frozen, food service product, 'Old Fashion Stuff'n'	1 oz	70	1	7	142	1	4.0	1

STUFFING MIX

Food Name	Serv. Size	Total Cal.	Prot. gms	Carbs gms	Sod. mgs	Fiber gms	Fat gms	Chol. mgs
(Brownberry) sage and onion, mix only	1 serving	255	9	47	1126	4	3.4	na
(Pepperidge Farm)								
apple and raisin, mix only	1/2 cup	140	4	27	520	2	1.5	0
country garden and herb, mix only	1/2 cup	150	4	22	360	2	5.0	0
harvest vegetable and herb, mix only	1/2 cup	140	5	23	300	2	3.0	0
(Stove Top)								
chicken-flavored, 'Flexible Serving' prepared	1/2 cup	120	3	19	460	1	3.0	0
chicken flavored, 'Flexible Serving' prepared								
w/margarine....................................	1/2 cup	170	4	20	510	1	9.0	0
cornbread, 'Flexible Serving' prepared	1/2 cup	110	3	19	500	1	2.5	0
cornbread, 'Flexible Serving' prepared w/margarine	1/2 cup	170	3	21	580	1	8.0	0
for beef, prepared w/margarine	1/2 cup	180	4	22	540	1	9.0	0
for turkey, prepared w/margarine	1/2 cup	170	4	20	530	1	9.0	0

STURGEON

Food Name	Serv. Size	Total Cal.	Prot. gms	Carbs gms	Sod. mgs	Fiber gms	Fat gms	Chol. mgs
mixed species, baked, broiled, grilled, or microwaved	3 oz	115	18	0	59	0	4.4	65
mixed species, baked, broiled, grilled, or microwaved,								
flaked	1 cup	184	28	0	94	0	7.0	105
mixed species, raw	3 oz	89	14	0	46	0	3.4	51
mixed species, smoked	3 oz	147	27	0	628	0	3.7	68
mixed species, smoked	1 oz	49	9	0	210	0	1.2	23

SUCCOTASH. See under VEGETABLE DISH/ENTRÉE.
SUCKER, WHITE

Food Name	Serv. Size	Total Cal.	Prot. gms	Carbs gms	Sod. mgs	Fiber gms	Fat gms	Chol. mgs
baked, broiled, grilled, or microwaved	3 oz	101	18	0	43	0	2.5	45
raw	3 oz	78	14	0	34	0	2.0	35

SUET

Food Name	Serv. Size	Total Cal.	Prot. gms	Carbs gms	Sod. mgs	Fiber gms	Fat gms	Chol. mgs
beef, raw	4 oz	965	2	0	8	0	106.2	77
beef, raw	1 oz	242	0	0	2	0	26.6	19

SUGAR
BEET

Food Name	Serv. Size	Total Cal.	Prot. gms	Carbs gms	Sod. mgs	Fiber gms	Fat gms	Chol. mgs
granulated (Crystal)	1 tsp	16	0	4	0	0	0.0	0
granulated juice, organic (Sucanat)	1 tsp	12	0	3	0	0	0.0	0

CANE
Brown

Food Name	Serv. Size	Total Cal.	Prot. gms	Carbs gms	Sod. mgs	Fiber gms	Fat gms	Chol. mgs
dark brown 'Old Fashioned' (Domino)	1 tsp	16	0	4	0	0	0.0	0
golden brown, Hawaiian (C&H)	1 tsp	16	0	4	0	0	0.0	0
granulated	1 tsp	12	0	3	1	0	0.0	0
light brown, golden, packed (Domino)	1 tsp	16	0	4	0	0	0.0	0
light brown, granulated, 'Brownulated' (Domino)	1 tsp	12	0	3	0	0	0.0	0

Food Name	Serv. Size	Total Cal.	Prot. gms	Carbs gms	Sod. mgs	Fiber gms	Fat gms	Chol. mgs
packed	1 cup	827	0	214	86	0	0.0	0
packed	1 tsp	17	0	4	2	0	0.0	0
unpacked	1 cup	545	0	141	57	0	0.0	0
unpacked	1 tsp	11	0	3	1	0	0.0	0
White								
confectioner's, sifted, 10-X powdered *(Domino)*	1/2 cup	240	0	60	0	0	0.0	0
confectioner's/powdered	1 tsp	10	0	2	0	0	0.0	0
confectioner's/powdered, unsifted	1 cup	467	0	119	1	0	0.1	0
confectioner's/powdered, unsifted	1 tbsp	31	0	8	0	0	0.0	0
cubes	1 cube	19	0	5	0	0	0.0	0
cubes, 'Dots' *(Domino)*	1 cube	8	0	2	0	0	0.0	0
granulated	1 cup	774	0	200	2	0	0.0	0
granulated	1 tsp	16	0	4	0	0	0.0	0
granulated *(Crystal)*	1 tsp	16	0	4	0	0	0.0	0
granulated *(Domino)*	1 tsp	16	0	4	0	0	0.0	0
granulated, 'Packets' *(Domino)*	1 pkt	16	0	4	0	0	0.0	0
granulated juice, organic *(Succanat)*	1 tsp	12	0	3	0	0	0.0	0
superfine, instant-dissolving *(Domino)*	1 tsp	16	0	4	0	0	0.0	0
MAPLE								
	1 oz	100	0	26	3	0	0.1	0
	1 tsp	11	0	3	0	0	0.0	0
approx 1.75 x 1.25 x 1/2 inch pieces	1 piece	99	0	25	3	0	0.1	0
TURBINADO *(Hain)*	1 tbsp	50	0	12	0	0	0.0	0
SUGAR APPLE/sweetsop								
raw, pulp	1 cup	235	5	59	23	11	0.7	0
raw, whole, approx 2 7/8 inch diam	1 fruit	146	3	37	14	7	0.4	0
SUGAR CANE BATON								
(Frieda of California)	1 oz	21	0	50	0	0	0.1	0
(Sprinkle Sweet)	1 tsp	2	0	1	19	0	0.0	0
SUGAR SNAP PEAS. See PEAS, SNAP.								
SUGAR SUBSTITUTE								
(Featherweight)								
liquid	3 drops	0	0	0	0	0	0.0	0
saccharin grain tablet	1/4 tablet	0	0	0	2	0	0.0	0
(Nutra Taste) w/o saccharin	1 pkt	4	0	1	0	0	0.0	0
(NutraSweet)								
w/aspartame, 'Equal'	1 pkt	4	0	1	0	0	0.0	0
w/aspartame, 'Equal'	1 tsp	12	0	3	0	0	0.0	0
(S&W) liquid, 'Nutradiet'	1/8 tsp	0	0	0	0	0	0.0	0
(Splenda)	1 tsp	2	0	1	0	0	0.0	0
(Sprinkle Sweet)	1 tsp	2	0	1	0	0	0.0	0
(Sucanat) juice, organic	1 tsp	12	0	3	0	0	0.0	0
(Sugar Twin)								
w/saccharin	1 pkt	4	0	1	0	0	0.0	0
w/saccharin, 'Plus'	1 pkt	3	0	1	0	0	0.0	0
(Superose)								
liquid	1 tsp	0	0	0	0	0	0.0	0
	1 tsp	4	0	1	4	0	0.0	0
(Sweet 'n Low) saccharin-based	1 pkt	4	0	1	0	0	0.0	0
(Sweet 10)								
	1/8 tsp	0	0	0	2	0	0.0	0
liquid	1 tsp	0	0	0	0	0	0.0	0
(Sweet One)	1 pkt	4	0	1	0	0	0.0	0
(Sweet Plus) w/saccharin, equivalent to 2 tsp sugar	1 pkt	4	0	1	0	0	0.0	0
(TKI Foods) w/aspartame, 'Superose Plus'	1 serving	0	0	1	0	0	0.0	0
(Weight Watchers) 'Sweet'ner'	1 pkt	4	0	1	30	0	0.0	0

SUMMER SQUASH. See under SQUASH. See also ZUCCHINI.

Food Name	Serv. Size	Total Cal.	Prot. gms	Carbs gms	Sod. mgs	Fiber gms	Fat gms	Chol. mgs
SUNCHOKE. See JERUSALEM ARTICHOKE.								
SUNDAE. See under ICE CREAM BAR/DESSERT; ICE CREAM SUBSTITUTE BAR/DESSERT.								
SUNFISH/calico bass/crappie/pumpkinfish								
baked, broiled, grilled, or microwaved	3 oz	97	21	0	88	0	0.8	73
raw	3 oz	76	16	0	68	0	0.6	57
SUN-DRIED TOMATO. See under TOMATO.								
SUNFLOWER BUTTER								
....	1 oz	164	6	8	147	na	13.5	0
....	1 tbsp	93	3	4	83	na	7.6	0
unsalted	1 oz	164	6	8	1	na	13.5	0
unsalted	1 tbsp	93	3	4	0	na	7.6	0
(Maranatha Natural) roasted	2 tbsp	170	4	8	5	0	14.0	0
(Roaster Fresh)								
gourmet	1 oz	160	6	5	1	0	13.6	0
roasted, w/o salt, creamy	1 oz	160	6	5	1	0	14.0	0
SUNFLOWER SEED								
Dried								
(Frito-Lay's).....................................	1 oz	160	7	6	265	0	14.0	0
kernels *(Arrowhead Mills)*	1 oz	160	7	6	3	4	13.0	0
kernels	1 cup	821	33	27	4	15	71.4	0
kernels, in shell	1 cup	262	10	9	1	5	22.8	0
kernels, shelled *(National Sunflower)*	1/4 cup	205	8	6	1	4	18.0	0
natural, unsalted *(Flanigan Farms)*	1/4 cup	160	6	5	0	4	14.0	0
salted, in shell *(Fisher)*	1 oz	170	6	6	110	0	14.0	0
salted, in shell, 15–16 shelled seeds *(Fisher)*	1 oz	160	6	6	100	0	14.0	0
unsalted *(Fisher)*................................	1 oz	170	6	6	0	0	14.0	0
Dry-roasted								
(Fisher)	1 oz	170	6	6	200	0	15.0	0
(Planters)	1 oz	160	6	6	170	0	14.0	0
in shell *(Fisher)*	1 oz	170	6	6	110	0	15.0	0
kernels *(Flavor House)*	1 oz	180	8	4	200	0	15.0	0
kernels *(Pathmark)*	1 oz	180	5	7	150	0	14.0	0
kernels, hulled, unsalted	1 cup	745	25	31	4	14	63.7	0
kernels, salted..................................	1 cup	745	25	31	998	12	63.7	0
kernels, salted..................................	1 oz	165	5	7	221	3	14.1	0
kernels, shelled *(Pathmark)*	1 oz	180	5	7	150	0	14.0	0
kernels, unsalted................................	1 oz	165	5	7	1	3	14.1	0
w/tamari *(Eden Foods)*	1 oz	170	8	9	50	3	11.0	0
Oil-roasted								
(Fisher)	1 oz	170	6	4	170	0	16.0	0
(Planters)	1 oz	170	6	5	135	0	15.0	0
kernels, salted..................................	1 cup	830	29	20	814	9	77.6	0
kernels, salted..................................	1 oz	174	6	4	171	2	16.3	0
kernels, shelled, salted	1 cup	830	29	20	814	9	77.6	0
kernels, unsalted	1 cup	830	29	20	4	9	77.6	0
kernels, unsalted................................	1 oz	174	6	4	1	2	16.3	0
Roasted								
barbecue, salted, w/shell *(David's)*	3/4 cup	190	7	5	1350	2	15.0	0
barbecue, salted, shelled *(David's)*	3/4 cup	190	7	5	130	2	15.0	0
salted, shelled *(David's)*..........................	3/4 cup	190	7	5	130	2	15.0	0
salted, w/shell *(David's)*	3/4 cup	190	7	5	1350	2	15.0	0
salted *(Harmony)*	1/4 cup	170	9	11	290	3	13.0	0
Toasted								
kernels, salted..................................	1 cup	829	23	28	821	15	76.1	0
kernels, salted..................................	1 oz	175	5	6	174	3	16.1	0
kernels, unsalted................................	1 cup	829	23	28	4	15	76.1	0

Food Name	Serv. Size	Total Cal.	Prot. gms	Carbs gms	Sod. mgs	Fiber gms	Fat gms	Chol. mgs
kernels, unsalted	1 oz	175	5	6	1	3	16.1	0
SUNFLOWER SEED OIL								
(Hain)	1 tbsp	120	0	0	0	0	14.0	0
(IGA)	1 tbsp	120	0	0	0	0	14.0	0
(Kroger)	1 tbsp	122	0	0	0	0	13.6	0
(Pathmark)	1 tbsp	130	0	0	0	0	14.0	0
at least 60% linoleic	1 cup	1927	0	0	0	0	218.0	0
at least 60% linoleic	1 tbsp	120	0	0	0	0	13.6	0
less than 60% linoleic	1 cup	1927	0	0	0	0	218.0	0
less than 60% linoleic	1 tbsp	120	0	0	0	0	13.6	0
linoleic, hydrogenated	1 cup	1927	0	0	0	0	218.0	0
linoleic, hydrogenated	1 tbsp	120	0	0	0	0	13.6	0
pure pressed, organic *(Spectrum)*	1 tbsp	120	0	0	0	0	14.0	0
SURIMI. See under CRAB SUBSTITUTE; SCALLOP SUBSTITUTE.								
SURINAM CHERRY. See PITANGA.								
SWAMP CABBAGE. See CABBAGE, SKUNK.								
SWEET CHESTNUT. See CHESTNUT, EUROPEAN.								
SWEET PEPPER. See PEPPER, BELL.								
SWEET POTATO								
Fresh								
baked in skin	1 cup	206	3	49	20	6	0.2	0
baked in skin	1 large	185	3	44	18	5	0.2	0
baked in skin	1 medium	117	2	28	11	3	0.1	0
baked in skin	1 small	62	1	15	6	2	0.1	0
boiled, w/o skin	1 medium	159	2	37	20	3	0.5	0
boiled, w/o skin, mashed	1 cup	344	5	80	43	6	1.0	0
raw, approx 5-inch long long	1 potato	137	2	32	17	4	0.4	0
raw, cubed	1 cup	140	2	32	17	4	0.4	0
Canned								
cut, in water *(Allens)*	1/2 cup	70	1	16	20	0	1.0	0
mashed	1 cup	258	5	59	191	4	0.5	0
mashed *(Joan of Arc)*	1/2 cup	90	1	24	45	0	0.0	0
mashed *(Princella)*	1/2 cup	90	1	24	45	0	0.0	0
mashed *(Royal Prince)*	1/2 cup	90	1	24	45	0	0.0	0
mashed, vacuum pack	1 cup	232	4	54	135	5	0.5	0
pieces, vacuum pack	1 cup	182	3	42	106	4	0.4	0
syrup pack, drained	1 cup	212	3	50	76	6	0.6	0
syrup pack, w/liquid	1 cup	203	2	48	100	6	0.5	0
whole, vacuum pack *(Taylor's Brand)*	1 cup	210	4	55	56	0	0.0	0
Frozen								
cubes	1 cup	169	3	39	11	3	0.3	0
whipped, food service product *(Stouffer's)*	1 oz	40	0	7	92	1	1.4	0
SWEET POTATO LEAF								
Fresh								
raw, whole, 12.25-inch leaf	1 leaf	6	1	1	1	0	0.0	0
raw, chopped	1 cup	12	1	2	3	1	0.1	0
steamed, chopped	1 cup	22	1	5	8	1	0.2	0
SWEETBREAD. See BEEF, PANCREAS; BEEF THYMUS; LAMB, PANCREAS; VEAL, PANCREAS; VEAL, THYMUS.								
SWEETENER. See BARLEY MALT; CORN SYRUP; HONEY; SUGAR, BEET; SUGAR CANE BATON; SUGAR, MAPLE; SUGAR SUBSTITUTE; SYRUP.								
SWEETSOP. See SUGAR APPLE.								
SWISS CHARD/chard								
Fresh								
boiled, drained, chopped	1 cup	35	3	7	313	4	0.1	0
raw, chopped	1 cup	7	1	1	77	1	0.1	0
raw, whole	1 med leaf	9	1	2	102	1	0.1	0

Food Name	Serv. Size	Total Cal.	Prot. gms	Carbs gms	Sod. mgs	Fiber gms	Fat gms	Chol. mgs
SWORDFISH								
Fresh								
baked, broiled, grilled, or microwaved	3 oz	132	22	0	98	0	4.4	43
raw	3 oz	103	17	0	77	0	3.4	33
Frozen								
steaks, boneless, raw *(Peter Pan Seafoods)*	3.5 oz	118	19	0	102	0	4.0	39
steaks, w/o seasoning mix *(SeaPak)*	6-oz pkg	210	34	0	155	0	7.0	70
SYRUP								
BLACKBERRY *(Knott's Berry Farm)*	1 oz	120	0	30	0	0	0.0	0
BLUEBERRY								
(Estee) 'Breakfast'	1 tbsp	12	0	3	10	0	0.0	0
(Featherweight)	1 tbsp	16	0	4	35	0	0.0	0
(Knott's Berry Farm)								
....	1 oz	120	0	30	0	0	0.0	0
'Light'	1 oz	50	0	12	0	0	0.0	0
(Knudsen)	1 oz	75	1	19	0	0	1.0	0
(S&W) lower calorie	1/4 cup	60	0	15	105	0	0.0	0
BOYSENBERRY								
(Knott's Berry Farm)								
....	1 oz	120	0	30	0	0	0.0	0
'Light'	1 oz	50	0	12	0	0	0.0	0
BUTTER FLAVOR *(S&W)* lower calorie	1/4 cup	60	0	15	105	0	0.0	0
CHOCOLATE								
(Estee) 'Choco-Syp'	1 tbsp	20	0	5	5	0	0.0	0
(Hershey's) light, genuine chocolate	2 tbsp	50	1	12	48	1	0.1	0
(Nestlé) 'Quik'	2 tbsp	100	1	23	30	1	0.5	0
(Smucker's)	2 tbsp	130	1	27	35	0	2.0	0
FRUIT *(Smucker's)* all flavors	2 tbsp	100	0	26	0	0	0.0	0
MALT								
....	1 cup	1221	23.8	273.8	134	0	0.0	0
....	1 tbsp	76	1.5	17.1	8	0	0.0	0
(Eden Foods) barley, organic, w/sprouted barley	1 tbsp	60	1	14	0	0	0.0	0
MAPLE								
....	1 cup	825	0	212	28	0	0.6	0
....	1 tbsp	52	0	13	2	0	0.0	0
(Estee) 'Breakfast'	1 tbsp	12	0	3	35	0	0.0	0
(Knudsen) 'Fruit 'N Maple'	1 oz	105	1	26	0	0	1.0	0
(Maple House)								
100% pure	1 oz	100	0	61	4	0	0.0	0
no sugar	2 tbsp	110	0	27	50	0	0.0	0
(Maple Valley) no sugar, 'Lite'	2 tbsp	60	0	16	60	0	0.0	0
(Pillsbury)								
butter	1/4 cup	210	0	52	90	0	0.0	0
butter, lite	1/4 cup	100	0	24	180	1	0.0	0
lite	1/4 cup	100	0	24	180	1	0.0	0
regular	1/4 cup	210	0	52	90	0	0.0	0
(S&W) no sugar, saccharin sweetened	1 tsp	4	0	1	25	0	0.0	0
MAPLE FLAVOR *(S&W)* lower calorie	1/4 cup	60	0	15	105	0	0.0	0
PANCAKE								
cane and maple, 15% maple	1 cup	879	0	237	328	0	0.3	0
cane and maple, 15% maple	1 tbsp	56	0	15	21	0	0.0	0
cane and maple, 2% maple	1 cup	835	0	219	192	0	0.3	0
cane and maple, 2% maple	1 tbsp	53	0	14	12	0	0.0	0
(Aunt Jemima)								
'Butter Rich'	1/4 cup	210	0	52	170	0	0.0	0
'Butterlite'	1/4 cup	100	0	26	150	0	0.0	0
'Lite'	1 oz	54	0	13	92	0	0.1	0
lite, lower calorie, 3% real maple syrup	1/4 cup	100	0	27	160	0	0.0	0

Food Name	Serv. Size	Total Cal.	Prot. gms	Carbs gms	Sod. mgs	Fiber gms	Fat gms	Chol. mgs
'Original' rich maple taste	1 oz	100	0	26	60	0	0.0	0
pancake/waffle	1/4 cup	210	0	53	120	0	0.0	0
(Br'er Rabbit)								
dark	1 oz	120	0	31	0	0	0.0	0
light	1 oz	120	0	31	0	0	0.0	0
(Cary's) sugar-free, lower calorie, artificial maple	1/4 cup	35	0	9	105	0	0.0	0
(Estee)	1 tbsp	4	0	1	25	0	0.0	0
(Featherweight)	1 tbsp	16	0	4	25	0	0.0	0
(Hungry Jack)								
	2 tbsp	100	0	26	25	0	0.0	0
light, microwaveable	1/4 cup	100	0	24	180	1	0.0	0
lite	2 tbsp	50	0	14	105	0	0.0	0
microwaveable	1/4 cup	210	0	52	90	0	0.0	0
(Karo)	4 tbsp	234	0	59	83	0	0.0	0
(Knott's Berry Farm)								
	1 oz	110	0	28	0	0	0.0	0
'Country'	1 oz	110	0	27	0	0	0.0	0
'Light' microwavable	1 oz	45	0	11	70	0	0.0	0
lower calorie, microwave, 'Heat & Pour'	1 oz	45	0	11	70	0	0.0	0
microwave, 'Heat & Pour'	1 oz	110	0	28	90	0	0.0	0
w/30% real maple, microwaveable	1 oz	110	0	28	90	0	0.0	0
(Log Cabin)								
butter flavor, 'Country Kitchen'	1 oz	100	0	27	100	0	0.0	0
'Country Kitchen'	1 oz	100	0	26	20	0	0.0	0
lite, lower calorie	1 oz	50	0	13	90	0	0.0	0
'Pancake & Waffle'	1 oz	100	0	26	35	0	0.0	0
syrup product 'Country Kitchen Lite'	1 oz	50	0	13	85	0	0.0	0
(Mrs. Butterworth's)								
lower calorie	1/4 cup	100	0	25	100	0	0.0	0
thick and rich, 'Lite'	2 tbsp	60	0	15	65	0	0.0	0
(S&W)								
butter flavor, reduced calorie	1/4 cup	60	0	15	105	na	0.0	0
maple flavor, reduced calorie	1/4 cup	60	0	15	105	na	0.0	0
(Vermont Maid)	1 tbsp	50	0	13	5	0	0.0	0
(Weight Watchers) lower calorie	1 tbsp	25	0	7	40	0	0.0	0
RASPBERRY (Knudsen)	1 oz	75	1	18	0	0	1.0	0
RICE (Lundberg Family) organic 'Sweet Dreams'	1 tbsp	42	1	10	2	0	1.0	0
SORGHUM								
	1 cup	957	0	247	26	0	0.0	0
	1 tbsp	61	0	16	2	0	0.0	0
STRAWBERRY								
(Knott's Berry Farm)	1 oz	120	0	30	0	0	0.0	0
(Knudsen & Sons)	1 oz	75	1	18	0	0	1.0	0
(Nestlé) 'Quik'	2 tbsp	110	0	27	0	0	0.0	0
(S&W)								
lower calorie	1/4 cup	60	0	15	105	0	0.0	0
w/saccharin	1 tsp	4	0	1	25	0	0.0	0

T

Food Name	Serv. Size	Total Cal.	Prot. gms	Carbs gms	Sod. mgs	Fiber gms	Fat gms	Chol. mgs
TABBOULEH MIX. See under RICE DISH/ENTRÉE MIX.								
TACO								
(Owens)								
ham, refrigerated, 'Border Breakfasts'	2.17 oz	90	7	13	430	0	6.0	50
sausage, refrigerated, 'Border Breakfasts'	2.17 oz	190	7	11	345	0	12.0	65

Food Name	Serv. Size	Total Cal.	Prot. gms	Carbs gms	Sod. mgs	Fiber gms	Fat gms	Chol. mgs
TACO DINNER/ENTRÉE KIT								
(Pancho Villa)								
w/2 shells, seasoning, and sauce, mix only	1 serving	150	2	20	790	2	8.0	0
prepared	2 tacos	270	2	20	840	4	13.0	60
(Tio Sancho)								
taco sauce, 'Dinner Kit'	2 oz	62	2	13	750	1	0.2	0
taco seasoning, 'Dinner Kit'	1.25 oz	104	2	21	2500	2	1.4	0
taco shell, 'Dinner Kit'	1 shell	64	1	8	1	1	3.1	0
TACO FILLING								
(Hunt's) 'Manwich'	1/4 cup	31	1	7	587	1	0.1	0
(Chili Bowl) beef	1/4 cup	150	8	4	240	2	11.0	15
(McCarty) chicken	1.29 oz	80	7	1	181	0	5.1	75
TACO MIX								
(Del Monte) starter	8 oz	140	3	28	2180	0	1.0	0
(Natural Touch)								
	.3 tbsp	60	8	5	585	3	0.9	0
vegetarian	2 tbsp	90	10	6	0	0	2.0	0
(Old El Paso) prepared	1 taco	67	2	8	423	0	3.0	0
(Ortega) meat, prepared	1 oz	60	4	1	105	0	4.0	20
(Tio Sancho) 'Dinner Kit'	1 shell	64	1	8	1	1	3.1	0
TACO SALAD SEASONING. See under SEASONING MIX.								
TACO SEASONING MIX. See under SEASONING MIX.								
TACO SHELL								
baked	1 oz	133	2	18	104	2	6.4	0
baked, large, 6.5-inch dia	1 shell	98	2	13	77	2	4.7	0
baked, medium, 5-inch diam	1 shell	62	1	8	49	1	3.0	0
baked, mini, 3-inch diam	1 shell	23	0	3	18	0	1.1	0
baked, no salt added	1 oz	133	2	18	4	2	6.4	0
baked, no salt added, medium, 5-inch diam	1 shell	61	1	8	2	1	2.9	0
baked, no salt added, mini, 3-inch diam	1 shell	23	0	3	1	0	1.1	0
(Azteca)								
corn	1 shell	60	1	7	65	0	3.0	0
flour, for salad	1 shell	200	3	18	130	0	12.0	0
(Bearitos) blue corn	1 serving	130	3	17	0	na	7.0	0
(Chi-Chi's)	0.96 oz	140	2	17	5	0	7.0	0
(Gebhardt)	1 shell	52	1	6	2	1	2.8	0
(Lawry's)								
	1 shell	50	1	8	123	0	2.1	0
'Super'	1 shell	86	1	13	210	0	3.6	0
(Old El Paso)								
mini	3 shells	70	1	7	60	1	4.0	0
'Super'	2 shells	190	3	21	150	2	12.0	0
'Super Size'	1 shell	100	1	11	95	2	6.0	0
(Ortega)	1 shell	50	0	8	5	0	2.0	0
(Pancho Villa)	3 shells	190	2	19	0	3	11.0	0
(Rosarita)	1 serving	52	1	6	2	1	2.8	0
(Tio Sancho)								
	1 shell	64	1	8	1	1	3.1	0
'Super'	1 shell	94	2	11	2	1	4.7	0
TAFFY. See under CANDY.								
TAHINI. See SESAME BUTTER.								
TAHINI MIX								
(Arrowhead Mills) organic	1 oz	170	6	4	1	3	17.0	0
(Westbrae)								
Mid-Eastern, organic	2 tbsp	220	9	3	0	0	20.0	0
raw, organic	2 tbsp	210	8	1	0	0	19.0	0
toasted, organic	2 tbsp	220	8	3	0	0	19.0	0

Food Name	Serv. Size	Total Cal.	Prot. gms	Carbs gms	Sod. mgs	Fiber gms	Fat gms	Chol. mgs
TAMALE DINNER/ENTRÉE								
(Amy's Kitchen) pie, organic, frozen, 'Mexican'	8-oz pie	220	10	41	480	11	3.0	0
(Dennison's) in chili gravy, canned, 'Tamalito'	7.5 oz	310	6	37	1395	0	16.0	0
(Derby)								
beef, canned	6.561 oz	253	7	21	1034	4	17.4	23
beef, canned	2 tamales	160	8	15	570	1	7.0	24
(Gebhardt)								
	2 tamales	290	5	19	730	2	22.0	54
canned	5.75 oz	269	5	19	770	3	20.7	28
jumbo, canned	6.949 oz	332	6	24	930	3	25.2	34
jumbo, canned	1 serving	166	3	12	465	2	12.6	17
(Hormel)								
beef, canned	2 pieces	140	4	8	550	0	10.0	0
beef, canned, 'Hot'N Spicy'	2 pieces	140	4	9	612	0	10.0	0
beef, frozen	1 piece	140	6	13	555	0	7.0	0
canned	7.5 oz	280	6	19	990	0	20.0	35
hot-spicy, canned	7.5 oz	280	6	19	990	0	20.0	35
(Libby's) beef, w/sauce, canned	7.5 oz	408	9	26	1200	0	30.2	43
(Old El Paso) canned	2 pieces	190	5	16	380	0	12.0	20
(Patio) frozen	13 oz	470	12	58	1850	0	21.0	35
(Van Camp's) w/sauce, canned	1 cup	293	8	29	1132	2	16.2	0
(Wolf Brand) canned	7.75 oz	328	8	25	1181	2	24.5	0
TAMARI. See under SAUCE.								
TAMARIND/Indian date								
Fresh								
raw, pulp	1 cup	287	3	75	34	6	0.7	0
raw, whole, approx 1 x 3 inches	1 fruit	5	0	1	1	0	0.0	0
'Tamarindos' *(Frieda of California)*	3.5 oz	239	3	63	51	0	0.6	0
TANGERINE. See also MANDARIN ORANGE								
Fresh								
raw, sections	1 cup	86	1	22	2	4	0.4	0
raw, whole, large, approx 2.5-inch diam	1 fruit	43	1	11	1	2	0.2	0
raw, whole, medium, approx 2 3/8 inch diam	1 fruit	37	1	9	1	2	0.2	0
raw, whole, small, approx 2.25 inch diam	1 fruit	31	0	8	1	2	0.1	0
TANGERINE JUICE								
canned, sweetened	1 cup	125	1	30	2	0	0.5	0
canned, sweetened	1 fl oz	16	0	4	0	0	0.1	0
chilled, 'Pure & Light Mandarin Tangerine' *(Dole)*	6 fl oz	97	1	25	20	0	0.1	0
fresh, raw	1 cup	106	1	25	2	0	0.5	0
fresh, raw	1 fl oz	13	0	3	0	0	0.1	0
frozen concentrate, diluted	1 cup	111	1	27	2	na	0.3	0
frozen concentrate, diluted	1 fl oz	14	0	3	0	na	0.0	0
frozen concentrate, undiluted	6 fl oz	345	3	83	6	1	0.8	0
frozen or chilled *(Minute Maid)*	6 fl oz	90	1	23	0	0	0.0	0
TANNIA. See YAUTIA.								
TAPIOCA. See also under PUDDING.								
pearl, dry	1 cup	544	0	135	2	1	0.0	0
pearl, dry	1 oz	97	<0.1	25.1	tr	0.3	tr	0
TAQUITO beef, crispy, shredded *(Prima Rosa by Ruiz)*	5 taquitos	330	14	35	480	9	15.0	35
TARO								
cooked, sliced	1 cup	187	1	46	20	7	0.1	0
raw, sliced	1 cup	116	2	28	11	4	0.2	0
Tahitian, cooked, sliced	1 cup	60	6	9	74	na	0.9	0
Tahitian, raw, sliced	1 cup	55	3	9	63	na	1.2	0
TARO CHIPS								
	1 oz	141	1	19	97	2	7.1	0
	10 chips	115	1	16	79	2	5.7	0

Food Name	Serv. Size	Total Cal.	Prot. gms	Carbs gms	Sod. mgs	Fiber gms	Fat gms	Chol. mgs
salted *(Ray's)*	1 oz	139	2	20	167	0	6.0	0
unsalted *(Ray's)*	1 oz	139	2	20	15	0	6.0	0
TARO LEAF								
raw, chopped	1 cup	12	1	2	1	1	0.2	0
raw, whole, 11 x 6.5-inch leaf	1 leaf	4	0	1	0	0	0.1	0
steamed, chopped	1 cup	35	4	6	3	3	0.6	0
TARO SHOOT								
cooked, sliced	1 cup	20	1	4	3	na	0.1	0
raw, whole	1 med shoot	9	1	2	1	na	0.1	0
raw, sliced	1/2 cup	5	0	1	0	na	0.0	0
TARRAGON								
dried *(McCormick/Schilling)*	1 tsp	2	0	0	0	0	0.0	0
ground	1 tbsp	14	1	2	3	0	0.3	0
ground	1 tsp	5	0	1	1	0	0.1	0
ground *(Spice Islands)*	1 tsp	5	0	1	1	0	0.1	0
ground, fresh *(Durkee)*	1 tsp	10	0	0	0	0	0.0	0
ground, fresh *(Laurel Leaf)*	1 tsp	10	0	0	0	0	0.0	0
TEA								
BLACK								
Brewed								
decaffeinated, prepared w/tap water	6 fl oz	2	0	1	5	0	0.0	0
decaffeinated, prepared w/tap water	8 fl oz	2	0	1	7	0	0.0	0
regular, prepared w/distilled water	6 fl oz	2	0	1	0	0	0.0	0
regular, prepared w/tap water	6 fl oz	2	0	1	5	0	0.0	0
regular, prepared w/tap water	8 fl oz	2	0	1	7	0	0.0	0
(Bigelow)								
Darjeeling	5.25 fl oz	1	0	0	1	0	0.0	0
'Earl Grey'	5.25 fl oz	1	0	0	1	0	0.0	0
'English Teatime'	5.25 fl oz	1	0	0	0	0	0.0	0
(Celestial Seasonings)								
'Classic English Breakfast'	8 fl oz	3	0	0	1	0	0.0	0
decaffeinated	8 fl oz	4	0	1	5	0	0.0	0
'Extraordinary Earl Grey'	8 fl oz	3	0	1	1	0	0.0	0
(Exotica)								
'Assam Breakfast'	8 fl oz	0	0	0	0	0	0.0	0
'Ceylon Earl Grey'	8 fl oz	0	0	0	0	0	0.0	0
'Champagne Oolong'	8 fl oz	0	0	0	0	0	0.0	0
'China White'	8 fl oz	0	0	0	0	0	0.0	0
'Darjeeling'	8 fl oz	0	0	0	0	0	0.0	0
'Dragonwell'	8 fl oz	0	0	0	0	0	0.0	0
'Osmanthus'	8 fl oz	0	0	0	0	0	0.0	0
'Reserve Blend'	8 fl oz	0	0	0	0	0	0.0	0
'Silver Jasmine'	8 fl oz	0	0	0	0	0	0.0	0
(Lipton)								
black, regular	6 fl oz	0	0	0	0	0	0.0	0
black, w/lemon flavor	6 fl oz	3	0	1	1	0	0.0	0
(Stash's)								
'American'	8 fl oz	0	0	0	0	0	0.0	0
'China Black'	8 fl oz	0	0	0	0	0	0.0	0
'Earl Grey' decaffeinated	8 fl oz	0	0	0	0	0	0.0	0
'English Breakfast' decaffeinated	8 fl oz	0	0	0	0	0	0.0	0
'English Breakfast'	8 fl oz	0	0	0	0	0	0.0	0
'Oolong'	8 fl oz	0	0	0	0	0	0.0	0
'Orange Pekoe'	8 fl oz	0	0	0	0	0	0.0	0
Instant								
powder, unsweetened	1 tsp	2	0	0	1	0	0.0	0
powder, unsweetened, prepared	8 fl oz	2	0	0	7	0	0.0	0

Food Name	Serv. Size	Total Cal.	Prot. gms	Carbs gms	Sod. mgs	Fiber gms	Fat gms	Chol. mgs
(Lipton) decaffeinated, prepared	6 fl oz	0	0	0	0	0	0.0	0
GREEN, brewed *(Bigelow)* 'Chinese Fortune'	5.25 fl oz	1	0	0	1	0	0.0	0
HERBAL/FLAVORED								
Bagged								
(Good Earth)								
'Good Night' caffeine-free	1 bag	1	0	1	0	0	0.0	0
apple and spice, caffeine-free	1 bag	1	0	1	5	0	0.0	0
chamomile, caffeine-free	1 bag	1	0	0	0	0	0.0	0
fruit and spice, caffeine-free	1 bag	1	0	1	0	0	0.0	0
ginseng, caffeine-free	1 bag	1	0	0	0	0	0.0	0
lemon twist, caffeine-free	1 bag	2	0	1	0	0	0.0	0
orange spice, caffeine-free	1 bag	1	0	1	0	0	0.0	0
original flavor, caffeine-free	1 bag	4	0	0	0	0	0.0	0
original spice, caffeine-free	1 bag	4	0	1	0	0	0.0	0
(Super Dieters Tea)								
apricot, caffeine-free	1 bag	3	1	1	5	0	1.0	0
cinnamon spice, caffeine-free	1 bag	3	1	1	5	0	1.0	0
lemon mint, caffeine-free	1 bag	0	0	0	0	0	0.0	0
original flavor, caffeine-free	1 bag	3	1	1	5	0	1.0	0
peppermint, caffeine-free	1 bag	3	1	1	5	0	1.0	0
Brewed								
chamomile, brewed	6 fl oz	2	0	0	2	0	0.0	0
chamomile, brewed	8 fl oz	2	0	0	2	0	0.0	0
herbal, all types, except chamomile, brewed	6 fl oz	2	0	0	2	0	0.0	0
herbal, all types, except chamomile, brewed	8 fl oz	2	0	0	2	0	0.0	0
(Bigelow)								
almond orange	5 fl oz	1	0	0	1	0	0.0	0
'Apple Orchard'	5.25 fl oz	5	0	1	1	0	0.0	0
apple spice	5 fl oz	1	0	0	1	0	0.0	0
chamomile	5 fl oz	1	0	0	2	0	0.0	0
chamomile mint	5 fl oz	1	0	0	1	0	0.0	0
cinnamon orange	5 fl oz	1	0	0	1	0	0.0	0
'Cinnamon Stick'	5.25 fl oz	1	0	0	1	0	0.0	0
'Constant Comment'	5.25 fl oz	1	0	0	1	0	0.0	0
cranberry apple	5 fl oz	1	0	0	1	0	0.0	0
'Fruit & Almond'	5.25 fl oz	1	0	0	1	0	0.0	0
grains, roasted, w/carob	5 fl oz	3	0	1	1	0	0.0	0
hibiscus, w/rose hips	5 fl oz	1	0	0	1	0	0.0	0
'I Love Lemon'	5.25 fl oz	1	0	0	1	0	0.0	0
'Lemon & C'	5 fl oz	1	0	0	1	0	0.0	0
'Lemon Lift'	5.25 fl oz	1	0	0	1	0	0.0	0
'Mint Blend'	5 fl oz	1	0	0	3	0	0.0	0
'Mint Medley'	5.25 fl oz	1	0	0	1	0	0.0	0
'Orange & C'	5 fl oz	1	0	0	1	0	0.0	0
'Orange & Spice'	5.25 fl oz	1	0	0	1	0	0.0	0
peppermint	5 fl oz	1	0	0	2	0	0.1	0
'Plantation Mint'	5.25 fl oz	1	0	0	1	0	0.0	0
'Raspberry Royale'	5.25 fl oz	1	0	0	1	0	0.0	0
red raspberry	5 fl oz	1	0	0	1	0	0.0	0
spearmint	5 fl oz	1	0	0	1	0	0.0	0
'Specially Strawberry'	5 fl oz	1	0	0	1	0	0.0	0
'Sweet Dreams'	5.25 fl oz	1	0	0	1	0	0.0	0
'Take-A-Break'	5.25 fl oz	1	0	1	1	0	0.0	0
(Celestial Seasonings)								
'Almond Sunset'	8 fl oz	3	0	1	2	0	0.0	0
'Amaretto Nights'	8 fl oz	3	0	1	1	0	0.0	0
apple spice, 'Fruit & Tea'	8 fl oz	3	0	0	1	0	0.0	0

Food Name	Serv. Size	Total Cal.	Prot. gms	Carbs gms	Sod. mgs	Fiber gms	Fat gms	Chol. mgs
'Bavarian Chocolate Orange'	8 fl oz	7	0	2	5	0	0.0	0
chamomile	8 fl oz	2	0	1	5	0	0.0	0
'Cinnamon Apple Spice'	8 fl oz	3	0	0	1	0	0.0	0
'Cinnamon Rose'	8 fl oz	2	0	1	1	0	0.0	0
'Cinnamon Vienna'	8 fl oz	2	0	0	2	0	0.0	0
'Country Peach Spice'	8 fl oz	3	0	1	3	0	0.0	0
'Cranberry Cove'	8 fl oz	3	0	1	1	0	0.0	0
'Darjeeling Gardens'	8 fl oz	3	0	1	1	0	0.0	0
'Emperor's Choice'	8 fl oz	4	0	1	2	0	0.1	0
'Ginseng Plus'	8 fl oz	3	0	1	4	0	0.0	0
'Grandma's Tummy Mint'	8 fl oz	2	0	0	7	0	0.0	0
'Irish Cream Mist'	8 fl oz	3	0	1	1	0	0.0	0
lemon, 'Fruit & Tea'	8 fl oz	3	0	1	1	0	0.0	0
'Lemon Mist'	8 fl oz	2	0	1	3	0	0.0	0
'Lemon Zinger'	8 fl oz	4	0	1	1	0	0.0	0
'Mandarin Orange Spice'	8 fl oz	5	0	1	2	0	0.0	0
'Mellow Mint'	8 fl oz	2	0	0	4	0	0.0	0
'Mint Magic'	8 fl oz	1	0	0	3	0	0.0	0
'Mo's 24'	8 fl oz	2	0	0	4	0	0.0	0
'Morning Thunder'	8 fl oz	3	0	0	1	0	0.0	0
orange spice, 'Fruit & Tea'	8 fl oz	3	0	0	1	0	0.0	0
'Orange Zinger'	8 fl oz	5	0	1	1	0	0.0	0
peppermint	8 fl oz	2	0	1	8	0	0.0	0
raspberry, 'Fruit & Tea'	8 fl oz	2	0	1	1	0	0.0	0
'Raspberry Patch'	8 fl oz	4	0	1	1	0	0.0	0
'Red Zinger'	8 fl oz	4	0	1	2	0	0.0	0
'Roastaroma'	8 fl oz	11	0	2	4	0	0.1	0
'Sleepytime'	8 fl oz	5	0	1	2	0	0.0	0
spearmint	8 fl oz	5	0	0	6	0	0.1	0
'Strawberry Fields'	8 fl oz	4	0	1	1	0	0.0	0
'Sunburst C'	8 fl oz	3	0	1	6	0	0.0	0
'Swiss Mint'	8 fl oz	3	0	0	1	0	0.0	0
'Wild Forest Blackberry'	8 fl oz	2	0	2	1	0	0.0	0
(Glenny's) ginseng, 100% natural	42 grams	180	2	58	20	4	7.0	0
(Lipton)								
'Almond Pleasure'	8 fl oz	4	0	1	0	0	0.0	0
chamomile	8 fl oz	4	0	1	0	0	0.0	0
cinnamon apple	8 fl oz	2	0	1	0	0	0.0	0
'Citrus Sunset'	8 fl oz	4	0	1	0	0	0.0	0
'Gentle/Tangy Orange'	8 fl oz	4	0	1	0	0	0.0	0
'Lemon Soother'	8 fl oz	4	0	1	0	0	0.0	0
'Toasty Spice'	8 fl oz	6	0	1	0	0	0.0	0
(Stash's)								
'Apple Cinnamon'	8 fl oz	0	0	0	0	0	0.0	0
'Black Currant Ice'	8 fl oz	0	0	0	0	0	0.0	0
'Caravan'	8 fl oz	0	0	0	0	0	0.0	0
'Chamomile'	8 fl oz	0	0	0	0	0	0.0	0
'Citrus Spice'	8 fl oz	0	0	0	0	0	0.0	0
'Crepe Faire'	8 fl oz	0	0	0	0	0	0.0	0
'Estate'	8 fl oz	0	0	0	0	0	0.0	0
'Herbal Peach'	8 fl oz	0	0	0	0	0	0.0	0
'Irish Breakfast'	8 fl oz	0	0	0	0	0	0.0	0
'Jasmine Spice'	8 fl oz	0	0	0	0	0	0.0	0
'Lemon Blossom'	8 fl oz	0	0	0	0	0	0.0	0
'Lemon Spice'	8 fl oz	0	0	0	0	0	0.0	0
'Licorice Spice'	8 fl oz	0	0	0	0	0	0.0	0
'Moroccan Mint'	8 fl oz	0	0	0	0	0	0.0	0

Food Name	Serv. Size	Total Cal.	Prot. gms	Carbs gms	Sod. mgs	Fiber gms	Fat gms	Chol. mgs
'Orange Spice' decaffeinated	8 fl oz	0	0	0	0	0	0.0	0
'Orange Spice'	8 fl oz	0	0	0	0	0	0.0	0
'Oregon Mint'	8 fl oz	0	0	0	0	0	0.0	0
'Oriental Rose'	8 fl oz	0	0	0	0	0	0.0	0
'Peach'	8 fl oz	0	0	0	0	0	0.0	0
'Peppermint'	8 fl oz	0	0	0	0	0	0.0	0
'Premium Green'	8 fl oz	0	0	0	0	0	0.0	0
'Ruby Mist'	8 fl oz	0	0	0	0	0	0.0	0
'Sandman'	8 fl oz	0	0	0	0	0	0.0	0
'Tangerine'	8 fl oz	0	0	0	0	0	0.0	0
'Tropical Fruit'	8 fl oz	0	0	0	0	0	0.0	0
'Tropical Mist'	8 fl oz	0	0	0	0	0	0.0	0
'Wild Black Currant'	8 fl oz	0	0	0	0	0	0.0	0
'Wild Raspberry'	8 fl oz	0	0	0	0	0	0.0	0
'Wintermint'	8 fl oz	0	0	0	0	0	0.0	0
(Tetley)								
'Apple Freeze'	8 fl oz	79	0	20	1	0	0.0	0
'Classic'	8 fl oz	69	0	17	1	0	0.0	0
'Classic Lemon'	8 fl oz	108	0	27	1	0	0.0	0
'Diet Lemon Frost'	8 fl oz	10	0	2	1	0	0.0	0
'Diet Raspberry Blizzard'	8 fl oz	10	0	2	1	0	0.0	0
'Lemon Frost'	8 fl oz	89	0	22	1	0	0.0	0
'Orange Glazier'	8 fl oz	79	0	20	1	0	0.0	0
'Peach Chiller'	8 fl oz	79	0	20	1	0	0.0	0
'Raspberry Blizzard'	8 fl oz	95	0	24	1	0	0.0	0
Instant								
(Nature's Plus)								
Chinese herbal, citrus-flavored	1 tsp	24	0	6	0	0	0.0	0
Chinese herbal, decaffeinated, citrus-flavored, 'Chi'	1 tsp	24	0	6	0	0	0.0	0
TEA, ICED								
BLACK								
(Clinical Resource) 'Lemon Iced Tea'	8 fl oz	180	9	36	70	na	0.0	0
(Lipton)								
regular, w/natural lemon flavor	8.45 fl oz	96	2	24	20	0	0.3	0
w/lemon, sugar-free	8 fl oz	1	0	0	10	0	0.0	0
(Nestea)								
diet	8 fl oz	4	0	1	35	0	0.0	0
regular	8 fl oz	90	0	22	35	0	0.0	0
sweetened	16 fl oz	97	0	27	0	0	0.0	0
w/lemon, sugar-free	8 fl oz	2	0	1	0	0	0.0	0
w/lemon, sugar-sweetened	8 fl oz	70	0	17	0	0	0.0	0
natural	16 fl oz	180	2	44	50	0	0.0	0
natural	6 fl oz	66	1	17	18	0	0.0	0
(Shasta)	12 fl oz	124	0	34	28	0	0.0	0
(10-K)	8 fl oz	60	0	15	55	0	0.0	0
(Tetley)								
regular	8 fl oz	74	0	19	20	0	0.0	0
sweetened	8 fl oz	74	0	19	20	0	0.0	0
w/lemon	8 fl oz	74	0	19	20	0	0.0	0
(Thick & Easy)								
honey consistency	1/2 cup	70	0	17	20	0	0.0	0
nectar consistency	1/2 cup	60	0	16	15	0	0.0	0
(Veryfine) w/lemon	8 fl oz	80	1	16	10	0	0.0	0
HERBAL/FLAVORED								
(Fruitopia)								
'Born Raspberry'	16 fl oz	162	0	44	0	0	0.0	0
'Lemon Berry Intuition'	16 fl oz	166	0	44	0	0	0.0	0

Food Name	Serv. Size	Total Cal.	Prot. gms	Carbs gms	Sod. mgs	Fiber gms	Fat gms	Chol. mgs
'Peaceable Peach'	16 fl oz	162	0	44	0	0	0.0	0
(Knudsen)								
hibiscus, 'Iced Tea Cooler'	1 cup	90	0	23	40	0	0.0	0
blacklemon, 'Iced Tea Cooler'	1 cup	90	0	23	40	0	0.0	0
blackmango, 'Iced Tea Cooler'	1 cup	90	0	23	40	0	0.0	0
blackorange, 'Iced Tea Cooler'	1 cup	90	0	23	40	0	0.0	0
blackraspberry, 'Iced Tea Cooler'	1 cup	90	0	23	40	0	0.0	0
(Nestea)								
apple spice	16 fl oz	180	2	44	50	0	0.0	0
apple spice	6 fl oz	66	1	17	18	0	0.0	0
peach	16 fl oz	180	2	44	50	0	0.0	0
peach	6 fl oz	66	1	17	18	0	0.0	0
raspberry	16 fl oz	180	2	44	50	0	0.0	0
raspberry	6 fl oz	66	1	17	18	0	0.0	0
tropical	16 fl oz	180	2	44	50	0	0.0	0
tropical	6 fl oz	66	1	17	18	0	0.0	0
(Wyler's) 'Fruit Tea Punch'	12 fl oz	118	0	30	1	0	0.0	0

TEA, ICED, MIX
BLACK

Food Name	Serv. Size	Total Cal.	Prot. gms	Carbs gms	Sod. mgs	Fiber gms	Fat gms	Chol. mgs
(Crystal Light)								
decaffeinated, sugar-free, prepared	8 fl oz	4	0	0	0	0	0.0	0
sugar-free, prepared	8 fl oz	4	0	0	0	0	0.0	0
(Lipton)								
decaffeinated, sugar-free, prepared	8 fl oz	1	0	0	5	0	0.0	0
lemon flavor, decaffeinated, prepared	6 fl oz	55	0	14	1	0	0.0	0
lemon flavor, prepared	6 fl oz	55	0	14	1	0	0.0	0
lemon flavor, w/NutraSweet, prepared	8 fl oz	5	0	1	2	0	0.0	0
sugar-free, prepared	8 fl oz	1	0	0	6	0	0.0	0
sweet, no lemon, mix only	1 2/3 tbsp	70	0	17	0	0	0.0	0
sweet, sugar-free, no lemon, mix only	1 tbsp	0	0	1	0	0	0.0	0
(Nestea)								
decaffeinated, '100%' prepared	8 fl oz	0	0	0	0	0	0.0	0
lemon flavor, decaffeinated, sugar-free, mix only	2 tsp	6	0	1	0	0	0.0	0
lemon flavor, sugar-free, prepared	8 fl oz	4	0	1	0	0	0.0	0
'100%' mix only	1 tsp	2	0	0	0	0	0.0	0
'100%' prepared	8 fl oz	2	0	0	0	0	0.0	0
sugar-free, prepared	8 fl oz	6	0	1	5	0	0.0	0
w/sugar and lemon, prepared	8 fl oz	70	0	19	0	0	0.0	0
(Pathmark)								
lemon flavor, mix only	1 tsp	6	0	1	0	0	0.0	0
lemon flavor, artificially sweetened, mix only	1 tsp	4	0	1	20	0	0.0	0
lemon flavor, decaffeinated, low-calorie, prepared	8 fl oz	4	0	1	0	0	0.0	0
lemon flavor, decaffeinated, sugar-sweetened, mix only	2 tbsp	80	0	20	0	0	0.0	0
lemon flavor, low-calorie, prepared	8 fl oz	4	0	1	0	0	0.0	0
'No Frills' mix only	0.75 oz	70	0	21	75	0	0.0	0

HERBAL/FLAVORED

Food Name	Serv. Size	Total Cal.	Prot. gms	Carbs gms	Sod. mgs	Fiber gms	Fat gms	Chol. mgs
(Lipton)								
tropical flavor, sugar-free, mix only	1 tbsp	5	0	1	0	0	0.0	0
tropical flavor, w/sugar, mix only	1 2/3 tbsp	90	0	22	0	0	0.0	0
(Nestea) all flavors, 'Ice Teasers' prepared	8 fl oz	6	0	1	0	0	0.0	0
(Soothing Moments)								
cinnamon apple, caffeine-free, mix only	1/2 tsp	5	0	1	0	0	0.0	0
gentle orange, caffeine-free, mix only	1/2 tsp	5	0	1	0	0	0.0	0
lemon soother, caffeine-free, mix only	1/2 tsp	5	0	1	0	0	0.0	0

TEASEED OIL

Food Name	Serv. Size	Total Cal.	Prot. gms	Carbs gms	Sod. mgs	Fiber gms	Fat gms	Chol. mgs
	1 cup	1927	0	0	0	0	218.0	0
	1 tbsp	120	0	0	0	0	13.6	0

Food Name	Serv. Size	Total Cal.	Prot. gms	Carbs gms	Sod. mgs	Fiber gms	Fat gms	Chol. mgs
TEFF FLOUR. See under FLOUR.								
TEFF SEED (Arrowhead Mills)	2 oz	200	7	41	6	8	1.0	0
TEMPEH								
	1 cup	320	31	16	15	na	17.9	0
(White Wave)								
5-grain, vegetarian	1 piece	140	12	15	0	4	4.0	0
original, soy, vegetarian	1 piece	150	16	10	0	6	6.0	0
sea veggie, vegetarian	1 piece	120	12	11	25	8	3.0	0
soy rice, vegetarian	1 piece	140	12	13	0	5	5.0	0
wild rice, vegetarian	1 piece	140	13	12	10	6	4.0	0
TENDERGREEN. See MUSTARD SPINACH.								
TEQUILA								
80 proof	1 fl oz	65	0	0	0	0	0.0	0
86 proof	1 fl oz	70	0	0	0	0	0.0	0
90 proof	1 fl oz	74	0	0	0	0	0.0	0
94 proof	1 fl oz	77	0	0	0	0	0.0	0
100 proof	1 fl oz	83	0	0	0	0	0.0	0
TERIYAKI STIR-FRY ENTRÉE (Lunch Express)	1 entrée	260	15	39	550	4	5.0	30
TERRAPIN, diamondback, raw	100 gm	111	18.6	0.0	50	0	3.5	50
THYME, DRIED								
dried (McCormick/Schilling)	1 tsp	17	0	1	0	0	0.0	0
fresh	1 tsp	1	0	0	0	0	0.0	0
fresh	1/2 tsp	0	0	0	0	0	0.0	0
ground (Spice Islands)	1 tsp	5	0	1	1	0	0.1	0
ground	1 tbsp	12	0	3	2	2	0.3	0
ground	1 tsp	4	0	1	1	1	0.1	0
ground, fresh (Durkee)	1 tsp	5	0	0	0	0	0.0	0
ground, fresh (Laurel Leaf)	1 tsp	5	0	0	0	0	0.0	0
TILEFISH								
baked, broiled, grilled, or microwaved	3 oz	125	21	0	50	0	4.0	54
raw	3 oz	82	15	0	45	0	2.0	43
TOASTER BISCUIT. See BISCUIT, TOASTER.								
TOASTER PASTRY. See PASTRY, TOASTER.								
TOFU								
fried	1 oz	77	5	3	5	1	5.7	0
fuyu, salted and fermented	1 block	13	1	1	316	na	0.9	0
fuyu, salted and fermented, prepared w/calcium								
sulfate	1 block	13	1	1	316	na	0.9	0
okara	1 cup	94	4	15	11	na	2.1	0
(Nasoya)								
five-spice	1 piece	70	8	0	70	0	4.0	0
French country	1 piece	70	8	0	130	0	4.0	0
(White Wave) less fat	1 piece	90	10	4	5	2	4.0	0
EXTRA FIRM								
w/nigari	1/5 block	87	9	2	9	0	5.7	0
(Azumaya) Chinese style	3.5 oz	0	11	2	5	0	4.0	0
(Mori-Nu)								
silken	1 slice	46	6	2	53	0	1.6	0
silken	3 oz	55	7	2	60	1	2.0	0
silken, light	1 slice	32	6	1	82	0	0.6	0
silken, light	3 oz	35	6	1	80	na	1.0	0
(Nasoya)	1 piece	93	9	1	9	0	5.0	0
FIRM								
nigan	1/2 cup	97	10	4	10	1	5.6	0
prepared w/calcium sulfate	1/2 cup	183	20	5	18	3	11.0	0
(Azumaya) Japanese style	3.5 oz	70	7	4	5	0	2.5	0
(Kikkoman)	3 oz	50	6	2	30	0	2.5	0

Food Name	Serv. Size	Total Cal.	Prot. gms	Carbs gms	Sod. mgs	Fiber gms	Fat gms	Chol. mgs
(Mori-Nu)								
silken	1/2 pkg	90	10	4	50	0	4.0	0
silken	1 slice	52	6	2	30	0	2.3	0
silken	3 oz	50	6	2	30	1	2.5	0
silken, light	3 oz	35	5	1	70	1	1.0	0
silken, light	1 slice	31	5	1	71	0	0.7	0
(Nasoya)	1 piece	76	9	2	8	0	3.8	0
FREEZE-DRIED/koyadofu	1 oz	136	13.6	4.1	2	>0.1	8.6	0
REGULAR, prepared w/calcium sulfate	1/2 cup	94	10	2	9	0	5.9	0
SOFT								
(Azumaya) Kinugoshi	3.5 oz	50	4	5	5	0	4.0	0
(Kikkoman)	3 oz	45	4	2	5	0	2.5	0
(Mori-Nu)								
silken	1/2 pkg	80	7	4	10	0	4.0	0
silken	1 slice	46	4	2	4	0	2.3	0
silken	3 oz	45	4	2	5	1	2.5	0
(Nasoya)								
	1 piece	64	7	2	7	0	3.0	0
silken	1 piece	48	5	2	12	0	2.2	0
nigan	1 cubic inch	11	1	0	1	0	0.6	0
TOFU SPREAD								
(Natural Touch)								
green chili, canned, 'Tofu Topper'	2 tbsp	50	2	2	0	0	4.0	0
herb and spice, canned, 'Tofu Topper'	2 tbsp	50	2	2	0	0	4.0	0
Mexican, canned, 'Tofu Topper'	2 tbsp	60	2	2	0	0	5.0	0
TOM COLLINS. See under COCKTAIL; COCKTAIL MIX.								
TOMATILLO/ground husk tomato								
raw, chopped or diced	1/2 cup	21	1	4	1	1	0.7	0
raw, whole	1 medium	11	0	2	0	1	0.3	0
TOMATO. See also TOMATO DISH.								
Canned								
(A&P)	1/2 cup	25	1	6	220	0	1.0	0
(Featherweight)	1/2 cup	20	1	4	1	0	0.0	0
'Choice Cut' *(Hunt's)*	1/2 cup	22	1	5	325	1	0.2	0
chopped, food service product *(Angela Mia)*	1/2 cup	24	2	4	254	1	0.4	0
crushed *(Angela Mia)*	1/2 cup	27	2	6	380	2	0.2	0
crushed *(Contadina)*	1/4 cup	20	1	4	150	1	0.0	0
crushed *(Hunt's)*	1/2 cup	29	1	7	286	2	0.3	0
crushed *(Pathmark)*	1/2 cup	40	1	9	210	0	0.0	0
crushed *(Progresso)*	1/4 cup	20	1	4	95	1	0.0	0
crushed *(S&W)*	1/4 cup	20	1	4	95	1	0.0	0
crushed, 'No Frills' *(Pathmark)*	1 cup	90	3	20	510	0	0.0	0
crushed, chunky, food service product *(Angela Mia)*	1/2 cup	26	2	5	317	2	0.3	0
crushed, concentrated, food service product								
(Angela Mia)	1/4 cup	30	2	6	25	1	0.4	0
crushed, food service product *(Angela Mia)*	1/2 cup	32	1	7	317	1	0.4	0
crushed, Italian flavored *(Hunt's)*	1/2 cup	40	2	9	460	1	1.0	0
crushed, organic, no salt added *(Eden Foods)*	1/2 cup	35	2	6	0	0	0.0	0
cut, peeled, 'Ready-Cut' *(S&W)*	1/2 cup	25	1	6	220	0	0.0	0
diced, in juice *(Hunt's)*	1/2 cup	20	1	4	477	1	0.1	0
diced, in juice, no salt added *(Hunt's)*	1/2 cup	20	1	4	8	1	0.1	0
diced, in purée, food service product *(Hunt's)*	1/2 cup	23	1	5	304	1	0.1	0
diced, in rich purée *(S&W)*	1/2 cup	35	1	8	290	0	0.0	0
diced, Italian style *(Muir Glen)*	1/2 cup	25	1	4	190	1	0.0	0
diced, organic *(Eden Foods)*	1/2 cup	30	1	6	5	2	0.0	0
diced, peeled *(Libby's)*	1/2 cup	25	1	4	300	1	0.0	0
diced, w/green chilies *(Eden Foods)*	1/2 cup	30	2	5	35	2	0.0	0

Food Name	Serv. Size	Total Cal.	Prot. gms	Carbs gms	Sod. mgs	Fiber gms	Fat gms	Chol. mgs
diced, w/green chilies *(Ro-Tel)*	1/2 cup	20	0	4	370	1	0.0	0
diced, w/Italian herbs, 'Choice Cut' *(Hunt's)*	1/2 cup	24	1	5	600	1	0.0	0
diced, w/roasted garlic, 'Choice Cut' *(Hunt's)*	1/2 cup	24	1	5	505	1	0.0	0
dried, chopped, marinated *(Parmalat)*	3 pieces	35	1	3	5	1	2.5	0
in aspic, supreme *(S&W)*	1/2 cup	60	1	16	860	0	0.0	0
in juice, no salt added *(S&W)*	1/2 cup	25	1	4	30	1	0.0	0
Italian style *(Contadina)*	1/2 cup	35	1	8	250	0	1.0	0
Mexican style *(S&W)*	1/2 cup	40	1	8	360	0	0.0	0
'No Frills' *(Pathmark)*	1 cup	50	2	11	440	0	0.0	0
organic, diced *(Muir Glen)*	1/2 cup	25	1	4	170	1	0.0	0
'Pasta Ready' *(Contadina)*	1/2 cup	40	1	5	620	1	2.0	0
pear-shaped *(Hunt's)*	1/2 cup	20	1	4	360	1	0.1	0
pear-shaped, Italian flavored *(Hunt's)*	1/2 cup	20	1	5	320	1	1.0	0
peeled *(Contadina)*	1/2 cup	25	1	4	220	1	0.0	0
peeled, 'Choice Cut' *(Hunt's)*	1/2 cup	20	1	5	460	1	1.0	0
peeled, whole, in juice *(DiNapoli)*	1/2 cup	25	1	6	220	0	0.0	0
plum, w/basil sauce *(Contadina)*	1/2 cup	70	2	8	450	3	3.0	0
primavera 'Pasta Ready' *(Contadina)*	1/2 cup	50	1	8	600	1	1.5	0
'Recipe Ready' *(Contadina)*	1/2 cup	25	1	5	200	1	0.0	0
sliced *(A&P)*	1/2 cup	35	1	8	350	0	1.0	0
sliced *(Finast)*	1/2 cup	35	1	9	355	0	0.0	0
sliced *(Pathmark)*	1/2 cup	35	1	9	360	0	0.0	0
sliced *(S&W)*	1/2 cup	35	1	9	355	0	0.0	0
sliced, Italian *(S&W)*	1/2 cup	35	1	9	355	0	0.0	0
w/basil, peeled *(Progresso)*	1/2 cup	25	1	4	220	1	0.0	0
w/crushed red pepper 'Pasta Ready' *(Contadina)*	1/2 cup	60	1	8	690	1	3.0	0
w/green chilies *(Old El Paso)*	1/4 cup	14	0	3	480	0	0.0	0
w/jalapeños *(Contadina)*	1/2 cup	35	1	8	250	0	1.0	0
w/jalapeños *(Ortega)*	1 oz	8	0	1	120	0	0.0	0
w/mushrooms 'Pasta Ready' *(Contadina)*	1/2 cup	50	1	9	640	1	1.5	0
w/olives 'Pasta Ready' *(Contadina)*	1/2 cup	60	1	8	638	1	3.0	0
w/three cheeses 'Pasta Ready' *(Contadina)*	1/2 cup	70	1	8	650	1	4.0	1
wedges, w/liquid *(Del Monte)*	1/2 cup	30	1	8	355	0	0.0	0
whole *(Hunt's)*	2 tomatoes	22	2	4	404	1	0.1	0
whole *(Stokely)*	1/2 cup	25	1	5	190	0	0.0	0
whole, 'Nutradiet' *(S&W)*	1/2 cup	25	1	5	20	0	0.0	0
whole, Italian flavored *(Hunt's)*	1/2 cup	25	1	6	420	1	1.0	0
whole, no salt added *(Hunt's)*	2 tomatoes	22	1	5	3	1	0.5	0
whole, peeled *(Finast)*	1/2 cup	25	1	6	195	0	0.0	0
whole, peeled *(Hunt's)*	4.83 oz	21	2	4	373	1	0.1	0
whole, peeled *(Libby's)*	1/2 cup	25	1	4	220	1	0.0	0
whole, peeled *(Progresso)*	1/2 cup	25	1	4	220	1	0.0	0
whole, peeled *(S&W)*	1/2 cup	20	2	4	90	1	0.0	0
whole, peeled, food service product *(Hunt's)*	1 serving	11	1	2	202	0	0.1	0
whole, peeled, no salt added *(Hunt's)*	4.83 oz	21	2	4	9	1	0.1	0
whole, peeled, no salt added *(Pathmark)*	1/2 cup	25	1	6	20	0	0.0	0
whole, peeled, organic *(Muir Glen)*	1/2 cup	30	1	5	260	1	0.0	0
whole, peeled, w/liquid *(Del Monte)*	1/2 cup	25	1	5	220	0	0.0	0
whole, peeled, w/tomato juice *(Pathmark)*	1/2 cup	25	1	6	220	0	0.0	0
Dried *(Melissa's)*	5 pieces	55	3	10	15	2	0.5	0
Fresh, raw, ripe								
cherry, red, ripe, June–October	1 cup	31	1	7	13	2	0.5	0
cherry, red, ripe, June–October, medium	1 tomato	4	0	1	2	0	0.1	0
cherry, red, ripe, November–May	1 cup	31	1	7	13	2	0.5	0
cherry, red, ripe, November–May, medium	1 tomato	4	0	1	2	0	0.1	0
cherry, red, ripe, year-round average	1 cup	31	1	7	13	2	0.5	0
cherry, red, ripe, year-round average, medium	1 tomato	4	0	1	2	0	0.1	0

Food Name	Serv. Size	Total Cal.	Prot. gms	Carbs gms	Sod. mgs	Fiber gms	Fat gms	Chol. mgs
green, raw, chopped	1 cup	43	2	9	23	2	0.4	0
green, raw, whole, large	1 tomato	44	2	9	24	2	0.4	0
green, raw, whole, medium	1 tomato	30	1	6	16	1	0.2	0
green, raw, whole, small	1 tomato	22	1	5	12	1	0.2	0
orange, raw, chopped	1 cup	25	2	5	66	1	0.3	0
orange, raw, whole, medium	1 tomato	18	1	4	47	1	0.2	0
plum, red, ripe, raw, June–October, medium	1 tomato	13	1	3	6	1	0.2	0
plum, red, ripe, raw, November–May, medium	1 tomato	13	1	3	6	1	0.2	0
plum, red, ripe, raw, year-round average, whole, medium	1 tomato	13	1	3	6	1	0.2	0
plum/Italian, raw, June–October, medium	1 tomato	13	1	3	6	1	0.2	0
red, ripe, boiled	1 cup	65	3	14	26	2	1.0	0
red, ripe, boiled, medium	2 tomatoes	66	3	14	27	2	1.0	0
red, ripe, raw, June–October, chopped	1 cup	38	2	8	16	2	0.6	0
red, ripe, raw, June–October, medium	1 tomato	26	1	6	11	1	0.4	0
red, ripe, raw, June–October, 1/2-inch slices, medium	1 slice	6	0	1	2	0	0.1	0
red, ripe, raw, June–October, 1/4-inch slices, medium	1 slice	4	0	1	2	0	0.1	0
red, ripe, raw, June–October, quartered, medium	1/4 tomato	7	0	1	3	0	0.1	0
red, ripe, raw, June–October, whole, 3 inch diam	1 tomato	38	2	8	16	2	0.6	0
red, ripe, raw, June–October, whole, 2 3/5 inch diam	1 tomato	26	1	6	11	1	0.4	0
red, ripe, raw, June–October, whole, 2 2/5 inch diam	1 tomato	19	1	4	8	1	0.3	0
red, ripe, raw, November–May, chopped or sliced	1 cup	38	2	8	16	2	0.6	0
red, ripe, raw, November–May, medium	1 tomato	26	1	6	11	1	0.4	0
red, ripe, raw, November–May, quartered, medium	1/4 tomato	7	0	1	3	0	0.1	0
red, ripe, raw, November–May, 1/2 inch slices, medium	1 slice	6	0	1	2	0	0.1	0
red, ripe, raw, November–May, 1/4 inch slices, medium	1 slice	4	0	1	2	0	0.1	0
red, ripe, raw, November–May, whole, 3 inch diam	1 large	38	2	8	16	2	0.6	0
red, ripe, raw, November–May, whole, 2 3/5 inch diam	1 tomato	26	1	6	11	1	0.4	0
red, ripe, raw, year-round average, chopped or sliced	1 cup	38	2	8	16	2	0.6	0
red, ripe, raw, year-round average, quartered, medium	1/4 tomato	7	0	1	3	0	0.1	0
red, ripe, raw, year-round average, 1/2 inch slices, medium	1 slice	6	0	1	2	0	0.1	0
red, ripe, raw, year-round average, 1/4 inch slices, medium	1 slice	4	0	1	2	0	0.1	0
red, ripe, raw, year-round average, whole, 3-inch diam	1 large	38	2	8	16	2	0.6	0
red, ripe, raw, year-round average, whole, 2 3/5-inch diam	1 tomato	26	1	6	11	1	0.4	0
red, ripe, raw, year-round average, whole, 2 2/5-inch diam	1 tomato	19	1	4	8	1	0.3	0
red, ripe, stewed	1 cup	80	2	13	460	2	2.7	0
yellow, raw, chopped	1 cup	21	1	4	32	1	0.4	0
yellow, raw, whole, medium	1 tomato	32	2	6	49	1	0.6	0
Pickled *(Claussen)* kosher, in jars, approx. 1.7 oz	1 piece	9	0	2	571	0	0.0	0
Sun-dried								
	1 cup	139	8	30	1131	7	1.6	0
	1 piece	5	0	1	42	0	0.1	0
in oil and herbs *(Bella Sun Luci)*	2/3 oz	60	2	6	20	2	3.0	0
packed in oil, drained	1 cup	234	6	26	293	6	15.5	0
packed in oil, drained	1 piece	6	0	1	8	0	0.4	0
sun-ripened, 2-3 pieces *(Mezzetta)*	1/5 oz	15	1	3	5	1	0.0	0
yellow, in olive oil, 3 pieces *(Trader Joe's)*	1/5 oz	15	1	3	5	1	0.0	0

Food Name	Serv. Size	Total Cal.	Prot. gms	Carbs gms	Sod. mgs	Fiber gms	Fat gms	Chol. mgs
TOMATO DISH								
(Contadina)								
stewed, canned	1/2 cup	40	1	9	250	1	0.0	0
stewed, Italian style, canned	1/2 cup	40	1	8	260	1	0.0	0
stewed, Mexican style, canned	1/2 cup	40	1	9	220	1	0.0	0
(Del Monte)								
stewed, canned	1/2 cup	35	1	8	355	0	0.0	0
stewed, no salt added, canned	1/2 cup	35	1	8	45	0	0.0	0
stewed, original recipe, no salt added, canned	1/2 cup	35	1	9	50	2	0.0	0
(Green Giant)								
stewed, classic recipe, canned	1/2 cup	35	1	7	360	2	0.0	0
stewed, Italian recipe, canned	1/2 cup	30	1	7	360	2	0.0	0
stewed, Mexican recipe, canned	1/2 cup	35	1	7	400	2	0.0	0
(Hunt's)								
stewed, canned	1/2 cup	33	1	7	357	2	0.3	0
stewed, canned, food service product	1/2 cup	29	1	7	262	1	0.1	0
stewed, Italian flavored, canned	1/2 cup	35	1	8	400	1	1.0	0
stewed, no salt added, canned	1/2 cup	29	1	7	21	1	0.1	0
stewed, no salt added, canned	1/2 cup	33	1	7	31	2	0.3	0
(Muir Glen) whole, stewed, organic, canned	1/2 cup	25	1	4	190	1	0.0	0
(S&W)								
stewed, 50% reduced salt, canned	1/2 cup	35	1	9	180	0	0.0	0
stewed, no salt	1/2 cup	35	1	7	15	2	0.0	0
(Stokely) stewed, canned	1/2 cup	35	1	8	220	0	0.0	0
TOMATO JUICE. See also FRUIT JUICE BLEND.								
canned	1 cup	41	2	10	877	1	0.1	0
canned	6 fl oz	31	1	8	657	1	0.1	0
canned, no salt added	1 cup	41	2	10	24	2	0.1	0
canned, no salt added	6 fl oz	31	1	8	18	1	0.1	0
canned, no salt added	1 fl oz	5	0	1	3	0	0.0	0
(A&P)	6 fl oz	30	1	7	550	0	0.0	0
(Biotta)	6 fl oz	28	1	6	277	0	0.1	0
(Campbell's)	8 fl oz	50	2	9	860	1	0.0	0
(Del Monte)								
	8 fl oz	40	3	7	550	0	0.0	0
from concentrate	8 fl oz	50	2	10	760	1	0.0	0
(Featherweight)	6 fl oz	35	1	8	10	0	0.0	0
(Hunt's)								
	8 fl oz	34	2	8	689	2	0.3	0
food service product	8 fl oz	35	2	7	610	1	0.1	0
no salt added	8 fl oz	34	2	8	12	2	0.3	0
(Knudsen) organic	8 fl oz	50	1	10	0	0	0.0	0
(Libby's)								
bottled or canned	6 fl oz	35	2	7	500	0	0.0	0
canned	5.5 fl oz	35	2	6	460	0	0.0	0
(Pathmark)								
	6 fl oz	30	1	6	510	0	0.0	0
frozen, diluted	6 fl oz	35	1	8	450	0	0.0	0
(S&W)								
	5.5 fl oz	30	2	5	380	0	0.0	0
'California'	6 fl oz	35	1	8	600	0	0.0	0
'Nutradiet'	6 fl oz	35	1	8	20	0	0.0	0
(Stokely)	4 fl oz	20	1	4	330	0	0.0	0
(Welch's)	6 fl oz	35	1	7	550	0	0.0	0
TOMATO PASTE								
	6-oz can	139	6	33	1343	7	0.9	0
	1/2 cup	107	5	25	1035	5	0.7	0

Food Name	Serv. Size	Total Cal.	Prot. gms	Carbs gms	Sod. mgs	Fiber gms	Fat gms	Chol. mgs
no salt added	1 cup	215	10	51	231	11	1.4	0
no salt added	6-oz can	139	6	33	150	7	0.9	0
no salt added	1 tbsp	13	1	3	14	1	0.1	0
(Contadina)								
	2 tbsp	30	2	6	20	1	0.0	0
Italian style	2 tbsp	40	1	7	320	1	1.0	0
(Hunt's) no salt added	2 tbsp	30	1	6	7	2	0.5	0
(Progresso)	2 tbsp	30	2	6	20	1	0.0	0
(S&W)	2 tbsp	30	2	6	20	1	0.0	0
TOMATO PURÉE								
	1 cup	100	4	24	998	5	0.4	0
no salt added	1 cup	100	4	24	85	5	0.4	0
(Angela Mia)	2.19 oz	16	1	3	21	0	0.3	0
(Contadina)								
	1/4 cup	20	1	4	15	1	0.0	0
w/crushed tomatoes	1/2 cup	30	1	6	350	0	1.0	0
(Hunt's)								
	1/4 cup	24	1	5	98	2	0.3	0
food service product	1/4 cup	26	3	5	22	1	0.4	0
(Progresso) thick style	1/4 cup	25	1	5	15	1	0.0	0
TOMATO SAUCE								
(A&P) canned	1/2 cup	45	2	9	600	0	1.0	0
(Buitoni) marinara	1/2 cup	70	1	11	570	0	3.0	0
(Contadina)								
	1/4 cup	20	1	4	280	1	0.0	0
chunky, light	1/2 cup	45	2	8	470	2	0.5	0
four-cheese	4 oz	300	8	7	400	0	27.0	80
garden vegetable	5 oz	80	2	9	580	0	3.0	0
Italian sausage	5 oz	110	5	8	570	0	6.0	15
Italian style	1/4 cup	15	1	4	320	1	0.0	0
marinara, refrigerated, 'Fresh'	7.5 oz	100	4	12	700	0	4.0	0
pesto	2.33 oz	350	7	5	440	0	34.0	10
plum	5 oz	80	2	8	420	0	4.0	5
plum, w/basil, refrigerated, 'Fresh'	7.5 oz	100	3	14	700	0	4.0	5
refrigerated, 'Light'	0.5 oz	50	2	9	570	0	0.0	0
thick and zesty	1/4 cup	20	1	3	340	1	0.0	0
(Del Monte)								
canned	1 cup	70	3	16	1330	0	1.0	0
no salt added	1 cup	70	3	16	50	0	1.0	0
no salt added	1/4 cup	20	0	4	20	1	0.0	0
w/onions	1 cup	100	3	23	1150	0	1.0	0
(Eden Foods) lightly seasoned, organic	1/4 cup	25	1	5	45	1	0.0	0
(Finast)								
	1/2 cup	45	2	9	650	0	0.0	0
no salt added	8 oz	90	4	18	10	0	0.0	0
(Health Valley)								
	1 cup	70	2	13	460	0	0.5	0
no salt added	1 cup	70	2	13	43	0	0.5	0
(Hunt's)								
	1/4 cup	16	1	3	366	1	0.2	0
canned 'Special'	4 oz	35	1	8	320	0	0.0	0
canned	4 oz	30	1	7	730	0	0.0	0
'Casera'	2.19 oz	22	1	5	293	1	0.1	0
chunky tomato	2.19 oz	13	1	3	405	1	0.1	0
food service product	1/4 cup	15	1	3	360	1	0.2	0
hot, 'Maya'	1.06 oz	6	0	1	174	0	0.2	0
Italian style	1/4 cup	33	1	5	210	1	1.2	0

Food Name	Serv. Size	Total Cal.	Prot. gms	Carbs gms	Sod. mgs	Fiber gms	Fat gms	Chol. mgs
Italian style	4 oz	60	2	11	520	0	2.0	0
'Meatloaf Fixin's'	2 oz	20	1	5	580	1	1.0	0
no salt added	1/4 cup	16	1	3	12	1	0.2	0
w/garlic	4 oz	70	2	10	480	2	2.0	0
w/herbs	1/4 cup	32	1	5	271	1	1.0	0
w/mushrooms	4 oz	25	1	6	710	2	1.0	0
w/onions	4 oz	40	1	9	650	2	1.0	0
w/tomato bits	4 oz	30	1	7	620	2	1.0	0
(Old El Paso)								
w/green chilies	1/4 cup	14	1	3	480	0	1.0	0
w/jalapeños	1/4 cup	11	1	2	150	0	1.0	0
(Pathmark)								
	1/2 cup	40	2	9	620	0	0.0	0
marinara, 'No Frills'	1/2 cup	80	1	12	620	0	3.0	0
no salt added	1/2 cup	45	2	9	25	0	0.0	0
(Progresso)	1/4 cup	20	1	4	260	1	0.0	0
(Rokeach)								
Italian style	3 oz	60	1	8	243	0	2.0	0
low-sodium	3 oz	50	1	8	124	0	2.0	0
marinara	3 oz	60	1	9	257	0	2.0	0
(S&W)	1/4 cup	20	1	4	300	1	0.0	0
(Stokely)	1/2 cup	30	2	7	810	0	0.0	0
TOMATOSEED OIL								
	1 cup	1927	0	0	0	0	218.0	0
	1 tbsp	120	0	0	0	0	13.6	0

TONIC WATER. See under SOFT DRINKS AND MIXERS.
TOPPING. See individual listings.
TORSK. See CUSK.

TORTELLINI DISH/ENTRÉE

Food Name	Serv. Size	Total Cal.	Prot. gms	Carbs gms	Sod. mgs	Fiber gms	Fat gms	Chol. mgs
(Bernardi)								
cheese	1 cup	260	13	40	400	4	6.0	20
cheese, w/spinach pasta	1 cup	280	13	40	320	2	8.0	30
cheese, tortelloni	1 cup	260	13	40	400	4	6.0	20
meat filled, precooked	1 cup	250	11	38	490	2	6.0	40
meat filled, w/raw pasta	1 cup	280	12	41	460	1	8.0	20
(Contadina)								
cheese	3/4 cup	261	13	39	331	3	6.0	45
cheese and basil	1 cup	360	16	49	380	3	11.0	65
chicken and prosciutto, tortelloni	1 cup	360	15	46	440	3	13.0	75
chicken and vegetable	3/4 cup	259	10	39	219	2	7.0	45
garlic and cheese, light	1 cup	280	15	50	390	3	5.0	55
sausage and bell pepper, tortelloni, spicy	1 cup	330	13	47	290	3	10.0	90
(Mona's) cheese, frozen	1 cup	370	17	50	490	1	11.0	30
(Weight Watchers) cheese, frozen	9 oz	310	14	50	570	0	6.0	15
(Stouffer's) cheese, w/Alfredo sauce, frozen	8 7/8 oz	580	26	35	830	0	37.0	0
(Tofutti) meatless, frozen	2 oz	220	12	38	110	0	2.0	0

TORTELLONI ENTRÉE. See under TORTELLINI DISH/ENTRÉE.

TORTILLA

Food Name	Serv. Size	Total Cal.	Prot. gms	Carbs gms	Sod. mgs	Fiber gms	Fat gms	Chol. mgs
corn, no salt added, ready to bake or fry	1 oz	63	2	13	3	1	0.7	0
corn, no salt added, ready-to-bake or fry, 6-inch diam	1 tortilla	58	1	12	3	1	0.7	0
corn, ready-to-bake or fry	1 oz	63	2	13	46	1	0.7	0
corn, ready-to-bake or fry, 6-inch diam	1 tortilla	58	1	12	42	1	0.7	0
flour, ready to bake or fry, 12-inch diam	1 tortilla	380	10	65	559	4	8.3	0
flour, ready to bake or fry, 10-inch diam	1 tortilla	234	6	40	344	2	5.1	0
flour, ready to bake or fry, 7–8-inch diam	1 tortilla	159	4	27	234	2	3.5	0
flour, ready to bake or fry, 6-inch diam	1 tortilla	104	3	18	153	1	2.3	0
flour, ready to bake or fry	1 oz	92	2	16	136	1	2.0	0

Food Name	Serv. Size	Total Cal.	Prot. gms	Carbs gms	Sod. mgs	Fiber gms	Fat gms	Chol. mgs
(Azteca)								
corn	1 tortilla	45	1	9	10	0	0.0	0
flour, 7-inch diam	1 tortilla	80	2	14	110	0	2.0	0
flour, 9-inch diam	1 tortilla	130	3	23	180	0	3.0	0
(Fry's) flour, fajita style, extra soft	1 tortilla	100	2	17	160	0	2.0	0
(Garcia's)								
flour, burrito style	1 tortilla	220	5	37	220	2	5.0	0
flour, fajita style	1 tortilla	100	2	17	220	1	2.5	0
wheat, 8-inch diam	1 tortilla	160	4	24	360	2	5.0	0
(LA LA'S) flour	1 tortilla	160	4	28	350	1	3.0	0
(La Tortilla)								
flour, burrito sized, 99% fat free	1 tortilla	120	4	25	350	10	0.5	0
flour, fat free	1 tortilla	60	2	13	180	6	0.0	0
whole wheat, 99% fat free	1 tortilla	60	2	12	180	9	0.0	0
(Mission)								
flour, burrito size 'Premium'	1 tortilla	230	6	40	395	0	6.0	0
flour, light	1 tortilla	70	2	16	280	4	1.0	0
flour, soft, taco size, 8-inch diam	1 tortilla	146	4	25	249	na	3.1	na
(Old El Paso)								
corn	1 tortilla	60	1	10	170	0	1.0	0
flour	1 tortilla	150	4	27	360	0	3.0	0
(Tyson)								
flour, burrito style	1 tortilla	173	5	29	40	0	4.0	0
flour, burrito style, large, heat pressed	1 tortilla	182	5	33	90	0	4.0	0
flour, burrito style, small, hand stretched	1 tortilla	106	3	19	50	0	2.0	0
flour, fajita style	1 tortilla	84	3	18	20	0	2.0	0
flour, soft, taco size	1 tortilla	121	4	20	30	0	3.0	0
TORTILLA CHIPS. See also CORN CHIPS AND SNACKS.								
(Bachman)								
....	1 oz	140	2	19	140	0	6.0	0
nacho cheese	1 oz	140	2	18	210	0	6.0	0
no salt	1 oz	140	2	19	0	0	6.0	0
(Barbara's Bakery)								
yellow corn, no salt added, organic	1 oz	140	2	18	15	0	7.0	0
yellow corn, regular, organic	1 oz	140	2	18	120	0	7.0	0
(Bearitos)								
blue corn, organic	1 oz	146	3	17	29	1	7.0	0
blue corn, organic, unsalted	1 oz	137	3	17	3	1	6.5	0
no salt added	1 oz	140	2	16	5	2	7.0	1
yellow corn, no salt added, organic	1 oz	148	2	17	2	1	7.2	0
yellow corn, organic	1 oz	143	2	18	58	1	6.4	0
(Bravos)								
nacho cheese flavored, round	1 oz	150	2	18	180	0	8.0	0
nacho cheese flavored, strips	1 oz	140	2	18	220	0	7.0	0
nacho cheese and jalapeño	1 oz	150	2	19	170	0	7.0	0
(Buenitos)								
no salt added	1 oz	150	2	18	1	4	8.0	0
'Tortilla Chips'	1 oz	150	2	18	80	4	8.0	0
(Doritos)								
approx 18 chips	1 oz	140	2	19	230	0	6.0	0
cool ranch	1 oz	140	2	18	160	1	7.0	0
cool ranch, approx 16 chips	1 oz	140	2	18	170	2	7.0	0
cool ranch, light	1 oz	120	2	21	240	0	4.0	0
'Jumpin' Jack' approx 16 chips	1 oz	140	2	18	220	2	7.0	0
nacho, spicy	1 oz	140	2	18	210	1	7.0	0
nacho cheese, approx 15 chips	1 oz	140	2	18	240	0	7.0	0
nacho cheese 'Light'	1 oz	120	2	21	290	0	4.0	0

Food Name	Serv. Size	Total Cal.	Prot. gms	Carbs gms	Sod. mgs	Fiber gms	Fat gms	Chol. mgs
'Nacho Cheesier'	1 oz	140	2	17	190	1	7.0	0
salsa and cheese, 'Thins'	1 oz	150	2	17	180	0	8.0	0
'Salsa Rio' approx 16 chips	1 oz	140	2	18	190	2	7.0	0
salsa verde	1 oz	150	2	20	210	1	7.0	0
taco, approx 16 chips	1 oz	140	2	18	250	2	7.0	0
'Taco Bell'	1 oz	150	2	21	170	1	7.0	0
toasted corn, approx 16 chips	1 oz	140	2	19	80	2	7.0	0
toasted	1 oz	140	2	18	120	1	7.0	0
white corn, lightly salted, 'Thins'	1 oz	140	2	19	135	0	7.0	0
(Eagle) ranch	1 oz	140	2	17	190	0	8.0	1
(Featherweight)								
low-salt, round	1 oz	150	2	18	10	0	8.0	0
nacho cheese, low-salt	1 oz	150	2	18	45	0	8.0	0
(Garden of Eden)								
black bean, organic	10 chips	150	3	18	55	1	7.0	0
blue corn and sunflower seed, organic	10 chips	160	3	16	70	1	8.0	0
blue corn, hot and spicy, organic	10 chips	140	2	3	80	2	7.0	0
blue corn, organic, no salt added	10 chips	150	2	18	0	1	7.0	0
blue corn, salted, organic	10 chips	150	2	18	55	1	7.0	0
chipotle, hot and smoky, organic	10 chips	120	2	23	80	1	2.0	0
unsalted, no oil added, organic	10 chips	110	2	23	10	1	1.0	0
w/jalapeño, organic	10 chips	140	2	18	80	2	7.0	0
yogurt and green onion, organic	10 chips	120	2	23	70	1	2.0	0
(Guiltless Gourmet)								
baked, original	1 oz	110	2	22	160	2	1.0	0
blue corn	1 oz	110	3	22	140	2	1.0	0
chili lime	1 oz	110	2	22	200	2	1.0	0
nacho, baked	1 oz	110	3	22	200	2	1.0	0
original, no salt added	1 oz	110	2	22	26	2	1.0	0
ranch	1 oz	110	3	22	200	2	1.0	0
white corn	1 oz	110	3	22	140	2	1.0	0
yellow corn, baked, no salt added, approx 24 chips	1 oz	110	3	22	26	3	1.0	0
yellow corn, baked, w/salt, approx 24 chips	1 oz	110	3	22	160	3	1.0	0
(Hain)								
sesame	1 oz	140	2	19	190	0	7.0	0
sesame, cheese	1 oz	160	2	20	270	0	8.0	5
sesame, no salt added	1 oz	140	2	19	0	0	7.0	5
taco	1 oz	160	2	15	320	0	11.0	5
(Keebler)								
cinnamon crispana, flour, 'Chacho's'	1 oz	140	2	19	70	0	7.0	0
original, restaurant style 'Chacho's'	1 oz	140	3	18	180	0	7.0	5
(Kettle Tias)								
blue corn, lightly salted	1 oz	140	3	18	80	2	6.0	0
blue corn, no salt added	1 oz	140	3	18	2	2	6.0	0
yellow corn, lightly salted	1 oz	140	2	19	80	2	7.0	0
yellow corn, no salt added	1 oz	140	2	19	3	2	7.0	0
(La Famous)								
no salt added	1 oz	140	2	18	5	0	7.0	0
regular	1 oz	140	2	18	180	0	7.0	0
(Laura Scudder's)								
nacho cheese, jalapeño, 'Strips'	1 oz	150	2	19	170	0	7.0	0
nacho cheese, 'Triangles'	1 oz	140	2	18	220	0	7.0	0
picante, 'Restaurant Style Strips'	1 oz	150	2	19	190	0	7.0	0
restaurant style, lightly salted	1 oz	140	2	18	90	0	7.0	0
(Louise's) 95% nonfat	1 oz	120	2	23	170	1	1.5	0
(Mexi-Snax)								
hot	12 chips	140	2	21	70	0	5.0	0

Food Name	Serv. Size	Total Cal.	Prot. gms	Carbs gms	Sod. mgs	Fiber gms	Fat gms	Chol. mgs
no salt added	12 chips	140	2	21	0	0	6.0	0
vegetable medley	12 chips	140	2	21	114	0	5.0	0
(Mi Ranchito)								
jalapeño cheddar	10 chips	140	2	20	170	1	7.0	0
spicy red chili, 'Rojo's'	10 chips	140	2	20	100	1	7.0	0
(Michael Season's)								
white corn, lightly salted	1 oz	135	3	17	120	na	6.0	0
yellow corn, lightly salted, organic	1 oz	135	2	19	120	na	5.0	0
yellow corn, organic	1 oz	135	2	19	80	na	5.0	0
(Old El Paso)								
crispy, approx 16 chips	1 oz	150	2	17	105	1	8.0	0
'NaChips' approx 9 chips	1 oz	150	2	18	80	2	7.0	0
white corn, low-sodium, round, 'NaChips'	1 oz	160	2	17	5	0	9.0	0
(Planters)								
nacho cheese	1 oz	150	2	18	160	0	8.0	0
traditional	1 oz	150	2	18	150	0	8.0	0
(Santitas)								
food service product, 'Restaurant Strips'	1 oz	140	2	19	60	1	6.0	0
100% white corn	1 oz	140	2	19	80	1	6.0	0
restaurant style	1 oz	140	2	19	50	1	6.0	0
(Slimchips) nonfat, approx 10 chips	0.4 oz	44	1	10	60	1	0.5	0
(Tio Sancho) 'Microwave Snacks'	4 oz	567	9	74	590	4	26.1	0
(Tostitos)								
approx 11 chips	1 oz	140	2	18	170	0	8.0	0
baked	1 oz	110	2	24	200	2	1.0	0
bite-size	1 oz	140	2	17	110	1	8.0	0
lime and chile	1 oz	150	2	17	180	1	7.0	0
nacho cheese, sharp, approx 11 chips	1 oz	150	2	17	200	0	8.0	0
restaurant style	1 oz	140	2	19	110	1	6.0	0
rounds	1 oz	150	1	18	85	1	8.0	0
unsalted	1 oz	110	3	24	0	2	1.0	0
white corn, baked, 'Cool Ranch'	1 oz	130	2	21	170	0	3.0	0
(Vera Cruz)								
tortilla rounds, baked	1 oz	120	2	22	78	2	1.5	0
tortilla rounds, baked, unsalted	1 oz	120	2	22	0	2	1.5	0
(Wise) nacho cheese flavored, crispy, round	1 oz	150	2	18	180	0	8.0	0
TORULA YEAST. See under YEAST.								
TOSTACO SHELL *(Old El Paso)*	1 shell	100	1	11	10	1	5.0	0
TOSTADA CHIPS								
(Michael Season's) yellow corn, lightly salted, bite-sized	1 oz	135	2	19	120	na	5.0	0
TOSTADA SHELL								
(Bearitos) yellow corn	1 shell	140	2	17	0	2	7.0	0
(Lawry's)	1 shell	73	1	10	147	0	3.5	0
(Ortega)	1 shell	50	0	8	5	0	2.0	0
(Pancho Villa)	1 shell	55	1	6	65	0	3.0	0
(Rosarita)								
	1 shell	63	1	9	10	0	2.4	18
1-oz shell	2 shells	138	2	17	88	4	7.6	0
(Tio Sancho)	1 shell	67	1	8	1	1	3.2	0
TOWELGOURD. See GOURD, DISHCLOTH.								
TRAIL MIX SNACK								
(Harmony)								
'Deluxe Super'	1/4 cup	150	3	23	35	3	7.0	0
nut and berry mix	1/4 cup	160	5	21	0	3	8.0	0
(Maranatha Natural)								
'Deluxe'	1/4 cup	150	5	13	5	3	9.0	0
'Mountain Delight'	1/4 cup	140	5	15	30	3	8.0	0

Food Name	Serv. Size	Total Cal.	Prot. gms	Carbs gms	Sod. mgs	Fiber gms	Fat gms	Chol. mgs
'Nature Trail'	1/4 cup	150	4	15	0	2	9.0	0
'Snack Attack'	1/4 cup	140	2	16	0	2	8.0	0
(Pacific Shores) all fruit	1/4 cup	110	0	21	20	2	2.0	0
(Pilgram Joe's) cranberry	1/4 cup	150	5	12	5	3	9.0	0
(Trader Joe's)								
'Muir Trail Mix'	1/4 cup	180	7	11	0	2	13.0	0
w/carob chips, 'Mt. Baldy Mix'	1/4 cup	190	0	15	5	3	14.0	0
TREE FERN								
cooked, chopped	1/2 cup	28	0	8	4	3	0.1	0
cooked, whole, 6.5-inch long	1 frond	12	0	3	2	1	0.0	0
TREE MUSHROOM. See MUSHROOM, OYSTER.								
TRITICALE	1 cup	645	25	138	10	na	4.0	0
TROUT								
MIXED SPECIES								
baked, broiled, grilled, or microwaved	3 oz	162	23	0	57	0	7.2	63
raw	3 oz	126	18	0	44	0	5.6	49
RAINBOW								
farmed, baked, broiled, grilled, or microwaved	3 oz	144	21	0	36	0	6.1	58
farmed, raw	3 oz	117	18	0	30	0	4.6	50
wild, baked, broiled, grilled, or microwaved	3 oz	128	19	0	48	0	4.9	59
wild, raw	3 oz	101	17	0	26	0	2.9	50
SEA								
mixed species, baked, broiled, grilled, or microwaved	3 oz	113	18	0	63	0	3.9	90
mixed species, raw	3 oz	88	14	0	49	0	3.1	71
TUNA								
Canned								
in oil, drained	3 oz	158	23	0	337	0	6.9	26
in water, drained	3 oz	99	22	0	287	0	0.7	26
in water, no salt added, drained	3 oz	99	22	0	43	0	0.7	26
solid, in olive oil (Progresso)	1/4 cup	160	0	0	250	0	12.0	30
very low sodium (Chicken of the Sea)	2 oz	60	13	0	35	0	0.5	25
Frozen, steak, w/o seasoning mix (SeaPak)	6 oz pkg	180	40	0	65	0	2.0	75
ALBACORE								
Canned								
solid white, in soybean oil, drained (Bumble Bee)	2 oz	100	14	0	310	0	8.0	30
solid white, in soybean oil, drained (Finast)	2 oz	145	14	1	320	0	10.0	0
solid white, in soybean oil, drained (S&W)	2 oz	160	13	0	450	0	12.0	0
solid white, in soybean oil, drained (Star-Kist)	2 oz	140	14	1	310	0	10.0	25
solid white, in spring water, fancy (Chicken of the Sea)	2 oz	60	14	1	250	0	1.0	0
solid white, in water, drained (A&P)	2 oz	70	15	1	310	0	1.0	0
solid white, in water, drained (Bumble Bee)	2 oz	60	14	0	310	0	2.0	30
solid white, in water, drained (Finast)	2 oz	70	15	1	310	0	1.0	0
solid white, in water, drained (Pathmark)	2 oz	70	15	0	310	0	2.0	0
solid white, in water, drained (Star-Kist)	2 oz	70	15	1	310	0	1.0	25
solid white, in water, drained (Weight Watchers)	2 oz	70	15	1	210	0	1.0	25
Frozen								
steak, white, boneless/skinless, raw								
(Peter Pan Seafoods)	3.5 oz	102	19	0	51	0	4.9	54
BLUEFIN								
Fresh								
baked, broiled, grilled, or microwaved	3 oz	156	25	0	43	0	5.3	42
raw	3 oz	122	20	0	33	0	4.2	32
CHUNK LIGHT								
Canned								
in Canola oil (Chicken of the Sea)	2 oz	110	13	0	250	0	6.0	30
in oil (S&W)	3 oz	167	21	0	349	0	9.1	46
in vegetable oil, w/liquid (Chicken of the Sea)	2 oz	160	12	1	250	0	12.0	0

Food Name	Serv. Size	Total Cal.	Prot. gms	Carbs gms	Sod. mgs	Fiber gms	Fat gms	Chol. mgs
in soybean oil, drained *(Bumble Bee)*	2 oz	110	12	0	310	0	12.0	30
in soybean oil, drained *(Finast)*	2 oz	150	13	1	310	0	13.0	0
in soybean oil, drained *(Star-Kist)*	2 oz	150	13	1	310	0	13.0	25
in soybean oil, drained, 'Fancy' *(S&W)*	2 oz	140	13	0	450	0	10.0	0
in water *(Captains Choice)*	3 oz	90	18	0	465	0	2.0	0
in water *(Chicken of the Sea)*	2 oz	60	13	0	250	0	0.5	30
in water *(S&W)*	3 oz	106	23	0	349	0	0.8	53
in water, diet, drained *(Star-Kist)*	2 oz	65	14	1	35	0	1.0	25
in water, drained *(Bumble Bee)*	2 oz	50	12	0	310	0	1.0	30
in water, drained *(Featherweight)*	2 oz	60	13	0	30	0	1.0	30
in water, drained *(Finast)*	2 oz	60	13	1	310	0	1.0	0
in water, drained *(Pathmark)*	2 oz	70	15	0	310	0	2.0	0
in water, drained *(Star-Kist)*	2 oz	60	13	1	310	0	1.0	25
in water, drained, 'Fancy' *(S&W)*	2 oz	60	13	0	500	0	1.0	0
in water, low-sodium *(Chicken of the Sea)*	2 oz	60	14	0	90	0	0.5	30
in water, no salt added, drained *(Weight Watchers)*	2 oz	60	14	1	210	0	1.0	25
in water, 60% less salt, drained *(Star-Kist)*	2 oz	65	14	1	120	0	1.0	25
CHUNK WHITE								
Canned								
in soybean oil, drained *(Bumble Bee)*	2 oz	110	12	0	310	0	12.0	30
in water *(Chicken of the Sea)*	2 oz	60	13	0	250	0	1.0	25
in water, diet, drained *(Star-Kist)*	2 oz	70	15	1	30	0	1.0	25
in water, drained *(A&P)*	2 oz	100	12	1	310	0	5.0	0
in water, drained *(Bumble Bee)*	2 oz	60	12	0	310	0	2.0	30
in water, 60% less salt, drained *(Star-Kist)*	2 oz	70	15	1	120	0	1.0	25
LIGHT								
Canned								
in oil, drained	3 oz	168	25	0	301	0	7.0	15
in oil, no salt added, drained	3 oz	168	25	0	43	0	7.0	15
in soybean oil, drained *(A&P)*	2 oz	150	13	1	310	0	13.0	0
in water, drained *(A&P)*	2 oz	60	13	1	310	0	1.0	0
in water, drained *(Empress)*	2 oz	60	12	0	310	0	1.0	0
SKIPJACK/aku/katsuo/oceanic bonito								
Fresh								
baked, broiled, grilled, or microwaved	3 oz	112	24	0	40	0	1.1	51
raw	3 oz	88	19	0	31	0	0.9	40
SOLID LIGHT								
Canned								
in Canola oil *(Chicken of the Sea)*	2 oz	90	14	0	250	0	3.0	25
in oil *(S&W)*	3 oz	121	26	0	349	0	2.3	30
in soybean oil, drained *(Star-Kist)*	2 oz	150	13	1	310	0	13.0	25
in soybean oil, drained, solid *(Progresso)*	1/3 cup	150	13	1	400	0	13.0	0
in water *(Chicken of the Sea)*	2 oz	70	15	0	250	0	1.0	25
in water, drained *(Star-Kist)*	2 oz	60	14	1	310	0	1.0	25
in water, drained, 'Prime Catch' *(Star-Kist)*	2 oz	60	14	1	310	0	1.0	25
SOLID WHITE								
Canned								
in soybean oil, drained *(Star-Kist)*	2 oz	140	14	1	310	0	10.0	25
in water *(Captains Choice)*	2 oz	70	15	0	250	0	1.0	25
WHITE								
Canned								
in oil, no salt added, drained	3 oz	158	23	0	43	0	6.9	26
in soybean oil, drained *(A&P)*	2 oz	150	13	1	310	0	10.0	0
in water, drained	3 oz	109	20	0	320	0	2.5	36
in water, no salt added, drained	3 oz	109	20	0	43	0	2.5	36
YELLOWFIN/ahi								
Fresh								
baked, broiled, grilled, or microwaved	3 oz	118	25	0	40	0	1.0	49

Food Name	Serv. Size	Total Cal.	Prot. gms	Carbs gms	Sod. mgs	Fiber gms	Fat gms	Chol. mgs
raw	3 oz	92	20	0	31	0	0.8	38
raw boneless	1 oz	31	7	0	10	0	0.3	13
Frozen								
steak, boneless, skinless, raw *(Peter Pan Seafoods)*	3.5 oz	131	23	0	61	0	4.1	45
TUNA DISH/ENTRÉE								
(Banquet) pie, frozen	7 oz	540	17	44	810	0	33.0	30
(Marie Callender's) chunky tuna and noodles	12 oz	960	18	43	1570	6	35.0	55
(Stouffer's)								
tuna-noodle casserole	1 entrée	320	20	37	1130	0	10.0	40
tuna-noodle casserole, frozen, food service product	1 oz	35	2	3	126	0	1.9	4
(Weight Watchers) tuna-noodle casserole	1 entrée	270	13	39	590	4	7.0	35
TUNA DISH/ENTRÉE MIX								
(Tuna Helper)								
au gratin meal, mix only	1/2 cup	190	6	34	730	1	3.5	3
au gratin meal, prepared	1 cup	300	13	37	890	1	11.0	20
buttery rice, prepared	1/5 pkg	160	4	32	830	0	2.0	0
cheesy pasta meal, mix only	3/4 cup	170	5	29	710	1	3.0	3
cheesy pasta meal, prepared	1 cup	280	14	32	890	1	11.0	20
creamy broccoli, prepared	1/5 pkg	200	6	35	800	0	4.0	0
creamy mushroom, prepared	1/5 pkg	140	5	28	580	0	1.0	0
creamy pasta meal, mix only	3/4 cup	190	5	29	730	1	6.0	3
creamy pasta meal, prepared	1 cup	300	14	31	910	1	13.0	20
fettuccine Alfredo meal, mix only	3/4 cup	170	5	30	730	1	3.5	0
fettuccine Alfredo meal, prepared	1 cup	310	14	32	950	1	14.0	15
pasta salad, prepared	1/5 pkg	140	5	28	580	0	1.0	0
pot pie, prepared	1/2 cup	340	5	35	920	1	20.0	0
pot pie, prepared	1/6 pkg	290	4	31	730	0	17.0	0
Romanoff meal, mix only	2/3 cup	210	7	38	650	1	3.0	5
Romanoff meal, prepared	1 cup	280	15	38	800	1	8.0	20
tetrazzini meal, mix only	2/3 cup	180	7	32	790	1	3.0	5
tetrazzini meal, prepared	1 cup	310	17	33	1010	1	12.0	20
TUNA SALAD SPREAD *(Libby's)* 'Spreadables'	1/3 cup	130	7	6	370	3	8.0	15
TUNA SUBSTITUTE								
(Natural Touch) vegetarian, 'Tuno'	1/3 cup drained	60	7	2	360	1	2.0	0
(Worthington)								
vegetarian, 'Tuno' 12-oz can	1/3 cup drained	80	7	4	380	1	4.0	0
vegetarian, 'Tuno' 12-oz roll	1/2 cup drained	80	6	2	290	1	6.0	0
TUNKA. See GOURD, WHITE.								
TURBOT, EUROPEAN								
baked, broiled, grilled, or microwaved	3 oz	104	17	0	163	0	3.2	53
raw	3 oz	81	14	0	128	0	2.5	41
TURKEY								
BACK								
Fresh								
all classes, meat and skin, raw	1 lb	896	81.6	0.0	304	0	59.2	336
all classes, meat and skin, raw	1 oz	56	5.1	0.0	19	0	3.7	21
all classes, meat and skin, roasted	4 oz	276	30.2	0.0	83	0	16.3	103
fryer/roaster, meat and skin, raw	4 oz	173	22.5	0	69	0	8.3	98
fryer/roaster, meat and skin, roasted	4 oz	233	30.0	0	80	0	11.7	123
fryer/roaster, meat only, raw	4 oz	137	23.6	0	75	0	4.0	85
fryer/roaster, meat only, roasted	4 oz	194	32.0	0	83	0	6.5	109
young hen, meat and skin, raw	4 oz	252	20.1	0	71	0	18.4	79
young hen, meat and skin, roasted	4 oz	290	30.0	0	79	0	17.9	97
young tom, meat and skin, raw	4 oz	205	21.2	0	81	0	12.7	90
young tom, meat and skin, roasted	4 oz	272	30.7	0	88	0	15.6	107
BREAST								
Fresh								
all classes, meat and skin, raw	1 lb	720	99.2	0.0	272	0	32.0	288

Food Name	Serv. Size	Total Cal.	Prot. gms	Carbs gms	Sod. mgs	Fiber gms	Fat gms	Chol. mgs
all classes, meat and skin, raw	1 oz	45	32.6	0.0	71	0	8.4	84
all classes, meat and skin, roasted	4 oz	214	32.6	0.0	71	0	8.4	84
fryer/roaster, meat and skin, raw	4 oz	152	27.2	0	55	0	3.0	80
fryer/roaster, meat and skin, roasted	4 oz	175	33.2	0	60	0	3.7	103
fryer/roaster, meat and skin, pre-basted, roasted	4 oz	114	25.7	0	454	0	4.0	48
young hen, meat and skin, raw	4 oz	191	24.7	0	63	0	9.5	71
young hen, meat and skin, roasted	4 oz	222	33.0	0	66	0	9.0	82
young tom, meat and skin, raw	4 oz	173	25.1	0	72	0	7.2	77
young tom, meat and skin, roasted	4 oz	216	32.7	0	77	0	8.4	86
Frozen or refrigerated								
barbecue, quartered *(Mr. Turkey)*	3.5 oz	95	21	1	901	0	0.8	35
cooked *(Land O'Lakes)*	3 oz	100	20	0	55	0	1.0	50
cooked *(Louis Rich)*	1 oz	47	8	0	21	0	1.5	21
cooked, 'Cook-N-Bag' *(Longacre)*	1 oz	38	8	1	85	0	1.0	15
cooked, 'Fresh Turkey Cuts' *(Louis Rich)*	1 oz	45	8	1	20	0	2.0	20
8% self-basting solution *(Jennie-O)*	4 oz	160	22	0	200	0	8.0	65
hen, cooked, w/o wings *(Louis Rich)*	1 oz	50	8	0	19	0	2.0	19
hickory smoked, cooked *(Louis Rich)*	1 oz	33	5	1	346	0	1.0	13
honey roasted, cooked *(Louis Rich)*	1 oz	33	5	1	318	0	0.8	12
oven-roasted, cooked *(Louis Rich)*	1 oz	31	5	0	296	0	0.9	13
raw, 'Cook-N-Bag' *(Longacre)*	1 oz	27	6	1	120	0	1.0	10
raw, 'Ready-to-Cook' *(Longacre)*	1 oz	39	8	0	150	0	1.0	0
raw, 'Tasti-Lean Tenders' *(Norbest)*	4 oz	135	28	0	81	0	2.0	0
roast, cooked *(Louis Rich)*	1 oz	42	8	0	20	0	0.8	19
roast, cooked, 'Fresh Turkey Cuts' *(Louis Rich)*	1 oz	40	8	1	20	0	1.0	20
slices, cooked *(Louis Rich)*	1 oz	39	8	0	24	0	0.5	17
smoked, cooked *(Louis Rich)*	1 oz	33	6	0	268	0	1.0	11
smoked, cooked, no bone *(Norbest)*	1 oz	42	6	0	218	0	1.6	0
steaks, cooked *(Louis Rich)*	1 oz	39	8	0	24	0	0.5	17
steaks, cooked, 'Fresh Turkey Cuts' *(Louis Rich)*	1 oz	40	8	1	25	0	1.0	20
steaks, cubed, raw *(Norbest)*	4 oz	135	28	0	81	0	2.0	0
strips and tips, raw, 'Tasti-Lean' *(Norbest)*	4 oz	135	28	0	81	0	2.0	0
tenderloins, cooked *(Louis Rich)*	1 oz	39	9	0	24	0	0.5	18
tenderloins, cooked, 'Fresh Turkey Cuts' *(Louis Rich)*	1 oz	40	8	1	25	0	1.0	20
COMPOSITE CUTS								
Canned								
chunk *(Hormel)*	6 3/4 oz	230	37	0	1278	0	10.0	0
chunk *(Swanson)*	1 cup	360	64	16	880	4	8.0	140
in broth, drained	5-oz can	231	34	0	663	0	9.7	94
puréed *(Bryan Foods)*	1/3 cup	160	13	0	45	na	11.0	50
CUTLET								
Frozen or refrigerated, raw, 'Tasti-Lean' *(Norbest)*	4 oz	135	28	0	81	0	2.0	0
DARK MEAT								
Fresh								
all classes, meat and skin, raw	1 lb	720	86.4	0.0	320	0	40.0	320
all classes, meat and skin, raw	1 oz	45	5.4	0.0	20	0	2.5	20
all classes, meat and skin, roasted	4 oz	251	31.2	0.0	86	0	13.1	101
all classes, meat only, raw	1 lb	560	91.2	0.0	352	0	19.2	320
all classes, meat only, raw	1 oz	35	5.7	0.0	22	0	1.2	20
all classes, meat only, roasted	4 oz	212	32.4	0.0	90	0	8.2	96
all classes, meat only, roasted, chopped or diced	1 cup	262	40.0	0.0	111	0	10.1	119
fryer/roaster, meat and skin, raw	4 oz	147	23.0	0	75	0	5.5	99
fryer/roaster, meat and skin, roasted	4 oz	208	31.8	0	87	0	8.1	134
fryer/roaster, meat only, raw	4 oz	114	23.4	0	79	0	3.1	93
fryer/roaster, meat only, roasted	4 oz	184	32.7	0	90	0	5.0	128
fryer/roaster, meat only, roasted, chopped or diced	1 cup	227	40.0	0	111	0	6.0	157
young hen, meat and skin, raw	4 oz	196	21.1	0	77	0	11.7	74

Food Name	Serv. Size	Total Cal.	Prot. gms	Carbs gms	Sod. mgs	Fiber gms	Fat gms	Chol. mgs
young hen, meat and skin, roasted .... 4 oz		265	31.3	0	82	0	14.6	96
young hen, meat only, raw .... 4 oz		149	22.9	0	84	0	5.5	71
young hen, meat only, roasted .... 4 oz		220	22.9	0	62	0	6.3	65
young hen, meat only, roasted, chopped or diced .... 1 cup		269	40.0	0	105	0	10.9	112
young tom, meat and skin, raw .... 4 oz		174	21.8	0	86	0	9.0	88
young tom, meat and skin, roasted .... 4 oz		235	31.0	0	91	0	12.4	104
young tom, meat only, raw .... 4 oz		141	23.2	0	91	0	4.7	86
young tom, meat only, roasted .... 4 oz		212	33.0	0	94	0	8.0	100
GIBLETS								
Fresh								
all classes, raw .... 4 oz		150	22	2.4	101	0	4.8	328
all classes, raw .... 1/2 oz		21	3	0	14	0	0.7	45
all classes, w/fat, simmered .... 0.35 oz		17	3	0	6	0	0.5	42
all classes, w/fat, simmered, chopped or diced .... 1 cup		242	39	3	86	0	7.4	606
GIZZARD								
Fresh								
all classes, raw .... 1 med gizzard		132	22	1	90	0	4.2	179
all classes, raw .... 1/4 oz		8	1	0	6	0	0.3	11
all classes, simmered .... 0.14 oz		7	1	0	2	0	0.2	9
all classes, simmered, chopped or diced .... 1 cup		236	43	1	78	0	5.6	336
GROUND								
Fresh								
all classes, breaded, battered, fried .... 3.33-oz patty		266	13	15	752	0	16.9	58
all classes, breaded, battered, fried .... 2.25-oz patty		181	9	10	512	0	11.5	40
all classes, cooked .... 4-oz patty		193	22	0	88	0	10.8	84
all classes, raw .... 4-oz patty		170	20	0	107	0	9.4	90
Frozen or refrigerated								
(Louis Rich) .... 4 oz		190	20	0	140	0	12.0	90
(Mr. Turkey) .... 1 oz		54	5	0	27	0	4.0	20
burger patty (Shelton's) .... 1 serving		170	20	0	110	0	10.0	90
cooked (Hudson) .... 1 oz		55	5	0	35	0	3.7	0
cooked (Longacre) .... 1 oz		60	5	0	20	0	4.0	30
extra lean, 97% fat-free (Turkey Store) .... 4 oz		120	27	0	75	0	1.5	55
lean, 7% fat, w/natural flavorings (Turkey Store) .... 4 oz		160	23	0	80	0	8.0	70
raw (Norbest) .... 1 oz		45	5	0	34	0	2.6	0
w/natural flavoring (Louis Rich) .... 1 oz		50	8	0	33	0	2.2	24
HEART								
Fresh								
all classes, raw .... 1 med heart		41	5	0	25	0	2.0	33
all classes, simmered, chopped or diced .... 1 cup		257	39	3	80	0	8.8	328
HINDQUARTER								
Frozen or refrigerated, roast (Land O'Lakes) .... 3 oz		140	17	0	80	0	8.0	0
LEG								
Fresh								
all classes, meat and skin, raw .... 1 lb		656	88.0	0.0	336	0	30.4	320
all classes, meat and skin, raw .... 1 oz		41	5.5	0.0	21	0	1.9	320
all classes, meat and skin, roasted .... 4 oz		236	31.6	0.0	87	0	11.1	96
fryer/roaster, meat and skin, raw .... 4 oz		135	23	0	78	0	4.0	99
fryer/roaster, meat and skin, roasted .... 4 oz		194	32.7	0	91	0	6.2	80
fryer/roaster, meat only, raw .... 4 oz		123	23.3	0	81	0	2.7	96
fryer/roaster, meat only, roasted .... 4 oz		182	33.2	0	92	0	4.3	136
young hen, meat and skin, raw .... 4 oz		173	21.8	0	81	0	8.6	72
young hen, meat and skin, roasted .... 4 oz		235	32.7	0	91	0	11.0	103
Frozen or refrigerated								
(Land O'Lakes). .... 3 oz		120	17	0	85	0	5.0	0
cooked (Louis Rich) .... 1 oz		56	8	0	22	0	2.6	27
cooked, 'Fresh Turkey Cuts' (Louis Rich) .... 1 oz		55	8	1	25	0	3.0	30

Food Name	Serv. Size	Total Cal.	Prot. gms	Carbs gms	Sod. mgs	Fiber gms	Fat gms	Chol. mgs
LIGHT MEAT								
Canned								
chunk white, in water, 97% fat-free *(Valley Fresh)*	2 oz	80	16	0	150	0	1.5	55
white meat *(Swanson)*	2.5 oz	80	17	1	260	0	1.0	0
Fresh								
all classes, meat and skin, raw	1 lb	720	97.6	0.0	272	0	33.6	288
all classes, meat and skin, raw	1 oz	45	6.1	0.0	17	0	2.1	18
all classes, meat and skin, roasted	4 oz	223	32.4	0.0	71	0	9.4	86
all classes, meat only, raw	1 lb	528	107.2	0.0	288	0	6.4	272
all classes, meat only, raw	1 oz	33	6.7	0.0	18	0	0.4	17
all classes, meat only, roasted	4 oz	178	33.9	0.0	73	0	3.7	78
all classes, meat only, roasted, chopped or diced	1 cup	220	41.9	0.0	90	0	4.5	97
fryer/roaster, meat and skin, raw	4 oz	152	26.5	0	57	0	4.4	87
fryer/roaster, meat and skin, roasted	4 oz	188	33	0	65	0	5.2	109
fryer/roaster, meat only, raw	4 oz	123	27.6	0	59	0	0.6	75
fryer/roaster, meat only, roasted	4 oz	160	34.1	0	64	0	1.3	98
fryer/roaster, meat only, roasted, chopped or diced	1 cup	196	42	0	78	0	1.7	120
young hen, meat and skin, raw	4 oz	189	24.8	0	63	0	9.3	71
young hen, meat and skin, roasted	4 oz	237	32.5	0	66	0	10.8	84
young hen, meat only, raw	4 oz	133	27.2	0	68	0	1.9	66
young hen, meat only, roasted	4 oz	184	34.6	0	68	0	4.3	78
young hen, meat only, roasted, chopped or diced	1 cup	225	42.0	0	84	0	5.2	95
young tom, meat and skin, raw	4 oz	179	25.0	0	72	0	8.0	77
young tom, meat and skin, roasted	4 oz	218	32.8	0	76	0	8.8	86
young tom, meat only, raw	4 oz	131	26.7	0	76	0	1.8	71
young tom, meat only, roasted	4 oz	176	34.1	0	78	0	3.3	79
LIVER								
Fresh								
all classes, raw	3.5 oz	140	20	4	98	0	4.0	475
all classes, raw	0.25 oz	10	1	0	7	0	0.3	33
all classes, simmered	0.18 oz	8	1	0	3	0	0.3	31
all classes, simmered, chopped or diced	1 cup	237	34	5	90	0	8.3	876
NECK								
Fresh								
all classes, raw	1 lb	608	91.2	0.0	416	0	24.0	352
all classes, raw	1 oz	38	5.7	0.0	26	0	1.5	22
all classes, simmered	4 oz	204	30.4	0.0	64	0	8.2	138
PATTY								
Frozen or refrigerated, kosher *(Empire Kosher)*	1 patty	200	13	14	280	1	10.0	5
SKIN								
Fresh								
all classes, raw	1 lb	1760	57.6	0.0	160	0	168.0	576
all classes, raw	1 oz	110	3.6	0.0	10	0	10.5	26
all classes, roasted	1 oz	125	5.6	0.0	15	0	11.2	32
fryer/roaster, raw	4 oz	325	18.0	0	39	0	26.8	159
fryer/roaster, roasted	4 oz	343	23.5	0	71	0	26.6	165
young hen, raw	4 oz	476	13.5	0	37	0	46.4	93
young hen, roasted	4 oz	551	21.6	0	50	0	50.8	121
young tom, raw	4 oz	421	15.7	0	45	0	39.4	108
young tom, roasted	4 oz	482	21.4	0	68	0	42.5	132
THIGH								
Frozen or refrigerated								
(Land O'Lakes).	3 oz	150	17	0	75	0	10.0	0
cooked *(Louis Rich)*	1 oz	64	8	0	20	0	3.7	27
cooked, 'Fresh Turkey Cuts' *(Louis Rich)*	1 oz	65	7	1	20	0	4.0	30
WHOLE								
Frozen or refrigerated								
barbecue, kosher *(Empire Kosher)*	5 oz	250	35	0	320	0	12.0	100

Food Name	Serv. Size	Total Cal.	Prot. gms	Carbs gms	Sod. mgs	Fiber gms	Fat gms	Chol. mgs
cooked, excluding giblets, 'Fresh Whole Turkey'								
(Louis Rich)	1 oz	50	8	1	25	0	2.0	25
cooked, no bone (Norbest)	1 oz	42	6	0	105	0	1.5	0
cooked, w/o giblets (Louis Rich)	1 oz	52	8	0	23	0	2.3	22
young (Land O'Lakes) frozen/refrig., young	3 oz	130	17	1	55	0	7.0	65
young, butter-basted (Land O'Lakes)	3 oz	140	17	1	135	0	8.0	85
young, self-basting, broth (Land O'Lakes)	3 oz	120	18	1	145	0	5.0	77
young, 3% self-basting solution, 'Natural Choice'								
(Jennie-O)	4 oz	170	22	0	120	0	8.0	85

WING

Fresh

Food Name	Serv. Size	Total Cal.	Prot. gms	Carbs gms	Sod. mgs	Fiber gms	Fat gms	Chol. mgs
all classes, meat and skin, raw	1 lb	896	91.2	0.0	256	0	56.0	320
all classes, meat and skin, raw	1 oz	56	5.7	0.0	16	0	3.5	20
all classes, meat and skin, roasted	4 oz	260	31.0	0.0	69	0	14.1	92
fryer/roaster, meat and skin, raw	3 oz	136	19.0	0	48	0	6.7	83
fryer/roaster, meat and skin, roasted	3 oz	178	24	0	62	0	8.6	99
fryer/roaster, meat only, raw	3 oz	92	19.8	0	56	0	1.0	69
fryer/roaster, meat only, roasted	3 oz	141	25.2	0	66	0	3.0	9
young hen, meat and skin, raw	3 oz	181	16.7	0	43	0	11.9	55
young hen, meat and skin, roasted	3 oz	205	24.5	0	49	0	11.6	67
young tom, meat and skin, raw	3 oz	160	17.1	0	51	0	9.7	63
young tom, meat and skin, roasted	3 oz	188	24.5	0	57	0	9.8	69

Frozen or refrigerated

Food Name	Serv. Size	Total Cal.	Prot. gms	Carbs gms	Sod. mgs	Fiber gms	Fat gms	Chol. mgs
(Land O'Lakes).	3 oz	120	18	0	65	0	5.0	0
cooked (Louis Rich)	1 oz	54	7	0	20	0	2.7	31
cooked, 'Drumettes' (Louis Rich)	1 oz	51	8	0	20	0	2.2	29
cooked, 'Fresh Turkey Cuts' (Louis Rich)	1 oz	55	7	1	20	0	3.0	30
portions, cooked (Louis Rich)	1 oz	54	7	0	17	0	2.9	29

TURKEY DINNER/ENTRÉE

Food Name	Serv. Size	Total Cal.	Prot. gms	Carbs gms	Sod. mgs	Fiber gms	Fat gms	Chol. mgs
(Armour) w/dressing and gravy, frozen, 'Classics'	11.5 oz	320	19	34	1280	0	12.0	50
(Banquet)								
pie, frozen	7 oz	510	16	39	860	0	31.0	40
pie, frozen, 'Supreme Microwave'	7 oz	430	15	30	740	0	27.0	35
sliced, w/gravy, frozen, 'Cookin' Bags'	5 oz	100	7	5	0	0	6.0	0
sliced, w/gravy, frozen, 'Family Entrées'	8 oz	150	12	8	0	0	8.0	0
turkey entrée, frozen	1 entrée	280	14	34	1060	3	10.0	55
turkey entrée, frozen	10.5 oz	390	18	35	1110	0	20.0	40
turkey entrée, frozen, 'Extra Helping'	19 oz	750	29	68	1980	0	42.0	65
w/dressing, potatoes, corn, in sauce	1 entrée	280	14	34	1061	3	9.9	52
w/gravy and dressing, frozen, 'Healthy Balance'	11.25 oz	270	16	41	750	0	5.0	40
w/mashed potatoes and corn, in seasoned sauce	1 serving	280	14	34	1061	3	9.9	52
(Budget Gourmet)								
breast, Dijon, frozen	11.2 oz	340	20	37	860	0	12.0	65
breast, sliced, frozen	11.1 oz	290	16	36	1200	0	9.0	45
turkey à la king, w/rice, frozen	10 oz	390	20	36	740	0	18.0	75
turkey entrée, glazed, frozen, 'Light'	1 entrée	250	15	38	730	2	4.0	30
w/escalloped noodles 'Special Selections'	1 entrée	440	19	44	840	2	20.0	115
(Butterball)								
breast, hickory-smoked, no skin, 99% fat-free	3 oz	80	17	1	710	0	1.0	35
breast, roasted, no skin, 99% fat-free	3 oz	80	16	2	750	0	1.0	30
breast, roasted, w/honey, no skin, 99% fat-free	3 oz	90	16	3	690	0	1.0	35
(Dinty Moore)								
w/dressing and gravy, 'Micro Meal'	1 bowl	280	23	32	1120	4	7.0	35
w/dressing and gravy, packaged, 'American Classics'	10 oz	290	28	33	910	0	5.0	40
(Empire Kosher) pie, kosher	1 pie	470	21	46	820	11	23.0	25
(Freezer Queen)								
croquettes, breaded, w/gravy, frozen	7 oz	250	13	19	940	0	13.0	0

Food Name	Serv. Size	Total Cal.	Prot. gms	Carbs gms	Sod. mgs	Fiber gms	Fat gms	Chol. mgs
sliced, frozen	10 oz	280	16	36	1210	0	8.0	0
sliced, w/gravy and dressing, frozen, 'Single Serve'	9 oz	230	17	32	1130	0	5.0	0
sliced, w/gravy, frozen, 'Cook-In-Pouch'	5 oz	70	7	6	880	0	2.0	0
sliced, w/gravy, frozen, 'Family Suppers'	7 oz	110	9	8	1160	0	5.0	0
w/gravy and dressing, frozen, 'Deluxe Family'	7 oz	160	12	18	1130	0	5.0	0
(Healthy Choice)								
breast medallions and vegetables, frozen, 'Classics'	12.5 oz	350	29	45	480	0	6.0	60
breast, 'Traditional'	1 entrée	290	22	40	460	5	4.5	45
breast, sliced, w/gravy and dressing, frozen	10 oz	270	27	30	530	0	4.0	50
breast, traditional, frozen	1 meal	280	22	40	460	7	3.0	45
'Country Inn Roast'	1 entrée	250	20	28	530	4	6.0	40
country roast, w/mushrooms, gravy, rice	1 entrée	223	19	28	437	3	3.9	26
roasted, w/mushrooms and gravy, frozen	8.5 oz	200	18	26	380	0	3.0	40
tetrazzini, frozen	12.6 oz	340	23	49	490	0	6.0	40
turkey and vegetables, 'Hearty Handfuls'	1 entrée	320	18	51	590	5	5.0	20
w/mushrooms, 'Country Roast'	1 entrée	230	19	26	440	2	5.0	45
w/vegetables, lowfat, frozen, 'Homestyle'	9.5 oz	230	24	28	470	0	3.0	35
(Hormel) w/vegetable, microwave, 'Health Selections'	7.25 oz	220	15	35	420	0	2.0	20
(Hudson) sliced, extra lean	1 slice	30	5	0	280	0	0.5	10
(Hungry Man)								
pot pie	1 pie	650	21	65	1510	5	34.0	45
turkey entrée, mostly white meat, frozen	1 entrée	510	29	64	1620	9	15.0	55
(Jennie-O)								
white and dark meat, roasted, w/gravy	4 oz	150	19	3	780	0	7.0	70
white meat, roasted, w/gravy	4 oz	150	19	3	780	0	7.0	55
(Le Menu)								
breast, sliced, w/mushroom gravy, frozen	10.5 oz	300	22	38	1020	0	7.0	0
glazed, frozen, 'LightStyle'	8.25 oz	260	18	34	720	0	6.0	35
sliced, frozen, 'LightStyle'	10 oz	210	21	21	540	0	5.0	30
turkey divan, frozen, 'LightStyle'	10 oz	260	25	23	420	0	7.0	60
white meat, w/gravy and stuffing, frozen	8 oz	200	19	19	610	0	5.0	25
(Lean Cuisine)								
breast, sliced, in mushroom sauce w/rice, frozen	8 oz	230	17	24	540	0	7.0	35
breast, sliced, w/dressing, frozen	7 7/8 oz	200	16	23	590	0	5.0	25
Dijon, frozen	9.5 oz	210	20	20	590	0	6.0	45
homestyle	1 entrée	230	18	26	590	3	6.0	50
homestyle, w/vegetables and pasta, frozen	9 3/8 oz	230	21	25	550	0	5.0	50
pot pie	1 entrée	300	20	34	590	3	9.0	50
tenderloins, glazed	1 entrée	240	14	37	590	5	5.0	30
(Libby's) w/gravy and dressing, microwave, 'Diner'	7 oz	170	11	15	830	1	7.0	35
(Louis Rich)								
breast, roasted, 99% fat-free	2 oz	50	11	1	620	0	0.5	25
breast, roasted, dinner slices, 99% fat-free	1 slice	70	16	1	910	0	1.0	35
nuggets/sticks, breaded	1 serving	235	12	13	577	0	14.9	34
nuggets/sticks, breaded	1 piece	77	4	4	190	0	4.9	11
patty, white meat, breaded	1 serving	220	12	13	550	0	13.0	35
(Marie Callender's)								
grilled breast and rice pilaf	11.7 oz	320	22	34	940	4	10.0	35
pot pie	1 pie	610	15	57	1070	3	36.0	15
turkey w/gravy and dressing, frozen	14 oz	500	31	52	2040	4	19.0	80
w/gravy and dressing, w/broccoli	1 entrée	504	31	52	2037	na	19.0	79
(Morton) turkey entrée, frozen	10 oz	230	15	28	1300	0	6.0	45
(Mountain House) tetrazzini, freeze-dried, prepared	1 cup	200	13	20	0	0	8.0	0
(Mrs. Paterson's)								
pie, w/broccoli, hand held, frozen, 'Aussie Pie'	5.5 oz	460	16	42	790	0	26.0	95
(Norbest)								
breast, w/gravy, raw	4 oz	115	21	1	492	0	2.4	0

Food Name	Serv. Size	Total Cal.	Prot. gms	Carbs gms	Sod. mgs	Fiber gms	Fat gms	Chol. mgs
w/gravy, raw	4 oz	115	20	1	600	0	2.7	0
(Pierre)								
nuggets, product 1936	1 piece	70	4	2	103	0	5.2	11
nuggets, product 1937	1 piece	49	3	1	81	0	3.7	8
patty, breaded, flame-broiled, product 1939	1 piece	287	15	8	453	0	21.3	42
patty, flame-broiled, frozen, product 9719	1 piece	86	12	0	362	0	3.9	47
patty, flame-broiled, frozen, product 9721	1 piece	105	15	0	446	0	4.8	58
patty, strip-shaped, frozen, product 1938	1 piece	94	5	3	153	0	7.0	15
(Pillsbury) casserole, frozen, 'Microwave Classic'	1 pkg	430	20	31	880	0	25.0	0
(Right Course)								
sliced, in mild curry sauce, w/rice pilaf, frozen	8.75 oz	320	23	40	570	0	8.0	50
(Shelton's)								
pot pie, white flour crust	1 serving	220	15	18	360	1	10.0	50
pot pie, whole wheat crust	1 serving	220	16	18	360	3	10.0	50
(Stouffer's)								
breast, roasted, w/gravy and stuffing, frozen	7 7/8 oz	270	19	27	920	0	9.0	0
pot pie	1 entrée	530	21	36	1040	3	33.0	65
roasted, w/stuffing, 'Homestyle'	1 entrée	280	19	25	950	1	11.0	40
tetrazzini......................................	1 entrée	360	19	33	1060	1	17.0	55
tetrazzini, frozen, food service product	1 oz	36	2	3	99	0	2.0	7
(Sunday House)								
young turkey, w/broth and caramel color	3 oz	110	16	0	560	0	5.0	60
(Swanson)								
breast, w/pasta, frozen	11.25 oz	310	22	36	670	0	9.0	35
pot pie	1 pie	400	10	42	700	3	21.0	25
turkey and dressing, mostly white meat, w/gravy	1 entrée	240	13	30	830	2	9.0	20
turkey entrée, frozen	11.5 oz	350	21	42	1090	0	11.0	0
turkey entrée, frozen, 'Hungry Man'	17 oz	550	36	61	1810	0	18.0	0
turkey entrée, mostly white meat, frozen	1 entrée	320	20	42	1030	4	8.0	35
(Turkey By George)								
hickory barbecue, packaged	5 oz	190	28	8	840	0	5.0	65
Italian Parmesan, packaged	5 oz	170	28	3	860	0	5.0	70
lemon pepper, packaged	5 oz	160	28	4	830	0	4.0	60
mustard tarragon, packaged.......................	5 oz	180	29	3	830	0	6.0	80
(Tyson)								
pie, frozen.....................................	9 oz	370	13	39	981	0	18.0	34
turkey entrée, frozen, 'Gourmet Selection'	11.5 oz	380	19	51	1350	0	11.0	0
w/dressing, frozen, 'Elmer Fudd'	6.55 oz	260	10	40	510	0	7.0	18
w/gravy, frozen, 'Gourmet Selections'	9.5 oz	320	19	34	900	0	12.0	35
(Ultra Slim-Fast)								
glazed, w/dressing, frozen	10.5 oz	340	28	49	570	0	5.0	50
medallions, in herb sauce, frozen	12 oz	280	23	33	950	0	6.0	40
(Weight Watchers)								
breast, stuffed.................................	1 entrée	230	17	28	680	6	5.0	15
medallions, roasted, w/mushroom sauce, frozen, 'Smart Ones'	8.5 oz	200	13	35	440	0	1.0	25
medallions, 'Smart Ones'	1 entrée	190	10	34	530	4	2.0	20
w/mushroom, rice, vegetable, 'Smart Ones'	1 entrée	214	15	35	504	3	1.7	24
(Wonderbites)								
fajita, flame-broiled, product 2196, 'Dippers'	1 piece	34	5	1	132	0	1.3	14
TURKEY FAT								
....	1 cup	1846	0	0	0	0	204.6	209
....	1 tbsp	115	0	0	0	0	12.8	13
....	1 tsp	39	0	0	0	0	4.3	4
TURKEY JERKY *(Shelton's)*	1/2 oz	50	9	1	125	0	0.5	25

TURKEY SEASONING. See under SEASONING MIX.

Food Name	Serv. Size	Total Cal.	Prot. gms	Carbs gms	Sod. mgs	Fiber gms	Fat gms	Chol. mgs
TURKEY SNACK STICKS								
(Turkey Store)								
breast meat, cheese, 'Gobble Stix' .... 1 stick		30	6	1	0	0	0.8	10
breast meat, smoked, 'Gobble Stix' .... 1 stick		25	5	0	0	0	0.2	10
TURKEY SPREAD								
(Libby's) turkey salad, 'Spreadables' .... 1/3 cup		150	7	7	310	2	10.0	25
(Underwood) chunky 'Light' .... 2 1/8 oz		75	11	2	330	0	2.0	25
TURKEY SUBSTITUTE								
(Worthington)								
canned, drained .... 2 slices		120	8	3	0	0	8.0	0
slices .... 3 slices		193	13	3	580	2	14.0	2
smoked, roll, frozen .... 4 slices		180	13	5	820	0	12.0	0
vegetarian, 'Meatless Smoked Turkey' .... 3 slices		140	10	3	620	2	10.0	0
vegetarian, 'Turkee Slices' .... 3 slices		170	13	3	580	2	12.0	0
TURMERIC								
dried *(McCormick/Schilling)* .... 1 tsp		8	0	2	0	0	0.0	0
ground .... 1 tbsp		24	1	4	3	1	0.7	0
ground .... 1 tsp		8	0	1	1	0	0.2	0
ground *(Durkee)* .... 1 tsp		9	0	0	0	0	0.0	0
ground *(Laurel Leaf)* .... 1 tsp		9	0	0	0	0	0.0	0
ground *(Spice Islands)* .... 1 tsp		7	0	1	1	0	0.2	0
TURNIP. See also RUTABAGA.								
Canned								
(Stokely) .... 1/2 cup		20	2	3	350	0	0.0	0
diced *(Allens)* .... 1/2 cup		16	2	2	25	0	1.0	0
Fresh								
boiled, drained, cubed .... 1 cup		33	1	8	78	3	0.1	0
boiled, drained, mashed .... 1 cup		48	2	11	115	5	0.2	0
raw, cubed .... 1 cup		35	1	8	87	2	0.1	0
Frozen								
cubes, boiled, drained .... 1 cup		33	1	8	446	3	0.1	0
diced *(Southern)* .... 3.5 oz		17	1	3	50	0	0.2	0
mashed, boiled, drained .... 1 cup		48	2	11	658	5	0.2	0
mashed, unprepared .... 10-oz pkg		45	3	8	71	5	0.5	0
w/greens, boiled, drained .... 1 cup		28	3	5	24	3	0.3	0
w/greens, unprepared .... 10-oz pkg		60	7	10	51	7	0.5	0
TURNIP, CABBAGE. See KOHLRABI.								
TURNIP GREENS								
Canned								
chopped *(Allens)* .... 1/2 cup		21	2	3	15	0	1.0	0
chopped *(Bush's Best)* .... 1/2 cup		20	2	3	310	0	0.0	0
chopped, w/diced turnips *(Allens)* .... 1/2 cup		19	2	1	15	0	1.0	0
seasoned w/pork *(Luck's)* .... 1 cup		35	1	5	240	2	1.5	0
w/diced turnips *(Bush's Best)* .... 1/2 cup		25	1	4	370	2	0.0	0
w/diced turnips *(Stokely)* .... 1/2 cup		20	2	0	340	0	0.0	0
w/liquid .... 1/2 cup		16	2	3	324	2	0.4	0
Fresh								
boiled, drained, chopped .... 4 oz		23	1.3	4.9	33	3.5	0.3	0
boiled, drained, chopped .... 1/2 cup		14	0.8	3.1	21	2.2	0.2	0
raw, chopped .... 1 cup		15	1	3	22	2	0.2	0
Frozen								
boiled, drained .... 10-oz pkg		66	7	11	33	7	0.9	0
chopped *(Flav-R-Pac)* .... 1/3 cup		30	2	2	20	2	0.0	0
chopped *(Frosty Acres)* .... 3.3 oz		20	2	4	10	1	0.0	0
chopped *(Seabrook)* .... 3.3 oz		20	2	4	11	1	0.0	0
chopped *(Southern)* .... 3.5 oz		25	3	4	70	0	0.3	0
TURNIP-ROOTED PARSLEY. See PARSLEY ROOT.								

Food Name	Serv. Size	Total Cal.	Prot. gms	Carbs gms	Sod. mgs	Fiber gms	Fat gms	Chol. mgs
chopped, boiled, drained	1 cup	29	2	6	42	5	0.3	0
chopped, unprepared	10-oz pkg	62	7	10	34	7	0.9	0
chopped, w/diced turnips (Flav-R-Pac)	1/3 cup	30	2	2	20	2	0.0	0
chopped or diced, unprepared	1/2 cup	18	2	3	10	2	0.3	0
w/diced turnips (Seabrook)	3.3 oz	20	3	3	0	0	0.0	0

TURNOVER. See under PASTRY.
TURTLE, GREEN

canned	3.5 oz	106	23.4	0.0	68	0	0.7	50
raw	3.5 oz	89	19.8	0.0	68	0	0.5	50

TUSCAN PEPPER. See PEPPER, TUSCAN.
TUSK. See CUSK.

U

Food Name	Serv. Size	Total Cal.	Prot. gms	Carbs gms	Sod. mgs	Fiber gms	Fat gms	Chol. mgs
UCUHUBA BUTTER OIL								
	1 cup	1927	0	0	0	0	218.0	0
	1 tbsp	120	0	0	0	0	13.6	0

UDON. See under NOODLE, JAPANESE.
UMEBOSHI/Japanese plum

peeled and seeded	1 oz	13	0.1	3.4	<1	0.1	0.1	0
raw, approx 0.6 oz	1 medium	5	<0.1	1.2	tr	0.1	<0.1	0
untrimmed	1 lb	132	1.2	34.1	3	1.4	0.6	0

V

Food Name	Serv. Size	Total Cal.	Prot. gms	Carbs gms	Sod. mgs	Fiber gms	Fat gms	Chol. mgs
VANILLA EXTRACT								
	1 cup	599	0	26	19	0	0.1	0
	1 tbsp	37	0	2	1	0	0.0	0
	1 tsp	12	0	1	0	0	0.0	0
pure (Virginia Dare)	1 tsp	10	0	0	0	0	0.0	0
VANILLA EXTRACT SUBSTITUTE								
imitation	1 tbsp	7	0	2	0	0	0.0	0
imitation	1 tsp	2	0	1	0	0	0.0	0
imitation, w/alcohol	1 tbsp	31	0	0	1	0	0.0	0
imitation, w/alcohol	1 tsp	10	0	0	0	0	0.0	0
VANILLA, BAKING chips, vanilla milk (Hershey's)	1/4 cup	240	3	25	65	0	14.0	0

VEAL
(NOTE: TRIMMED = Lean; separable fat removed after cooking. UNTRIMMED = Separable fat not removed.)
BRAIN

braised	3 oz	116	10	0	133	0	8.2	2635
pan-fried	3 oz	181	12	0	150	0	14.2	1802
raw	4 oz	134	12	0	144	0	9.3	1803

BREAST

Trimmed, whole, boneless, braised	3 oz	185	26	0	58	na	8.3	99
Untrimmed								
plate half, boneless, braised	3 oz	240	22	0	54	na	16.1	95
point half, boneless, braised	3 oz	211	24	0	56	na	12.0	97
whole, boneless, braised	3 oz	226	23	0	55	na	14.3	96

GROUND

broiled	3 oz	146	21	0	71	0	6.4	88
raw	4 oz	163	22	0	93	0	7.7	93

Food Name	Serv. Size	Total Cal.	Prot. gms	Carbs gms	Sod. mgs	Fiber gms	Fat gms	Chol. mgs
HEART								
braised	3 oz	158	25	0	49	0	5.7	150
raw	4 oz	125	19	0	87	0	4.5	118
KIDNEY								
braised	3 oz	139	22	0	94	0	4.8	672
raw	4 oz	112	18	1	202	0	3.5	413
LEG								
Trimmed								
top round, braised	3 oz	173	31	0	57	0	4.3	115
top round, breaded, pan-fried	3 oz	175	24	8	387	0	5.3	96
top round, pan-fried	3 oz	156	28	0	65	0	3.9	91
top round, raw	1 oz	30	6	0	18	0	0.5	22
top round, roasted	3 oz	128	24	0	58	0	2.9	88
Untrimmed								
top round, braised	3 oz	179	31	0	57	0	5.4	114
top round, breaded, pan-fried	3 oz	194	23	8	386	0	7.8	95
top round, pan-fried	3 oz	179	27	0	65	0	7.1	89
top round, raw	1 oz	33	6	0	18	0	0.9	22
top round, roasted	3 oz	136	24	0	58	0	4.0	88
LEG AND SHOULDER								
Trimmed								
cubed for stew, braised	3 oz	160	30	0	79	0	3.7	123
cubed for stew, raw	1 oz	31	6	0	24	0	0.7	24
LIVER								
braised	3 oz	140	18	2	45	0	5.9	477
pan-fried	3 oz	208	25	3	112	0	9.7	281
raw	4 oz	152	20	5	70	0	5.0	350
LOIN								
Trimmed								
braised	3 oz	192	29	0	71	0	7.8	106
raw	1 oz	33	6	0	26	0	0.9	23
roasted	3 oz	149	22	0	82	0	5.9	90
Untrimmed								
braised	3 oz	241	26	0	68	0	14.6	100
raw	1 oz	46	5	0	24	0	2.6	22
roasted	3 oz	184	21	0	79	0	10.5	88
LUNGS								
braised	3 oz	88	16	0	48	0	2.2	224
raw	4 oz	102	18	0	122	0	2.6	260
PANCREAS								
braised	3 oz	218	25	0	58	0	12.4	na
raw	4 oz	206	17	0	76	0	14.9	196
RIB								
Trimmed								
braised	3 oz	185	29	0	84	0	6.6	122
raw	1 oz	34	6	0	27	0	1.1	24
roasted	3 oz	150	22	0	82	0	6.3	98
Untrimmed								
braised	3 oz	213	28	0	81	0	10.7	118
raw	1 oz	46	5	0	25	0	2.6	23
roasted	3 oz	194	20	0	78	0	11.9	94
SHANK								
Trimmed								
fore and hind, braised	3 oz	150	27	0	80	0	3.7	107
fore and hind, raw	1 oz	31	5	0	24	na	0.8	21
Untrimmed								
fore and hind, braised	3 oz	162	27	0	79	na	5.3	105

Food Name	Serv. Size	Total Cal.	Prot. gms	Carbs gms	Sod. mgs	Fiber gms	Fat gms	Chol. mgs
fore and hind, raw	1 oz	32	5	0	24	na	1.0	21
SHOULDER								
Trimmed								
arm, braised	3 oz	171	30	0	77	0	4.5	132
arm, raw	1 oz	30	6	0	24	0	0.6	24
arm, roasted	3 oz	139	22	0	77	0	4.9	93
blade, braised	3 oz	168	28	0	86	0	5.5	134
blade, raw	1 oz	32	6	0	28	0	0.9	26
blade, roasted	3 oz	145	22	0	87	0	5.8	101
whole, arm and blade, braised	3 oz	169	29	0	82	0	5.2	111
whole, arm and blade, raw	1 oz	32	6	0	26	0	0.9	24
whole, arm and blade, roasted	3 oz	145	22	0	82	0	5.6	97
Untrimmed								
arm, braised	3 oz	201	29	0	74	0	8.7	126
arm, raw	1 oz	37	5	0	24	0	1.5	23
arm, roasted	3 oz	156	22	0	77	0	7.0	92
blade, braised	3 oz	191	27	0	83	0	8.6	130
blade, raw	1 oz	37	5	0	27	0	1.5	26
blade, roasted	3 oz	158	21	0	85	0	7.4	99
whole, arm and blade, braised	3 oz	194	27	0	81	0	8.6	107
whole, arm and blade, raw	1 oz	37	5	0	26	0	1.5	25
whole, arm and blade, roasted	3 oz	156	22	0	82	0	7.2	96
SIRLOIN								
Trimmed								
braised	3 oz	173	29	0	69	0	5.5	96
raw	1 oz	31	6	0	23	0	0.7	22
roasted	3 oz	143	22	0	72	0	5.3	88
Untrimmed								
braised	3 oz	214	27	0	67	0	11.2	92
raw	1 oz	43	5	0	22	0	2.2	22
roasted	3 oz	172	21	0	71	0	8.9	87
SPLEEN								
braised	3 oz	110	20	0	49	0	2.5	380
raw	4 oz	111	21	0	110	0	2.5	386
THYMUS								
braised	3 oz	148	27	0	56	0	3.6	399
raw	4 oz	112	20	0	94	0	2.8	304
TONGUE								
braised	3 oz	172	22	0	54	0	8.6	202
raw	4 oz	149	19	2	93	0	6.2	70
VEAL DINNER/ENTRÉE								
(Armour) parmigiana, frozen, 'Classics'	11.25 oz	400	18	34	1320	0	22.0	55
(Banquet)								
parmigiana	1 entrée	360	13	35	960	7	19.0	25
parmigiana, breaded patty, frozen, 'Cookin' Bags'	4 oz	230	10	20	0	0	11.0	0
parmigiana, w/tomato sauce, potato. peas in sauce	1 entrée	362	13	35	964	7	19.0	26
(Contadina) Parmigiana, frozen	1 oz	42	3	3	165	na	2.3	8
(Freezer Queen)								
parmigiana, breaded, frozen, 'Cook-In-Pouch'	5 oz	220	11	17	560	0	12.0	0
parmigiana, breaded, frozen, 'Deluxe Family Suppers'	7 oz	300	17	22	820	0	15.0	0
parmigiana, platter, frozen	10 oz	400	22	32	870	0	20.0	0
(Hormel)								
steak, breaded, frozen	4 oz	240	17	13	0	0	13.0	0
steak, frozen	4 oz	130	22	2	0	0	4.0	0
(Le Menu)								
Marsala, frozen, 'LightStyle'	10 oz	230	22	28	700	0	3.0	75
parmigiana, frozen	11.5 oz	390	24	36	840	0	17.0	0

Food Name	Serv. Size	Total Cal.	Prot. gms	Carbs gms	Sod. mgs	Fiber gms	Fat gms	Chol. mgs
(Morton) Parmigiana, frozen	10 oz	260	10	35	1510	0	8.0	35
(Pierre) veal and beef patty, Italian, frozen, product 1905	1 piece	279	14	12	591	1	19.6	36
(Stouffer's) Parmigiana, w/spaghetti, 'Homestyle'	1 entrée	420	20	43	1200	6	19.0	75
(Swanson)								
Parmigiana	1 entrée	390	19	40	1060	5	18.0	85
Parmigiana, 'Hungry Man'	1 entrée	640	34	74	1990	6	23.0	70
Parmigiana, frozen, 'Homestyle Recipe'	10 oz	330	19	33	960	0	13.0	0
(Weight Watchers)								
Parmigiana, breaded patty, frozen, 'Ultimate 200'	8.2 oz	150	22	5	550	0	4.0	50
VEGETABLE CHIPS								
(Eden Foods)	1-oz bag	130	1	22	200	0	4.0	0
sea vegetable *(Eden Foods)*	1-oz bag	130	1	22	200	0	5.0	0
VEGETABLE DISH/ENTRÉE See also individual listings.								
(Amy's Kitchen)								
pot pie	1 serving	360	7	44	540	4	18.0	45
shepherd's pie	1 serving	160	5	27	490	5	4.0	0
(Budget Gourmet)								
w/chicken, Chinese style, frozen	10 oz	280	11	47	590	0	7.0	10
w/chicken, Italian style, frozen	10.25 oz	310	14	50	690	0	8.0	30
(Dinty Moore) stew, canned	8 oz	155	5	20	850	0	6.0	14
(Flav-R-Pac)								
stir-fry w/asparagus, frozen	1 cup	25	1	4	25	2	0.0	0
stir-fry w/noodles, frozen	1 cup	50	2	9	25	2	0.0	0
stir-fry w/rice, frozen	1 cup	80	3	18	15	2	0.0	0
succotash, frozen	2/3 cup	100	4	22	50	2	1.0	0
vegetarian dinner blend	3/4 cup	25	1	4	20	2	0.0	0
(Frosty Acres) succotash, frozen	3.3 oz	100	4	19	47	1	0.0	0
(Gardenburger)								
vegetable patty, vegetarian, roasted, 'Gourmet'	2.5 oz	120	7	17	270	2	2.8	10
(Green Giant)								
broccoli, cauliflower, carrots, in cheese sauce	2/3 cup	80	3	11	560	2	2.5	5
four vegetables in butter sauce w/pasta								
(Green Giant)	3/4 cup	70	3	11	280	2	2.0	5
w/sauce, 'Garden Gourmet Fettuccine								
Primavera'	9.5 oz serving	307	13	34	734	2	13.3	14
(Hanover) rice and vegetables w/soy sauce, 'Stir Fry 2'	1 cup	130	5	27	636	2	0.4	na
(La Choy)								
chow mein, contains no meat	3/4 cup	35	2	6	820	2	0.4	0
chow mein, meatless, canned	1 cup	55	3	10	854	1	0.7	0
chow mein, vegetable, frozen, food service product	1 cup	108	2	20	1135	5	2.3	0
(Morningstar Farms)								
vegetarian, 'Garden Grille'	1 patty	120	6	18	280	4	2.5	<5
vegetarian, 'Garden Veggie Patties'	1 patty	100	10	3	350	4	2.5	0.0
(Morton)								
w/beef, frozen	7 oz	430	11	27	740	0	31.0	30
w/chicken, frozen	7 oz	420	14	27	740	0	28.0	35
w/turkey, frozen	7 oz	420	14	27	740	0	28.0	40
(Mountain House) stew, w/beef, freeze-dried, prepared	1 cup	230	11	27	77	0	7.0	0
(Natural Touch)								
vegetarian, 'Dinner Entrée'	1 pattie	220	19	2	380	2	15.0	0
vegetarian, 'Garden Veggie Pattie'	1 pattie	100	10	8	280	3	2.5	0
vegetarian, 'Okara Patties'	1 pattie	110	11	4	360	3	5.0	0
(S&W) succotash, canned, 'Country Style'	1/2 cup	80	4	16	250	1	1.0	0
(Seabrook) succotash, frozen	3.3 oz	100	4	19	47	1	0.0	0

Food Name	Serv. Size	Total Cal.	Prot. gms	Carbs gms	Sod. mgs	Fiber gms	Fat gms	Chol. mgs
(Shanghai) stir-fry, frozen	5.1 oz	75	6	11	510	0	1.0	0
(Stokely) succotash, canned	1/2 cup	90	3	20	300	0	0.0	0
(Stouffer's)								
chow mein, frozen, food service product	1 oz	14	0	2	156	0	0.7	0
lasagna, frozen, food service product	1 oz	45	2	4	114	na	2.6	3
(Tofu Classics) chow mein, Mandarin, prepared w/tofu	1/2 cup	110	8	14	390	0	6.0	0
(Ultra Slim-Fast) and beef tips, country style	12 oz	230	21	26	960	0	5.0	45
(Worthington)								
vegetarian, 'Multigrain Cutlets' 50-oz can	1 slice	80	12	4	300	3	1.5	0
vegetarian, 'Multigrain Cutlets' 20-oz can	2 slices	100	15	5	390	4	2.0	0
vegetarian, 'Vegetarian Cutlets'	1 slice	70	11	3	340	2	1.0	0
VEGETABLE FLAKES *(French's)* dehydrated	1 tbsp	12	0	3	20	0	0.0	0
VEGETABLE JUICE DRINK								
(Biotta)								
'Breuss Juice'	6 fl oz	67	2	13	147	0	0.1	0
'Cocktail'	6 fl oz	50	2	10	497	0	0.1	0
(Knudsen)								
'Very Veggie' blend, low-salt	8 fl oz	50	3	10	32	na	1.0	0
'Very Veggie' fruit juice sweetened	8 fl oz	50	3	10	32	2	1.0	0
'Very Veggie' low-sodium	8 fl oz	40	2	8	32	0	0.0	0
'Very Veggie' organic	8 fl oz	40	2	8	0	0	0.0	0
'Very Veggie' original	8 fl oz	40	2	8	560	0	0.0	0
'Very Veggie' spicy	8 fl oz	40	2	8	560	0	0.0	0
(Sacramento)	8 fl oz	30	3	9	850	2	0.0	0
(Smucker's)								
hearty	8 fl oz	58	1	13	714	0	0.1	0
hot and spicy	8 fl oz	58	1	13	650	0	0.1	0
(V8)								
low-salt	8 fl oz	60	2	11	140	2	0.0	0
100% juice	8 fl oz	50	1	10	620	1	0.0	0
100% juice, lightly tangy	8 fl oz	60	2	11	340	1	0.0	0
picante	11.5 fl oz	70	2	14	990	2	0.0	0
spicy hot	8 fl oz	50	2	10	780	1	0.0	0
(Veryfine) '100%'	6 fl oz	32	2	6	600	0	0.0	0
VEGETABLE OIL. See also individual listings.								
salad or cooking	1 cup	1927	0	0	0	0	218.0	0
salad or cooking	1 tbsp	120	0	0	0	0	13.6	0
(Blue Plate)	1 tbsp	130	0	0	0	na	14.0	na
(Crisco) Canola and corn oil blend	1 tbsp	120	0	0	0	0	14.0	0
(Finast)	1 tbsp	120	0	0	0	0	14.0	0
(Hain)								
'All Blend'	1 tbsp	120	0	0	0	0	14.0	0
w/garlic, 'Garlic & Oil'	1 tbsp	120	0	0	0	0	14.0	0
(Kroger)	1 tbsp	122	0	0	0	0	13.6	0
(Mazola) Canola and corn oil blend, 'Right Blend'	1 tbsp	120	0	0	0	0	14.0	0
(Pathmark)								
	1 tbsp	120	0	0	0	0	14.0	0
'No Frills'	1 tbsp	130	0	0	0	0	14.0	0
(Puritan)	1 tbsp	120	0	0	0	0	14.0	0
(Wesson)								
	1 tbsp	122	0	0	0	0	13.6	0
butter flavor	1 tbsp	122	0	0	0	0	13.6	0
Canola and vegetable oil blend, 'Best Blend'	1 tbsp	120	0	0	0	0	14.0	0

VEGETABLE OIL SPREAD. See MARGARINE; MARGARINE SPREAD; MARGARINE SUBSTITUTE.
VEGETABLE OYSTER. See SALSIFY.
VEGETABLE SPONGE. See GOURD, DISHCLOTH.

Food Name	Serv. Size	Total Cal.	Prot. gms	Carbs gms	Sod. mgs	Fiber gms	Fat gms	Chol. mgs
VEGETABLES, MIXED								
Canned								
(A&P)								
'Eastern'	1/2 cup	45	2	8	330	0	1.0	0
no salt added	1/2 cup	40	1	9	20	0	1.0	0
'Western'	1/2 cup	40	1	9	380	0	1.0	0
(Bush's Best) greens, mixed	1/2 cup	20	2	3	300	0	0.0	0
(Chun King) chow mein	1/2 cup	10	1	2	15	1	0.0	0
(Featherweight)	1/2 cup	40	2	8	25	0	0.0	0
(Finast)								
	1/2 cup	40	1	8	390	0	0.0	0
no salt added	1/2 cup	40	2	8	25	0	0.0	0
(Freshlike)								
water packed, no salt added	1/2 cup	35	2	8	25	0	0.0	0
water packed, no sugar or salt added	1/2 cup	35	2	8	25	0	0.0	0
(Green Giant)								
	1/2 cup	60	2	12	460	2	0.0	0
'Garden Medley'	1/2 cup	35	1	9	350	1	0.0	0
'Pantry Express'	1/2 cup	35	1	8	300	1	1.0	0
(La Choy)								
Chinese	1/2 cup	12	1	2	30	1	0.1	0
Chinese, food service product	2/3 cup	15	1	3	32	1	0.1	0
chop suey	1/2 cup	9	1	2	330	1	0.1	0
chop suey vegetables	1/2 cup	14	1	3	323	1	0.1	0
chop suey vegetables, food service product	1/2 cup	11	1	2	439	1	0.4	0
fancy	2/3 cup	9	1	1	32	1	0.1	0
(P&Q)								
'Chunky Eastern'	1/2 cup	40	2	8	330	0	1.0	0
'Chunky Western'	1/2 cup	40	1	9	380	0	1.0	0
(Pathmark)								
	1/2 cup	35	2	8	320	0	0.0	0
no salt added	1/2 cup	35	2	7	25	0	0.0	0
(S&W) 'Old Fashioned Harvest'	1/2 cup	35	1	6	380	0	0.0	0
(Stokely)								
	1/2 cup	40	2	8	300	0	0.0	0
no salt or sugar added	1/2 cup	40	2	8	25	0	0.0	0
(Veg-All)								
large cut, 'Homestyle'	1/2 cup	35	2	9	380	0	0.0	0
lite	1/2 cup	35	2	8	25	0	0.0	0
original	1/2 cup	35	2	8	320	0	0.0	0
Frozen								
(A&P)								
	3.3 oz	65	3	13	55	0	1.0	0
California blend	3.3 oz	25	2	5	25	0	1.0	0
Italian style blend	3.3 oz	40	2	8	35	0	1.0	0
Oriental style blend	3.3 oz	25	2	5	15	0	1.0	0
winter blend	3.3 oz	24	2	6	190	0	1.0	0
(Birds Eye)								
	3.3 oz	60	3	13	40	2	0.0	0
broccoli, cauliflower, carrots, 'Farm Fresh'	4 oz	35	2	7	40	3	0.0	0
broccoli, cauliflower, red peppers, 'Farm Fresh'	4 oz	30	3	5	25	3	0.0	0
broccoli, corn, red peppers, 'Farm Fresh'	4 oz	60	3	14	15	3	1.0	0
broccoli, green beans, pearl onions, red peppers	4 oz	35	2	7	15	3	0.0	0
broccoli, red peppers, bamboo shoots, mushrooms	4 oz	30	3	5	20	3	0.0	0
Brussels sprouts, cauliflower, carrots	4 oz	40	3	8	30	4	0.0	0
cauliflower, baby carrots, snow pea pods	4 oz	40	2	8	35	3	0.0	0

Food Name	Serv. Size	Total Cal.	Prot. gms	Carbs gms	Sod. mgs	Fiber gms	Fat gms	Chol. mgs
cauliflower, whole baby carrots, snow pea pods . . . . 4 oz		40	2	8	35	3	0.0	0
cauliflower, zucchini, carrots, red peppers . . . . 4 oz		30	2	6	25	2	0.0	0
Chinese style, 'Stir-Fry' . . . . 3.3 oz		35	2	8	540	2	0.0	0
Italian style, 'International Recipes' . . . . 3.3 oz		100	2	11	490	2	5.0	0
Japanese style, 'International Recipes' . . . . 3.3 oz		90	2	10	420	2	5.0	0
Japanese style, 'Stir-Fry' . . . . 3.3 oz		30	2	7	510	2	0.0	0
New England style, 'International Recipes' . . . . 3.3 oz		130	3	14	430	2	7.0	0
Oriental style, 'International Recipes' . . . . 3.3 oz		70	2	8	300	1	4.0	0
pepper stir-fry, 'Farm Fresh Mixtures' . . . . 1 cup		25	1	5	15	2	0.0	0
San Francisco style, 'International Recipes' . . . . 3.3 oz		100	2	11	400	1	5.0	0
sugar snap peas, baby carrots, water chestnuts . . . . 3.2 oz		50	2	11	20	4	0.0	0
(C&W)								
corn, broccoli, red peppers, 'Vegetable Stand' . . . . 2/3 cup		60	2	14	10	1	0.5	0
peas, corn, green beans, baby carrots . . . . 3/4 cup		60	3	11	45	2	0.0	0
petite peas and baby carrots, 'Early Harvest' . . . . 3.3 oz		60	4	12	95	0	0.0	0
red, green, and yellow bell pepper strips . . . . 1/2 cup		20	1	4	10	2	0.0	0
(Flav-R-Pac)								
Capri . . . . 3/4 cup		25	1	4	25	1	0.0	0
fajita blend . . . . 3/4 cup		20	1	5	10	1	0.0	0
fiesta . . . . 2/3 cup		60	4	10	131	6	0.0	0
five vegetables . . . . 2/3 cup		60	3	12	50	2	0.5	0
four vegetables . . . . 2/3 cup		50	2	9	45	2	0.0	0
Italian, frozen . . . . 2/3 cup		30	1	5	30	2	0.0	0
Italian, w/buttery sauce . . . . 1/2 cup		50	2	8	410	3	2.0	0
Mexicali . . . . 2/3 cup		80	3	18	75	3	0.5	0
omelette blend . . . . 3/4 cup		25	1	5	15	2	0.0	0
Oriental . . . . 3/4 cup		25	1	4	15	2	0.0	0
Scandinavian . . . . 3/4 cup		40	2	7	45	2	0.0	0
stew vegetables . . . . 2/3 cup		40	1	9	45	1	0.0	0
stew/soup vegetables . . . . 2/3 cup		40	1	9	45	1	0.0	0
stir-fry blend, frozen . . . . 3/4 cup		25	1	5	20	2	0.0	0
stir-fry blend, frozen, deluxe . . . . 3/4 cup		30	1	5	20	2	0.0	0
w/buttery sauce, frozen . . . . 1/2 cup		90	4	16	540	4	2.5	0
winter . . . . 1 cup		25	2	4	25	2	0.0	0
(Freshlike)								
. . . . 3.3 oz		70	3	13	45	0	0.0	0
'California Blend' . . . . 3.3 oz		30	2	6	20	0	0.0	0
'Chuckwagon Blend' . . . . 3.3 oz		70	2	16	5	0	1.0	0
'Country Blend' . . . . 3.3 oz		50	2	12	15	0	0.0	0
for soup . . . . 3.3 oz		50	2	11	40	0	0.0	0
for stew, 4-ways . . . . 3.3 oz		50	1	11	40	0	0.0	0
for stew, 5-ways . . . . 3.3 oz		50	1	12	40	0	0.0	0
'Italian Blend' food service product . . . . 3.3 oz		25	1	5	20	0	0.0	0
'Italian Blend' . . . . 3.3 oz		30	2	7	20	0	0.0	0
'Midwestern Blend' . . . . 3.3 oz		40	2	8	30	0	0.0	0
'Oriental Blend' . . . . 3.3 oz		25	3	5	10	0	0.0	0
'Scandinavian Blend' . . . . 3.3 oz		45	2	9	30	0	0.0	0
'Winter Blend' . . . . 3.3 oz		25	3	5	25	0	0.0	0
(Frosty Acres)								
. . . . 3.3 oz		65	3	13	50	1	0.0	0
Dutch style . . . . 3.2 oz		30	2	5	30	0	0.0	0
Italian style . . . . 3.2 oz		40	3	8	20	0	0.0	0
Oriental style . . . . 3.2 oz		25	2	5	15	0	0.0	0
(Green Giant)								
. . . . 1/2 cup		40	2	9	40	2	0.0	0
broccoli, cauliflower, carrots 'One Serving' . . . . 1 pkg		30	3	7	40	3	0.0	0

Food Name	Serv. Size	Total Cal.	Prot. gms	Carbs gms	Sod. mgs	Fiber gms	Fat gms	Chol. mgs
California style, 'American Mixtures'	1/2 cup	25	2	6	40	2	0.0	0
five vegetables in butter sauce	3/4 cup	60	2	8	300	2	2.0	5
heartland style, 'American Mixtures'	1 cup	30	2	6	35	3	0.0	0
LeSueur style, 'Valley Combinations'	1/2 cup	70	4	12	400	2	2.0	0
Manhattan style, 'American Mixtures'	1 cup	25	2	4	15	2	0.0	0
New England style, 'American Mixtures'	2/3 cup	70	2	13	70	3	1.5	0
'Plain Polybag'	1/2 cup	40	2	9	40	2	0.0	0
'Portion Pack'	3 oz	50	2	12	35	2	0.0	0
San Francisco style, 'American Mixtures'	3/4 cup	30	1	6	20	2	0.0	0
Santa Fe style, 'American Mixtures'	3/4 cup	60	2	13	10	2	0.0	0
Seattle style, 'American Mixtures'	3/4 cup	25	1	5	15	2	0.0	0
Western style, 'American Mixtures'	3/4 cup	50	1	9	10	2	1.5	0
(Health Valley)	1/2 cup	68	3	14	39	2	0.0	0
(La Choy) stir-fry vegetables, food service product	1/2 cup	34	3	6	2	1	0.1	0
(Pictsweet)								
'California'	3/4 cup	20	1	4	25	1	0.0	0
'Cantonese'	3.2 oz	35	2	7	25	0	0.0	0
'Chinese Stir-Fry'	3/4 cup	30	1	5	200	2	0.0	0
'Del Sol'	3.2 oz	30	2	6	25	0	0.0	0
'Grande'	3/4 cup	45	2	10	15	2	0.5	0
'Japanese'	3.2 oz	15	2	5	10	0	1.0	0
low-sodium, vitamins A and C	3.2 oz	60	3	12	40	0	0.0	0
'Oriental Stir-Fry'	3/4 cup	30	1	5	310	1	0.0	0
peas, carrots	2/3 cup	50	3	9	75	3	0.0	0
(Seabrook)	3.3 oz	65	3	13	50	1	0.0	0
(Southern)	3.5 oz	69	3	14	60	0	0.0	0
(Stokely)								
broccoli, cauliflower, baby carrots 'Singles'	3 oz	25	2	5	25	0	1.0	0
'Singles'	3 oz	60	3	12	40	0	1.0	0
(Trader Joe's) red, yellow, and green pepper strips, 'Melange a Trois'	1/3 cup	20	0	4	10	2	0.0	0
(Veg-All)								
	3.3 oz	70	3	13	45	0	0.0	0
'California Blend'	3.3 oz	30	2	6	20	0	0.0	0
'Chuckwagon Blend'	3.3 oz	70	2	16	5	0	1.0	0
'Country Blend'	3.3 oz	50	2	12	15	0	0.0	0
for soup	3.3 oz	50	2	11	40	0	0.0	0
for stew, 4-ways	3.3 oz	50	1	11	40	0	0.0	0
for stew, 5-ways	3.3 oz	50	1	12	40	0	0.0	0
'Italian Blend' food service product	3.3 oz	25	1	5	20	0	0.0	0
'Italian Blend'	3.3 oz	30	2	7	20	0	0.0	0
large cut	1/2 cup	45	1	9	350	2	0.0	0
'Midwestern Blend'	3.3 oz	40	2	8	30	0	0.0	0
'Oriental Blend'	3.3 oz	25	3	5	10	0	0.0	0
'Scandinavian Blend'	3.3 oz	45	2	9	30	0	0.0	0
'Winter Blend'	3.3 oz	25	3	5	25	0	0.0	0

VEGETARIAN FOODS. See individual listings.
VEGGIE BURGER. See under BEEF SUBSTITUTE DINNER/ENTRÉE.
VENISON. See CARIBOU; DEER; ELK; MOOSE.
VERMOUTH
(Gallo)

dry	2 fl oz	56	0	1	0	0	0.0	0
sweet	2 fl oz	90	0	9	0	0	0.0	0
(Gambarelli & Davitto)								
dry	2 fl oz	64	0	2	4	0	0.0	0
sweet	2 fl oz	77	0	8	4	0	0.0	0

Food Name	Serv. Size	Total Cal.	Prot. gms	Carbs gms	Sod. mgs	Fiber gms	Fat gms	Chol. mgs
(Lejon)								
dry	2 fl oz	64	0	2	4	0	0.0	0
sweet	2 fl oz	77	0	8	4	0	0.0	0
VICHY WATER. See under SOFT DRINKS AND MIXERS.								
VIENNA SAUSAGE. See under SAUSAGE.								
VINE SPINACH. See SPINACH, VINE.								
VINEGAR								
APPLE CIDER								
	1 cup	34	0	14	2	0	0.0	0
	1 tbsp	2	0	1	0	0	0.0	0
(Hain)	1 tbsp	2	0	4	1	0	0.0	0
(Heinz)	0.51 oz	2	0	0	1	0	0.0	0
(Indian Summer)	1 cup	40	1	14	5	0	1.0	0
(Lucky Leaf)								
pure	1 oz	4	0	2	0	0	0.0	0
(Musselman's)								
pure	1 oz	4	0	2	0	0	0.0	0
(S&W)	1 tbsp	0	0	0	0	0	0.0	0
(White House)								
distilled, colored or white, distilled	1 oz	4	0	2	5	0	0.0	0
MALT								
(Heinz) gourmet, 'Decanter'	0.51 oz	4	0	0	5	0	0.0	0
(S&W) malt ale, 'International'	1 tbsp	0	0	0	0	0	0.0	0
FLAVORED								
(Great Impressions)								
basil wine	1 tbsp	7	0	1	1	0	0.0	0
garlic wine	1 tbsp	7	0	1	1	0	0.0	0
hot paprika wine	1 tbsp	6	0	1	1	0	0.0	0
raspberry wine	1 tbsp	7	0	1	1	0	0.0	0
red wine	1 tbsp	6	0	1	1	0	0.0	0
(Heinz)								
garlic wine, gourmet, 'Decanter'	0.51 oz	4	0	0	0	0	0.0	0
tarragon, gourmet, 'Decanter'	0.51 oz	2	0	0	0	0	0.0	0
(S&W)								
garlic wine, 'International'	1 tbsp	0	0	0	0	0	0.0	0
Italian herb, 'International'	1 tbsp	0	0	0	0	0	0.0	0
tarragon, 'International'	1 tbsp	0	0	0	0	0	0.0	0
SALAD *(Heinz)* gourmet, 'Decanter'	0.51 oz	2	0	0	0	0	0.0	0
WHITE								
(Heinz) white, distilled	1 tbsp	2	0	0	1	0	0.0	0
(Indian Summer) white, distilled	1 cup	30	1	12	5	0	1.0	0
(Lucky Leaf) white, distilled	1 oz	4	0	2	0	0	0.0	0
(Musselman's) white, distilled	1 oz	4	0	2	0	0	0.0	0
(S&W) white, distilled	1 tbsp	0	0	0	0	0	0.0	0
WINE								
(Heinz) gourmet wine 'Decanter'	0.51 oz	4	0	0	0	0	0.0	0
(Lucky Leaf) red	1 oz	0	0	0	0	0	0.0	0
(Musselman's) red	1 oz	0	0	0	0	0	0.0	0
(Regina)								
all varieties	1 oz	4	0	0	0	0	0.0	0
red	1 oz	4	0	0	0	0	0.0	0
(S&W) red, 'International'	1 tbsp	0	0	0	0	0	0.0	0
VODKA								
80 proof	1 fl oz	64	0	0	0	0	0.0	0
86 proof	1 fl oz	70	0	0	0	0	0.0	0
90 proof	1 fl oz	73	0	0	0	0	0.0	0

Food Name	Serv. Size	Total Cal.	Prot. gms	Carbs gms	Sod. mgs	Fiber gms	Fat gms	Chol. mgs
94 proof	1 fl oz	76	0	0	0	0	0.0	0
100 proof	1 fl oz	82	0	0	0	0	0.0	0

W

Food Name	Serv. Size	Total Cal.	Prot. gms	Carbs gms	Sod. mgs	Fiber gms	Fat gms	Chol. mgs
WAFFLE								
(Aunt Jemima)								
apple cinnamon, frozen	1 waffle	176	5	29	616	2	5.6	6
buttermilk, frozen	1 waffle	179	4	29	615	1	5.8	7
low-fat, frozen	2 waffles	160	5	32	540	1	1.5	0
oat bran, frozen	2.5 oz	154	6	29	676	3	2.8	0
original, frozen, 2.5 oz	1 waffle	173	4	28	591	2	5.6	6
Quaker Oats, original, frozen	1 serving	197	5	30	563	na	6.0	12
whole-grain wheat, frozen	5 oz waffle	154	6	29	676	3	2.8	0
(Downyflake)								
apple and cinnamon, frozen 'Crisp & Healthy'	1 waffle	80	2	16	180	1	1.0	0
butter, frozen, 'Hot-N-Buttery'	2 waffles	180	4	27	620	0	6.0	0
buttermilk, frozen	2 waffles	190	5	32	750	0	5.0	0
buttermilk, frozen, 'Jumbo'	2 waffles	170	4	30	630	0	4.0	0
frozen, 'Jumbo'	2 waffles	170	4	30	570	0	4.0	0
frozen, blueberry, frozen	2 waffles	180	4	32	570	0	4.0	0
multigrain, frozen	2 waffles	250	6	28	500	4	4.0	0
oat bran, frozen	2 waffles	260	6	30	650	3	13.0	0
plain, frozen, 'Crisp & Healthy'	1 waffle	80	2	16	180	1	1.0	0
regular, frozen	2 waffles	120	3	20	420	0	3.0	0
rice bran, frozen	2 waffles	210	5	25	230	4	11.0	0
(Eggo)								
apple, 'Fruit Top'	3.1 oz	190	3	32	250	0	6.0	0
apple cinnamon	1 waffle	130	3	18	250	0	5.0	0
banana bread, 'Kellogg's Nutri-Grain'	1 serving	212	5	32	280	2	7.4	0
blueberry, frozen	1 waffle	130	3	18	250	0	5.0	0
blueberry, frozen, 'Fruit Top'	3.1 oz	190	3	32	250	0	6.0	0
blueberry, low-fat, 'Kellogg's Nutri-Grain'	1 serving	146	4	30	414	2	2.0	0
blueberry, low-fat, round, 'Kellogg's Nutri-Grain'	1 waffle	73	2	15	207	1	1.0	0
buttermilk, frozen	1 waffle	120	3	16	250	0	5.0	10
cinnamon toast, mini, sets of four	3 sets	280	5	45	470	0	9.0	25
golden oat	1 serving	139	5	26	270	2	2.3	1
golden oat, round	1 waffle	69	2	13	135	1	1.1	0
homestyle	1 waffle	120	3	16	250	0	5.0	10
homestyle, low-fat	1 serving	165	5	31	309	1	2.5	18
homestyle, mini, frozen, sets of four	3 sets	240	6	34	520	0	8.0	25
homestyle, round	1 waffle	83	2	15	155	0	1.2	9
'Kellogg's Nutri-Grain'	1 waffle	130	3	18	250	2	5.0	0
low-fat, 'Kellogg's Nutri-Grain'	1 serving	142	4	28	430	3	2.2	0
low-fat, round, 'Kellogg's Nutri-Grain'	1 waffle	71	2	14	215	1	1.1	0
multi-bran, 'Kellogg's Nutri-Grain'	2 waffles	180	5	32	400	6	6.0	0
nonfat, 'Kellogg's Special K'	2 waffles	140	6	29	250	0	0.0	0
nut and honey, frozen	2 waffles	240	6	32	430	0	10.0	25
oat bran, 'Common Sense'	1 waffle	110	3	16	220	2	4.0	0
oat bran, w/fruit and nut, 'Common Sense'	1 waffle	120	3	17	220	2	5.0	0
peach, 'Fruit Top'	3.1 oz	190	3	30	240	0	6.0	0
raisin and bran, 'Kellogg's Nutri-Grain'	1 waffle	130	3	18	250	2	5.0	0
strawberry	1 waffle	130	3	18	250	0	5.0	0
strawberry, 'Fruit Top'	1 waffle	190	3	31	230	0	6.0	0

Food Name	Serv. Size	Total Cal.	Prot. gms	Carbs gms	Sod. mgs	Fiber gms	Fat gms	Chol. mgs
wheat, whole grain, 'Kellogg's Nutri-Grain'	2 waffles	190	5	30	430	4	6.0	0
(Krusteaz)								
blueberry, frozen	1 waffle	110	3	19	210	2	3.0	3
buttermilk, frozen	1 waffle	100	3	16	190	2	2.0	4
buttermilk, frozen	1 waffle	100	3	16	190	2	2.0	4
golden, frozen	1 waffle	100	2	16	190	2	2.0	3
(Med Diet) Belgian, low-protein	1 serving	237	0	46	14	0	7.0	0
(Roman Meal) frozen	2 waffles	280	5	33	680	3	14.0	4
(Van's)								
apple cinnamon, frozen	1 waffle	75	3	8	68	3	2.0	0
Belgian, 7-grain, frozen	1 waffle	88	3	10	81	0	2.0	0
Belgian, oat bran, frozen	1 waffle	89	3	11	124	0	2.0	0
Belgian, original, frozen	1 waffle	86	3	14	54	0	2.0	0
honey almond, frozen	1 waffle	75	3	8	68	3	2.0	0
multigrain, frozen	1 waffle	75	3	8	68	3	2.0	0
WAFFLE DISH/MEAL								
(Swanson)								
Belgian, w/sausage, frozen, 'Great Starts'	2.85 oz	280	7	21	420	0	19.0	0
Belgian, w/sausage and strawberries, frozen	3.5 oz	210	3	31	240	0	8.0	0
w/bacon, frozen, 'Great Starts'	2.2 oz	230	7	19	710	0	14.0	0
WAFFLE MIX. See also PANCAKE/WAFFLE MIX.								
(Krusteaz) Belgian, prepared, 4-inch diam	1 waffle	170	5	22	350	0	7.0	45
WAKAME. See under SEA VEGETABLE.								
WALLEYE. See under PIKE; POLLACK								
WALNUT								
ALL TYPES								
chopped, natural, unsalted *(Flanigan Farms)*	1 oz	180	4	4	na	na	19.0	0
halves and pieces *(Azar)*	2 oz	360	8	10	5	3	35.0	0
halves and pieces, natural, unsalted *(Flanigan Farms)*	1/4 cup	180	7	5	0	2	18.0	0
BLACK								
Dried								
	1 oz	172	7	3	0	1	16.0	0
	1 tbsp	47	2	1	0	0	4.4	0
(Planters)	1 oz	180	7	3	0	0	17.0	0
chopped	1 cup	759	30	15	1	6	70.7	0
shelled *(Fisher)*	1 oz	170	7	3	0	0	16.0	0
Raw *(Planters)*	1 oz	180	7	3	0	0	17.0	0
ENGLISH								
Dried								
in shell, whole, 7 med nuts	1 cup	183	4	4	1	2	18.3	0
shelled *(Diamond)*	1 oz	192	5	4	0	0	19.0	0
shelled, chopped *(Fisher)*	1 oz	180	4	5	0	0	18.0	0
shelled, chopped	1 cup	785	18	16	2	8	78.3	0
shelled, ground	1 cup	523	12	11	2	5	52.2	0
shelled, ground *(Fisher)*	1 oz	180	4	5	0	0	18.0	0
shelled, halved *(Planters)*	1 oz	190	4	3	0	0	20.0	0
shelled, halved, 50 halves	1 cup	654	15	14	2	7	65.2	0
shelled, pieces *(Planters)*	1 oz	190	4	3	0	0	20.0	0
shelled, pieces or chips	1 cup	785	18	16	2	8	78.3	0
shelled, whole *(Planters)*	1 oz	190	4	3	0	0	20.0	0
Raw *(Fisher)*	1 oz	180	4	5	0	0	18.0	0
PERSIAN								
Dried								
shelled *(Diamond)*	1 oz	192	5	4	0	0	19.0	0
shelled, halves *(Planters)*	1 oz	190	4	3	0	0	20.0	0
shelled, pieces *(Planters)*	1 oz	190	4	3	0	0	20.0	0
shelled, whole *(Planters)*	1 oz	190	4	3	0	0	20.0	0

Food Name	Serv. Size	Total Cal.	Prot. gms	Carbs gms	Sod. mgs	Fiber gms	Fat gms	Chol. mgs
WALNUT OIL								
....	1 cup	1927	0	0	0	0	218.0	0
....	1 tbsp	120	0	0	0	0	13.6	0
(Hain)	1 tbsp	120	0	0	0	0	14.0	0
(International Collection)	1 tbsp	120	0	0	0	0	14.0	0
California, 100% pure *(Loriva)*	1 tbsp	125	0	0	0	0	14.0	0
pure pressed, organic *(Spectrum)*	1 tbsp	120	0	0	0	0	14.0	0
WASABI CHIPS								
(Eden Foods)								
....	1-oz bag	130	1	22	200	0	4.0	0
hot and spicy	1 oz bag	130	1	22	200	0	4.0	0
WASABI ROOT/Japanese horseradish								
raw, sliced	1 cup	142	6	31	22	10	0.8	0
raw, whole	1 med root	184	8	40	29	13	1.1	0
WATER								
FLAVORED. See also under SOFT DRINKS AND MIXERS.								
(Cascadia)								
cherry blackberry, sparkling, w/juice	6 fl oz	2	0	0	0	0	0.0	0
grapefruit, sparkling, w/juice	6 fl oz	2	0	0	0	0	0.0	0
guava berry, sparkling, w/juice	6 fl oz	2	0	0	0	0	0.0	0
lemonade, sparkling, w/juice	6 fl oz	2	0	0	0	0	0.0	0
(Clearly Canadian)								
sparkling, 'Coastal Cranberry'	6 fl oz	70	0	16	10	0	0.0	0
sparkling, 'Country Raspberry' sparkling	6 fl oz	70	0	16	10	0	0.0	0
sparkling, 'Mountain Blackberry'	6 fl oz	70	0	16	10	0	0.0	0
sparkling, 'Orchard Peach'	6 fl oz	70	0	16	10	0	0.0	0
sparkling, 'Western Loganberry'	6 fl oz	70	0	16	10	0	0.0	0
sparkling, 'Wild Cherry'	6 fl oz	70	0	16	10	0	0.0	0
(H2OH!)								
lemon-lime, sparkling	6 fl oz	0	0	0	0	0	0.0	0
natural berry, sparkling	6 fl oz	0	0	0	0	0	0.0	0
(Quest)								
black cherry, sparkling, 'Refresher'	8 fl oz	2	0	0	35	0	0.0	0
peach citrus, sparkling, 'Refresher'	8 fl oz	2	0	0	35	0	0.0	0
raspberry, sparkling, 'Refresher'	8 fl oz	2	0	0	35	0	0.0	0
red raspberry, sparkling, 'Refresher'	8 fl oz	2	0	0	35	0	0.0	0
strawberry-kiwi, sparkling, 'Refresher'	8 fl oz	2	0	0	35	0	0.0	0
tangerine lime, sparkling, 'Refresher'	8 fl oz	2	0	0	35	0	0.0	0
UNFLAVORED								
(Perrier)	8 fl oz	0	0	0	2	0	0.0	0
(Poland Spring)	8 fl oz	0	0	0	2	0	0.0	0
distilled *(Arrowhead)*	1 liter	0	0	0	0	0	0.0	0
drinking *(Arrowhead)*	1 liter	0	0	0	16	0	0.0	0
fluoridated *(Arrowhead)*	1 liter	0	0	0	16	0	0.0	0
mineral *(Perrier)*	1 liter	0	0	0	19	0	0.0	0
municipal	8 fl oz	0	0	0	7	0	0.0	0
sparkling, natural *(Clearly Canadian)*	6 fl oz	0	0	0	3	0	0.0	0
spring *(Arrowhead)*	1 liter	0	0	0	9	0	0.0	0
spring, 'Arizona Tule' *(Arrowhead)*	1 liter	0	0	0	7	0	0.0	0
Vichy *(Schweppes)*	6 fl oz	0	0	0	76	0	0.0	0
WATER BUFFALO								
raw	1 oz	28	6	0	15	0	0.4	13
roasted	3 oz	111	23	0	48	0	1.5	52
roasted, diced	1 cup	183	37.6	0.0	78	0	2.5	85
WATER CHESTNUT								
Canned								
Chinese *(LaChoy)*	1.28 oz	18	0	5	3	0	0.1	0

Food Name	Serv. Size	Total Cal.	Prot. gms	Carbs gms	Sod. mgs	Fiber gms	Fat gms	Chol. mgs
Chinese, sliced, w/liquid	1/2 cup	35	1	9	6	2	0.0	0
Chinese, whole, w/liquid	4 medium	14	0	3	2	1	0.0	0
chopped (LaChoy)	0.63 oz	9	0	2	2	1	0.1	0
sliced (China Boy)	1/2 cup	45	1	11	10	4	0.0	0
sliced (Chun King)	1 oz	12	1	2	5	0	1.0	0
sliced (La Choy)	2 tbsp	11	0	3	3	1	0.1	0
sliced, food service product (La Choy)	2 tbsp	11	0	3	3	1	0.1	0
whole (La Choy)	2 medium	10	0	2	2	1	0.1	0
whole, food service product (La Choy)	2 medium	10	0	2	2	1	0.1	0
Fresh								
Chinese, matai, raw, sliced	1/2 cup	60	1	15	9	2	0.1	0
Chinese, matai, raw, whole	4 medium	35	1	9	5	1	0.0	0
WATER CONVOLVULUS. See CABBAGE, SKUNK.								
WATERCRESS								
Fresh								
raw, chopped	1 cup	4	1	0	14	1	0.0	0
raw, whole sprigs	10 medium	3	1	0	10	0	0.0	0
raw, whole sprigs	1 medium	0	0	0	1	0	0.0	0
WATERMELON								
raw, balls	1 cup	49	1	11	3	1	0.7	0
raw, balls	10 balls	39	1	9	2	1	0.5	0
raw, diced	1 cup	49	1	11	3	1	0.7	0
raw, sliced, 1/16 of 10-inch diam melon	1 slice	92	2	21	6	1	1.2	0
WATERMELON SEED								
dried, kernels	1 cup	602	31	17	107	na	51.2	0
dried, kernels	1 oz	158	8	4	28	na	13.4	0
WAX BEAN. See BEAN, WAX.								
WAX GOURD. See GOURD, WAX.								
WELSH RAREBIT. See under CHEESE DISH/ENTRÉE.								
WEST INDIAN CHERRY. See ACEROLA.								
WESTERN ENTRÉE								
(Banquet) frozen	11 oz	630	28	40	720	0	41.0	90
(Morton) frozen	10 oz	290	14	29	1450	0	14.0	35
(Swanson) frozen	11.5 oz	430	22	43	1060	0	19.0	0
WHEAT								
BULGAR, gluten-free, 'Old World' (Ener-G Foods)	1/4 cup	181	5	39	2	8	0.6	0
DURUM	1 cup	651	26	137	4	na	4.7	0
HARD RED								
spring	1 cup	632	30	131	4	23	3.7	0
spring or winter, whole grain (Arrowhead Mills)	2 oz	190	8	41	1	8	1.0	0
winter	1 cup	628	24	137	4	23	3.0	0
HARD WHITE	1 cup	657	22	146	4	na	3.3	0
SOFT RED								
whole grain, for pastry (Arrowhead Mills)	2 oz	190	8	41	1	8	1.0	0
winter	1 cup	556	17	125	3	21	2.6	0
SOFT WHITE	1 cup	571	18	127	3	21	3.3	0
SPROUTED	1 cup	214	8	46	17	1	1.4	0
WHEAT BRAN								
crude	1 cup	125	9	37	1	25	2.5	0
crude (Arrowhead Mills)	2 oz	50	10	30	3	24	2.0	0
unprocessed (Quaker)	2 tbsp	8	1	4	0	3	0.2	0
unprocessed, miller's bran, dry (Hodgson Mill)	1/4 cup	30	2	10	0	7	0.0	0
unprocessed, natural (Miller's)	6 tbsp	70	4	17	2	12	1.0	0
WHEAT CAKE (Quaker) lightly salted	1 cake	35	1	7	45	1	0.0	0
WHEAT FLOUR. See under FLOUR.								
WHEAT GERM								
crude	1 cup	414	27	60	14	15	11.2	0

Food Name	Serv. Size	Total Cal.	Prot. gms	Carbs gms	Sod. mgs	Fiber gms	Fat gms	Chol. mgs
toasted, plain, ready to eat	1 cup	432	33	56	5	15	12.1	0
toasted, plain, ready to eat	1 oz	108	8	14	1	4	3.0	0
(Arrowhead Mills) raw	2 oz	210	15	26	1	7	6.0	0
(Hodgson Mill) untoasted, 25% protein, dry	2 tbsp	55	4	7	0	4	1.0	0
(Kretschmer)	2 tbsp	50	4	6	0	2	1.0	0
honey crunch	1 2/3 tbsp	52	4	8	2	1	1.1	0
honey crunch, sodium-free, cholesterol-free	1 oz	110	8	15	0	3	3.0	0
sodium-free, cholesterol-free	2 tbsp	50	4	6	0	2	1.0	0
WHEAT GERM NUTS (Anacon Foods)	1/2 oz	100	2	2	13	1	9.3	0
WHEAT GERM OIL								
	1 cup	1927	0	0	0	0	218.0	0
	1 tbsp	120	0	0	0	0	13.6	0
WHEAT GLUTEN								
(Arrowhead Mills) Vita 1	1 oz	100	15	9	1	1	1.0	0
(Hodgson Mill) Vital w/Vit-C	1 tbsp	30	6	2	0	1	0.0	0
WHEAT SNACKS								
wheat nuts, flavored, no salt added, all flavors except macadamia	1 oz	183	4	6	26	1	17.7	0
wheat nuts, formulated, unflavored, salted	1 oz	176	4	7	143	1	16.4	0
(Ralston)								
'Delicious'	16 crackers	140	2	23	220	1	4.0	na
full fat, 'Delicious'	16 crackers	140	3	20	120	2	6.0	0
full fat, 'Grand Union'	16 crackers	140	3	20	120	2	6.0	0
full fat, 'Stop & Shop'	16 crackers	140	3	20	120	2	6.0	0
full fat, unsalted, 'Stop & Shop'	16 crackers	140	3	20	80	2	6.0	na
'Grand Union'	16 crackers	140	2	23	220	1	4.0	na
less fat	16 crackers	140	2	23	220	1	4.0	0
unsalted tops, 'Stop & Shop'	16 crackers	140	2	23	85	1	4.0	na
WHEATGRASS								
powder (Pines)	1 tsp	13	1	2	1	1	0.0	0
tablets (Pines)	7 tablets	13	1	2	1	1	0.0	0
WHELK								
boiled, poached, or steamed	3 oz	234	41	13	350	0	0.7	111
raw	3 oz	116	20	7	175	0	0.3	55
WHEY								
acid, dried	1 cup	193	7	42	552	0	0.3	2
acid, dried	1 tbsp	10	0	2	28	0	0.0	0
acid, fluid	1 quart	235	7	50	473	0	0.9	5
acid, fluid	1 cup	59	2	13	118	0	0.2	1
sweet, dried	1 cup	512	19	108	1565	0	1.6	9
sweet, dried	1 tbsp	26	1	6	81	0	0.1	0
sweet, fluid	1 quart	263	8	51	526	0	3.5	20
sweet, fluid	1 cup	66	2	13	132	0	0.9	5
WHIPPED TOPPING. See CREAM TOPPING.								
WHISKEY								
80 proof	1 fl oz	64	0	0	0	0	0.0	0
86 proof	1 fl oz	70	0	0	0	0	0.0	0
90 proof	1 fl oz	73	0	0	0	0	0.0	0
94 proof	1 fl oz	76	0	0	0	0	0.0	0
100 proof	1 fl oz	82	0	0	0	0	0.0	0
WHISKEY SOUR. See under COCKTAIL; COCKTAIL MIX.								
WHITE ACRE PEAS, canned, fresh (Allens)	1/2 cup	90	7	14	440	0	1.0	0
WHITE BEAN. See BEAN, WHITE.								
WHITE CURRANT. See under CURRANT.								
WHITE GOURD. See CHINESE WATERMELON.								
WHITE MUSHROOM. See MUSHROOM, WHITE.								

Food Name	Serv. Size	Total Cal.	Prot. gms	Carbs gms	Sod. mgs	Fiber gms	Fat gms	Chol. mgs
WHITE PEPPER. See under PEPPER, GROUND.								
WHITE RICE. See under RICE.								
WHITE SUCKER. See SUCKER, WHITE.								
WHITEFISH								
mixed species, baked, broiled, grilled, or microwaved ..... 3 oz		146	21	0	55	0	6.4	65
mixed species, raw .... 3 oz		114	16	0	43	0	5.0	51
mixed species, smoked........................... 3 oz		92	20	0	866	0	0.8	28
mixed species, smoked, flaked .... 1 cup		147	32	0	1386	0	1.3	45
WHITE-FLOWERED GOURD. See GOURD, BOTTLE.								
WHITING/silver hake								
Fresh								
mixed species, baked, broiled, grilled, or microwaved ..... 3 oz		99	20	0	112	0	1.4	71
mixed species, raw .... 3 oz		77	16	0	61	0	1.1	57
Frozen, 'Individually Wrapped' *(Booth)* .... 4 oz		80	19	0	85	0	1.0	0
WILD RICE. See RICE, WILD.								
WINE. See also SHERRY; VERMOUTH; WINE, COOKING; WINE COOLER.								
(Mission Bell)								
'Arriba' .... 2 fl oz		95	0	7	4	0	0.0	0
'Diamond Red' .... 2 fl oz		95	0	7	4	0	0.0	0
'Silver Satin' .... 2 fl oz		83	0	5	4	0	0.0	0
'Silver Satin Bitter Lemon' .... 2 fl oz		83	0	6	4	0	0.0	0
'Swiss Up' .... 2 fl oz		84	0	6	4	0	0.0	0
BARBERA, white *(Colony)* .... 4 fl oz		91	0	4	4	0	0.0	0
BURGUNDY								
(Bravo) red .... 4 fl oz		91	0	2	4	0	0.0	0
(Carlo Rossi) red .... 4 fl oz		92	0	2	0	0	0.0	0
(Colony)								
red 'Classic' .... 4 fl oz		90	0	1	4	0	0.0	0
white, 'Classic' .... 4 fl oz		80	0	1	4	0	0.0	0
(Gallo)								
red .... 4 fl oz		88	0	1	0	0	0.0	0
red, 'Hearty' .... 4 fl oz		92	0	2	0	0	0.0	0
(Gambarelli & Davitto) red 'Parma' .... 4 fl oz		91	0	2	4	0	0.0	0
(Petri) red .... 4 fl oz		91	0	2	4	0	0.0	0
CABERNET SAUVIGNON								
(Colony) .... 4 fl oz		88	0	1	4	0	0.0	0
(Gallo) .... 4 fl oz		88	0	0	0	0	0.0	0
CARBONATED								
(Jacques Bonet)								
almond.. 4 fl oz		104	0	8	4	0	0.0	0
apricot .... 4 fl oz		111	0	10	4	0	0.0	0
cherry .... 4 fl oz		106	0	8	4	0	0.0	0
(Carlo Rossi) 'Paisano' .... 4 fl oz		92	0	2	0	0	0.0	0
(Jacques Bonet)								
peach .... 4 fl oz		111	0	10	4	0	0.0	0
raspberry .... 4 fl oz		106	0	8	4	0	0.0	0
CHABLIS								
(Bravo) .... 4 fl oz		86	0	2	4	0	0.0	0
(Carlo Rossi)								
pink .... 4 fl oz		92	0	4	0	0	0.0	0
white .... 4 fl oz		84	0	2	0	0	0.0	0
(Colony)								
.... 4 fl oz		98	0	5	4	0	0.0	0
'Classic' .... 4 fl oz		84	0	2	4	0	0.0	0
emerald .... 4 fl oz		102	0	5	4	0	0.0	0
gold .... 4 fl oz		97	0	4	4	0	0.0	0
ruby .... 4 fl oz		104	0	6	4	0	0.0	0

Food Name	Serv. Size	Total Cal.	Prot. gms	Carbs gms	Sod. mgs	Fiber gms	Fat gms	Chol. mgs
(Gallo)								
....	4 fl oz	80	0	4	0	0	0.0	0
'Blanc'	4 fl oz	80	0	1	0	0	0.0	0
(Petri)								
....	4 fl oz	98	0	5	4	0	0.0	0
'Chablis Blanc'	4 fl oz	86	0	2	4	0	0.0	0
(Gambarelli & Davitto) 'Parma'	4 fl oz	86	0	2	4	0	0.0	0
CHAMPAGNE								
(Jacques Bonet)								
brut	4 fl oz	92	0	2	4	0	0.0	0
extra dry	4 fl oz	97	0	3	4	0	0.0	0
pink	4 fl oz	98	0	4	4	0	0.0	0
(Lejon)								
brut	4 fl oz	92	0	3	4	0	0.0	0
extra dry	4 fl oz	97	0	2	4	0	0.0	0
pink	4 fl oz	98	0	4	4	0	0.0	0
CHENIN BLANC								
(Colony)	4 fl oz	86	0	2	4	0	0.0	0
(Gallo)	4 fl oz	88	0	2	0	0	0.0	0
CHIANTI								
(Carlo Rossi) 'Light'	4 fl oz	92	0	2	0	0	0.0	0
(Petri)	4 fl oz	91	0	2	4	0	0.0	0
COLD DUCK								
(Jacques Bonet)	4 fl oz	108	0	6	4	0	0.0	0
(Lejon)	4 fl oz	108	0	6	4	0	0.0	0
FRENCH COLOMBARD								
(Colony)	4 fl oz	84	0	2	4	0	0.0	0
(Gallo)	4 fl oz	88	0	2	0	0	0.0	0
GEWÜRZTRAMINER *(Gallo)*	4 fl oz	88	0	2	0	0	0.0	0
MARSALA *(Gambarelli & Davitto)*.	4 fl oz	77	0	4	4	0	0.0	0
MOSELLE *(Colony)* 'Rhineskeller'	4 fl oz	97	0	4	4	0	0.0	0
MUSCATEL *(Italian Swiss Colony)*	2 fl oz	122	0	6	4	0	0.0	0
PASTOSO *(Petri)*	4 fl oz	92	0	2	4	0	0.0	0
PORT								
(Gallo)								
....	2 fl oz	64	0	2	0	0	0.0	0
tawny, 'Livingston Cellars'	2 fl oz	86	0	6	0	0	0.0	0
white	2 fl oz	86	0	6	0	0	0.0	0
(Italian Swiss Colony)								
....	2 fl oz	85	0	6	4	0	0.0	0
white	2 fl oz	86	0	6	4	0	0.0	0
RED TABLE	3.5 fl oz	74	0	2	5	0	0.0	0
RHINE								
(Bravo)	4 fl oz	97	0	4	4	0	0.0	0
(Carlo Rossi)	4 fl oz	84	0	4	0	0	0.0	0
(Colony) 'Classic'	4 fl oz	89	0	4	4	0	0.0	0
(Gallo)	4 fl oz	80	0	4	0	0	0.0	0
(Gambarelli & Davitto) 'Parma'	4 fl oz	92	0	1	4	0	0.0	0
(Petri)	4 fl oz	97	0	4	4	0	0.0	0
RIESLING *(Gallo)* 'Johannisberg'	4 fl oz	84	0	2	0	0	0.0	0
ROSÉ								
(Bravo)	4 fl oz	92	0	3	4	0	0.0	0
(Carlo Rossi) 'Vin Rose'	4 fl oz	88	0	3	0	0	0.0	0
(Colony) 'Classic'	4 fl oz	89	0	3	4	0	0.0	0
(Gallo)								
'Grenache'	4 fl oz	88	0	2	0	0	0.0	0
'Red Rose'	4 fl oz	112	0	6	0	0	0.0	0

Food Name	Serv. Size	Total Cal.	Prot. gms	Carbs gms	Sod. mgs	Fiber gms	Fat gms	Chol. mgs
'Vin Rose'	4 fl oz	88	0	3	0	0	0.0	0
(Gambarelli & Davitto) 'Parma'	4 fl oz	92	0	3	4	0	0.0	0
(Petri)	4 fl oz	92	0	3	4	0	0.0	0
SAUVIGNON BLANC (Gallo)	4 fl oz	80	0	1	0	0	0.0	0
TOKAY (Italian Swiss Colony)	2 fl oz	82	0	5	4	0	0.0	0
WHITE TABLE	3.5 fl oz	70	0	1	5	0	0.0	0
WINE, COOKING								
(Holland House)								
Marsala	1 fl oz	9	0	2	186	0	0.0	0
red	1 fl oz	6	0	2	186	0	0.0	0
sherry	1 fl oz	5	0	1	186	0	0.0	0
vermouth	1 fl oz	2	0	1	186	0	0.0	0
white	1 fl oz	2	0	1	186	0	0.0	0
(Regina)								
Burgundy	1/4 cup	2	1	1	365	0	1.0	0
Sauternes	1/4 cup	2	1	1	365	0	1.0	0
sherry	1/4 cup	20	1	5	70	0	1.0	0
WINE COOLER								
(Bartles & Jaymes)								
berry cooler, 'Light'	12 fl oz	150	0	32	0	0	0.0	0
black cherry cooler, 'Light'	12 fl oz	139	0	30	0	0	0.0	0
citrus cooler, 'Light'	6 fl oz	67	1	12	0	0	1.0	0
tropical cooler, 'Light'	12 fl oz	151	0	32	0	0	0.0	0
WINGED BEAN. See BEAN, WINGED.								
WINTER RADISH. See under RADISH.								
WINTER SQUASH. See SQUASH, WINTER.								
WOLF FISH/ocean catfish								
Fresh								
Atlantic, baked, broiled, or grilled	3 oz	105	19	0	93	0	2.6	50
Atlantic, raw	3 oz	82	15	0	72	0	2.0	39
Frozen (Booth)	4 oz	115	20	0	85	0	20.0	0
WONTON WRAPPER								
including egg roll wrappers	1 oz	82	3	16	162	1	0.4	3
including egg roll wrappers, 7-inch square	1 wrapper	93	3	19	183	1	0.5	3
including egg roll wrappers, 3.5-inch square	1 wrapper	23	1	5	46	0	0.1	1
(Nasoya)	1 wrapper	23	1	5	19	0	0.0	0

Y

Food Name	Serv. Size	Total Cal.	Prot. gms	Carbs gms	Sod. mgs	Fiber gms	Fat gms	Chol. mgs
YAM								
Fresh								
boiled, drained, cubed	1 cup	158	2	38	11	5	0.2	0
boiled, drained, cubed	1/2 cup	79	1	19	5	3	0.1	0
raw, cubed	1 cup	177	2	42	14	6	0.3	0
Canned								
(Bush's Best)	1/2 cup	120	1	28	20	0	0.0	0
cut, in light syrup (Princella)	2/3 cup	160	0	40	35	3	0.5	0
orange pineapple (Royal Prince)	1/2 cup	210	1	43	30	3	0.5	0
CHINESE. See JICAMA.								
MOUNTAIN/HAWAIIAN								
Fresh								
raw, whole	1 medium	281	6	69	55	na	0.4	0
raw, cubed	1/2 cup	46	1	11	9	na	0.1	0
steamed, cubed	1 cup	119	3	29	17	na	0.1	0

Food Name	Serv. Size	Total Cal.	Prot. gms	Carbs gms	Sod. mgs	Fiber gms	Fat gms	Chol. mgs
YAM DISH								
(Flav-R-Pac) yam patties . . . . 2 pieces		150	1	33	200	3	1.0	0
(Stouffer's) yam and apples, frozen, food service product . . . 1 oz		37	0	8	26	0	0.7	0
YAMBEAN TUBER. See JICAMA.								
YARDLONG BEAN. See BEAN, YARDLONG.								
YAUTIA/tannia								
Fresh								
raw, sliced . . . . 1 cup		132	2	32	28	2	0.5	0
raw, whole . . . . 1 med root		299	4	72	64	5	1.2	0
YEAST								
BAKER'S								
active, dry . . . . 1 tbsp		35	5	5	6	3	0.6	0
active, dry . . . . 1 tsp		12	2	2	2	1	0.2	0
active dry *(Red Star)* . . . . 0.25 oz		15	2	2	5	0	0.0	0
active dry, 'RapidRise' *(Fleischmann's)* . . . . 0.25 oz		20	3	3	10	0	0.0	0
compressed . . . . 0.6-oz cake		18	1	3	5	1	0.3	0
BREWER'S								
debittered . . . . 1 oz		79	10.9	10.8	34	>0.5	0.3	0
debittered . . . . 1 tbsp		23	3.1	3.1	10	>0.1	0.1	0
torula . . . . 1 oz		78	10.8	10.4	4	>0.9	0.3	0
YELLOW BEAN. See BEAN, YELLOW.								
YELLOW MOMBIN. See JOBO.								
YELLOW PEPPER. See PEPPER, BANANA; PEPPER, BELL.								
YELLOW SQUASH. See under SQUASH.								
YELLOW EYE BEANS. See under BAKED BEANS, CANNED.								
YELLOWFIN TUNA. See under TUNA.								
YELLOWTAIL								
mixed species, baked, broiled, grilled, or microwaved . . . . . 3 oz		159	25	0	43	0	5.7	60
mixed species, raw . . . . 3 oz		124	20	0	33	0	4.5	47
YOGURT								
(Crowley) all flavors, 'Swiss Style' . . . . 1 cup		240	8	48	150	0	2.0	10
(Light n' Lively) all flavors except strawberry,								
nonfat, 'Free' . . . . 4.4 oz		50	4	8	60	0	0.0	0
(Ripple) all flavors, fat-free, '70' . . . . 6 oz		70	5	13	85	0	0.0	5
(Yoplait)								
all fruit flavors, custard style . . . . 6 oz		190	7	32	100	0	3.5	15
all fruit flavors, light . . . . 6 oz		90	5	16	75	0	0.0	0
all fruit flavors, nonfat . . . . 6 oz		90	5	16	75	0	0.0	0
all fruit flavors, original, 99% fat-free . . . . 6 oz		180	6	34	80	0	1.5	10
APPLE CINNAMON *(Dannon)* low-fat . . . . 1 container		240	9	46	140	1	3.0	15
APPLE CRISP *(New Country)* low-fat . . . . 6 oz		150	5	30	85	0	2.0	0
BANANA								
(Yoplait) custard style . . . . 6 oz		180	7	30	105	0	3.0	0
(Dannon) lowfat, 'Sprinkl'ins' . . . . 4.1 oz		140	5	24	80	0	2.0	5
BANANA BERRY								
(Light n' Lively) berry, low-fat, 1% milk fat, cultured . . . . 4.4 oz		130	5	24	75	0	1.0	10
BERRY *(Yoplait)* w/wheat, raisins, walnuts, 'Breakfast' . . . . 6 oz		200	8	39	125	0	2.0	0
BLACK CHERRY								
(Alta Dena)								
blended . . . . 8 oz		190	8	38	140	0	1.0	0
fruit on the bottom . . . . 1 cup		240	12	40	150	0	4.0	0
(Breyers) low-fat . . . . 8 oz		260	9	49	120	0	3.0	10
(Knudsen) nonfat, 'Cal 70' . . . . 6 oz		70	5	12	75	0	0.0	5
(Light n' Lively)								
. . . . 8 oz		230	9	44	125	0	2.0	15
nonfat, '100' . . . . 8 oz		100	8	17	100	0	0.0	0
(Mountain High) natural, 'Honey Light' . . . . 8 oz		190	9	35	140	0	1.0	5

Food Name	Serv. Size	Total Cal.	Prot. gms	Carbs gms	Sod. mgs	Fiber gms	Fat gms	Chol. mgs
BLUEBERRY								
(Alta Dena) fruit on the bottom, 'Maya'	1 cup	280	11	39	170	0	9.0	0
(Breyers) low-fat	8 oz	250	9	48	120	0	2.0	10
(Dannon)								
low-fat	1 container	240	9	46	140	1	3.0	15
nonfat, blended	3/4 cup	160	7	33	105	0	0.0	5
nonfat, light	8 oz	100	9	19	135	0	0.0	5
(Knudsen) nonfat, 'Cal 70'	6 oz	70	6	11	80	0	0.0	5
(Light n' Lively)								
	8 oz	240	8	46	130	0	2.0	10
nonfat, 'Free'	4.4 oz	50	4	8	60	0	0.0	0
nonfat, '100'	8 oz	90	8	15	110	0	0.0	0
(Mountain High) natural, 'Honey Light'	8 oz	190	9	35	140	0	1.0	5
(New Country) 'Supreme'	6 oz	150	5	31	90	0	2.0	0
(White Wave) nondairy	1 serving	150	5	31	55	1	1.0	0
(Yoplait)								
fruit on the bottom	6 oz	170	7	35	105	0	0.0	5
light	6 oz	90	5	16	70	0	0.0	5
99% fat-free, original	6 oz	180	8	32	130	0	2.0	0
BLUEBERRIES AND CREAM								
(Weight Watchers) 'Ultimate 90'	1 cup	90	8	14	140	3	0.0	0
BLUEBERRY AND VANILLA *(Yoplait)* parfait style	6 oz	200	8	34	120	0	3.0	0
BLUEBERRY CHEESECAKE *(Yogi)* w/gelatin, 'Sundae'	5.6 oz	50	6	14	75	0	1.0	4
BOYSENBERRY								
(Dannon) low-fat	1 container	240	9	45	150	1	3.0	15
(Yoplait) 99% fat-free, original	6 oz	180	8	32	130	0	2.0	0
CAPPUCCINO								
(Dannon) light	8 oz	100	9	16	135	0	0.0	5
(Weight Watchers) 'Ultimate 90'	1 cup	90	8	14	140	0	0.0	0
CHERRIES JUBILEE *(Weight Watchers)* 'Ultimate 90'	1 cup	90	8	14	140	0	0.0	0
CHERRY								
(Dannon)								
low-fat	1 container	240	9	45	140	1	3.0	15
low-fat, 'Sprinkl'ins'	4.1 oz	140	5	24	80	0	2.0	5
(Light n' Lively)	4.4 oz	140	5	27	70	0	1.0	5
(New Country) 'Supreme'	6 oz	150	5	32	90	0	2.0	0
(Yoplait)								
custard style	6 oz	180	7	30	95	0	4.0	20
light	6 oz	90	5	16	70	0	0.0	5
99% fat-free, original	6 oz	180	8	32	130	0	2.0	0
triple cherry, 'Trix'	6 oz	190	9	31	120	0	3.0	0
w/almonds, 'Breakfast'	6 oz	200	8	38	90	2	3.0	10
CHERRY VANILLA								
(Dannon)								
'Light'	8 oz	100	9	18	135	0	0.0	5
low-fat, 'Sprinkl'ins'	4.1 oz	140	5	24	95	0	2.0	5
nonfat, light	8 oz	100	9	18	135	0	0.0	5
(Lite-Line) 1% fat, 'Swiss Style'	1 cup	240	10	45	150	0	2.0	0
(Yogi) w/gelatin, 'Sundae'	5.6 oz	50	6	14	75	0	1.0	4
(Yoplait)								
light, custard style	6 oz	90	6	17	85	0	0.0	5
parfait style	6 oz	200	8	34	120	0	3.0	0
COFFEE								
(Bison) low-fat	1 cup	210	11	33	160	0	4.0	10
(Dannon)	8 oz	200	10	34	140	0	3.0	10
(Friendship) low-fat	1 cup	210	11	35	170	0	3.0	14

Food Name	Serv. Size	Total Cal.	Prot. gms	Carbs gms	Sod. mgs	Fiber gms	Fat gms	Chol. mgs
CRANBERRY RASPBERRY								
(Weight Watchers) 'Ultimate 90'	1 cup	90	8	14	140	0	0.0	0
FRUIT CRUNCH *(New Country)* low-fat	6 oz	150	5	30	90	0	2.0	0
GRAPE								
(Dannon) lowfat, 'Sprinkl'ins'	4.1 oz	140	5	24	110	0	2.0	5
(Light n' Lively)	4.4 oz	130	6	24	70	0	1.0	10
LEMON								
(Alta Dena) fruit on the bottom	1 cup	240	12	40	150	0	4.0	0
(Bison) low-fat	1 cup	210	11	33	160	0	4.0	10
(Dannon)								
......	8 oz	200	10	34	140	0	3.0	10
low-fat	1 container	210	10	36	160	0	3.0	15
(Knudsen) nonfat, 'Cal 70'	6 oz	70	6	12	125	0	0.0	0
(Light n' Lively) nonfat, '100'	8 oz	100	9	16	150	0	0.0	5
(Mountain High) natural	8 oz	220	10	31	140	0	6.0	0
(New Country) 'Supreme'	6 oz	150	5	31	90	0	2.0	0
(Yoplait) 99% fat-free, original	6 oz	180	8	32	130	0	2.0	0
LEMON CHIFFON								
(Dannon)								
blended	6 oz	150	8	30	110	0	0.0	5
'Light'	8 oz	100	9	15	135	0	0.0	5
(Weight Watchers) 'Ultimate 90'	1 cup	90	8	14	140	1	0.0	0
(Yogi) w/gelatin, 'Sundae'	5.6 oz	50	6	14	75	0	1.0	4
MIXED BERRIES								
(Alta Dena) blended	8 oz	190	8	39	140	0	1.0	0
(Breyers) low-fat	8 oz	250	9	48	120	0	2.0	10
(New Country) low-fat	6 oz	150	5	31	85	0	2.0	0
(Yoplait) custard style	6 oz	180	7	30	95	0	4.0	20
ORANGE								
(Dannon) low-fat	1 container	240	9	45	135	0	3.0	15
(New Country) 'Supreme'	6 oz	150	5	31	90	0	2.0	0
ORANGE-PINEAPPLE *(Yogi)* w/gelatin, 'Sundae'	5.6 oz	50	6	14	75	0	1.0	4
PEACH								
(Alta Dena) fruit on the bottom	1 cup	240	12	40	150	0	4.0	0
(Breyers) low-fat	8 oz	250	9	48	120	0	2.0	10
(Carnation) fruit on the bottom, 'Smooth'n Creamy'	8 oz	250	8	47	130	0	3.0	0
(Dannon)								
low-fat	1 container	240	9	45	140	1	3.0	15
nonfat, light	8 oz	100	9	17	135	0	0.0	5
(Knudsen) nonfat, 'Cal 70'	6 oz	70	6	11	95	0	0.0	0
(Light n' Lively)								
......	8 oz	240	9	46	120	0	2.0	15
nonfat, '100'	8 oz	100	9	16	115	0	0.0	5
(Lite-Line) 1% fat, 'Swiss Style'	1 cup	230	10	42	150	0	2.0	0
(Mountain High) natural	8 oz	220	10	31	140	0	6.0	0
(Weight Watchers) 'Ultimate 90'	1 cup	90	8	14	140	0	0.0	0
(Yogi) peachy, w/gelatin, 'Sundae'	5.6 oz	50	6	14	75	0	1.0	4
(Yoplait)								
99% fat-free, original	6 oz	180	8	32	130	0	2.0	0
nonfat, light, custard style	6 oz	90	6	17	85	0	0.0	5
nonfat, fruit on the bottom	6 oz	170	7	35	105	0	0.0	5
nonfat, w/granola, 'Crunch 'N Yogurt'	7 oz	220	8	43	125	0	2.0	5
PEACH AND VANILLA *(Yoplait)* parfait style	6 oz	200	8	34	120	0	3.0	0
PEACHES AND CREAM *(New Country)* low-fat	6 oz	150	5	31	90	0	2.0	0
PIÑA COLADA *(Yoplait)* 99% fat-free, original	6 oz	180	8	32	130	0	2.0	0
PINEAPPLE								
(Breyers) low-fat	8 oz	250	9	50	120	0	2.0	10

Food Name	Serv. Size	Total Cal.	Prot. gms	Carbs gms	Sod. mgs	Fiber gms	Fat gms	Chol. mgs
(Knudsen) nonfat, 'Cal 70'	6 oz	70	6	12	125	0	0.0	0
(Light n' Lively)	8 oz	230	9	47	120	0	2.0	10
(Yoplait) 99% fat-free, original	6 oz	180	8	32	130	0	2.0	0
PLAIN								
(Alta Dena)	1 cup	100	13	13	160	0	1.0	0
(Bison)								
low-fat	1 cup	150	12	17	180	0	4.0	10
nonfat	1 cup	120	12	16	170	0	0.0	0
(Breyers) low-fat	8 oz	140	12	16	170	0	3.0	20
(Crowley)								
	1 cup	160	10	14	150	0	8.0	30
low-fat	1 cup	140	12	17	180	0	2.0	10
nonfat	1 cup	120	13	17	180	0	1.0	1
(Dannon)								
low-fat	8 oz	140	10	16	160	0	4.0	15
nonfat	8 oz	110	11	16	160	0	0.0	5
(Friendship) low-fat, 1.5% fat	1 cup	150	12	17	190	0	3.0	14
(Knudsen)								
	8 oz	200	12	16	170	0	9.0	35
low-fat	8 oz	160	12	17	180	0	5.0	25
(Lite-Line) 1.5% fat, 'Swiss Style'	1 cup	140	12	18	150	0	2.0	0
(Meadow Gold) low-fat, 2% milk fat	1 cup	160	12	16	160	0	5.0	0
(Mountain High) plain	1 cup	200	12	16	140	0	9.0	0
(Weight Watchers) 'Ultimate 90'	1 cup	90	8	14	150	0	0.0	0
(White Wave) nondairy	1 serving	180	12	18	70	5	7.0	0
(Yoplait)								
98% fat-free, original	6 oz	120	10	15	150	0	2.0	15
nonfat	8 oz	120	13	18	160	0	0.0	5
RAINBOW PUNCH *(Yoplait)* 'Trix'	6 oz	190	9	31	120	0	3.0	0
RASPBERRIES AND CREAM								
(Weight Watchers) 'Ultimate 90'	1 cup	90	8	14	140	0	0.0	0
RASPBERRY								
(Alta Dena)								
blended	8 oz	180	8	37	140	0	1.0	0
fruit on the bottom	1 cup	240	12	40	150	0	4.0	0
(Breyers) low-fat	8 oz	250	9	48	120	0	2.0	10
(Dannon)								
low-fat	1 container	240	9	45	150	1	3.0	15
nonfat, blended	6 oz	150	8	30	110	0	0.0	5
nonfat, 'Light'	8 oz	100	9	18	135	0	0.0	5
(Knudsen) nonfat, 'Cal 70'	6 oz	70	6	11	80	0	0.0	5
(Light n' Lively)								
nonfat, '100'	8 oz	90	8	15	105	0	0.0	0
red	8 oz	230	9	43	130	0	2.0	10
red, nonfat, 'Free'	4.4 oz	50	4	8	60	0	0.0	0
(Meadow Gold)								
low-fat, natural, 'Sundae Style'	1 cup	250	10	42	160	0	4.0	0
red, low-fat, 1.5% milk fat	1 cup	250	10	42	160	0	4.0	0
(Mountain High) natural, 'Honey Light'	8 oz	190	9	35	140	0	1.0	5
(New Country) red, 'Supreme'	6 oz	150	5	31	90	0	2.0	0
(Yoplait)								
light	6 oz	90	5	16	70	0	0.0	5
99% fat-free, original	6 oz	180	8	32	130	0	2.0	0
nonfat, fruit on the bottom	6 oz	170	7	35	105	0	0.0	5
STRAWBERRY								
(Alta Dena)								
blended	8 oz	180	8	37	140	0	1.0	0

Food Name	Serv. Size	Total Cal.	Prot. gms	Carbs gms	Sod. mgs	Fiber gms	Fat gms	Chol. mgs
fruit on the bottom	1 cup	240	12	40	150	0	4.0	0
fruit on the bottom, 'Maya'	1 cup	280	11	39	170	0	9.0	0
(Breyers)								
	8 oz	218	9	41	118	0	1.8	20
low-fat	8 oz	250	9	48	120	0	2.0	10
nonfat, w/aspartame and fructose sweeteners	8 oz container	125	8	22	102	0	0.5	11
'Smooth & Creamy'	8 oz	232	9	45	125	1	2.0	20
(Carnation) 'Smooth 'n Creamy'	8 oz	230	8	44	115	0	3.0	0
(Crowley) nonfat	1 cup	190	12	35	190	0	1.0	1
(Dannon)								
low-fat	1 container	240	9	46	135	1	3.0	15
low-fat, 'Sprinkl'ins'	4.1 oz	140	5	24	95	0	2.0	5
nonfat, blended	6 oz	150	8	30	110	0	0.0	5
nonfat, light	8 oz	100	9	17	135	0	0.0	5
(Knudsen)								
low-fat	8 oz	250	10	45	135	0	4.0	15
nonfat, 'Cal 70'	6 oz	70	6	11	85	0	0.0	0
(Light n' Lively)								
	8 oz	240	9	45	130	0	2.0	15
	4.4 oz	135	4	27	56	0	1.0	11
nonfat	4.4 oz	70	4	12	55	0	0.0	0
nonfat, '100'	8 oz	90	8	15	105	0	0.0	5
(Lite-Line) low-fat, 1% fat	1 cup	240	10	46	150	0	2.0	0
(Mountain High) natural, 'Honey Light'	8 oz	190	9	35	140	0	1.0	5
(New Country) 'Supreme'	6 oz	150	5	30	90	0	2.0	0
(Sara Lee) 'Free & Light'	1/10 pkg	120	2	26	90	0	1.0	0
(Weight Watchers) 'Ultimate 90'	1 cup	90	8	14	140	2	0.0	0
(White Wave) nondairy	1 serving	150	5	30	40	3	1.0	0
(Yoplait) custard style	6 oz	180	7	30	105	0	3.0	0
99% fat-free, original	6 oz	180	8	32	130	0	2.0	0
nonfat, fruit on the bottom	6 oz	170	7	35	105	0	0.0	5
nonfat, light	6 oz	90	5	16	70	0	0.0	5
nonfat, light, custard style	6 oz	90	6	17	85	0	0.0	5
STRAWBERRY AND VANILLA *(Yoplait)* parfait style	6 oz	200	8	34	120	0	3.0	0
STRAWBERRY CHEESECAKE								
(Yogi) w/gelatin, 'Sundae'	5.6 oz	50	6	14	75	0	1.0	4
STRAWBERRY FRUIT BASKET								
(Knudsen) nonfat, 'Cal 70'	6 oz	70	6	11	75	0	0.0	5
STRAWBERRY FRUIT CUP								
(Dannon) light	8 oz	100	9	17	135	0	0.0	5
(Light n' Lively)								
	8 oz	240	9	47	120	0	2.0	15
nonfat, 'Free'	4.4 oz	50	4	8	55	0	0.0	0
'100'	8 oz	90	8	15	100	0	0.0	0
(New Country) low-fat	6 oz	150	5	30	85	0	2.0	0
STRAWBERRY-ALMOND *(Yoplait)* 'Breakfast Yogurt'	6 oz	200	8	38	90	2	3.0	10
STRAWBERRY-BANANA								
(Alta Dena) fruit on the bottom	1 cup	180	12	35	128	0	1.0	0
(Breyers) low-fat	8 oz	250	9	50	120	0	2.0	10
(Carnation) 'Smooth 'n Creamy'	8 oz	240	9	42	125	0	4.0	0
(Dannon)								
light	8 oz	100	9	17	135	0	0.0	5
low-fat	1 container	240	9	43	140	1	3.0	15
low-fat, 'Sprinkl'ins'	4.1 oz	140	5	24	95	0	2.0	5
(Knudsen) nonfat, 'Cal 70'	6 oz	70	6	12	80	0	0.0	0
(Light n' Lively)								
	8 oz	260	9	52	120	0	2.0	10

Food Name	Serv. Size	Total Cal.	Prot. gms	Carbs gms	Sod. mgs	Fiber gms	Fat gms	Chol. mgs
nonfat, 'Free'	4.4 oz	50	4	8	60	0	0.0	0
(Mountain High) natural, 'Honey Light'	8 oz	190	9	35	140	0	1.0	5
(New Country)	6 oz	150	5	31	85	0	2.0	0
(Weight Watchers) 'Ultimate 90'	1 cup	90	8	14	140	2	0.0	0
(Yoplait)								
bash, 'Trix'	6 oz	190	9	31	120	0	3.0	0
fruit on the bottom	6 oz	170	7	35	105	0	0.0	5
light	6 oz	90	5	16	70	0	0.0	5
99% fat-free, original	6 oz	180	8	32	130	0	2.0	0
w/wheat and walnuts, 'Breakfast'	6 oz	200	8	40	110	0	2.0	0
STRAWBERRY-RHUBARB (Yoplait)	6 oz	190	8	32	110	0	3.0	10
TROPICAL FRUIT								
(Dannon) nonfat, light	8 oz	100	9	18	135	0	0.0	5
(Weight Watchers) nonfat, 'Ultimate 90'	1 cup	90	10	13	120	0	0.0	5
(Yoplait) w/wheat, raisin, nuts, 'Breakfast'	6 oz	200	8	41	110	0	3.0	0
VANILLA								
(Bison) low-fat	1 cup	210	11	33	160	0	4.0	10
(Breyers) low-fat	8 oz	230	11	41	150	0	3.0	20
(Crowley) low-fat	1 cup	200	12	33	170	0	2.0	10
(Dannon)								
French, fat-free, blended	3/4 cup	150	7	31	100	0	0.0	5
low-fat	1 container	210	10	36	160	0	3.0	15
nonfat, light	8 oz	100	9	16	135	0	0.0	5
w/wheat, 'Hearty Nuts & Raisins'	8 oz	270	9	48	120	0	5.0	10
(Friendship) low-fat	1 cup	210	11	35	170	0	3.0	14
(Knudsen)								
low-fat	8 oz	240	11	43	135	0	4.0	15
nonfat, 'Cal 70'	6 oz	70	6	11	90	0	0.0	0
(New Country) French, low-fat	6 oz	150	5	31	90	0	2.0	0
(Weight Watchers) 'Ultimate 90'	1 cup	90	8	14	140	0	0.0	0
(White Wave) nondairy	1 serving	140	6	23	45	1	2.5	0
(Yoplait)								
	6 oz	180	9	29	120	0	3.0	15
custard style	6 oz	180	7	30	110	0	4.0	20
fat-free	6 oz	150	8	28	110	0	0.0	5
nonfat, light, custard style	6 oz	90	6	17	85	0	0.0	5
nonfat, w/granola, 'Crunch 'N Yogurt'	7 oz	220	8	43	125	0	2.0	5
WILD BERRY								
(Light n' Lively) low-fat, 1% milk fat, cultured	4.4 oz	140	5	28	70	0	1.0	5
YOGURT, FROZEN								
(Alta Dena) apricot mango	4 oz	90	3	20	210	0	0.0	0
(Ben & Jerry's)								
black raspberry swirl	1/2 cup	150	4	32	65	0	0.0	0
cappuccino	1/2 cup	140	4	30	75	0	0.0	0
chocolate	1/2 cup	130	3	29	50	1	0.0	0
vanilla fudge swirl	1/2 cup	140	5	31	75	1	0.0	0
(Bison) chocolate	3.5 oz	94	3	18	50	0	2.0	5
(Breyers)								
black cherry	1/2 cup	120	3	24	50	0	1.0	10
chocolate	1/2 cup	120	3	24	65	0	1.0	10
peach	1/2 cup	110	3	22	50	0	1.0	10
red raspberry	1/2 cup	120	3	23	50	0	1.0	10
strawberry	1/2 cup	110	3	22	45	0	1.0	10
strawberry-banana	1/2 cup	110	3	22	45	0	1.0	10
vanilla	1/2 cup	120	3	23	55	0	1.0	15
(Cascadian Farm)								
chocolate, organic	1/2 cup	105	4	20	54	1	2.0	7

Food Name	Serv. Size	Total Cal.	Prot. gms	Carbs gms	Sod. mgs	Fiber gms	Fat gms	Chol. mgs
strawberry, organic	1/2 cup	102	4	19	57	1	1.0	6
vanilla, organic	1/2 cup	109	4	20	65	0	2.0	7
(Crowley)								
banana, soft-serve, 'Peaks of Perfection'	1/2 cup	100	3	19	50	0	2.0	5
cherry	3 oz	80	2	16	40	0	1.0	5
chocolate	3 oz	80	2	15	40	0	2.0	10
chocolate, soft-serve, 'Peaks of Perfection'	1/2 cup	100	4	19	60	0	2.0	5
lemon, soft-serve, 'Peaks of Perfection'	1/2 cup	100	3	19	50	0	2.0	5
peach	3 oz	80	2	16	40	0	1.0	5
plain, 'Peaks of Perfection'	1/2 cup	90	2	20	40	0	1.0	5
raspberry	3 oz	80	2	16	40	0	1.0	5
raspberry, soft-serve, 'Peaks of Perfection'	1/2 cup	100	3	19	50	0	2.0	5
strawberry	3 oz	80	2	16	40	0	1.0	5
strawberry, soft-serve, 'Peaks of Perfection'	1/2 cup	100	3	19	50	0	2.0	5
vanilla	3 oz	80	2	15	40	0	2.0	10
vanilla, soft-serve, 'Peaks of Perfection'	3.5 oz	100	3	19	50	0	2.0	5
(Dannon)								
blueberry, soft-serve	1/2 cup	100	3	18	50	0	2.0	5
butter pecan, soft-serve	1/2 cup	100	3	18	55	0	2.0	5
cappuccino, light	4 oz	80	4	19	70	0	0.0	0
cappuccino, soft-serve	1/2 cup	100	3	18	55	0	2.0	5
caramel pecan, 'Pure Indulgence'	4 oz	180	4	22	70	0	8.0	20
cheesecake, soft-serve	1/2 cup	100	4	18	55	0	2.0	5
chocolate, light	4 oz	80	4	19	70	0	1.0	0
chocolate, 'Pure Indulgence'	3 oz	130	5	24	75	0	3.0	10
chocolate, soft-serve	1/2 cup	120	5	23	65	0	2.0	5
chocolate nut, chunky, 'Pure Indulgence'	4 oz	190	5	24	60	0	9.0	20
cookies and cream, 'Pure Indulgence'	4 oz	180	4	18	95	0	7.0	20
Heath Bar crunch, 'Pure Indulgence'	4 oz	170	4	25	100	0	7.0	25
lemon meringue, soft-serve	1/2 cup	100	4	18	55	0	2.0	5
mixed berry, low-fat	1 container	240	9	45	150	1	3.0	15
peach, light	4 oz	80	4	19	70	0	0.0	0
peach, soft-serve	1/2 cup	100	4	18	55	0	2.0	5
piña colada, soft-serve	1/2 cup	100	4	18	55	0	2.0	5
raspberry soft-serve	1/2 cup	100	3	18	50	0	2.0	5
red raspberry	4 oz	90	3	21	65	0	0.0	0
red raspberry, soft-serve, nonfat	1/2 cup	90	3	21	65	0	0.0	0
strawberry, light	4 oz	80	4	19	70	0	0.0	0
strawberry-banana	1/2 cup	100	3	18	50	0	2.0	5
vanilla, 'Pure Indulgence'	3 oz	130	5	25	50	0	3.0	10
vanilla, light	4 oz	80	4	20	70	0	0.0	0
(Dreyers)								
blueberry, 'Inspirations'	3 oz	80	2	15	40	0	1.0	5
cherry, 'Inspirations'	3 oz	80	2	15	40	0	1.0	5
cherry vanilla, fat-free	1/2 cup	90	3	19	45	na	0.0	0
cherry vanilla, nonfat, 'Inspirations'	4 oz	90	4	19	80	0	0.0	0
chocolate, 'Inspirations'	3 oz	80	2	15	40	0	1.0	5
(Dreyers) chocolate fudge, fat-free	1/2 cup	100	3	22	75	na	0.0	0
'Perfectly Peach' 'Inspirations'	3 oz	80	2	15	40	0	1.0	5
raspberry, 'Inspirations'	3 oz	80	2	15	40	0	1.0	5
strawberry, 'Inspirations'	3 oz	80	2	15	40	0	1.0	5
strawberry-banana, 'Inspirations'	3 oz	80	2	15	40	0	1.0	5
vanilla, fat-free	1/2 cup	80	3	18	45	na	0.0	0
vanilla and chocolate, fat-free	1/2 cup	80	3	18	65	na	0.0	0
vanilla chocolate swirl, 'Inspirations'	4 oz	90	4	19	85	0	0.0	0
vanilla raspberry swirl, 'Inspirations'	3 oz	80	2	15	45	0	1.0	5
(Edys)								
cherry vanilla	1/2 cup	90	3	19	45	na	0.0	0

Food Name	Serv. Size	Total Cal.	Prot. gms	Carbs gms	Sod. mgs	Fiber gms	Fat gms	Chol. mgs
chocolate fudge	1/2 cup	100	3	22	75	na	0.0	0
vanilla	1/2 cup	80	3	18	45	na	0.0	0
vanilla and chocolate	1/2 cup	80	3	18	65	na	0.0	0
(Elan) chocolate almond	1/2 cup	160	5	23	65	0	7.0	0
(Haagen-Dazs)								
banana, soft-serve, nonfat	1 oz	25	1	5	15	0	0.0	0
chocolate, soft-serve	1 oz	30	1	4	13	0	1.0	3
chocolate, soft-serve, nonfat	1 oz	30	1	6	20	0	0.0	0
peach	3 oz	120	4	20	30	0	3.0	31
'Praline Pandemonium' 'Extras'	4 oz	240	7	33	115	0	9.0	45
raspberry, soft-serve	1 oz	30	1	5	15	0	1.0	3
strawberry	3 oz	120	4	21	30	0	3.0	29
strawberry, soft-serve	1 oz	25	1	5	10	0	0.0	0
strawberry, soft-serve, nonfat	1 oz	25	1	5	10	0	0.0	0
'Strawberry Cheesecake Craze' 'Extras'	4 oz	210	7	31	100	0	7.0	50
vanilla almond crunch	3 oz	150	5	22	65	0	5.0	33
(Sealtest)								
black cherry, nonfat, 'Free'	1/2 cup	110	2	24	50	0	0.0	0
chocolate, nonfat, 'Free'	1/2 cup	110	3	24	55	0	0.0	0
peach, nonfat, 'Free'	1/2 cup	100	2	23	35	0	0.0	0
red raspberry, nonfat, 'Free'	1/2 cup	100	2	23	40	0	0.0	0
strawberry, nonfat, 'Free'	1/2 cup	100	2	22	35	0	0.0	0
(Stars)								
butter pecan	1/2 cup	210	5	18	110	0	14.0	30
cappuccino fudge, fruit-sweetened	1/2 cup	110	4	22	65	0	0.0	0
carob-peppermint, nonfat, fruit-sweetened	1/2 cup	110	4	22	65	0	0.0	0
chocolate	1/2 cup	170	5	20	70	0	8.0	30
dark chocolate, nonfat, fruit sweetened	1/2 cup	110	4	23	55	0	0.0	0
espresso almond fudge	1/2 cup	200	5	23	110	1	10.0	30
fruit, nonfat, fruit-sweetened, 'Black Leopard'	1/2 cup	100	4	20	60	0	0.0	0
mango raspberry, nonfat, fruit sweetened	1/2 cup	100	4	23	55	0	0.0	0
mint chip	1/2 cup	210	5	18	110	0	14.0	30
peanut butter cup	1/2 cup	200	5	23	110	1	10.0	30
'Vanilla Bean'	1/2 cup	170	5	20	70	0	8.0	30
'Very Berry Blueberry' nonfat,	1/2 cup	110	4	23	55	0	0.0	0
(Stonyfield Farm)								
apricot mango, nonfat, natural	4 oz	110	5	22	70	0	0.0	5
(Stonyfield Farm)								
chocolate mint chip	4 oz	140	6	24	75	5	3.0	5
chocolate peanut butter swirl	4 oz	210	9	20	70	1	10.0	5
chocolate walnut amaretto	4 oz	150	7	21	80	1	5.0	5
coffee, French roast, decaffeinated	4 oz	100	6	20	85	0	0.0	5
coffee hazelnut fudge	4 oz	150	6	23	80	1	4.0	5
'Double Raspberry'	4 oz	120	5	25	65	0	0.0	0
'Double Strawberry'	4 oz	100	5	21	65	0	0.0	5
Dutch chocolate, nonfat	4 oz	110	6	21	80	0	0.0	5
mocha fudge, nonfat	4 oz	120	5	24	85	0	0.0	5
'Very Vanilla'	4 oz	100	6	20	80	0	0.0	5
(TCBY Treats)								
all flavors, regular	1/2 cup	140	4	23	60	0	3.0	15
all flavors, hand-dipped, 96% nonfat	1/2 cup	110	3	22	65	1	2.5	5
all flavors, hand-dipped, nonfat	1/2 cup	100	3	22	55	1	0.0	0
all flavors, nonfat, no sugar added	1/2 cup	80	4	20	35	0	0.0	0
all flavors, soft-serve, nonfat	1/2 cup	110	4	23	60	0	0.0	0
(Yoplait)								
caramel turtle fudge	1/2 cup	120	2	24	105	0	2.0	5
chocolate fudge brownie	1/2 cup	110	3	24	75	1	1.5	5

Food Name	Serv. Size	Total Cal.	Prot. gms	Carbs gms	Sod. mgs	Fiber gms	Fat gms	Chol. mgs
mixed berry	6 oz	180	8	32	130	0	2.0	0
vanilla	1/2 cup	100	3	20	70	0	1.5	5
YOGURT BAR, FROZEN								
(Cascadian Farm)								
blackberry, organic	1 bar	80	3	14	45	1	1.0	5
chocolate, organic	1 bar	80	3	15	40	1	1.5	5
vanilla, organic	1 bar	80	3	15	50	0	1.0	5
(Dole)								
cherry, 'Fruit & Yogurt'	1 bar	80	2	17	22	0	1.0	0
raspberry, 'Fruit & Yogurt'	1 bar	70	1	17	18	0	1.0	0
strawberry, 'Fruit & Yogurt'	1 bar	70	1	17	16	0	1.0	0
(Haagen-Dazs)								
peach	1 bar	100	2	18	20	0	1.0	15
'Strawberry Daiquiri'	1 bar	100	2	20	20	0	1.0	20
'Tropical Orange Passion'	1 bar	100	2	21	30	0	1.0	20
(Yoplait)								
'Vanilla Orange Creme', lowfat	1 bar	30	1	8	25	0	0.5	0
vanilla/chocolate/strawberry, w/dark chocolate coating	1 bar	110	2	11	35	0	6.0	5
YOGURT DRINK. See under SPORTS AND DIET/NUTRITION DRINKS.								
YOKAN	1 oz	74	0.9	17.2	24	0	(tr)	0
YUCA. See CASSAVA.								

Z

Food Name	Serv. Size	Total Cal.	Prot. gms	Carbs gms	Sod. mgs	Fiber gms	Fat gms	Chol. mgs
ZANTE CURRANT. See under CURRANT.								
ZITI. See under PASTA.								
ZITI DISH/ENTRÉE. See under PASTA DISH/ENTRÉE.								
ZUCCHINI								
Canned, Italian style *(Progresso)*	1/2 cup	50	1	8	540	2	2.0	1
Fresh								
baby, raw, whole	1 large	3	0	0	0	0	0.1	0
baby, raw, whole	1 medium	2	0	0	0	0	0.0	0
w/skin, boiled, drained, mashed	1/2 cup	19	1	5	4	2	0.1	0
w/skin, boiled, drained, sliced	1 cup	29	1	7	5	3	0.1	0
w/skin, raw, chopped	1 cup	17	1	4	4	1	0.2	0
w/skin, raw, sliced	1 cup	16	1	3	3	1	0.2	0
w/skin, raw, whole	1 large	45	4	9	10	4	0.5	0
w/skin, raw, whole	1 medium	27	2	6	6	2	0.3	0
w/skin, raw, whole	1 small	17	1	3	4	1	0.2	0
Frozen								
(Seabrook)	3.3 oz	16	1	3	2	1	0.0	0
(Southern)	3.5 oz	18	1	4	20	0	0.1	0
breaded, kosher *(Empire Kosher)*	1 piece	100	5	18	280	1	0.0	0
breaded, 'Quick Krisp' *(Stilwell)*	3.3 oz	200	4	24	410	0	10.0	15
sliced *(Flav-R-Pac)*	2/3 cup	15	1	2	15	1	0.0	0
w/skin, boiled, drained	1 cup	38	3	8	4	3	0.3	0
w/skin, unprepared	3-lb pkg	231	16	49	27	18	1.8	0
w/skin, unprepared	10-oz pkg	48	3	10	6	4	0.4	0

Fast-Food/Chain Restaurant Values

Food Name	Serv. Size	Total Cal.	Prot. gms	Carbs gms	Sod. mgs	Fiber gms	Fat gms	Chol. mgs
ARBY'S								
BACON	2 strips	90	5	0	220	0	7.0	10
BISCUIT								
w/margarine	2.8 oz	270	5	26	750	0	16.0	0
CATSUP/KETCHUP	1 pkt	10	na	3	90	0	0.0	0
CHEESE								
Swiss	1 slice	45	3	0	220	0	3.0	10
CROISSANT								
	2.2 oz	260	6	28	300	0	16.0	20
DRESSING								
bleu cheese	2.5 oz	390	3	3	770	0	39.0	30
buttermilk ranch	2.5 oz	210	0	2	600	0	49.0	5
buttermilk ranch, reduced calorie	2 oz	50	0	12	710	0	0.0	0
honey French	2.5 oz	350	0	24	530	0	27.0	0
Italian, lower calorie	2.19 oz	20	0	4	1110	0	1.0	0
Thousand Island	2.5 oz	350	0	11	580	0	33.0	15
EGG								
scrambled	1.8 oz	70	6	0	70	0	5.0	220
FINGER MEAL								
chicken	10.7 oz	880	35	81	2240	0	47.0	60
FINGER SNACK								
chicken	7.4 oz	610	20	62	1610	0	32.0	30
jalapeño bites	3.9 oz	330	7	29	670	2	21.0	40
mozzarella sticks	4.8 oz	470	18	34	1330	2	29.0	60
onion petals	4 oz	410	4	43	300	2	24.0	0
FRENCH FRIES								
cheddar curly	6 oz	450	8	52	1420	0	25.0	5
curly, large	7 oz	600	8	75	1710	0	30.0	0
curly, medium	4.5 oz	380	5	49	1100	0	19.0	0
curly, small	3.8 oz	320	4	40	910	0	16.0	0
homestyle, large	7.5 oz	630	8	86	1240	6	29.0	0
homestyle, medium	5 oz	420	5	57	830	4	19.0	0
homestyle, small	4 oz	340	4	46	660	3	15.0	0
FRENCH TOASTIX, w/o powdered sugar or syrup	3 hotcakes	370	7	48	440	4	17.0	0
HAM	1.5 oz	50	7	1	830	0	3.0	30
HOT CHOCOLATE	8.6 oz	110	2	23	120	0	1.0	0
MAPLE SYRUP	1.5 oz	220	0	54	50	0	0.0	0
MUSTARD								
German	1 pkt	5	0	0	60	0	0.0	0
honey	1 oz	130	0	5	170	0	12.0	10
ORANGE JUICE	10 oz	140	1	34	0	0	0.0	0
SAUCE								
Arby's	1 pkt	15	0	3	110	0	0.0	0
barbecue dipping	1 oz	40	0	10	350	0	0.0	0
beef stock aus jus	2 oz	10	0	0	440	0	0.0	0
bronco berry	1.5 oz	90	0	23	35	0	0.0	0
horsey	1 pkt	60	0	3	100	0	5.0	0
marinara sauce	1.5 oz	35	1	4	260	0	1.5	0
tangy Southwest	1.52 oz	250	0	3	280	0	25.0	30
SANDWICH								
Arby-Q	6.6 oz	380	19	42	990	3	15.0	30
Beef 'N Cheddar	7 oz	510	26	45	1250	3	28.0	50
chicken, bacon 'n Swiss	7.8 oz	610	37	52	1620	5	30.0	75
chicken breast fillet	7.6 oz	560	30	49	1080	6	28.0	55
chicken cordon bleu	8.9 oz	650	40	50	2120	5	34.0	90
fish fillet sandwich	7.9 oz	540	23	51	880	2	27.0	40
French dip sub	7.1 oz	490	30	43	1440	3	22.0	56
grilled chicken, lowfat	6.3 oz	280	30	33	920	4	5.0	50
grilled chicken deluxe	8.7 oz	420	30	42	930	3	16.0	60

Food Name	Serv. Size	Total Cal.	Prot. gms	Carbs gms	Sod. mgs	Fiber gms	Fat gms	Chol. mgs
hot ham 'n Swiss sub	9.7 oz	570	30	47	2660	2	31.0	100
Italian sub	10.3 oz	800	28	49	2610	2	54.0	85
Philly beef 'n Swiss sub	11.1 oz	780	39	52	2140	4	48.0	90
roast beef, big Montana	11 oz	720	50	44	2270	7	40.0	110
roast beef, giant	8.1 oz	550	34	43	1560	5	28.0	70
roast beef, junior	4.6 oz	340	18	36	790	3	16.0	30
roast beef, regular	5.6 oz	400	23	36	1030	3	20.0	40
roast beef, super	8.7 oz	530	24	50	1190	5	27.0	40
roast beef melt w/cheddar	5.4 oz	380	19	38	960	3	19.0	30
roast beef sub	10.7 oz	770	32	48	2170	3	49.0	70
roast chicken club	8.4 oz	540	37	39	1590	3	29.0	70
roast chicken deluxe, low-fat	7 oz	260	23	32	950	4	5.0	40
roast turkey deluxe, lowfat	6.9 oz	230	19	33	870	4	5.0	25
turkey sub	10.7 oz	670	29	49	2130	2	39.0	60
POTATO, BAKED								
broccoli 'n cheddar	13.6 oz	550	14	71	730	7	25.0	50
chicken broccoli	15.8 oz	830	35	68	970	7	47.0	60
cool ranch	12.3 oz	500	8	67	150	6	23.0	25
deluxe	12.3 oz	610	14	68	860	6	31.0	80
jalapeño	14.6 oz	660	15	72	930	6	36.0	50
Philly chicken	15.8 oz	880	32	75	1020	7	53.0	70
w/butter and sour cream	11.3 oz	500	8	65	170	6	24.0	60
POTATO CAKES	2 cakes	220	2	21	460	3	14.0	0
SALAD								
garden, w/one crouton packet, 2 saltine crackers	10.2 oz	110	9	16	150	1	3.0	0
grilled chicken, low-fat	14.2 oz	190	25	16	530	1	4.0	40
roast chicken, lowfat	14.2 oz	200	25	16	800	1	5.0	40
w/one crouton packet, 2 saltine crackers	5.4 oz	90	5	12	130	0	3.0	0
SAUSAGE PATTY	1.4 oz	200	7	1	290	0	19.0	60
SHAKE								
chocolate	10.3 oz	390	8	69	270	0	9.0	10
jamocha	10.3 oz	380	8	66	300	0	9.0	10
strawberry	10.3 oz	380	8	67	270	0	9.0	10
vanilla	10.3 oz	380	8	67	270	0	9.0	12
TURNOVER								
iced apple	3.4 oz	360	4	54	180	6	14.0	0
iced cherry	3.5 oz	350	4	53	190	0	14.0	0

ARTHUR TREACHER'S

Food Name	Serv. Size	Total Cal.	Prot. gms	Carbs gms	Sod. mgs	Fiber gms	Fat gms	Chol. mgs
CHICKEN PATTIES	2 patties	369	27	17	495	0	21.6	65
COD FILLET, 'Bake'n Broil' tail shape	5 oz	245	20	10	144	0	14.2	0
COLESLAW	3 oz	123	1	11	266	0	8.2	7
DESSERT, Lemon Luv	1 serving	276	3	35	314	0	13.9	1
FISH FILLET	5.2 oz	355	19	25	450	0	19.8	56
FRENCH FRIES, chips	4 oz	276	4	35	39	0	13.2	5
HUSHPUPPY, 'Krunch Pup'	1 piece	203	5	12	446	0	14.8	25
SANDWICH								
chicken	1 sandwich	413	16	44	708	0	19.2	32
fish	1 sandwich	440	16	39	836	0	24.0	42
SHRIMP	7 pieces	381	13	27	538	0	24.4	93

AU BON PAIN

Food Name	Serv. Size	Total Cal.	Prot. gms	Carbs gms	Sod. mgs	Fiber gms	Fat gms	Chol. mgs
BAGEL								
cinnamon	1 bagel	395	14	86	605	4	2.0	0
onion	1 bagel	390	16	81	665	4	2.0	0
plain	1 bagel	380	15	79	665	3	2.0	0
sesame	1 bagel	425	17	81	665	4	5.0	0

Food Name	Serv. Size	Total Cal.	Prot. gms	Carbs gms	Sod. mgs	Fiber gms	Fat gms	Chol. mgs
BREAD								
baguette	1 loaf	810	27	166	1830	0	2.0	0
cheese	1 loaf	1670	70	269	4140	0	29.0	75
four-grain	1 loaf	1420	57	262	3050	0	11.0	1
multigrain	2 slices	391	16	77	2040	0	3.0	1
onion herb	1 loaf	1430	52	263	2390	0	13.0	0
pita pocket	2 slices	80	3	18	0	0	1.0	0
ponsienne	1 loaf	1490	49	166	3380	0	4.0	0
rye	2 slices	374	14	73	2170	0	4.0	0
CHICKEN POT PIE	1 serving	440	18	46	1109	0	21.0	45
COOKIE								
chocolate chip	1 cookie	280	2	37	70	0	15.0	25
chocolate chunk, w/pecan, 'Gourmet'	1 cookie	290	3	37	200	0	17.0	10
cookie, oatmeal, oatmeal raisin, 'Gourmet'	1 cookie	250	4	41	230	0	9.0	10
peanut butter, 'Gourmet'	1 cookie	290	7	33	250	0	15.0	10
shortbread, 'Gourmet'	1 cookie	425	5	46	385	0	26.0	68
white chocolate chunk, w/pecan, 'Gourmet'	1 cookie	300	3	37	200	0	17.0	10
CROISSANT								
almond	1 croissant	420	8	41	250	0	25.0	95
apple	1 croissant	250	4	38	150	0	10.0	25
blueberry cheese	1 croissant	380	7	44	280	0	20.0	60
chocolate	1 croissant	400	5	46	220	0	24.0	35
cinnamon raisin	1 croissant	390	7	60	240	0	13.0	35
coconut pecan	1 croissant	440	7	51	290	0	23.0	45
croissant, plain	1 croissant	220	5	29	240	0	10.0	25
hazelnut chocolate	1 croissant	480	6	56	220	0	28.0	35
raspberry cheese	1 croissant	400	7	49	280	0	20.0	60
strawberry cheese	1 croissant	400	7	49	280	0	20.0	60
sweet cheese	1 croissant	420	8	45	310	0	23.0	70
MUFFIN								
blueberry, gourmet	1 muffin	390	8	66	410	0	4.0	40
bran, gourmet	1 muffin	390	7	73	940	0	11.0	20
carrot, gourmet	1 muffin	450	7	58	610	0	22.0	15
corn, gourmet	1 muffin	460	8	71	510	0	17.0	25
cranberry walnut, gourmet	1 muffin	350	7	53	730	0	13.0	15
oat bran apple gourmet	1 muffin	400	7	71	590	0	2.0	0
pumpkin gourmet	1 muffin	410	6	63	500	0	16.0	20
whole grain, gourmet	1 muffin	440	10	68	310	0	16.0	30
PASTRY								
cheese Danish	1 Danish	390	8	43	530	2	22.0	78
cherry Danish	1 Danish	335	7	42	480	2	16.0	50
cherry dumpling Danish	1 Danish	360	5	59	255	1	13.0	0
raspberry Danish	1 Danish	335	6	43	480	2	16.0	50
ROLL								
'Alpine'	1 roll	220	8	43	810	0	3.0	0
braided	1 roll	387	10	64	1540	0	11.0	34
country seed	1 roll	220	9	37	460	0	4.0	0
croissant	1 roll	300	7	38	240	0	14.0	35
French	1 roll	320	10	65	710	0	1.0	0
hearth	1 roll	370	16	69	600	0	3.0	0
'Petit Pain'	1 roll	220	7	44	490	0	1.0	0
pumpernickel	1 roll	210	8	42	1005	0	2.0	0
raisin	1 roll	250	8	46	480	0	4.0	0
rye	1 roll	230	8	44	0	0	2.0	0
soft	1 roll	310	8	50	410	0	8.0	0
vegetable	1 roll	230	6	40	410	0	5.0	0
SALAD								
garden, small	1 salad	20	5	5	10	0	1.0	0

Food Name	Serv. Size	Total Cal.	Prot. gms	Carbs gms	Sod. mgs	Fiber gms	Fat gms	Chol. mgs
garden w/grilled chicken	1 salad	110	14	9	330	0	2.0	30
garden w/shrimp	1 salad	102	11	8	193	0	2.0	105
garden w/tuna	1 salad	350	21	11	480	0	25.0	40
Italian, low-calorie	1 salad	68	0	3	360	0	6.0	5
SANDWICH								
chicken, cracked pepper, on French roll	1 sandwich	440	33	66	1390	0	3.0	50
chicken, cracked pepper, on hearth roll	1 sandwich	490	39	70	1280	0	5.0	50
chicken, cracked pepper, on soft roll	1 sandwich	430	31	51	1090	0	10.0	50
chicken, grilled, on French roll	1 sandwich	450	33	66	1320	0	5.0	60
chicken, grilled, on hearth roll	1 sandwich	500	39	70	1210	0	7.0	60
chicken, grilled, on soft roll	1 sandwich	440	31	51	1020	0	12.0	60
chicken, tarragon, on French roll	1 sandwich	590	34	68	1014	0	16.0	70
chicken, tarragon, on hearth roll	1 sandwich	640	40	72	904	0	18.0	70
chicken, tarragon, on soft roll	1 sandwich	580	32	53	714	0	23.0	70
ham, on French roll	1 sandwich	470	27	68	1680	0	8.0	115
ham, on hearth roll	1 sandwich	520	33	72	1570	0	10.0	115
ham, on soft roll	1 sandwich	460	25	53	1380	0	15.0	115
ham and cheese croissant, hot, filled	1 sandwich	370	10	38	280	0	20.0	55
roast beef, on French roll	1 sandwich	500	34	66	1020	0	9.0	60
roast beef, on hearth roll	1 sandwich	550	40	70	910	0	11.0	60
roast beef, on soft roll	1 sandwich	490	32	51	720	0	16.0	60
spinach and cheese croissant, hot, filled	1 sandwich	290	9	29	310	0	16.0	45
turkey and cheddar croissant, hot, filled	1 sandwich	410	16	38	680	0	22.0	70
turkey and havarti croissant, hot, filled	1 sandwich	410	17	38	630	0	21.0	70
turkey sandwich, smoked, on French roll	1 sandwich	420	32	65	1660	0	2.0	35
turkey sandwich, smoked, on hearth roll	1 sandwich	470	38	69	1550	0	4.0	35
turkey sandwich, smoked, on soft roll	1 sandwich	410	30	50	1360	0	9.0	35
SANDWICH FILLING								
boursin cheese	1 serving	290	6	2	390	0	29.0	90
brie cheese	1 serving	300	18	3	510	0	24.0	85
provolone cheese	1 serving	155	10	1	180	0	12.6	36
SOUP								
beef barley	1 bowl	112	9	15	901	0	3.0	18
beef barley	1 cup	75	6	10	600	0	2.0	12
broccoli, cream of	1 bowl	302	8	18	219	0	26.0	54
broccoli, cream of	1 cup	201	5	12	146	0	17.0	36
chicken, w/noodle	1 bowl	119	12	14	743	0	1.7	26
chicken, w/noodle	1 cup	79	8	9	495	0	1.0	17
chili, vegetarian	1 bowl	208	9	37	763	0	4.0	0
chili, vegetarian	1 cup	139	6	24	508	0	3.0	0
clam chowder	1 bowl	433	17	36	1029	0	27.0	90
clam chowder	1 cup	289	11	24	687	0	18.0	60
minestrone	1 cup	105	5	20	265	0	2.0	1
split pea	1 bowl	264	18	45	453	0	2.0	1
split pea	1 cup	176	12	30	303	0	1.0	1
tomato Florentine	1 bowl	92	4	15	221	0	1.7	0
tomato Florentine	1 cup	61	3	10	147	0	1.0	0
vegetarian, garden	1 bowl	44	2	9	92	0	1.0	0
vegetarian, garden	1 cup	29	1	6	61	0	1.0	0

BASKIN-ROBBINS

ICE

Food Name	Serv. Size	Total Cal.	Prot. gms	Carbs gms	Sod. mgs	Fiber gms	Fat gms	Chol. mgs
grape	1/2 cup	100	0	27	10	0	0.0	0
margarita	1/2 cup	110	0	28	10	0	0.0	0
ICE CREAM								
'Berries 'n Banana,' sugarless	1/2 cup	80	4	15	55	0	1.0	5
'Call Me Nuts,' sugarless	1/2 cup	110	3	21	55	1	2.0	5
'Cappuccino Blast,' w/whipped cream	1 serving	160	3	22	60	0	7.0	30
'Caramel Banana Surprise,' nonfat	1/2 cup	110	3	24	95	0	0.0	0

Food Name	Serv. Size	Total Cal.	Prot. gms	Carbs gms	Sod. mgs	Fiber gms	Fat gms	Chol. mgs
caramel praline, soft serve, nonfat	1/2 cup	120	4	25	85	0	0.0	0
'Cherry Cordial,' sugarless	1/2 cup	100	3	18	55	0	2.0	5
chocolate chip, 'Chillyburger'	1 serving	220	4	27	100	1	11.0	25
chocolate chip, sugarless	1/2 cup	100	4	17	70	0	2.5	6
chocolate chip, sugarless, 'Low, Lite 'n Luscious'	1 serving	100	3	20	0	0	2.0	4
chocolate marshmallow, nonfat	1/2 cup	110	4	26	75	1	0.0	0
chocolate vanilla twist, nonfat	1/2 cup	100	4	21	100	0	0.0	0
'Chocolate Wonder,' nonfat	1/2 cup	90	4	20	70	1	0.0	0
'Chunky Banana,' sugarless	1/2 cup	90	3	16	55	0	1.5	5
coconut fudge, sugarless	1/2 cup	110	3	20	60	1	1.5	5
'Double Raspberry,' light	1/2 cup	90	3	16	40	0	2.0	10
espresso, light	1/2 cup	110	3	18	55	0	4.0	10
'Jamoca Swirl,' nonfat	1/2 cup	110	3	23	105	0	0.0	0
'Jamoca Swiss Almond,' sugarless	1/2 cup	100	3	16	65	0	2.5	5
'Just Chocolate Vanilla' dairy, nonfat	1/2 cup	100	4	21	60	0	0.0	0
'Just Peachy' dairy, nonfat	1/2 cup	100	3	22	60	0	0.0	0
'Kookaberry Kiwi,' nonfat	1/2 cup	90	3	20	90	0	0.0	0
'Mocha Cappuccino Blast,' nonfat	1 serving	120	3	26	75	0	0.0	0
peach, nonfat	1/2 cup	100	3	22	90	0	0.0	0
peanut butter cream, nonfat	1/2 cup	100	4	21	110	0	0.0	0
pineapple cheesecake, nonfat	1/2 cup	110	3	24	100	0	0.0	0
pineapple coconut, sugarless	1/2 cup	90	3	16	60	0	1.5	5
'Pistachio Creme Chip,' light	1/2 cup	120	4	17	55	0	4.0	10
'Pralines 'n Cream'	1 scoop	280	4	35	180	0	14.0	36
praline, light	1/2 cup	120	3	18	65	0	4.0	10
'Raspberry Revelation' sugarless	1/2 cup	100	3	20	55	1	1.0	5
'Rocky Path,' light	1/2 cup	130	4	19	55	1	4.0	10
strawberry, sugarless, 'Low, Lite 'n Luscious'	1 serving	80	2	17	70	0	1.0	3
'Strawberry Royal,' light	1/2 cup	110	2	19	120	0	3.0	9
vanilla, soft serve, nonfat	1/2 cup	120	5	25	85	0	0.0	0
'Thin Mint,' sugarless	1/2 cup	100	3	16	65	0	2.5	5
'Vanilla Bean,' nonfat	1/2 cup	100	4	20	110	0	0.0	0
'Vanilla Swiss Almond,' sugarless	1/2 cup	110	3	20	60	1	2.0	5
ICE CREAM BAR								
'Sundae Bars' chocolate, caramel ribbon, light	1 bar	150	3	24	75	0	5.0	11
'Cappuccino Blast'	1 bar	120	2	18	35	0	5.0	20
ICE CREAM CONE								
waffle, cone and cup, plain	1 cone	140	3	28	5	0	2.0	0
sugar, cone and cup, plain	1 cone	60	1	11	45	0	1.0	0
SHERBET								
orange	1/2 cup	120	1	26	25	0	1.5	5
rainbow	1/2 cup	120	1	26	25	0	1.5	5
SORBET								
fruit whip, nonfat	1 serving	80	0	24	20	0	0.0	0
raspberry cranberry	1/2 cup	110	0	29	10	0	0.0	0
red raspberry	1/2 cup	120	0	30	10	0	0.0	0
strawberry, soft-serve, nonfat	1 serving	100	0	20	20	0	0.0	0
TOPPING								
butterscotch	1 oz	100	1	24	80	0	1.0	3
hot fudge	1 oz	100	1	17	45	0	3.0	0
hot fudge, nonfat, sugar-free	1 oz	90	2	20	96	1	0.0	0
praline caramel	1 oz	90	0	19	105	0	0.0	0
strawberry	1 oz	60	0	14	5	0	0.0	0
YOGURT, FROZEN								
black cherry, nonfat	1/2 cup	110	3	24	50	0	0.0	0
blueberry, lowfat	1/2 cup	120	4	24	70	0	1.5	5
cheesecake, lowfat	1/2 cup	120	4	21	75	0	1.5	10
chocolate, lowfat	1/2 cup	120	5	23	75	0	1.5	5
chocolate, lowfat, large	9 oz	315	9	54	90	0	9.0	9

Food Name	Serv. Size	Total Cal.	Prot. gms	Carbs gms	Sod. mgs	Fiber gms	Fat gms	Chol. mgs
chocolate, lowfat, medium	7 oz	246	7	42	70	0	7.0	7
chocolate mint, nonfat	1/2 cup	100	4	23	60	1	0.0	0
coconut, nonfat, large	9 oz	180	9	45	90	0	0.0	0
coconut, nonfat, medium	7 oz	140	7	35	70	0	0.0	0
coconut, nonfat, small	5 oz	100	5	25	50	0	0.0	0
Dutch chocolate, nonfat	1/2 cup	100	4	23	60	1	0.0	0
'For Heaven's Cake,' low-fat	1/2 cup	120	3	24	75	0	2.0	10
'Have Your Cake,' low-fat	1/2 cup	110	4	22	100	0	1.0	4
Kahlua frozen, nonfat	1/2 cup	100	3	21	55	0	0.0	0
key lime nonfat	1/2 cup	100	3	22	55	0	0.0	0
'Mango in Paradise,' nonfat	1/2 cup	130	4	28	70	1	0.0	0
maple walnut, nonfat	1/2 cup	100	3	22	55	0	0.0	0
peach, nonfat	1/2 cup	100	3	22	50	0	0.0	0
'Peppermint Twist,' nonfat	1/2 cup	100	3	22	55	0	0.0	0
piña colada, nonfat	1/2 cup	110	3	22	50	0	0.0	0
raspberry, nonfat	1/2 cup	100	3	22	55	0	0.0	0
raspberry, nonfat, large	9 oz	225	9	45	90	0	0.0	0
raspberry, nonfat, medium	7 oz	164	7	35	70	0	0.0	0
raspberry, nonfat, small	5 oz	125	5	25	50	0	0.0	0
strawberry, low-fat, large	9 oz	270	9	54	90	0	9.0	9
strawberry, low-fat, medium	7 oz	211	7	42	70	0	7.0	7
strawberry, low-fat, small	5 oz	150	5	30	50	0	5.0	5
strawberry, nonfat	1/2 cup	100	3	23	55	0	0.0	0
strawberry, nonfat, large	9 oz	225	9	45	90	0	0.0	0
strawberry, nonfat, medium	7 oz	176	7	35	70	0	0.0	0
vanilla, low-fat	1/2 cup	120	4	22	75	0	2.0	10
vanilla, low-fat, large	9 oz	270	9	54	90	0	9.0	9
vanilla, low-fat, medium	7 oz	211	7	42	70	0	7.0	7
vanilla, nonfat	1/2 cup	110	4	23	65	0	0.0	0

BIG BOY RESTAURANT
DESSERT

Food Name	Serv. Size	Total Cal.	Prot. gms	Carbs gms	Sod. mgs	Fiber gms	Fat gms	Chol. mgs
'No-no' frozen	1 serving	75	2	17	36	0	0.0	0
yogurt, frozen, nonfat	1 serving	72	2	16	31	0	0.0	0

ENTRÉE

Food Name	Serv. Size	Total Cal.	Prot. gms	Carbs gms	Sod. mgs	Fiber gms	Fat gms	Chol. mgs
chicken and vegetable stir-fry	1 serving	562	43	68	750	0	14.0	68
chicken breast, w/salad, no dressing, oat bran bread	1 serving	349	38	20	342	0	13.0	65
chicken breast, w/mozzarella, salad, no dressing, bread	1 serving	370	42	24	353	0	12.0	76
chicken, Cajun, w/salad, no dressing, oat bran bread	1 serving	349	38	20	612	0	13.0	65
cod, baked, w/salad, no dressing, oat bran bread	1 serving	364	43	20	371	0	12.0	68
cod, Dijon, baked, w/salad, no dressing, bread	1 serving	427	44	21	567	0	18.0	68
cod, broiled, w/salad, no dressing, oat bran bread	1 serving	364	43	20	371	0	12.0	68
cod, Dijon, broiled, w/salad, no dressing, bread	1 serving	427	44	21	567	0	18.0	68
cod, Cajun, w/salad, no dressing, oat bran bread	1 serving	364	43	20	461	0	12.0	68
spaghetti marinara, w/salad, no dressing, oat bran bread	1 serving	450	15	87	761	0	6.0	8
vegetable stir-fry	1 serving	408	9	74	703	0	10.0	0

SALAD

Food Name	Serv. Size	Total Cal.	Prot. gms	Carbs gms	Sod. mgs	Fiber gms	Fat gms	Chol. mgs
chicken breast, Dijon	1 salad	391	42	31	415	0	11.0	65
dinner, no dressing	1 salad	19	1	4	11	0	0.0	0

SALAD DRESSING, buttermilk

Food Name	Serv. Size	Total Cal.	Prot. gms	Carbs gms	Sod. mgs	Fiber gms	Fat gms	Chol. mgs
SALAD DRESSING, buttermilk	1 serving	36	0	4	151	0	2.0	10

SANDWICH

Food Name	Serv. Size	Total Cal.	Prot. gms	Carbs gms	Sod. mgs	Fiber gms	Fat gms	Chol. mgs
chicken w/mozzarella, on pita, 'Heart Smart'	1 sandwich	404	42	26	421	0	13.0	76
turkey, on pita, 'Heart Smart'	1 sandwich	224	22	24	833	0	5.0	75

SIDE DISH

Food Name	Serv. Size	Total Cal.	Prot. gms	Carbs gms	Sod. mgs	Fiber gms	Fat gms	Chol. mgs
corn	1 serving	90	3	21	1	0	1.0	0

Food Name	Serv. Size	Total Cal.	Prot. gms	Carbs gms	Sod. mgs	Fiber gms	Fat gms	Chol. mgs
mixed vegetables	1 serving	27	2	5	42	0	0.0	0
potato, baked	1 serving	163	5	37	7	0	0.0	0
rice	1 serving	114	3	25	633	0	0.0	0
roll	1 roll	139	3	30	187	0	0.0	2
SOUP								
cabbage	1 bowl	43	2	9	727	0	1.0	1
cabbage	1 cup	37	2	8	623	0	0.0	1
BOJANGLES								
BISCUIT.	1 serving	239	4	30	588	0	11.0	1
CHICKEN								
breast, no skin, 'Southern'	3.5 oz	239	25	10	766	0	11.5	92
breast, no skin, 'Southern'	4 oz	271	28	11	869	0	13.0	104
leg, no skin, 'Southern'	1.8 oz	128	7	5	312	0	12.0	54
leg, no skin, 'Southern'	3.5 oz	251	14	10	611	0	23.5	106
thigh, no skin, 'Southern'	3.5 oz	291	21	11	653	0	18.7	97
thigh, no skin, 'Southern'	3.2 oz	264	19	10	592	0	17.0	88
SANDWICH, chicken fillet, grilled, no mayo	1 sandwich	329	27	37	418	0	7.0	59
SIDE DISH								
coleslaw	1 serving	105	1	19	406	0	4.0	0
dirty rice	1 serving	167	5	21	397	0	7.0	12
pinto bean, Cajun	1 serving	124	6	25	463	0	0.0	0
BONANZA RESTAURANTS								
HALIBUT FILLET								
	6 oz	139	26	3	128	0	2.0	60
	3.5 oz	82	15	2	75	0	1.2	35
RIBEYE STEAK								
	5.5 oz	196	28	1	563	0	8.0	50
	3.5 oz	126	18	1	361	0	5.1	32
BOSTON MARKET								
CHICKEN								
drumstick, Tabasco barbecue	1 drumstick	130	14	4	190	0	6.0	50
1/4 chicken, dark meat, w/o skin	1/4 chicken	190	22	1	440	0	10.0	115
1/4 chicken, dark meat, w/skin	1/4 chicken	320	30	2	500	0	21.0	155
1/4 chicken, teriyaki, dark meat, w/skin	1/4 chicken	340	40	17	890	0	12.0	135
1/4 chicken, teriyaki, dark meat, w/skin	1/4 chicken	380	30	17	870	0	21.0	155
1/4 chicken, w/skin	1/4 chicken	590	70	4	1010	0	33.0	280
1/4 chicken, w/wing, white meat, w/skin	1/4 chicken	280	0	2	510	0	12.0	135
1/4 chicken, w/o wing, white meat, w/o skin	1/4 chicken	170	33	2	480	0	4.0	85
Southwest, savory	1 portion	400	40	26	1670	4	15.0	100
triple topped	1 portion	470	50	20	1350	1	22.0	155
wing, Tabasco barbecue	1 wing	110	9	4	170	0	7.0	30
CHICKEN POT PIE.	1 pie	780	32	61	1480	4	46.0	135
CORNBREAD	1 loaf	200	3	33	390	1	6.0	25
DESSERT								
brownie	1 piece	450	6	47	190	3	27.0	80
chocolate chip cookie	1 cookie	340	4	48	240	1	17.0	25
cinnamon apple pie	1/5 pie	390	2	46	250	2	23.0	0
GRAVY, chicken	1 oz	15	0	2	170	0	1.0	0
HAM, Boston hearth, lean	5 oz	210	25	9	1490	0	9.0	75
MEAT LOAF								
w/brown gravy	7 oz	390	30	19	1040	1	22.0	120
w/chunky tomato sauce	8 oz	370	30	22	1170	2	18.0	120
SALAD								
Caesar, entrée	10 oz	510	17	17	1130	3	42.0	35
Caesar, side	4 oz	200	7	7	450	1	17.0	15
Caesar, w/o dressing	8 oz	230	16	14	500	3	12.0	20
chicken, chunky	3/4 cup	370	28	3	800	1	27.0	120

Food Name	Serv. Size	Total Cal.	Prot. gms	Carbs gms	Sod. mgs	Fiber gms	Fat gms	Chol. mgs
chicken Caesar	13 oz	650	43	17	1580	3	45.0	105
tossed, individual, w/Caesar dressing	1 salad	380	5	18	810	3	31.0	15
tossed, individual, w/fat-free ranch dressing	1 salad	160	5	29	940	4	2.5	0
tossed, individual, w/old Venice dressing	1 salad	340	4	20	1110	3	27.0	0
SANDWICH								
barbecue chicken	1 sandwich	540	30	84	1690	3	9.0	75
barbecue chicken pastry	1 sandwich	640	17	56	1260	1	39.0	60
broccoli chicken cheddar pastry	1 sandwich	690	21	45	1050	2	47.0	85
chicken, w/cheese and sauce sandwich	1 sandwich	750	41	72	1860	5	33.0	135
chicken, w/o cheese and sauce	1 sandwich	430	34	62	910	4	4.5	65
chicken salad	1 sandwich	680	39	63	1360	4	30.0	120
ham, w/cheese and sauce	1 sandwich	750	38	72	1730	5	34.0	100
ham and cheddar pastry	1 sandwich	640	19	47	1560	1	41.0	60
ham sub, w/o cheese and sauce	1 sandwich	440	25	66	1450	4	8.0	45
Italian chicken pastry	1 sandwich	630	21	43	910	2	41.0	60
meatloaf, w/cheese	1 sandwich	860	46	95	2270	6	33.0	165
meatloaf, w/o cheese	1 sandwich	690	40	86	1610	6	21.0	120
turkey, open faced	1 sandwich	500	37	61	2170	3	12.0	80
turkey, w/cheese and sauce	1 sandwich	710	45	68	1390	4	28.0	110
turkey club	1 sandwich	650	39	64	1590	4	26.0	105
turkey sub, w/o cheese and sauce	1 sandwich	400	45	61	1070	4	3.5	60
SIDE DISH								
applesauce, cinnamon	3/4 cup	250	0	56	45	3	4.5	0
applesauce, cinnamon, low-fat, chunky	3/4 cup	250	1	62	30	2	0.0	0
barbecue baked beans	3/4 cup	270	8	48	540	12	5.0	0
black rice and beans	1 cup	300	8	45	1050	5	10.0	0
broccoli cauliflower au gratin	3/4 cup	200	9	14	600	3	11.0	20
broccoli rice casserole	3/4 cup	240	5	26	800	2	12.0	40
broccoli w/red peppers	3/4 cup	60	3	5	130	3	3.5	0
butternut squash, low-fat	3/4 cup	160	2	25	580	3	6.0	15
carrots, honey glazed	3/4 cup	280	1	35	80	4	15.0	0
chili, chicken	1 cup	220	18	21	1000	6	7.0	40
coleslaw	3/4 cup	300	2	30	540	3	19.0	20
corn, whole kernel	3/4 cup	180	5	30	170	2	4.0	0
coyote bean salad	3/4 cup	190	4	24	210	9	9.0	0
cranberry relish, low-fat	3/4 cup	370	2	84	5	5	5.0	0
fruit salad	3/4 cup	70	1	15	10	1	0.5	0
green beans	3/4 cup	80	1	5	200	3	6.0	0
green bean casserole	3/4 cup	130	2	10	440	2	9.0	20
macaroni and cheese	3/4 cup	280	13	32	830	1	11.0	30
potato, baked, sweet low-fat	1 potato	460	6	94	510	10	7.0	0
potato, mashed, homestyle	2/3 cup	190	3	24	570	1	9.0	25
potato, mashed, homestyle, w/gravy	3/4 cup	210	4	26	740	1	10.0	25
potato, new, low-fat	3/4 cup	130	3	25	150	2	2.5	0
potato planks, oven-roasted, low-fat	5 planks	180	3	32	370	3	5.0	0
potato salad, old-fashioned	3/4 cup	340	2	30	870	2	24.0	30
red beans and rice, low-fat	1 cup	260	8	45	1050	4	5.0	5
rice pilaf	2/3 cup	180	5	32	600	2	5.0	0
spinach, creamed	3/4 cup	260	9	11	740	2	20.0	55
squash casserole	3/4 cup	330	7	20	1110	3	24.0	70
stuffing, savory	3/4 cup	310	6	44	1140	3	12.0	0
sweet potato casserole	3/4 cup	280	3	39	190	2	18.0	10
vegetables, steamed, low-fat	2/3 cup	35	2	7	35	3	0.5	0
zucchini marinana, low-fat	3/4 cup	60	1	7	330	2	3.0	0
SOUP								
chicken noodle	1 cup	130	11	12	1310	2	4.5	40
chicken tortilla	1 cup	220	10	19	1410	2	11.0	35
potato	1 cup	270	8	24	1020	2	16.0	40
tomato bisque	1 cup	280	4	16	1280	2	23.0	50
TURKEY, breast, rotisserie, skinless, low-fat	5 oz	170	36	1	850	0	1.0	100

Food Name	Serv. Size	Total Cal.	Prot. gms	Carbs gms	Sod. mgs	Fiber gms	Fat gms	Chol. mgs
BRAUM'S								
....	1 serving	180	3	16	35	0	3.0	0
diet, sugarless, w/NutraSweet	1 serving	90	3	13	0	0	3.0	0
nonfat	1 serving	90	4	20	55	0	0.0	0
'Premium Light'	1 serving	102	3	15	0	56	3.0	0
BRAZIER. See DAIRY QUEEN/BRAZIER.								
BRESLER'S								
ICE CREAM, 'Royal Lites,' all flavors	1 serving	132	5	9	70	0	5.0	16
SHERBET, all flavors	1 serving	160	1	34	0	0	2.0	6
YOGURT, FROZEN								
gourmet, all flavors	1 serving	116	4	22	0	0	2.0	7
nonfat, all flavors	1 serving	108	4	24	0	0	0.0	0
BURGER CHEF								
BREAKFAST								
sausage biscuit	1 serving	418	16	33	1313	0	25.0	45
scrambled eggs and bacon platter	1 serving	567	21	50	1108	0	31.0	0
scrambled eggs and sausage platter	1 serving	668	26	50	1411	0	40.0	479
'Sunrise' w/bacon	1 serving	392	19	30	978	0	21.0	384
'Sunrise' w/sausage	1 sandwich	526	26	30	1412	0	33.0	419
CHEESEBURGER								
regular	1 serving	278	14	28	641	0	12.0	37
double patty	1 serving	402	23	28	835	0	22.0	74
DESSERT, apple turnover	1 serving	237	2	38	0	0	9.0	0
HAMBURGER								
'Big Chef'	1 serving	556	22	37	840	0	36.0	78
mushroom, single patty	1 serving	520	28	34	744	0	29.0	92
regular	1 serving	235	11	27	480	0	9.0	27
'Super Chef'	1 serving	604	27	35	1088	0	39.0	99
'Top Chef'	1 serving	541	30	29	1007	0	33.0	100
HAMBURGER MEAL, 'Funmeal'	1 serving	514	14	85	513	0	19.0	27
SANDWICH								
chicken club	1 sandwich	521	36	33	0	0	25.0	0
'Fisherman's Fillet'	1 sandwich	534	26	41	0	0	32.0	0
SIDE DISH								
french fries, large	1 serving	285	4	36	456	0	14.0	0
french fries, regular	1 serving	204	3	26	327	0	10.0	0
'Hash Rounds'	1 serving	235	3	26	349	0	14.0	0
salad, lettuce	1 salad	11	1	3	8	0	0.0	0
BURGER KING								
BEVERAGE								
chocolate shake, medium	1 serving	440	12	75	330	4	10.0	30
chocolate shake, medium, syrup added	1 serving	570	14	105	520	3	10.0	30
chocolate shake, small	1 serving	330	9	58	250	3	7.0	25
chocolate shake, small, syrup added	1 serving	390	10	72	350	2	7.0	20
'Coca-Cola Classic,' medium	22 fl oz	280	0	70	na	0	0.0	0
coffee	12 fl oz	5	0	1	5	0	0.0	0
'Diet Coke,' medium	22 fl oz	1	0	0	na	0	0.0	0
orange juice,'Tropicana'	10 fl oz	140	2	33	0	0	0.0	0
milk, 2%.	8 fl oz	130	8	12	120	0	5.0	20
'Sprite,' medium	22 fl oz	260	0	66	na	0	0.0	0
strawberry shake, medium, syrup added	1 medium	550	13	104	350	2	9.0	30
strawberry shake, small, syrup added	1 serving	390	10	72	260	1	7.0	20
vanilla shake, medium	1 medium	430	13	73	330	2	9.0	30
vanilla shake, small	1 small	330	10	56	250	1	7.0	20

Food Name	Serv. Size	Total Cal.	Prot. gms	Carbs gms	Sod. mgs	Fiber gms	Fat gms	Chol. mgs
BREAKFAST								
bacon	3 pieces	40	3	0	170	na	3.0	10
biscuit	1 serving	300	6	35	830	1	15.0	0
biscuit w/egg	1 sandwich	380	11	37	1010	1	21.0	140
biscuit w/sausage	1 sandwich	490	13	36	1240	1	33.0	35
biscuit w/sausage, egg and cheese	1 sandwich	620	20	37	1650	1	43.0	185
'Cini-Minis' w/vanilla icing	1 serving	110	0	20	40	na	3.0	0
'Cini-Minis' w/o vanilla icing	4 rolls	440	6	51	710	1	23.0	25
'Croissan'wich' w/sausage and cheese	1 sandwich	450	13	21	940	1	35.0	45
'Croissan'wich' w/sausage, egg, and cheese	1 sandwich	530	18	23	1120	1	41.0	185
French toast sticks	5 sticks	440	7	51	490	3	23.0	2
ham	1 serving	35	6	0	770	na	1.0	15
hash brown rounds, large	1 serving	410	3	42	750	4	26.0	0
hash brown rounds, small	1 serving	240	2	25	440	2	15.0	0
BUN								
hamburger	1 serving	130	5	24	250	na	2.0	0
'Whopper'	1 serving	220	8	39	370	na	4.0	0
CHEESE, American, processed	2 slices	90	6	0	420	na	8.0	25
CHEESEBURGER								
bacon double	1 serving	620	41	28	1230	1	38.0	125
bacon	1 serving	400	24	27	940	1	22.0	70
double patty	1 serving	580	38	27	1060	1	36.0	120
regular	1 serving	360	21	27	760	1	19.0	60
'Double Whopper'	1 serving	1010	55	47	1460	3	67.0	180
'Double Whopper' w/o mayo	1 serving	850	55	47	1460	3	50.0	180
'Whopper'	1 serving	760	35	47	1380	3	48.0	110
'Whopper' w/o mayo	1 serving	600	35	47	1380	3	31.0	110
'Whopper Jr.'	1 serving	450	22	28	770	2	28.0	65
'Whopper Jr.' w/o mayo	1 serving	370	22	28	770	2	19.0	65
CHICKEN BREAST PATTY, 'BK Broiler'	1 serving	140	21	4	570	na	4.0	90
CHICKEN TENDERS								
	5 pieces	230	14	11	590	0	14.0	40
	4 pieces	180	11	9	470	0	11.0	30
CONDIMENTS								
barbecue sauce, 'Bull's Eye'	1/2 oz	20	0	5	140	na	0.0	0
butter, whipped, 'Land O' Lakes Classic Blend'	1 serving	65	0	0	75	na	7.0	0
catsup	1/2 oz	15	0	4	180	na	0.0	0
dip, 'A.M. Express'	1 serving	80	0	21	20	na	0.0	0
dipping sauce	1 serving	170	0	2	200	na	17.0	0
dipping sauce, barbecue	1 serving	35	0	9	400	na	0.0	0
dipping sauce, honey flavored	1 serving	90	0	23	10	na	0.0	0
dipping sauce, honey mustard	1 serving	90	0	10	150	na	6.0	10
dipping sauce, sweet and sour	1 serving	45	0	11	50	na	0.0	0
jam, grape, 'A.M. Express'	1 serving	30	0	7	0	na	0.0	0
jam, strawberry, 'A.M. Express'	1 serving	30	0	8	0	na	0.0	0
'King Sauce'	1/2 oz	70	0	2	70	na	7.0	4
mustard	1/9 oz	0	0	0	40	na	0.0	0
tartar sauce	1.5 oz	260	0	0	330	na	29.0	20
DESSERT, Dutch apple pie	1 serving	300	3	39	230	2	15.0	0
HAMBURGER								
'Big King'	1 burger	640	38	28	980	1	42.0	125
'Double Whopper' w/o mayo	1 serving	760	49	47	980	3	42.0	155
'Double Whopper'	1 serving	920	49	47	980	3	59.0	155
regular	1 serving	320	19	27	520	1	15.0	50
'Whopper Jr.' w/o mayo	1 serving	320	19	28	530	2	15.0	55
'Whopper Jr.'	1 serving	400	19	28	530	2	24.0	55
'Whopper' w/o mayo	1 serving	510	29	47	900	3	23.0	85
'Whopper'	1 serving	660	29	47	900	3	40.0	85

Food Name	Serv. Size	Total Cal.	Prot. gms	Carbs gms	Sod. mgs	Fiber gms	Fat gms	Chol. mgs
HAMBURGER PATTY								
regular	1 serving	170	14	0	55	na	13.0	50
'Whopper'	1 serving	250	20	0	85	na	19.0	70
LETTUCE.	3/4 oz	0	0	0	0	na	0.0	0
ONION.	1/2 oz	5	0	1	0	na	0.0	0
PICKLE.	4 slices	0	0	0	140	na	0.0	0
SANDWICH								
'Chick 'N Crisp'	1 sandwich	460	16	37	890	3	27.0	35
'Chick 'N Crisp' w/o mayo	1 sandwich	360	16	37	890	3	16.0	35
chicken	1 sandwich	710	26	54	1400	2	43.0	60
chicken, w/o mayo	1 sandwich	500	26	54	1400	2	20.0	60
chicken, 'BK Broiler'	1 sandwich	530	29	45	1060	2	26.0	105
chicken, 'BK Broiler' w/o mayo	1 sandwich	370	29	45	1060	2	9.0	105
fish, 'BK Big'	1 sandwich	720	23	59	1180	3	43.0	80
SIDE DISH								
French fries, king size, salted	1 serving	590	5	74	1110	5	30.0	0
French fries, medium, salted	1 serving	400	3	50	820	4	21.0	0
French fries, medium, unsalted	1 serving	400	3	50	760	4	21.0	0
French fries, small, salted	1 serving	250	2	32	550	2	13.0	0
French fries, small, unsalted	1 serving	250	2	32	480	2	13.0	0
onion rings, king size, salted	1 serving	600	8	74	880	6	30.0	4
onion rings, medium	1 serving	380	5	46	550	4	19.0	2
TOMATO	2 slices	5	0	1	0	na	0.0	0
CAPTAIN D'S								
CONDIMENTS								
salad dressing, Italian, nonfat, low-calorie	2 tbsp	9	0	2	568	0	0.0	0
sweet and sour sauce	2 tbsp	52	0	13	5	0	0.0	0
ENTRÉE								
chicken, w/rice, green beans, breadstick, salad	1 serving	414	30	55	2615	0	8.0	71
fish, baked, w/rice, green beans, breadstick, coleslaw	1 serving	659	36	62	1767	0	30.0	54
orange roughy, w/rice, green beans, breadstick, salad	1 serving	537	35	56	2156	0	19.0	39
shrimp, w/rice, green beans, breadstick, salad	1 serving	457	56	34	2194	0	10.0	191
SIDE DISH								
breadstick, plain	1 stick	91	3	17	210	0	1.0	0
green beans, seasoned	1 serving	46	2	5	752	0	2.0	4
rice	serving	124	3	28	9	0	0.0	0
salad, dinner, no dressing	1 salad	27	1	3	67	0	1.0	1
white bean	1 serving	126	8	22	99	0	1.0	2
CARL'S JR.								
BACON.	2 strips	50	3	0	140	0	4.0	10
BEVERAGE								
chocolate shake	13.5 fl oz	390	9	74	280	0	7.0	30
'Coca-Cola Classic' regular	16 fl oz	200	0	54	25	0	0.0	0
coffee	12 fl oz	5	1	1	5	0	0.0	0
'Diet Coke,' regular	16 fl oz	0	0	0	40	0	0.0	0
'Diet 7-Up,' regular	16 fl oz	0	0	0	80	0	0.0	0
'Dr. Pepper,' regular	16 fl oz	200	0	52	70	0	0.0	0
hot chocolate	12 fl oz	110	2	22	80	1	2.0	0
iced tea, regular	16 fl oz	5	0	0	55	0	0.0	0
lemonade, 'Minute Maid' original style, regular	16 fl oz	190	0	52	95	0	0.0	0
milk, 1%.	10 fl oz	150	14	18	180	0	3.0	15
'Nestea,' raspberry, regular	16 fl oz	160	0	42	40	0	0.0	0
orange juice	10 fl oz	140	2	33	30	0	0.0	0
orange soda, 'Minute Maid' regular	16 fl oz	210	0	58	20	0	0.0	0
root beer, 'Barq's,' regular	16 fl oz	220	0	60	70	0	0.0	0

Food Name	Serv. Size	Total Cal.	Prot. gms	Carbs gms	Sod. mgs	Fiber gms	Fat gms	Chol. mgs
'Sprite,' regular	16 fl oz	190	0	54	65	0	0.0	0
strawberry shake	13.5 fl oz	400	9	77	240	0	7.0	30
vanilla shake	13.5 fl oz	330	11	54	250	0	8.0	35
BREADSTICK.	1 stick	35	1	7	60	1	0.5	0
BREAKFAST								
burrito	1 burrito	480	27	26	750	2	30.0	465
cheese Danish	1 serving	400	5	49	390	1	22.0	15
English muffin, w/margarine	1 muffin	210	5	27	300	2	9.0	0
French toast dips, w/o syrup	1 serving	370	6	42	430	1	20.0	0
hash brown nuggets	1 serving	330	3	32	470	3	21.0	0
quesadilla	1 quesadilla	310	14	27	670	2	16.0	230
scrambled egg	1 egg	160	13	1	125	0	11.0	425
'Sunrise Sandwich' no bacon or sausage	1 sandwich	360	14	28	700	2	21.0	225
CHEESE								
American	1 slice	60	3	0	280	0	5.0	15
Swiss	1 slice	50	4	0	250	0	3.5	10
CHEESEBURGER								
double Western bacon	1 burger	900	51	64	1770	2	49.0	155
Western bacon	1 burger	650	32	63	1430	2	30.0	80
CHICKEN STARS.	1 serving	280	12	15	330	0	19.0	40
CONDIMENTS. See also Salad Dressing.								
barbecue sauce	1 pkt	50	1	11	270	0	0.0	0
croutons, salad bar item	1 crouton	35	0	5	65	0	1.0	0
honey sauce	1 pkt	90	0	22	0	0	0.0	0
jam, strawberry	1 pkt	35	0	9	0	0	0.0	0
jelly, grape	1 pkt	35	0	9	0	0	0.0	0
mustard sauce	1 serving	50	0	11	210	0	0.0	0
salsa	1 serving	10	0	2	160	0	0.0	0
sweet and sour sauce	1 serving	50	0	12	80	0	0.0	0
syrup, table	1 serving	90	0	21	0	0	0.0	0
DESSERT								
chocolate cake	1 cake	300	3	49	260	4	10.0	23
chocolate chip cookie	1 cookie	370	3	49	350	1	19.0	25
strawberry swirl cheesecake	1 serving	290	6	30	230	0	17.0	55
HAMBURGER								
'Famous Star'	1 burger	580	25	49	910	2	32.0	70
'Jr.'	1 burger	330	18	34	480	1	13.0	45
'Super Star'	1 burger	790	42	50	970	2	46.0	130
SALAD								
'Salad-To-Go,' charbroiled chicken	1 salad	200	25	12	440	3	7.0	75
'Salad-To-Go,' gardeb	1 salad	50	3	4	60	2	2.5	10
SALAD DRESSING								
blue cheese	1 pkt	320	2	1	370	0	35.0	25
French, nonfat	1 pkt	60	0	16	660	0	0.0	0
house	1 pkt	220	1	3	440	0	22.0	20
Italian, nonfat	1 pkt	15	0	4	770	0	0.0	0
Thousand Island	1 pkt	230	1	5	420	0	23.0	20
SANDWICH								
bacon Swiss crispy chicken	1 sandwich	690	31	60	1560	4	36.0	75
barbecue chicken	1 sandwich	280	25	37	830	2	3.0	60
chicken club	1 sandwich	460	32	33	1110	2	22.0	90
fish, 'Carl's Catch'	1 sandwich	510	18	50	1030	1	27.0	80
ranch crispy chicken	1 sandwich	590	24	59	1170	4	29.0	50
Santa Fe chicken	1 sandwich	510	28	32	1240	2	31.0	95
SAUSAGE PATTY.	1 patty	200	8	2	480	1	19.0	30
SIDE DISH								
baked potato, w/bacon and cheese	1 serving	630	20	76	1700	6	29.0	35
baked potato, w/broccoli and cheese	1 serving	530	11	74	950	7	21.0	15
baked potato, plain	1 serving	290	6	68	20	6	0.0	0
baked potato, w/sour cream and chives	1 serving	430	7	70	135	6	14.0	10

Food Name	Serv. Size	Total Cal.	Prot. gms	Carbs gms	Sod. mgs	Fiber gms	Fat gms	Chol. mgs
French fries	1 serving	290	5	37	170	3	14.0	0
French fries, criss cut	1 serving	410	5	43	950	4	24.0	0
onion rings	1 serving	430	7	53	700	3	21.0	0
zucchini	1 serving	340	5	37	860	2	19.0	0
CARVEL								
ICE CREAM								
'Caravella'	1 serving	164	4	16	92	0	8.0	61
'Thinny-Thin'	1 serving	92	4	16	80	0	0.0	4
ICE CREAM CONE								
plain	1 cone	25	1	5	25	0	0.0	0
sugar	1 cone	45	1	10	30	0	1.0	0
YOGURT, FROZEN								
'Lo-Yo'	1 serving	124	4	20	76	0	4.0	16
sugarless, low-fat	1 serving	104	4	20	80	0	4.0	8
CHICK-FIL-A								
BEVERAGE								
'Coca-Cola Classic' small	1 serving	110	0	28	10	0	0.0	0
'Diet Coke' small	1 serving	0	0	0	10	0	0.0	0
iced tea, sweetened, small	1 serving	150	0	38	50	0	0.0	0
iced tea, unsweetened, small	1 serving	0	0	0	50	0	0.0	0
lemonade, small	1 serving	90	0	23	4	0	0.0	0
lemonade, diet, small	1 serving	5	0	2	4	0	0.0	0
CHICKEN PIECES								
'Chick-N-Strips' 4 per serving	1 strip	230	29	10	380	0	8.0	20
nuggets, fried, 8 per serving	1 serving	290	28	12	770	0	14.0	60
DESSERT								
brownie, fudge nut	1 brownie	350	10	41	650	0	16.0	30
cheesecake	1 slice	300	6	23	200	0	21.0	115
'Ice Dream Cone' small	1 serving	140	11	16	240	0	4.0	40
lemon pie	1 slice	280	1	19	550	0	22.0	5
SALAD								
chargrilled chicken garden	1 salad	190	26	12	800	4	5.0	83
'Chick-N-Strips'	1 salad	370	32	21	724	4	17.0	113
chicken Caesar	1 salad	230	31	5	940	2	10.0	85
side	1 salad	70	5	13	0	1	0.0	0
SANDWICH								
chicken	1 sandwich	290	24	29	870	1	9.0	50
chicken, chargrilled	1 sandwich	280	27	36	640	1	3.0	40
chicken club	1 sandwich	390	33	38	980	2	12.0	70
chicken salad	1 sandwich	320	25	42	810	1	5.0	10
SIDE DISH								
carrot and raisin salad	1 cup	150	5	28	650	2	2.0	6
coleslaw	1 cup	130	6	11	430	1	6.0	15
French fries, potato waffle, small	1 serving	290	1	49	960	0	10.0	5
SOUP, breast of chicken, hearty	1 cup	110	16	10	760	1	1.0	45
CHURCH'S FRIED CHICKEN								
CHICKEN								
breast, fried	4.3 oz serving	278	21	9	560	0	17.0	0
breast, fried	3.5 oz	228	17	7	459	0	13.9	0
breast, w/o bone	3.5 oz	252	24	5	642	0	15.6	82
breast, w/o bone	2.8 oz	200	19	4	510	0	12.4	65
breast fillet	1 serving	608	27	46	725	0	34.0	0
breast fillet, w/cheese	1 serving	661	30	47	921	0	38.0	0
leg	3.5 oz	179	16	6	348	0	10.9	0
leg	2.9-oz serving	147	13	5	286	0	9.0	0
leg, w/o bone	3.5 oz	247	22	4	282	0	16.1	79
leg, w/o bone	2 oz	140	13	2	160	0	9.1	45

Food Name	Serv. Size	Total Cal.	Prot. gms	Carbs gms	Sod. mgs	Fiber gms	Fat gms	Chol. mgs
thigh	4.2-oz serving	306	19	9	448	0	22.0	0
thigh	3.5 oz	257	16	8	376	0	18.5	0
thigh, w/o bone	3.5 oz	290	20	7	655	0	20.4	101
thigh, w/o bone	2.8 oz	230	16	5	520	0	16.2	80
wing, fried	4.8-oz serving	303	22	9	583	0	20.0	0
wing, fried	3.5 oz	223	16	7	428	0	14.7	0
wing, w/o bone	3.5 oz	284	21	9	614	0	18.3	68
wing, w/o bone	3.1 oz	250	19	8	540	0	16.1	60
DESSERT								
apple pie	3.1 oz	280	2	41	340	1	12.3	5
frozen dessert	1 serving	180	4	27	65	0	6.0	0
FISH								
fillet	1 serving	430	20	45	675	0	18.0	0
fillet, w/cheese	1 serving	483	23	46	870	0	22.0	0
HOT DOG								
super	1 serving	520	17	44	1365	0	27.0	0
w/cheese	1 serving	330	15	21	990	0	21.0	0
w/cheese, super	1 serving	580	22	45	1605	0	34.0	0
w/chili	1 serving	320	13	23	985	0	20.0	0
w/chili, super	1 serving	570	21	47	1595	0	32.0	0
SIDE DISH								
biscuit	2.1 oz	250	2	26	640	1	16.4	5
Cajun rice	3.5 oz	148	1	18	296	1	8.0	6
Cajun rice	3.1 oz	130	1	16	260	1	7.0	5
coleslaw	3 oz	92	4	8	230	2	5.5	0
corn on the cob	5.7 oz	190	8	32	15	4	5.4	0
corn on the cob, w/butter oil	1 med ear	237	4	33	20	0	9.0	0
French fries	2.7 oz	210	3	29	60	2	10.5	0
French fries, large	1 serving	320	3	40	185	0	16.0	0
hushpuppy	2 pieces	156	3	23	110	0	6.0	0
mashed potatoes, w/gravy	3.7 oz	90	1	14	520	1	3.3	0
mashed potatoes, w/gravy	3.5 oz	86	1	13	496	1	3.1	0
okra	2.8 oz	210	3	19	520	4	16.1	0
onion rings	1 serving	280	4	31	140	0	16.0	0

COLOMBO
YOGURT, FROZEN

Food Name	Serv. Size	Total Cal.	Prot. gms	Carbs gms	Sod. mgs	Fiber gms	Fat gms	Chol. mgs
French vanilla	8 oz	215	8	30	140	0	7.0	0
'Gourmet'								
Bavarian chocolate chunk	3 oz	120	3	18	40	0	4.0	10
caramel pecan chunk	3 oz	120	4	19	150	0	3.0	10
dream	3 oz	90	3	16	45	0	2.0	10
'Heath Bar Crunch'	3 oz	130	3	19	75	0	5.0	15
mocha Swiss almond	3 oz	120	3	17	45	0	5.0	10
peanut butter cup	3 oz	140	4	16	90	0	7.0	5
'Strawberry Passion'	3 oz	100	1	18	40	0	2.0	5
wild raspberry cheesecake	3 oz	100	2	18	40	0	2.0	5
low-fat	4 oz	99	3	18	35	0	2.0	10
nonfat	4 oz	95	4	21	70	0	0.0	0
'Sundae Style'								
banana split, 'Sundae Style'	3 oz	100	2	20	50	0	1.0	5
caramel fudge sundae, low-fat, 'Sundae Style'	3 oz	100	3	21	60	0	1.0	5
chocolate peanut butter twist, 'Sundae Style'	3 oz	110	3	18	65	0	3.0	5

COUSIN'S SUBS
BACON

Food Name	Serv. Size	Total Cal.	Prot. gms	Carbs gms	Sod. mgs	Fiber gms	Fat gms	Chol. mgs
BACON	3 strips	50	3	1	145	na	4.0	8
BREAD								
Italian	1 oz	85	4	12	410	0	2.0	1
wheat, 2 3/4 oz per half sub	1 oz	85	5	11	450	0	2.0	1

Food Name	Serv. Size	Total Cal.	Prot. gms	Carbs gms	Sod. mgs	Fiber gms	Fat gms	Chol. mgs
CONDIMENT, tzatziki sauce	1 serving	50	1	1	110	na	4.0	20
DESSERT								
chocolate chip cookie	1 cookie	210	2	25	190	na	11.0	20
cranberry walnut cookie	1 cookie	187	2	24	66	na	8.4	na
PEPPERONI	6 slices	70	5	0	180	na	6.0	25
SALAD								
chef, low-fat	1 salad	194	25	6	998	na	7.9	109
garden, low-fat	1 salad	136	15	6	383	na	5.9	65
Italian	1 salad	288	26	6	1063	na	17.9	106
seafood, low-fat	1 salad	176	21	12	1043	na	5.9	65
side, low-fat	1 salad	71	8	0	198	na	4.2	39
tuna	1 salad	306	26	6	483	na	19.9	85
SANDWICH								
Cold								
bacon, lettuce, and tomato sub	1/2 sub	593	20	34	1418	na	39.8	48
bacon, lettuce, and tomato sub, w/o mayo	1/2 sub	337	20	34	1418	na	13.5	18
cheese sub	1/2 sub	664	31	30	1636	na	46.3	87
cheese sub, mini	1/2 sub	354	17	16	872	na	24.7	46
cheese sub, mini, w/o mayo	1/2 sub	228	17	16	872	na	10.7	30
cheese sub, w/o mayo	1/2 sub	427	31	30	1636	na	20.1	57
club sub	1/2 sub	730	50	30	2828	na	45.4	173
club sub, w/o mayo	1/2 sub	494	50	30	2828	na	19.2	143
'Cousins Special' sub, mini	1/2 sub	290	13	25	680	na	14.0	6
ham and cheese sub	1/2 sub	622	35	30	1748	na	40.1	107
ham and cheese sub, mini	1/2 sub	332	19	16	932	na	21.4	57
ham and cheese sub, mini, w/o mayo	1/2 sub	206	19	16	932	na	7.4	41
ham and cheese sub, w/o mayo	1/2 sub	386	35	30	1748	na	13.8	77
ham sub	1/2 sub	547	29	30	1441	na	34.3	85
ham sub, low-fat, mini, w/o mayo	1/2 sub	167	16	16	768	na	4.3	29
ham sub, low-fat, w/o mayo	1/2 sub	311	29	30	1441	na	8.0	55
ham sub, mini	1/2 sub	292	16	16	768	na	18.3	45
Italian cappacolla and cheese sub	1/2 sub	567	35	30	1850	na	33.9	73
Italian cappacolla and Genoa sub	1/2 sub	567	32	30	1771	na	35.5	58
Italian Cousins Special sub	1/2 sub	731	43	30	2490	na	48.6	111
Italian Genoa and cheese sub	1/2 sub	668	37	30	2023	na	44.5	75
Italian sub, regular	1/2 sub	622	35	30	2008	na	40.0	79
meatball and cheese sub, mini	1/2 sub	365	23	16	1927	na	23.1	55
roast beef sub	1/2 sub	598	41	30	1571	na	34.8	54
roast beef sub, w/o mayo	1/2 sub	361	41	30	1571	na	8.5	24
seafood w/crab sub	1/2 sub	555	25	38	1747	na	33.6	35
seafood w/crab sub, mini	1/2 sub	296	13	20	932	na	17.9	19
tuna sub	1/2 sub	756	30	32	1450	na	54.3	95
tuna sub, made w/o added mayo on bread	1/2 sub	500	30	32	1450	na	28.0	65
tuna sub, mini	1/2 sub	495	14	22	670	na	37.0	56
tuna sub, mini, made w/o added mayo on bread	1/2 sub	290	14	22	670	na	16.0	32
turkey sub	1/2 sub	561	32	30	2021	na	34.8	102
turkey sub, low-fat, mini, w/o mayo	1/2 sub	172	17	16	1078	na	4.4	38
turkey sub, low-fat, w/o mayo	1/2 sub	325	32	30	2021	na	8.5	72
turkey sub, mini	1/2 sub	299	17	16	1078	na	18.5	54
veggie sub	1/2 sub	360	26	33	1590	na	14.3	35
Hot								
cheese steak sub	1/2 sub	470	33	46	540	na	17.0	40
chicken breast sub	1/2 sub	556	37	30	1391	na	31.8	33
chicken breast sub, w/o mayo	1/2 sub	320	37	30	1391	na	5.5	3
double cheese steak sub	1/2 sub	550	44	35	640	na	26.0	61
gyro sub	1/2 sub	550	28	57	650	na	23.0	36
Italian sausage sub	1/2 sub	816	44	30	5204	na	57.5	35
meatball and cheese sub	1/2 sub	685	44	30	3613	na	43.3	104
pepperoni melt sub	1/2 sub	702	41	30	1908	na	46.1	131

Food Name	Serv. Size	Total Cal.	Prot. gms	Carbs gms	Sod. mgs	Fiber gms	Fat gms	Chol. mgs
pepperoni melt sub, w/o mayo	1/2 sub	466	41	30	1908	na	19.8	101
Philly cheese steak sub	1/2 sub	510	32	43	430	na	23.0	45
steak sub	1/2 sub	425	28	51	360	na	12.0	40
veggie sub	1/2 sub	380	21	48	320	na	11.0	0
SIDE DISH								
French fries, large	1 serving	525	7	72	464	na	24.5	21
French fries, medium	1 serving	400	5	55	353	na	18.7	16
French fries, small	1 serving	275	4	38	243	na	12.8	11
SOUP								
cheese, large	1 serving	330	11	23	1760	na	22.0	28
cheese, regular	1 serving	210	7	15	1120	na	14.0	18
cheese broccoli, large	1 serving	261	8	22	1224	na	16.5	21
cheese broccoli, regular	1 serving	166	5	14	779	na	10.5	13
chicken noodle, low-fat, large	1 serving	165	10	21	1444	na	4.1	28
chicken noodle, low-fat, regular	1 serving	105	6	13	919	na	2.6	18
chicken w/wild rice, large	1 serving	289	11	23	1691	na	16.5	28
chicken w/wild rice, regular	1 serving	184	7	15	1076	na	10.5	18
chili, large	1 serving	344	25	32	1485	na	13.8	62
chili, low-fat, regular	1 serving	219	16	20	945	na	8.8	39
clam chowder, low-fat, large	1 serving	248	12	30	1004	na	8.3	21
clam chowder, low-fat, regular	1 serving	158	8	19	639	na	5.3	13
potato, cream of, large	1 serving	261	7	30	1031	na	12.4	7
potato, cream of, low-fat, regular	1 serving	166	4	19	656	na	7.9	4
red rice and beans, low-fat, large	1 serving	179	7	36	1059	na	2.1	0
red rice and beans, low-fat, regular	1 serving	114	4	23	674	na	1.3	0
tomato basil, low-fat, large	1 serving	138	4	21	949	na	4.1	7
tomato basil, low-fat, regular	1 serving	88	3	13	604	na	2.6	4
vegetable beef, low-fat, large	1 serving	110	7	19	1403	na	2.1	14
vegetable beef, low-fat, regular	1 serving	70	4	12	893	na	1.3	9

DAIRY QUEEN/BRAZIER

Food Name	Serv. Size	Total Cal.	Prot. gms	Carbs gms	Sod. mgs	Fiber gms	Fat gms	Chol. mgs
BEVERAGE								
chocolate milkshake, large	1 serving	990	19	168	360	0	26.0	70
chocolate milkshake, regular	14 fl oz	540	12	94	290	0	14.0	45
malted, 'Queen' large	21 fl oz	889	16	157	304	0	21.0	60
milkshake, 'Queen' large	21 fl oz	831	16	140	304	0	22.0	60
vanilla malt	14.7 fl oz	610	13	106	230	0	14.0	45
vanilla malt milkshake	14.7 fl oz	610	13	106	230	0	14.0	45
vanilla milkshake, large	16.3 fl oz	600	13	101	260	0	16.0	50
vanilla milkshake, regular	14 fl oz	520	12	88	230	0	14.0	45
DESSERT								
Banana split	1 serving	510	8	96	180	3	12.0	30
'Blizzard'								
Heath	14.3 oz	820	16	114	410	0	36.0	60
Heath	10.3 oz	560	11	79	280	0	23.0	40
Heath	3.5 oz	202	4	28	101	0	8.9	15
strawberry	13.5 oz	740	13	92	230	0	16.0	50
strawberry	9.4 oz	500	9	64	160	0	12.0	35
strawberry	3.5 oz	193	3	24	60	0	4.2	13
'Brownie Delight'								
hot fudge	10.8-oz serving	710	11	102	340	0	29.0	35
hot fudge	3.5 oz	232	4	33	111	0	9.5	11
'Breeze'								
Heath	13.4 oz	680	15	113	360	0	21.0	15
Heath	9.6 oz	450	11	78	230	0	12.0	10
Heath	3.5 oz	179	4	30	95	0	5.5	4
strawberry	12.5 oz	590	12	90	170	0	1.0	5
strawberry	8.7 oz	400	9	63	115	0	1.0	5
strawberry	3.5 oz	166	3	25	48	0	0.3	1

Food Name	Serv. Size	Total Cal.	Prot. gms	Carbs gms	Sod. mgs	Fiber gms	Fat gms	Chol. mgs
'Buster Bar'								
.... 3.5 oz		299	7	27	146	0	19.3	10
.... 5.3 oz		450	11	40	220	0	29.0	15
'Chipper Sandwich' .... 1 serving		318	5	56	170	0	7.0	13
'Dilly Bar'								
.... 3.5 oz		247	4	25	59	0	15.3	12
.... 3 oz		210	3	21	50	0	13.0	10
'Double Delight' .... 1 serving		490	9	69	150	0	20.0	25
'DQ Frozen Cake'								
undecorated .... 3.5 oz		231	4	30	128	0	10.9	12
undecorated .... 5.8 oz		380	6	50	210	0	18.0	20
'DQ Sandwich' .... 1 serving		140	3	24	40	0	4.0	5
'Fudge Nut Bar' .... 1 serving		406	8	40	167	0	25.0	10
Ice cream cone								
chocolate .... 3.5 oz		162	4	25	81	0	4.9	14
chocolate .... 5 oz		230	6	36	115	0	7.0	20
chocolate .... 7.5 oz		350	8	54	170	0	11.0	30
chocolate, chocolate dipped .... 1 serving		525	9	61	145	0	24.0	30
chocolate, chocolate dipped .... 5.5 oz		330	6	40	100	0	16.0	20
chocolate, 'Queen's Choice' .... 1 serving		326	5	40	84	0	16.0	52
vanilla .... 3 oz		140	4	22	60	0	4.0	15
vanilla .... 3.5 oz		162	4	25	67	0	4.9	14
vanilla .... 5 oz		230	6	36	95	0	7.0	20
vanilla .... 7.5 oz		340	9	53	140	0	10.0	30
vanilla, 'Queen's Choice' .... 1 serving		322	4	40	71	0	16.0	52
'Mr. Misty Float' .... 1 serving		390	5	74	95	0	7.0	20
'Mr. Misty Freeze' .... 1 serving		500	9	91	140	0	12.0	30
'Mr. Misty'								
large .... 1 serving		340	0	84	10	0	0.0	0
regular .... 11.6 oz serving		250	0	63	10	0	0.0	0
'Nutty Double Fudge'								
.... 3.5 oz		211	4	31	62	0	8.0	13
.... 9.7 oz		580	10	85	170	0	22.0	55
'Peanut Buster Parfait'								
.... 10.8 oz		710	16	94	410	0	32.0	30
.... 3.5 oz		232	5	31	134	0	10.4	10
'QC Big Scoop'								
chocolate .... 4.5 oz		310	5	40	100	0	14.0	35
chocolate .... 3.5 oz		243	4	31	78	0	11.0	27
vanilla .... 4.5 oz		300	5	39	100	0	14.0	35
vanilla .... 3.5 oz		235	4	31	78	0	11.0	27
Strawberry shortcake .... 1 serving		540	10	100	215	0	11.0	25
Sundae								
chocolate .... 6.2 oz		300	6	54	100	0	7.0	20
chocolate .... 3.5 oz		171	3	31	57	0	4.0	11
chocolate, large .... 1 serving		440	8	78	165	0	10.0	30
strawberry, waffle cone .... 3.5 oz		202	5	32	127	0	6.9	12
strawberry, waffle cone .... 6.1 oz		350	8	56	220	0	12.0	20
Yogurt, frozen								
.... 7 oz		230	8	49	100	0	1.0	5
cone, large .... 7.5 oz		260	9	56	115	0	1.0	5
cone, regular .... 5 oz		180	6	38	80	0	1.0	5
cup, regular .... 5 oz		170	6	35	70	0	1.0	5
strawberry sundae .... 12.5 oz		200	6	43	80	0	1.0	5
CHEESEBURGER								
double patty .... 3.5 oz		251	16	14	472	0	15.0	53
double patty .... 8 oz		570	37	31	1070	0	34.0	120
regular .... 3.5 oz		234	13	19	513	0	11.5	39

Food Name	Serv. Size	Total Cal.	Prot. gms	Carbs gms	Sod. mgs	Fiber gms	Fat gms	Chol. mgs
regular	5.5 oz	365	20	30	800	0	18.0	60
triple patty	1 serving	820	58	34	1010	0	50.0	140
CHICKEN NUGGETS, all white meat	1 serving	276	16	13	505	0	18.0	39
HAMBURGER								
double patty	3.5 oz	232	16	15	317	0	12.6	48
double patty	7 oz	460	31	29	630	0	25.0	95
'Homestar Ultimate'	3.5 oz	255	16	11	404	0	17.1	51
'Homestar Ultimate'	9.7 oz	700	43	30	1110	0	47.0	140
regular	3.5 oz	219	12	20	409	0	9.2	32
regular	5 oz	310	17	29	580	0	13.0	45
triple patty	1 serving	710	51	33	690	0	45.0	135
HOT DOG								
'DQ Hounder' w/cheese	1 serving	533	19	22	1995	0	40.0	89
'DQ Hounder' w/chili	1 serving	575	22	25	1900	0	41.0	89
'DQ Hounder'	1 serving	480	16	21	1800	0	36.0	80
'Super Dog' w/cheese	1 serving	580	22	45	1605	0	34.0	100
'Super Dog' w/chili	1 serving	570	21	47	1595	0	32.0	100
'Super Dog'	3.5 oz	297	10	21	685	0	19.1	30
'Super Dog'	7 oz	590	20	41	1360	0	38.0	60
SALAD								
garden, w/o dressing	10 oz	200	13	7	240	0	13.0	185
side, w/o dressing	4.8 oz	25	1	4	15	0	0.0	0
SALAD DRESSING								
French, diet	2 oz	90	1	11	450	0	5.0	0
Thousand Island	2 oz	225	1	10	570	0	21.0	25
SANDWICH								
barbecue beef	3.5 oz	176	9	27	549	0	3.1	16
barbecue beef	4.5 oz	225	12	34	700	0	4.0	20
chicken fillet, breaded	3.5 oz	226	13	19	400	0	10.5	29
chicken fillet, breaded	6.7 oz	430	24	37	760	0	20.0	55
chicken fillet, breaded, w/cheese	3.5 oz	235	13	19	480	0	12.3	34
chicken fillet, breaded, w/cheese	7.2 oz	480	27	38	980	0	25.0	70
chicken fillet, grilled	6.5 oz	300	25	33	800	0	8.0	50
chicken fillet, grilled	3.5 oz	163	14	18	434	0	4.3	27
fish fillet	3.5 oz	218	9	23	370	0	9.4	27
fish fillet	6 oz	370	16	39	630	0	16.0	45
fish fillet, w/cheese	3.5 oz	228	10	22	461	0	11.4	33
fish fillet, w/cheese	6.5 oz	420	19	40	850	0	21.0	60
SIDE DISH								
French fries	3.5 oz	300	4	40	160	0	14.0	0
French fries, large	4.5 oz	390	5	52	200	0	18.0	0
onion rings	3 oz	240	4	29	135	0	12.0	0
DEL TACO								
BURRITO								
beef, deluxe	1 serving	440	23	43	878	0	20.0	63
'Big Del'	1 serving	453	22	49	1047	0	20.0	59
breakfast	1 burrito	256	9	30	409	0	11.0	90
chicken	1 serving	264	13	32	771	0	10.0	36
chicken, spicy	1 serving	480	23	65	1620	8	16.0	40
chicken fajita, 'Deluxe'	1 serving	435	22	41	944	0	22.0	84
combination	1 serving	413	21	46	1035	0	17.0	49
combo	1 serving	490	26	53	1380	8	21.0	55
combo, deluxe	1 serving	530	27	56	1390	9	25.0	60
'Del Beef'	1 serving	590	32	45	1110	4	33.0	95
'Del Beef' deluxe	1 serving	550	31	42	1090	3	30.0	90
green	1 serving	229	9	32	714	0	8.0	15
green, large	1 serving	330	14	46	1149	0	11.0	22
red	1 serving	235	10	32	656	0	8.0	17

Food Name	Serv. Size	Total Cal.	Prot. gms	Carbs gms	Sod. mgs	Fiber gms	Fat gms	Chol. mgs
red, large	1 serving	342	14	46	1149	0	11.0	22
'The Works'	1 serving	480	18	69	1500	9	18.0	25
CHEESEBURGER	1 serving	284	14	26	852	0	13.0	42
CONDIMENTS								
guacamole	2 tbsp	60	1	2	130	0	6.0	0
hot sauce	1 tbsp	2	0	1	38	0	0.0	0
salsa	4 tbsp	14	1	3	308	0	0.0	1
HAMBURGER	1 serving	231	11	26	649	0	8.0	29
QUESADILLA								
cheese	1 serving	260	10	24	530	1	12.0	30
chicken	1 serving	580	33	41	1240	2	31.0	104
SALAD								
chicken, deluxe	1 serving	710	31	75	2130	14	32.0	65
taco, deluxe	1 salad	760	31	76	2010	14	37.0	70
SIDE DISH								
French fries	1 serving	242	3	32	136	0	11.0	0
refried beans, w/cheese	1 serving	122	7	17	890	0	7.0	9
TACO								
	1 serving	160	7	11	150	1	10.0	20
beef	1 serving	210	11	11	240	1	13.0	35
beef, double, deluxe	1 serving	240	11	13	250	1	16.0	40
beef, double, soft, deluxe	1 serving	250	12	18	440	1	14.0	40
beef, soft	1 serving	210	12	16	430	1	11.0	35
chicken fajita, deluxe	1 serving	211	11	18	492	0	10.0	53
chicken fajita, soft, deluxe	1 serving	210	11	16	520	1	12.0	30
regular	1 serving	211	9	19	320	0	10.0	32
soft	1 serving	146	5	17	223	0	6.0	16
TOSTADA	1 serving	210	9	24	640	6	9.0	15

DENNY'S
APPETIZER

Food Name	Serv. Size	Total Cal.	Prot. gms	Carbs gms	Sod. mgs	Fiber gms	Fat gms	Chol. mgs
'Kids Heads N' Tails Cracker'	0.5 oz	70	2	9	165	0	3.0	0
mozzarella sticks, 8 sticks	8 oz	710	36	49	5220	6	41.0	48
sampler	17 oz	1405	47	124	5305	4	80.0	75
BEVERAGE								
'Blender Blaster' Butterfinger	13 oz	768	13	97	345	0	38.0	106
'Blender Blaster' kids jr	7 oz	370	7	46	175	0	18.0	49
apple juice	10 fl oz	125	0	33	24	0	0.0	0
coffee, French vanilla flavored	8 fl oz	76	0	16	4	0	1.0	2
coffee, hazelnut flavored	8 fl oz	66	0	14	4	0	1.0	2
coffee, Irish cream flavored	8 fl oz	73	0	16	4	0	1.0	2
cola float	12 oz	280	3	47	109	0	10.0	39
grapefruit juice	10 fl oz	115	1	29	0	0	0.0	0
hot chocolate	8 fl oz	90	4	18	155	0	2.0	0
iced tea, raspberry flavored	16 fl oz	78	0	21	0	0	0.0	0
lemonade, w/ice	16 fl oz	150	0	35	38	0	0.0	0
milk, chocolate, whole milk	10 fl oz	235	9	30	189	0	9.0	37
milk, 2%	5 fl oz	90	5	7	70	0	5.0	19
milkshake, malted, vanilla, or chocolate	12 oz	583	12	82	278	0	26.0	100
milkshake, vanilla or chocolate	12 oz	560	11	76	272	0	26.0	100
orange juice	10 fl oz	125	2	31	31	0	0.0	0
orange-strawberry-banana juice drink, 10% juice	10 fl oz	137	0	38	0	0	0.0	0
root beer float	12 oz	280	3	47	109	0	10.0	39
tomato juice	10 fl oz	55	2	11	921	2	0.0	0
BREAKFAST MEAL. See also individual listings.								
'All American Slam' w/o bread, choice of potato or grits	13 oz	712	38	9	1281	1	62.0	686
'Cinnamon Swirl Slam'	13 oz	1105	38	68	1374	2	78.0	635
'Country Slam'	18 oz	1000	41	61	2727	1	66.0	467
'Farmer's Slam'	19 oz	1200	51	82	3204	3	80.0	704

Food Name	Serv. Size	Total Cal.	Prot. gms	Carbs gms	Sod. mgs	Fiber gms	Fat gms	Chol. mgs
'French Slam'	14 oz	1029	44	58	1428	2	71.0	777
'Kids Frenchtastic Slam' w/o bread, potato, or meat	6 oz	452	19	22	664	1	33.0	311
'Kids Junior Grand Slam' w/o bread, potato, or meat	5 oz	397	17	33	1118	1	25.0	230
'Moons Over My Hammy' w/o bread, choice of potato or grits	12 oz	807	44	46	2247	2	48.0	430
'Original Grand Slam'	10 oz	795	34	65	2237	2	50.0	460
'Play It Again Slam'	15 oz	1192	51	98	3555	3	75.0	690
'Sausage Lover's Slam'	17 oz	960	31	33	1934	9	68.0	480
'Scram Slam'	18 oz	740	39	14	1293	3	62.0	686
'Senior Belgian Waffle Slam' w/o syrup, margarine	6 oz	399	16	12	612	0	33.0	302
'Senior Triple Play' w/o bread, potato, or meat	8 oz	537	20	64	1445	2	25.0	409
sirloin steak and eggs, w/o bread, choice of potato or grits	9 oz	622	43	1	632	1	49.0	572
'Slim Slam' w/o topping	12 oz	495	34	98	1746	1	12.0	34
'Southern Slam'	13 oz	1065	37	47	2449	0	84.0	484
T-bone steak and eggs, w/o bread, choice of potato or grits	14 oz	991	73	1	1003	1	77.0	657
BREAD AND ROLLS. See also French Toast.								
bagel, w/o added condiments	3 oz	235	9	46	495	0	1.0	0
biscuit, w/butter	3 oz	272	5	39	790	0	11.0	0
English muffin, 1 muffin, w/o added condiments	4 oz	125	5	24	198	1	1.0	0
toast, dry, 1 slice	1 oz	90	3	17	166	1	1.0	0
toast, herb	2 oz	170	2	15	325	1	11.0	1
BUFFALO CHICKEN BURGER								
burger only, w/o added condiments	13 oz	803	37	67	2143	5	45.0	77
BUFFALO WINGS, 12 wings	15 oz	940	80	3	2126	2	68.0	460
CEREAL, ready to eat, 'Kellogg's' average dry	1 oz	100	2	23	276	1	0.0	0
CHEESE	8 oz	293	6	13	895	4	23.0	19
CHEESEBURGER								
classic, burger only, w/o added condiments	13 oz	836	47	43	1595	3	53.0	137
'Kids The Big Cheese' w/o fries or substitute	3 oz	334	9	28	828	2	20.0	24
w/bacon, burger only, w/o added condiments	14 oz	875	53	58	1672	5	52.0	163
CHICKEN DINNER								
breast, grilled, w/o salad dressing, bread	4 oz	130	24	0	560	0	4.0	67
Charleston, w/o choice of side dishes	6 oz	327	25	16	993	1	18.0	65
'Senior Grilled Chicken Breast Dinner' w/o bread, soup, salad, fruit, vegetable	6 oz	200	25	15	824	1	5.0	67
CHICKEN NUGGETS								
'Kids Dennysaur' w/o fries or substitute	2 oz	190	9	9	340	0	13.0	30
CHICKEN STRIPS DINNER								
5 strips, w/o choice of side dishes	10 oz	720	7	56	1666	0	33.0	95
Buffalo, 5 strips, w/o choice of side dishes	10 oz	734	48	43	1673	0	42.0	96
CHILI, with cheese topping	11 oz	401	26	21	1039	7	19.0	57
CONDIMENTS								
bacon, 4 strips	1 oz	162	12	1	640	0	18.0	36
bacon, peppered, 4 strips	1 oz	175	12	2	930	0	13.0	38
barbecue sauce	1.5 oz	47	0	11	595	0	1.0	0
cream cheese	1 oz	100	2	1	90	0	10.0	31
guacamole	1.5 oz	74	1	4	264	1	6.0	0
honey	0.5 oz	40	0	12	1	0	0.0	0
margarine, whipped	0.5 oz	87	0	0	117	0	10.0	0
marinara sauce	1.5 oz	48	1	7	206	1	2.0	0
mushroom, grilled	2 oz	14	2	2	0	1	0.0	0
raisins	0.75 oz	65	1	17	3	1	0.0	0
salsa	1.5 oz	14	0	1	241	0	0.0	0
sour cream	1.5 oz	91	1	2	23	0	9.0	19
sugar, brown	1 oz	110	0	30	10	0	0.0	0
syrup, blueberry flavored	1.5 oz	102	0	26	15	0	0.0	0

Food Name	Serv. Size	Total Cal.	Prot. gms	Carbs gms	Sod. mgs	Fiber gms	Fat gms	Chol. mgs
syrup, maple flavored, 3 tbsp	1.5 oz	143	0	36	26	0	0.0	0
syrup, maple flavored, sugar free	1.5 oz	23	0	9	71	0	0.0	0
syrup, strawberry flavored	1.5 oz	91	0	23	36	0	0.0	0
tartar sauce	1.5 oz	230	0	5	185	0	24.0	17
tomato, sliced, 3 slices	2 oz	13	1	3	6	1	0.0	0
DESSERT								
apple pie, 1/6 pie	7 oz	470	3	64	470	1	24.0	0
banana royale	10 oz	548	6	80	184	6	25.0	64
banana split	19 oz	894	15	121	177	6	43.0	78
'Butterfinger Hot Fudge Sundae'	9 oz	780	9	106	333	1	38.0	71
cheescake, w/o topping	4 oz	470	6	48	280	0	27.0	90
cherry pie, 1/6 pie	7 oz	630	3	101	550	2	25.0	0
chocolate layer cake	3 oz	275	4	42	62	0	12.0	26
chocolate peanut butter pie, 1/6 pie	6 oz	653	15	64	319	3	39.0	27
chocolate silk pie, 1/6 pie	6 oz	650	10	60	220	2	43.0	165
Dutch apple pie, 1/6 pie	7 oz	440	10	65	290	1	19.0	0
hot fudge cake	7 oz	620	7	73	170	1	35.0	60
key lime pie, 1/6 pie	6 oz	600	6	79	300	0	27.0	35
'Kids Jr. Butterfinger Hot Fudge Sundae'	4 oz	341	3	46	141	0	17.0	25
Oreo cookies and creme pie, 1/6 pie	6 oz	590	10	73	390	3	30.0	20
rainbow sherbet	4 oz	120	1	25	30	0	1.5	5
sundae, double scoop, w/o topping	6 oz	375	6	29	86	0	27.0	74
sundae, single scoop, w/o topping, 'Delicious Dip'	3 oz	188	3	14	43	0	14.0	37
yogurt, frozen, chocolate chocolate chip, low-fat	4 oz	110	4	19	60	1	2.0	5
EGGS BENEDICT, w/o choice of potato or grits	15 oz	695	34	34	1718	1	46.0	515
FISH DINNER								
	9 oz	732	30	48	1335	3	47.0	105
'Senior Fish Dinner' w/o bread, soup, salad, fruit, vegetable	5 oz	465	15	25	743	1	34.0	68
FRENCH TOAST								
plain, w/o choice of meat, fruit topping or syrup, margarine	2 pieces	507	16	54	594	3	24.0	219
cinnamon swirl, w/o choice of meat, fruit topping or syrup, margarine	12 oz	1030	23	124	675	4	49.0	280
GARDEN BURGER, burger only, w/o added condiments	11 oz	665	18	75	1051	8	33.0	36
GRAVY								
biscuit and sausage	7 oz	398	8	45	1267	0	21.0	12
brown	1 oz	13	0	2	184	0	0.0	0
chicken	1 oz	14	0	2	139	0	0.5	2
country	1 oz	17	0	2	93	0	1.0	0
sausage	4 oz	126	3	6	477	0	10.0	12
HAM, grilled, grilled slice	3 oz	94	15	2	761	0	3.0	23
HAMBURGER								
'Big Texas Barbecue' burger only, w/o added condiments	14 oz	929	53	53	2271	3	58.0	163
'Classic' burger only, w/o added condiments	11 oz	673	37	42	1142	3	40.0	106
'Double Decker' burger only, w/o added condiments	15 oz	1247	55	82	2200	4	80.0	125
'Garlic Mushroom Swiss' burger only, w/o added condiments	15 oz	872	48	58	1529	5	51.0	116
'Kid's Burgerlicious' w/cheese, w/o fries or substitute	4 oz	341	15	24	580	1	20.0	40
'Kid's Burgerlicious' w/o fries or substitute	4 oz	296	13	24	368	1	17.0	28
HOT DOG MEAL, 'Kids Pig in a Blanket'	5 oz	479	16	63	1684	2	21.0	32
HOTCAKES								
buttermilk, w/o choice of meat, fruit topping or syrup, margarine	3 hotcakes	491	12	95	1818	3	7.0	0
'Kids Smiley-Face Hotcakes' w/meat, w/o syrup, margarine	6 oz	463	14	63	1410	2	22.0	38

Food Name	Serv. Size	Total Cal.	Prot. gms	Carbs gms	Sod. mgs	Fiber gms	Fat gms	Chol. mgs
'Kids Smiley-Face Hotcakes' w/o meat, w/o syrup, margarine	4 oz	344	7	62	1014	2	9.0	13
OATMEAL								
'Quaker'	4 oz	100	5	18	175	3	2.0	0
and fixings, w/o juice, bread	20 oz	535	13	115	95	7	6.0	12
OMELET								
farmer's, w/o bread, choice of potato or grits	14 oz	650	29	17	1158	1	51.0	655
ham and cheddar, w/o bread, choice of potato or grits	10 oz	581	37	4	1180	0	45.0	672
'Senior Omelette' w/o bread, potato, or meat	9 oz	429	25	8	755	2	20.0	515
'Ultimate' w/o bread, choice of potato or grits	13 oz	564	30	9	939	2	47.0	639
'Veggie-Cheese' w/o bread, choice of potato or grits	12 oz	480	26	9	535	2	39.0	644
PIZZA MEAL, 'Kids Pizza Party'	6 oz	400	18	47	1090	7	15.0	10
POT ROAST DINNER								
w/gravy	7 oz	292	42	5	927	0	11.0	87
'Senior Pot Roast Dinner' w/o bread, soup, salad, fruit, vegetable	4 oz	160	25	3	512	0	6.0	48
POTATO PANCAKE, w/o meat, w/o choice of fruit topping or syrup, margarine	13 oz	530	14	59	1125	6	27.0	253
SALAD								
Buffalo chicken, w/o dressing, bread	16 oz	516	33	26	1197	4	35.0	79
Caesar, side, w/dressing, w/o bread	6 oz	362	11	20	913	3	26.0	23
California grilled chicken, w/o dressing, bread	13 oz	277	33	10	720	4	12.0	89
fried chicken, w/o dressing, bread	15 oz	438	33	26	1030	4	26.0	78
garden, side, w/o dressing, bread	7 oz	113	3	16	147	3	4.0	0
'Garden Chicken Delight' w/o dressing, bread	16 oz	277	30	30	785	6	5.0	67
grilled chicken Caesar, w/dressing, w/o bread	13 oz	600	37	19	1792	4	41.0	101
SALAD DRESSING								
blue cheese	1 oz	163	1	1	205	0	18.0	20
Caesar	1 oz	133	1	1	380	0	14.0	2
French	1 oz	106	0	3	274	0	10.0	7
honey mustard, nonfat	1 oz	38	0	9	121	0	0.0	0
Italian, lower calorie, reduced calorie	1 oz	15	0	3	385	0	0.5	0
ranch	1 oz	101	1	1	215	0	11.0	8
Thousand Island	1 oz	118	0	5	170	0	11.0	15
SALMON DINNER								
Alaskan salmon, grilled, w/o salad dressing, bread	6 oz	210	43	1	103	0	4.0	101
SANDWICH								
bacon, lettuce and tomato, sandwich only, w/o added condiments	6 oz	634	18	37	1116	2	46.0	54
Charleston chicken, sandwich only, w/o added condiments	11 oz	632	35	53	1967	4	32.0	81
club, sandwich only, w/o added condiments	11 oz	718	32	62	1666	3	38.0	75
grilled cheese, sandwich only	7 oz	510	19	40	1360	3	30.0	54
grilled chicken, fit-fare, sandwich only	14 oz	434	35	56	1705	4	9.0	82
grilled chicken, sandwich only, w/o added condiments	11 oz	520	35	64	1613	3	14.0	77
ham and swiss, on rye, sandwich only, w/o added condiments	9 oz	533	23	40	1638	5	31.0	36
ham and swiss, sandwich only, w/o added condiments	9 oz	497	22	34	1537	4	30.0	36
Reuben, sandwich only, w/o added condiments	9 oz	580	27	37	2726	5	35.0	69
'Super Bird' sandwich only, w/o added condiments	9 oz	620	35	48	1880	2	32.0	60
turkey breast, on multigrain bread, sandwich only, w/o added condiments	9 oz	476	23	39	1107	5	26.0	57
turkey sub, sandwich only	9 oz	476	23	39	1107	5	26.0	57
SHRIMP DINNER								
'Kids Shrimpsational Basket' w/o fries or substitute	5 oz	291	10	27	774	2	16.0	68
fried	8 oz	558	19	49	1114	3	32.0	135
SIDE DISH								
applesauce, 'Musselmans'	3 oz	60	0	15	13	1	0.0	0
banana, slices	4 oz	100	1	27	0	3	0.0	0

Food Name	Serv. Size	Total Cal.	Prot. gms	Carbs gms	Sod. mgs	Fiber gms	Fat gms	Chol. mgs
banana, whole	4 oz	110	1	29	0	4	0.0	0
baked potato, plain, w/skin	7 oz	220	5	51	16	5	0.0	0
broccoli, w/butter	4 oz	65	3	7	280	3	3.0	5
carrots, w/honey glaze	4 oz	80	1	12	220	3	3.0	0
corn, w/butter	4 oz	120	3	19	260	5	4.0	5
cottage cheese	3 oz	72	9	2	281	0	3.0	10
country fried potato	6 oz	515	3	23	805	9	35.0	8
French fries, chili cheese	12 oz	816	29	77	917	3	44.0	74
French fries, unsalted	4 oz	323	5	44	130	0	14.0	0
fries, seasoned	4 oz	261	5	35	556	0	12.0	0
fries, smothered cheese	9 oz	767	27	69	875	0	48.0	78
fruit mix	3 oz	36	1	9	16	1	0.0	0
grapefruit, 1/2 grapefruit	5 oz	60	1	16	0	6	0.0	0
grapes	3 oz	55	1	15	0	1	1.0	0
green beans, w/bacon	4 oz	60	1	6	390	3	4.0	5
green peas, w/butter	4 oz	100	5	14	360	4	3.0	5
grits	4 oz	80	2	18	520	0	0.0	0
hash browns	4 oz	218	2	20	424	2	14.0	0
hash browns, covered	6 oz	318	9	21	604	2	23.0	30
hash browns, covered and smothered	8 oz	359	9	26	790	2	26.0	30
hash browns, doubled, covered, smothered	13 oz	460	12	48	1213	5	26.0	30
mashed potato, plain	6 oz	105	3	21	378	2	1.0	0
melon, cantaloupe, 1/4 melon	3 oz	32	1	8	16	1	0.0	0
melon, honeydew, 1/4 melon	3 oz	31	1	8	22	1	0.0	0
onion rings	4 oz	381	5	38	1003	1	23.0	6
sausage link, 1 link	3 oz	354	16	0	944	0	32.0	64
sausage patty, 2 patties	3 oz	300	10	1	466	0	28.0	56
strawberry-banana medley	4 oz	108	1	27	6	2	1.0	0
stuffing, bread, plain	3 oz	100	3	19	405	1	1.0	0
vegetable rice pilaf	3 oz	85	2	16	325	1	1.0	0
SKILLET MEAL								
'Big Texas Chicken Fajita' w/o bread	17 oz	1217	49	25	1817	8	70.0	518
'Meat Lover's' w/o bread	15 oz	1147	41	24	2507	7	93.0	460
'Sausage Supreme' w/o bread	16 oz	1054	17	30	1740	8	83.0	430
SOUP								
broccoli, cream of	8 oz	193	4	15	818	2	12.0	0
chicken noodle	8 oz	60	2	8	640	0	2.0	10
clam chowder	8 oz	214	5	22	903	1	11.0	5
potato, cream of	8 oz	222	4	23	761	2	12.0	0
split pea	8 oz	146	8	18	819	2	6.0	5
vegetable beef	8 oz	79	6	11	820	2	1.0	5
STEAK MEAL								
chicken-fried steak and eggs, w/o choice of bread, potato or grits	8 oz	430	22	9	861	4	36.0	440
'Senior Chicken-Fried Steak Dinner' w/o bread, soup, salad, fruit, or vegetable	8 oz	341	16	29	943	2	18.0	27
sirloin	6 oz	271	22	0	273	0	21.0	62
T-bone	12 oz	642	45	1	719	0	50.0	170
chicken-fried steak	7 oz	495	29	24	1150	1	32.0	53
steak and shrimp dinner	9 oz	645	36	31	1143	2	42.0	150
STIR-FRY								
grilled chicken, w/o bread	18 oz	524	34	72	1886	11	11.0	43
vegetable, w/o bread	20 oz	470	13	90	1780	16	6.0	0
TOPPING								
blueberry	3 oz	106	0	26	15	0	0.0	0
blueberry	2 oz	71	0	17	10	0	0.0	0
cherry	3 oz	86	0	21	5	0	0.0	0
cherry	2 oz	57	0	14	3	0	0.0	0
chocolate	2 oz	317	2	27	83	0	25.0	0

Food Name	Serv. Size	Total Cal.	Prot. gms	Carbs gms	Sod. mgs	Fiber gms	Fat gms	Chol. mgs
fudge	2 oz	201	1	30	96	1	10.0	3
nut, 1 tsp	0.3 oz	42	1	1	0	0	4.0	0
strawberry	3 oz	115	1	26	12	1	1.0	0
strawberry	2 oz	77	1	17	8	1	1.0	0
whipped cream, 2 tbsp	0.3 oz	23	0	2	3	0	2.0	7
TURKEY DINNER								
roast turkey and stuffing, w/gravy, w/o salad dressing, bread	14 oz	388	46	38	2467	2	3.0	116
'Senior Turkey and Stuffing Dinner' w/o bread, soup, salad, fruit, vegetable	8 oz	220	25	25	1378	1	2.0	60
WAFFLE								
'Kids Wacky Waffles' w/o syrup or margarine	5 oz	215	4	23	102	0	12.0	78
w/o choice of meat, fruit topping or syrup, and margarine	1 waffle	304	7	23	200	0	21.0	146
D'LITES OF AMERICA								
CHEESE, light	1 slice	53	5	2	0	0	3.0	0
CHEESEBURGER								
w/bacon, on multigrain bun	1 serving	370	32	20	0	0	18.0	0
w/bacon, on sesame seed bun	1 serving	370	32	20	0	0	18.0	0
CONDIMENTS								
salad dressing, lower calorie	1 tbsp	40	0	1	0	0	4.0	0
salad dressing, mayonnaise type mayonnaise, light	1 tbsp	40	0	1	0	0	4.0	0
tartar sauce, light	1 tbsp	60	0	2	0	0	6.0	0
DESSERT								
frozen, 'Chocolate D'Lite'	1 serving	203	6	36	0	0	4.0	0
HAMBURGER								
'Double D'Lite' on multigrain bun	1 serving	450	44	19	0	0	22.0	0
'Double D'Lite' on sesame seed bun	1 serving	450	44	19	0	0	22.0	0
'Junior D'Lite' on multigrain bun	1 serving	200	15	19	0	0	7.0	0
'Junior D'Lite' on sesame seed bun	1 serving	200	15	19	0	0	7.0	0
'Quarter Pound D'Lite' on multigrain bun	1 serving	280	25	19	0	0	12.0	0
'Quarter Pound D'Lite' on sesame seed bun	1 serving	280	25	19	0	0	12.0	0
SANDWICH								
chicken fillet, on multigrain bun	1 sandwich	280	23	24	0	0	11.0	0
chicken fillet, on sesame seed bun	1 sandwich	280	23	24	0	0	11.0	0
fish fillet, on multigrain bun	1 sandwich	390	22	29	0	0	21.0	0
fish fillet, on sesame bun	1 sandwich	390	22	29	0	0	21.0	0
ham and cheese, on multigrain bun	1 sandwich	280	27	26	0	0	8.0	0
ham and cheese, on sesame seed bun	1 sandwich	280	27	26	0	0	8.0	0
vegetarian, 'Vegetarian D'Lite'	1 sandwich	270	16	20	0	0	14.0	0
SIDE DISH								
baked potato	10-oz serving	230	6	50	0	0	1.0	0
baked potato	3.5 oz	81	2	18	0	0	0.3	0
baked potato, 'Mexican'	1 serving	510	27	61	0	0	18.0	0
baked potato, w/bacon and cheddar	1 serving	490	25	52	0	0	20.0	0
baked potato, w/broccoli and cheddar	1 serving	410	15	51	0	0	16.0	0
French fries, large	1 serving	320	4	42	0	0	15.0	0
French fries, regular	1 serving	260	3	34	0	0	12.0	0
potato skin, 'Mexi-Skins'	1 piece	99	4	6	0	0	7.0	0
salad bar platter	1 salad	130	10	9	0	0	6.0	0
SOUP								
broccoli, cream of	1 serving	180	8	21	0	0	7.0	0
'D'Lite'	1 serving	130	14	10	0	0	4.0	0
DOMINO'S								
BREADSTICK	1 piece	116	3	18	152	1	4.0	0

Food Name	Serv. Size	Total Cal.	Prot. gms	Carbs gms	Sod. mgs	Fiber gms	Fat gms	Chol. mgs
BUFFALO WINGS								
barbecue	1 piece	50	6	2	175	0	2.0	26
hot	1 piece	45	5	1	354	0	2.0	26
CHEESY BREAD	1 piece	142	4	18	183	1	6.0	6
PIZZA								
Deep-dish								
cheese, individual, 6-inch	1 serving	598	23	68	1341	4	28.0	36
cheese, large, 14-inch diam	2 slices	677	26	80	1575	5	30.0	41
cheese, medium, 12-inch diam	2 slices	482	19	56	1123	3	22.0	30
ham, individual, 6-inch diam	1 serving	615	25	69	1497	4	28.0	43
ham, large, 14-inch diam	2 slices	708	31	81	1868	5	31.0	53
ham, medium, 12-inch diam	2 slices	505	22	57	1338	3	23.0	39
pepperoni, individual, 6-inch diam	1 serving	647	25	69	1524	4	32.0	47
pepperoni, large, 14-inch diam	2 slices	775	31	81	1940	5	38.0	61
pepperoni, medium, 12-inch diam	2 slices	556	22	56	1397	3	28.0	45
sausage, individual, 6-inch diam	1 serving	642	25	70	1478	4	31.0	45
sausage, large, 14-inch diam	2 slices	787	31	83	1917	5	38.0	64
sausage, medium, 12-inch diam	2 slices	559	22	58	1362	4	28.0	45
vegetable, w/mushrooms, green peppers, onions, olives, individual, 6-inch diam	1 serving	616	23	70	1399	5	29.0	36
vegetable, w/mushrooms, green peppers, onions, olives, large, 14-inch diam	2 slices	697	27	83	1636	5	31.0	41
vegetable, w/mushrooms, green peppers, onions, olives, medium, 12-inch diam	2 slices	498	19	58	1172	4	23.0	30
Hand-tossed								
cheese, medium, 12-inch diam	2 slices	375	15	55	776	3	11.0	23
cheese, large, 14-inch diam	2 slices	516	21	75	1080	4	15.0	32
ham, medium, 12-inch diam	2 slices	398	19	55	990	3	12.0	32
ham, large, 14-inch diam	2 slices	547	26	76	1372	4	17.0	44
pepperoni, medium, 12-inch diam	2 slices	448	19	55	1049	3	17.0	38
pepperoni, large, 14-inch diam	2 slices	614	26	75	1444	4	24.0	52
sausage, medium, 12-inch diam	2 slices	452	19	57	1015	3	17.0	39
sausage, large, 14-inch diam	2 slices	626	26	78	1422	5	24.0	54
vegetable, w/mushrooms, green peppers, onions, olives, medium, 12-inch diam	2 slices	391	16	57	824	4	12.0	23
vegetable, w/mushrooms, green peppers, onions, olives, large, 14-inch diam	2 slices	536	22	77	1141	5	17.0	32
Thin crust								
cheese, medium, 12-inch diam	1/4 of pizza	273	12	31	835	2	12.0	23
cheese, large, 14-inch diam	1/4 of pizza	382	17	43	1172	2	17.0	32
ham, medium, 12-inch diam	1/4 of pizza	296	15	31	1050	2	13.0	32
ham, large, 14-inch diam	1/4 of pizza	414	21	44	1464	2	18.0	44
pepperoni, medium, 12-inch diam	1/4 of pizza	347	15	31	1109	2	18.0	38
pepperoni, large, 14-inch diam	1/4 of pizza	481	21	44	1536	2	25.0	52
sausage, medium, 12-inch diam	1/4 of pizza	350	15	33	1074	2	18.0	39
sausage, large, 14-inch diam	1/4 of pizza	492	22	47	1513	3	25.0	54
vegetable, w/mushrooms, green peppers, onions, olives, medium, 12-inch diam	1/4 of pizza	289	12	33	884	2	13.0	23
vegetable, w/mushrooms, green peppers, onions, olives, large, 14-inch diam	1/4 of pizza	402	17	46	1232	3	18.0	32
DRUTHER'S								
BISCUITS AND GRAVY	8.1-oz serving	331	6	42	1233	1	14.7	3
BREAKFAST MEAL								
bacon and fried egg platter	1 serving	721	25	62	1224	2	41.9	500
bacon and scrambled egg platter	1 serving	742	26	64	1243	2	43.0	501
biscuit, bacon, and egg	3.1-oz serving	258	12	15	653	1	16.3	253
biscuit, ham, and egg	3.5-oz serving	217	13	15	796	1	11.2	256
ham and fried egg platter	1 serving	681	29	62	1622	2	35.3	511

Food Name	Serv. Size	Total Cal.	Prot. gms	Carbs gms	Sod. mgs	Fiber gms	Fat gms	Chol. mgs
ham and scrambled egg platter	1 serving	762	27	64	1408	2	44.6	515
sausage and biscuit platter, two of each	3.4-oz serving	358	12	26	894	1	22.3	34
sausage and egg biscuit	3.3-oz serving	246	11	15	674	1	15.1	257
sausage and fried egg platter	1 serving	741	26	63	1390	2	43.4	515
sausage and scrambled egg platter	1 serving	742	26	64	1243	2	43.0	501
CHEESEBURGER								
'Deluxe Quarter'	8.7 oz	660	33	46	768	1	37.6	127
double patty	6.4 oz	500	29	35	618	0	26.1	105
regular	4.7 oz	380	19	35	585	0	17.8	69
CHICKEN								
12 pieces	3.9 lbs	5496	319	637	12904	16	171.2	902
8 pieces	2.6 lbs	3664	213	425	8558	11	114.1	601
breast, w/wing, dinner or snack	2 pieces	595	48	28	1607	1	30.7	154
leg, w/thigh, dinner or snack	2 pieces	549	38	29	1205	1	29.8	152
thigh and leg, dinner or snack	3 pieces	1281	78	90	2566	2	66.9	273
thigh and wing, dinner or snack	3 pieces	1309	80	87	2465	2	70.3	271
CHICKEN ENTRÉE								
breast and wing, w/potatoes and coleslaw	2 pieces	970	54	76	1899	2	49.9	159
leg and thigh, w/potatoes and coleslaw	2 pieces	925	44	77	1530	2	49.0	157
FISH ENTRÉE								
	13.3-oz entrée	770	43	79	1306	4	31.3	117
fried, w/fries	11.2 oz	729	42	71	1292	4	29.8	112
FISH SANDWICH	4.8 oz	349	22	33	821	2	14.4	56
HAMBURGER	4.4 oz	327	16	35	382	0	13.4	55
DUNKIN' DONUTS								
BAGEL								
blueberry	1 bagel	340	10	75	670	0	1.0	0
cinnamon raisin	1 bagel	340	10	74	480	1	1.0	0
egg	1 bagel	350	11	72	610	0	1.5	25
everything	1 bagel	360	11	74	710	0	2.0	0
garlic	1 bagel	360	11	76	720	0	1.0	0
onion	1 bagel	330	10	70	660	0	1.0	0
plain	1 bagel	340	10	73	710	0	1.0	0
poppyseed	1 bagel	360	11	74	710	0	2.5	0
pumpernickel	1 bagel	350	11	75	560	2	1.5	0
salt	1 bagel	340	10	73	3030	0	1.0	0
sesame	1 bagel	380	12	74	720	0	4.5	0
wheat	1 bagel	330	12	73	670	4	1.5	0
BEVERAGE								
'Coolatta' coffee w/cream	16 fl oz	410	3	51	65	0	22.0	75
'Coolatta' coffee w/milk	16 fl oz	260	4	52	75	0	4.0	15
'Coolatta' coffee w/skim milk	16 fl oz	230	4	52	80	0	0.0	0
'Coolatta' coffee w/2% milk	16 fl oz	240	4	52	80	0	2.0	10
'Coolatta' orange mango fruit	16 fl oz	290	0	71	30	0	0.0	0
'Coolatta' pink lemonade	16 fl oz	350	0	88	30	0	0.0	0
'Coolatta' raspberry lemonade	16 fl oz	280	0	68	35	0	0.0	0
'Coolatta' strawberry fruit	16 fl oz	280	0	70	30	1	0.0	0
'Coolatta' vanilla	16 fl oz	450	1	94	170	0	7.0	0
'Dunkaccino'	18.75 fl oz	480	4	67	470	1	22.0	20
'Dunkaccino'	10 fl oz	250	2	34	240	0	11.0	10
'Dunkaccino'	14 fl oz	360	3	51	360	1	17.0	15
'Dunkaccino'	20 fl oz	510	4	71	500	1	23.0	20
hot cocoa	18.75 fl oz	440	4	75	610	3	15.0	0
hot cocoa	10 fl oz	230	2	38	310	2	8.0	0
hot cocoa	14 fl oz	330	3	57	460	2	11.0	0
hot cocoa	20 fl oz	470	5	79	640	3	16.0	0
BREAKFAST SANDWICH								
'Omwich' bagel, w/bacon and cheddar	1 sandwich	600	26	79	1630	0	21.0	295

Food Name	Serv. Size	Total Cal.	Prot. gms	Carbs gms	Sod. mgs	Fiber gms	Fat gms	Chol. mgs
'Omwich' bagel, Spanish, cheese .... 1 sandwich		570	24	79	1370	0	18.0	280
'Omwich' bagel, three cheese .... 1 sandwich		610	25	78	1630	0	22.0	305
'Omwich' croissant, w/bacon and cheddar .... 1 sandwich		560	21	33	1190	1	38.0	295
'Omwich' croissant, Spanish, cheese .... 1 sandwich		530	19	33	930	1	36.0	285
'Omwich' croissant, three cheese .... 1 sandwich		560	20	33	1200	1	39.0	305
'Omwich' English muffin, w/bacon and cheddar .... 1 sandwich		400	21	33	1440	2	21.0	295
'Omwich' English muffin, Spanish, cheese .... 1 sandwich		370	18	34	1180	2	18.0	280
'Omwich' English muffin, three cheese .... 1 sandwich		400	19	33	1450	2	22.0	305
'Omwich' ham, egg, cheese .... 1 sandwich		320	22	31	1340	2	12.0	195
CINNAMON BUN .... 1 bun		510	8	85	420	0	15.0	10
COOKIE								
chocolate chocolate chunk .... 1 cookie		210	3	26	110	2	11.0	35
chocolate chunk .... 1 cookie		220	3	28	105	1	11.0	35
chocolate chunk w/nuts .... 1 cookie		230	3	27	110	1	12.0	35
chocolate-white chocolate chunk .... 1 cookie		230	3	28	120	1	12.0	35
oatmeal raisin pecan .... 1 cookie		220	3	29	110	1	10.0	30
peanut butter chocolate chunk w/nuts .... 1 cookie		240	4	24	125	2	14.0	25
peanut butter w/nuts .... 1 cookie		240	5	24	150	1	14.0	30
CREAM CHEESE								
chive .... 1 packet		190	3	3	220	0	19.0	55
garden vegetable .... 1 packet		180	3	3	310	0	17.0	45
lite .... 1 packet		130	5	3	250	0	11.0	30
plain .... 1 packet		200	4	3	230	0	19.0	60
salmon .... 1 packet		180	5	2	150	0	17.0	50
CROISSANT								
almond .... 1 croissant		350	6	34	270	2	22.0	5
chocolate .... 1 croissant		400	5	37	240	2	25.0	5
plain .... 1 croissant		290	5	26	270	0	18.0	5
DOUGHNUT								
apple crumb .... 1 donut		230	3	34	270	0	10.0	0
apple fritter .... 1 donut		300	4	41	360	1	14.0	0
apple n' spice .... 1 donut		200	3	29	270	0	8.0	0
Bavarian kreme .... 1 donut		210	3	30	270	0	9.0	0
Bismark, chocolate-iced .... 1 donut		340	3	50	290	0	15.0	0
black raspberry .... 1 donut		210	3	32	280	0	8.0	0
blueberry cake .... 1 donut		290	3	35	400	0	16.0	10
blueberry crumb .... 1 donut		240	3	36	260	0	10.0	0
Boston kreme .... 1 donut		240	3	36	280	0	9.0	0
bow tie .... 1 donut		300	4	34	340	0	17.0	0
butternut cake ring .... 1 donut		300	3	36	360	0	16.0	0
cake, glazed .... 1 donut		270	3	33	360	0	15.0	0
chcolate cake glazed .... 1 donut		290	3	33	370	1	16.0	0
chocolate coconut cake .... 1 donut		300	4	31	370	1	19.0	0
chocolate cruller, glazed .... 1 donut		280	3	35	360	1	15.0	0
chocolate kreme-filled .... 1 donut		270	3	35	260	0	13.0	0
chocolate-frosted cake .... 1 donut		300	3	38	370	0	16.0	0
chocolate-frosted .... 1 donut		200	3	29	260	0	9.0	0
cinnamon cake .... 1 donut		270	3	31	360	0	15.0	0
coconut cake .... 1 donut		290	3	33	360	0	17.0	0
coffee roll .... 1 donut		270	4	33	340	1	14.0	0
coffee roll, chocolate-frosted .... 1 donut		290	4	36	340	1	15.0	0
coffee roll, maple frosted .... 1 donut		290	4	36	340	1	14.0	0
cruller, glazed .... 1 donut		290	3	37	350	0	15.0	0
double chocolate cake .... 1 donut		310	3	37	370	2	17.0	0
dunkin' .... 1 donut		240	3	25	340	0	15.0	0
éclair .... 1 donut		270	3	39	290	0	11.0	0
fritter, glazed .... 1 donut		260	4	31	330	1	14.0	0
glazed .... 1 donut		180	3	25	250	0	8.0	0
jelly stick .... 1 donut		290	3	44	390	0	12.0	0

Food Name	Serv. Size	Total Cal.	Prot. gms	Carbs gms	Sod. mgs	Fiber gms	Fat gms	Chol. mgs
jelly-filled	1 donut	210	3	32	280	0	8.0	0
lemon	1 donut	200	3	28	270	0	9.0	0
maple frosted	1 donut	210	3	30	260	0	9.0	0
marble frosted	1 donut	200	3	29	260	0	9.0	0
old fashioned cake	1 donut	250	3	26	360	0	15.0	0
plain cruller	1 donut	240	3	25	340	0	15.0	0
powdered cake	1 donut	270	3	32	350	0	15.0	0
powdered cruller	1 donut	270	3	30	340	0	15.0	0
strawberry	1 donut	210	3	32	260	0	8.0	0
strawberry-frosted	1 donut	210	3	30	260	0	9.0	0
sugar cruller	1 donut	250	3	27	340	0	15.0	0
sugar raised	1 donut	170	3	22	250	0	8.0	0
sugared cake	1 donut	250	3	27	350	0	15.0	0
toasted coconut cake	1 donut	300	3	35	370	0	17.0	0
vanilla kreme-filled	1 donut	270	3	36	250	0	13.0	0
vanilla-frosted	1 donut	210	3	30	260	0	9.0	0
whole wheat glazed cake	1 donut	310	4	32	380	2	19.0	0
DOUGHNUT HOLE								
'Munchkin' cake butternut	3 munchkins	200	2	25	240	0	11.0	0
'Munchkin' cake chocolate glazed	3 munchkins	200	2	26	250	0	10.0	0
'Munchkin' cake cinnamon	4 munchkins	250	3	30	330	0	14.0	0
'Munchkin' cake coconut	3 munchkins	200	2	23	240	0	12.0	0
'Munchkin' cake glazed	3 munchkins	200	2	27	250	0	10.0	0
'Munchkin' cake plain	4 munchkins	220	2	22	310	0	14.0	0
'Munchkin' cake powdered	4 munchkins	250	2	29	310	0	14.0	0
'Munchkin' cake sugared	4 munchkins	240	2	28	310	0	14.0	0
'Munchkin' cake toasted coconut	3 munchkins	200	2	24	250	0	11.0	0
'Munchkin' yeast glazed	5 munchkins	200	3	27	220	0	9.0	0
'Munchkin' yeast jelly filled	5 munchkins	210	3	30	240	0	9.0	0
'Munchkin' yeast lemon filled	4 munchkins	170	2	23	190	0	8.0	0
'Munchkin' yeast sugar raised	7 munchkins	220	4	26	290	0	12.0	0
MUFFIN								
apple and spice, low-fat	1 muffin	240	4	54	460	0	1.5	0
apple cinnamon pecan	1 muffin	510	8	74	590	1	21.0	70
apple n' spice	1 muffin	350	5	57	390	2	12.0	35
banana nut	1 muffin	360	7	52	490	3	15.0	35
banana, low-fat	1 muffin	250	4	57	430	0	1.5	0
blueberry, 4-oz muffin	1 muffin	320	6	49	480	3	12.0	35
blueberry, 6-oz muffin	1 muffin	490	8	76	610	2	17.0	75
blueberry, lower fat reduced fat	1 muffin	450	8	77	590	2	12.0	65
blueberry, low-fat	1 muffin	250	4	55	430	1	1.5	0
bran	1 muffin	390	11	60	620	3	12.0	20
bran, low-fat	1 muffin	240	4	57	430	4	1.0	0
cherry	1 muffin	340	6	53	510	2	12.0	40
cherry, low-fat	1 muffin	250	4	56	430	0	1.5	0
chocolate chip, 4 oz muffin	1 muffin	400	6	58	440	4	17.0	35
chocolate chip, 6 oz muffin	1 muffin	590	9	88	560	3	24.0	75
chocolate hazelnut chunk	1 muffin	610	10	87	610	3	26.0	70
chocolate, low-fat	1 muffin	250	4	53	470	2	2.5	0
corn, 4 oz muffin	1 muffin	390	8	57	590	2	15.0	55
corn, 6 oz muffin	1 muffin	500	10	78	920	1	16.0	80
corn, low-fat	1 muffin	240	3	52	480	0	2.5	45
corn, reduced fat	1 muffin	460	10	79	900	1	11.0	75
cranberry orange	1 muffin	470	8	76	600	2	15.0	75
cranberry orange nut	1 muffin	350	6	52	500	3	15.0	35
cranberry orange, low-fat	1 muffin	240	4	55	430	1	1.5	0
honey bran raisin	1 muffin	490	7	84	880	5	16.0	30

Food Name	Serv. Size	Total Cal.	Prot. gms	Carbs gms	Sod. mgs	Fiber gms	Fat gms	Chol. mgs
lemon poppyseed	1 muffin	360	5	56	530	1	13.0	35
oat bran	1 muffin	370	11	55	620	3	13.0	20

EL POLLO LOCO

BEANS
pinto	6 oz	185	11	29	744	8	4.0	0
black, smoky	5 oz	255	6	29	609	4	13.0	11
black, smoky, bowl	16 oz	604	29	75	1955	6	23.0	54

BEVERAGE
smoothie, kiwi strawberry	9.5 oz	357	5	66	141	2	7.0	23
smoothie, 'Minute Maid' orange	20 oz	526	9	99	198	0	4.0	44
smoothie, 'Minute Maid' orange	16 oz	457	8	84	176	0	4.0	41
smoothie, strawberry banana	11 oz	367	3	68	136	2	7.0	23

BURRITO
black bean, smoky	8 oz	515	15	71	1197	9	20.0	21
'BRC'	7 oz	440	15	64	1105	9	14.0	15
chicken, classic	11 oz	580	31	66	1595	9	22.0	108
chicken, Southwest	12 oz	627	30	69	1795	5	27.0	60
chicken Caesar, Mexican	11 oz	734	36	65	1214	2	35.0	79
'Chicken Grande'	14 oz	648	33	72	1705	10	26.0	120
'Chicken Lovers'	9 oz	476	29	47	1373	8	19.0	143
'Ultimate Chicken'	12.8 oz	633	92	66	1237	5	23.0	89

CHICKEN
breast, flame-broiled, w/o bone	3 oz	160	26	0	390	0	6.0	110
leg, flame-broiled, w/o bone	1.75 oz	90	11	0	150	0	5.0	75
thigh, flame-broiled, w/o bone	2 oz	180	16	0	230	0	12.0	130
wing, flame-broiled, w/o bone	1.5 oz	110	12	0	220	0	6.0	80
CHICKEN NUGGETS, 'Dinosaur Chicken Bites' 4 oz	4 pieces	185	12	11	345	2	10.4	64
CHURROS	1.75 oz	179	3	18	221	1	11.0	5

CONDIMENTS. See also Salad Dressing.
gravy	1 oz	14	0	2	139	0	0.0	2
guacamole	1.75 oz	52	0	5	280	0	3.0	0
jalapeño hot sauce, 0.5 oz	1 pkt	5	0	1	110	0	0.0	0
salsa, avocado	1 oz	12	0	1	204	0	1.0	0
salsa, house	1 oz	6	0	1	96	0	0.0	0
salsa, pico de gallo	1 oz	11	0	2	131	0	0.5	0
salsa, spicy chipotle	1 oz	7	0	1	179	0	0.0	0
sour cream, light	1 oz	45	2	2	25	0	3.0	12

DESSERT
banana split	15 oz	717	12	107	310	3	28.0	56
cheesecake	3.5 oz	310	8	30	228	0	18.0	58
'Foster's Freeze' w/o topping	4.6 oz	180	4	30	100	0	5.0	20

SALAD
'Pollo Bowl'	17 oz	469	30	66	1868	8	11.0	42
bowl, flame-broiled chicken	12 oz	357	25	39	1079	4	13.0	42
bowl, Mexican Caesar chicken	11 oz	491	25	32	1170	2	30.0	55
bowl, Southwest chicken	13 oz	529	25	40	1332	4	31.0	52
garden, large	14 oz	225	14	17	214	4	13.0	30
garden, regular	4 oz	105	5	7	99	1	7.0	15
tostada, w/o shell and sour cream	14 oz	304	29	28	1175	4	11.0	57

SALAD DRESSING
blue cheese	2 oz	300	2	2	590	0	32.0	50
cilantry, creamy	1.75 oz	266	1	1	306	0	29.0	13
Italian, light	2 oz	25	0	3	990	0	1.0	0
ranch	2 oz	350	1	2	500	0	39.0	5
Southwest	1.75 oz	301	0	2	443	0	32.0	18
Thousand Island	2 oz	270	1	9	460	0	27.0	30

Food Name	Serv. Size	Total Cal.	Prot. gms	Carbs gms	Sod. mgs	Fiber gms	Fat gms	Chol. mgs
SIDE DISH. See also Beans.								
coleslaw	5 oz	206	2	12	358	2	16.0	11
corn cobbette	3 oz	80	3	18	10	1	1.0	0
French fries	5.5 oz	444	6	61	605	0	19.0	0
macaroni and cheese	1 serving	330	14	32	1290	4	16.0	30
mashed potato	5 oz	97	3	21	369	2	1.0	0
potato salad	6 oz	256	3	30	527	3	14.0	15
Spanish rice	4 oz	130	2	24	397	1	3.0	0
vegetables, fresh	4 oz	57	2	8	79	3	2.0	0
TACO								
'Al Carbon'	3 oz	164	13	14	21	1	6.0	68
chicken, soft	4.5 oz	237	17	15	629	0	12.0	74
taquito, chicken	5 oz	370	15	43	690	3	17.0	25
TORTILLA								
corn, 6-inch diam	1 oz	70	1	14	35	1	1.0	0
corn, 4.5-inch diam	0.5 oz	32	1	6	21	0	0.5	0
flour, 11-inch diam	3 oz	260	7	42	583	6	7.0	0
flour, 6-inch diam	1 oz	90	3	13	224	0	3.0	0
spicy tomato	3 oz	254	7	42	577	2	6.0	0
TORTILLA CHIPS, no salt	5 oz	760	9	86	22	7	42.0	0
TOSTADA SHELL	5.6 oz	440	7	42	610	0	27.0	0
EVERYTHING YOGURT								
YOGURT, FROZEN								
low-fat	1 serving	95	3	18	30	0	1.0	5
nonfat	1 serving	80	3	17	40	0	0.0	0
GODFATHER'S PIZZA								
PIZZA								
Cheese								
golden crust, large	1/10 pizza	261	8	31	314	0	11.0	23
golden crust, medium	1/8 pizza	229	8	28	272	0	9.0	19
golden crust, small	1/6 pizza	213	8	27	258	0	8.0	19
original crust, large	1/10 pizza	271	12	37	329	0	8.0	28
original crust, medium	1/8 pizza	242	10	35	285	0	7.0	22
original crust, mini	1/4 pizza	138	6	20	159	0	4.0	13
original crust, small	1/6 pizza	239	10	32	289	0	7.0	25
thin crust, large	1/10 pizza	228	11	28	464	0	7.0	16
thin crust, medium	1/8 pizza	210	10	26	410	0	7.0	14
thin crust, small	1/6 pizza	180	9	21	370	0	6.0	10
Combo								
golden crust, large	1/10 pizza	322	14	33	602	0	15.0	34
golden crust, medium	1/8 pizza	283	13	30	526	0	13.0	29
golden crust, small	1/6 pizza	273	13	29	542	0	12.0	31
original crust, large	1/10 pizza	332	16	39	617	0	12.0	39
original crust, medium	1/8 pizza	318	16	37	569	0	12.0	38
original crust, mini	1/4 pizza	164	8	21	287	0	5.0	17
original crust, small	1/6 pizza	299	15	34	573	0	11.0	37
thin crust, large	1/10 pizza	336	17	31	870	0	16.0	27
thin crust, medium	1/8 pizza	310	15	29	790	0	14.0	25
thin crust, small	1/6 pizza	270	13	23	710	0	13.0	25
STUFFED PIZZA								
cheese, large	1/10 pizza	381	16	44	677	0	16.0	32
cheese, medium	1/8 pizza	350	14	42	610	0	13.0	25
cheese, small	1/6 pizza	310	13	38	560	0	11.0	25
combo, large	1/10 pizza	521	23	47	1204	0	26.0	48
combo, medium	1/8 pizza	480	21	45	1105	0	23.0	43
combo, small	1/6 pizza	430	19	41	1000	0	20.0	40

Food Name	Serv. Size	Total Cal.	Prot. gms	Carbs gms	Sod. mgs	Fiber gms	Fat gms	Chol. mgs
GOLDEN CORRAL								
BREAD, 'Texas Toast'	1 serving	170	5	26	230	0	6.0	0
CHICKEN								
fillet, 'Golden Fried'	1 serving	370	37	14	570	0	19.0	85
fillet, 'Golden Grilled'	1 serving	170	32	0	520	0	5.0	100
POTATO, baked	1 serving	220	5	46	60	0	2.0	0
RIBEYE STEAK, regular	1 serving	450	34	0	220	0	35.0	120
SHRIMP, 'Golden Fried'	1 serving	250	12	24	470	0	12.0	90
SIRLOIN STEAK								
	5-oz serving	230	27	0	270	0	14.0	85
chopped	4-oz serving	320	28	0	160	0	23.0	100
tips, w/onions and pepper	8.2-oz serving	290	30	8	260	0	13.0	120
HARDEE'S								
BEVERAGE								
chocolate shake	12.3 fl oz	370	13	67	270	na	5.0	30
orange juice	10 fl oz	140	2	34	5	na	0.0	0
vanilla shake	12.3 fl oz	350	12	65	300	na	5.0	20
BISCUIT								
and gravy	1 serving	530	10	56	1550	na	30.0	15
apple cinnamon n' raisin	1 serving	250	2	42	350	na	8.0	0
jelly	1 serving	440	6	57	1000	na	21.0	0
chicken	1 sandwich	590	24	62	1820	na	27.0	45
country ham	1 sandwich	440	14	44	1710	na	22.0	30
egg and cheese	1 sandwich	520	17	45	1420	na	30.0	210
ham	1 sandwich	410	13	45	1200	na	20.0	25
'Made From Scratch'	1 serving	390	6	44	1000	na	21.0	0
omelet	1 sandwich	550	20	45	1350	na	32.0	225
plain or buttermilk	1 biscuit	353	6	47	1020	1	16.0	2
sausage and egg	1 sandwich	620	19	45	1370	na	41.0	225
sausage biscuit	1 sandwich	550	12	44	1310	na	36.0	25
steak	1 sandwich	580	15	56	1580	na	32.0	30
CHICKEN								
breast, w/o bone	1 serving	370	29	29	1190	na	15.0	75
leg, w/o bone	1 serving	170	13	15	570	na	7.0	45
thigh, w/o bone	1 serving	330	19	30	1000	na	15.0	60
wing, w/o bone	1 serving	200	10	23	740	na	8.0	30
DESSERT								
apple turnover	1 serving	270	4	38	250	na	12.0	0
cone, twist	1 serving	180	4	34	120	na	2.0	10
peach cobbler	1 serving	310	2	60	360	na	7.0	0
GRAVY	1 serving	20	0	3	260	na	0.0	0
HAMBURGER								
'All-Star'	1 burger	660	29	41	1260	na	43.0	100
'Famous Star'	1 burger	570	24	41	860	na	35.0	80
'Frisco Burger'	1 burger	720	31	37	1180	na	49.0	95
'Monster Burger'	1 burger	1060	49	37	1860	na	79.0	185
regular	1 burger	270	13	29	550	na	11.0	35
'Super Star'	1 burger	790	40	41	970	na	53.0	145
HOT DOG, w/condiments	1 serving	450	15	25	1240	na	32.0	55
SANDWICH								
bacon Swiss crispy chicken	1 sandwich	670	24	45	1600	na	44.0	55
chicken fillet	1 sandwich	480	24	44	1190	na	23.0	55
chicken, grilled	1 sandwich	350	23	28	860	na	16.0	65
'Fisherman's Fillet'	1 sandwich	530	25	45	1280	na	28.0	75
'Frisco Ham'	1 sandwich	450	22	42	1290	na	22.0	225
ham and cheese, hot	1 sandwich	300	16	34	1390	na	12.0	50
roast beef, big	1 sandwich	410	24	26	1140	na	24.0	40
roast beef, monster	1 sandwich	610	35	26	1940	na	39.0	105
roast beef, regular	1 sandwich	310	17	26	800	na	16.0	40

Food Name	Serv. Size	Total Cal.	Prot. gms	Carbs gms	Sod. mgs	Fiber gms	Fat gms	Chol. mgs
SIDE DISH								
coleslaw	1 serving	240	2	13	340	na	20.0	10
crispy curl potatoes, large	1 serving	520	7	62	1450	na	28.0	0
crispy curl potatoes, medium	1 serving	340	5	41	950	na	18.0	0
crispy curl potatoes, monster	1 serving	590	8	70	1640	na	31.0	0
French fries, large	1 serving	440	5	59	520	na	21.0	0
French fries, monster	1 serving	510	6	67	590	na	24.0	0
French fries, regular	1 serving	340	4	45	390	na	16.0	0
hash rounds, regular	1 serving	230	3	24	560	na	14.0	0
mashed potato, small	1 serving	70	2	14	330	na	0.0	0
HARVEY'S FOODS								
BREAKFAST								
pancake	1 serving	89	2	17	0	0	1.0	8
sausage	1 serving	167	9	3	0	0	14.0	12
toast, plain	1 serving	250	8	48	0	0	3.0	0
CHEESEBURGER	1 serving	415	22	41	0	0	18.0	30
CHICKEN FINGERS	1 serving	240	15	18	0	0	12.0	57
DESSERT, apple turnover	1 serving	179	1	28	0	0	7.0	7
HAMBURGER								
double	1 burger	530	31	44	0	0	26.0	34
regular	1 burger	355	18	40	0	0	14.0	17
super	1 burger	477	37	38	0	0	19.0	112
HOT DOG	1 serving	332	12	32	0	0	15.0	50
MUFFIN								
blueberry	1 muffin	254	4	45	0	0	6.0	0
bran	1 muffin	301	5	42	0	0	13.0	0
SANDWICH								
chicken	1 sandwich	419	19	46	0	0	16.0	110
'Western'	1 sandwich	347	15	58	0	0	10.0	265
SIDE DISH								
French fries	1 serving	478	10	56	0	0	24.0	5
hash browns	1 serving	146	2	15	0	0	9.0	2
onion rings	1 serving	288	4	36	0	0	14.0	5
HUNGRY HUNTER								
CHICKEN, breast, teriyaki, boneless, charbroiled	1 serving	413	71	9	237	0	8.0	193
CRAB								
Alaskan king, w/1 tbsp butter	1 serving	432	73	0	3436	0	13.0	194
Alaskan king, w/o butter	1 serving	332	73	0	3319	0	2.0	163
STEAK								
filet mignon	8 oz	539	69	0	150	0	27.0	203
filet mignon, choice	3.5 oz	238	30	0	66	0	11.9	90
LOBSTER								
cooked, w/o butter	1 serving	139	29	2	539	0	1.0	102
cooked, w/1 tbsp. butter	1 serving	241	29	2	657	0	12.0	133
SIDE DISH								
baked potato	1 serving	185	4	43	13	4	0.0	0
rice pilaf	1 serving	142	4	26	223	1	2.0	0
SNAPPER, RED, fresh, cooked in 1/2 oz. butter	1 serving	329	47	0	262	0	15.0	114
IN-N-OUT								
BEVERAGE								
chocolate shake	15 fl oz	690	9	83	350	0	36.0	95
'Coca-Cola Classic'	16 fl oz	198	0	54	12	0	0.0	0
coffee	10 fl oz	5	0	1	3	0	0.0	0
'Diet Coke'	16 fl oz	0	0	0	20	0	0.0	0
'Dr. Pepper'	16 fl oz	200	0	52	0	0	0.0	0
iced tea	16 fl oz	0	0	0	0	0	0.0	0
lemonade	16 fl oz	180	0	40	20	0	0.0	0

Food Name	Serv. Size	Total Cal.	Prot. gms	Carbs gms	Sod. mgs	Fiber gms	Fat gms	Chol. mgs
milk	10 fl oz	180	12	18	190	0	6.0	30
root beer	16 fl oz	222	0	60	48	0	0.0	0
'Seven-Up'	16 fl oz	220	0	52	40	0	0.0	0
strawberry shake	15 fl oz	690	8	91	280	2	33.0	85
vanilla shake	15 fl oz	680	9	78	390	2	37.0	90
CHEESEBURGER								
'Protein Style' w/lettuce leaves, w/o bun	1 serving	330	18	11	720	2	25.0	60
regular	1 serving	480	22	39	1000	3	27.0	60
w/o spread, w/mustard and ketchup	1 serving	400	22	41	1080	3	18.0	55
HAMBURGER								
'Double Double'	1 serving	670	37	40	1430	3	41.0	120
'Double Double' protein style, w/lettuce leaves, w/o bun	1 serving	520	33	11	1160	2	39.0	120
'Double Double' w/o spread, w/mustard and ketchup	1 serving	590	37	42	1510	3	32.0	115
regular	1 serving	390	16	39	640	3	19.0	40
regular, protein style, w/lettuce leaves, w/o bun	1 serving	240	12	10	370	2	17.0	40
regular, w/o spread, w/mustard and ketchup	1 serving	310	16	41	720	3	10.0	35
SIDE DISH, French fries	1 serving	400	7	54	245	2	18.0	0

JACK IN THE BOX

Food Name	Serv. Size	Total Cal.	Prot. gms	Carbs gms	Sod. mgs	Fiber gms	Fat gms	Chol. mgs
BEVERAGE								
cappuccino ice cream shake, regular	16 fl oz	630	11	80	320	0	29.0	90
chocolate ice cream shake, regular	16 fl oz	630	11	85	330	0	27.0	85
'Coca-Cola Classic' regular	20 fl oz	170	0	46	8	0	0.0	0
coffee, regular	12 fl oz	5	0	1	5	0	0.0	0
'Diet Coke' regular	20 fl oz	0	0	0	15	0	0.0	0
'Dr. Pepper' regular	20 fl oz	190	0	49	25	0	0.0	0
iced tea, regular	20 fl oz	0	0	0	0	0	0.0	0
lemonade, 'Minute Maid' regular	20 fl oz	190	0	65	100	0	0.0	0
milk, 2%	8 fl oz	130	9	14	85	0	5.0	25
orange juice	10 fl oz	150	2	34	20	1	0.0	0
Oreo cookie ice cream shake, regular	16 fl oz	740	13	91	490	2	36.0	95
root beer, 'Barq's' regular	20 fl oz	180	0	50	40	0	0.0	0
'Sprite' regular	20 fl oz	160	0	41	40	0	0.0	0
BREAKFAST								
'Breakfast Jack'	1 sandwich	280	17	28	750	1	12.0	190
French toast sticks, w/bacon	1 serving	470	12	53	700	2	23.0	30
pancake, w/bacon	1 serving	370	12	59	1020	3	9.0	30
sausage croissant	1 sandwich	700	21	38	1000	0	51.0	240
'Supreme Croissant'	1 sandwich	530	22	37	960	0	32.0	225
'Ultimate Breakfast Sandwich'	1 sandwich	600	34	39	1470	2	34.0	400
CHEESE								
American	1 slice	45	2	1	230	0	4.0	10
Swiss style	1 slice	40	2	1	210	0	4.0	10
CHEESEBURGER								
'Bacon Ultimate'	1 burger	1020	58	37	1740	1	71.0	210
double patty	1 burger	460	24	32	1090	2	27.0	80
'Jumbo Jack'	1 burger	680	31	39	1130	2	45.0	115
regular	1 burger	320	14	30	720	2	16.0	40
'Ultimate'	1 burger	950	52	37	1370	1	66.0	195
CHICKEN, breast pieces	5 pieces	360	27	24	970	1	17.0	80
CHICKEN MEAL								
chicken teriyaki bowl	1 serving	670	26	128	1730	3	4.0	15
4 chicken pieces, w/French fries	1 serving	730	26	79	1690	5	34.0	65
CONDIMENTS. See also Salad Dressing.								
barbecue dipping sauce	1 serving	45	1	11	310	0	0.0	0
buttermilk dipping house sauce	1 serving	130	1	3	240	1	13.0	10
catsup	1 serving	10	0	2	105	0	0.0	0
croutons, salad bar item	1 serving	50	1	8	105	0	2.0	0

Food Name	Serv. Size	Total Cal.	Prot. gms	Carbs gms	Sod. mgs	Fiber gms	Fat gms	Chol. mgs
jelly, grape	1 serving	40	0	10	5	0	0.0	0
margarine-like spread, 'Country Crock'	1 serving	25	0	0	45	0	2.5	0
salsa	1 serving	10	0	2	200	0	0.0	0
sour cream	1 serving	60	1	1	30	0	6.0	20
soy sauce	1 serving	5	1	1	480	0	0.0	0
sweet and sour sauce	1 serving	45	1	11	160	0	0.0	0
syrup	1 serving	130	0	30	5	0	0.0	0
tartar sauce	1 serving	210	1	2	340	0	22.0	30
DESSERT								
apple turnover, hot	1 serving	340	4	41	510	2	18.0	0
carrot cake	1 serving	370	3	54	340	2	16.0	40
double fudge cake	1 serving	300	3	50	320	1	10.0	50
cheesecake	1 serving	320	7	32	220	1	18.0	65
strawberry ice cream, regular	16 fl oz	640	10	85	300	0	28.0	85
vanilla ice cream, regular	16 fl oz	610	12	73	320	0	31.0	95
FISH AND CHIPS	1 serving	780	19	86	1740	6	39.0	45
HAMBURGER								
'Jumbo Jack'	1 burger	590	27	39	670	2	37.0	90
regular	1 burger	280	12	30	490	2	12.0	30
'Sourdough Jack'	1 burger	690	34	37	1180	2	45.0	105
SALAD								
chicken garden	1 salad	200	23	8	420	3	9.0	65
side	1 salad	50	2	3	75	1	3.0	10
SALAD DRESSING								
blue cheese	1 serving	210	1	11	750	0	15.0	25
house, buttermilk	1 serving	290	1	6	560	0	30.0	20
Italian, low-calorie	1 serving	25	0	2	670	0	1.5	0
Thousand Island	1 serving	250	1	10	570	0	24.0	35
SANDWICH								
chicken	1 sandwich	420	16	39	950	2	23.0	40
chicken, 'Jack's Spicy'	1 sandwich	570	24	52	1020	2	29.0	50
'Chicken Fajita Pita'	1 sandwich	280	24	25	840	3	9.0	75
chicken fillet, grilled	1 sandwich	480	27	39	1110	4	24.0	65
'Chicken Supreme'	1 sandwich	830	33	67	2130	3	48.0	75
'Philly Cheesesteak'	1 sandwich	580	33	56	1860	1	16.0	80
'Sourdough Breakfast'	1 sandwich	450	21	36	1040	2	24.0	205
SIDE DISH								
eggroll	3 egg rolls	440	15	40	1020	4	24.0	35
French fries, curly, chili cheese	1 serving	650	14	60	1760	4	41.0	25
French fries, curly, seasoned	1 serving	410	6	45	1010	4	23.0	0
French fries, jumbo	1 serving	430	4	58	890	4	20.0	0
French fries, regular	1 serving	350	4	46	710	3	16.0	0
French fries, super scoop	1 serving	610	6	82	1250	5	28.0	0
hash browns	1 serving	170	1	14	250	1	12.0	0
jalapeños, stuffed	7 jalapeños	530	14	46	1730	3	31.0	60
onion rings	1 serving	410	6	45	1010	4	23.0	0
potato, bacon cheddar wedges	1 serving	800	20	49	1470	4	58.0	55
TACO								
monster	1 serving	270	12	19	670	4	17.0	30
regular	1 serving	170	7	12	460	2	10.0	20

KENTUCKY FRIED CHICKEN

Food Name	Serv. Size	Total Cal.	Prot. gms	Carbs gms	Sod. mgs	Fiber gms	Fat gms	Chol. mgs
BISCUIT	1 biscuit	180	4	20	560	0	10.0	0
CHICKEN								
breast, extra crispy, w/o bone, 5.9 oz	1 breast	470	39	17	874	1	28.0	160
breast, hot and spicy, w/o bone, 6.5 oz	1 breast	505	38	23	1170	1	29.0	162
breast, original recipe, w/o bone, 5.4 oz	1 breast	400	29	16	1116	1	24.0	135
drumstick, extra crispy, w/o bone, 2.4 oz	1 drumstick	195	15	7	375	1	12.0	77
drumstick, hot and spicy, w/o bone, 2.3 oz	1 drumstick	175	13	9	360	1	10.0	77
drumstick, original recipe, w/o bone, 2.2 oz	1 drumstick	140	13	4	422	0	9.0	75

Food Name	Serv. Size	Total Cal.	Prot. gms	Carbs gms	Sod. mgs	Fiber gms	Fat gms	Chol. mgs
popcorn, large	6.0 oz	620	30	36	1046	0	40.0	73
popcorn, small	3.5 oz	362	17	21	610	0	23.0	43
thigh, extra crispy, w/o bone, 4.2 oz	1 thigh	380	21	14	625	1	27.0	118
thigh, hot and spicy, w/o bone, 3.8 oz	1 thigh	355	19	13	630	1	26.0	126
thigh, original recipe, w/o bone, 3.2 oz	1 thigh	250	16	6	747	1	18.0	95
wing, honey barbecue	6 pieces	607	33	33	1145	1	38.0	193
wing, hot	6 pieces	471	27	18	1230	2	33.0	150
wing, whole, extra crispy, w/o bone, 1.9 oz	1 wing	220	10	10	415	1	15.0	55
wing, whole, hot and spicy, w/o bone, 1.9 oz	1 wing	210	10	9	360	1	15.0	55
wing, whole, original recipe, w/o bone, 1.6 oz	1 wing	140	9	5	414	0	10.0	55
CHICKEN POT PIE, chunky	13 oz	770	29	69	2160	5	42.0	70
CHICKEN SANDWICH								
honey barbecue, w/sauce, 5.3 oz	1 sandwich	310	28	37	560	2	6.0	125
original recipe, w/o sauce, 6.6 oz	1 sandwich	360	28	3	890	1	13.0	60
original recipe, w/sauce, 7.3 oz	1 sandwich	450	29	33	940	2	22.0	70
'Tender Roast' w/o sauce, 6.2 oz	1 sandwich	270	31	26	690	1	5.0	65
'Tender Roast' w/sauce, 7.4 oz	1 sandwich	350	32	23	880	1	15.0	75
'Triple Crunch Zinger' w/o sauce, 6.2 oz	1 sandwich	390	25	39	650	2	15.0	50
'Triple Crunch Zinger' w/sauce, 7.4 oz	1 sandwich	550	28	36	830	2	32.0	85
'Triple Crunch' w/o sauce, 6.2 oz	1 sandwich	390	25	39	650	2	15.0	50
'Triple Crunch' w/o sauce, 6.6 oz	1 sandwich	490	28	29	710	2	29.0	70
CHICKEN STRIPS								
crispy	3 strips	300	26	18	1165	1	16.0	56
crispy, spicy	3 strips	335	25	23	1140	1	15.0	70
DESSERT								
apple pie, 4.0 oz	1 slice	310	2	44	280	0	14.0	0
double chocolate chip, 2.7 oz	1 serving	320	4	41	230	1	16.0	55
'Little Bucket Parfait' chocolate creme, 4.0 oz	1 serving	290	3	37	330	2	15.0	15
'Little Bucket Parfait' fudge brownie, 3.5 oz	1 serving	280	3	44	190	1	10.0	145
'Little Bucket Parfait' lemon creme, 4.5 oz	1 serving	410	7	62	290	4	14.0	20
'Little Bucket Parfait' strawberry shortcake, 3.5 oz	1 serving	200	1	33	220	1	7.0	10
pecan pie, 4.0 oz	1 slice	490	5	66	510	2	23.0	65
strawberry creme pie, 2.7 oz	1 slice	280	4	32	130	2	15.0	15
SIDE DISH								
barbecue baked beans	5.5 oz	190	6	33	760	6	3.0	5
coleslaw	5 oz	232	2	26	284	3	13.5	8
corn on the cob	5.7 oz	150	5	35	20	2	1.5	0
macaroni and cheese	5.4 oz	180	7	21	860	2	8.0	10
mashed potato, w/gravy	4.8 oz	120	1	17	440	2	6.0	1
potato salad	5.6 oz	230	4	23	540	3	14.0	15
potato wedges	4.8 oz	280	5	28	750	5	13.0	5
KRYSTAL								
BREAKFAST								
bacon biscuit	3.6 oz	355	9	36	1055	0	20.0	14
egg biscuit	4.8 oz	372	10	36	813	0	21.0	133
gravy biscuit	8.2 oz	445	9	43	1306	0	26.0	13
plain biscuit	3.2 oz	289	5	35	777	0	14.0	1
sausage biscuit	4.3 oz	429	10	37	987	0	27.0	29
'Sunriser'	3.6 oz	264	13	17	551	0	17.0	157
CHEESEBURGER								
regular	1 serving	189	11	16	456	0	10.0	30
w/bacon	6.4 oz	583	36	34	935	0	35.0	114
'Burger Plus'	7 oz	545	33	37	962	0	31.0	105
double patty	1 serving	214	11	22	674	0	8.0	16
CHILI								
large	12-oz serving	322	17	33	1012	0	11.0	25
regular	8-oz serving	214	11	22	674	0	8.0	16
CORN DOG, 'Corn Pup'	2.3 oz	214	6	17	566	0	14.0	24

Food Name	Serv. Size	Total Cal.	Prot. gms	Carbs gms	Sod. mgs	Fiber gms	Fat gms	Chol. mgs
DESSERT								
apple pie	4.5 oz	320	3	45	420	0	14.0	0
lemon meringue pie	4 oz	340	7	60	130	0	9.0	45
pecan pie	4 oz	450	5	61	290	0	24.0	55
DOUGHNUT								
plain	1.3 oz	100	1	17	130	0	9.0	6
w/chocolate icing	1.8 oz	162	1	27	149	0	11.0	6
w/vanilla icing	1.8 oz	148	1	29	130	0	9.0	6
HAMBURGER								
'Big K'	7.3 oz	608	40	35	1281	0	36.0	125
'Burger Plus'	6.4 oz	488	30	36	709	0	27.0	90
double patty	4 oz serving	276	18	24	532	0	14.0	43
small	2.2 oz serving	158	9	15	339	0	7.0	21
HOT DOG								
'Chili Cheese Pup'	2.6 oz	203	8	15	623	0	13.0	24
'Chili Pup'	2.5 oz	184	7	14	593	0	12.0	19
plain	1.9 oz	164	6	14	469	0	10.0	15
MILKSHAKE, chocolate	12.8 fl oz	271	8	41	175	0	10.0	32
SANDWICH								
chicken, 6.4 oz	1 sandwich	392	21	44	707	0	16.0	33
country ham, 4.5 oz	1 sandwich	379	15	36	1488	0	19.0	23
SIDE DISH								
French fries, crisscut, 'Krys Kross'	2.6 oz	242	3	33	589	0	11.0	10
French fries, crisscut, 'Krys Kross' w/cheese	3.6 oz	292	4	35	789	0	15.0	11
French fries, regular, large	5 oz serving	615	5	111	191	0	17.0	15
French fries, regular, medium	3.9 oz serving	474	4	86	147	0	13.0	12
French fries, regular, small	2.8 oz serving	338	3	61	105	0	9.0	8
LITTLE CAESARS								
BREAD, 'Crazy Bread'	1 serving	98	4	18	119	0	1.0	2
CONDIMENTS, 'Crazy Sauce'	1 serving	63	3	11	360	0	1.0	0
PIZZA								
'Baby Pan! Pan!'	1 serving	525	28	53	1180	0	22.0	60
cheese, single slice, 2.2 oz	1 slice	170	9	20	285	0	6.0	10
pepperoni combination, single slice	1 serving	190	10	20	340	1	7.0	15
'Pizza! Pizza!' large	1 serving	169	11	18	240	0	6.0	15
'Pizza! Pizza!' medium	1 serving	154	10	16	220	0	5.0	15
'Pizza! Pizza!' small	1 serving	138	9	14	200	0	5.0	15
'Pizza! Pizza!' square, large	1 serving	188	10	22	380	0	6.0	20
'Pizza! Pizza!' square, medium	1 serving	185	10	22	370	0	6.0	20
PIZZA MEAL								
cheese pizza, hand-tossed, w/individual tossed salad	1 serving	600	30	73	1605	3	21.0	35
vegetable pizza, w/individual tossed salad	1 serving	640	34	76	1715	4	22.0	40
SALAD								
antipasto, w/low-calorie dressing	12 oz serving	170	10	12	1145	0	9.0	40
Greek, w/low-calorie dressing	11 oz serving	140	8	8	1075	0	8.0	25
tossed, small	1 serving	37	2	7	85	0	1.0	0
tossed, w/low-calorie dressing	11 oz serving	80	4	11	745	0	2.0	0
SANDWICH								
ham and cheese	1 sandwich	520	28	55	1045	1	21.0	45
submarine, Italian	1 sandwich	590	29	55	1230	2	28.0	60
tuna melt	1 sandwich	700	34	58	825	1	37.0	65
turkey	1 sandwich	450	24	49	1590	0	17.0	45
vegetarian	1 sandwich	620	30	58	1000	1	30.0	55
LONG JOHN SILVER'S								
CHICKEN								
batter-dipped, 2 oz	1 piece	120	8	11	400	3	6.0	15

Food Name	Serv. Size	Total Cal.	Prot. gms	Carbs gms	Sod. mgs	Fiber gms	Fat gms	Chol. mgs
'FlavorBaked'	2.6 oz	110	19	1	600	1	3.0	55
CLAMS, batter-dipped	3 oz	300	11	31	670	5	17.0	40
CONDIMENTS. See also Salad Dressing.								
catsup	0.32 oz	10	0	2	110	0	0.0	0
honey mustard sauce	0.42 oz	20	0	5	60	na	0.0	0
malt vinegar	0.28 oz	0	0	0	15	na	0.0	0
margarine	0.18 oz	35	0	0	35	na	4.0	0
shrimp sauce	0.42 oz	15	0	3	180	na	0.0	0
sour cream	1 oz	60	1	1	15	na	6.0	15
sweet and sour sauce	0.42 oz	20	0	5	45	na	0.0	0
tartar sauce	0.42 oz	35	0	5	35	na	1.5	0
FISH								
batter-dipped, 2.98 oz	1 piece	170	11	12	470	5	11.0	30
'Flavorbaked' 2.3 oz	1 piece	90	14	1	320	0	2.5	35
SALAD								
garden	1 salad	45	3	9	25	4	0.0	0
grilled chicken	1 salad	140	20	10	260	4	2.5	45
ocean chef	1 salad	130	14	15	540	4	2.0	60
side	4.3 oz	25	1	4	15	1	0.0	0
SALAD DRESSING								
French, fat-free	1.5 oz	50	0	14	360	na	0.0	0
Italian	1 oz	130	0	2	280	na	14.0	0
ranch	1 oz	170	0	1	260	na	18.0	5
ranch, nonfat	1.5 oz	50	2	13	380	na	0.0	0
Thousand Island	1 oz	110	0	5	280	na	10.0	15
SANDWICH								
fish, batter-dipped, no sauce	5.4 oz	320	17	40	800	6	13.0	20
fish, 'Ultimate'	6.4 oz	430	18	44	1340	3	21.0	35
chicken, 'Flavorbaked'	5.8 oz	290	24	27	970	2	10.0	60
fish, 'Flavorbaked'	6 oz	320	23	28	930	2	14.0	55
SHRIMP, batter-dipped, 0.4 oz	1 piece	35	1	2	95	0	2.5	10
SIDE DISH								
baked potato	8 oz	210	4	49	10	3	0.0	0
cheese sticks	1.6 oz	160	6	12	360	1	9.0	10
coleslaw	3.4 oz	140	1	20	260	3	6.0	0
corn cobbette, w/butter	3.3 oz	140	3	19	0	0	8.0	0
corn cobbette w/o butter	3.05 oz	80	3	19	0	0	0.5	0
French fries	3 oz	250	3	28	500	3	15.0	0
green beans	3.5 oz	30	2	5	310	2	0.5	5
hushpuppy, 0.8 oz	1 piece	60	1	9	25	0	2.5	0
rice pilaf	3 oz	140	3	26	210	1	3.0	0

MAZZIO'S

Food Name	Serv. Size	Total Cal.	Prot. gms	Carbs gms	Sod. mgs	Fiber gms	Fat gms	Chol. mgs
CHICKEN PARMESAN, noodles chicken Parmesan	17.5 oz	590	39	68	1600	0	19.0	50
FETTUCCINE ALFREDO, small	1 serving	440	14	34	680	0	28.0	55
GARLIC BREAD, w/cheese	2 slices	700	21	74	1280	0	35.0	15
LASAGNA, meat, small	1 serving	460	24	26	1370	0	25.0	95
NACHOS, meat	4.5 oz	500	21	21	1200	0	37.0	75
PIZZA								
cheese, deep pan	1 serving	350	17	42	620	0	8.0	15
cheese, original, medium	2 slices	260	14	33	450	0	8.0	10
cheese, thick crust	1 serving	220	13	22	440	0	9.0	15
combination, deep pan, medium	1 slice	410	19	42	930	0	18.0	20
combination, original, medium	1 slice	320	17	34	780	0	13.0	25
'Light' medium	1 slice	240	10	30	460	0	8.0	20
pepperoni, deep pan, medium	1 slice	380	18	38	740	0	17.0	25
pepperoni, original, medium	1 slice	280	16	30	600	0	11.0	30
sausage, deep pan, medium	1 slice	430	21	41	1040	0	21.0	25
sausage, original, medium	1 slice	350	18	34	890	0	16.0	20

Food Name	Serv. Size	Total Cal.	Prot. gms	Carbs gms	Sod. mgs	Fiber gms	Fat gms	Chol. mgs
SANDWICH								
barbecue beef and cheddar	1 sandwich	580	39	53	1260	0	24.0	95
chicken and cheddar	1 sandwich	570	33	56	1350	0	24.0	70
ham and cheese sandwich	1 sandwich	790	40	71	1900	0	39.0	85
SPAGHETTI ENTRÉE, small	1 serving	290	11	39	800	0	10.0	5
MCDONALD'S								
BEVERAGE								
apple bran muffin, low-fat	1 serving	300	6	61	380	3	3.0	0
chocolate shake, small	1 small	360	11	60	250	1	9.0	40
'Coca-Cola Classic' medium	21 fl oz	310	0	58	20	0	0.0	0
'Diet Coke' medium	21 fl oz	0	0	0	40	0	0.0	0
English muffin	1 serving	140	4	25	210	1	2.0	0
orange drink, 'Hi-C' medium	21 fl oz	240	0	64	40	0	0.0	0
milk, 1%	8 fl oz	100	8	13	115	0	2.5	10
orange juice	6 fl oz	80	0	20	20	0	0.0	0
'Sprite' medium	21 fl oz	210	0	56	80	0	0.0	0
strawberry shake, small	1 serving	360	11	60	180	0	9.0	40
vanilla shake, small	1 serving	360	11	59	250	0	9.0	40
BREAKFAST								
apple Danish	1 serving	340	5	47	340	2	15.0	20
bacon, egg, and cheese biscuit	1 sandwich	540	21	36	1550	1	34.0	250
biscuit, plain or buttermilk	1 serving	262	4	35	757	1	11.9	2
breakfast burrito	1 serving	320	13	21	660	1	20.0	195
cheese Danish	1 serving	400	7	45	400	2	21.0	40
cinnamon roll	1 serving	390	6	50	310	2	18.0	65
hash browns	1 serving	130	1	14	330	1	8.0	0
hotcakes, plain	1 serving	340	9	58	630	3	8.0	20
hotcakes, w/margarine and syrup	1 serving	600	9	104	770	3	17.0	20
sausage biscuit	1 sandwich	470	11	35	1080	1	31.0	35
sausage and egg biscuit	1 sandwich	550	18	35	1160	1	37.0	245
'Egg McMuffin'	1 sandwich	290	17	27	790	1	12.0	235
ham, egg, and cheese bagel	1 sandwich	550	26	58	1490	9	23.0	255
sausage	1 serving	170	6	0	290	0	16.0	35
'Sausage McMuffin'	1 sandwich	360	13	26	740	1	23.0	45
'Sausage w/Egg McMuffin'	1 sandwich	440	19	27	890	1	28.0	255
scrambled eggs	2 eggs	160	13	1	170	0	11.0	425
Spanish omelette bagel	1 sandwich	690	27	59	1560	10	38.0	275
steak, egg, and cheese bagel	1 sandwich	660	36	57	1300	9	31.0	285
CHEESEBURGER								
'Big Xtra!'	1 burger	810	29	52	1870	4	55.0	120
'Quarter Pounder with Cheese'	1 burger	530	28	38	1310	2	30.0	95
regular	1 burger	320	16	35	830	2	13.0	40
CHICKEN NUGGETS								
'Chicken McNuggets'	4 pieces	190	10	13	360	1	11.0	35
'Chicken McNuggets'	6 piece	290	15	20	540	2	17.0	55
'Chicken McNuggets'	9 piece	430	23	29	810	2	25.0	80
CONDIMENTS. See also Salad Dressing.								
barbecue sauce	1 pkg	45	0	10	250	0	0.0	0
croutons, salad bar item	1 pkg	50	1	9	105	1	1.0	0
honey	1 pkg	45	0	12	0	0	0.0	0
honey mustard sauce	1 pkg	50	0	3	85	0	4.5	10
hot mustard sauce	1 pkg	60	1	7	240	0	3.5	5
mayonnaise, light	1 pkg	40	0	0	80	0	4.0	5
sweet and sour sauce	1 pkg	50	0	11	140	0	0.0	0
DESSERT								
apple pie, baked	1 serving	260	3	34	200	0	13.0	0
chocolate chip cookie	1 serving	170	2	22	120	1	10.0	20
ice cream cone, vanilla, reduced fat	1 serving	150	4	23	75	0	4.5	20

Food Name	Serv. Size	Total Cal.	Prot. gms	Carbs gms	Sod. mgs	Fiber gms	Fat gms	Chol. mgs
'McDonaldland'	1 pkg	180	3	32	190	1	5.0	0
'McFlurry' Butterfinger	1 serving	620	16	90	260	0	22.0	70
'McFlurry' M&M	1 serving	630	16	90	210	1	23.0	75
'McFlurry' Nestlé Crunch	1 serving	630	16	89	230	0	24.0	75
'McFlurry' Oreo	1 serving	570	15	82	280	0	20.0	70
nut topping, for sundae	1 serving	40	2	2	55	0	3.5	0
sundae, hot caramel	1 serving	360	7	61	180	0	10.0	35
sundae, hot fudge	1 serving	340	8	52	170	1	12.0	30
sundae, strawberry	1 serving	290	7	50	95	0	7.0	30
HAMBURGER								
'Big Mac'	1 burger	570	26	45	1100	3	32.0	85
'Big Xtra!'	1 burger	710	24	51	1400	4	46.0	95
'Quarter Pounder'	1 burger	430	23	37	840	2	21.0	70
regular	1 burger	270	13	35	600	2	8.0	30
SALAD								
shaker, chef	1 salad	150	17	5	740	2	8.0	95
shaker, garden	1 salad	100	7	4	120	2	6.0	75
shaker, grilled chicken Caesar	1 salad	100	17	3	240	2	2.5	40
SALAD DRESSING								
Caesar	1 pkg	150	2	5	390	0	13.0	15
herb vinaigrette, nonfat	1 pkg	30	0	7	220	0	0.0	0
honey mustard	1 pkg	150	1	13	290	0	11.0	15
ranch	1 pkg	170	0	2	480	0	18.0	10
red ranch, reduced calorie	1 pkg	130	0	18	370	0	6.0	0
Thousand Island	1 pkg	130	0	11	360	0	9.0	15
SANDWICH								
chicken, crispy	1 sandwich	550	23	54	1180	2	27.0	50
'Chicken McGrill'	1 sandwich	450	26	46	970	2	18.0	60
'Chicken McGrill' w/o mayo	1 sandwich	340	26	45	890	2	7.0	50
'Fillet-O-Fish'	1 sandwich	470	15	45	890	1	26.0	50
SIDE DISH								
French fries, large	1 serving	540	8	68	350	6	26.0	0
French fries, medium	1 serving	450	6	57	290	5	22.0	0
French fries, small	1 serving	210	3	26	135	2	10.0	0
French fries, super size	1 serving	610	9	77	390	7	29.0	0
MRS. WINNER								
BISCUIT								
	1 serving	245	4	45	503	0	5.0	0
CHICKEN								
breast, fried, no skin	4 oz	280	23	14	480	0	15.0	115
fillet, baked	1 serving	120	10	0	360	0	2.0	33
leg, fried, no skin	1.7 oz	110	10	5	115	0	6.0	50
HAM, country	1 serving	60	4	0	565	0	1.0	14
ROLL, honey yeast	1 roll	200	8	35	290	0	4.0	7
SALAD								
chicken	1 salad	583	9	39	875	0	8.0	3
seafood	1 salad	553	5	41	756	0	9.0	4
tossed	1 salad	6	1	1	439	0	0.0	1
SANDWICH								
chicken, breaded	1 sandwich	203	19	12	1000	0	10.0	37
chicken fillet	1 sandwich	379	12	45	541	0	7.0	28
chicken salad	1 sandwich	313	10	33	599	0	6.0	1
steak	1 sandwich	429	11	43	644	0	11.0	21
SAUSAGE, patty	1 serving	200	6	0	400	0	10.0	8
SIDE DISH								
coleslaw	1 serving	188	1	9	549	0	16.0	1
French fries	1 serving	225	6	27	214	0	9.0	1
mashed potato, w/gravy	1 serving	148	3	22	823	0	3.0	2

Food Name	Serv. Size	Total Cal.	Prot. gms	Carbs gms	Sod. mgs	Fiber gms	Fat gms	Chol. mgs
potato wedges, oven roasted	1 serving	139	4	31	132	0	1.0	1
STEAK ENTRÉE, country fried	1 serving	220	12	0	205	0	14.0	7
PERKINS								
BROCCOLI, raw	4 oz	31	3	6	31	0	0.4	0
CHICKEN ENTRÉE								
lemon pepper, w/rice pilaf, broccoli, salad	1 serving	620	59	60	1364	0	12.5	136
FRUIT CUP, w/cantaloupe, honeydew,								
blueberries	4.5 oz serving	48	1	12	12	0	0.3	0
HASH BROWNS	3 oz	101	2	17	28	0	2.6	0
MUFFIN								
apple	1 muffin	543	9	76	728	0	24.0	95
banana nut	1 muffin	586	9	75	702	0	29.0	92
blueberry	1 muffin	506	7	71	671	0	23.0	88
bran	1 muffin	478	9	83	572	0	17.0	0
carrot	1 muffin	560	7	88	780	0	23.0	81
chocolate chocolate chip	1 muffin	546	10	73	629	0	26.0	83
corn	1 muffin	683	12	121	1550	0	17.0	33
cranberry nut	1 muffin	558	9	71	671	0	28.0	88
oat bran	1 muffin	513	10	87	588	0	16.0	0
plain	1 muffin	586	9	81	797	0	26.0	104
plain, low-fat	1 muffin	495	12	111	802	0	1.2	5
OMELET								
'Country Club'	1 serving	932	47	6	1134	1	79.1	1154
'Country Club' w/3 oz hash browns	1 serving	1033	49	23	1162	1	81.7	1154
'Deli Ham and Lotsa Cheese'	1 serving	962	53	8	1832	1	79.1	864
'Deli Ham and Lotsa Cheese' w/3 oz hash browns	1 serving	1063	55	25	1860	1	81.7	864
'Denver' w/fruit cup	1 serving	235	23	22	795	0	6.5	154
'Everything'	1 serving	697	45	9	870	0	53.4	814
'Everything' w/3 oz hash browns	1 serving	798	46	25	898	2	56.0	814
'Granny's Country'	1 serving	941	43	7	786	1	81.5	810
'Granny's Country' w/9 oz hash browns	1 serving	1245	48	57	869	1	89.2	810
ham and cheese	1 serving	644	41	3	832	1	51.3	743
ham and cheese, w/3 oz hash browns	1 serving	745	42	19	860	1	53.9	743
mushroom and cheese	1 serving	687	32	5	925	1	59.9	744
mushroom and cheese, w/3 oz hash browns	1 serving	788	34	22	953	1	62.5	744
seafood, w/fruit cup	1 serving	271	29	28	595	0	5.7	197
ORANGE ROUGHY ENTRÉE,								
w/rice pilaf, broccoli, salad	1 serving	467	33	60	1387	0	7.0	133
PANCAKE								
buttermilk	3 pancakes	442	13	70	988	0	12.0	24
'Harvest Grain' w/1.5 oz low-cal syrup	5 pancakes	473	11	93	1640	0	3.4	0
'Short Stack Harvest Grain'	3 pancakes	268	7	56	1020	0	2.0	0
PIE								
apple	1 slice	521	3	72	457	0	26.0	0
apple, w/Equal sugar substitute	1 slice	420	3	55	371	0	24.0	0
cherry	1 slice	571	4	84	702	0	26.0	0
cherry, w/Equal sugar substitute	1 slice	425	4	55	513	0	24.0	0
coconut cream	1 slice	437	6	56	488	0	33.0	5
French silk	1 slice	551	4	59	478	0	37.0	53
lemon meringue	1 slice	395	2	63	528	0	16.0	0
peanut butter brownie	1 slice	455	9	44	436	0	35.0	29
pecan	1 slice	669	7	106	670	0	26.0	17
SALAD								
chef, mini	1 salad	214	23	7	643	0	11.0	55
dinner, 'Lite and Healthy'	1 salad	103	3	15	496	0	2.1	0
SYRUP, low-calorie	1.5 oz	26	0	7	0	0	0.0	0
TOAST, w/.5 oz margarine, grape jelly	0.75-oz slice	219	2	28	224	1	12.2	8
VEGETABLE STIR-FRY, w/mixed vegetables	6 oz	49	3	10	23	0	0.4	0

Food Name	Serv. Size	Total Cal.	Prot. gms	Carbs gms	Sod. mgs	Fiber gms	Fat gms	Chol. mgs
VEGETABLE SANDWICH								
stir-fry, on pita	1 sandwich	308	44	41	752	0	9.2	26
stir-fry, on pita, w/coleslaw	1 sandwich	441	45	54	877	0	17.8	36
stir-fry, on pita, w/coleslaw and pasta salad	1 sandwich	626	49	63	1395	0	32.5	37
stir-fry, on pita, w/pasta salad	1 sandwich	493	48	50	1270	0	23.9	27
PETER PIPER PIZZA								
PIZZA								
Beef								
extra large	1 slice	280	15	36	446	0	8.0	20
large	1 slice	296	15	39	482	0	8.0	20
express lunch	1 slice	165	9	21	257	0	5.0	13
medium	1 slice	222	12	29	359	0	6.0	15
small	1 slice	194	10	25	319	0	5.0	14
Cheese								
extra large	1 pizza	3078	160	437	3113	0	73.0	211
extra large	1 slice	257	13	36	260	0	6.1	18
large	1 pizza	2159	112	311	2176	0	49.4	140
large	1 slice	270	14	39	271	0	6.2	18
express lunch pizza	1 pizza	608	32	83	609	0	16.0	47
express lunch pizza	1 slice	152	8	21	152	0	4.0	12
medium	1 pizza	1622	84	235	1614	0	37.0	105
medium	1 slice	203	11	29	201	0	5.0	13
small	1 pizza	1059	60	152	1073	0	25.0	70
small	1 slice	177	9	25	179	0	4.0	12
w/black olive, large	1 slice	259	24	22	407	0	8.0	12
w/black olive, medium	1 slice	193	18	17	303	0	6.0	9
w/black olive, small	1 slice	171	16	15	276	0	6.0	8
w/green pepper, large	1 slice	245	24	22	339	0	7.0	12
w/green pepper, medium	1 slice	183	18	17	256	0	5.0	9
w/green pepper, small	1 slice	163	16	15	283	0	4.0	8
w/ham, large	1 slice	258	26	22	473	0	7.0	17
w/ham, medium	1 slice	194	19	16	356	0	6.0	13
w/ham, small	1 slice	172	17	15	317	0	5.0	11
w/jalapeño, large	1 slice	244	24	22	424	0	7.0	12
w/jalapeño, medium	1 slice	183	18	17	319	0	5.0	9
w/jalapeño, small	1 slice	163	16	15	283	0	4.0	8
w/mushroom, large	1 slice	245	24	22	379	0	7.0	12
w/mushroom, medium	1 slice	183	18	17	283	0	5.0	9
w/mushroom, small	1 slice	162	16	15	245	0	4.0	8
w/onion, large	1 slice	243	24	22	341	0	7.0	12
w/onion, medium	1 slice	183	18	17	257	0	5.0	9
w/onion, small	1 slice	162	16	15	228	0	4.0	8
w/pineapple, large	1 slice	246	23	23	341	0	7.0	12
w/pineapple, medium	1 slice	185	18	17	256	0	5.0	8
w/pineapple, small	1 slice	164	16	15	228	0	4.0	8
Salami								
express lunch	1 slice	164	9	21	199	0	5.0	15
extra large	1 slice	273	14	37	322	0	7.5	22
large	1 slice	288	15	39	342	0	8.0	23
medium	1 slice	216	11	29	254	0	6.0	17
small	1 slice	189	8	25	223	0	5.0	15
PIZZA HUT								
BREADSTICK	1 serving	130	3	20	170	1	4.0	0
BREADSTICK DIPPING SAUCE	1 serving	30	1	5	170	1	0.5	0
CHICKEN								
Buffalo wings, hot	4 pieces	210	22	4	900	0	12.0	130
Buffalo wings, mild	5 pieces	200	23	1	510	0	12.0	150

Food Name	Serv. Size	Total Cal.	Prot. gms	Carbs gms	Sod. mgs	Fiber gms	Fat gms	Chol. mgs
GARLIC BREAD	1 slice	150	3	16	240	1	8.0	0
PASTA								
cavatini	1 serving	480	21	66	1170	9	14.0	8
'Cavatini Supreme'	1 serving	560	24	73	1400	10	19.0	10
spaghetti, w/marinara sauce	1 serving	490	18	91	730	8	6.0	0
spaghetti, w/meat sauce	1 serving	600	23	98	910	9	13.0	8
spaghetti, w/meatballs	1 serving	850	37	120	1120	10	24.0	17
PIZZA								
Apple, dessert	1 slice	250	3	48	230	2	4.5	0
Beef								
hand-tossed, medium	1 slice	347	16	44	943	4	12.0	21
pan, medium	1 slice	399	15	45	773	4	18.0	20
Sicilian, medium	1 slice	282	13	31	824	3	12.0	19
stuffed crust, medium	1 slice	466	23	46	1137	3	22.0	30
thin and crispy, medium	1 slice	305	14	28	814	3	15.0	24
Cheese								
'Big New Yorker'	1 slice	393	20	42	1099	3	16.6	19
hand-tossed, medium	1 slice	309	14	43	848	3	9.0	11
pan, medium	1 slice	361	13	44	678	3	15.0	11
pan, personal	1 pizza	813	31	110	1581	8	27.0	24
Sicilian, medium	1 slice	295	12	32	815	3	13.0	11
stuffed crust, medium	1 slice	445	22	46	1090	3	19.0	24
thin and crispy, medium	1 slice	243	11	27	653	2	10.0	11
Cherry, dessert	1 slice	250	3	47	220	3	4.5	0
'Chicken Supreme'								
hand-tossed, medium	1 slice	291	15	44	841	4	6.0	17
pan, medium	1 slice	343	15	45	671	3	12.0	16
Sicilian, medium	1 slice	269	13	32	732	3	10.0	15
stuffed crust, medium	1 slice	432	24	47	1111	3	17.0	32
'The New Edge' medium	1 slice	90	7	9	290	1	3.5	15
thin and crispy, medium	1 slice	232	13	29	681	3	7.0	19
Ham								
hand-tossed, medium	1 slice	279	13	43	857	3	6.0	15
pan, medium	1 slice	331	12	44	687	3	12.0	15
Sicilian, medium	1 slice	257	11	30	745	3	10.0	14
stuffed crust, medium	1 slice	404	24	45	1190	2	22.0	39
thin and crispy, medium	1 slice	212	10	27	662	2	7.0	15
Italian sausage								
hand-tossed, medium	1 slice	363	16	44	975	4	14.0	26
pan, medium	1 slice	415	15	45	805	3	20.0	26
Sicilian, medium	1 slice	333	13	31	855	3	18.0	24
stuffed crust, medium	1 slice	478	22	46	1164	3	23.0	35
thin and crispy, medium	1 slice	325	14	28	865	3	18.0	32
'Meat Lover's'								
thin and crispy, medium	1 slice	339	15	28	970	3	19.0	35
hand-tossed, medium	1 slice	376	17	44	1077	4	15.0	30
pan, medium	1 slice	428	16	45	607	3	21.0	29
Sicilian, medium	1 slice	344	14	31	948	3	18.0	27
stuffed crust, medium	1 slice	543	26	46	1427	3	29.0	48
'The New Edge' medium	1 slice	160	7	8	440	1	11.0	20
Pepperoni								
'Big New Yorker'	1 slice	380	18	42	1116	3	16.0	22
hand-tossed, medium	1 slice	301	13	43	867	3	8.0	15
pan, medium	1 slice	353	12	44	791	3	14.0	14
pan, personal	1 pizza	810	30	111	1661	8	28.0	32
Sicilian, medium	1 slice	227	11	31	754	3	113.0	13
stuffed crust, medium	1 slice	438	21	45	1116	2	19.0	27
thin and crispy, medium	1 slice	235	10	27	672	2	10.0	14

Food Name	Serv. Size	Total Cal.	Prot. gms	Carbs gms	Sod. mgs	Fiber gms	Fat gms	Chol. mgs
'Pepperoni Lover's'								
hand-tossed, medium	1 slice	372	17	43	1123	3	14.0	26
pan, medium	1 slice	370	13	44	767	3	16.0	18
Sicilian, medium	1 slice	321	13	31	899	3	16.0	19
stuffed crust, medium	1 slice	525	26	46	1413	3	26.0	40
thin and crispy, medium	1 slice	289	13	28	859	2	14.0	22
Pork								
hand-tossed, medium	1 slice	342	16	44	990	4	12.0	20
pan, medium	1 slice	394	15	45	820	4	18.0	20
Sicilian, medium	1 slice	314	13	31	868	3	16.0	18
stuffed crust, medium	1 slice	461	22	46	1176	3	21.0	29
thin and crispy, medium	1 slice	298	14	28	875	3	15.0	23
'Super Supreme'								
hand-tossed, medium	1 slice	359	16	45	1024	4	12.0	23
pan, medium	1 slice	401	15	46	854	4	18.0	22
Sicilian, medium	1 slice	323	13	32	911	3	16.0	21
stuffed crust, medium	1 slice	505	25	46	1371	3	25.0	44
thin and crispy, medium	1 slice	304	14	29	902	3	15.0	26
'Supreme'								
'Big New Yorker'	1 slice	459	10	44	1310	4	22.3	33
hand-tossed, medium	1 slice	333	15	44	927	4	11.0	18
pan, medium	1 slice	385	14	45	757	4	17.0	18
pan, personal	1 pizza	808	30	111	1579	8	27.0	28
Sicilian, medium	1 slice	307	13	32	815	3	15.0	17
stuffed crust, medium	1 slice	487	24	47	1227	3	23.0	33
thin and crispy, medium	1 slice	284	13	29	784	3	13.0	20
Taco								
beef, hand-tossed, medium	1 slice	270	13	35	870	3	8.0	15
beef, pan, medium	1 slice	300	12	36	770	3	12.0	15
beef, thin and crispy, medium	1 slice	260	13	29	850	2	10.0	20
chicken, hand-tossed, medium	1 slice	290	12	35	940	3	11.0	15
chicken, pan, medium	1 slice	320	12	36	830	3	15.0	15
chicken, thin and crispy, medium	1 slice	260	11	26	850	2	12.0	20
hand-tossed, medium	1 slice	280	12	34	870	3	11.0	15
meatless, hand-tossed, medium	1 slice	250	11	35	790	3	8.0	10
meatless, pan, medium	1 slice	290	10	36	680	3	12.0	10
meatless, thin and crispy, medium	1 slice	230	9	27	700	2	8.0	10
pan, medium	1 slice	310	12	36	800	3	13.0	15
pan, personal	1 pizza	780	27	90	1900	7	35.0	30
thin and crispy, medium	1 slice	260	12	27	860	2	11.0	20
'The Works' 'The New Edge' medium	1 slice	110	5	9	270	1	6.0	10
'Veggie Lover's'								
hand-tossed, medium	1 slice	281	12	45	771	4	6.0	7
pan, medium	1 slice	333	11	46	601	4	12.0	7
Sicilian, medium	1 slice	252	10	32	627	3	10.0	7
stuffed crust, medium	1 slice	421	20	48	1039	3	17.0	19
'The New Edge' medium	1 slice	70	4	9	180	1	3.0	5
thin and crispy, medium	1 slice	222	9	30	621	3	8.0	7
SANDWICH								
ham and cheese	1 sandwich	550	33	57	2150	4	21.0	22
'Supreme'	1 sandwich	640	34	62	2150	4	28.0	28

PONDEROSA

CHICKEN ENTRÉE

	Serv. Size	Total Cal.	Prot. gms	Carbs gms	Sod. mgs	Fiber gms	Fat gms	Chol. mgs
breast	5.5 oz	98	20	1	400	0	2.1	54
wing	2 pieces	213	11	11	610	0	9.0	75

CONDIMENTS. See also Salad Bar Items; Salad Dressing.

	Serv. Size	Total Cal.	Prot. gms	Carbs gms	Sod. mgs	Fiber gms	Fat gms	Chol. mgs
cheese sauce	2 oz	52	1	6	355	0	2.0	4
cheese topping, herb and garlic	1 tbsp	100	0	0	120	0	10.0	0

Food Name	Serv. Size	Total Cal.	Prot. gms	Carbs gms	Sod. mgs	Fiber gms	Fat gms	Chol. mgs
gravy, brown	2 oz	25	1	4	167	0	1.0	0
gravy, turkey	2 oz	25	1	5	228	0	0.2	0
margarine, liquid	1 tbsp	100	0	0	110	0	11.0	0
margarine, whipped	1 tbsp	34	0	0	65	0	1.2	0
tartar sauce	1 oz	85	0	11	477	0	10.9	9
DESSERT								
dougnut, winter mix	3.5 oz	25	2	4	371	0	0.0	0
gelatin dessert, plain, nonfat	4 oz	71	1	17	73	0	0.0	0
ice milk, chocolate	3.5 oz	152	4	30	70	0	3.0	22
ice milk, vanilla	3.5 oz	150	4	30	58	0	3.0	20
mousse, chocolate	4 oz	312	0	28	72	0	18.0	0
mousse, chocolate	1 oz	78	0	7	18	0	4.4	0
mousse, strawberry	4 oz	297	0	25	68	0	18.0	0
mousse, strawberry	1 oz	74	0	6	17	0	4.6	0
pudding, banana	4 oz	207	1	27	114	0	10.0	0
vanilla wafer cookie, peanut butter	2 wafers	35	0	6	25	0	1.0	5
DESSERT TOPPING								
caramel	1 oz	100	0	26	72	0	0.7	2
chocolate	1 oz	89	1	24	37	0	0.3	0
peanut, granulated	.2 oz	30	1	1	0	0	2.3	0
strawberry	1 oz	71	0	24	29	0	0.2	0
strawberry glaze	1 oz	37	0	10	4	0	0.0	0
whipped	1 oz	80	0	5	16	0	7.0	0
FISH. See also individual listings.								
nuggets	1 piece	31	2	2	52	0	1.7	8
baked, 'Bake 'R Broil' baked	5.2 oz	230	19	10	330	0	13.0	50
fried	3.2 oz	190	9	17	170	0	9.0	15
HALIBUT, broiled	6 oz	170	35	0	68	0	2.4	0
HOT DOG	1.6 oz	144	5	1	460	0	13.0	27
MEATBALLS	2 pieces	115	5	2	16	0	4.0	21
ORANGE ROUGHY, broiled	5 oz	139	0	21	88	0	5.0	28
ROLL								
dinner	1 piece	184	5	33	311	0	3.0	0
sourdough	1 piece	110	4	22	230	0	1.0	0
SALAD BAR ITEMS								
banana chips	.2 oz	25	0	3	0	0	1.3	0
banana	1 medium	87	1	23	1	0	0.2	0
breadstick, Italian	1 stick	100	4	19	200	0	1.0	0
breadstick, sesame	2 sticks	35	1	6	60	0	0.0	0
broccoli, raw	1 oz	9	1	2	4	0	0.9	0
cabbage, green	1 oz	9	1	2	7	0	0.0	0
cheese, imitation, shredded	1 oz	90	6	1	420	0	7.0	5
chicken macaroni salad	3.5 oz	335	8	49	431	0	12.0	9
chicken salad	3.5 oz	212	11	8	334	0	15.0	42
chow mein noodles	.2 oz	25	1	3	42	0	1.2	0
coconut, shredded	.2 oz	25	0	2	14	0	1.9	0
croutons	1 oz	115	4	18	351	0	4.0	0
fruit cocktail	4 oz	97	1	25	7	0	0.2	0
granola	.2 oz	24	1	3	0	0	1.0	0
grapes	10 grapes	34	0	9	2	0	0.2	0
ham, diced	2 oz	120	9	1	780	0	10.0	76
lemon	1 wedge	3	0	1	0	0	0.1	0
macaroni salad	3.5 oz	335	8	49	431	0	11.7	9
onion, green	1 piece	7	0	2	1	0	0.1	0
onion, yellow	1 oz	11	0	3	3	0	0.0	0
orange	1 piece	45	1	11	1	0	0.1	0
pasta salad	3.5 oz	268	6	34	441	0	12.0	0
pickle chips, sweet	.14 oz	4	0	1	1	0	0.0	0

Food Name	Serv. Size	Total Cal.	Prot. gms	Carbs gms	Sod. mgs	Fiber gms	Fat gms	Chol. mgs
pickle spear, dill	.14 oz	1	0	0	54	0	0.0	0
potato salad	3.5 oz	126	2	16	300	0	6.0	7
turkey ham salad	3.5 oz	186	8	10	654	0	13.0	12
turkey, julienne	1 oz	29	5	1	192	0	1.0	15
yogurt, frozen, fruit flavor	4 oz	115	5	23	70	0	1.0	5
yogurt, frozen, vanilla	4 oz	110	5	18	75	0	2.0	6
SALAD DRESSING								
blue cheese	1 oz	130	1	1	266	0	14.0	27
coleslaw	1 oz	150	0	6	284	0	14.0	31
creamy Italian	1 oz	103	0	3	373	0	10.0	0
cucumber, lower calorie	1 oz	69	0	3	315	0	6.0	0
Italian, lower calorie	1 oz	31	0	1	371	0	3.0	0
oil	1 tbsp	120	0	0	0	0	14.0	0
Parmesan pepper	1 oz	150	1	2	281	0	15.0	9
ranch	1 oz	147	0	1	297	0	15.0	3
sweet-n-tangy	1 oz	122	0	8	347	0	10.0	1
Thousand Island	1 oz	113	0	8	405	0	10.0	9
SALMON, broiled	6 oz	192	37	3	72	0	3.0	60
SCROD, baked	7 oz	120	27	0	80	0	1.0	65
SHRIMP								
fried	7 pieces	230	22	31	612	0	1.0	105
mini	6 pieces	47	5	6	125	0	1.0	22
SIDE DISH								
baked beans	4 oz	170	6	21	330	0	6.0	0
baked potato	7.2 oz	145	4	33	6	0	0.0	0
corn	3.5 oz	90	3	21	5	0	0.4	0
French fries	3 oz	120	2	17	39	0	4.0	3
green beans	3.5 oz	20	1	3	391	0	0.0	0
macaroni and cheese	1 oz	17	1	4	80	0	0.5	1
macaroni salad	3.5 oz	335	8	49	431	0	11.7	9
mashed potato	4 oz	62	2	13	191	0	0.0	20
okra, breaded	4 oz	124	3	23	483	0	1.0	1
onion rings, breaded	4 oz	213	3	30	620	0	9.0	2
pasta/noodles	2 oz	78	2	16	1	0	0.3	0
potato wedges	3.5 oz	130	3	16	170	0	6.0	0
rice pilaf	4 oz	160	4	26	450	0	4.0	22
spinach	1 oz	7	1	1	20	0	0.1	0
stuffing	4 oz	230	6	27	800	0	11.0	22
SPAGHETTI, w/sauce	6 oz	188	5	33	520	0	5.0	0
STEAK								
chopped	4 oz	225	19	1	150	0	16.0	80
kabobs, meat only	3 oz	153	26	2	280	0	5.0	67
Kansas City strip	5 oz	138	21	1	850	0	5.7	76
New York strip, choice	8 oz	314	45	1	570	0	10.5	50
Porterhouse, choice	16 oz	640	57	3	1130	0	30.9	82
Porterhouse, non-graded	13 oz	440	43	1	1844	0	30.0	67
ribeye, choice	6 oz	282	29	1	570	0	14.0	60
ribeye, non-graded	5 oz	219	25	1	1130	0	13.0	75
sirloin, choice	7 oz	241	35	1	570	0	11.0	63
sirloin tips, choice	5 oz	197	29	1	280	0	8.0	71
T-bone, choice	10 oz	444	44	2	850	0	18.0	80
T-bone, non-graded	8 oz	178	25	2	850	0	8.5	71
teriyaki	5 oz	174	32	5	1420	0	3.0	64
STEAK SANDWICH	4 oz	208	20	2	850	0	11.0	62
SWORDFISH, broiled	5.9 oz	271	44	0	0	0	10.0	84
TROUT	5 oz	228	30	1	51	0	4.0	110

POPEYES

Food Name	Serv. Size	Total Cal.	Prot. gms	Carbs gms	Sod. mgs	Fiber gms	Fat gms	Chol. mgs
BISCUIT, plain or buttermilk	1 biscuit	233	4	31	673	1	10.6	2

Food Name	Serv. Size	Total Cal.	Prot. gms	Carbs gms	Sod. mgs	Fiber gms	Fat gms	Chol. mgs
CHICKEN								
breast, mild, w/o bone	3.7 oz	270	23	9	660	2	15.9	60
breast, spicy, w/o bone	3.7 oz	270	23	9	590	2	15.9	60
leg, mild, w/o bone	1.7 oz	120	10	4	240	0	7.3	40
leg, spicy, w/o bone	1.7 oz	120	10	4	240	0	7.3	40
nuggets, fried	4.2 oz	410	17	18	660	3	31.9	55
thigh, mild, w/o bone	3.1 oz	300	15	9	620	1	22.7	70
thigh, spicy, w/o bone	3.1 oz	300	15	9	450	1	22.7	70
wing, mild, w/o bone	1.6 oz	160	9	7	290	0	10.7	40
wing, spicy, w/o bone	1.6 oz	160	9	7	290	0	10.7	40
DESSERT								
apple pie	3.1 oz	290	3	37	820	2	15.8	10
SHRIMP	2.8 oz	250	16	13	650	3	16.4	110
SIDE DISH								
Cajun rice	3.9 oz	150	10	17	1260	3	5.4	25
coleslaw	4 oz	149	1	14	271	3	11.2	3
corn on the cob	5.2 oz	90	4	21	20	9	2.9	0
French fries	3 oz	240	4	31	610	3	12.2	10
mashed potato, w/gravy	3.8 oz	100	5	11	460	3	6.0	5
onion rings	3.1 oz	310	5	31	210	2	19.3	25
red beans and rice	5.9 oz	270	8	30	680	7	16.9	10
QUINCY'S								
CATFISH, fillet, 2 pieces	6.9-oz serving	309	26	19	101	0	12.0	0
CHEESEBURGER, 1/4 lb precooked	1 serving	451	28	32	432	0	23.0	0
CHICKEN								
breast, grilled	5-oz serving	145	35	0	140	0	0.4	72
strips, 4 pieces	4.5 oz	318	39	4	0	0	15.0	0
CHILI, w/beans	9.2-oz serving	346	20	32	1380	0	16.0	0
CORNBREAD	1.9-oz serving	178	4	28	263	0	6.0	0
HAMBURGER, 1/4 lb precooked	1 serving	403	25	32	284	0	19.0	0
MUSHROOM SAUCE	3-oz serving	27	1	5	366	0	1.0	0
SHRIMP, 7 pieces	3.9-oz serving	248	22	11	205	0	12.0	0
SIDE DISH								
baked potato, w/o butter	8.8-oz serving	181	5	41	8	0	1.0	0
coleslaw	2.1-oz serving	60	1	4	75	0	5.0	0
green beans	4.3-oz serving	40	2	7	500	0	1.0	0
peppers and onions	4-oz serving	80	1	8	11	0	5.0	0
steak fries	5.5-oz serving	426	7	56	90	0	21.0	0
SOUP								
broccoli, cream of	9.2-oz serving	193	3	13	1045	0	14.0	0
clam chowder	9.2-oz serving	198	6	15	1185	0	14.0	0
vegetable beef soup	8.6-oz serving	78	5	10	1045	0	2.0	0
STEAK								
chopped, luncheon	4-oz serving	350	30	0	72	0	25.0	0
country style, w/mushroom sauce	6-oz serving	288	18	17	315	0	19.0	0
fillet	5.6-oz serving	331	51	0	159	0	12.0	0
ribeye	7.3-oz serving	665	31	0	205	0	60.0	0
sirloin club	4.8-oz serving	283	44	0	160	0	10.0	0
sirloin tips	4-oz serving	236	37	0	113	0	9.0	0
sirloin	5.9-oz serving	649	38	0	206	0	54.0	0
sirloin, large	7.7-oz serving	852	50	0	241	0	70.0	0
sirloin, petite	4-oz serving	446	26	0	118	0	37.0	0
T-bone	7.8-oz serving	1045	43	0	222	0	95.0	0
RALLY'S								
CHEESEBURGER								
'Rallyburger w/Cheese'	1 burger	486	24	33	1185	0	29.4	79
'Bacon Cheeseburger'	1 burger	622	33	35	1629	0	40.3	99

Food Name	Serv. Size	Total Cal.	Prot. gms	Carbs gms	Sod. mgs	Fiber gms	Fat gms	Chol. mgs
'Double Cheeseburger'	1 burger	733	42	34	1473	0	49.1	92
CHEESEBURGER MEAL								
'Large Combo' w/soft drink	1 meal	1018	29	129	1645	0	45.0	89
'Small Combo' w/soft drink	1 meal	764	33	85	1416	0	37.2	84
CHICKEN SANDWICH	1 sandwich	531	18	40	364	0	30.8	18
CHILI	8 oz	340	22	21	1199	0	19.0	67
FRENCH FRIES								
large	1 serving	317	5	39	439	0	15.6	10
regular	1 serving	158	3	20	219	0	7.8	5
HAMBURGER 'Rallyburger'	1 burger	436	21	33	955	0	24.9	67
HAMBURGER MEAL								
'Large Combo' w/soft drink	1 meal	968	26	129	1415	0	40.5	76
'Small Combo' w/soft drink	1 meal	714	24	84	1186	0	32.7	71
SAUSAGE								
'Smokin' Sausage'	1 serving	724	28	31	1998	0	55.0	40
'Smokin' Sausage' w/chili	1 serving	830	35	35	2163	0	62.0	67
TACO, soft	1 taco	223	12	17	377	0	9.9	36
RAX								
BEEF, roast beef	2.8 oz	140	14	1	524	0	9.0	36
BREADSTICK, sesame, salad bar item	1 oz	150	3	13	405	0	10.0	0
CHEESE, American, processed, slices	0.5 oz	60	3	1	180	0	5.0	15
CONDIMENTS. See also SALAD DRESSING.								
Alfredo sauce, pasta bar item	3.5 oz	80	2	12	70	0	3.0	10
banana pepper, Mexican bar item	1 tbsp	2	1	1	20	0	1.0	0
barbecue meat topping	3.25 oz	140	13	13	898	0	4.0	24
celery, salad bar item	1 tbsp	1	1	1	10	0	1.0	0
cheese sauce, regular, Mexican bar item	3.5 oz	420	10	58	365	0	17.0	11
chili topping	3 oz	80	8	8	221	0	2.0	18
chow mein noodles, salad bar item	1 oz	140	4	17	242	0	6.0	1
coconut, salad bar item	1 oz	160	1	15	1	0	11.0	0
croutons, salad bar item	0.5 oz	40	2	8	155	0	1.0	1
green onion, Mexican bar item	1/4 cup	10	1	2	1	0	1.0	0
margarine, liquid	1 tbsp	100	1	1	100	0	11.0	0
mushroom sauce	1 oz	16	1	1	113	0	1.0	0
nacho cheese sauce, Mexican bar item	3.5 oz	470	10	57	190	0	22.0	11
onion, diced	0.5 oz	10	1	1	1	0	1.0	0
pickle	1 spear	8	1	2	928	0	1.0	0
sour topping	3.5 oz	130	3	5	79	0	11.0	1
spaghetti sauce, pasta bar item	3.5 oz	80	1	19	635	0	1.0	1
spaghetti sauce, w/meat, pasta bar item	3.5 oz	150	7	12	419	0	8.0	1
spicy meat sauce, Mexican bar item	3.5 oz	80	5	6	751	0	4.0	12
sunflower seeds and raisins, salad bar item	1 oz	130	5	6	5	0	10.0	0
taco sauce, Mexican bar item	3.5 oz	30	1	6	806	0	1.0	0
taco shell, Mexican bar item	1 shell	40	1	6	53	0	2.0	0
turkey bits, salad bar item	2 oz	70	10	1	686	0	3.0	49
DESSERT								
butterscotch pudding, salad bar item	3.5 oz	141	2	20	151	0	6.0	2
chocolate chip cookie	1 cookie	130	1	17	65	0	6.0	1
chocolate pudding, salad bar item	3.5 oz	141	2	20	121	0	6.0	2
lime gelatin, salad bar item	1/2 cup	90	2	20	90	0	1.0	0
strawberry gelatin, salad bar item	1/2 cup	90	2	20	90	0	1.0	0
vanilla pudding, salad bar item	3.5 oz	141	2	20	121	0	6.0	2
DESSERT TOPPING, whipped	1 dollop	50	1	4	6	0	4.0	2
PASTA								
rainbow rotini, pasta bar item	3.5 oz	180	6	30	9	0	4.0	2
shells, pasta bar item	3.5 oz	170	7	27	2	0	4.0	0
spaghetti, pasta bar item	3.5 oz	140	3	23	1	0	4.0	0
vegetable, pasta bar item	3.5 oz	100	4	12	11	0	4.0	0

Food Name	Serv. Size	Total Cal.	Prot. gms	Carbs gms	Sod. mgs	Fiber gms	Fat gms	Chol. mgs
SALAD								
chef, w/o dressing	12.5-oz serving	230	22	4	1048	0	14.0	322
garden, gourmet, 'Lighterside'	1 serving	134	7	13	350	0	6.0	2
garden, w/o dressing	10.5-oz serving	160	12	4	362	0	11.0	273
SALAD DRESSING								
blue cheese	1 tbsp	50	1	1	110	0	5.0	8
blue cheese, 'Lite'	1 tbsp	35	1	2	240	0	3.0	3
French	1 tbsp	60	1	6	140	0	4.0	0
Italian	1 tbsp	50	1	3	159	0	4.0	0
Italian, 'Lite'	1 tbsp	30	1	1	152	0	3.0	0
oil	1 tbsp	130	1	1	1	0	14.0	0
poppyseed	1 tbsp	60	1	5	107	0	4.0	6
ranch	1 tbsp	45	1	1	103	0	5.0	5
Thousand Island	1 tbsp	70	1	6	110	0	6.0	8
Thousand Island, 'Lite'	1 tbsp	40	1	3	143	0	3.0	5
vinegar	1 tbsp	2	1	1	5	0	1.0	0
SANDWICH								
barbecue	5.7-oz serving	420	21	53	1343	0	14.0	24
beef, bacon, and chicken, 'BBC'	8-oz serving	720	30	40	1873	0	49.0	137
fish	7-oz serving	460	14	58	935	0	17.0	1
ham and Swiss	7.9-oz serving	430	23	42	1737	0	23.0	37
Philly beef and cheese	8.25-oz serving	480	25	44	1346	0	22.0	49
roast beef, large	8-oz serving	570	22	41	1169	0	35.0	36
roast beef, regular	5.25-oz serving	320	20	33	969	0	11.0	36
roast beef, 'Uncle Al' small	3.1-oz serving	260	12	21	562	0	14.0	19
turkey bacon club	9-oz serving	670	29	41	1878	0	43.0	87
SIDE DISH								
baked potato, barbecue, w/2 oz cheese	1 serving	730	24	104	1071	0	24.0	18
baked potato, cheese and bacon	3-oz serving	780	22	110	910	0	28.0	23
baked potato, cheese and broccoli	3-oz serving	760	19	112	489	0	26.0	11
baked potato, chili, w/2 oz cheese	1 serving	700	22	101	599	0	23.0	25
baked potato, plain	8.8-oz serving	270	8	60	70	0	1.0	0
baked potato, w/margarine	9.3-oz serving	370	8	60	170	0	11.0	0
baked potato, w/sour cream topping	1 serving	400	11	65	149	0	11.0	0
broccoli, salad bar item	1/2 cup	16	2	2	7	0	1.0	0
coleslaw, salad bar item	3.5 oz	70	1	8	187	0	4.0	1
French fries, large, salted	4.5-oz serving	390	3	50	104	0	20.0	16
French fries, large, unsalted	4.5-oz serving	390	3	50	66	0	20.0	16
French fries, regular, salted	3-oz serving	260	2	33	69	0	13.0	10
French fries, regular, unsalted	3-oz serving	260	2	33	44	0	13.0	10
grapefruit sections, salad bar item	1 cup	80	2	18	10	0	1.0	0
grapes, salad bar item	1 cup	100	1	25	5	0	1.0	0
kale, salad bar item	1 oz	16	2	2	21	0	1.0	0
kidney beans, salad bar item	1 cup	220	14	40	8	0	1.0	0
macaroni salad, salad bar item	3.5 oz	160	2	21	216	0	7.0	1
pasta salad, salad bar item	3.5 oz	80	2	16	322	0	1.0	1
potato salad, salad bar item	1 cup	260	7	41	0	0	7.0	7
refried beans, Mexican bar item	3 oz	120	6	16	375	0	4.0	2
Spanish rice, Mexican bar item	3.5 oz	90	3	20	442	0	1.0	0
three-bean salad	1/2 cup	100	3	23	450	0	1.0	0
SOUP								
broccoli, cream of	3.5 oz	50	1	6	219	0	2.0	1
chicken soup w/noodles, pasta bar item	3.5 oz	40	2	8	1040	0	1.0	10
RED LOBSTER								
CALAMARI								
breaded, fried, dinner portion	10 oz	720	26	60	2300	0	42.0	280
breaded, fried, lunch portion	5 oz	360	13	30	1150	0	21.0	140

Food Name	Serv. Size	Total Cal.	Prot. gms	Carbs gms	Sod. mgs	Fiber gms	Fat gms	Chol. mgs
CATFISH								
dinner portion	10 oz	340	40	0	100	0	20.0	170
lunch portion	5 oz	170	20	0	50	0	10.0	85
CHICKEN, breast	4-oz serving	120	24	0	60	0	3.0	65
CLAMS								
cherrystone, dinner portion	10 oz	260	36	22	1080	0	4.0	160
cherrystone, lunch portion	5 oz	130	18	11	540	0	2.0	80
COD								
Atlantic, fillet, dinner portion	10 oz	200	46	0	400	0	2.0	140
Atlantic, fillet, lunch portion	5 oz	100	23	0	200	0	1.0	70
CRAB								
king, legs, 1 lb	1 serving	170	32	6	900	0	2.0	100
snow, legs, 1 lb	1 serving	150	33	1	1630	0	2.0	130
FLOUNDER								
dinner portion	10 oz	200	42	2	190	0	2.0	140
lunch portion	5 oz	100	21	1	95	0	1.0	70
GROUPER								
dinner portion	10 oz	220	52	0	140	0	2.0	130
lunch portion	5 oz	110	26	0	70	0	1.0	65
HADDOCK								
dinner portion	10 oz	220	48	4	360	0	2.0	170
lunch portion	5 oz	110	24	2	180	0	1.0	85
HALIBUT								
dinner portion	10 oz	220	50	2	210	0	2.0	120
lunch portion	5 oz	110	25	1	105	0	1.0	60
HAMBURGER, 1/3 lb before cooked	1 serving	320	27	0	70	0	23.0	105
LANGOSTINO								
dinner portion	10 oz	240	52	4	820	0	2.0	420
lunch portion	5 oz	120	26	2	410	0	1.0	210
LOBSTER								
Maine, cooked, 1 1/4 lb	1 serving	240	36	5	550	0	8.0	310
rock, tail, cooked	1 serving	230	49	2	1090	0	3.0	200
MACKEREL								
dinner portion	10 oz	380	2	40	500	0	24.0	200
raw weight	5 oz	190	1	20	250	0	12.0	100
MONKFISH								
dinner portion	10 oz	220	0	48	190	0	2.0	160
lunch portion	5 oz	110	0	24	95	0	1.0	80
MUSSELS	3-oz serving	70	9	3	150	0	2.0	50
OCEAN PERCH								
Atlantic, dinner portion	10 oz	260	48	2	380	0	8.0	150
Atlantic, lunch portion	5 oz	130	24	1	190	0	4.0	75
OYSTERS, on half shell	6 oysters	110	8	11	90	0	4.0	60
POLLACK								
dinner portion	10 oz	240	56	2	180	0	2.0	180
lunch portion	5 oz	120	28	1	90	0	1.0	90
RED ROCKFISH								
dinner portion	10 oz	180	42	0	190	0	2.0	170
lunch portion	5 oz	90	21	0	95	0	1.0	85
RED SNAPPER								
dinner portion	10 oz	220	50	0	280	0	2.0	140
lunch portion	5 oz	110	25	0	140	0	1.0	70
SALMON								
Norwegian, dinner portion	10 oz	460	54	6	120	0	24.0	160
Norwegian, lunch portion	5 oz	230	27	3	60	0	12.0	80
sockeye, dinner portion	10 oz	320	56	6	120	0	8.0	100
sockeye, lunch portion	5 oz	160	28	3	60	0	4.0	50

Food Name	Serv. Size	Total Cal.	Prot. gms	Carbs gms	Sod. mgs	Fiber gms	Fat gms	Chol. mgs
SCALLOPS								
calico, dinner portion	10 oz	360	64	16	320	0	4.0	230
calico, lunch portion	5 oz	180	32	8	260	0	2.0	115
deep sea, dinner portion	10 oz	260	52	4	520	0	4.0	100
deep sea, lunch portion	5 oz	130	26	2	260	0	2.0	50
SHARK								
blacktip, dinner portion	10 oz	300	70	0	180	0	2.0	120
blacktip, lunch portion	5 oz	150	35	0	90	0	1.0	60
mako, dinner portion	10 oz	280	68	0	120	0	2.0	200
mako, lunch portion	5 oz	140	34	0	60	0	1.0	100
SHRIMP, 8-12 pieces	1 serving	120	25	0	110	0	2.0	230
SOLE								
w/lemon, dinner portion	10 oz	240	54	2	180	0	2.0	130
w/lemon, lunch portion	5 oz	120	27	1	90	0	1.0	65
STEAK, strip	7 oz	690	29	0	70	0	64.0	140
SWORDFISH								
dinner portion	10 oz	200	34	0	280	0	8.0	200
lunch portion	5 oz	100	17	0	140	0	4.0	100
TILEFISH								
dinner portion	10 oz	200	40	0	120	0	4.0	160
lunch portion	5 oz	100	20	0	60	0	2.0	80
TROUT								
rainbow, dinner portion	10 oz	340	46	0	180	0	18.0	180
rainbow, lunch portion	5 oz	170	23	0	90	0	9.0	90
TUNA								
yellowfin, dinner portion	10 oz	360	64	0	140	0	12.0	140
yellowfin, lunch portion	5 oz	180	32	0	70	0	6.0	70
ROUND TABLE								
PIZZA								
'Alfredo Contempo'								
pan crust	1 slice	220	12	27	240	1	7.4	25
thin crust	1 slice	170	9	17	210	1	6.5	25
'Bacon Super Deli'								
pan crust	1 slice	260	12	26	380	0	13.5	25
thin crust	1 slice	200	9	16	360	0	12.6	25
Cheese								
pan	1 slice	210	10	26	250	1	7.2	20
thin crust	1 slice	170	8	17	330	1	5.6	25
Chicken and garlic								
pan, gourmet	1 slice	230	11	27	310	1	8.1	25
thin crust, gourmet	1 slice	170	9	17	280	0	7.2	25
'Classic Pesto'								
pan	1 slice	230	9	27	240	1	8.8	15
thin crust	1 slice	170	7	18	210	1	7.9	15
'Garden Delight'								
pan crust	1 slice	200	9	27	250	1	6.2	15
thin crust	1 slice	150	7	18	250	1	5.6	15
'Garden Pesto'								
pan crust	1 slice	230	9	28	230	1	8.6	15
thin crust	1 slice	170	7	18	200	1	7.7	15
'Gourmet Veggie'								
pan crust	1 slice	220	9	28	230	1	7.4	20
thin crust	1 slice	160	7	18	200	1	6.5	15
Italian Garlic Supreme'								
pan crust	1 slice	250	10	27	240	1	10.5	25
thin crust	1 slice	200	8	17	220	0	10.4	25
'King Arthur's Supreme'								
pan crust	1 slice	240	10	27	320	1	9.8	25

Food Name	Serv. Size	Total Cal.	Prot. gms	Carbs gms	Sod. mgs	Fiber gms	Fat gms	Chol. mgs
thin crust	1 slice	200	9	18	340	1	10.1	25
Pepperoni								
pan crust	1 slice	220	9	26	240	1	8.1	20
thin crust	1 slice	170	8	17	240	0	8.0	20
'Salute Chicken Cashew'								
pan crust	1 slice	200	9	31	260	1	4.5	15
thin crust	1 slice	150	7	21	240	1	4.1	15
'Salute Chicken and Garlic'								
pan crust	1 slice	200	9	28	270	1	5.8	20
thin crust	1 slice	150	8	18	250	1	5.4	20
'Salute Veggie'								
pan crust	1 slice	190	8	28	190	1	5.1	10
thin crust	1 slice	140	6	19	170	1	4.7	10
'Santa Fe Chicken'								
pan crust	1 slice	240	11	27	360	1	9.2	30
thin crust	1 slice	180	9	17	310	1	7.8	25
ROY ROGERS								
BISCUIT	1 serving	231	4	26	575	0	12.0	5
BREAKFAST								
crescent, regular	1 serving	408	13	28	820	0	27.0	207
crescent, w/bacon	1 serving	446	15	28	982	0	30.0	212
crescent, w/ham	1 serving	456	20	29	1243	0	29.0	227
crescent, w/sausage	1 serving	564	19	28	1145	0	42.0	248
apple swirl Danish	1 serving	328	5	62	279	0	7.0	0
cheese swirl Danish	1 serving	383	8	54	369	0	15.0	0
cinnamon rod pastry,	1 serving	376	5	55	339	0	15.0	0
egg platter, w/bacon and biscuit	1 serving	607	21	44	1236	0	39.0	424
egg platter, w/biscuit, regular	1 serving	557	18	44	1020	0	34.0	417
egg platter, w/ham and biscuit,	1 serving	605	25	44	1442	0	36.0	437
egg platter, w/sausage and biscuit	1 serving	713	25	44	1345	0	49.0	458
pancake platter, regular, w/syrup and butter, regular	1 serving	386	5	63	547	0	13.0	51
pancake platter, w/bacon, w/syrup and butter	1 serving	436	8	63	763	0	17.0	58
pancake platter, w/ham, w/syrup and butter	1 serving	434	11	64	969	0	15.0	71
pancake platter, w/sausage, w/syrup and butter	1 serving	542	11	63	872	0	28.0	92
CHEESEBURGER								
'Express'	1 serving	613	30	42	1122	0	37.0	82
'Express' w/bacon	1 serving	641	33	36	1317	0	41.0	89
regular	1 serving	525	29	37	830	0	29.0	76
regular, w/bacon	1 sandwich	520	24	32	1620	na	33.0	72
small	1 serving	275	15	24	558	0	13.0	36
CHICKEN								
breast, fried	1 serving	412	33	17	609	0	24.0	118
breast and wing, fried	1 serving	604	44	25	894	0	37.0	165
breast and wing, w/o skin, 'Roy's Roaster'	1 serving	190	32	2	0	0	6.0	0
dark meat, 1/4 'Roy's Roaster'	1 serving	490	43	2	1120	0	34.0	225
dark meat, w/o skin, 1/4 'Roy's Roaster'	1 serving	190	24	1	400	0	10.0	110
leg, fried	1 serving	140	12	6	190	0	8.0	40
leg and thigh, fried	1 serving	436	30	17	596	0	28.0	125
nuggets, fried, 9 pieces	9 pieces	435	18	30	915	na	27.0	23
nuggets, fried, 6 pieces	6 pieces	290	12	20	610	na	18.0	15
thigh, fried	1 serving	296	18	12	406	0	20.0	85
white meat, 1/4 'Roy's Roaster'	1 serving	500	56	3	1450	0	29.0	240
white meat, w/o skin, '1/4 Roy's Roaster'	1 serving	190	32	2	700	0	6.0	100
wing, fried	1 serving	192	11	9	285	0	13.0	47
CONDIMENTS. See also Salad Dressing.								
Chinese noodles, salad bar item	1/4 cup	55	2	7	113	0	3.0	1
croutons, salad bar item	2 tbsp	14	1	3	50	0	0.0	0
granola, salad bar item	1/4 cup	65	2	9	8	0	3.0	0

Food Name	Serv. Size	Total Cal.	Prot. gms	Carbs gms	Sod. mgs	Fiber gms	Fat gms	Chol. mgs
grapes, salad bar item	5 grapes	20	0	5	1	0	0.0	0
onion, chopped, salad bar item	2 tbsp	7	0	2	0	0	0.0	0
DESSERT								
caramel sundae	1 serving	293	7	52	193	0	9.0	23
chocolate sundae	1 serving	358	8	61	290	0	10.0	37
gelatin parfait, salad bar item	1/4 cup	50	1	10	23	0	2.0	0
hot fudge sundae	1 serving	337	7	53	186	0	13.0	23
strawberry shortcake	1 serving	440	8	39	420	na	19.0	15
strawberry sundae	1 serving	216	6	33	99	0	7.0	23
vanilla sundae	1 serving	306	8	45	282	0	11.0	40
HAMBURGER								
'Express'	1 serving	561	27	42	899	0	32.0	70
regular	1 serving	472	26	37	607	0	25.0	64
'Roy Rogers Bar'	1 serving	573	36	38	1252	0	31.0	96
small	1 serving	222	12	23	336	0	9.0	26
ROLL, crescent	1 serving	287	5	27	547	0	18.0	5
SALAD, grilled chicken	1 salad	120	18	2	520	0	4.0	60
SALAD DRESSING								
Thousand Island	2 tbsp	160	0	4	150	0	16.0	0
bacon and tomato	2 tbsp	136	0	6	150	0	12.0	0
blue cheese	2 tbsp	150	2	2	153	0	16.0	0
Italian, low-calorie	2 tbsp	70	0	2	100	0	6.0	0
ranch	2 tbsp	155	0	4	100	0	14.0	0
SANDWICH								
chicken, 'Gold Rush'	1 sandwich	558	22	51	1326	na	30.0	35
fish	1 sandwich	514	18	58	857	0	24.0	62
roast beef	1 sandwich	329	31	29	875	na	10.0	62
roast beef, large	1 sandwich	373	35	31	840	0	12.0	82
roast beef, w/cheese	1 sandwich	403	29	37	954	0	15.0	70
roast beef, w/cheese, large	1 sandwich	427	38	31	1062	0	17.0	94
SIDE DISH								
baked potato, plain, 'Hot Topped'	1 serving	211	6	48	65	0	0.0	0
broccoli, salad bar item	1/4 cup	6	1	1	6	0	0.0	0
coleslaw	1 serving	110	1	11	261	0	7.0	5
French fries, large	5.5 oz serving	440	6	54	225	0	22.0	19
French fries, regular	4 oz serving	320	4	39	164	0	16.0	13
French fries, small	3 oz serving	238	3	29	122	0	12.0	10
fruit cocktail, salad bar item	1/4 cup	46	0	12	1	0	0.0	0
Greek noodles, salad bar item	1/4 cup	159	3	19	328	0	9.0	0
lettuce, Romaine, salad bar item	1 cup	9	1	1	5	0	0.0	0
macaroni salad, salad bar item	1/4 cup	93	2	10	301	0	5.0	0
potato salad, salad bar item	1/4 cup	54	1	5	348	0	3.0	0

SCHLOTZSKY'S DELI

Food Name	Serv. Size	Total Cal.	Prot. gms	Carbs gms	Sod. mgs	Fiber gms	Fat gms	Chol. mgs
BEVERAGE								
'Coca-Cola' regular	20 fl oz	248	na	68	15	na	0.0	na
'Diet Coke' regular	20 fl oz	0	na	0	25	na	0.0	na
iced tea, regular	20 fl oz	na	na	na	na	na	na	na
lemonade, 'All Natural' regular	20 fl oz	183	na	43	14	0	0.0	0
'Mr. Pibb' regular	20 fl oz	243	na	65	35	na	0.0	na
orange, 'Minute Maid' regular	20 fl oz	265	na	73	0	na	0.0	na
root beer, 'Barq's' regular	20 fl oz	278	na	75	60	na	0.0	na
'Sprite' regular	20 fl oz	243	na	65	55	na	na	na
CHILI, 'Timberline'	8 oz cup	210	14	24	814	7	7.0	32
CONDIMENTS. See also Salad Dressing.								
croutons, garlic cheese, salad bar item	1 crouton	46	1	5	142	0	2.0	0
chow mein noodles	1 serving	74	2	9	111	1	4.0	0
DESSERT								
fudge brownie cake	1 serving	410	5	46	135	3	25.0	35

Food Name	Serv. Size	Total Cal.	Prot. gms	Carbs gms	Sod. mgs	Fiber gms	Fat gms	Chol. mgs
cookies and creme cheesecake	1 serving	330	6	36	320	1	18.0	35
chocolate chip cookie	1 cookie	160	2	23	150	0	7.0	10
chocolate chunk cookie	1 cookie	160	2	23	150	1	7.0	10
chocolate pecan chunk cookie	1 cookie	170	2	23	140	1	8.0	10
fudge chocolate chunk cookie	1 cookie	170	2	22	170	1	8.0	10
New York style cheesecake	1 serving	310	7	31	230	0	18.0	60
oatmeal raisin cookie	1 cookie	150	2	1	na	na	1.0	200
peanut butter cookie	1 cookie	170	2	21	190	1	8.0	10
peanut butter chocolate cookie	1 cookie	170	2	21	160	1	8.0	10
strawberry swirl cheesecake	1 serving	300	6	30	230	0	17.0	55
sugar cookie	1 cookie	160	2	23	180	0	6.0	15
white chocolate macadamia cookie	1 cookie	170	2	22	140	0	8.0	10
PIZZA								
bacon, tomato, and mushroom, sourdough crust, 8-inch	1 pizza	635	27	78	1891	4	24.0	38
barbecue chicken, sourdough crust, 8-inch	1 pizza	653	38	78	2103	3	20.0	74
chicken and pesto, sourdough crust, 8-inch	1 pizza	649	40	78	2187	4	19.0	74
double cheese and pepperoni, sourdough crust, 8-inch	1 pizza	744	32	77	2206	4	34.0	62
double cheese, sourdough crust, 8-inch	1 pizza	603	26	77	1772	4	21.0	34
fresh tomato and pesto, sourdough crust, 8-inch	1 pizza	539	23	76	1670	4	16.0	27
Mediterranean, sourdough crust, 8-inch	1 pizza	564	24	84	1787	3	19.0	36
New Orleans, sourdough crust, 8-inch	1 pizza	666	40	79	2493	4	20.0	74
original combination, sourdough crust, 8-inch	1 pizza	648	26	79	1994	5	25.0	41
smoked turkey and jalapeño, sourdough crust, 8-inch	1 pizza	647	38	81	2591	4	19.0	62
Southwestern, sourdough crust, 8-inch	1 pizza	635	38	76	2015	4	19.0	71
Thai chicken, sourdough crust, 8-inch	1 pizza	681	40	88	2303	5	19.0	72
vegetarian special, sourdough crust, 8-inch	1 pizza	551	24	76	1757	4	17.0	27
SALAD								
Caesar, w/o dressing, croutons, chow mein noodles	1 salad	152	11	11	505	4	8.0	15
chef's, ham and turkey, dressing, croutons, chow mein noodles	1 salad	248	23	15	1442	3	11.0	51
chef's, smoked turkey, w/o dressing, croutons, chow mein noodles	1 salad	243	24	15	1275	3	10.0	53
chicken Caesar, w/o dressing, croutons, chow mein noodles	1 salad	254	28	13	935	4	10.0	63
chicken, Chinese, w/o dressing, croutons, chow mein noodles	1 salad	150	20	11	448	3	3.0	47
garden, small, w/o dressing, croutons, chow mein noodles	1 salad	25	1	3	55	1	1.0	0
garden, w/o dressing, croutons, chow mein noodles	1 salad	61	3	8	119	3	1.0	0
Greek, w/o dressing, croutons, chow mein noodles	1 salad	220	13	25	563	4	12.0	27
SALAD DRESSING								
Caesar, 'Olde World'	1 pkt	260	2	1	250	0	27.0	25
Greek balsamic vinaigrette	1 pkt	170	0	2	330	0	17.0	0
Italian, light	1 pkt	90	0	3	690	0	8.0	0
ranch, spicy	1 pkt	230	1	2	310	0	25.0	15
ranch, spicy, light	1 pkt	140	1	9	350	0	11.0	15
ranch, traditional	1 pkt	270	0	1	370	0	29.0	5
sesame ginger vinaigrette	1 pkt	170	1	8	370	0	15.0	0
Thousand Island	1 pkt	220	0	6	360	0	21.0	30
SANDWICH								
Bacon, lettuce and tomato								
large, on sourdough bun	1 sandwich	1141	41	140	3066	6	46.0	80
regular, on sourdough bun	1 sandwich	578	21	70	1548	3	24.0	41
small, on sourdough bun	1 sandwich	379	13	47	1010	2	15.0	26
Cheese								
large, on sourdough bun	1 sandwich	1857	87	159	4365	8	98.0	180

Food Name	Serv. Size	Total Cal.	Prot. gms	Carbs gms	Sod. mgs	Fiber gms	Fat gms	Chol. mgs
regular, on sourdough bun	1 sandwich	854	38	79	2107	4	44.0	72
small, on sourdough bun	1 sandwich	596	27	53	1432	3	31.0	54
Chicken								
breast, large, on sourdough bun	1 sandwich	1008	72	158	4522	6	15.0	155
breast, regular, on sourdough bun	1 sandwich	535	37	81	2365	3	10.0	85
breast, small, on sourdough bun	1 sandwich	363	25	55	1596	2	7.0	58
Chicken club								
large, on sourdough bun	1 sandwich	1351	88	149	4678	8	45.0	209
medium on sourdough bun	1 sandwich	686	44	75	2403	4	23.0	106
small, on sourdough bun	1 sandwich	458	29	50	1591	3	15.0	71
Corned beef								
large, on sourdough bun	1 sandwich	1134	81	139	4751	6	25.0	167
regular, on dark rye bun	1 sandwich	587	40	70	2488	4	15.0	84
small, on dark rye bun	1 sandwich	388	27	47	1625	3	10.0	56
'Deluxe Original'								
large, on sourdough bun	1 sandwich	2638	143	173	10762	8	152.0	451
regular, on sourdough bun	1 sandwich	1296	69	87	5405	4	75.0	217
small, on sourdough bun	1 sandwich	1044	55	60	4275	3	65.0	192
Dijon chicken								
large, on sourdough bun	1 sandwich	972	74	150	3981	8	10.0	137
regular, on wheat bun	1 sandwich	497	38	74	2091	6	6.0	68
small, on wheat bun	1 sandwich	330	25	50	1373	4	4.0	46
Ham and cheese								
original, large, on sourdough bun	1 sandwich	1625	93	163	6807	8	67.0	183
original, regular, on sourdough bun	1 sandwich	789	44	82	3428	4	32.0	83
original, small, on sourdough bun	1 sandwich	537	30	55	2298	3	22.0	58
'Original'								
large, on sourdough bun	1 sandwich	1917	90	161	6155	8	102.0	246
regular, on sourdough bun	1 sandwich	941	42	81	3166	4	50.0	122
small, on sourdough bun	1 sandwich	713	32	55	2327	3	41.0	100
Pastrami and Swiss								
large, on sourdough bun	1 sandwich	1681	114	148	7211	6	69.0	304
regular, on dark rye bun	1 sandwich	861	57	74	3718	4	37.0	152
small, on dark rye bun	1 sandwich	570	38	49	2445	3	24.0	101
Pesto chicken								
large, on sourdough bun	1 sandwich	999	73	145	3799	7	15.0	141
regular, on sourdough bun	1 sandwich	512	37	73	1927	4	9.0	71
small, on sourdough bun	1 sandwich	346	25	49	1297	2	6.0	48
Philly								
large, on sourdough bun	1 sandwich	1709	121	157	4477	7	66.0	244
regular, on sourdough bun	1 sandwich	824	57	78	2189	4	32.0	113
small, on sourdough bun	1 sandwich	559	39	52	1467	2	22.0	78
Reuben								
corned beef, large, on sourdough bun	1 sandwich	1594	102	147	6944	7	62.0	262
corned beef, regular, on dark rye bun	1 sandwich	833	51	74	3514	4	35.0	132
corned beef, small, on dark rye bun	1 sandwich	528	32	50	2269	3	21.0	80
pastrami, large, on sourdough bun	1 sandwich	1777	113	152	7765	7	77.0	308
pastrami, regular, on dark rye bun	1 sandwich	924	56	77	3924	4	43.0	155
pastrami, small, on dark rye bun	1 sandwich	619	38	51	2679	3	29.0	103
turkey, large, on sourdough bun	1 sandwich	1656	101	159	7704	7	69.0	247
turkey, regular, on dark rye bun	1 sandwich	863	50	80	3893	4	39.0	124
turkey, small, on dark rye bun	1 sandwich	579	33	54	2659	3	26.0	83
Roast beef								
large, on sourdough bun	1 sandwich	1185	87	145	3362	6	28.0	164
regular, on sourdough bun	1 sandwich	617	43	73	1733	3	17.0	83
small, on sourdough bun	1 sandwich	413	29	49	1162	2	11.0	55
Roast beef and cheese								
large, on sourdough bun	1 sandwich	1749	120	163	4987	8	70.0	255

Food Name	Serv. Size	Total Cal.	Prot. gms	Carbs gms	Sod. mgs	Fiber gms	Fat gms	Chol. mgs
regular, on sourdough bun	1 sandwich	848	57	82	2451	4	34.0	119
small, on sourdough bun	1 sandwich	580	39	55	1666	3	24.0	83
Santa Fe chicken								
large, on sourdough bun	1 sandwich	1182	82	155	4232	9	29.0	185
regular, on jalapeño cheese bun	1 sandwich	642	43	77	2302	4	19.0	106
small, on jalapeño cheese bun	1 sandwich	431	29	52	1547	3	13.0	72
'Texas Schlotzsky's'								
large, on sourdough bun	1 sandwich	1544	84	155	6446	6	65.0	184
regular, on jalapeño cheese bun	1 sandwich	816	43	76	3357	3	37.0	98
small, on jalapeño cheese bun	1 sandwich	561	30	51	2263	2	26.0	69
Tuna								
albacore, large, on sourdough bun	1 sandwich	1000	59	147	3099	6	26.0	122
albacore, regular, on wheat bun	1 sandwich	533	31	74	1655	4	16.0	69
albacore, small, on wheat bun	1 sandwich	361	21	50	1122	3	11.0	47
Tuna melt								
albacore, large, on sourdough bun	1 sandwich	1631	93	158	4474	7	77.0	214
albacore, regular, on wheat bun	1 sandwich	818	45	79	2293	5	40.0	106
albacore, small, on wheat bun	1 sandwich	562	31	53	1552	3	28.0	74
Turkey								
breast, smoked, large, on sourdough bun	1 sandwich	988	68	150	4229	6	13.0	118
breast, smoked, regular, on sourdough bun	1 sandwich	498	34	75	2123	3	7.0	60
breast, smoked, small, on sourdough bun	1 sandwich	335	23	50	1426	2	5.0	40
original, large, on sourdough bun	1 sandwich	2083	123	166	7535	8	104.0	324
original, regular, on sourdough bun	1 sandwich	1017	58	83	3744	4	51.0	154
original, small, on sourdough bun	1 sandwich	763	43	56	2789	3	41.0	125
Turkey bacon club								
large, on sourdough bun	1 sandwich	1790	108	161	6086	7	80.0	240
regular, on wheat bun	1 sandwich	874	52	79	3009	5	40.0	113
small, on wheat bun	1 sandwich	596	35	53	2012	3	27.0	78
Turkey guacamole								
large, on sourdough bun	1 sandwich	1317	73	166	5255	6	42.0	118
regular, on sourdough bun	1 sandwich	683	36	84	2680	3	24.0	60
small, on sourdough bun	1 sandwich	448	24	56	1764	2	15.0	40
Vegetable club								
large, on sourdough bun	1 sandwich	1112	39	151	2716	9	41.0	46
regular, on sourdough bun	1 sandwich	584	19	76	1435	5	24.0	24
small, on sourdough bun	1 sandwich	393	13	50	962	3	16.0	17
Vegetarian								
large, on sourdough bun	1 sandwich	966	34	150	2398	8	26.0	48
regular, on wheat bun	1 sandwich	519	18	75	1329	5	17.0	32
small, on wheat bun	1 sandwich	351	12	51	889	4	11.0	22
Western, large, on sourdough bun	1 sandwich	1261	35	150	2235	8	61.0	125
Western, regular, on sourdough bun	1 sandwich	651	18	75	1161	4	33.0	62
Western, small, on sourdough bun	1 sandwich	449	12	51	790	3	23.0	47
SIDE DISH								
coleslaw, country style	5 oz	225	1	16	288	1	16.0	5
coleslaw, shredded	5 oz	225	1	16	388	1	16.0	19
macaroni salad	5 oz	338	4	23	619	1	23.0	9
potato salad, 'Choice'	5 oz	253	2	18	525	1	18.0	9
potato salad, diced, w/egg	5 oz	216	3	18	600	1	13.0	38
potato salad, mustard/egg	5 oz	225	2	17	534	1	15.0	5
seven bean medley	8 oz cup	145	7	24	1260	8	2.0	0
SOUP								
Boston clam chowder	8 oz cup	233	5	24	1062	1	15.0	10
broccoli cheese	8 oz cup	252	7	23	1104	1	17.0	17
broccoli, cream of	8 oz cup	206	4	25	1152	1	13.0	15
cauliflower cheese	8 oz cup	252	3	24	993	1	19.0	11
chicken gumbo	8 oz cup	110	4	13	1114	2	5.0	20
chicken noodle, old-fashioned	8 oz cup	122	8	18	1104	1	2.0	39

Food Name	Serv. Size	Total Cal.	Prot. gms	Carbs gms	Sod. mgs	Fiber gms	Fat gms	Chol. mgs
chicken tortilla	8 oz cup	167	10	24	1026	3	3.0	22
chicken, w/wild rice	8 oz cup	378	10	24	1201	1	28.0	78
corn chowder	8 oz cup	284	2	38	1010	1	17.0	6
creamy turkey vegetable	8 oz cup	218	7	21	871	1	14.0	22
French onion	8 oz cup	78	3	9	1716	0	3.0	0
minestrone	8 oz cup	89	3	17	1048	3	1.0	0
potato, cream of, w/bacon	8 oz cup	226	2	31	1209	2	13.0	5
ravioli tomato	8 oz cup	111	6	21	1115	1	2.0	17
red beans and rice	8 oz cup	167	8	32	934	4	1.0	0
tomato Florentine	8 oz cup	100	3	19	1182	1	1.0	0
vegetable beef barley	8 oz cup	100	6	12	1160	2	3.0	11
vegetable cheese	8 oz cup	289	6	24	1338	2	19.0	28
vegetable, lumberjack	8 oz cup	133	3	19	1482	6	6.0	6
vegetable, vegetarian	8 oz cup	138	3	20	1536	6	6.0	6
Wisconsin cheese	8 oz cup	319	4	26	1104	1	25.0	22

SHAKEY'S PIZZA
CHICKEN ENTRÉE

fried, w/potatoes	3 pieces	947	57	51	2293	0	56.0	0
fried, w/potatoes	5 pieces	1700	97	130	5327	0	90.0	0

PIZZA
Cheese

homestyle pan crust, 12-inch pie	1/10 pie	303	14	31	591	0	13.7	21
thick crust, 'Shakey's Special' 12-inch pie	1/10 pie	208	13	22	423	0	8.3	18
thick crust, regular, 12-inch pie	1/10 pie	170	9	22	421	0	4.8	13
thin crust, 'Shakey's Special' 12-inch pie	1/10 pie	171	13	14	475	0	8.7	16
thin crust, regular, 12-inch pie	1/10 pie	133	8	13	323	0	5.2	14
Ham and cheese, 'Hot Ham and Cheese'	1 serving	550	36	56	2135	0	21.0	0

Pepperoni

homestyle pan crust 12-inch pie	1/10 pie	343	16	31	740	0	15.4	27
thick crust, 12-inch pie	1/10 pie	185	10	22	422	0	6.4	17
thin crust, 12-inch pie	1/10 pie	148	8	13	403	0	6.9	14

Sausage and mushroom

homestyle pan crust, 12-inch pie	1/10 pie	343	16	31	677	0	16.9	24
thick crust, 12-inch pie	1/10 pie	179	10	22	420	0	5.6	15
thin crust, 12-inch pie	1/10 pie	141	9	13	336	0	6.0	13

Sausage and pepperoni

homestyle pan crust, 12-inch pie	1/10 pie	374	17	31	676	0	19.9	24
thick crust, 12-inch pie	1/10 pie	177	11	22	424	0	8.0	19
thin crust, 12-inch pie	1/10 pie	166	9	13	397	0	8.4	17

'Sausage Supreme'

homestyle pan crust, vegetable, 12-inch pie	1/10 pie	320	15	32	652	0	14.7	21
'Special' homestyle pan crust, 12-inch pie	1/10 pie	384	18	32	878	0	20.7	29
'Thai Chicken' thick crust, 12-inch pie	1/10 pie	162	9	22	418	0	4.1	13
POTATO, wedges	15 pieces	950	17	120	3703	0	36.0	0

SANDWICH

'Hot Ham and Cheese'	1 sandwich	550	36	56	2135	0	21.0	0
'Super Hot Hero'	1 sandwich	810	36	67	2688	0	44.0	0
SPAGHETTI ENTRÉE, w/meat sauce and garlic bread	1 serving	940	26	134	1904	0	33.0	0

SHONEY'S

BISCUIT	1 serving	170	3	22	364	0	8.1	0
BREAD, Grecian	1 serving	80	2	13	94	0	2.2	0

BREAKFAST

bacon	3 strips	109	6	0	303	0	9.4	16
croissant, plain	1 serving	260	5	22	260	0	16.0	2
egg, fried	1 egg	159	6	1	69	0	14.7	274
ham	2 slices	59	7	1	526	0	2.1	28
honey bun	1 bun	265	4	32	33	0	14.0	3

Food Name	Serv. Size	Total Cal.	Prot. gms	Carbs gms	Sod. mgs	Fiber gms	Fat gms	Chol. mgs
pancake, 6-inch	1 cake	91	2	20	522	0	0.2	0
sausage	1 patty	103	4	0	161	0	9.6	17
syrup, low calorie	2.2 oz	98	0	24	0	0	0.0	0
toast, w/butter	2 slices	163	4	25	296	1	5.2	0
CHEESEBURGER, 'Mushroom/Swiss Burger'	1 burger	616	32	29	1135	1	41.7	106
CHICKEN ENTRÉE								
charbroiled, 'LightSide'	1 serving	239	39	1	592	0	7.0	85
tenders, 'America's Favorites'	1 serving	388	35	17	239	0	20.4	64
COMBINATION ENTRÉE								
'Fish N' Shrimp'	1 serving	487	28	37	644	0	25.5	127
'Italian Feast'	1 serving	500	38	44	369	1	19.6	74
ribeye steak and chicken, charbroiled	1 serving	605	35	0	211	0	50.5	141
sirloin and chicken, charbroiled	1 serving	357	32	0	160	0	24.5	99
steak and chicken, charbroiled	8-oz serving	435	31	0	280	0	34.4	123
'Steak N' Shrimp' charbroiled shrimp	1 serving	361	37	1	198	0	22.6	141
'Steak N' Shrimp' fried shrimp	1 serving	507	37	15	249	0	32.7	150
CONDIMENTS. See also Salad dressing.								
gravy, country	3 oz	114	1	6	358	0	9.8	2
onion, sautéed	2.5-oz serving	37	1	4	221	1	2.1	0
sweet and sour sauce, souffle cup	1 cup	58	0	15	5	0	0.0	0
tartar sauce, souffle cup	1 cup	84	0	4	177	0	7.7	11
DESSERT								
apple pie, à la mode	1 serving	492	6	67	574	0	23.0	35
brownie, walnut, à la mode	1 serving	576	10	61	435	0	33.7	35
carrot cake	1 serving	500	9	56	476	0	26.0	37
hot fudge cake	1 serving	522	7	82	485	0	19.7	27
hot fudge sundae	1 serving	451	7	60	226	0	22.0	60
strawberry pie	1 serving	332	2	45	247	2	16.7	0
strawberry sundae	1 serving	380	6	48	145	0	19.0	69
FISH								
baked, 'LightSide'	1 serving	170	35	2	1641	0	1.0	83
fried, 'Light'	1 serving	297	20	22	536	0	14.4	65
FISH ENTRÉE, fried, w/fries	1 serving	639	32	50	873	3	34.8	103
HAMBURGER								
'All-American'	1 burger	501	25	27	597	1	32.6	86
'Old Fashioned'	1 burger	470	25	26	681	1	28.2	82
'Shoney Burger'	1 burger	498	23	22	782	0	35.7	79
w/bacon	1 burger	591	29	29	801	1	40.0	86
HAMBURGER PATTY, beef, light	1 serving	289	21	0	187	0	22.9	82
LASAGNA ENTRÉE								
'America's Favorites'	1 serving	297	8	45	870	3	9.8	26
light, 'LightSide'	1 serving	297	8	45	870	0	10.0	26
LIVER ENTRÉE, w/onions, 'America's Favorites'	1 serving	411	35	15	321	1	22.9	529
SALAD DRESSING								
Thousand Island	2 tbsp	130	1	2	179	0	13.0	12
Biscayne, low-calorie	2 tbsp	62	6	1	334	0	1.0	0
blue cheese	2 tbsp	113	0	0	109	0	13.0	15
French	2 tbsp	124	2	2	204	0	12.0	12
French rue	2 tbsp	122	5	2	364	0	10.0	0
honey mustard	2 tbsp	165	2	2	5	0	17.0	18
Italian, creamy	2 tbsp	135	0	1	454	0	15.0	0
Italian, golden	2 tbsp	141	0	1	302	0	15.0	0
Italian, nonfat	2 tbsp	10	0	2	615	0	0.0	0
Ranch	2 tbsp	95	0	0	10	0	10.0	15
SANDWICH								
cheese and bacon, grilled	1 sandwich	440	18	28	1200	1	28.2	36
cheese, grilled	1 sandwich	454	17	29	1519	0	29.0	0
chicken fillet	1 sandwich	464	30	39	585	1	21.2	51

Food Name	Serv. Size	Total Cal.	Prot. gms	Carbs gms	Sod. mgs	Fiber gms	Fat gms	Chol. mgs
chicken, charbroiled	1 sandwich	451	43	28	1002	1	17.0	90
fish	1 sandwich	323	12	41	740	0	12.7	21
ham club, on whole wheat	1 sandwich	642	37	45	2105	11	35.5	78
ham, baked	1 sandwich	290	19	28	1263	2	10.3	42
patty melt	1 sandwich	640	39	30	826	7	41.7	121
Philly steak	1 sandwich	673	32	37	1242	0	44.0	103
Reuben	1 sandwich	596	33	32	3873	6	34.7	138
'Slim Jim'	1 sandwich	484	27	40	1620	1	23.9	57
steak, country fried	1 sandwich	588	25	67	1501	1	25.8	29
turkey club, on whole wheat	1 sandwich	635	44	44	1289	10	32.7	100
SEAFOOD PLATTER ENTRÉE	1 serving	566	33	46	893	0	28.0	127
SHRIMP								
bite-sized	1 serving	387	16	25	1266	0	24.7	140
charbroiled	1 serving	138	25	3	170	0	3.0	162
SHRIMP ENTRÉE								
boiled	1 serving	93	20	0	210	0	1.0	182
sampler	1 serving	412	26	26	783	0	22.7	217
'Shrimper's Feast' regular	1 serving	383	17	30	216	0	22.2	125
'Shrimper's Feast' large	1 serving	575	25	45	324	0	33.3	188
SIDE DISH								
ambrosia salad	1/4 cup	75	1	12	167	1	3.3	0
apple grape surprise salad	1/4 cup	19	0	5	2	0	0.0	0
baked potato	10-oz serving	264	6	61	16	7	0.3	0
beet-onion salad	1/4 cup	25	1	3	167	1	1.3	0
broccoli-cauliflower-ranch salad	1/4 cup	65	1	2	12	1	6.4	9
carrot-apple salad	1/4 cup	99	1	4	10	1	9.1	8
coleslaw	1/4 cup	69	1	5	106	1	5.1	7
cucumber salad, lite	1/4 cup	12	0	3	344	0	0.1	0
'Don's Pasta Salad'	1/4 cup	82	2	9	223	0	4.6	0
French fries	3-oz serving	189	3	29	273	3	7.5	0
French fries	4-oz serving	252	4	39	364	4	9.9	0
'Fruit Delight Salad'	1/4 cup	54	1	10	2	1	1.6	0
grits	3 oz	57	1	6	62	0	3.2	0
grits, instant	100 grams	67	1	7	73	0	3.8	0
hash browns	3 oz	90	2	14	50	0	3.1	0
home fries	3 oz	115	2	19	53	0	3.7	0
Italian vegetable salad	1/4 cup	11	0	3	110	1	0.1	0
kidney bean salad	1/4 cup	55	3	7	154	2	2.1	2
macaroni salad	1/4 cup	207	4	17	382	0	13.9	14
mixed squash salad	1/4 cup	49	1	2	230	0	4.1	0
mushroom, sauteed	3-oz serving	75	2	4	968	1	6.5	0
onion rings	1 ring	52	1	5	102	0	3.1	2
Oriental salad	1/4 cup	79	1	13	31	1	2.7	1
pea salad	1/4 cup	73	3	4	89	2	5.5	42
rice	3.5-oz serving	137	2	23	765	0	3.7	1
rotelli pasta	1/4 cup	78	1	9	82	0	4.0	0
seigan salad	1/4 cup	72	2	8	122	1	3.6	5
snow salad	1/4 cup	72	1	9	18	0	4.1	0
spaghetti salad	1/4 cup	81	2	9	20	0	4.6	0
spring salad	1/4 cup	38	1	2	162	1	2.9	0
summer salad	1/4 cup	114	1	2	233	1	11.6	0
three-bean salad	1/4 cup	96	1	12	189	1	5.1	0
Waldorf salad	1/4 cup	81	1	9	68	1	5.2	2
SOUP								
bean	6 oz	63	4	10	479	1	1.1	4
beef, w/cabbage	6 oz	86	6	9	503	2	3.0	13
broccoli, cream of	6 oz	75	2	11	415	0	4.6	1
cauliflower	6 oz	124	4	12	560	1	9.2	12

Food Name	Serv. Size	Total Cal.	Prot. gms	Carbs gms	Sod. mgs	Fiber gms	Fat gms	Chol. mgs
Cheddar chowder	6 oz	91	3	14	948	0	2.3	0
cheese Florentine, w/ham	6 oz	110	4	12	890	1	7.8	11
chicken, cream of	6 oz	136	5	14	1164	0	8.9	11
chicken gumbo	6 oz	60	4	7	1050	0	2.0	0
chicken noodle	6 oz	62	3	9	127	0	1.4	14
chicken vegetable, cream of	6 oz	79	4	13	714	0	1.3	0
chicken w/rice	6 oz	72	3	13	117	1	0.5	6
clam chowder	6 oz	94	2	10	66	0	5.4	0
corn chowder	6 oz	148	4	22	510	0	4.7	0
onion	6 oz	29	1	2	88	0	2.0	1
potato	6 oz	102	1	17	335	2	3.4	0
tomato, w/vegetable	6 oz	46	2	10	314	0	0.3	0
tomato Florentine	6 oz	63	2	11	683	0	1.1	0
vegetable beef	6 oz	82	4	14	1254	0	1.5	5
SPAGHETTI ENTRÉE								
'America's Favorites'	1 serving	496	24	63	387	2	16.3	55
SPAGHETTI ENTRÉE, LIGHT								
light, 'LightSide'	1 serving	248	12	32	194	0	8.0	28
STEAK, sirloin, charbroiled	6 oz	357	32	0	160	0	24.5	99
STEAK ENTRÉE, country fried steak								
'America's Favorites'	1 serving	449	19	34	1177	1	27.2	27
SIZZLER								
BEEF								
roast beef, sliced	2/3 oz	17	3	0	276	0	0.3	8
steak, New York strip	12 oz	600	70	5	200	0	35.0	180
steak, sirloin	6.25 oz	447	55	0	245	0	34.0	120
BEEF PATTY	8 oz	530	42	0	150	0	38.0	156
BREAD, focaccia	2 pieces	108	2	9	134	0	7.0	1
BREADSTICK, garlic, soft	1 oz	75	2	15	112	0	0.5	0
CHICKEN								
breast, lemon herb	5 oz	151	27	27	0	0	4.0	0
wing	1 oz	73	4	4	136	0	4.0	20
wing, Cajun	3 oz	201	16	2	435	0	14.4	111
wing, Southern	1 oz	73	5	4	135	0	6.0	20
wing, whole, Southern	1 oz	74	4	4	285	0	4.8	18
CHICKEN ENTRÉE, w/noodles	6 oz	164	13	20	524	0	4.0	40
CHICKEN PATTY, 'Malibu'	1 patty	368	27	12	0	0	25.0	0
CHILI, 'Grande' w/beans	6 oz	100	5	18	1190	0	1.0	0
CONDIMENTS								
buttery dipping sauce	1.5 oz	330	0	0	0	0	37.0	0
guacamole	1 oz	42	0	2	425	0	4.0	0
guacamole, extra chunky	3.5 oz serving	285	3	7	0	0	18.4	0
hibachi sauce	1.5 oz	57	0	11	707	0	0.0	0
Malibu sauce	1.5 oz	283	0	0	354	0	31.0	28
margarine, whipped	1.5 tbsp	105	0	0	146	0	12.0	0
marinade	1 oz	13	0	3	90	0	0.0	0
nacho cheese sauce	2 oz	120	5	3	600	0	10.0	30
pepper, bell, salad bar item	2 oz	8	1	2	1	1	0.0	0
salsa	1 oz	7	0	2	156	0	0.0	0
tartar sauce	1.5 oz	170	0	6	453	0	17.0	14
turkey ham, salad bar item	1 oz	62	4	0	376	0	5.0	19
CORNED BEEF, sliced	1 oz	45	8	0	55	0	1.5	0
CRAB, snow, legs and claws,	3.5 oz	91	21	0	539	0	1.1	55
CRAB, IMITATION, shredded	3.5 oz serving	104	12	14	864	0	1.0	22
CROISSANT, mini	1 croissant	120	2	12	95	0	8.0	4
DESSERT								
'Parfait Salad'	3.5 oz serving	84	2	17	66	0	1.7	0
yogurt, frozen, chocolate, soft-serve	4 oz	136	1	24	100	0	4.0	0

Food Name	Serv. Size	Total Cal.	Prot. gms	Carbs gms	Sod. mgs	Fiber gms	Fat gms	Chol. mgs
yogurt, frozen, vanilla, soft-serve .... 4 oz		136	1	24	100	0	4.0	0
DESSERT TOPPING								
chocolate syrup .... 1 oz		90	0	21	15	0	0.0	0
strawberry, nonfat .... 1 oz		70	0	18	5	0	0.0	0
whipped .... 1 tbsp		12	0	1	0	0	1.0	0
FISH NUGGETS .... 1 oz		40	4	5	100	0	0.0	10
HALIBUT, steak .... 6 oz		180	36	0	103	0	2.0	86
HAMBURGER, w/lettuce and tomato .... 1 serving		626	45	36	335	1	33.0	142
LASAGNA								
w/meat .... 8 oz		327	21	23	657	0	13.0	37
vegetable .... 8 oz		245	15	29	553	0	8.0	19
MACARONI AND CHEESE .... 6 oz		214	10	22	590	0	9.0	26
MEATBALL .... 4 meatballs		157	9	5	461	1	11.0	30
PASTA								
fettuccine .... 2 oz		80	3	15	5	0	1.0	5
fettuccine, whole egg, dry .... 2 oz		210	9	40	8	0	1.0	0
ravioli, cheese .... 4 oz		260	10	47	270	0	4.0	20
spaghetti .... 2 oz		80	3	16	1	1	0.0	0
POLLACK, breaded .... 4 oz		140	14	18	280	0	1.0	35
SALAD DRESSING								
bacon, hot .... 1 tbsp		40	0	58	90	0	20.0	0
blue cheese .... 1 oz		111	1	1	168	0	12.0	8
honey mustard .... 1 oz		160	0	4	110	0	16.0	10
Italian, lite .... 1 oz		14	0	2	350	0	0.0	0
Italian, Parmesan .... 1 oz		100	0	2	450	0	10.0	0
Japanese rice vinegar, nonfat .... 1 oz		10	0	2	172	0	0.0	0
Malibu .... 1 tbsp		100	0	0	125	0	11.0	10
ranch .... 1 oz		120	0	2	240	0	12.0	10
ranch, lower calorie .... 1 oz		90	0	4	270	0	8.0	10
sour .... 1.5 oz		89	0	0	44	0	9.0	0
sour .... 2 tbsp		60	0	0	30	0	6.0	0
Thousand Island .... 1 oz		143	0	3	125	0	15.0	11
SALMON .... 8 oz		247	32	0	232	0	12.0	41
SCALLOP, breaded, approx 30-40 .... 4 oz		160	14	24	393	0	1.0	18
SHRIMP								
broiled .... 5 oz		150	23	0	377	0	6.0	218
butterfly, breaded, approx 16-20 .... 3.5 oz		220	10	16	440	0	13.0	50
butterfly, breaded, approx 10-12 .... 3.5 oz		145	10	14	280	0	0.1	0
butterfly, Cajun, breaded, approx 16-20 .... 3.5 oz		145	10	24	280	0	0.1	0
butterfly, lemon pepper, breaded, approx 21-25 .... 2 oz		190	5	38	211	0	1.0	5
Cajun, breaded, approx 80-90 .... 3.5 oz		140	10	22	198	0	0.9	0
mini, breaded, approx 50-60 .... 3.5 oz		140	10	22	198	0	0.9	0
mini, Cajun, breaded, approx 40-50 .... 3.5 oz		141	10	22	200	0	0.9	0
scampi .... 5 oz		143	27	0	386	0	3.0	150
tempura-battered, approx 21-25 .... 3 oz		155	10	13	442	0	8.0	74
SIDE DISH								
avocado, salad bar item .... 1/2 avocado		153	2	6	11	3	15.0	0
baked potato, flesh only .... 4 oz		105	2	24	6	2	0.0	0
broccoli, salad bar item .... 1/2 cup		12	1	2	12	1	0.0	0
carrot-raisin salad .... 2 oz		130	1	10	104	1	10.0	10
cauliflower, battered, not fried .... 3.5 oz serving		184	3	21	49	0	10.3	0
cheese toast .... 1 piece		273	6	16	494	1	21.0	5
Chinese chicken salad .... 2 oz		54	4	6	119	1	2.0	10
corn nuggets .... 3 oz		117	3	22	325	0	8.4	0
cottage cheese, low-fat .... 1/2 cup		100	14	4	390	0	2.0	8
French fries .... 4 oz		358	5	45	245	4	12.0	0
four-bean salad .... 3.5 oz serving		104	3	19	226	0	2.5	0
grapes, salad bar item .... 1/2 cup		29	0	8	1	1	0.0	0
jicama, salad bar item .... 2 oz		13	1	3	1	0	0.0	0

Food Name	Serv. Size	Total Cal.	Prot. gms	Carbs gms	Sod. mgs	Fiber gms	Fat gms	Chol. mgs
jicama salad, spicy	2 oz	16	0	4	28	0	0.0	0
kidney beans, salad bar item	1/4 cup	52	3	10	222	4	0.0	0
kiwifruit, salad bar item	2 oz	35	1	8	3	2	0.0	0
lettuce, Romaine, salad bar item	1 cup	9	1	1	4	1	0.0	0
macaroni and cheddar salad	3.5 oz serving	185	3	16	476	0	12.5	14
Mediterranean Minted fruit salad	2 oz	29	1	7	11	0	0.0	1
'Mexican Fiesta Salad'	2 oz	54	2	10	99	1	1.0	0
okra, breaded, not fried	3.5 oz serving	105	3	24	503	0	0.5	1
onion rings, steak cut, breaded, not fried	.5 oz serving	395	5	39	558	0	24.4	0
'Oriental Pasta Salad'	3.5 oz serving	114	4	23	781	0	1.6	1
potato and egg salad	3.5 oz serving	140	2	16	340	0	7.8	28
potato salad, 'Old Fashioned'	2 oz	84	1	10	231	1	5.0	8
potato salad, 'Old Fashioned'	3.5 oz serving	150	2	17	416	0	8.7	23
potato salad, red, herb	2 oz	121	1	9	271	1	9.0	9
potato salad, red, herb	3.5 oz serving	213	2	15	437	0	16.2	15
potato skin	2 oz	160	2	22	463	3	8.0	0
refried beans	3 oz	120	5	16	320	0	4.0	2
rice pilaf	6 oz	256	4	47	866	1	5.0	0
'Seafood Louis' pasta salad	2 oz	64	3	9	139	1	2.0	17
seafood salad	2 oz	56	3	4	255	0	3.0	7
shell pasta salad	3.5 oz serving	112	3	19	591	0	2.7	1
spinach, salad bar item	1/2 cup	6	1	1	22	1	0.0	0
teriyaki beef salad	2 oz	49	4	5	136	1	2.0	7
tuna pasta salad	2 oz	133	6	6	188	0	10.0	10
tuna salad	3.5 oz serving	353	8	7	296	0	32.9	44
SOUP								
broccoli cheese soup	4 oz	139	3	10	355	0	9.0	8
chicken w/noodle	4 oz	31	2	4	495	0	1.0	7
clam chowder	4 oz	118	3	11	511	0	6.0	6
minestrone, nonfat	4 oz	36	1	7	443	2	0.0	1
vegetable, vegetarian	6 oz	50	2	6	630	0	1.0	0
vegetable sirloin soup	4 oz	60	6	6	364	0	2.0	10
SWORDFISH	8 oz	315	45	0	331	0	14.0	89
TACO SHELL	1 shell	50	1	7	20	1	2.0	0
TUNA, yellowfin	3.5 oz serving	125	15	0	50	0	4.0	65
SKIPPER'S								
CHICKEN ENTRÉE								
'Lite Catch' 3 pieces, w/small green salad	1 serving	305	26	17	673	0	15.0	58
tenderloin strips, 5 pieces, w/fries	1 serving	793	44	69	798	0	38.0	77
CHICKEN STRIPS, 'Create A Catch'	1 serving	82	8	4	150	0	4.0	15
CLAM ENTRÉE, 'Basket' strips w/fries	1 serving	1003	22	90	569	0	70.0	14
COD ENTRÉE								
3 pieces, thick cut, w/fries	1 serving	665	27	68	1054	0	32.0	38
4 pieces, thick cut w/fries	1 serving	759	34	74	1388	0	36.0	50
5 pieces, thick cut, w/fries	1 serving	853	42	80	1723	0	41.0	62
COMBINATION ENTRÉE								
'Combos' clam strips, 1 piece fish, fries	1 serving	868	25	81	667	0	54.0	61
'Combos' jumbo shrimp, 1 piece fish, fries	1 serving	720	24	75	1268	0	36.0	91
'Combos' original shrimp, 1 piece fish, fries	1 serving	728	24	77	943	0	37.0	105
'Combos' oysters, 1 piece fish, fries	1 serving	885	25	95	809	0	44.0	80
'Lite Catch' 1 piece fish, 2 pieces chicken, small green salad	1 serving	399	29	24	880	0	21.0	96
3-piece, chicken strip, fish, fries	1 serving	805	80	72	858	0	40.0	100
3-piece, chicken strip, shrimp, fries	1 serving	800	36	77	1036	0	39.0	97
DESSERT								
gelatin, nonfat, 'Jell-O' 'Create A Catch'	1 serving	55	1	12	35	0	0.0	0
root beer float	1 serving	302	3	33	66	0	10.0	10

Food Name	Serv. Size	Total Cal.	Prot. gms	Carbs gms	Sod. mgs	Fiber gms	Fat gms	Chol. mgs
FISH								
fillet, 'Create A Catch'	1 serving	175	11	11	357	0	10.0	53
FISH ENTRÉE								
1 fish fillet, w/fries	1 serving	558	17	51	408	0	28.0	55
2 fish fillets, w/fries	1 serving	733	28	71	765	0	38.0	108
3 fish fillets, w/fries	1 serving	908	39	82	1122	0	48.0	160
'Lite Catch' 2 pieces, w/small green salad	1 serving	409	25	27	937	0	23.0	119
FISH SANDWICH								
'Create A Catch'	1 sandwich	524	19	43	1191	0	33.0	86
'Create A Catch' double	1 sandwich	698	30	54	1548	0	73.0	139
OYSTER ENTRÉE, w/fries 'Basket'	1 serving	1038	28	118	853	0	51.0	52
SALAD								
green, small, 'Lite Catch'	1 salad	59	3	6	223	0	3.0	13
shrimp and seafood	1 salad	167	23	15	657	0	3.0	80
side	1 salad	24	0	4	8	0	0.0	0
SALAD DRESSING								
salad dressing, blue cheese, premium	1 pouch	222	1	4	240	0	23.0	8
salad dressing, Italian, gourmet	1 pouch	140	0	2	200	0	15.0	0
salad dressing, Italian, low-calorie	1 pouch	17	0	2	680	0	1.0	0
salad dressing, ranch house	1 pouch	188	1	2	302	0	20.0	0
salad dressing, Thousand Island	1 pouch	160	0	8	415	0	14.0	6
tartar sauce	1 tbsp	65	0	0	102	0	7.0	4
SALMON, baked	4.4 oz	270	39	1	504	0	11.0	70
SEAFOOD ENTRÉE, w/fries 'Skipper's Platter Basket'	1 serving	1038	32	97	1202	0	63.0	111
SHRIMP ENTRÉE								
w/fries, 'Basket'	1 serving	723	20	82	1121	0	36.0	102
w/fries, jumbo, 'Basket'	1 serving	707	20	79	911	0	35.0	73
w/seafood salad, 'Lite Catch'	1 serving	167	23	15	657	0	3.0	80
SIDE DISH								
baked potato	1 serving	145	4	32	6	0	0.0	0
coleslaw	.5 oz serving	289	2	10	329	0	27.0	50
French fries, 'Create A Catch'	1 serving	383	6	50	51	0	18.0	2
SOUP								
clam chowder, 'Create A Catch' cup	1 serving	100	3	14	525	0	3.5	12
clam chowder, 'Create A Catch' pint	1 serving	200	5	19	1050	0	7.0	24
salmon chowder, 'Alder Smoked Salmon'	6 oz	166	13	14	73	0	7.0	0
SONIC								
CHEESEBURGER								
#1	1 serving	70	4	0	267	0	5.8	18
#2	1 serving	70	4	0	267	0	5.8	18
w/bacon	1 serving	548	28	23	839	0	38.6	87
jalapeño, double meat and cheese	1 serving	638	44	22	1358	0	40.6	136
mini	1 serving	281	17	20	644	0	14.4	45
CHILI PIE	1 serving	327	12	20	313	0	22.6	28
CORN DOG	1 sandwich	280	7	30	700	0	15.0	35
HAMBURGER								
#1	1 serving	409	20	23	444	0	26.6	58
#2	1 serving	323	20	23	549	0	15.7	50
hickory	1 serving	314	20	23	459	0	15.7	50
mini	1 serving	246	14	20	510	0	11.5	36
'Super Sonic' double meat and cheese, w/mayo	1 serving	730	44	24	1023	0	51.5	144
'Super Sonic' double meat and cheese, w/mustard	1 serving	644	44	24	1128	0	40.7	136
HOT DOG								
'Cheese Coney' extra long	1 serving	635	24	45	632	0	39.0	65
'Cheese Coney' w/onions, extra long	1 serving	640	25	47	632	0	39.2	65
'Cheese Coney' regular	1 serving	358	14	23	341	0	23.3	40
regular	1 serving	258	8	21	241	0	15.3	23
'Cheese Coney' regular, w/onions	1 serving	361	14	24	341	0	23.3	40

Food Name	Serv. Size	Total Cal.	Prot. gms	Carbs gms	Sod. mgs	Fiber gms	Fat gms	Chol. mgs
SANDWICH								
bacon, lettuce, tomato	1 sandwich	327	8	27	600	0	19.3	9
cheese, grilled	1 sandwich	288	12	25	841	0	17.0	36
chicken	1 sandwich	319	21	41	890	0	9.0	47
chicken, breaded	1 sandwich	455	23	36	755	0	24.7	42
chicken, grilled, no dressing	1 sandwich	215	21	23	716	0	4.3	63
fish	1 sandwich	277	17	38	655	0	7.0	6
steak	1 sandwich	631	19	46	1047	0	41.6	50
SIDE DISH								
French fries, large	1 serving	315	5	50	67	0	11.2	11
French fries, regular	1 serving	233	3	37	50	0	8.0	8
French fries, w/cheese, large	1 serving	420	11	51	468	0	20.2	38
onion rings, large	1 serving	577	8	54	532	0	37.8	0
onion rings, regular	1 serving	404	5	38	372	0	26.5	0
potato pieces, 'Tater Tots'	1 serving	150	2	19	330	0	7.0	10
potato pieces, 'Tater Tots' w/cheese	1 serving	220	6	19	569	0	13.0	28
SPAGHETTI WAREHOUSE								
MARINADE, dinner serving	1 serving	403	13	75	303	5	5.0	0
MINESTRONE SOUP	1 serving	56	3	8	155	2	1.0	3
TOMATO SAUCE, dinner serving	1 serving	410	13	76	454	6	5.0	0
STEAK 'N SHAKE								
CHEESEBURGER								
'Steakburger'	1 serving	353	23	33	658	0	13.0	na
'Steakburger' super	1 serving	451	35	33	680	0	18.0	na
'Steakburger' triple patty	1 serving	626	52	34	934	0	30.0	na
CHILI								
'Chili Mac' w/4 saltines	1 serving	310	15	34	1301	0	12.0	na
'Chili 3 Ways' w/4 saltines	1 serving	411	19	45	1734	0	16.0	na
w/oyster crackers	1 serving	337	16	37	1157	0	14.0	na
DESSERT								
apple Danish	1 piece	391	6	35	352	0	24.0	na
apple pie à la mode	1 serving	549	4	76	525	0	25.0	na
brownie	1 brownie	258	3	39	165	0	12.0	na
cheesecake	1 serving	368	7	61	294	0	11.0	na
cheesecake, w/strawberries	1 serving	386	7	65	294	0	11.0	na
cherry pie à la mode	1 serving	476	6	63	314	0	22.0	na
'Coca-Cola Float'	1 serving	514	16	76	230	0	17.0	na
fudge brownie sundae	1 serving	645	7	81	262	0	35.0	na
hot fudge nut sundae	1 serving	530	5	51	121	0	34.0	na
'Lemon Float'	1 serving	555	18	82	248	0	19.0	na
'Lemon Freeze'	1 serving	548	15	69	213	0	25.0	na
'Orange Float'	1 serving	502	16	74	224	0	17.0	na
'Orange Freeze'	1 serving	516	14	63	198	0	24.0	na
'Root Beer Float'	1 serving	529	17	78	237	0	17.0	na
strawberry sundae	1 serving	330	2	29	81	0	22.0	na
HAMBURGER								
'Steakburger'	1 serving	277	18	33	425	0	7.0	na
'Steakburger' super	1 serving	375	30	33	447	0	12.0	na
'Steakburger' triple patty	1 serving	474	43	33	468	0	17.0	na
SALAD								
chef	1 salad	313	41	6	1582	0	18.0	na
lettuce and tomato, w/1 oz Thousand Island dressing	1 salad	168	1	7	223	0	15.0	na
SANDWICH								
cheese, toasted	1 sandwich	250	9	24	606	0	13.0	na
egg	1 sandwich	275	12	33	490	0	10.0	na
ham, baked	1 sandwich	451	29	37	1858	0	22.0	na
ham and egg	1 sandwich	434	36	33	1850	0	17.0	na

Food Name	Serv. Size	Total Cal.	Prot. gms	Carbs gms	Sod. mgs	Fiber gms	Fat gms	Chol. mgs
SIDE DISH								
baked beans	1 serving	173	9	27	656	0	4.0	na
French fries	1 serving	211	3	28	297	0	10.0	na
STEAK PLATTER, low calorie	1 serving	293	37	3	242	0	14.0	na
SUBWAY								
BEVERAGE								
'Berry 'Lishus Fruizle Smoothie'	12 oz	154	1	40	9	3	0.3	0
'Berry Blitz Fruizle Smoothie'	12 oz	129	1	37	7	7	0.0	0
'Berry Breeze Fruizle Smoothie'	12 oz	120	0	32	7	2	0.1	0
'Island Berry Fruizle Smoothie'	12 oz	120	0	32	7	2	0.1	0
'Island Fever Fruizle Smoothie'	12 oz	137	0	36	7	1	0.2	0
'Peach Paradise Fruizle Smoothie'	12 oz	119	0	32	7	1	0.1	0
'Peach Pizazz Fruizle Smoothie'	12 oz	126	0	33	10	1	0.0	0
'Pineapple Delite Fruizle Smoothie'	12 oz	142	1	38	6	1	0.3	0
'Pineapple Passion Fruizle Smoothie'	12 oz	140	1	38	6	1	0.2	0
'Sunrise Energizer Fruizle Smoothie'	12 oz	160	1	42	8	2	0.3	0
'Tropical Trio Fruizle Smoothie'	12 oz	138	0	36	7	1	0.2	0
'Wild Berries Fruizle Smoothie'	12 oz	130	1	36	8	5	0.1	0
BREAD								
Italian, 12-inch	1 large	380	14	76	840	0	2.0	0
Italian, 6-inch	1 small	190	7	38	420	0	1.0	0
wheat, 12-inch	1 serving	420	16	78	860	6	5.0	0
wheat, 6-inch	1 serving	210	8	39	430	3	3.0	0
wrap, 10.5-inch	1 wrap	200	0	45	720	1	2.0	0
CONDIMENTS								
bacon, 'Optional Fixin's'	2 slices	42	3	0	160	0	3.0	9
cheese	2 triangles	41	2	0	204	0	3.0	10
lettuce, deli style, 'Standard Fixin's'	1 serving	2	0	0	1	0	0.0	0
lettuce, 'Standard Fixin's'	1 serving	4	0	1	3	0	0.0	0
mayonnaise, regular, 'Optional Fixin's'	1 tsp	37	0	0	27	0	4.0	3
mayonnaise, light, 'Optional Fixin's'	1 tsp	18	0	0	33	0	2.0	2
vinegar, 'Optional Fixin's'	1 tsp	1	0	0	0	0	0.0	0
mustard, 'Optional Fixin's'	2 tsp	7	0	1	115	0	0.0	0
oil, 'Optional Fixin's'	1 tsp	45	0	0	0	0	5.0	0
olives, deli style, 'Standard Fixin's'	2 rings	2	0	0	6	0	0.0	0
olives, 'Standard Fixin's'	2 rings	2	0	0	6	0	0.0	0
onion, deli style, 'Standard Fixin's'	1 serving	2	0	1	0	0	0.0	0
onion 'Standard Fixin's'	1 serving	5	0	1	0	0	0.0	0
peppers, deli style 'Standard Fixin's'	2 strips	1	0	0	0	na	0.0	0
peppers, 'Standard Fixin's'	2 strips	1	0	0	0	0	0.0	0
pickle, deli style, 'Standard Fixin's'	2 chips	1	0	0	92	0	0.0	0
pickle, 'Standard Fixin's'	3 chips	2	0	0	139	0	0.0	0
tomato, deli style, 'Standard Fixin's'	2 slices	8	0	2	4	0	0.0	0
tomato, 'Standard Fixin's'	2 slices	6	0	1	2	0	0.0	0
COOKIE								
Brazil nut	1 cookie	215	2	29	153	1	10.0	14
chocolate chip, 'M&M's'	1 cookie	212	2	29	144	1	10.0	13
chocolate chip	1 cookie	214	3	29	144	1	10.0	12
chocolate chunk	1 cookie	215	2	29	144	1	10.0	13
macadamia nut	1 cookie	222	2	28	144	1	11.0	12
oatmeal raisin	1 cookie	199	3	29	159	1	8.0	14
oatmeal raisin, low-fat	1 cookie	168	3	33	171	2	3.0	15
peanut butter	1 cookie	223	3	27	214	1	12.0	0
sugar	1 cookie	225	2	28	180	0	12.0	18
ROLL, deli style	1 serving	170	6	31	350	1	2.0	0
SALAD								
chicken breast, roasted, w/o dressing, cheese, condiments	1 salad	162	20	13	693	1	4.0	48

Food Name	Serv. Size	Total Cal.	Prot. gms	Carbs gms	Sod. mgs	Fiber gms	Fat gms	Chol. mgs
'Classic Italian BMT, w/o dressing, cheese, condiments	1 salad	269	14	11	1305	1	19.0	52
'Cold Cut Trio' w/o dressing, cheese, condiments	1 salad	193	12	12	1162	1	12.0	47
ham, w/o dressing, cheese, condiments	1 salad	112	12	11	1068	1	3.0	25
meatball, w/o dressing, cheese, condiments	1 salad	232	13	17	751	3	13.0	35
roast beef, w/o dressing, cheese, condiments	1 salad	115	12	11	654	1	3.0	20
seafood and crab, w/light mayo, w/o dressing	1 salad	157	7	17	761	2	7.0	14
steak and cheese, w/o dressing	1 salad	182	17	13	887	2	8.0	37
'Subway Club' w/o dressing, cheese, condiments	1 salad	123	14	12	965	1	3.0	26
'Subway Melt' w/o dressing	1 salad	190	16	12	1346	1	9.0	41
tuna, made w/light mayo, w/o dressing, cheese, condiments	1 salad	198	11	11	669	1	12.0	32
turkey and ham, w/o dressing, cheese, condiments	1 salad	107	11	11	982	1	2.0	23
turkey breast, w/o dressing, cheese, condiments	1 salad	101	11	12	896	1	2.0	20
'Veggie Delite, w/o dressing, cheese, condiments	1 salad	51	2	10	308	1	1.0	0
SANDWICH								
Bacon and egg								
deli style sub	1 sandwich	323	14	33	569	1	14.0	185
6-inch sub	1 sandwich	363	16	41	649	3	15.0	185
wrap	1 sandwich	353	8	47	939	1	14.0	185
Bologna, deli style sub, w/o cheese, condiments	1 sandwich	283	11	37	785	1	10.0	19
Cheese and egg								
deli style sub	1 sandwich	323	14	33	613	1	14.0	187
6-inch sub	1 sandwich	363	16	41	693	3	15.0	187
wrap	1 sandwich	353	8	47	983	1	14.0	187
Chicken breast								
roasted, 6-inch hot sub, w/o cheese, condiments	1 sandwich	342	26	46	966	3	6.0	48
roasted, super, 6-inch hot sub, w/o cheese, condiments	1 sandwich	453	44	49	1351	4	9.0	96
Chicken Parmesan wrap	1 sandwich	333	17	56	1393	2	5.0	45
'Classic Italian BMT'								
6-inch sub, w/o cheese, condiments	1 sandwich	450	21	45	1579	3	21.0	52
super, 6-inch sub, w/o cheese, condiments	1 sandwich	668	33	47	2576	3	39.0	104
'Cold Cut Trio'								
6-inch sub, w/o cheese, condiments	1 sandwich	374	19	45	1435	3	14.0	47
super, 6-inch sub, w/o cheese, condiments	1 sandwich	517	29	47	2289	3	24.0	93
Ham and egg								
deli style sub	1 sandwich	312	16	33	789	1	12.0	189
6-inch sub	1 sandwich	352	18	41	869	3	13.0	189
wrap	1 sandwich	342	10	47	1159	1	12.0	189
Ham								
deli style sub, w/o cheese, condiments	1 sandwich	224	12	37	827	1	3.0	12
6-inch sub, w/o cheese, condiments	1 sandwich	293	18	45	1342	3	5.0	25
super, 6-inch sub, w/o cheese, condiments	1 sandwich	354	27	47	2101	3	7.0	50
Meatball								
6-inch hot sub, w/o cheese, condiments	1 sandwich	413	19	50	1025	5	15.0	35
super, 6-inch hot sub, w/o cheese, condiments	1 sandwich	594	30	58	1468	7	27.0	70
Roast beef								
deli style sub, w/o cheese, condiments	1 sandwich	236	14	37	678	1	4.0	13
6-inch sub, w/o cheese, condiments	1 sandwich	296	19	45	928	3	5.0	20
super, 6-inch sub, w/o cheese, condiments	1 sandwich	360	29	47	1273	3	7.0	40
Seafood and crab								
super, w/light mayo, 6-inch sub	1 sandwich	444	18	58	1486	5	15.0	27
w/light mayo, 6-inch sub	1 sandwich	338	14	51	1034	4	9.0	14
Steak and cheese								
6-inch hot sub	1 sandwich	363	24	47	1160	4	10.0	37
super, 6-inch sub	1 sandwich	495	39	50	1739	5	17.0	75
wrap	1 sandwich	353	16	53	1450	2	9.0	37

Food Name	Serv. Size	Total Cal.	Prot. gms	Carbs gms	Sod. mgs	Fiber gms	Fat gms	Chol. mgs
'Subway Club'								
6-inch sub, w/o cheese, condiments	1 sandwich	304	21	46	1239	3	5.0	26
super, 6-inch sub, w/o cheese, condiments	1 sandwich	377	32	48	1895	3	7.0	52
'Subway Melt'								
6-inch hot sub	1 sandwich	370	23	46	1619	3	11.0	41
super, 6-inch hot sub	1 sandwich	509	36	48	2657	3	19.0	83
Tuna								
w/light mayo, deli style sub, w/o cheese, condiments	1 sandwich	267	12	37	627	1	8.0	16
w/light mayo, 6-inch sub, w/o cheese, condiments	1 sandwich	378	18	45	942	3	14.0	32
w/light mayo, super, 6-inch sub, w/o cheese, condiments	1 sandwich	525	27	46	1303	3	26.0	64
Turkey and ham								
6-inch sub, w/o cheese, condiments	1 sandwich	288	18	45	1256	3	4.0	23
super, 6-inch sub, w/o cheese, condiments	1 sandwich	343	27	47	1929	3	6.0	45
Turkey bacon wrap, deluxe	1 sandwich	355	14	52	1823	1	10.0	39
Turkey breast								
deli style sub, w/o cheese, condiments	1 sandwich	227	13	37	678	1	4.0	13
6-inch sub, w/o cheese, condiments	1 sandwich	282	17	45	1170	3	4.0	20
super, 6-inch sub, w/o cheese, condiments	1 sandwich	333	26	47	1758	3	4.0	40
'Veggie Delite' 6-inch sub, w/o cheese, condiments	1 sandwich	232	9	43	582	3	3.0	0
Western egg								
deli style sub	1 sandwich	311	14	36	603	2	12.0	182
6-inch sub	1 sandwich	351	16	44	683	4	12.0	182
wrap	1 sandwich	341	8	50	973	2	12.0	182

SWENSEN'S
ICE CREAM

Food Name	Serv. Size	Total Cal.	Prot. gms	Carbs gms	Sod. mgs	Fiber gms	Fat gms	Chol. mgs
'Almond Praline Delight' low-fat	1/2 cup	130	3	25	85	0	2.0	5
caramel apple crisp, low-fat	1/2 cup	130	3	26	75	0	1.0	5
caramel turtle fudge, light	1 serving	120	3	18	50	0	4.0	10
caramel turtle fudge, low-fat	1/2 cup	140	3	26	70	0	2.5	5
chocolate chocolate chip cheesecake, low-fat	1/2 cup	130	3	26	80	0	2.5	5
chocolate fudge brownie, low-fat	1/2 cup	120	3	24	70	0	2.5	5
cookies and cream, light	1 serving	130	3	20	60	0	4.0	10
ice cream, cookies and cream, low-fat	1/2 cup	130	3	25	80	0	2.5	5
vanilla, light	1 serving	110	3	15	50	0	4.0	10

YOGURT, FROZEN

Food Name	Serv. Size	Total Cal.	Prot. gms	Carbs gms	Sod. mgs	Fiber gms	Fat gms	Chol. mgs
Black Forest cake	1 serving	95	3	21	130	0	1.0	5
Black Forest cake, low-fat	1/2 cup	110	4	22	55	1	1.5	0
blueberry and cream, gourmet, sugar-free	1 serving	110	3	17	90	0	4.0	10
butter pecan, low-fat	1/2 cup	120	4	20	55	0	3.0	5
cherry, nonfat	1/2 cup	90	3	20	45	0	0.0	0
chocolate raspberry truffle, gourmet, sugar-free	1 serving	130	3	18	80	0	5.0	8
coconut pineapple	1 serving	120	4	26	65	0	1.0	5
hazelnut amaretto, low-fat	1/2 cup	120	4	20	50	0	3.0	0
mocha chip, low-fat	1/2 cup	110	4	22	50	0	1.5	0
strawberry banana and cream, nonfat	1/2 cup	90	3	20	45	0	0.0	0
triple chocolate, low-fat	1/2 cup	120	4	24	50	1	1.5	0
triple chocolate, nonfat	1 serving	100	4	21	65	0	0.0	0
vanilla Swiss almond, gourmet, sugar-free	1 serving	140	4	15	100	0	7.0	10
vanilla, nonfat	1/2 cup	90	3	20	60	0	0.0	0

SWISS CHALET
CHICKEN

Food Name	Serv. Size	Total Cal.	Prot. gms	Carbs gms	Sod. mgs	Fiber gms	Fat gms	Chol. mgs
CHICKEN	1/2 chicken	634	72	1	0	0	38.0	0

DESSERT

Food Name	Serv. Size	Total Cal.	Prot. gms	Carbs gms	Sod. mgs	Fiber gms	Fat gms	Chol. mgs
apple pie	1 serving	394	3	45	0	0	23.0	0
Black Forest cake	1 piece	278	3	36	0	0	14.0	0
chocolate éclair	1 serving	205	2	27	0	0	10.0	0
coconut pie	1 serving	292	2	40	0	0	14.0	0

Food Name	Serv. Size	Total Cal.	Prot. gms	Carbs gms	Sod. mgs	Fiber gms	Fat gms	Chol. mgs
fudge nut cake	1 piece	346	4	48	0	0	16.0	0
vanilla ice cream	1 serving	195	3	16	0	0	14.0	0
GRAVY, sandwich	1 serving	35	1	5	0	0	1.0	0
ROLL	1 roll	116	3	24	0	0	1.0	0
SALAD, chicken	1 salad	500	42	23	0	0	42.0	0
SANDWICH								
chicken	1 sandwich	360	33	42	0	0	5.0	0
chicken, hot	1 sandwich	310	30	30	0	0	6.0	0
SIDE DISH								
baked potato	1 serving	227	8	52	0	0	0.0	0
coleslaw, 'Chalet'	1 serving	56	2	10	0	0	1.0	0
French fries	1 serving	478	10	57	0	0	24.0	0
SOUP, chicken, 'Chalet'	1 serving	97	9	11	0	0	2.0	0

TCBY
YOGURT, FROZEN

Food Name	Serv. Size	Total Cal.	Prot. gms	Carbs gms	Sod. mgs	Fiber gms	Fat gms	Chol. mgs
nonfat, giant	31.6 oz	869	32	182	356	0	0.0	0
nonfat, kiddie	3.2 oz	88	3	18	36	0	0.0	0
nonfat, large	10.5 oz	289	10	60	118	0	0.0	0
nonfat, medium	8.2 oz	226	8	47	92	0	0.0	0
nonfat, small	5.9 oz	162	6	34	66	0	0.0	0
nonfat, super	15.2 oz	418	15	87	171	0	0.0	0
regular, giant	31.6 oz	1027	32	182	474	0	24.0	79
regular, kiddie	3.2 oz	104	3	18	48	0	2.0	8
regular, large	10.5 oz	342	10	60	156	0	8.0	26
regular, medium	8.2 oz	267	8	47	126	0	6.0	20
regular, small	5.9 oz	192	6	34	90	0	4.0	15
regular, super	15.2 oz	494	15	87	228	0	11.0	38
strawberry	8 oz	220	9	43	150	0	2.0	0
sugarless, nonfat, giant	31.6 oz	632	32	142	316	0	0.0	0
sugarless, nonfat, kiddie	3.2 oz	64	3	14	32	0	0.0	0
sugarless, nonfat, large	10.5 oz	210	10	47	105	0	0.0	0
sugarless, nonfat, medium	8.2 oz	164	8	37	82	0	0.0	0
sugarless, nonfat, small	5.9 oz	118	6	27	59	0	0.0	0
sugarless, nonfat, super	15.2 oz	304	15	68	152	0	0.0	0

TACO BELL
BURRITO

Food Name	Serv. Size	Total Cal.	Prot. gms	Carbs gms	Sod. mgs	Fiber gms	Fat gms	Chol. mgs
bacon and egg, double, 6.25 oz	1 serving	480	18	39	1240	2	27.0	400
bean, 7 oz	1 serving	370	13	54	1080	12	12.0	10
'Big Beef Supreme' 10.5 oz	1 serving	510	23	52	1500	11	23.0	60
'Big Beef' 7 oz	1 serving	400	19	43	1320	6	17.0	50
'Big Chicken Supreme' 9 oz	1 serving	460	27	50	1200	3	17.0	70
chicken, grilled, 7 oz	1 serving	390	19	49	1240	3	13.0	40
chili cheese, 5 oz	1 serving	330	13	40	900	4	13.0	25
'Country Breakfast' 4 oz	1 serving	270	8	26	690	2	14.0	195
'Fiesta Breakfast' 3.5 oz	1 serving	280	9	25	580	2	16.0	25
'Grande Breakfast' 6.25 oz	1 serving	420	13	43	1050	3	22.0	205
7-layer, 10 oz	1 serving	520	16	65	1270	13	22.0	25
'Supreme' 9 oz	1 serving	430	17	50	1210	9	18.0	40
CHALUPA								
'Baja Beef' 5.5 oz	1 serving	420	14	30	760	3	27.0	35
'Baja Chicken' 5.5 oz	1 serving	400	17	28	660	2	24.0	40
'Baja Steak' 5.5 oz	1 serving	400	17	27	680	2	24.0	30
beef, supreme, 5.5 oz	1 serving	380	14	29	580	3	23.0	40
chicken, supreme, 5.5 oz	1 serving	360	17	28	490	2	20.0	45
'Santa Fe Beef' 5.5 oz	1 serving	440	14	31	660	4	29.0	35
'Santa Fe Chicken' 5.5 oz	1 serving	420	17	30	560	2	26.0	40
'Santa Fe Steak' 5.5 oz	1 serving	430	18	29	580	2	27.0	35
steak, supreme, 5.5 oz	1 serving	360	17	27	500	2	20.0	35

Food Name	Serv. Size	Total Cal.	Prot. gms	Carbs gms	Sod. mgs	Fiber gms	Fat gms	Chol. mgs
CINNAMON TWIST, 1 oz	1 serving	180	1	25	290	1	8.0	0
DESSERT, chaco taco ice cream, 4 oz	1 serving	310	3	37	100	1	17.0	20
GORDITA								
'Baja Beef' 5.5 oz	1 serving	360	13	29	810	4	21.0	35
'Baja Chicken' 5.5 oz	1 serving	340	16	28	710	3	18.0	40
'Baja Steak' 5.5 oz	1 serving	340	17	27	730	3	18.0	30
beef, supreme, 5.5 oz	1 serving	300	17	27	550	3	14.0	35
chicken, supreme, 5.5 oz	1 serving	300	16	28	530	3	13.0	45
'Santa Fe Beef' 5.5 oz	1 serving	380	14	31	700	5	23.0	35
'Santa Fe Chicken' 5.5 oz	1 serving	370	17	30	610	3	20.0	40
'Santa Fe Steak' 5.5 oz	1 serving	370	17	29	620	3	20.0	35
steak, supreme, 5.5 oz	1 serving	300	17	27	550	3	14.0	35
MEXIMELT, big beef, 4.75 oz	1 serving	290	15	22	830	4	15.0	45
NACHOS								
'Bellegrande' 11 oz	1 serving	760	20	83	1300	17	39.0	35
'Big Beef Supreme' 7 oz	1 serving	440	14	44	800	9	24.0	35
chicken, 'Bellegrande' 11 oz	1 serving	740	23	82	1200	15	36.0	40
regular, 3.5 oz	1 serving	320	5	34	560	3	18.0	5
steak, 'Bellegrande' 11 oz	1 serving	740	24	81	1220	15	37.0	35
PIZZA								
Mexican, 7.75 oz	1 serving	540	20	42	1030	7	35.0	45
Mexican beef, 7.75 oz	1 serving	530	24	39	950	6	33.0	45
Mexican chicken, 7.75 oz	1 serving	520	23	41	940	6	32.0	50
QUESADILLA								
cheese, 4.25 oz	1 serving	350	16	31	860	3	18.0	50
cheese, breakfast, 5.5 oz	1 serving	380	15	33	1010	1	21.0	280
chicken, 6 oz	1 serving	400	25	33	1050	3	19.0	75
w/bacon, breakfast, 6 oz	1 serving	450	19	33	1200	2	27.0	290
w/sausage, breakfast, 6 oz	1 serving	430	17	33	1090	1	25.0	285
SALAD								
taco, w/salsa, 19 oz	1 salad	850	30	69	2250	16	52.0	70
taco, w/salsa, w/o shell, 16.5 oz	1 salad	430	25	36	1990	15	22.0	70
SIDE DISH								
hash brown nuggets, 3.5 oz	1 serving	280	2	29	570	1	18.0	0
Mexican rice, 4.75 oz	1 serving	190	5	23	750	1	9.0	15
pintos and cheese, 4.5 oz	1 serving	180	9	18	640	10	8.0	15
TACO								
'Double Decker' 5.75 oz	1 serving	330	14	37	740	9	15.0	30
'Double Decker Supreme' 7 oz	1 serving	380	15	39	760	9	18.0	40
'Supreme' 4 oz	1 serving	210	9	14	350	3	14.0	40
grilled chicken, soft, 4.5 oz	1 serving	200	14	20	530	2	7.0	35
grilled steak, soft, 4.5 oz	1 serving	200	14	19	570	2	7.0	25
grilled steak, soft, 'Supreme' 5.75 oz	1 serving	240	15	21	580	2	11.0	35
regular, 2.75 oz	1 serving	170	9	12	340	3	10.0	30
soft, 'Supreme' 5 oz	1 serving	260	11	22	590	3	13.0	40
soft, 3.5 oz	1 serving	210	11	20	570	3	10.0	30
TOSTADA, 6.25 oz	1 serving	250	10	27	640	11	12.0	15

TACO JOHN'S
BURRITO

Food Name	Serv. Size	Total Cal.	Prot. gms	Carbs gms	Sod. mgs	Fiber gms	Fat gms	Chol. mgs
bean	5 oz	249	10	36	636	0	6.0	0
beef	5 oz	355	16	25	666	0	18.0	0
chicken, super, w/o sour cream, cheese	1 serving	366	30	40	844	0	14.0	0
chicken, w/o sour cream, cheese	1 serving	227	27	19	639	0	10.0	0
combination	5 oz	302	11	30	651	0	12.0	0
super	8.3 oz	434	17	66	1022	0	11.0	0
super, w/o sour cream, cheese	1 serving	389	18	51	856	0	16.0	0
Texas chili	12.3 oz	518	23	48	746	0	24.0	0
w/green chili	12.3 oz	405	18	38	995	0	24.0	0

Food Name	Serv. Size	Total Cal.	Prot. gms	Carbs gms	Sod. mgs	Fiber gms	Fat gms	Chol. mgs
w/green chili, w/o sour cream, cheese .... 1 serving		367	20	40	998	0	18.0	0
CHILI, Texas .... 9.5 oz		430	23	35	1580	0	22.0	0
CHIMICHANGA .... 12 oz		487	16	54	1226	0	19.0	0
ENCHILADA .... 7 oz		379	19	33	431	0	18.0	0
NACHOS								
regular .... 4 oz		407	11	42	307	0	19.0	0
super .... 11.25 oz		657	23	57	857	0	34.0	0
PASTRY								
'Apple Grande' Danish .... 3 oz		257	5	44	231	0	8.0	0
churro .... 1.2 oz		122	2	12	153	0	7.0	0
SALAD								
chicken taco, super, w/o dressing, sour cream .... 1 salad		377	26	56	882	0	15.0	0
taco, w/o shell, dressing, sour cream, cheese .... 1 salad		228	13	30	440	0	13.0	0
taco, super .... 12.3 oz		450	16	48	880	0	18.0	0
SANDWICH, chicken fillet, 'Sierra' .... 8.5 oz		500	31	46	1493	23	21.0	41
SIDE DISH								
'Potato Ole' large .... 6 oz		414	6	96	1595	0	6.0	0
refried beans .... 9.5 oz		331	19	79	1195	0	6.0	0
Mexican rice .... 1 serving		340	7	59	1280	0	8.0	0
TACO								
'Taco Bravo' w/o sour cream .... 1 serving		319	16	42	658	0	14.0	0
'Taco Bravo' super .... 8 oz		485	18	51	1006	0	20.0	0
chicken, soft shell .... 1 serving		180	18	20	490	0	8.0	0
regular .... 4.3 oz		228	11	15	347	0	13.0	0
soft .... 5 oz		276	13	23	505	0	13.0	0
TACOBURGER .... 6 oz		332	14	31	660	0	14.0	0
TOSTADA .... 4.3 oz		228	11	15	347	0	13.0	0
TACO TIME								
BEEF, shredded .... 2.5 oz		70	1	1	31	0	0.0	0
BURRITO								
bean, crisp .... 5.25 oz		427	15	53	453	9	18.0	12
bean, soft, double .... 9.5 oz		506	23	77	860	19	12.0	22
bean, soft, single, 'Value' .... 6.75 oz		380	16	58	715	13	10.0	15
chicken, crisp .... 4.75 oz		422	17	32	795	2	25.0	54
combination, soft, double .... 9.5 oz		617	39	66	1343	18	23.0	63
meat, 'Casita' .... 12 oz		647	40	54	1233	16	31.0	89
meat, crisp .... 5.25 oz		552	34	39	1000	7	30.0	58
meat, soft, double .... 9.5 oz		726	57	55	1809	17	33.0	99
meat, soft, single, 'Value' .... 6.75 oz		491	31	48	1197	12	21.0	56
veggie .... 11 oz		491	21	70	643	10	16.0	24
CHEESE, Cheddar .... 0.75 oz		86	5	0	132	0	7.0	22
CHEESEBURGER, taco, meat .... 7.5 oz		633	31	48	1291	7	36.0	66
CHICKEN .... 2.5 oz		109	11	2	402	0	6.0	33
CHIPS .... 2 oz		266	4	35	461	3	12.0	0
CRUSTOS .... 3.5 oz		373	9	47	86	na	15.0	0
CONDIMENTS								
enchilada sauce .... 1 oz		12	0	3	133	1	0.0	0
guacamole .... 1 oz		29	0	2	94	1	2.0	0
hot sauce .... 1 oz		10	0	2	120	0	0.0	0
salad dressing, sour cream .... 1.5 oz		137	1	2	207	0	14.0	8
salad dressing, Thousand Island .... 1 oz		160	0	4	220	0	16.0	10
salsa, ranchero .... 2 oz		21	1	3	192	1	1.0	0
sour cream .... 1 oz		55	1	1	11	0	5.0	19
EMPANADA, cherry .... 4 oz		250	5	37	46	na	9.0	0
LETTUCE .... 0.5 oz		2	0	0	1	0	0.0	0
NACHOS								
deluxe .... 15.25 oz		1048	46	91	2252	17	57.0	109
regular .... 10.5 oz		680	26	61	1250	11	38.0	78

Food Name	Serv. Size	Total Cal.	Prot. gms	Carbs gms	Sod. mgs	Fiber gms	Fat gms	Chol. mgs
QUESADILLA, cheese	3.25 oz	205	11	17	255	1	11.0	30
SALAD								
chicken taco, w/o dressing	9 oz	370	19	27	861	3	21.0	48
taco, regular, w/o dressing	7.5 oz	479	30	30	895	7	28.0	63
'Tostada Delight' w/meat	9.75 oz	628	36	48	1004	13	33.0	82
SIDE DISH								
French fries, 'Mexi'	8 oz	532	6	54	1598	na	34.0	0
French fries, 'Mexi' regular	4 oz	266	3	27	799	na	17.0	0
Refritos	7 oz	326	18	44	525	13	10.0	22
Mexican rice	4 oz	159	3	30	530	1	2.0	0
TACO								
chicken, soft	7 oz	387	21	41	933	7	16.0	48
crisp	4 oz	295	22	16	609	5	17.0	48
flour, soft, rolled	7 oz	512	33	46	1111	12	23.0	63
meat	2.5 oz	208	22	7	576	5	11.0	38
meat, natural, 'Super'	11.25 oz	627	41	60	915	14	27.0	82
shredded beef, soft, 'Super'	8 oz	368	12	38	556	7	11.0	22
soft, 'Value'	5.25 oz	316	24	23	599	5	15.0	48
TACO SHELL, 6-inch	1.25 oz	110	2	14	48	2	6.0	0
TOMATO	0.5 oz	3	0	1	1	0	0.0	0
TORTILLA								
flour, 10-inch	2.75 oz	213	6	31	393	6	4.0	0
flour, 8-inch	1.25 oz	107	5	16	33	2	3.0	0
flour, 7-inch	1.75 oz	88	4	16	42	1	1.0	0
flour, fried, 10-inch	2.75 oz	318	6	37	315	2	16.0	0
flour, fried, 8-inch	1.3 oz	205	4	24	203	1	11.0	0
wheat, 11-inch	3.5 oz	175	8	33	84	2	3.0	0
WENDY'S								
BACON	1 slice	20	2	0	65	0	1.5	5
BEVERAGE								
coffee	6 fl oz	0	0	1	0	0	0.0	0
coffee, decaffeinated	6 fl oz	0	0	1	0	0	0.0	0
cola, diet, small	8 fl oz	0	0	0	20	0	0.0	0
cola, small	8 fl oz	90	0	24	10	0	0.0	0
'Frosty' large	20 oz	540	14	91	320	0	14.0	60
'Frosty' medium	16 oz	440	11	73	260	0	11.0	50
'Frosty' small	12 oz	330	8	56	200	0	8.0	35
hot chocolate	6 fl oz	80	1	15	135	0	3.0	0
lemonade, small	8 fl oz	90	0	24	5	0	0.0	0
lemon-lime soft drink	8 fl oz	90	0	24	25	0	0.0	0
milk, 2%	8 fl oz	110	8	11	115	0	4.0	15
tea, hot or iced	6 fl oz	0	0	0	0	0	0.0	0
BREAD, pita, 'Classic Greek'	1 pita	440	15	50	1050	4	20.0	35
BREADSTICK, soft	1 stick	130	4	23	250	1	3.0	5
BUN								
Kaiser	1 bun	190	6	36	340	2	3.0	0
sandwich	1 bun	160	5	29	280	2	2.5	0
CHEESE								
American	1 slice	70	3	1	320	0	5.0	15
American, junior	1 slice	45	2	0	220	0	3.5	10
Cheddar, shredded	2 tbsp	70	4	1	110	0	6.0	15
imitation, shredded, salad bar item	2 tbsp	50	3	1	260	0	4.0	0
CHEESEBURGER								
junior	1 burger	320	17	34	830	2	13.0	45
bacon, junior	1 burger	380	20	34	850	2	19.0	60
deluxe, junior	1 burger	360	18	36	890	3	17.0	50
kid's meal	1 burger	320	17	33	830	2	13.0	45

Food Name	Serv. Size	Total Cal.	Prot. gms	Carbs gms	Sod. mgs	Fiber gms	Fat gms	Chol. mgs
CHICKEN								
fillet, breaded	1 piece	230	22	10	490	0	12.0	55
fillet, grilled	1 fillet	110	22	0	450	0	3.0	60
fillet, spicy	1 piece	210	22	10	920	0	9.0	60
nuggets, fried	5 pieces	210	14	7	460	0	14.0	45
nuggets, fried	4 pieces	170	11	5	370	0	11.0	35
CHILI								
large	12 oz	310	23	32	1190	7	10.0	45
small	8 oz	210	15	21	800	5	7.0	30
CONDIMENTS. See also Salad Dressing.								
bacon bits, salad bar item	2 tbsp	45	6	0	550	0	2.5	10
barbecue sauce	1 packet	45	1	10	160	0	0.0	0
buffalo wing sauce, spicy	1 packet	25	0	4	210	0	1.0	0
catsup	1 tsp	10	0	2	75	0	0.0	0
croutons, salad bar item	2 tbsp	14	1	4	65	0	1.0	0
honey mustard sauce	1 packet	130	0	6	220	0	12.0	10
honey mustard, lower calorie	1 tsp	25	0	2	45	0	1.5	0
lettuce	1 leaf	0	0	0	0	0	0.0	0
lettuce, iceberg/Romaine, salad bar item	1 cup	10	0	2	5	1	0.0	0
margarine, whipped	1 packet	60	0	0	115	0	7.0	0
mayonnaise	1 tsp	30	0	1	60	0	3.0	5
mustard	1 tsp	0	0	0	50	0	0.0	0
onion, red, sliced, salad bar item	3 rings	0	0	1	0	0	0.0	0
onion, sliced	4 rings	5	0	1	0	0	0.0	0
Parmesan blend, grated, salad bar item	2 tbsp	70	4	5	290	0	4.0	10
pepperoni, sliced, salad bar item	6 slices	30	1	0	70	0	3.0	5
pickle	4 slices	0	0	0	140	0	0.0	0
salad oil	1 tbsp	120	0	0	0	0	14.0	0
sour cream	1 packet	60	1	1	15	0	6.0	10
sunflower seeds and raisins, salad bar item	2 tbsp	80	0	5	0	1	5.0	0
sweet and sour sauce	1 packet	50	0	12	120	0	0.0	0
tomato, sliced	1 slice	5	0	1	0	0	0.0	0
tomato, wedges, salad bar item	1 piece	5	0	1	0	0	0.0	0
turkey ham, diced, salad bar item	2 tbsp	50	3	0	280	0	4.0	25
COOKIE, chocolate chip	1 cookie	270	3	36	120	1	13.0	30
CRACKERS, saltine	2 crackers	25	1	4	80	0	0.5	0
HAMBURGER								
'Big Bacon Classic'	1 burger	580	34	46	1460	3	30.0	100
junior	1 burger	270	15	34	610	2	10.0	30
kid's meal	1 burger	270	15	33	610	2	10.0	30
single, plain	1 burger	360	24	31	580	2	16.0	65
w/everything	1 burger	420	25	37	920	3	20.0	70
HAMBURGER PATTY								
regular	2 oz	100	9	0	150	0	7.0	30
quarter-pound	0.25 lb	200	19	0	290	0	14.0	65
SALAD								
Caesar, side	1 salad	100	8	8	620	1	4.0	10
chicken Caesar	1 salad	260	26	17	1170	2	9.0	60
chicken, grilled	1 salad	200	25	9	720	3	8.0	50
garden, deluxe	1 salad	110	7	9	350	3	6.0	0
side	1 salad	60	4	5	180	2	3.0	0
taco	1 salad	380	26	28	1040	7	19.0	65
SALAD DRESSING								
blue cheese	2 tbsp	180	1	0	180	0	19.0	15
Caesar vinaigrette, pita dressing	1 tbsp	70	0	1	170	0	7.0	0
French	2 tbsp	120	0	6	330	0	10.0	0
French, nonfat	2 tbsp	35	0	8	150	0	0.0	0
garden ranch, pita dressing	1 tbsp	50	0	1	125	0	4.5	10

Food Name	Serv. Size	Total Cal.	Prot. gms	Carbs gms	Sod. mgs	Fiber gms	Fat gms	Chol. mgs
Italian Caesar	2 tbsp	150	1	1	240	0	16.0	20
Italian, reduced fat	2 tbsp	40	0	2	340	0	3.0	0
ranch, 'Hidden Valley'	2 tbsp	100	1	1	220	0	10.0	10
ranch, reduced fat, 'Hidden Valley'	2 tbsp	60	1	2	240	0	5.0	10
Thousand Island	2 tbsp	90	0	2	125	0	8.0	10
wine vinegar	1 tbsp	0	0	0	0	0	0.0	0
SANDWICH								
chicken, breaded	1 sandwich	440	28	44	840	2	18.0	60
chicken, grilled	1 sandwich	310	27	35	790	2	8.0	65
chicken, spicy	1 sandwich	410	28	43	1280	2	15.0	65
chicken Caesar pita	1 pita	490	34	48	1320	4	18.0	65
chicken club	1 sandwich	470	31	44	970	2	20.0	70
'Garden Ranch Chicken Pita'	1 pita	480	30	51	1180	5	18.0	70
'Garden Veggie Pita'	1 pita	400	11	52	760	5	17.0	20
SIDE DISH								
applesauce, salad bar item	2 tbsp	30	0	7	0	0	0.0	0
baked potato, plain	10 oz	310	7	71	25	7	0.0	0
baked potato, w/bacon and cheese	1 serving	530	17	78	1390	7	18.0	20
baked potato, w/broccoli and cheese	1 serving	470	9	80	470	9	14.0	5
baked potato, w/cheese	1 serving	570	14	78	640	7	23.0	30
baked potato, w/chili and cheese	1 serving	630	20	83	770	9	24.0	40
baked potato, w/sour cream and chives	1 serving	380	8	74	40	8	6.0	15
cantaloupe, sliced, salad bar item	1 piece	15	0	4	0	0	0.0	0
chicken salad, salad bar item	2 tbsp	70	4	2	135	0	5.0	0
cottage cheese, salad bar item	2 tbsp	30	4	1	125	0	1.5	5
cucumbers, salad bar item	2 slices	0	0	0	0	0	0.0	0
egg, hard cooked, salad bar item	2 tbsp	40	3	0	30	0	3.0	110
French fries, 'Biggie'	5.6 oz	470	6	61	150	6	23.0	0
French fries, 'Great Biggie'	6.7 oz	570	8	73	180	7	27.0	0
French fries, small	3.2 oz	270	4	35	85	3	13.0	0
green peas, salad bar item	2 tbsp	15	1	3	25	1	0.0	0
green peppers, salad bar item	2 pieces	0	0	1	0	0	0.0	0
orange, sliced, salad bar item	2 slices	15	0	4	0	1	0.0	0
pasta salad, salad bar item	2 tbsp	35	1	4	180	1	1.5	0
peaches, sliced, salad bar item	1 piece	15	0	4	0	0	0.0	0
potato salad, salad bar item	2 tbsp	80	0	5	180	0	7.0	5
watermelon, wedges, salad bar item	1 piece	20	0	4	0	0	0.0	0
TACO CHIPS	15 chips	210	3	24	180	2	11.0	0
WHATABURGER								
BACON	1 slice	38	2	0	106	na	3.3	6
BEVERAGE								
'Cherry Coke' medium	1 serving	227	0	60	11	na	0.0	0
chocolate shake, junior	1 serving	364	9	61	172	na	9.3	36
'Coca-Cola Classic' medium	1 serving	211	0	56	19	na	0.0	0
coffee, small	1 serving	5	0	1	5	na	0.0	0
'Diet Coke' medium	1 serving	2	0	1	26	na	0.0	0
'Dr. Pepper' medium	1 serving	207	0	52	51	na	0.0	0
iced tea, 'Lipton' medium	1 serving	5	0	2	15	na	0.0	0
orange juice, 'Tropicana'	10 fl oz	140	2	33	0	na	0.0	0
milk, 2%	1 serving	113	8	11	113	na	4.3	18
'Sprite' medium	1 serving	211	0	48	45	na	0.0	0
strawberry shake, junior	1 serving	352	9	60	168	na	8.9	35
root beer, medium	1 serving	237	0	63	25	na	0.0	0
vanilla shake, junior	1 serving	325	9	51	172	na	9.5	37
BISCUIT, plain	1 serving	280	5	37	509	na	13.4	3
BREAKFAST								
bacon biscuit	1 sandwich	359	10	37	730	na	20.2	15

Food Name	Serv. Size	Total Cal.	Prot. gms	Carbs gms	Sod. mgs	Fiber gms	Fat gms	Chol. mgs
bacon, egg, and cheese biscuit	1 sandwich	511	18	38	1010	na	32.9	213
'Breakfast on a Bun' w/bacon biscuit	1 sandwich	365	18	29	815	na	19.4	210
Breakfast on a Bun' w/sausage biscuit	1 sandwich	455	20	30	886	na	28.1	232
cinnamon roll	1 serving	320	4	39	190	na	16.0	10
egg and cheese biscuit	1 sandwich	434	14	38	797	na	26.3	202
egg omelet sandwich	1 sandwich	288	13	29	602	na	12.8	198
pancake	3 pancakes	259	11	40	842	na	5.8	0
pancake, 3 pancakes w/2 slices bacon	1 serving	335	15	40	1074	na	12.4	12
pancake, 3 pancakes w/1 sausage patty	1 serving	426	18	40	1127	na	21.1	34
platter, w/bacon, scrambled eggs, biscuit, hash browns	1 serving	695	22	54	1162	na	44.0	389
platter, w/sausage, scrambled eggs, biscuit, hash browns	1 serving	785	25	54	1234	na	52.7	412
sausage and gravy biscuit	1 sandwich	479	9	48	1253	na	27.4	20
sausage biscuit	1 sandwich	446	12	37	794	na	28.7	37
sausage, egg, and cheese biscuit	1 sandwich	601	21	38	1081	na	41.6	236
toast, Texas	1 slice	147	4	22	250	na	4.5	0
CHEESE, large slice	1 slice	89	5	0	338	na	7.4	22
CHICKEN STRIPS	2 strips	300	16	15	630	na	20.0	35
COOKIE								
chocolate chunk	1 serving	247	4	28	75	na	16.0	36
white chocolate macadamia nut	1 serving	269	3	31	80	na	16.0	34
FAJITA								
beef	1 serving	326	22	34	670	na	11.9	28
chicken, grilled	1 serving	272	18	35	691	na	6.7	33
GRAVY, peppered	3 oz	75	0	8	375	na	4.5	0
HAMBURGER								
'Justaburger'	1 burger	298	15	30	598	na	13.0	42
'Whataburger'	1 burger	598	30	61	1096	na	26.0	84
'Whataburger' double meat	1 burger	823	49	62	1298	na	42.4	168
'Whataburger' on small bun, w/o oil	1 burger	407	25	34	839	na	18.8	84
'Whataburger Jr.'	1 burger	322	16	35	603	na	13.3	42
MUFFIN, blueberry	1 serving	239	6	36	538	na	7.9	0
SALAD								
garden	1 salad	56	3	11	32	na	0.6	0
chicken, grilled	1 salad	150	23	14	434	na	1.2	49
SANDWICH								
chicken, grilled	1 sandwich	442	34	48	1103	na	14.2	66
chicken, grilled, on small white bun, w/mustard, w/o oil, dressing	1 sandwich	300	33	35	994	na	3.2	66
chicken, grilled, w/o dressing	1 sandwich	385	34	46	989	na	8.5	66
chicken, grilled, w/o dressing, oil	1 sandwich	358	34	46	989	na	5.5	66
fish, 'Whatacatch'	1 sandwich	467	18	43	636	na	25.0	33
SIDE DISH								
French fries, junior	1 serving	221	4	25	139	na	12.1	0
French fries, large	1 serving	442	7	49	227	na	24.2	0
French fries, regular	1 serving	332	5	37	208	na	18.1	0
onion rings, large	1 serving	498	8	51	893	na	28.7	0
onion rings, regular	1 serving	329	5	34	596	na	19.1	0
TAQUITO								
bacon and egg	1 serving	335	15	32	761	na	16.1	286
potato and egg	1 serving	446	14	48	883	na	21.8	281
sausage and egg	1 serving	443	20	32	790	na	25.9	315
TURNOVER, apple, fried	1 serving	215	2	27	241	na	10.8	0

WHITE CASTLE
BEVERAGE

Food Name	Serv. Size	Total Cal.	Prot. gms	Carbs gms	Sod. mgs	Fiber gms	Fat gms	Chol. mgs
chocolate shake	14 fl oz	220	8	32	140	0	7.0	25

Food Name	Serv. Size	Total Cal.	Prot. gms	Carbs gms	Sod. mgs	Fiber gms	Fat gms	Chol. mgs
'Coca-Cola Classic'	14 fl oz	120	0	32	12	0	0.0	0
coffee, black, small	1 serving	6	0	1	5	0	0.0	0
'Diet Coke'	14 fl oz	1	0	0	13	0	0.0	0
tea, iced	14 fl oz	45	0	12	15	0	0.0	0
vanilla shake	14 fl oz	230	8	35	150	0	7.0	25
BREAKFAST, egg, sausage, cheese on bun	1 sandwich	340	14	17	900	0	25.0	130
CHEESEBURGER								
double patty	1 sandwich	285	14	16	430	5	18.0	30
regular	1 sandwich	160	7	11	250	2	9.0	15
w/bacon	1 sandwich	200	10	12	400	3	13.0	25
CHICKEN RINGS	6 rings	310	16	14	620	0	21.0	70
CHILI	12 oz	375	30	45	1635	0	15.0	0
HAMBURGER								
double	1 burger	235	11	16	200	4	14.0	20
regular	1 burger	135	6	11	135	2	7.0	10
SANDWICH								
chicken	1 sandwich	190	8	21	360	0	8.0	20
fish	1 sandwich	160	8	18	220	0	6.0	15
SIDE DISH								
cheese sticks	3 sticks	290	15	19	730	0	17.0	0
French fries, small	1 serving	115	0	15	15	2	6.0	0
onion rings	8 rings	540	8	69	1300	0	26.0	0